THE UPPER EXTREMITY
IN SPORTS MEDICINE

THE UPPER EXTREMITY
IN SPORTS MEDICINE

Edited by

JAMES A. NICHOLAS, M.D.

Founder and Director
Nicholas Institute of Sports Medicine and Athletic Trauma
Director Emeritus, Department of Orthopaedic Surgery, Lenox Hill Hospital
Consulting Physician, Hospital for Special Surgery
Chairman, Medical Staff, and Team Physician
New York Jets Football Club
New York, New York

ELLIOTT B. HERSHMAN, M.D.

Executive Associate Director, Department of Orthopaedic Surgery
Consultant, Nicholas Institute of Sports Medicine and Athletic Trauma
Associate Orthopaedic Surgeon, Lenox Hill Hospital
Team Orthopaedist, New York Jets Football Club
Team Physician, Hunter College Athletic Program
New York, New York

with

MARTIN A. POSNER, M.D.
editor of Hand Section

Associate Clinical Professor of Orthopaedics, Mount Sinai School of Medicine
Chief of Hand Services, Lenox Hill Hospital
Hospital for Joint Diseases and Orthopaedic Institute, Mount Sinai Hospital
Consultant Hand Surgeon for Nicholas Institute of Sports Medicine
and Athletic Trauma, Blythdale Children's Hospital
New York Jets Football Club, New York Knicks Basketball Team
New York Rangers Hockey Team
New York, New York

SECOND EDITION

with 1570 *illustrations and* 12 *color plates*

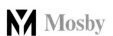 Mosby

St. Louis Baltimore Boston Carlsbad Chicago Naples New York Philadelphia Portland
London Madrid Mexico City Singapore Sydney Tokyo Toronto Wiesbaden

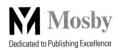
Dedicated to Publishing Excellence

A Times Mirror
Company

Publisher: Alison Miller
Acquisition Editor: Robert Hurley
Developmental Editor: Kathryn H. Falk
Project Manager: Patricia Tannian
Senior Production Editor: Suzanne C. Fannin
Manufacturing Supervisor: Betty Richmond
Book and Cover Designer: Gail Morey Hudson

SECOND EDITION

Copyright © 1995 by Mosby–Year Book, Inc.

Previous edition copyrighted 1990

Printed in the United States of America
Composition by Clarinda Company
Printing/binding by Maple-Vail Book Mfg. Group

Mosby–Year Book, Inc.
11830 Westline Industrial Drive
St. Louis, Missouri 63146

Library of Congress Cataloging in Publication Data

The upper extremity in sports medicine / edited by James A. Nicholas.
  Elliott B. Hershman ; with Martin A. Posner, editor of hand section.
  —2nd ed.
      p. cm.
    Companion v. to: The lower extremity and spine in sports medicine.
    Includes bibliographical references and index.
    ISBN 0-8151-6392-4 (alk. paper)
    1. Arm—Wounds and injuries. 2. Sports injuries.   I. Nicholas,
James A., 1921– . II. Hershman. Elliott B. III. Posner, Martin
A. IV. Lower extremity and spine in sports medicine.
    [DNLM: 1. Arm Injuries. 2. Athletic Injuries. WE 805 U683 1995]
  RD557.U67 1995
  617.5'7044—dc20
  DNLM/DLC
  for Library of Congress   95-6355
                                                                 CIP

95 96 97 98 99 / 9 8 7 6 5 4 3 2 1

Contributors

FRED L. ALLMAN, Jr., M.D.

Director, Atlanta Sports Medicine Clinic
Former Orthopaedic Consultant
University of Georgia and Georgia Tech Athletes
Atlanta, Georgia

THOMAS E. ANDERSON, M.D.

Orthopaedic Surgeon
Section of Sports Medicine
Department of Orthopaedics
Cleveland Clinic Foundation
Team Physician
Chagrin Falls High School
Chagrin Falls, Ohio
Cleveland Browns
Cleveland State University
Cleveland, Ohio

JAMES R. ANDREWS, M.D.

Medical Director, American Sports Medicine Institute
Birmingham, Alabama
Clinical Professor of Orthopaedics and Sports Medicine
University of Virginia Medical School
Charlottesville, Virginia
Team Physician
Auburn University
Auburn, Alabama

JACK T. ANDRISH, M.D.

Orthopaedic Surgeon
Section of Sports Medicine
Section of Pediatric Orthopaedics
Department of Orthopaedics
Cleveland Clinic Foundation
Orthopaedic Consultant, Cleveland Cavaliers
Team Physician, Orange High School
Cleveland, Ohio

GEORGE H. BELHOBEK, M.D.

Chairman, Department of Diagnostic Radiology—Clinic
Section of Musculoskeletal Radiology
Cleveland Clinic Foundation
Cleveland, Ohio

JAMES B. BENNETT, M.D.

Clinical Professor
Department of Orthopaedic Surgery
Baylor College of Medicine
Fondren Orthopedic Group
Texas Orthopedic Hospital
Consultant
Houston Oilers
Houston Rockets
Houston Astros
Houston, Texas

JOHN A. BERGFELD, M.D.

Head, Section of Sports Medicine
Cleveland Clinic Foundation
Team Physician, Cleveland Browns and Cleveland Cavaliers
Physician, Cleveland Ballet
Cleveland, Ohio

GEORGE P. BOGUMILL, Ph.D., M.D.

Professor of Orthopaedic Surgery
Georgetown University Hospital
Washington, D.C.
Consultant in Hand Surgery
Walter Reed Army Medical Center
Clinical Professor of Surgery
Uniformed Services University of Health Sciences
Bethesda, Maryland

CHRISTINA BONCI, M.S., A.T., C.

Assistant Athletic Director for Sports Medicine
Head Athletic Trainer
Intercollegiate Athletics for Women
University of Texas, Austin
Austin, Texas

JOHN J. BREMS, M.D.

Cleveland Clinic Foundation
Section of Upper Extremity
Cleveland, Ohio
Assistant Professor, Department of Surgery
Ohio State University
Columbus, Ohio
Team Physician, Lake Catholic High School
Cleveland, Ohio

v

MICHAEL G. BROWNE, M.D.

Fellow
Nicholas Institute of Sports Medicine and Athletic Trauma
Department of Orthopaedic Surgery, Lenox Hill Hospital
New York, New York

T. PEPPER BURRUSS, P.T., A.T., C.

Head Athletic Trainer, Green Bay Packers
Green Bay, Wisconsin

CAROLYN A. CARLSON, P.T.

Director of Rehabilitation Services
Rehab Associates of Atlanta
Atlanta, Georgia

DARRYL CONWAY, A.T., C.

Assistant Athletic Trainer, New York Jets
New York, New York

FRANK A. CORDASCO, M.D.

Assistant Clinical Professor of Orthopaedic Surgery
Columbia University, College of Physicians and Surgeons
Assistant Attending Orthopaedic Surgeon
St. Lukes—Roosevelt Hospital Center
Columbia—Presbyterian Medical Center
New York, New York

VINCENT DiSTEFANO, M.D.

Associate Clinical Professor of Orthopaedic Surgery
University of Pennsylvania
Chairman, Department of Orthopaedic Surgery
Director, Orthopaedic Sports Medicine Fellowship
Program
Graduate Hospital
Consultant, Philadelphia Eagles
Philadelphia, Pennsylvania

PIERCE J. FERRITER, M.D.

Adjunct Orthopaedic Surgeon
Lenox Hill Hospital
Consultant, Nicholas Institute of Sports Medicine and
Athletic Trauma
New York, New York

PETER J. FOWLER, M.D., F.R.C.S.(C.)

Professor of Orthopaedic Surgery
University of Western Ontario
Head, Section of Sports Medicine
Department of Orthopaedics
University Hospital
London, Ontario, Canada

RALPH A. GAMBARDELLA, M.D.

Associate, Kerlan-Jobe Orthopaedic Clinic
Inglewood, California
Associate Clinical Professor
Department of Orthopaedics
University of Southern California, School of Medicine
Orthopaedic Consultant
Los Angeles Dodgers
University of Southern California Department of Athletics
Loyola Marymount Department of Athletics
Los Angeles, California

RONALD E. GLOUSMAN, M.D.

Assistant Clinical Professor of Orthopaedics
University of Southern California
Los Angeles, California
Assistant Instructor Sports Medicine
Rancho Los Amigos Medical Center
Downey, California
Team Physician, Anaheim Mighty Ducks
Anaheim, California
Orthopaedic Consultant
Los Angeles Lakers
Los Angeles Dodgers
Los Angeles Angels
Los Angeles Kings
Los Angeles, California

KAREN M. GRIFFIN, P.T., A.T., C.

Clinical Supervisor
Sports Rehabilitation
The Sports Medicine Center at Baptist Hospital
Nashville, Tennessee

ELLIOTT B. HERSHMAN, M.D.

Executive Associate Director, Department of Orthopaedic
Surgery
Consultant, Nicholas Institute of Sports Medicine and
Athletic Trauma
Associate Orthopaedic Surgeon, Lenox Hill Hospital
Team Orthopaedist, New York Jets Football Club
Team Physician, Hunter College Athletic Program
New York, New York

JOHN A. HURLEY, M.D.

Attending Surgeon
Department of Orthopaedic Surgery
Morristown Memorial Hospital
Morristown, New Jersey
Associate Clinical Professor
Orthopaedic Surgery
University of Medicine and Dentistry of New Jersey
Newark, New Jersey

JOHN F. JENNINGS, M.D.

Attending Hand Surgeon
Department of Plastic Surgery
Grandview Hospital
Sellersville, Pennsylvania

FRANK W. JOBE, M.D.

Associate, Kerlan-Jobe Orthopaedic Clinic
Inglewood, California
Clinical Professor
Department of Orthopaedics
University of Southern California, School of Medicine
Orthopaedic Consultant
Los Angeles, California
Los Angeles Dodgers
PGA Tour
Senior PGA Tour

VI A. MAYER, O.T.R.

Clinical Instructor
Division of Hand Surgery and Sports Medicine
Department of Orthopaedics
University of Virginia
Charlottesville, Virginia

JOHN R. McCARROLL, M.D.

Orthopaedic Surgeon
Methodist Sports Medicine Center
Indianapolis, Indiana
Orthopaedic Consultant
Indiana University Athletic Department
Bloomington, Indiana

FRANK C. McCUE, III, M.D.

Alfred R. Shands Professor of Orthopaedic Surgery and
Plastic Surgery of the Hand
Director, Division of Sports Medicine and Hand Surgery
Team Physician, University of Virginia
Department of Athletics
University of Virginia
Charlottesville, Virginia

CHARLES P. MELONE, Jr., M.D., F.A.C.S.

Clinical Professor, Orthopaedic Surgery
Director, Orthopaedic Hand Surgery
New York University Medical Center
Medical Advisory Board
New York State Athletic Commission
Hand Surgery Consultant
New York Yankees
New York Islanders
New Jersey Nets
New Jersey Devils
New York State Athletic Commission
New York City Public School Athletic League
New York Golden Gloves
New York, New York

FRANCIS X. MENDOZA, M.D.

Associate Orthopaedic Surgeon
Chief, Shoulder and Elbow Section
Department of Orthopaedic Surgery
Consultant, Nicholas Institute of Sports Medicine and
Athletic Trauma
Lenox Hill Hospital
New York, New York

JEFFREY MINKOFF, M.D.

Clinical Professor of Orthopaedics
New York University Medical Center
Attending Orthopaedic Surgeon
Lenox Hill Hospital
Beth Israel North Hospital
North Shore University Hospital
Team Physician, New York Islanders
New York, New York
New Jersey Nets
East Rutherford, New Jersey

C. ALEXANDER MOSKWA, Jr., M.D.

Orthopaedic Surgeon
Sports Medicine Princeton
Orthopaedic Associates of Princeton
Princeton, New Jersey

JAMES A. NICHOLAS, M.D.

Founder and Director
Nicholas Institute of Sports Medicine and Athletic Trauma
Director Emeritus, Department of Orthopaedic Surgery,
Lenox Hill Hospital
Consulting Physician, Hospital for Special Surgery
Chairman, Medical Staff, and Team Physician
New York Jets Football Club
New York, New York

STEPHEN J. NICHOLAS, M.D.

Associate Director
Nicholas Institute of Sports Medicine and Athletic Trauma
Department of Orthopaedic Surgery
Lenox Hill Hospital
Associate Team Orthopaedist
New York Jets Football Club
New York, New York

ROBERT P. NIRSCHL, M.D.

Director of Virginia Sports Medicine Institute
Arlington, Virginia
Clinical Assistant Professor, Orthopaedics
Georgetown University School of Medicine
Washington, D.C.

TOM R. NORRIS, M.D.

Attending Physician
Department of Orthopaedic Surgery
California Pacific Medical Center
San Francisco, California

PATRICK F. O'LEARY, M.D.

Clinical Associate Professor of Surgery
Cornell University Medical College
Director, Spine Service
The Hospital for Special Surgery
Chief, Spine Service
Lenox Hill Hospital
New York, New York

MICHAEL J. PAGNANI, M.D.

Attending Orthopaedic Surgeon
The Lipscomb Clinic
Clinical Assistant Professor
Department of Orthopaedics and Rehabilitation
Vanderbilt University School of Medicine
Associate Team Physician
Tennessee State University
Orthopaedic Consultant, Nashville Sounds Baseball
Nashville, Tennessee

RICHARD D. PARKER, M.D.

Medical Director, Sports/Orthopaedic Rehabilitation
Staff Physician, Section of Sports Medicine
Department of Orthopaedics
Cleveland Clinic Foundation
Team Physician, St. Edwards High School
Cleveland, Ohio

JAMES C. PARKES, II, M.D.

Associate Clinical Professor of Orthopaedic Surgery
Columbia University, College of Physicians and Surgeons
Attending Surgeon
St. Lukes—Roosevelt Hospital Center
New York, New York

JOSEPH PATTEN, A.T.C.

Assistant Head Athletic Trainer, New York Jets
New York, New York

CLAYTON A. PEIMER, M.D.

Chief of Hand Surgery
Millard Fillmore Hospital
Associate Professor of Orthopaedic Surgery
Clinical Assistant Professor of Anatomical Sciences and
Rehabilitation Medicine
University at Buffalo
State University of New York
Buffalo, New York

JACQUELIN PERRY, M.D.

Professor of Orthopaedics
Professor of Biokinesiology and Physical Therapy
University of Southern California
Los Angeles, California
Chief, Pathokinesiology Service
Chief, Polio Service
Rancho Los Amigos Medical Center
Downey, California
Consultant, Centinela Biomechanics Laboratory
Inglewood, California

FRANK A. PETTRONE, M.D.

Associate Clinical Professor
Department of Orthopaedics
Georgetown University Hospital
Washington, D.C.

GEORGE PIANKA, M.D.

Adjunct Orthopaedic Surgeon
Consultant Hand Surgeon
Nicholas Institute of Sports Medicine and Athletic Trauma
Lenox Hill Hospital
Hospital for Joint Diseases, Orthopaedic Institute
New York, New York
New York Hospital Medical Center, Queens
Queens, New York

MARTIN A. POSNER, M.D.

Associate Clinical Professor of Orthopaedics
Mount Sinai School of Medicine
Chief of Hand Services
Lenox Hill Hospital
Hospital for Joint Diseases and Orthopaedic Institute
Consultant Hand Surgeon
Nicholas Institute of Sports Medicine and Athletic Trauma
Blythdale Children's Hospital
New York Jets
New York Knicks
New York Rangers
New York, New York

MAHVASH RAFII, M.D.

Professor of Clinical Radiology
New York University School of Medicine
Attending Radiologist
New York University Medical Center
Bellevue Hospital
New York, New York

ROBERT C. REESE, Jr., A.T.C.

Consultant, Nicholas Institute of Sports Medicine and
Athletic Trauma
Lenox Hill Hospital
Head Athletic Trainer, New York Jets
New York, New York

ALLEN B. RICHARDSON, M.D., F.A.C.S.

Associate Professor of Surgery
Division of Orthopaedic Surgery
John A. Burns School of Medicine
Team Physician, University of Hawaii
Chief Medical Officer
United States Swimming, Inc.
Chairman, Medical Committee
Federation Internationale Natation Amateur
Honolulu, Hawaii

ANDREW K. SANDS, M.D.

Attending Staff
Department of Orthopaedic Surgery
Beth Israel Hospital
New York, New York

SCOTT P. SCHEMMEL, M.D.

Orthopaedic Physician
Sports Medicine Center
Dubuque, Iowa
Consultant
Loras College
Clarke College
Team Physician
University of Wisconsin
Platteville, Wisconsin

DANIEL W. SCHMOLL, M.D.

Village Family Practice
Prairie Village, Kansas

LAWRENCE H. SCHNEIDER, M.D.

Clinical Professor of Orthopaedic Surgery
Director, Division of Hand Surgery
Jefferson Medical College
Thomas Jefferson University
Philadelphia, Pennsylvania

BETH SLOANE, P.T.

Physical Trainer and Athletic Trainer
Seacoast Sports Medicine and Rehabilitation Center
Newbury Port, Massachusetts

JANET SOBEL, R.P.T.

Private Practice
Member, United States Tennis Association (U.S.T.A.)
Chevy Chase, Maryland

HOWARD J. SWEENEY, M.D.

Director, Center for Arthroscopic Surgery
Evanston Hospital
Evanston, Illinois
Head Team Physician
Northwestern University
Associate Clinical Professor of Orthopaedic Surgery
Northwestern University Medical School
Chicago, Illinois

LAURA A. TIMMERMAN, M.D.

Assistant Professor
Department of Orthopaedics
University of California, Davis, School of Medicine
University of California, Davis, Medical Center
Sacramento, California
Team Physician
University of California
Berkeley, California

ANDREW H. TURTEL, M.D.

Attending Orthopaedic Surgeon
Lenox Hill Hospital
Beth Israel North Hospital
Hospital for Joint Diseases
New York, New York
Team Physician, New Jersey Nets
East Rutherford, New Jersey

RUSSELL F. WARREN, M.D.

Surgeon in Chief
The Hospital for Special Surgery
Professor of Orthopaedic Surgery
Cornell University Medical College
New York, New York

KEITH WATSON, M.D.

Assistant Director of the Orthopedic Residency Program
Fort Worth Affiliated Hospitals
Fort Worth, Texas

GARRON G. WEIKER, M.D.

Vice Chairman, Division of Education
Administrative Head, Section of Sports Medicine
Cleveland Clinic Foundation
Cleveland, Ohio

TERRY L. WHIPPLE, M.D., F.A.C.S.

Clinical Professor of Orthopaedic Surgery
Bowman Gray School of Medicine
Winston-Salem, North Carolina
Clinical Associate Professor of Hand and Sports Medicine
University of Virginia School of Medicine
Charlottesville, Virginia
Clinical Associate Professor of Orthopaedic Surgery
Medical College of Virginia
Richmond, Virginia

JAMES A. WHITESIDE, M.D.

Director, Medical Aspects of Sports
Alabama Sports Medicine and Orthopaedic Center
American Sports Medicine Institute
Birmingham, Alabama
Team Physician
Troy State University
Troy, Alabama

E.F. SHAW WILGIS, M.D.

Associate Professor, Orthopaedic and Plastic Surgery
The Johns Hopkins Hospital
Chief, Division of Hand Surgery
Director, Raymond Curtis Hand Center
Union Memorial Hospital
Baltimore, Maryland

ADOLPH J. YATES, Jr., M.D.
Assistant Professor
Division of Orthopedics and Rehabilitation
Oregon Health Sciences University
Assistant Chief of Orthopedic Surgery
Portland VAMC
Portland, Oregon

JOHN G. YOST, Jr., M.D.
Associate Clinical Professor of Orthopaedic Surgery
Truman Medical Center
University of Missouri
Kansas City, Missouri
Team Physician
Baker University
Baldwin City, Kansas
Orthopaedic Consultant
Northwest Missouri State University
Maryville, Missouri

To

Christiana, Tatiana, Charles, and Marina

our next generation of athletes

To

Susan

the heart of my love and life

Foreword

In 1986 Drs. Nicholas and Hershman published the first edition of *The Lower Extremity and Spine in Sports Medicine.* The second, completely updated, and revised edition of these monumental and well-received volumes was published in 1995. In his forward to these books, Dr. Robert Larson described Dr. Nicholas' treatment philosophy: with any injury there are alterations in the function of adjacent joints in the athlete as a whole. This "linkage mechanism" serves as a unifying theme to both books. Dr. Nicholas has stressed a multidisciplinary approach to athletic injuries.

The Upper Extremity in Sports Medicine, first published in 1990, completed the task of providing the sports medicine practitioner with a comprehensive resource on sports injuries of the musculoskeletal system. The publication of this second edition is extremely timely. The explosion of information on the knee in the 1970s and early 1980s was followed by a similar phenomenon for the shoulder in the late 1980s and early 1990s. This revised and totally updated book consolidates and clearly presents the new information.

The chapters of this distinguished text reflect the wide experience and acknowledged expertise of the authors. The editors help the reader by summarizing the key points in each chapter throughout the text. Although this work enriches the entire field of sports medicine, the ultimate benefactor will be the individual athlete.

Bertram Zarins, M.D.

Preface
to the second edition

The popularity of sports reflects society's abiding interest in them, both as entertainment and leisure time activities. The pursuit of sports is integrated into daily life to such a degree that sports medicine has become an important ingredient in successful and safe athletic participation.

The technology explosion is progressing so rapidly that constant updates are needed in the diagnostic, surgical, clinical, and rehabilitative aspects of sports medicine. Advances in these areas over the past few years, coupled with technologic breakthroughs in imaging, have yielded earlier and more accurate diagnoses. Surgical techniques improve as many procedures give way to arthroscopic or minimally invasive protocols. Nonoperative care and rehabilitation benefit from well-controlled research, with improved and accelerated rehabilitation techniques forming part of the routine care of athletes. Clinical and basic science research enables athletes to safely and successfully extend their careers. New procedures and techniques should be viewed with healthy skepticism until meaningful data to support them are available; therefore sports medicine practitioners should continue to base their treatment on generally accepted principles. This text makes available to the sports medicine clinician the most current information extant in the field. We have added extensive material on the latest techniques in imaging, surgical procedures, nonoperative treatment, and rehabilitation.

The health care reform debate seeks to emphasize the role of primary care professionals as the initial contact to the injured athlete. As health care changes, up-to-date reference texts are vital to the ability of providers to care for athletes. Costs may be controlled by accurate diagnosis and early treatment. We have attempted to make our text a resource to meet the needs of the primary care provider and the specialist in sports medicine. The prevention of athletic trauma, given its high cost, cannot be stressed enough; we have included new information in this area as well.

We continue to emphasize the linkage relationship of movement. Integration of the entire musculoskeletal system into prevention and treatment is an integral part of sports medicine. The entire text is written with these concepts in mind.

We hope the reader finds these books a useful reference for the prevention, diagnosis, and treatment of injuries in athletes. If safe participation, speedy and successful recovery from injury, and enhanced quality of life from sports are achieved, we have met our goal—for our athletes.

James A. Nicholas
Elliott B. Hershman

Preface
to the first edition

To focus only on the area of injury and its treatment causes us to lose perspective on the injury's broader implications to the body's interrelated systems. In our companion volume, *The Lower Extremity and Spine in Sports Medicine*, we showed that function can be altered in sites distant both distally and proximally from the injury. In this volume on the upper extremity and cervical spine, we continue our efforts to show that all parts of the linkage system work together and therefore can be disrupted together. One must bear in mind that all systems and parts of the body are linked; damage to one system or part has implications for the other systems or parts. In the lower extremity, for example, an ankle injury can cause one to lose strength in proximal segments of muscle far removed from the injury site, such as those that govern hip abduction. When an injury is treated as an entity unto itself, without regard for the other physical systems that may be involved, other problems, such as contractures from disuse and immobilization, may develop. In the upper extremity, injury to the arm, for example, will cause residual disability in scapular and cervical muscle strength, or shoulder or elbow range of motion. Further effects of such weakness and disability can impact on the ability to use and consume oxygen, which will disrupt the economy of motion and impede efficient cardiorespiratory function. One goes on from there to an athlete's stress reactions about inability to perform, which affects his psychologic well-being.

One injury can have wide-ranging effects throughout the body, and disciplines such as anatomy, physiology, pathology, biomechanics, cardiology, kinesiology, and others become united in the sense of each having an answer to the question, "what is wrong?" Therefore in athletic injuries, the whole body must be involved in rehabilitation; power development must not be restricted to just the injured hand, or elbow, or shoulder. It must be a total-body approach, since the body itself is a total and linked system.

Not only the musculoskeletal system is affected by an orthopaedic injury. When muscle weakness causes a person to strain in an activity, the cardiorespiratory system perceives an extra load; this extra load puts maximum demands on the heart and can cause cardiac problems. When the demands of an activity cannot be satisfied, a person can injure himself, even to the point of a heart attack.

We like to conceptualize the comprehensive care of the athlete as the "7 Ps": performer, performance demand, pathology, practice, prescription, practitioner, and prevention. The performer must be aware of the performance demand of his activity, and practice to perfect his performance. As well, the practitioner, through awareness of pathologic conditions both inherent in the human body and peculiar to a particular athlete (history of injury, body type), formulates a prescription for that athlete's safe performance of the sport, and thereby encourages prevention of an injury. This concept recognizes the multidisciplinary aspects of sports medicine, and combines them into a total approach to treatment and rehabilitation.

We at the Nicholas Institute of Sports Medicine and Athletic Trauma, the first hospital-based institute of its kind in the country, have worked for many years to develop the concept of linkage as part of our treatment program. At the Institute, patients are given a program of treatment that encompasses the entire physical system, not just the injury. For example, a hand patient is given strengthening exercises for the arm, shoulder, and chest. The body as an integrated system means that the level action in joints such as the elbow and shoulder also involve links in the cervical spine, the upper back, and torso. Motion in the elbow, for example, translates into the shoulder and scapular muscles. Malfunction of any of the links necessarily affects smooth translation, in effect turning a ripple into a tidal wave and disrupting normal movement throughout the linkage. What this means is that an elbow injury that prevents normal elbow movement can cause problems in the scapular region. A whole spectrum of disabilities can flourish throughout the linkage system of the body, caused by one injury affecting one joint in one area. Viewing the body dimensionally as an x y z axis, one can understand how an injury in x can reverberate to y and then into z in linked fashion.

Exercise programs must be tailored to meet the ultimate demands of sport, and rehabilitation must involve the total linkage system, including the athlete's psychologic profile. Such an approach will not only be cost-effective in terms of care, but will also serve the patient well in his daily life.

James A. Nicholas
Elliott B. Hershman

Acknowledgments

Our deep appreciation and gratitude:

To our contributing authors, who continue to write up-to-date, authoritative, and well-researched chapters. We cannot thank them enough for their efforts in completing this project.

To Suzanne VanderSanden whose unsurpassed organizational and leadership skills enabled clinical schedules and responsibilities to mesh with didactic, research, and writing commitments. Her daily administrative efforts keep the office afloat.

To Trish Naso and Pat Kennemur, who ably and diligently handled our correspondence and communication.

To Jeannette Gudino, Peggy Pappas, Shirley Bekas, and Mary DiRado for their energetic and gracious assistance throughout the publication process.

To George Tanis and Sophie Bedmarz of the Lenox Hill Hospital Department of Medical Photography for their outstanding work in the production of many of the fine photographs used throughout the text.

To our editors at Mosby–Year Book, Bob Hurley, Kathy Falk, Ellen Baker-Geisel, and Suzanne Fannin. They continued to guide and work untiringly on this text. Their patience and understanding are invaluable.

Contents

PART I Cervical Spine

CHAPTER 1

The Relationship Between Cervical Spine Injury and the Upper Extremity

Pierce J. Ferriter
Patrick F. O'Leary

Cervical spine injuries have been associated with all major sports, including water sports,[3] football,[28] skiing,[30] gymnastics,[10] rugby,[15] and ice hockey.[11,25] Although the incidence of injury to the cervical spine is much lower than injuries incurred to other parts of the body, the impact to the athlete can be much greater.

Sports with cervical spine injury reports

- Water sports
- Football
- Skiing
- Gymnastics
- Rugby
- Ice hockey

The clinical syndrome of acute cervical spine injury with nerve root compression manifests itself in the upper extremity. The first sign of injury is often radicular. Discomfort in the shoulder, arm, or hand with or without weakness may be the only symptom of severe cervical injury. Congenital lesions of the cervical spine (those that cause narrowing of the canal) may impinge on the spinal cord. This in turn can cause transient paralysis of the upper or lower extremities if unusual demands are placed on the neck during athletic performance.

The purpose of this chapter is to make the physician who treats athletes aware of cervical injuries. The implication of a neck injury is devastating to the patient, family, coaches, and fans alike. This chapter first deals with the epidemiology of cervical injuries and then proceeds to a discussion of the anatomy of the cervical spine. The authors then outline the various injuries that can occur in the cervical spine with their respective mechanisms. The chapter concludes with a discussion of prevention.

EPIDEMIOLOGY

The epidemiology of head and neck injuries was studied when the National Football Head and Neck Injury Registry was established in 1975.[33] To evaluate injury patterns (frequency and associations), comparison was made for two 5-year periods: 1959 to 1963 and 1971 to 1975. Initially, the Registry collected information retrospectively from 1971 through 1975.

During the 5-year period from 1959 to 1963, Schneider[28] reported 56 (1.4 per 100,000) injuries that involved a fracture and/or dislocation, and permanent cervical quadriplegia occurred in 30 athletes during that period (0.7 per 100,000). The Registry documented 259 (4.1 per 100,000) injuries involving a fracture and/or dislocation of the cervical spine in 99 (1.58 per 100,000) football injuries with associated permanent quadriplegia during the 1971 to 1975 seasons. These data indicate an increase in the number of individuals with cervical injuries during the latter 5-year period (Table 1-1).

These changes reflect the improvements in protective headgear for football players. During the same period,

FIG. 1-1. Incidence of cervical spine fractures, subluxations, and dislocations for all levels of participation in football underwent a dramatic decrease from 1976 to 1978 as a result of the rule changes. (Reproduced from Torg JS et al: *JAMA* 254[24]:3439, 1985.)

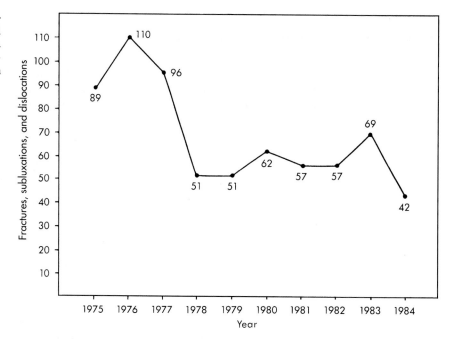

TABLE 1-1 Comparison of the occurrence of neck injuries between 1959 through 1963 and 1971 through 1975

Source (Year)	Cervical Spine Fractures/ Dislocations	Permanent Cervical Quadriplegics
Schneider (1959-1963)	56	30
Football Head and Neck Injury Registry (1971-1975)	259	99

Modified from Torg JS et al: *JAMA* 241:1477, 1979.

the incidence of intracranial injuries decreased dramatically. Because the athletes' heads were protected by the helmets, they were used more as battering rams in blocking and tackling. Therefore the number of neck injuries increased dramatically during this time, when the cervical spine was rendered more vulnerable to injuries. As a result of the Registry findings, the National Collegiate Athletic Association (NCAA) and the National Federation of State High-school Athletic Associations adopted rule changes intended to control spearing (head-first) techniques. The NCAA Football Rules Committee established these new rules beginning in the 1976 season: (1) no player shall intentionally strike a runner with the

Spearing rules

- No player shall intentionally strike a runner with the crown or top of the helmet
- No player shall deliberately use his helmet to butt or ram an opponent
- Spearing is the deliberate use of the helmet in an attempt to punish an opponent

crown or top of the helmet; (2) no player shall deliberately use his helmet to butt or ram an opponent; and (3) spearing is the deliberate use of the helmet in an attempt to punish an opponent.

As a result of these rules, Torg et al[33] demonstrated the decrease in both high school and college levels of cervical spine fractures, dislocations, and subluxations. In 1975, the season before the rule changes, there were 6.5 injuries per 100,000 participants and 29.3 per 100,000 at the high school and college levels, respectively. Over the ensuing 8 years, the incidence of cervical spine injury gradually declined until there were 1.9 per 100,000 and 6.7 per 100,000 at the high school and college level, respectively, in 1984. The number of cervical spine fractures, dislocations, and subluxations went from 110 in 1976 to 51 in 1978. This decrease has also been maintained from 1978 to 1984 (Fig. 1-1).[33]

Gymnastics also established patterns of injuries. The National Registry of Gymnastic Catastrophic Injuries was established in 1978. In its first 2 years, the National Registry documented 11 gymnastic injuries involving the cervical spine on the trampoline and minitramp across the nation.[4] Nine athletes developed permanent quadriplegia and two patients died (Table 1-2). Most of these participants were skilled, and some were participating under the direction of physical education instructors.

Subsequent to the study by the National Registry, guidelines have been published concerning the use of the trampoline in organized sports activities. The American Academy of Pediatrics has regarded the trampoline as a potentially dangerous apparatus when not used with precautions. The Academy has stated that *the trampoline has no place in competitive sports and should never be used at home or in recreational settings.* These guidelines dramatically decreased the number of serious injuries to participants.

TABLE 1-2 National incidence of gymnastic injuries, July 1978 through June 1980

Event	Sex	Person	Circumstances	Injury
1. Trampoline	M	Skilled teenager	Practice, gymnastics club	Quadriplegia
2. Trampoline	M	Young boy	Backyard recreation	Death
3. Trampoline	M	Skilled young adult	Backyard game of "horse"	Quadriplegia
4. Trampoline	M	Advanced beginner teen	Military base recreation	Quadriplegia
5. Trampoline	M	College assistant instructor	P.E. class demonstration	Quadriplegia
6. Minitramp	M	College cheerleader	Warmup for football game	Quadriplegia
7. Minitramp	M	High school gymnast	Practice for pep rally	Quadriplegia
8. Minitramp	F	High school cheerleader	Cheerleader practice	Death
9. Tumbling	M	College gymnast	Practicing high-bar dismount	Quadriplegia
10. Uneven bars	F	High school gymnast	Practicing routine	Quadriplegia
11. Minitramp	M	College cheerleader	Unscheduled practice	Quadriplegia

From Torg JS: *Athletic injuries to the head, neck, and face,* Philadelphia, 1982, Lea & Febiger.

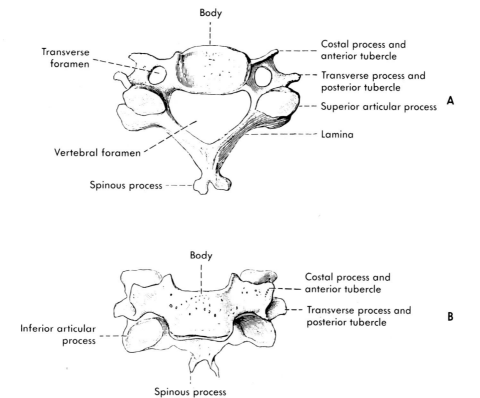

FIG. 1-2. A, Typical cervical vertebra with its spinous process, lamina, and vertebral body. **B,** Note the articular facets and shape of the vertebral bodies on the frontal view. (From Disse J: *K von Bardeleben's handbuch der Anatomie des Menschen,* Jena, Germany, 1896, Fischer.)

Catastrophic neurotrauma is rare but occurs with some degree of frequency in football and gymnastics. Such injuries occur in other sports, but not with the frequency to allow epidemiologic analysis.

Restructuring of the rules for trampoline use has resulted in a dramatic decrease in spinal injuries from this activity. By the same token, the ruling in 1976 to ban spearing and head-butting techniques in football tackling has also resulted in a drop in neurotrauma in this sport. The data available show that cervical injuries are most likely to result from improper technique and not from the activity itself. Therefore proper education of players, coaches, and teachers is most effective in controlling serious injuries.

ANATOMY

In the most simple description, the cervical spine is a column of seven vertebral bodies that connect the head to the thorax. Four of the vertebrae are typical (third to sixth) and three are more specialized (first, second, and seventh). The spinal cord is housed in the vertebral ca-

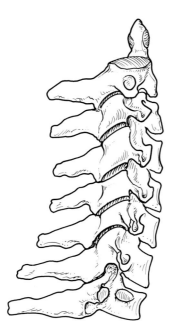

FIG. 1-3. Shingling effect of articular facets. The superior facets are directed dorsally and cranially, and the inferior facets are directed ventrally and caudally.

nal. A spinal nerve that innervates the upper limb exits through each of the vertebral foramina. Injuries to the cervical spine may produce signs and symptoms related to the upper extremity based on the level of injury, as well as on the amount of nervous tissue affected.

Lower Cervical Segments (C3, C4, C5, C6)

A typical lower cervical vertebra has a small vertebral body that is concave on its superior surface and convex on its inferior surface (Fig. 1-2). Projecting laterally from the body are the **transverse processes**. The **foramen transversarium** is a canal in the transverse process that transmits the vertebral artery except at C7, where the foramen contains the **accessory vertebral vein**. At the junction of the pedicle and the neural arch are located the **superoarticular and inferoarticular processes.** The articular facets are flat; the superior face dorsally and cranially. The inferior facets are directed ventrally and caudally (Fig. 1-3). These articulations form a shingling effect that should be preserved in a normal cervical spine. The facet joints of the lower cervical spine are diarthrodial joints with synovial membranes and fibrous capsules. The joint capsules are lax to permit increased motion. When subjected to excessive force, these joints may dislocate, leading to a unilateral or bilateral facet dislocation. The spinous processes of the third, fourth, and fifth cervical vertebrae are usually bifid, whereas those of the sixth and seventh are longer. The distance between the spinous processes is usually constant, and if a line were extended from each tip, they would tend to converge on a central point. Widening of the spinous processes indicates disruption of those ligaments between them and interrupts the converging lines (Fig. 1-4).

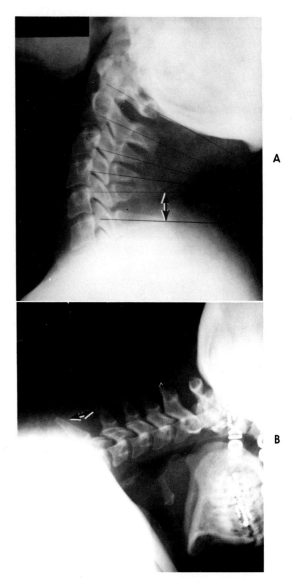

FIG. 1-4. A, Divergence of lines between C5 and C6 indicating disruption of the interspinous ligaments. **B,** Accentuated in flexion.

Atlantoaxial Complex (C1, C2)

The first two cervical vertebrae form a unique joint called the **atlantoaxial complex.** The atlas is a bony ring consisting of one posterior and one anterior arch connected by two lateral masses (Fig. 1-5). The lateral masses bear superoinferior and inferoarticular facets and transverse processes. The superoarticular facets are directed upward for the reception of the occipital condyles. Flexion of the head takes place with these joints. The inferoarticular facets face downward and articulate with the superoarticular facets of the axis.

The second cervical vertebra, or axis, provides a surface upon which the atlas may rotate. This is the **odontoid process,** or **dens** (Fig. 1-6). The dens represents the body of the atlas. Besides being a pivot joint for the atlas, the dens provides an insertion point for the transverse atlantal ligament.

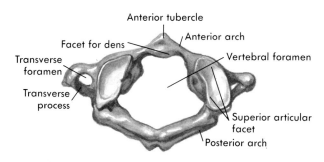

FIG. 1-5. Atlas consists of a ring with an anterior and posterior arch connected by two articular facets. (From Seeley RR, Stephens TD, Tate P: *Anatomy and physiology,* ed 2, St Louis, 1992, Mosby.)

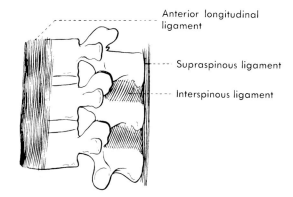

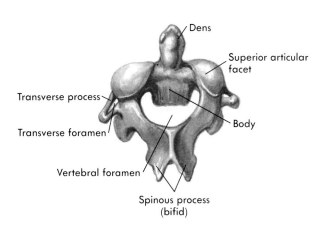

FIG. 1-6. Axis provides a surface from which the atlas can rotate. It contains the bony dens, which represents the body of the axis. (From Seeley RR, Stephens TD, Tate P: *Anatomy and physiology,* ed 2, St Louis, 1992, Mosby.)

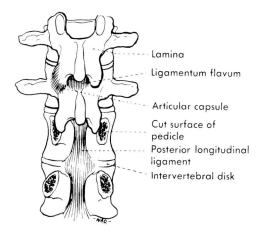

FIG. 1-7. Anterior and posterior longitudinal ligaments of the spine are its major stabilizers and prevent excessive flexion and extension. The ligamentum flavum connects adjacent lamina. (From Hollinshead WH: *Anatomy for surgeons: the back and limbs,* ed 3, Philadelphia, 1982, Harper & Row.)

Transitional Vertebra (C7)

The seventh cervical vertebra is a transitional vertebra because it is located between the very mobile cervical vertebral bodies (C1 through C6) and the thoracic vertebral bodies, which are generally much more stable. Its spinous process is longer than that of the other cervical vertebrae and is easily palpable. Its body is proportionally broader than the bodies of the vertebrae above. Because it is at the base of the cervical spine, the seventh vertebra is sometimes difficult to visualize radiographically, especially in patients with short necks and muscular chests.

Canal Size

Cervical spinal stenosis is a condition that narrows the spinal canal with the potential of compressing the spinal cord. Several authors[12,20,21,34] have shown that those patients with a narrow canal are much more prone to develop neurapraxia and/or transient quadriplegia when they sustain an acute hyperflexion or extension injury to the neck. Different methods of measuring the spinal canal have been advocated, and these consist of the **direct method**[21] and the **ratio method.**[34] Each author points out that, if the spinal canal is less than 14 mm in

diameter or has a ratio of less than 0.80 (which compares the sagittal diameter of the canal to the anteroposterior width of the vertebral body), then the patient is placed at great risk of neurologic injury if the cervical spine is stressed.

Soft Tissue

The ligaments and intervertebral disks maintain the normal alignment of the cervical spine. The **anterior and posterior longitudinal ligaments** are the major stabilizers of the spine and prevent excessive flexion and extension (Fig. 1-7). The anterior longitudinal ligament consists of longitudinal fibers that adhere to the intervertebral disks. It extends from the base of the skull to the sacrum. The posterior longitudinal ligament extends over the dorsal surface of the vertebral bodies within the vertebral canal. The ligament is composed of longitudinal fibers denser and more compact than the anterior longitudinal ligament. It fans out over the posterior surface of the intervertebral disks and prevents posterior extrusion. The intervertebral disk is interposed between adjacent vertebral bodies and forms a strong bond between them. Each disk consists of a gelatinous **nucleus pul-**

FIG. 1-10. A, T1 image of the cervical spine in a patient after trauma during a wrestling match. Magnetic resonance image demonstrates subluxation of C4 on C5 with a bulging disk and narrowing of the spinal canal. **B,** T2 image shows more clearly the compression of the spinal cord.

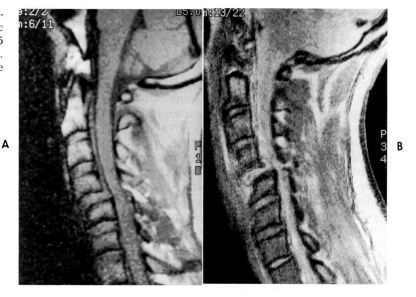

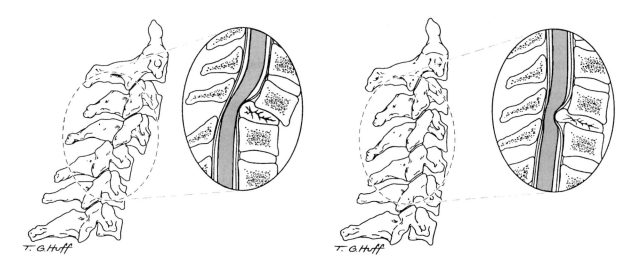

FIG. 1-11. Demonstrates possible mechanism of injury to the spinal cord when closed reduction is attempted. Disk may herniate when reduction maneuver is performed. MRI is necessary to rule out potential problem before reduction is contemplated. (From Doran S et al: *J Neurosurg* 79:342, 1993.)

The role of MRI in the evaluation of the trauma patient is evolving.[16] The development of MRI-compatible ventilation and monitoring devices has aided the physician's ability to examine the injured patient. It has been shown to be superior in detecting soft-tissue, disk, and nerve-tissue injury. It is especially useful in the evaluation of patients with negative plain radiographs who have experienced a neurologic loss.

Both T1- and T2-weighted sequences are necessary for detection of bony and soft tissue injury (Fig. 1-10). Bony elements such as vertebral body fractures are best assessed by T1-weighted images. Ligament injury can be identified by the presence of ligamentous discontinuity or hemorrhage in the soft tissue.

One of the most significant advances made possible by MRI is that injuries of the spinal cord can now be seen.[23] Cord edema and hemorrhage are readily detected on T2-weighted images. The area of edema is hyperintense, and hemorrhage is hypointense on T2-weighted images.[7]

MRI also enables assessment of the position of herniated disk material in the injured spine of patients with traumatic locked facets. Closed reduction and traction may result in increased spinal cord compression and neurologic deficit (Fig. 1-11).[16] Rizzolo et al[26] reported

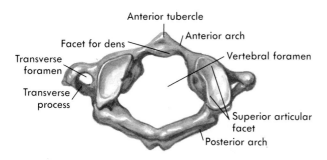

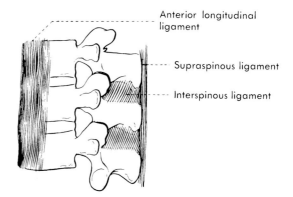

FIG. 1-5. Atlas consists of a ring with an anterior and posterior arch connected by two articular facets. (From Seeley RR, Stephens TD, Tate P: *Anatomy and physiology,* ed 2, St Louis, 1992, Mosby.)

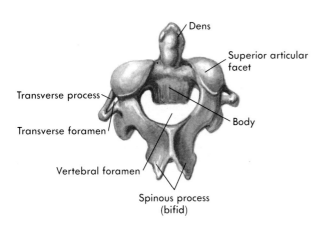

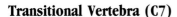

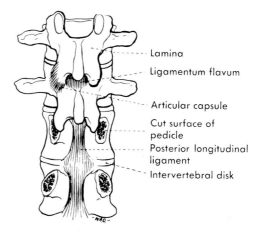

FIG. 1-6. Axis provides a surface from which the atlas can rotate. It contains the bony dens, which represents the body of the axis. (From Seeley RR, Stephens TD, Tate P: *Anatomy and physiology,* ed 2, St Louis, 1992, Mosby.)

FIG. 1-7. Anterior and posterior longitudinal ligaments of the spine are its major stabilizers and prevent excessive flexion and extension. The ligamentum flavum connects adjacent lamina. (From Hollinshead WH: *Anatomy for surgeons: the back and limbs,* ed 3, Philadelphia, 1982, Harper & Row.)

Transitional Vertebra (C7)

The seventh cervical vertebra is a transitional vertebra because it is located between the very mobile cervical vertebral bodies (C1 through C6) and the thoracic vertebral bodies, which are generally much more stable. Its spinous process is longer than that of the other cervical vertebrae and is easily palpable. Its body is proportionally broader than the bodies of the vertebrae above. Because it is at the base of the cervical spine, the seventh vertebra is sometimes difficult to visualize radiographically, especially in patients with short necks and muscular chests.

Canal Size

Cervical spinal stenosis is a condition that narrows the spinal canal with the potential of compressing the spinal cord. Several authors[12,20,21,34] have shown that those patients with a narrow canal are much more prone to develop neurapraxia and/or transient quadriplegia when they sustain an acute hyperflexion or extension injury to the neck. Different methods of measuring the spinal canal have been advocated, and these consist of the **direct method**[21] and the **ratio method.**[34] Each author points out that, if the spinal canal is less than 14 mm in diameter or has a ratio of less than 0.80 (which compares the sagittal diameter of the canal to the anteroposterior width of the vertebral body), then the patient is placed at great risk of neurologic injury if the cervical spine is stressed.

Soft Tissue

The ligaments and intervertebral disks maintain the normal alignment of the cervical spine. The **anterior and posterior longitudinal ligaments** are the major stabilizers of the spine and prevent excessive flexion and extension (Fig. 1-7). The anterior longitudinal ligament consists of longitudinal fibers that adhere to the intervertebral disks. It extends from the base of the skull to the sacrum. The posterior longitudinal ligament extends over the dorsal surface of the vertebral bodies within the vertebral canal. The ligament is composed of longitudinal fibers denser and more compact than the anterior longitudinal ligament. It fans out over the posterior surface of the intervertebral disks and prevents posterior extrusion. The intervertebral disk is interposed between adjacent vertebral bodies and forms a strong bond between them. Each disk consists of a gelatinous **nucleus pul-**

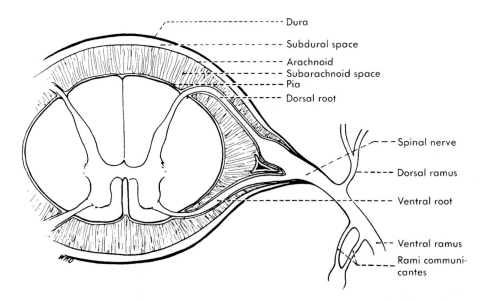

FIG. 1-8. Diagram of a spinal nerve as it exits the intervertebral foramen. (From Hollinshead WH: *Anatomy for surgeons: the back and limbs,* ed 3, Philadelphia, 1982, Harper & Row.)

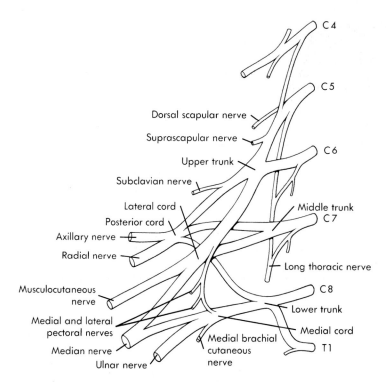

FIG. 1-9. Brachial plexus is formed by the ventral rami of C5 through T1. (From Seeley RR, Stephens TD, Tate P: *Anatomy and physiology,* St Louis, 1992, Mosby.)

posus, two cartilaginous **endplates,** and the **annulus fibrosis.** The intervertebral disks are important shock absorbers that resist axial loading. Under pressure the nucleus pulposus becomes flatter and distends the posterior longitudinal ligament.

The articulations of the vertebral arches are secured by the **articular capsule, supraspinous ligaments, interspinous ligaments,** and **ligamentum flavum.** The facet joints are enveloped by the articular capsules, which are thin and loose. These capsules prevent excessive gliding motion. The ligamentum flavum connects the lamina of each adjacent vertebra. They consist of strong elastic fibers that are important in resisting excessive flexion of the neck. The interspinous and supraspinous ligaments connect the adjoining processes and, along with the ligamentum flavum, resist hyperflexion (Fig. 1-7).

Neurologic Anatomy

A general knowledge of the neurologic anatomy of the cervical spine and the upper extremity is necessary for the assessment of neck injuries. Radicular symptoms may be the only finding in cervical fracture, dislocation, and disk herniations. Results of radiographic testing may be negative, and the physician must be aware of any neurologic deficit expressed by the patient.

The spinal nerves are formed by the union of the dorsal and ventral roots as they emanate from the spinal cord (Fig. 1-8). Outside the **intervertebral foramen,** the spinal nerve divides into a **dorsal ramus** and a **ventral ramus.** The ventral rami supply the skin and muscles of the upper extremity. The **brachial plexus** is then formed by the ventral rami of the spinal nerves C5 through T1 (Fig. 1-9).[13,14]

The ventral rami of C5 and C6 fuse to form the **superior trunk.** The C7 ventral ramus forms the middle trunk. The ventral rami of C8 and T1 form the inferior trunk. Each trunk divides into an anterior and posterior division. The anterior divisions of the superior and middle trunk form the lateral cord. The posterior cord is formed by the posterior division of the tree trunks. The medial cord is formed by the anterior division of the inferior trunk. The cords end by dividing into peripheral nerves. Deficits in the peripheral nerves in the upper extremity alert the examiner to a potential cervical spine injury.

Cervical spine injuries cause lesions proximal to the plexus at either the spinal cord or the spinal nerve level. The cutaneous and motor functions of the upper extremity follow a segmental pattern of innervation; therefore diagnosis of injuries can be made based on the peripheral nerve deficit. The segmental, sensory, and motor innervation of the upper extremity is noted in Tables 1-3 and 1-4. The deep tendon reflexes also follow a segmental distribution (Table 1-5).

IMAGING

The diagnostic evaluation of the cervical spine–injured patient begins with standard radiographs. After a preliminary diagnosis, other imaging modalities such as

TABLE 1-3 Segmental sensory distribution of the upper extremity

Spinal Nerve	Dermatomal Distribution
C4	Shoulder pad area
C5	Lateral aspect of arm
C6	Lateral aspect of forearm, hand, and the radial two digits
C7	Middle finger
C8	Ulnar two digits and medial aspect of hand and wrist
T1	Medial aspect of forearm
T2	Medial aspect of arm

From Torg JS: *Athletic injuries to the head, neck, and face,* Philadelphia, 1982, Lea & Febiger.

TABLE 1-4 Segmental motor innervation in the upper extremity

Spinal Nerve	Area of Innervation
C5, C6	Deltoid and other intrinsic muscles of the shoulder (abduction, hyperextension, and external rotation at shoulder)
C5, C6	Biceps, brachialis, and supinator (elbow flexion and supination of forearm)
C6, C7	Pronators of forearm
C7 (C6, C8)	Triceps and extensors of wrist and of fingers at the metacarpal joints
C8, T1	Intrinsic muscles of the hand

TABLE 1-5 Segmental levels of deep tendon reflexes

Reflex	Corresponding Nerve
Biceps	C5 (C6)
Triceps	C7 (C6)
Radial jerk (supinator reflex)	C5 (C6, C67)
Ulnar jerk (pronator reflex)	C6 (C7, C8)

computed tomography (CT) and magnetic resonance imaging (MRI) scans may be used before definitive treatment is rendered. A standard cervical spine series is considered to be a lateral radiograph showing the cervicothoracic junction (C7 to the top of T1), and anteroposterior (AP) and open-mouth odontoid views. It has been shown that 94% of errors leading to missed or delayed diagnosis of cervical spine injuries were due to the failure to obtain an adequate series of initial radiographs.[6] Other films such as obliques, pillar views, and flexion-extension x rays are ordered on an individual case basis.

CT scanning is best used to clarify fractures when they are detected on plain films. CT is preferable to conventional tomography because of its superior contrast resolution, decreased examination time, smaller radiation dose, diminished patient manipulation, and ability to perform multiplanar reconstruction.[23] CT can detect fractures of the lamina and facets more accurately than plain films. Spinal canal diameters can also be assessed using CT scanning.

FIG. 1-10. A, T1 image of the cervical spine in a patient after trauma during a wrestling match. Magnetic resonance image demonstrates subluxation of C4 on C5 with a bulging disk and narrowing of the spinal canal. **B,** T2 image shows more clearly the compression of the spinal cord.

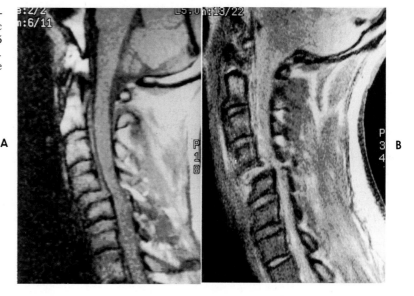

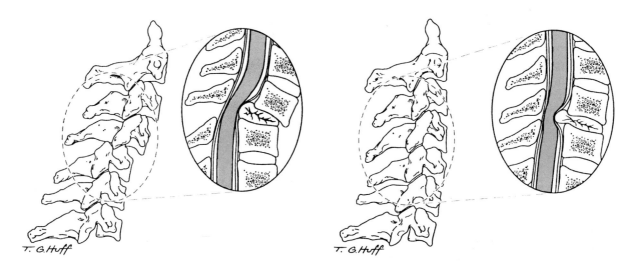

FIG. 1-11. Demonstrates possible mechanism of injury to the spinal cord when closed reduction is attempted. Disk may herniate when reduction maneuver is performed. MRI is necessary to rule out potential problem before reduction is contemplated. (From Doran S et al: *J Neurosurg* 79:342, 1993.)

The role of MRI in the evaluation of the trauma patient is evolving.[16] The development of MRI-compatible ventilation and monitoring devices has aided the physician's ability to examine the injured patient. It has been shown to be superior in detecting soft-tissue, disk, and nerve-tissue injury. It is especially useful in the evaluation of patients with negative plain radiographs who have experienced a neurologic loss.

Both T1- and T2-weighted sequences are necessary for detection of bony and soft tissue injury (Fig. 1-10). Bony elements such as vertebral body fractures are best assessed by T1-weighted images. Ligament injury can be identified by the presence of ligamentous discontinuity or hemorrhage in the soft tissue.

One of the most significant advances made possible by MRI is that injuries of the spinal cord can now be seen.[23] Cord edema and hemorrhage are readily detected on T2-weighted images. The area of edema is hyperintense, and hemorrhage is hypointense on T2-weighted images.[7]

MRI also enables assessment of the position of herniated disk material in the injured spine of patients with traumatic locked facets. Closed reduction and traction may result in increased spinal cord compression and neurologic deficit (Fig. 1-11).[16] Rizzolo et al[26] reported

TABLE 1-6 Mechanism of injury resulting in permanent cervical quadriplegia (1971-1975)

	Injuries Resulting in Quadriplegia (%) (n = 73)	Injuries not Resulting in Quadriplegia (%) (n = 136)
Hyperflexion	10	11
Hyperextension	3	8
Vertical compression (spearing)	52	39
Knee or thigh to head	15	17
Collision, pileup, or ground contact	11	19
Tackled	7	7
Machine-related	3	0
Face mask acting as lever	0	0

From Torg JS: *Athletic injuries to the head, neck, and face,* Philadelphia, 1982, Lea & Febiger.

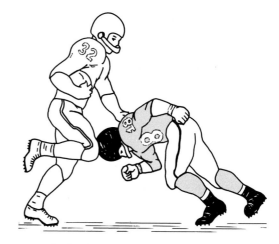

FIG. 1-12. The head is used as a battering ram during spearing. (Originally published in *Can Med Assoc J* 109:48, 1973.)

a 40% incidence of disk herniation in unilateral locked facets and an 80% incidence in bilateral locked facets in a review of 55 patients with cervical spine trauma. Eismont, Arena, and Green[9] found that six of 68 patients with facet dislocation also had a concurrent disk herniation. It is now recommended that an MRI scan be performed before attempting reduction of the locked facets. If a herniated disk is discovered, anterior diskectomy and arthrodesis is advised over attempts at closed reduction.

There are two limiting factors when attempting to obtain MRI in acutely spine-injured patients: (1) maintenance of spinal stabilization and (2) prolonged scan times on unmonitored patients. The maintenance of cervical traction during MRI requires the use of a nonferromagnetic skull traction device. With regard to time restraints, T1-weighted images are done first. They demonstrate cord transection and deformity. If time allows, T2-weighted images are done, which characteristically take longer.

The potential for MRI in acute spinal cord injury is promising. MRI allows visualization of the traumatized spinal cord. Such information may have important prognostic and therapeutic implications. It has also found to be extremely important before instituting various treatment modalities.

MECHANISMS OF INJURY

The evaluation of cervical spine injuries begins the moment the injury occurs. An understanding of the mechanism of injury can aid in arriving at the proper diagnosis. A variety of mechanisms has been shown to cause significant injury to the cervical spine, causing quadriplegia (Table 1-6).[32] Originally it was thought that in football the helmet acted as a guillotine in the hyperextension injury, severing the posterior cervical spinal cord. Virgin[37] has shown this not to be the case. Carter and Frankel[1] also have shown through static-free body analysis that the impact of the posterior rim of the hel-

met on the base of the neck is a rare cause of severe cervical spine injury.

A number of mechanisms have been implicated in causing fracture dislocations of the cervical spine. Accidental falls and diving into shallow water (resulting in hyperflexion) have resulted in a number of significant fractures of the cervical spine. On the playing field, however, **axial load** has been the most common mechanism causing cervical fractures. From 1971 through 1975, 52% of all cervical spine quadriplegias resulted from spearings, when the head was used as a battering ram in football (Fig. 1-12).[33] It must be remembered that, during forward flexion of the neck, the cervical spine is straightened, losing its normal cervical lordosis.[36] The resultant straight column of soft tissue, disk, and vertebral bodies must absorb the force. If the energy-absorbing capacity of this column is exceeded, muscle and ligament tears, disk herniation, and fractures can occur. Therefore it is not surprising that the most vulnerable position of the cervical spine is flexion. In football the highest percentage of injuries occurs in the defensive back position (Table 1-7).[32] The neck is placed under extreme load during a tackle.

INJURIES

A multiplicity of injuries may occur in the cervical spine during athletic competition. The purpose of this chapter is not to identify each injury, but rather to mention the most common injuries and to address how they affect the upper extremity.

In the evaluation of any cervical injury, the physical and radiographic findings are most important in the final treatment. The following are a number of acute cervical injuries that can occur in athletics. Emphasis is placed on those injuries that most commonly cause damage to the upper extremities. Cervical strains and muscle contusions are not addressed here because their clinical findings are most commonly localized to the neck.

TABLE 1-7 Injury by activity

	Permanent Cervical Quadriplegia, 1971-1975		Cervical Fracture Dislocations Without Quadriplegia, 1971-1975	
	High School (%) (n = 77)	College (%) (n = 18)	High School (%) (n = 105)	College (%) (n = 46)
Tackling	72	78	59	49
Tackled	14	22	15	24
Blocking	6	0	7	16
Drill	3	0	5	7
Collision pileup	3	0	12	4
Machine-related	2	0	2	0

From Torg JS: *Athletic injuries to the head, neck, and face*, Philadelphia, 1982, Lea & Febiger.

Cervical Burner

The most common cervical spine injury that refers symptoms to the upper extremity is the brachial plexus stretch neurapraxia, or **burner**.[31] Clancy et al[2] has reported a 49% incidence in college football players over their 4-year exposure. They classify the injuries into three grades, depending on the length of time that symptoms persist and the electromyographic (EMG) findings. The typical history is of a player who develops sharp and burning pain in the neck that radiates into the arm and hand following contact with the head, neck, or shoulder during a play.[18] There may be associated weakness or paresthesias in the hand. The mechanism of injury is that the athlete's head is laterally flexed away from the site of the injury, or the involved shoulder is driven downward or backward, thus placing traction on the brachial plexus.

The clinical manifestations of each grade of injury correspond to Seddon's classification of nerve injuries.[29]

A Grade I injury corresponds to a neurapraxia. This results in a transitory loss of motor and sensory function of the upper extremity that may last for minutes or hours. EMG results fail to demonstrate any signs of axonal injury.

A Grade II injury is one that produces significant motor weakness and sensory deficit lasting 2 weeks. EMG studies reveal changes consistent with axonotmesis. Most often affected is the upper trunk of the brachial plexus, which causes significant deltoid infraspinatus and supraspinatus and biceps muscle weakness. Again, the mechanism for the Grade II injuries puts a similar stretch on the brachial plexus when the shoulder is driving downward and away from the flexed neck.

A Grade III brachial plexus injury corresponds to Seddon's neurotmesis. This injury produces motor and sensory deficits for up to 1 year. Here the mechanism of injury is the same; however, the force is greater. This results in irreversible damage to the nerves, with resulting muscle loss.

Because most of these injuries are transient, no clinical treatment is necessary. For those patients who have more than a temporary loss of motor strength, the treatment consists of rehabilitation and prevention of atrophy of the involved muscles. Players should not involve themselves in contact sports until they have achieved full strength in the upper extremities. A routine cervical spine series should be performed on all patients sustaining a significant brachial plexus injury to rule out any osseous abnormalities.

The natural history and treatment of burners is discussed in Chapter 31.

Transient Quadriplegia

Transient quadriplegia is a neurologic syndrome that has serious implications for the young athlete. The symptoms include burning pain, numbness, tingling, and loss of sensation.[17,34] The extremities may be weak or even completely paralyzed. These findings are transient and usually resolve within minutes. This form of quadriplegia has been caused by hyperflexion and hyperextension, as well as by axial loading injuries to the cervical spine.[34]

The causes of transient quadriplegia have been varied, occurring in individuals with developmental stenosis of the cervical spine, congenital fusions, cervical instability, and protrusion of an intervertebral disk. When any of these entities occur in combination, there is a much higher risk of causing neurologic sequelae by narrowing of the canal diameter. The normal average diameter of the middle part of the cervical spine (between the third and sixth cervical vertebrae) has been reported to be 17 mm.[8,12] The standard method of measurement determines the distance from the midpoint of the posterior aspect of the vertebral body to the nearest point of the corresponding spinolaminar line. Torg et al[34] (Fig. 1-13) have devised a second method of measurement called the ratio method, which compares the sagittal diameter of the spinal canal to the anteroposterior width of the vertebral body. This method compensates for variations in radiographic technique. A canal measurement of 14 mm or less at any cervical segment falls below two standard deviations from the norm and puts the patient at risk.

One study reported the association between a narrowed sagittal diameter of the cervical spine and the development of myelopathy. Further compromise of the canal diameter can be caused by osteophytes, vertebral subluxation, or herniated disks. Penning[24] demonstrated the effects of flexion and extension on the sagittal diameter of the cervical spine. He coined the term *pinchers mechanism* when the cord is pinched by the processes of the two opposing bodies (Fig. 1-14). The degree of pinching is determined by the sagittal diameter of the spinal cord and the degree of extension or flexion (Fig. 1-15).

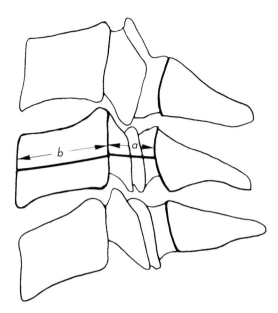

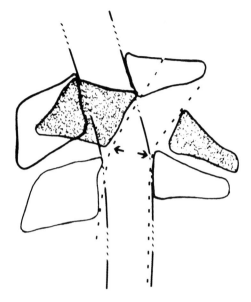

FIG. 1-13. *a,* Ratio of the spinal canal to the vertebral body is the distance from the midpoint of the posterior aspect of the vertebral body to the nearest point on the corresponding spinolaminar line. *b,* Divided by the anteroposterior width of the vertebral body. (From Torg JS et al: *J Bone Joint Surg* 68A[9]:1354, 1986.)

FIG. 1-14. The pinchers mechanism, as described by Panning, occurs between the posteroinferior aspect of the vertebral body and the anterosuperior aspect of the spinolaminar line of the subadjacent vertebra. (From Torg JS et al: *J Bone Joint Surg* 68A[9]: 1354, 1986.)

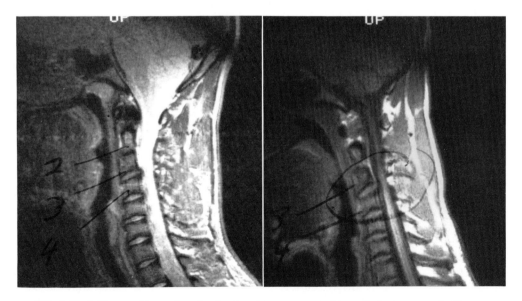

FIG. 1-15. A 19-year-old wrestler who developed temporary quadriparesis during a match. Note narrowing of the spinal canal at C3 and C4 by a disk herniation in flexion.

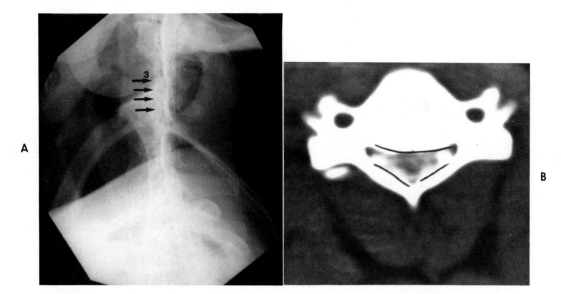

FIG. 1-16. A, Myelogram demonstrates significant narrowing of the dye column caused by spinal stenosis at C3 through C5. **B,** Contrast-enhanced computed tomography scan confirms narrowing of the canal.

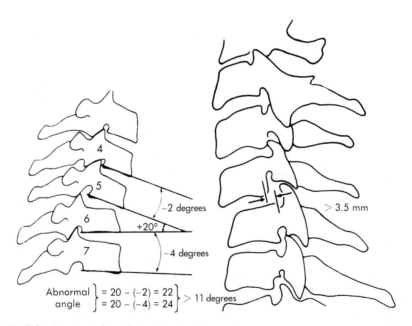

FIG. 1-17. White's criteria for stability. Vertebral body displacement should not exceed 3.5 mm and angular displacement less than 11 degrees. (From White AA et al: *Clin Orthop* 109:85, 1975.)

Patients who evidence clinical symptoms of transient quadriplegia after cervical spinal injury should be regarded with caution. A careful neurologic examination must be performed, recording the onset and resolution of symptoms. Permanent neurologic deficits, quadriplegia, or death may occur if the patient's complaints are ignored and a treatable condition is present. Patients should have an adequate work-up with myelography because this appears to be the best diagnostic tool at this time to rule out canal narrowing (Fig. 1-16).[17] Torg et al[34] reported no increased incidence of permanent neu-

rologic damage in 117 athletes who resumed sports activities after sustaining an episode of transient quadriplegia. They warned that patients with other factors contributing to cervical canal stenosis, such as cervical spondylosis, congenital abnormalities, or ligamentous instability, should be treated on an individual basis.[19]

Cervical Spine Fractures and Dislocations

Fractures and dislocations of the cervical spine are common injuries in today's athletic events. They have been documented in skiing, football, trampolining, and

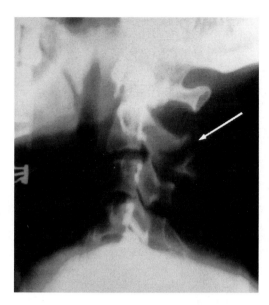

FIG. 1-18. Hangman's fracture through the neural arch of the second cervical vertebra.

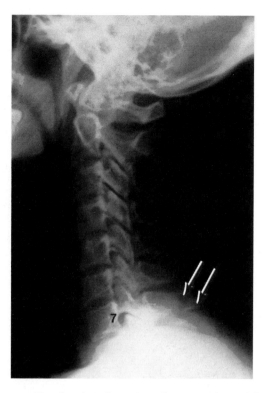

FIG. 1-19. Clay shoveler's fracture involves an avulsion of the spinous process of C7.

rugby. For simplicity's sake, they can be divided into fractures of the posterior elements and fractures of the anterior elements. Because of the proximity of the osseous fragments to the nerve roots and spinal cord, they are often associated with clinical findings referred to the upper extremity. Based on the segmental innervation of the sensory and motor elements of the upper extremity, the physician is able to document the level of injury.

Identifying a fracture of the cervical spine is the first step in treating this serious injury. Determining the stability of the fracture and/or dislocation may have far-reaching implications for the health of the athlete. Biomechanical studies have shown that normal ligaments permit little motion between vertebrae. White et al[38] have shown that, in the stable spine, horizontal displacement of one vertebral body onto another never exceeds 3.5 mm. Angular displacement greater than 11 degrees between each vertebra suggests instability of the cervical spine (Fig. 1-17). Only when ligaments were disrupted did such displacement exist. Therefore displacement of the cervical spine may be reduced, but it may remain unstable because of loss of the supporting ligaments.

Fractures of the Posterior Elements

Fractures of the neural arch of the second vertebra, or **Hangman's fracture,** occur when a vertical and hyperextension force is applied to the skull and cervical spine (Fig. 1-18). These fractures are usually stable, being adequately treated with a brace that controls flexion.[24] When there is subluxation of the second vertebra on the third, potential instability exists because of rupture of the anterior and posterior longitudinal ligaments as well as the cervical disks. In these cases halo immobilization is called for, and surgery may even be necessary when reduction cannot be accomplished. Neuro-

logic symptoms are rare in this injury because the canal is widened by the fracture.

Another fracture involving the posterior elements of the cervical spine is the **clay shoveler's fracture.** It involves the spinous process of C7, C6, or T1, in decreasing order (Fig. 1-19). Classified as an avulsion fracture, it is caused by distraction of the tight posterior ligaments when the neck is abruptly flexed. The pain is localized to the posterior aspect of the cervical spine; however, it does radiate into the shoulders. These are often difficult to identify on the lateral radiograph if the patient has a short neck or broad shoulders. A swimmer's view is often needed. These are stable fractures, and they do well with a short period of collar immobilization.

Dislocations of the cervical spine result from severe flexion and rotational forces. A unilateral or bilateral facet dislocation may occur. A **unilateral facet dislocation** occurs when the rotational forces tear the facet joint capsule. Lateral radiographs demonstrate moderate anterior displacement of the vertebral body (less than 50% of the vertebral body width). On the AP view the spinous process is deviated toward the locked facet (Fig. 1-20). These are stable injuries but often compress the nerve root as they exit the neural foramen. Motor weakness and sensory loss in the extremities are often associated with these injuries. Careful neurologic examination identifies the level. Treatment involves closed reduction using cervical traction and immobilization with a halo.

Bilateral facet dislocations are more severe inju-

FIG. 1-20. Unilateral facet dislocation of C4 on C5. Note displacement is less than 50%.

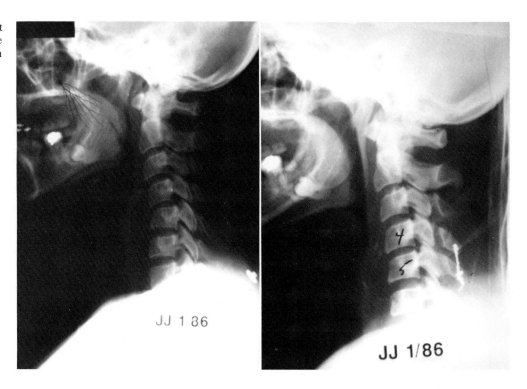

FIG. 1-21. A, Bilateral facet dislocation of C6 on C7. **B,** Solid posterior fusion 1 year later.

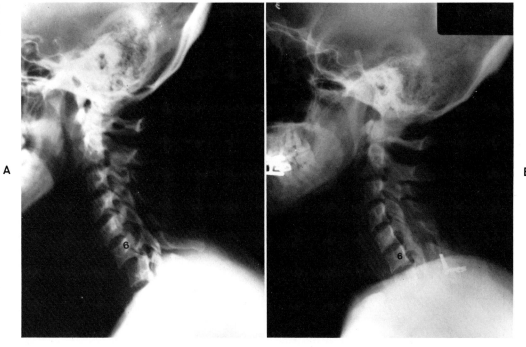

ries, resulting from purely flexion forces. They are often associated with neurologic deficit or complete quadriplegia. The facet capsules, posterior longitudinal ligament, and intervertebral disks are all disrupted. The lateral view demonstrates anterior displacement of the involved vertebra greater than 50% of the AP width (Fig. 1-21). Because these injuries are unstable, they require reduction and posterior fusion.

Fractures of the Anterior Elements

Fractures of the anterior portion of the vertebral bodies are caused by axial loading as well as flexion forces.[35] The pattern of the fracture and extent of disruption of the vertebral body depend on the amount of force applied to the neck at the moment of impact. Compression fractures are classified into four types based on the amount of bony disruption. Type I is the tear-drop fracture, which

ruptures the cortical endplate and breaks a chip off the anterior lip of the vertebral body; Type II occurs when the fracture involves the upper half of the vertebral body, and a larger fragment may be broken off anteriorly; Type III is a fracture of both the superior and the inferior endplates, with the fracture lines running throughout the vertebral body (the posterior cortex is intact); Type IV is a fracture of the vertebra likened to a burst fracture of the lumbar spine; this destroys the entire vertebral body with retropulsion of the fragments into the spinal canal. Types III and IV fractures are often associated with neurologic compromise (Fig. 1-22).

Type I and II fractures are treated with immobilization and do well. Type III and IV fractures are more serious; therefore treatment is often surgical. Flexion and extension radiographs are often necessary to detect instability, as measured by White's criteria.[38] CT scanning and myelography detect bony fragments in the spinal canal (Fig. 1-23). If surgery is necessary based on instability or neurologic injury, an anterior approach is necessary because the fracture is located anteriorly in the cervical spine. Decompression and fusion of the appropriate level are necessary.

Cervical Disk Herniation

Acute cervical disk herniation resulting from athletic injuries is a rare but reported event.[2] Roaf[27] has shown

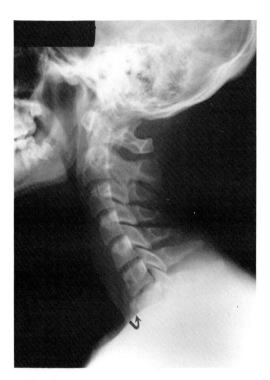

FIG. 1-22. Type II fracture of C7 in a gymnast.

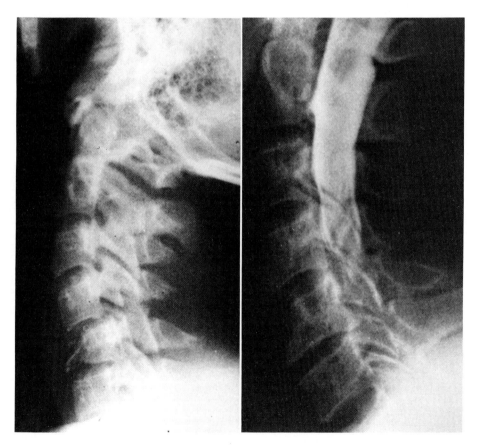

FIG. 1-23. Displaced anterior body fracture of C5. Myelogram demonstrates complete block of the dye column at C5. (From Weidner A: The cervical spine research society editorial committee. In Ubinder A: *The cervical spine,* Philadelphia, 1989, JB Lippincott.)

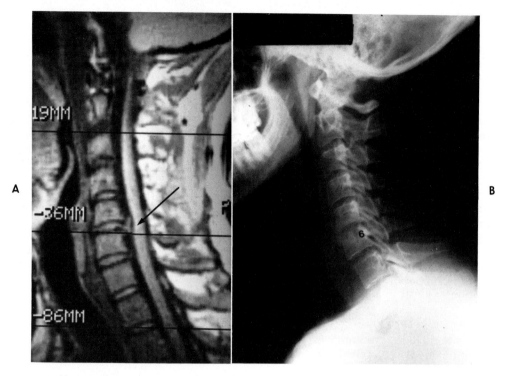

FIG. 1-24. A, Magnetic resonance image demonstrates cervical disk herniation at C5-C6. **B,** Cervical fusion at 10 weeks.

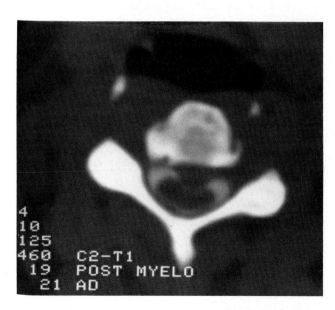

FIG. 1-25. Myelogram and computed tomography scan demonstrates herniated cervical disk at C3-C4.

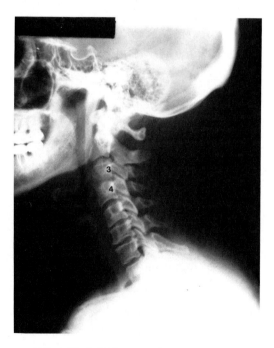

FIG. 1-26. Solid fusion at C3-C4 1 year later.

that compressive loading results in vertebral endplate fracture with extrusion of the nucleus pulposus into the vertebral body. If asymmetric compression occurs, the pressure tears the annulus, expressing the nucleus into the vertebral canal and foramen.

Cervical disk herniations that compress the nerve root characteristically cause neck, shoulder, and arm pain. The pain is often associated with motor weakness and sensory disturbances in the upper extremity, based on the segmental nerve distribution. A decreased reflex may also be noted. Conservative care is the rule. The athlete ceases competition and is placed at rest with a soft cervical collar and appropriate medications. When the symptoms persist or a significant neurologic deficit is present, a more detailed work-up is necessary. MRI has proved to be an excellent way to screen and detect cervical disk herniations. The extent of the herniation can be documented (Fig. 1-24). Myelography with CT scanning has stood the test of time and is also an excellent diagnostic tool, as well as a test done before surgery (Fig. 1-25). Cervical disk excision with fusion has lead to excellent results (Fig. 1-26).[5] Return to athletic participation after disk excision and fusion is decided on a case-by-case basis, based on age, activity level, and neurologic recovery.

INJURY PREVENTION

America has been enveloped by the fitness movement, with millions actively participating in some sport or exercise daily. Associated with this is a corresponding increase in the number of athletic injuries involving the cervical spine. Prevention of cervical spine injuries begins with education of the treating physicians, coaches, and players alike. It has been shown that modifying techniques and providing closer supervision during athletic events promotes reduction of serious injuries.

Coaches have an important role in the prevention of serious injuries because they come into daily contact with the players and supervise their activities. It has been shown that modifying sports techniques has produced dramatic reduction of serious cervical injuries in football. It is up to the coaches to enforce these techniques among their players. Closer supervision during activities such as diving and gymnastics has also been demonstrated to lessen the chances of significant cervical injuries.

And finally education must involve the players. The athletes must understand the proper techniques involving the sport in which they participate. They must wear protective equipment when necessary, and they should be educated to the dangers of their sports, such as spearing in football and improper techniques in diving, because of the high risks of injuries involved in these activities.

If such awareness exists among all personnel involved, a continuing decrease in severe injuries will follow.

SUMMARY

The physician must be aware of the variety of injuries that can occur in the cervical spine. Treatment of a patient with a cervical spine injury begins with the initial evaluation. A meticulous neurologic evaluation should be carried out to document evidence of paralysis, either sensory or motor. This examination must be repeated over hours and days to observe for recovery. If symptoms do not resolve, the physician must search for the cause with various tests, as outlined in this chapter. The physician's hardest role occurs when significant pathologic damage exists in the spine, whereupon the athlete may be advised to cease participation. Surgery is a career-ending procedure for most athletes, because further injury could be devastating. When significant neurologic injury exists, however, surgery could become necessary to alleviate symptoms.

A missed or improperly treated cervical spine injury can lead to a lifetime of severe disability for the athlete. The purpose of this chapter has been to present information about a variety of injuries that can occur in the cervical spine, along with their mechanisms and clinical presentations. Because the upper extremity is linked via its neurologic anatomy to the cervical spine, many injuries manifest themselves as pain, weakness, or sensory loss there. The physician who recognizes and understands this can prevent serious injury.

REFERENCES

1. Carter DR, Frankel VH: Biomechanics of hyperextension injuries to the cervical spine in football, *Am J Sports Med* 8:302, 1980.
2. Clancy WG Jr et al: Upper trunk brachial plexus injuries in contact sports, *Am J Sports Med* 5:209, 1977.
3. Clarke KS: A survey of sports-related spinal cord injuries in schools and colleges, 1973-1975, *J Safety Res* 9:140, 1977.
4. Clarke KS et al: *First annual gymnastics catastrophic injury report,* Washington, DC, 1980, U.S. Gymnastics Safety Association.
5. Cloward RB: Acute cervical spine injuries, *CIBA Clinical Symposia* 32(1):1, 1980.
6. Davis J et al: The etiology of missed cervical spine injuries, *J Trauma* 34:342, 1993.
7. Doran S et al: Magnetic resonance imaging documentation of coexistent traumatic locked facets of the cervical spine and disc herniation, *J Neurosurg* 79:341, 1993.
8. Edwards WC, LaRocca H: The developmental segmental sagittal diameter of the cervical spinal canal in patients with cervical spondylosis, *Spine* 8:20, 1983.
9. Eismont F, Arena M, Green B: Extrusion of an intervertebral disc associated with traumatic subluxation or dislocation to the facets, *J Bone Joint Surg* 73A:1555, 1991.
10. Ellis WG et al: The trampoline and serious neurological injuries: a report of five cases, *JAMA* 174:1673, 1960.
11. Feriencik K: Trends in ice hockey injuries: 1965 to 1977, *Phys Sportsmed* 7:81, 1979.
12. Gant TT, Puffer J: Cervical stenosis: a developmental anomaly with quadriparesis during football, *Am J Sports Med* 4:219, 1976.
13. Goss CM: *Gray's anatomy of the human body,* ed 29(American), Philadelphia, 1973, Lea & Febiger.
14. Hollinshead WH: *Anatomy for surgeons: the back and limbs,* ed 3, Philadelphia, 1982, Harper & Row.
15. Hoskins T: Rugby injuries to the cervical spine in English schoolboys, *Practitioner* 223:365, 1979.
16. Kalfas I et al: Magnetic resonance imaging in acute spinal cord trauma, *Neurosurgery* 23:295, 1988.
17. Ladd AL, Scranton PE: Congenital cervical stenosis presenting as transient quadriplegia in athletes, *J Bone Joint Surg* 68A(9):1371, 1986.

18. Markey KL, DiBenedetto M, Curl WW: Upper trunk brachial plexopathy: the stinger syndrome, *Am J Sports Med* 21(5):142, 1993.

19. Meyer SA et al: Cervical spinal stenosis and stingers in collegiate football players, *Am J Sports Med* 22:158, 1994.

20. Moiel RH et al: Central cord syndrome resulting from congenital narrowness of the cervical spine canal, *J Trauma* 10:502, 1970.

21. Murone I: The importance of the sagittal diameters of the cervical spine in relation to spondylosis and myelopathy, *J Bone Joint Surg* 56B(1):30, 1974.

22. Reference deleted in proofs.

23. Pathria M, Petersilge C: Spinal trauma, *Radiol Clin North Am* 29:847, 1991.

24. Penning L: Some aspects of plain radiography of the cervical spine in chronic myelopathy, *Neurology* 12:513, 1962.

25. Reynen PD, Clancy WG: Cervical spine injury, hockey helmets, and face masks, *Am J Sports Med* 22(2):167, 1994.

26. Rizzolo S et al: Intervertebral disc injury complicating cervical spine trauma, *Spine* 16:187, 1992.

27. Roaf R: A study of the mechanics of spinal injuries, *J Bone Joint Surg* 42B:8, 1960.

28. Schneider RC: Serious and fatal neurosurgical football injuries, *Clin Neurosurg* 12:226, 1966.

29. Seddon H: *Surgical disorders of the peripheral nerves,* Edinburgh, 1972, Churchill-Livingstone.

30. Shields CL Jr, Fox JM, Stauffer ES: Cervical cord injuries in sports, *Phys Sportsmed* 6(9):71, 1978.

31. Speer K, Bassett F: The prolonged burner syndrome, *Am J Sports Med* 18(6):591, 1990.

32. Torg JS: *Athletic injuries to the head, neck and face,* Philadelphia, 1982, Lea & Febiger.

33. Torg JS et al: National Football Head and Neck Injury Registry: report and conclusions 1978, *JAMA* 241:1477, 1979.

34. Torg JS et al: Neurapraxia of the cervical spine cord with transient quadriplegia, *J Bone Joint Surg* 68A(9):1354, 1986.

35. Torg JS et al: Axial loading injuries to the middle cervical spine segment: an analysis and classification of 25 cases, *Am J Sports Med* 19(1):6, 1991.

36. Torg JS et al: Spear tackler's spine: an entity precluding participation in tackle football and collision activities that expose the cervical spine to axial energy inputs, *Am J Sports Med* 21(5):640, 1993.

37. Virgin H: Cineradiographic study of football helmets and the cervical spine, *Am J Sports Med* 8:310, 1980.

38. White AA et al: Biomechanical analysis of clinical stability in the cervical spine, *Clin Orthop* 109:85, 1975.

PART II   Shoulder

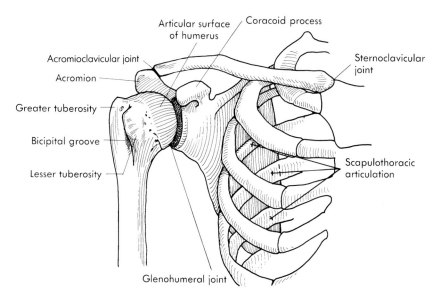

FIG. 2-1. Shoulder joint complex: the acromioclavicular joint, sternoclavicular joint, glenohumeral joint, and scapulothoracic articulation.

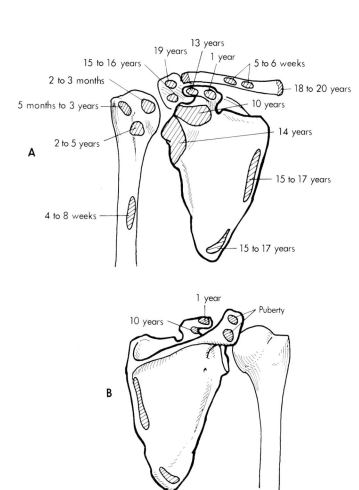

FIG. 2-2. Ossification centers. A, Scapula and humerus. B, Clavicle.

osity then fuses first to the lesser tuberosity, and these coalesce with the ossification center for the humeral head at approximately the fifth to the seventh year of age radiographically.[65] Ogden, Condogue, and Jensen[51] have noted microscopic evidence of fusion at an earlier stage. The proximal humerus fuses with the humeral shaft during the late teens for females and approximately 1 year later for males. In addition, the proximal humerus accounts for approximately 80% of the growth of the entire humerus, with the distal epiphysis accounting for the remaining 20%.[20,71]

Clavicle

The development of the clavicle also begins in the early fetal stage and is the first bone to ossify.[26,28,71] The clavicle develops from intramembranous bone, with the primary center for ossification occurring from two separate areas in the central portion of the shaft of the clavicle.[50] These fuse rapidly during early fetal development, somewhere between the fifth and sixth week of gestation. Epiphyses then appear at either end of the clavicle, with the medial or sternal epiphysis appearing at approximately 18 to 19 years of age (range 12 to 22 years) and usually fusing with the remainder of the clavicle during the early to middle twenties.[20,28,33,50] The medial or sternal growth plate contributes most to the longitudinal growth of the clavicle, accounting for approximately 80% of the entire length; the lateral or acromial growth place accounts for the other 20%.[50] The lateral epiphysis, although rare in occurrence, has been noted to appear at approximately 19 to 20 years of age; however, it fuses rapidly after its appearance with the remainder of the clavicle and therefore may not be as readily detectable radiographically as many of the other ossification centers.[67,71]

CHAPTER 2 Anatomy of the Shoulder

John A. Hurley

To describe the anatomy of the shoulder joint, it may be more accurate to use the term *the shoulder joint complex*. There are really four joints comprising the shoul-der joint complex—the glenohumeral, the acromiocla-vicular, the sternoclavicular, and the scapular thoracic articulation—rather than just the shoulder joint, which many people interpret as being just the glenohumeral joint (Fig. 2-1). The shoulder joint complex is unique in that it connects the axial skeleton and the remainder of the upper extremity. The concerted action of these four joints enables one to use the remainder of the upper ex-tremity with efficiency and accuracy. The shoulder joint complex, because of its bony configuration, flexibility, and gliding motions, gives one the ability to use the up-per extremity in a multitude of positions and motions. If for any reason one of these joints is injured, this can al-ter one's ability to use the remainder of the upper ex-tremity with any degree of precision.[54]

DEVELOPMENT OF THE SHOULDER JOINT COMPLEX

The development of the shoulder joint complex has been studied by several authors. It begins in utero from a number of ossification centers (Fig. 2-2).*

Humerus

The humerus begins to ossify in early intrauterine de-velopment somewhere between the fourth and ninth weeks of gestation.[13,25,30,33] The ossification centers that represent the humeral metaphysis as well as the diaph-ysis are ossified at the time of birth, whereas those of the proximal and distal epiphysis remain unossified.[25,71] The proximal humerus develops from three separate centers of ossification, the first one being for that of the head and the other two being for the greater and lesser tuberosi-ties. The ossification center for the humeral head appears at approximately 2 to 3 months after birth but at times may not be visualized until approximately the sixth month of postnatal development.[11,20,25,39,51] Approxi-mately 20% of newborn infants demonstrate radio-graphic evidence of ossification of the proximal humeral epiphysis at birth.[51,71] The ossification center for the greater tuberosity does not develop until some time be-tween the fifth month and third year of life; the center for the lesser tuberosity, appearing approximately 2 years after that for the greater tuberosity, usually appears some time in the third year of life.[11,20,51,65] The greater tuber-

---

*References 10, 25-27, 30, 39, 49, and 67.

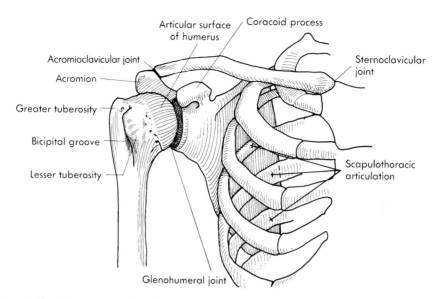

FIG. 2-1. Shoulder joint complex: the acromioclavicular joint, sternoclavicular joint, glenohumeral joint, and scapulothoracic articulation.

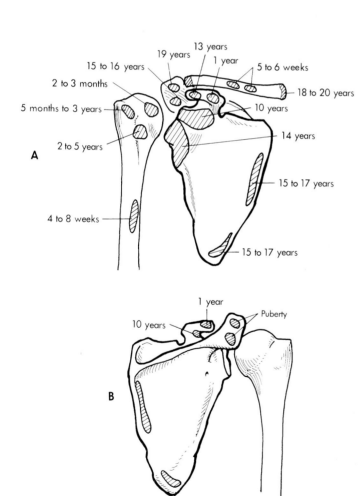

FIG. 2-2. Ossification centers. **A,** Scapula and humerus. **B,** Clavicle.

osity then fuses first to the lesser tuberosity, and these coalesce with the ossification center for the humeral head at approximately the fifth to the seventh year of age radiographically.[65] Ogden, Condogue, and Jensen[51] have noted microscopic evidence of fusion at an earlier stage. The proximal humerus fuses with the humeral shaft during the late teens for females and approximately 1 year later for males. In addition, the proximal humerus accounts for approximately 80% of the growth of the entire humerus, with the distal epiphysis accounting for the remaining 20%.[20,71]

Clavicle

The development of the clavicle also begins in the early fetal stage and is the first bone to ossify.[26,28,71] The clavicle develops from intramembranous bone, with the primary center for ossification occurring from two separate areas in the central portion of the shaft of the clavicle.[50] These fuse rapidly during early fetal development, somewhere between the fifth and sixth week of gestation. Epiphyses then appear at either end of the clavicle, with the medial or sternal epiphysis appearing at approximately 18 to 19 years of age (range 12 to 22 years) and usually fusing with the remainder of the clavicle during the early to middle twenties.[20,28,33,50] The medial or sternal growth plate contributes most to the longitudinal growth of the clavicle, accounting for approximately 80% of the entire length; the lateral or acromial growth place accounts for the other 20%.[50] The lateral epiphysis, although rare in occurrence, has been noted to appear at approximately 19 to 20 years of age; however, it fuses rapidly after its appearance with the remainder of the clavicle and therefore may not be as readily detectable radiographically as many of the other ossification centers.[67,71]

PART II Shoulder

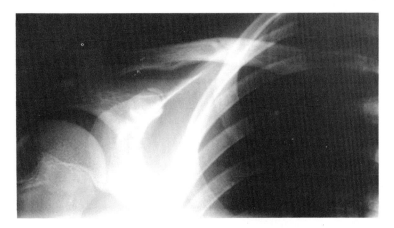

FIG. 2-3. Radiograph demonstrating ossification center at the tip of the coracoid, which may be interpreted as an avulsion fracture.

Scapula

The development of the scapula also begins in utero at approximately 2 months' gestation, with the scapular body being the only portion that is well ossified at the time of birth.[13,20,28,71] However, complete ossification of the scapula does not occur until well into the early twenties. The scapula develops from multiple ossification centers; one of the earliest is that of the middle portion of the coracoid process, which appears as early as 4 months of age but may not be apparent until 15 to 18 months of age.[13,62,65,71] The second ossification center appears at the base of the coracoid process, which becomes apparent at approximately age 10 to 11 years; this ossification center also contributes to the formation of the superior 25% of the glenoid fossa. The coracoid may also have several other ossification centers. One appears at the tip of the coracoid process during the middle teens. It resembles a shell-like pattern at the coracoid tip, which radiographically may be mistaken for an avulsion fracture (Fig. 2-3).[13,20,39,61,71]

The acromion also has two to five multiple ossification centers appearing during the early to middle teens. These have been named by various authors as the preacromion, mesoacromion, metaacromion, and basiacromion; they usually fuse first with each other and then with the remainder of the body of the scapula during the early to middle twenties.[20,33,62,71] However, at times they may remain unfused, leading to a condition known as *os acromiale*, which was originally noted by Liberson in 3% of the cases he studied, with bilateral involvement in 60%. Other authors have noted an incidence of somewhere between 7% and 15% (Fig. 2-4).[42,43,47,71]

Other ossification centers originating during scapular development appear along the vertebral border of the scapula and along the inferior angle of the scapula. Both of these appear during puberty and fuse with the remainder of the body during the late teens to early twenties. The final ossification center to be discussed in regard to the scapula, and perhaps most important, is that for the

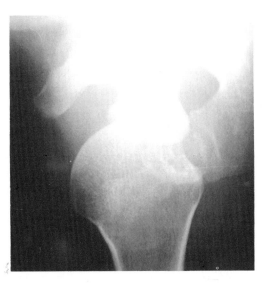

FIG. 2-4. Radiograph of os acromiale demonstrating failure of fusion between mesoacromion and metaacromion.

remainder of the glenoid. This is formed from a horseshoe-shaped epiphysis that forms the inferior three fourths of the glenoid fossa. This center appears at puberty and fuses with the remainder of the scapula during the late teens to early twenties.[62,65]

∎ ∎ ∎

Being aware of these many ossification centers and the time frames during which they appear and fuse may be helpful in evaluating radiographs of adolescents sustaining trauma, as well as in evaluating certain developmental deformities that may be congenital, secondary to growth arrest, or a maldevelopment of one of these ossification centers.

OSTEOLOGY OF THE SHOULDER JOINT COMPLEX
Clavicle

The initial bone to note in a discussion of the bony architecture of the shoulder joint complex is the clavicle because it serves as the connection between the axial skeleton and the appendicular skeleton of the upper extremity. The clavicle has an S-shaped configuration with a convex anterior border medially and a concave anterior border laterally. It has a cylindrical configuration medially, being somewhat thicker, although laterally it becomes flattened and narrow. The S-shaped configuration of the clavicle gives it some inherent stability and mobility during elevation of the upper extremity.

Sternoclavicular Joint

Medially, the clavicle articulates with the sternum as well as with the first rib, forming a synovial articulation. Laterally the clavicle articulates with the acromion to once again form a synovial joint. The articulation between the clavicle and the sternum medially and with the first rib is a relatively incongruent joint, with only 50% of the clavicle articulating with the manubrium and first rib and the remainder being prominent superiorly.[20]

Acromioclavicular Joint

A similar situation occurs laterally where the clavicle articulates with the acromion. This is a somewhat incongruous articulation. The clavicle serves as the origin and insertion for several muscles about the upper extremity that support it, with roughened surfaces appearing on both the superior and the anterior borders of the clavicle, which serve as attachment sites for these muscles. DePalma[17,19,20] described varying morphologies to the lateral end of the clavicle with regard to both its torsion and its articulation with the acromion. These could basically be broken down to three types: Type 1 has a relatively vertically oriented joint; Type 2 has a more oblique configuration sloping medially at its inferior surface; and Type 3 has an almost horizontal angulation between the acromion and clavicle (Fig. 2-5). Moseley[45] also described a variety of articulations between the lateral clavicle and acromion. One type of articulation overrides the place where the clavicle is superior to the acromion, similar to DePalma's Type 2. One has a vertical incongruency similar to DePalma's Type 1. A third type has an underriding articulation where the clavicle articulates on the undersurface of the acromion. The clinical significance of these according to DePalma was the fact that the majority of patients with degenerative changes at the acromioclavicular joint had Type 1 clavicles, which he believed was secondary to the increased shear forces acting on the articular surface in this type of joint. Also, the Type 1 joints were smaller in comparison to Types 2 and 3, thereby increasing their contact forces.

Scapula

The scapula is the other bone that makes up the shoulder joint complex. It comprises the scapular body, the scapular spine, the acromion, the scapular neck, the glenoid fossa, and the coracoid process.

Scapula components

- Body
- Neck
- Spine
- Glenoid
- Coracoid

Body

The body of the scapula is a large, flattened, triangular area situated on the posterior lateral aspect of the upper thorax between the second and seventh ribs, oriented 30 to 45 degrees anterior to the coronal plane of the body.[6] The costal surface is concave and is known as the *subscapular fossa,* whereas the dorsal surface is convex and divided by the spine of the scapula into a supraspinous and infraspinous fossa, with these latter two communicating by way of the spinoglenoid notch. At the superior border of the supraspinous fossa is the supraspinous notch through which travels the suprascapular nerve. The notch is turned into a closed space by the suprascapular ligament, which travels from the superior corners of the notch. Above the ligament travels the suprascapular artery (Fig. 2-11). The suprascapular nerve can become entrapped as it travels through the notch by thickening of the ligament secondary to trauma or fracture, and on occasion ganglia have been reported to cause compression of the nerve as it travels through the notch.[23,56]

Coracoid Process

The coracoid process is a bony projection off the anterior surface of the scapula just medial to the scapular neck (Fig. 2-1). The coracoid projects anteriorly and lat-

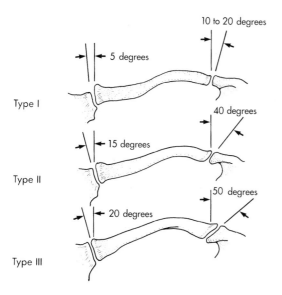

FIG. 2-5. Variations in the acromioclavicular and sternoclavicular articulations.

erally and has a hooked configuration; it serves as the origin and insertion of several muscles and ligaments that are discussed later. The coracoid process lies near the junction of the lateral and middle thirds of the clavicle and can generally be easily palpated along the medial border of the deltoid muscle. It serves as an important landmark in surgical procedures about the shoulder because the neurovascular structures travel along the inferior medial surface of the coracoid.

Acromion

The acromion has received a great deal of attention in regard to its configuration and orientation and the effect it has on various pathologic conditions that affect the shoulder. The slope of the acromion has been studied to evaluate its association with pathologic conditions of the rotator cuff.[2,7,44,48] Several investigators have examined the slope of the acromion by obtaining lateral radiographs of the scapula. They measure the angle formed by a line joining the posteroinferior aspect of the acromion and the anterior margin of the acromion with a line formed by joining the posteroinferior aspect of the acromion and the inferior tip of the coracoid process. From these measurements a system to classify the various **angles of inclination of the acromion** has been developed: Type 1 acromions have a relatively high angle or flat undersurface; Type 2 have a downward curve and a decreased angle of inclination; and Type 3 have almost a hooked configuration along the anterior portion of the acromion and a further reduction of the angle of inclination. According to these authors, the lower the angle of inclination the higher the association with pathologic conditions of the rotator cuff.

Acromion morphology

- Type 1—high angle and flat surface
- Type 2—downward curve and decreased angle of inclination
- Type 3—hooked configuration anteriorly and decreased angle of inclination

---

Glenoid Fossa

The glenoid has also been investigated to determine whether any abnormalities exist that may lead to the development of shoulder disorders.[15,16,35,41,57] The glenoid has a comma-shaped appearance, with the tail superior and the head inferior. Several investigators have evaluated whether an abnormal glenoid version existed in patients with instability patterns about the shoulder. Das, Saha, and Roy[16] were some of the earlier investigators, and they found the normal version of the glenoid to be retroverted approximately 2 to 12 degrees. Studies by these authors and others using computed tomography (CT) scans have noted a mean retroversion of between 2 and 7 degrees in a normal patient population.[15,35,41,57] Saha found that patients with anterior instability tended to have an increased anteversion of the glenoid; however, this has not been substantiated by other investiga-

tors.[15,16] Studies on posterior instability of the shoulder have also focused on the version of the glenoid, with one author noting an increased retroversion of −15 degrees on plain films of his patient population, with posterior instability of the shoulder. Studies by this author noted an increased retroversion in his patient population of between −9 and −10 degrees as determined by CT scans.[9,35] Therefore it appears that the glenoid may have varying version angles that may contribute to instability patterns about the shoulder, especially in patients with posterior instability.

Proximal Humerus

The final bone in the shoulder joint complex is the proximal humerus, which consists of the head, the anatomic neck, which is a slight constriction lateral to the articular surface, and the greater and lesser tuberosities.

Tuberosities

The **greater tuberosity** is the most lateral structure on the superior aspect of the humerus and projects superiorly as well as posteriorly; the **lesser tuberosity** is situated along the anterior margin of the proximal humerus. The tuberosities are separated by the intertubercular groove through which passes the biceps tendon. The proximal end of the humerus connects with the shaft of the humerus, via the surgical neck.

Glenohumeral Articulation

The humeral head that articulates with the glenoid has been studied by several investigators to determine normal anatomy. It has been found that the humeral head has a slight retroversion in relation to the humeral epicondyles measuring approximately 20 to 35 degrees, whereas the angle formed by the humeral head and shaft was found to be between 130 and 150 degrees.[15,20,36,64] Abnormalities in the version of the humeral head have not been found in conjunction with shoulder instability problems.[15,41,57] As previously mentioned, the proximal end of the humerus articulates with the glenoid in what one would assume is a perfect sphere. However, Saha[63] has noted a relative incongruency in this articulation, i.e., three different types of glenohumeral articulation being based on the relative size of the humeral head in comparison to the glenoid, with the size of the humeral head being smaller, equal to, or larger than the corresponding radius of curvature of the glenoid.[63,64] This may have some significance in relation to patients with instability patterns, as noted by one study in which patients with recurrent dislocations were noted to have a smaller glenoid diameter in relation to the humeral head, which therefore decreased the effective contact surface and made a somewhat more unstable configuration.[15,57,63]

Bicipital Groove

Finally, as previously mentioned, the bicipital groove travels between the greater and lesser tuberosities and lies along the anterior aspect of the surface of the humerus. The bicipital groove may demonstrate varying configurations, as noted by Hitchcock,[32] depending on

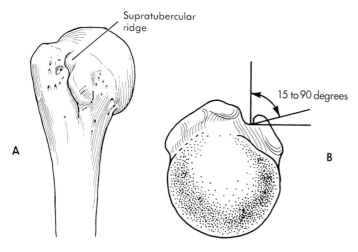

FIG. 2-6. A, Bicipital groove with supratubercular ridge. **B,** Angle of inclination of medial wall.

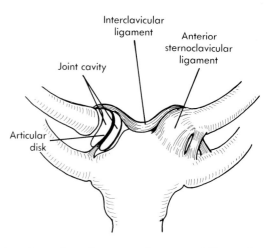

FIG. 2-7. Sternoclavicular joint with interposed fibrocartilaginous disk and surrounding ligaments.

the height of the medial wall of the groove, which is formed by the lesser tuberosity (Fig. 2-6).[20] In 70% of the specimens he studied, the medial wall had a height of about 60 to 90 degrees in relation to the floor of the groove, with the remaining specimens having a lower medial wall. DePalma[20] has also noted this, as well as the presence of a supratubercular ridge of bone in the superior portion of the groove, which projects from the lesser tuberosity. He thought that a combination of a supratubercular ridge and a decreased height of the medial wall may predispose an individual to instability of the bicipital tendon within the groove.

CAPSULAR AND LIGAMENTOUS SUPPORTS OF THE SHOULDER JOINT COMPLEX

The joints that make up the shoulder joint complex are relatively unconstrained and rely heavily on the surrounding soft-tissue structures for stability.

Sternoclavicular Joint

The sternoclavicular joint, as noted previously, is composed of two relatively incongruent surfaces, the medial end of the clavicle and the posterior lateral aspect of the manubrium and first rib (Fig. 2-7).[17] With only the inferior portion of the clavicle articulating with the manubrium and first rib, the presence of a **fibrocartilaginous**

Sternoclavicular joint supporting structures
■ Capsule
■ Anterior sternoclavicular ligament
■ Posterior sternoclavicular ligament
■ Costoclavicular ligament
■ Interclavicular ligament
■ Sternohyoid muscle
■ Sternothyroid muscle
■ Sternocleidomastoid muscle

---

disk between these two surfaces serves to improve their articular congruency. The fibrocartilaginous disk divides the joint almost completely in half and attaches superiorly to the upper medial end of the clavicle and passes downward between the articular surfaces to attach to the first costal cartilage.[5,17,19] In a small percentage of the specimens studied by DePalma,[18] there was a perforation within the substance of the disk. He thought that the disk acted as a buffer in protecting the joint from degenerative change, as well as in stabilizing the sternoclavicular joint. Degenerative changes in the sternoclavicular joint were not noted to significantly occur until somewhere in the seventh decade. The joint is further supported by the capsule, anterior and posterior sternoclavicular ligaments, interclavicular ligament, and costoclavicular ligaments. The **costoclavicular ligaments** extend from the undersurface of the proximal end of the clavicle to the superior surface of the first rib and are composed of an anterior and posterior fasciculus.[5,12,19] The anterior bundle travels upward and lateral from the first costal cartilage to the proximal end of the clavicle, whereas the posterior bundle travels upward and medially. These two bundles become unified along their lateral margins, and there is a bursa between the two bundles.[12,19] The **interclavicular ligament** runs across the superior aspect of the manubrium to join the medial ends of both clavicles. The **sternoclavicular ligaments** consist of an anterior and a posterior bundle with the posterior being the more important. Bearn[5] studied the anatomy of the sternoclavicular joint and assessed the various ligaments in regard to their stabilizing effect on the joint and in maintaining clavicular poise. He identified the capsule, the interclavicular ligaments, costoclavicular ligaments, sternoclavicular ligaments, and the fibrocartilaginous disk and did selective cutting studies to determine the effect each ligament had on maintaining the clavicular poise. It was not until he cut the capsule of joint and sternoclavicular ligaments that he found complete downward depression of the lateral end of the clavicle, and therefore he thought that this was the main sup-

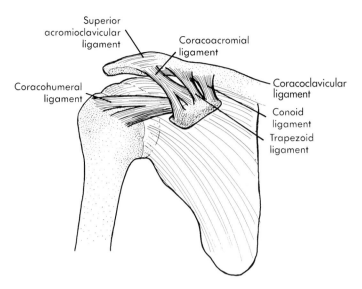

Superior acromioclavicular ligament
Coracoacromial ligament
Coracohumeral ligament
Coracoclavicular ligament
Conoid ligament
Trapezoid ligament

FIG. 2-8. Acromioclavicular joint with surrounding ligaments, including the coracoclavicular, coracoacromial, and coracohumeral.

porting structure of this joint, whereas cutting the remaining ligaments had little effect on clavicular poise. Cave,[12] on the other hand, thought that the costoclavicular ligaments were important in maintaining clavicular stability in the studies that he did.

The sternoclavicular joint is further supported by the sternohyoid and sternothyroid muscles, which attach immediately behind the sternoclavicular joint and the sternocleidomastoid muscle, which attaches in front. These muscles also act as important barriers to the great vessels that lie directly behind them.

Acromioclavicular Joint

The acromioclavicular joint is formed by the lateral end of the clavicle and acromion (Fig. 2-8). This articulation is also a relatively incongruent one for which nature, once again, has provided an intraarticular **fibrocartilaginous disk** to improve congruity. DePalma[17] noted that the disk undergoes degeneration and found a significant amount of it as well as articular cartilage changes in the bone as early as the second decade, with the disk almost completely degenerated by the fourth decade. The acromioclavicular joint is reinforced by the surrounding capsule and ligaments, containing an anterior, posterior, superior, and inferior component, in addition to the coracoclavicular ligaments, which are composed of two individual ligaments, the **conoid** and **trapezoid ligaments.** The acromioclavicular ligaments extend from the acromion to the clavicle circumferentially

around the joint, whereas the conoid and trapezoid ligaments extend from the undersurface of the clavicle to the tip of the coracoid process and function mainly as suspensory ligaments for the upper extremity. The conoid ligament is cone shaped and attaches on the posteromedial aspect of the coracoid, with its base being attached to the undersurface of the clavicle. The trapezoid ligament extends from the anterior lateral base of the coracoid to insert onto the undersurface of the clavicle also. The coracoclavicular ligaments attach along the posterior curve of the clavicle and are important in helping to rotate the clavicle on its long access with overhead activity.[20] Several investigators have studied the stabilizing effects that each set of ligaments has on the acromioclavicular joint.[22,61,70] Urist,[70] one of the original investigators, found that the coracoclavicular ligaments are important in controlling vertical stability, whereas the acromioclavicular ligaments function primarily in restraining posterior translation of the clavicle. Fukuda et al,[22] in biomechanical studies on the ligamentous system of the acromioclavicular joint, have confirmed Urist's findings and have also determined the important influence the acromioclavicular ligaments have on controlling posterior axial rotation of the clavicle in addition to posterior displacement. They also found that the conoid ligament was the primary restraint to anterior and superior displacement of the clavicle.

Glenohumeral Joint

The glenohumeral joint can be compared with a golf ball sitting on the tee with minimal restraints. It relies on the surrounding joint capsule and ligaments to provide static stability and also the surrounding muscles, i.e., the rotator cuff, to provide dynamic stability. The glenoid only articulates with approximately 30% of the humeral head, whereas this contact surface is increased to approximately 75% by the glenoid labrum.[53,64]

Labrum

The labrum was once thought to be a fibrocartilaginous structure surrounding the glenoid and providing further stability; however, studies by Moseley and Overgaard[46] and Cooper et al[14] have demonstrated it to be a redundant fold of capsular tissue with a minimal fibrocartilaginous component near its transitional zone. Cooper et al found, through cadaver dissection, that the superior and anterosuperior portion of the labrum is loosely attached to the glenoid, whereas the inferior labrum is firmly attached to the glenoid rim. The labrum, in and of itself, does not appear to provide much stability to the glenohumeral joint.[46,71] It is continuous with the articular cartilage of the glenoid and functions centrally and laterally as the insertion site for the glenohumeral ligament. DePalma, Callery, and Bennett[21] have shown, in cadaver dissections, that the superior portion of the labrum dissociates from the underlying glenoid with advancing age. Other authors have noted this phenomenon in athletes who participate in throwing sports; this has been attributed to the pull of the biceps tendon, which inserts into the superior labrum during the throwing arc.[1] However, in view of these cadaveric studies, unless

---

Acromioclavicular joint supporting structures

- Acromioclavicular ligaments
- Coracoclavicular ligaments

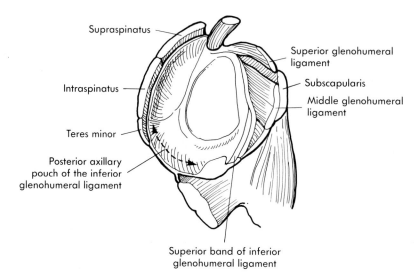

FIG. 2-9. Lateral view of glenoid with surrounding ligaments and muscles.

the superior labrum is torn or completely detached, a loose attachment may represent normal anatomy. The arterial supply to the labrum is provided by the suprascapular, circumflex scapular, and posterior circumflex humeral arteries.

Glenohumeral Ligaments

The glenohumeral ligaments have been studied by many investigators and have been described in *Gray's Anatomy* as being capsular thickenings.* The capsule of the glenohumeral joint is two times the surface area of the humeral head, which provides the ability to move the arm throughout a large arc of motion that is unique to the glenohumeral joint.[38] Studies on the strength of the glenohumeral joint capsule have shown it to be twice as strong as that of the elbow, as well as having a greater stretching capacity.[38] As previously mentioned, the ligaments insert onto the labrum and glenoid neck. Reeves[60] has shown in his studies that the weakest point of this attachment site in the young is at the labral site, whereas in the elderly the capsule and subscapularis tendon tear laterally in a dislocating shoulder.

Three ligaments have been defined anteriorly and are referred to as the **superior, middle,** and **inferior glenohumeral ligaments** (Fig. 2-9). Superiorly, the **coracohumeral ligament** also provides stability to the shoulder. The coracohumeral ligament extends from the base of the coracoid process to the top of the bicipital groove on the greater tuberosity. It covers the interval between the supraspinatus and subscapularis and has been found to provide stability to the joint when the arm is in a dependent position.[4] Underneath the coracohumeral ligament is the superior glenohumeral ligament, which originates from the upper segment of the glenoid labrum at the supraglenoid tubercle and base of the coracoid process to insert onto the upper segment of the lesser tu-

berosity at the anatomic neck. The superior glenohumeral ligament was identified in 90% of cadavers studied, but its size and integrity varied. It has been found to provide little stability to the glenohumeral joint. The middle glenohumeral ligament originates from the anterosuperior portion of the glenoid labrum down as far as the junction of the middle and inferior thirds of the glenoid and is directed slightly downward in an oblique direction to insert along the medial aspect of the lesser tuberosity.[69] The middle glenohumeral ligament lies underneath the subscapularis muscle and tendon; this relationship is well demonstrated during arthroscopy. It has been found to exist approximately 60% of the time in cadaver studies and its contribution to glenohumeral stability is variable.

The inferior glenohumeral ligament is the thickest of the ligaments. It reinforces the inferior capsule[52,69] and is the main static stabilizer in the abducted arm. The inferior glenohumeral ligament originates along the inferior border of the glenoid labrum and glenoid rim to attach onto the inferior neck of the humerus. It has been compared with a hammock in supporting the humeral head. The anterior superior edge is slightly thickened and has been referred to as the superior band of the inferior glenohumeral ligament, whereas the inferior portion of the ligament is somewhat thinner and has been referred to as the axillary pouch.[69] A posterior thickening has also been identified and referred to as the posterior band. With abduction and external rotation, the anterior band fans out to support the head while the portion band provides this support when the arm is internally rotated.

Turkel et al[69] have done studies on the stabilizing effect of the various ligaments about the shoulder, and they found the superior band of the inferior glenohumeral ligament to be the major stabilizer of the glenohumeral joint when the arm is in 90 degrees of abduction and external rotation. These authors also noted that in the neu-

---

*References 13, 14, 28, 38, 46, 52, 60, 68, 69, and 71.

tral position the subscapularis muscle and the middle glenohumeral ligament provided the majority of the stability to the shoulder. With further degrees of abduction, for example, 45 degrees, the stabilizers became the subscapularis, the middle glenohumeral ligament, and the superior portion of the inferior glenohumeral ligament. With further abduction the subscapularis was positioned superior to the humeral head, uncovering it somewhat anteriorly and inferiorly, thereby providing little stability in this position. Posteriorly the capsule is rather thin in comparison to the anterior capsule, therefore providing little restraining force to glenohumeral movement posteriorly.

Synovial Recesses

The anterior ligaments can insert directly onto the labrum or their insertion can occur further medially along the scapular neck, forming synovial recesses. These recesses were described by DePalma, Callery, and Bennett[21] and Moseley and Overgaard[46] and can have varying sizes, depending on how far medial along the neck of the scapula the ligaments insert and depending on their occurrence. These authors described several types of recesses, with Type 1 occurring above the middle glenohumeral ligament, Type 2 occurring as one synovial recess below this middle glenohumeral ligament, Type 3 appearing as one above and one below the middle glenohumeral, and Type 4 occurring as one large recess above the inferior glenohumeral ligament with the middle glenohumeral being absent. These recesses are clinically important in that they represent a discontinuity in the anterior capsule mechanism and ligamentous structures, which may predispose the shoulder to recurrent instability.[20] In addition, according to DePalma these recesses prevent the subscapularis tendon from coming close to the underlying scapular neck, therefore diminishing the dynamic stability provided anteriorly by the subscapularis. The most common of the recesses is that above the middle glenohumeral ligament. In addition to these recesses, many times an interval occurs between the superior and middle glenohumeral ligaments. This serves as the entrance to the subscapularis bursa from the glenohumeral joint and may be of variable size and occurrence. It has been implicated as a possible cause for recurrent instability.[13,20,21,46]

Synovial recesses

- Above middle glenohumeral ligament
- Below middle glenohumeral ligament
- Above inferior glenohumeral ligament

ROTATOR CUFF INTERVAL

The rotator cuff interval is found to exist between the superior border of the subscapularis tendon and the lower border of the supraspinatus tendon. It has its base at the coracoid process and its apex at the transverse hu-

meral ligament. The interval is thought to contain the coracohumeral ligament and superior glenohumeral ligament. It is believed to contribute significantly to glenohumeral motion and stability. Studies by Harryman et al[31] have found that, if the interval is imbricated, humeral head translation decreases posteriorly and inferiorly; release of this interval increases glenohumeral motion in flexion, external rotation, extension, and adduction.

CORACOACROMIAL ARCH

The coracoacromial arch is formed by yet another ligament about the glenohumeral joint, that being the **coracoacromial ligament** along with the acromion process (Fig. 2-8). The coracoacromial ligament is a triangular band containing two fascicles originating from the lateral border of the coracoid from its tip to its base; these then converge laterally to insert on the anterior aspect of the acromion just lateral to the acromioclavicular joint. The ligament extends posteriorly along the acromion to the lateral border of the acromial process.[32] The function of the coracoacromial ligament has not been clearly defined. The coracoacromial arch is a relatively unyielding structure that protects the humeral head from trauma and provides some stability against superior migration of the humeral head. Between the coracoacromial ligament and the underlying rotator cuff is the subacromial bursa, which is one of the larger bursae about the shoulder complex and gives the shoulder some inherent gliding ability. The bursa extends from the coracoid process medially to the greater tuberosity laterally with further extension posteriorly and anteriorly. Numerous other bursae surrounding the shoulder joint complex improve the gliding mechanics of the shoulder and can generally be found between tendons and the underlying bones.

MUSCLES OF THE SHOULDER COMPLEX

The muscles surrounding the shoulder joint complex provide the ability to generate motion while at the same time providing dynamic stability to the glenohumeral joint.* Muscles about the shoulder joint complex can basically be broken down into three categories: those attaching to the scapula with their origin from the axial skeleton; those that have their origin from the scapula and insert onto the humerus; and those that have their origin from the axial skeleton and insert onto the humerus.

Axial Skeleton to Scapula

The first group of muscles, those attaching to the scapula with their origin from the axial skeleton, include the trapezius, levator scapula, rhomboid major and minor, and serratus anterior (Fig. 2-10). The **trapezius muscle** originates from the superior nuchal line and the external occipital protuberance of the skull, the spinous processes of the seven cervical vertebrae, and the spi-

---

*References 3, 34, 36, 37, 53, 63, and 66.

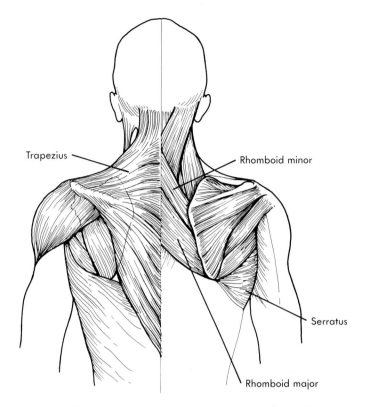

Trapezius

Rhomboid minor

Serratus

Rhomboid major

FIG. 2-10. Posterior view of superficial and deep muscles connecting the axial skeleton to the scapula.

nous processes of all the thoracic vertebrae and their intervening supraspinous ligaments. The upper fibers run obliquely downward to insert along the distal third of the clavicle, whereas the fibers of the lower cervical and upper thoracic region travel laterally to insert onto the acromion, with the fibers from the lower thoracic region traveling laterally and upward to insert along the spine of the scapula. The trapezius is innervated by the spinal accessory nerve, which travels along its undersurface. Lying beneath the trapezius are the levator scapula, rhomboid major and minor, and the serratus anterior.

Scapula to spine muscle attachments

- Trapezius
- Levator scapula
- Rhomboid major
- Rhomboid minor
- Serratus anterior

The **levator scapula** originates from the posterior tubercles of the transverse processes of the first through fourth cervical vertebrae. It inserts into the superior angle of the scapula and along the medial border of the scapula to approximately the level of the scapular spine. It receives its innervation from the cervical plexus and occasionally from the dorsal scapular nerve.

The **rhomboids** also lie deep to the trapezius, with the rhomboid minor arising from the spinous processes of the seventh cervical and thoracic vertebrae and the intervening supraspinous ligament. It inserts along the medial border of the scapula near the base of the scapular spine. The rhomboid major starts from the spinous processes of the second through fifth thoracic vertebrae and their respective supraspinous ligaments, and it inserts along the medial border of the scapula just below the insertion of the rhomboid minor. Both rhomboids are supplied by the dorsal scapular nerve, which travels on the deep surface of each of these respective muscles close to their scapular insertion.

The **serratus anterior** arises from the outer surface of the first eight ribs and follows the curvature of the ribs to insert along the medial aspect of the scapula on its costal surface. The upper portion of the muscle inserts along the medial border of the scapula, whereas the lower portion inserts at the inferior angle of the scapula, which is thought to be where this muscle has its main action. The serratus anterior is supplied by the long thoracic nerve that travels along the superficial portion of the muscle.

These five muscles act to move the scapula with some of them having more than one function because of the multitude of fibers that make up each muscle.[33,36] The trapezius acts to elevate as well as retract the scapula. The rhomboids and levator scapula primarily retract and rotate the scapula downward. The serratus anterior acts to rotate the scapula upward as well as to protract it. The

function of the serratus can be appreciated when there has been injury to the long thoracic nerve because winging of the scapula can be noticed. The most important function of the serratus is to rotate the scapula upward, which happens because of its insertion along the inferior angle of the scapula. Upward rotation of the scapula is also brought out by the trapezius by virtue of its fibers inserting onto the acromion. The concerted action of these two muscles therefore becomes important in rotating the acromion away from the humerus in forward elevation of the upper extremity, thereby avoiding impingement.

Scapular motion

Trapezius
- Elevates scapula
- Retracts scapula

Rhomboids
- Retract and rotate scapula downward

Serratus anterior
- Rotates scapula upward

Levator scapula
- Retracts and rotates scapula downward

The next muscle is the **pectoralis minor,** which is an anterior muscle originating from the axial skeleton in general from the second rib to the fifth rib, with some variability between these and the third through the sixth ribs. The pectoralis minor inserts onto the medial aspect of the coracoid process and is covered by the pectoralis major. It serves to protect the neurovascular structures that travel on its inferior surface. The pectoralis minor muscle is innervated by the medial and lateral pectoral nerves.

Axial Skeleton to Humerus

The next set of muscles, the latissimus dorsi and pectoralis major, begins from the axial skeleton and inserts onto the humerus.

Latissimus Dorsi

The **latissimus dorsi** starts from the spinous processes of the lower six thoracic vertebrae and all of the lumbar and upper cervical vertebrae. It also takes origin from the posterior iliac crest and the lower three ribs; the fibers of the muscle then converge to insert along the anterior surface of the proximal humerus between the pectoralis major and teres major at the crest of the lesser tubercle and the floor of the intertubercular groove. It receives its innervation from the thoracodorsal nerve, which travels on its undersurface; its main function is to adduct, medially rotate, and extend the arm.

The other muscle in this group is the **pectoralis major,** which begins at the medial third of the clavicle, lateral aspect of the manubrium, body of the sternum, and cartilages of the first six ribs. The upper fibers travel in a lateral direction, and the lower ones travel up and un-

---

Axial skeleton to humerus

Latissimus dorsi
- Adducts
- Medially rotates
- Extends

Pectoralis major
- Adducts
- Medially rotates

---

der the upper fibers, twisting as they go under the upper fibers to insert on the inferior border of the greater tuberosity at the lateral lip of the intertubercular groove. The pectoralis major is innervated by the lateral and medial pectoral nerves and serves to adduct and medially rotate the arm.

Scapula to Humerus

The next set of muscles originates from the scapula and inserts onto the humerus. The most superficial muscle in this group is the deltoid, whereas the deeper muscles include the rotator cuff (i.e., supraspinatus, infraspinatus, subscapularis, and teres minor) and the teres major.

Deltoid

The deltoid originates from the lateral third of the clavicle, the acromion, and the spine of the scapula and inserts into the deltoid tuberosity along the anterior lateral aspect of the proximal humerus. The middle portion of the deltoid that arises from the lateral aspect of the acromion is the most powerful portion of the muscle because of its interposed tendon-like septa that serve as both the origin and the insertion of numerous muscle fibers, giving the deltoid muscle a multipennate configuration. The deltoid receives its innervation from the axillary nerve, which winds around the humeral neck and then travels along the undersurface of the deltoid at approximately the level of the inferior aspect of the glenohumeral joint.

Scapula to humerus muscles

- Deltoid
- Supraspinatus
- Subscapularis
- Teres major
- Teres minor
- Infraspinatus

Rotator Cuff

Functional anatomy. The rotator cuff muscles act to dynamically stabilize the shoulder. This has been studied by many investigators in patients with recurrent instability of the shoulder.[*] The subscapularis muscle in particular has been identified as the cause of recurrent in-

*References 3, 4, 11, 29, 37, 54, 55, 63, and 66.

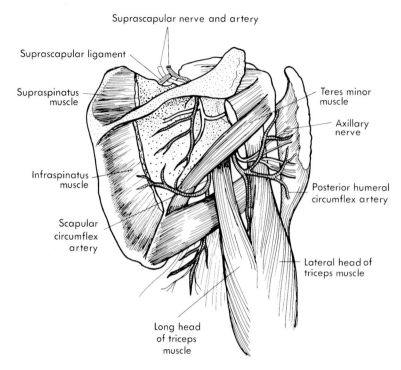

Suprascapular nerve and artery

Suprascapular ligament

Supraspinatus
muscle

Teres minor
muscle

Axillary
nerve

Infraspinatus
muscle

Posterior humeral
circumflex artery

Scapular
circumflex
artery

Lateral head of
triceps muscle

Long head
of triceps
muscle

FIG. 2-11. Posterior view of shoulder with quadrangular space containing the axillary nerve and posterior humeral circumflex artery; and triangular space containing the scapular circumflex artery.

stability by the fact that it becomes attenuated through repeated dislocations.[66] Jobe et al[37] have noted on electromyogram (EMG) analysis a misfiring of the subscapularis muscle in patients with anterior instability. Others have noted the ability to decrease the incidence of recurring instability with a rehabilitative program focused at strengthening the internal rotators, especially the subscapular.[3] Cain et al.[11] showed the importance of the posterior shoulder muscles (i.e., the infraspinatus and teres minor) in controlling external rotatory forces about the shoulder, thereby decreasing the strain on the inferior glenohumeral ligaments and adding a restraining force to anterior dislocation. Basmajian and Bazant[4] have noted the importance of the supraspinatus muscle and superior capsule in preventing downward subluxation of the humeral head with respect to the glenoid.[34] It therefore becomes apparent that the function of all the rotator cuff muscles is extremely important in dynamically stabilizing the glenohumeral joint.

Vascular anatomy. The blood supply to the rotator cuff has also been studied by various investigators who noted an arterial supply to the tendons of the rotator cuff coming from their respective muscle bellies; the supraspinatus is noted to have a relative area of avascularity approximately 1 cm from its insertion to the greater tuberosity. This was rather consistent in all the specimens at all ages studied by Rathbun and MacNab.[58] This zone of relative avascularity has been implicated as the cause for degeneration of the supraspinatus tendon and as one cause of rotator cuff tears.

Subscapularis muscle. The subscapularis muscle arises from the costal surface of the scapula, with its muscles converging into an anterior tendon that inserts onto the lesser tuberosity of the humerus. It is innervated by the subscapularis nerve.

Supraspinatus muscle. The supraspinatus muscle arises from the supraspinous fossa and passes laterally under the coracoacromial arch to attach to the greater tuberosity. It is supplied by the suprascapular nerve and vessels that travel on its undersurface.

Infraspinatus muscle. The infraspinatus muscle arises from the infraspinous fossa and travels laterally to insert on the posterior aspect of the greater tuberosity. It is also supplied by the suprascapular nerve and vessels.

Teres minor muscle. The teres minor muscle arises from the central third of the lateral border of the scapula below the scapular neck to pass behind the long head of the triceps and insert onto the lower posterior aspect of the greater tuberosity.

Teres major muscle. Finally, the teres major muscle arises from the lower third of the lateral border of the scapula and travels around the anterior aspect of the humerus and in front of the long head of the triceps to insert onto the crest of the lesser tubercle. The lower border of the teres minor posteriorly corresponds to the lower border of the subscapularis muscle anteriorly.

The upper border of the teres major along with the lower border of the teres minor and the long head of the triceps form the **triangular space,** through which travel the scapular circumflex vessels (Fig. 2-11).[13,28,32,71] Lat-

eral to this is the **quadrangular** or **quadrilateral space** formed by the lower border of the teres minor, the upper border of the teres major, the lateral border of the long head of the triceps, and the medial border of the humerus, through which travel the axillary nerve and the posterior humeral circumflex artery.[13,28,33,59,71] The teres minor and deltoid receive their innervation by the axillary nerve, whereas the teres major is supplied by the lower subscapular nerve.

Biceps

The last muscle-tendon unit of the shoulder joint complex to discuss is that of the biceps and biceps tendon. The biceps originates via its long head at the superior border of the labrum and by its short head from the coracoid process. These portions converge distally and finally insert into the bicipital tuberosity of the radius. The intracapsular portion of the biceps is tendinous; it travels distally to enter the intertubercular groove as it exits the glenohumeral joint. The synovial lining of the glenohumeral joint accompanies the biceps tendon as it exits into the intertubercular groove.[13,20,28,33,71] Because of its attachment to the superior labrum, it has been implicated as being a deforming force in causing superior labral tears in the athlete participating in throwing sports.[1] Its function is thought by some to act as a depressor of the humeral head when the arm is in external rotation because in this position it travels over the top of the humeral head.

NEUROVASCULAR SUPPLY TO THE SHOULDER JOINT COMPLEX
Arterial Supply

The arterial circulation to the shoulder joint complex is derived mainly from the axillary artery, which is a continuation of the subclavian artery into the axilla. As it continues into the arm, it becomes the brachial artery and finally divides into its two terminal branches, the radial and the ulnar arteries. The axillary artery gives off six main branches to supply the shoulder joint complex: the superior thoracic artery, the thoracoacromial artery, the lateral thoracic, the subscapularis, and the anterior and posterior circumflex humeral vessels (Fig. 2-11).[28] Proximal to the axillary artery in the region of the subclavian division, a branch is given off called the thyrocervical trunk; from this arises the suprascapular artery,

which supplies the supraspinatus and infraspinatus muscle. The main arteries traveling toward the shoulder joint complex itself are those composing the acromial branch of the thoracoacromial artery, which passes above the coracoacromial ligament. It is important to be aware of this branch when dissecting during surgery in this area that requires release of the coracoacromial ligament because it may lead to excessive bleeding if it is cut. The anterior and posterior humeral circumflex arteries arise at the lower border of the subscapularis muscle and can be injured in surgical dissections for recurrent dislocations, fractures, or joint replacement. The ascending branch of the anterior circumflex humeral artery is the main source of blood supply for the humeral head.[40] It enters the bone at the upper end of the bicipital groove and gives off branches to the greater and lesser tuberosity. The blood supply to the glenohumeral joint arises primarily from branches of the suprascapular, subscapular, and both humeral circumflex arteries.

Venous System

The venous system about the shoulder joint complex in general accompanies the arteries. Its termination is in the axillary vein, which is a continuation of the basilic vein. The cephalic vein enters into the axillary vein proximally and reaches the axillary vein by passing between the deltoid and the pectoralis major muscles. The cephalic vein and this muscle interval is an important landmark in anterior surgical approaches to the glenohumeral joint.

Venous drainage systems

- Axillary vein
- Basilic vein
- Cephalic vein

Nerve Supply

The nerve supply to the shoulder joint complex (Fig. 2-12) arises mainly from the fifth through the seventh cervical nerve roots via its formation into the brachial plexus. The plexus is formed by the fifth, sixth, seventh, and eighth cervical nerves and the first thoracic nerve. It then forms an upper, middle, and lower trunk, from which arise anterior and posterior divisions. These then realign into forming cords, which are named lateral, medial, and posterior because of their relationship to the axillary artery.

The important branches in regard to the shoulder joint complex are those of the lateral cord, which includes the lateral pectoral nerve, and the musculocutaneous nerve, which leaves the axilla by passing through the coracobrachialis several centimeters below its insertion. The musculocutaneous nerve is subject to injury during retraction of the conjoint tendon during anterior shoulder surgery.

Axillary artery branches

- Superior thoracic artery
- Thoracoacromial artery
- Lateral thoracic artery
- Subscapularis artery
- Anterior humeral circumflex artery
- Posterior humeral circumflex artery

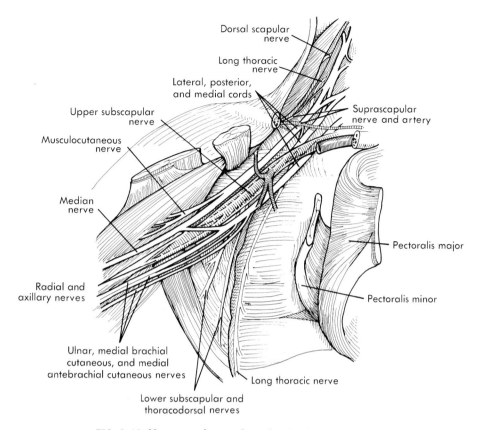

Dorsal scapular
nerve

Long thoracic
nerve

Lateral, posterior,
and medial cords

Upper subscapular
nerve

Suprascapular
nerve and artery

Musculocutaneous
nerve

Median
nerve

Pectoralis major

Pectoralis minor

Radial and
axillary nerves

Ulnar, medial brachial
cutaneous, and medial
antebrachial cutaneous nerves

Long thoracic nerve

Lower subscapular and
thoracodorsal nerves

FIG. 2-12. Neurovascular supply to the shoulder joint complex.

The posterior cord gives off the remaining important branches in regard to the shoulder joint complex. These are the upper subscapular nerve, which supplies the subscapular muscle, the thoracodorsal nerve, which travels along the lateral border of the scapula and supplies the latissimus dorsi, and the lower subscapular nerve, which gives off a branch of the subscapularis muscle and then continues along to innervate the teres major.

Finally, the axillary nerve travels along the inferior portion of the subscapularis muscle and then winds around the shoulder joint capsule and humeral neck where it divides into an anterior and posterior branch. The anterior branch travels around anteriorly to supply the middle and anterior deltoid, and the posterior branch supplies the posterior deltoid as well as the teres minor. The axillary nerve, as previously mentioned, is susceptible to injury during surgery about the shoulder, and studies by Bryan, Schauder, and Tullos[8] have noted the close relationship of the axillary nerve during surgical procedures about the shoulder. They found the nerve to be within 0.5 and 2.5 cm of a posterior arthroscopic portal; between 0.65 and 0.9 cm of an anterior shoulder approach; and within 0.32 cm of the incisions in the capsule during a capsular shift procedure.

The other important nerves about the shoulder joint complex include the long thoracic nerve, which travels along the medial wall of the axilla to supply the serratus anterior, and the suprascapular nerve, which arises from the upper trunk to travel along the superior border of the scapula in the suprascapular notch. The suprascapular nerve may be compressed by the transverse ligament, on top of which travels a suprascapular artery to go on to innervate the supraspinatus and infraspinatus muscles. The nerve supply to the glenohumeral joint arises primarily from the axillary nerve, suprascapular nerve, and lateral pectoral nerves.[24]

REFERENCES
1. Andrews JR, Carson WG, McCleod W: Glenoid labrum tears related to the long head of the biceps. *Am J Sports Med* 13:337, 1985.
2. Aoki M, Usui, Ishii M: *The slope of the acromion and rotator cuff impingement.* Paper presented to the Society of American Shoulder and Elbow Surgeons Second Open Meeting, New Orleans, 1986.
3. Aronen JG, Regan K: Decreasing the incidence of recurrence of first time anterior shoulder dislocations with rehabilitation, *Am J Sports Med* 12:283, 1984.
4. Basmajian JV, Bazant FJ: Factors preventing downward dislocation of the adducted shoulder joint, *J Bone Joint Surg* 41A:1182, 1959.
5. Bearn JG: Direct observations on the function of the capsule of the sternoclavicular joint in clavicle support, *J Anat* 101:159, 1967.
6. Bechtol C: Biomechanics of the shoulder, *Clin Orthop* 146:37, 1980.

7. Bigliani LJ, Morrison DS: *The morphology of the acromion and its relationship to rotator cuff tears,* Paper presented to the Society of American Shoulder and Elbow Surgeons Second Open Meeting, New Orleans, 1986.
8. Bryan WJ, Schauder K, Tullos H: The axillary nerve and its relationship to common sports medicine shoulder procedures, *Am J Sports Med* 14:113, 1986.
9. Brewer B, Wubben R, Carrera G: Excessive retroversion of the glenoid cavity, *J Bone Joint Surg* 68A:724, 1986.
10. Camp JO, Cilley EI: Diagrammatic chart showing time of appearance of the various centers of ossification and period of union, *Am J Roentgenol* 26:905, 1931.
11. Cain PR et al: Anterior stability of the glenohumeral joint: a dynamic model, *Am J Sports Med* 15:144, 1987.
12. Cave AJE: The nature and morphology of the costoclavicular ligament, *J Anat* 95:170, 1961.
13. Clemente CO: *Gray's anatomy,* ed 13 (American edition), Philadelphia, 1985, Lea & Febiger.
14. Cooper DE et al: Anatomy, histology and vascularity of the glenoid labrum, *J Bone Joint Surg* 74A:46, 1992.
15. Cyprien JM et al: Humeral retrotorsion and glenohumeral relationship in the normal shoulder and in recurrent anterior dislocation (scapulometry), *Clin Orthop* 175:8, 1983.
16. Das SP, Saha AK, Roy GS: Observations on the tilt of the glenoid cavity of scapula, *J Anat Soc India* 15:114, 1966.
17. DePalma AF: Degenerative changes in the sternoclavicular and acromioclavicular joints in various decades, Springfield, Ill, 1957, Charles C Thomas.
18. DePalma AF: The role of the disks of the sternoclavicular and acromioclavicular joints, *Clin Orthop* 13:222, 1959.
19. DePalma AF: Surgical anatomy of acromioclavicular and sternoclavicular joints, *Surg Clin North Am* 43:1541, 1963.
20. DePalma AF: *Surgery of the shoulder,* Philadelphia, 1983, JB Lippincott.
21. DePalma AF, Callery G, Bennett G: The variational anatomy and degenerative lesions of the shoulder joint, *Instr Course Lect* 6:255, 1949.
22. Fukuda K et al: Biomechanical study of the ligamentous system of the acromioclavicular joint. *J Bone Joint Surg* 68A:434, 1986.
23. Ganzhorn RW et al: Suprascapular nerve entrapment: a case report, *J Bone Joint Surg* 63A:492, 1981.
24. Gardner E: The innervation of the shoulder joint, *Anat Rec* 102:1, 1949.
25. Gardner E: The prenatal development of the human shoulder joint, *Surg Clin North Am* 43:1465, 1963.
26. Gardner E: The embryology of the clavicle, *Clin Orthop* 58:9, 1968.
27. Gardner E, Gray DJ: Prenatal development of the human shoulder and acromioclavicular joints, *Am J Anat* 92:219, 1953.
28. Gardner E, Gray DJ, O'Rahilly R: *Anatomy,* Philadelphia, 1975, WB Saunders.
29. Glousman R et al: *Dynamic EMG: analysis of the throwing shoulder with glenohumeral instability,* Paper presented to the Society of American Shoulder and Elbow Surgeons Third Open Meeting, San Francisco, 1987.
30. Gray DJ, Gardner E: The prenatal development of the humerus, *Am J Anat* 124:431, 1969.
31. Harryman DJ et al: The role of the rotator internal capsule in passive motion and stability of the shoulder, *J Bone Joint Surg* 74A:53, 1992.
32. Hitchcock HH: Painful shoulder: observation on role of tendon of long head of biceps brachii in its causation, *J Bone Joint Surg* 30A:263, 1948.
33. Hollinshead WH, Rosse C: *Textbook of anatomy,* ed 4, New York, 1985, Harper & Row.
34. Howell AB et al: Role of the supraspinatus muscle in shoulder function, *J Bone Joint Surg* 68A:398, 1986.
35. Hurley JA et al: *Posterior shoulder instability: results of operative vs. non-operative treatment,* Paper presented to the American Academy of Orthopaedic Surgeons, San Francisco, 1987.
36. Inman VT et al: Observations on the function of the shoulder joint, *J Bone Joint Surg* 26:1, 1944.
37. Jobe FW et al: An EMG analysis of the shoulder in throwing and pitching, *Am J Sports Med* 11:3, 1983.
38. Kaltsas DS: Comparative study of the properties of the shoulder joint capsule with those of other joint capsules, *Clin Orthop* 173:20, 1983.
39. Kohler A, Zimmer EA: *Borderlands of normal and early pathologic in skeletal roentgenology,* ed 11 (American edition), New York, 1968, Grune & Stratton.
40. Laing PG: The arterial supply of the adult humerus, *J Bone Joint Surg* 38A:1105, 1956.
41. Laumann U, Kramps HA: Computer tomography on recurrent shoulder dislocation. In Bateman JE (ed): *Surgery of the shoulder,* St Louis, 1984, Mosby.
42. Liberson R: Os acromiale: a contested anomaly, *J Bone Joint Surg* 19:683, 1937.
43. McClure JG, Raney B: Anomalies of the scapula, *Clin Orthop* 110:22, 1975.
44. Morrison DS, Bigliani LU: *The clinical significance of variations in acromial morphology,* Paper presented to the Society of American Shoulder and Elbow Surgeons Third Open Meeting, San Francisco, 1987.
45. Moseley HF: The clavicle: its anatomy and function, *Clin Orthop* 58:17, 1968.
46. Moseley HF, Overgaard B: The anterior capsular mechanism in recurrent anterior dislocation of the shoulder, *J Bone Joint Surg* 44B:913, 1962.
47. Mudge K et al: Rotator cuff tears associated with os acromiale, *J Bone Joint Surg* 68A:427, 1984.
48. Neer CS, Poppen NK: *Supraspinatus outlet,* Paper presented to the Society of American Shoulder and Elbow Surgeons Third Open Meeting, San Francisco, 1987.
49. O'Brien S et al: The anatomy and histology of the inferior glenohumeral ligament complex of the shoulder, *Am J Sports Med* 18:449, 1990.
50. Ogden JA, Conologue GS, Bronson ML: Radiology of post-natal skeletal development: the clavicle, *Skeletal Radiol* 4:196, 1979.
51. Ogden JA, Conologue GJ, Jenson P: Radiology of post-natal skeletal development: the proximal humerus, *Skeletal Radiol* 2:153, 1978.
52. Ouesen J, Nielsen S: Stability of the shoulder joint, *Acta Orthop Scand* 56:149, 1985.
53. Perry J: Anatomy and biomechanics of the shoulder in throwing, swimming, gymnastics and tennis, *Clin Sports Med* 2(2):247, 1983.
54. Poppen NK, Walker PS: Normal and abnormal motion of the shoulder, *J Bone Joint Surg* 58A:195, 1976.
55. Poppen NK, Walker PS: Forces at the glenohumeral joint in abduction, *Clin Orthop* 135:165, 1978.
56. Post M, Mayer V: Suprascapular nerve entrapment: diagnosis and treatment, *Clin Orthop* 223:126, 1987.
57. Randelli M, Gambrioli PL: Glenohumeral osteometry by computed tomography in normal and unstable shoulders, *Clin Orthop* 208:151, 1986.
58. Rathbun JB, MacNab I: The microvascular pattern of the rotator cuff, *J Bone Joint Surg* 52B:540, 1970.
59. Redler M, Ryland L, McCue F: Quadrilateral space syndrome in a throwing athlete, *Am J Sports Med* 14:511, 1986.
60. Reeves B: Anterior capsular strength of the shoulder, *J Bone Joint Surg* 50B:858, 1968.
61. Rockwood C, Green D: *Fractures in adults,* Philadelphia, 1984, JB Lippincott.
62. Rockwood C, Wilkins K, King R: *Fractures in children,* Philadelphia, 1984, JB Lippincott.
63. Saha AK: Dynamic stability of the glenohumeral joint, *Acta Orthop Scand* 42:491, 1971.
64. Sarrafian SK: Gross and functional anatomy of the shoulder, *Clin Orthop* 173:11, 1983.
65. Silverman F: *Caffey's pediatric x-ray diagnosis,* ed 8, Chicago, 1985, Yearbook Medical Publishers.

66. Symeonides PP: The significance of the subscapularis muscle in the pathogenesis of recurrent anterior dislocation of the shoulder, *J Bone Joint Surg* 54B:476, 1972.

67. Todd TW, DeErrico J Jr: The clavicular epiphyses, *Am J Anat* 41:25, 1928.

68. Townley CO: The capsular mechanism in recurrent dislocation of the shoulder, *J Bone Joint Surg* 32A:370, 1950.

69. Turkel SJ et al: Stabilizing mechanisms preventing anterior dislocation of the glenohumeral joint, *J Bone Joint Surg* 63A:1208, 1981.

70. Urist MR: Complete dislocation of the acromioclavicular joint: the nature of the traumatic lesion and effective methods of treatment with an analysis of 41 cases, *J Bone Joint Surg* 28:813, 1946.

71. Warwick R, Williams PL (eds): *Gray's anatomy,* ed 35 (British edition), Philadelphia, 1973, WB Saunders.

CHAPTER 3

History and Physical Examination of the Shoulder

Tom R. Norris

The most important aspect of the effective management of an athlete's painful shoulder is an accurate diagnosis. This is determined on the basis of an extensive knowledge of extrinsic and intrinsic causes of shoulder pain combined with a detailed history, a complete physical examination, and judicious use of ancillary testing. An understanding of shoulder anatomy, kinematics,[153] biomechanics, and familiarity with specialized use of the shoulder and arm in specific sports assists in identification of the complex derangements that can interfere with optimal shoulder function.

ETIOLOGY OF SHOULDER PAIN

Unfortunately, multiple problems may exist in the same athlete. It is common to see a combination of bone, muscle, tendon, ligament, and, more rarely, nerve and vascular injuries in the evaluation of shoulder dysfunction. Acromioclavicular arthritis may coexist with cervical radiculopathy. Shoulder impingement and rotator cuff tearing, commonly seen in the middle-aged or aging athlete,[67] are now being recognized from overuse in the younger athlete with shoulder instability.[80] Failure to appreciate these complex interrelationships may result

in incomplete or ill-conceived treatments and thus impede the athlete's return to optimal function.

Extrinsic Problems

The neck is the most common source of extrinsic pain radiating to the shoulder. This pain may be gradual in onset or result from acute trauma.

In football a spearhead tackle may fracture the cervical spine, leading to quadriplegia. A tackle that forces the head away from the shoulder with associated "burners" and "stingers"[102,135,140] stretches the upper cords of the brachial plexus and results in transient shoulder and arm weakness. Repeated episodes or more severe injuries cause permanent weakness.[144]

The brachial plexus is at risk with any falls that force the head and shoulder apart. The athlete is susceptible to these hard falls in gymnastics, wrestling, and higher speed sports such as bicycling, motorcycle racing, skiing, and hockey.

Cervical arthrosis with spondylosis, foraminal osteophytes, herniated disks, and more distal nerve entrapment syndromes should be considered in the neurologic evaluation, with screening ancillary tests performed as necessary. Electrodiagnostic studies, radiographs, computed tomography (CT), magnetic resonance imaging (MRI), and noninvasive vascular studies all have a role.

Extrinsic causes of shoulder pain

- Brachial plexus injury
- Cervical spondylosis
- Cervical disk herniation
- Syringomyelia
- Thoracic outlet syndrome
- Diaphragmatic irritation
- Lung tumor
- Brachial neuropathy
- Myocardial ischemia

The condition in an athlete with a C5-C6 disk injury is similar to that of a suprascapular nerve entrapment or a rotator cuff tear with spinatus atrophy and shoulder external rotation weakness.

Spinal cord injury in the cervical or even thoracolumbar region may be followed years later with shoulder pain and apparent arthritic dissolution of the humeral head. Although it has been stated that syringomyelia does not usually cause pain in the shoulder, the posttraumatic syrinx associated with advanced shoulder arthritis occurs in patients who initially manifest severe shoulder pain. Screening tests, with aspirations and cultures to rule out infection of the glenohumeral joint, and MRI have allowed identification of the previously missed posttraumatic syrinx. The treatment was altered to provide adequate syrinx shunting rather than local shoulder surgery.[124]

Shoulder pain can be misconstrued as primary neck injury. If for any reason an athlete has shoulder pain, there is a tendency to immobilize or protect the arm with adduction, internal rotation, and slight elevation of the shoulder. Muscle fatigue and spasms, primarily in the posterior trapezius and levator scapula insertion, result in secondary neck pain.

Thoracic outlet syndrome with proximal compression of the nerves and arteries is much less common than cervical radiculopathy and is more difficult to diagnose. Leffert[91] reports that a history of trauma is present in approximately 40% of those with thoracic outlet syndrome. Women of childbearing age are predilected in a ratio of 3.5:1 compared with men. The pain radiates to the medial arm and forearm and occasionally to the ring and small fingers, causing inability to use the arm above shoulder level because of fatigue. These same symptoms may be the initial symptoms with recurrent transient subluxations of the glenohumeral joint.[93,149,151] The differential is important. Repairing a shoulder subluxation or dislocation can eliminate the numbness, tingling, and positional fatigue in the combined clinical setting.

The history of onset is important. The atraumatic slow loss of the ability to raise the arm may occur from a viral plexitis. An arthrogram is normal, and the electromyogram (EMG) is helpful in making the diagnosis, whereas after sudden traumatic loss of the ability to raise the arm, the differential diagnosis indicates either a neck or brachial plexus injury with rotator cuff tear or fixed dislocation of the shoulder. That these can also occur in combination emphasizes the need for thorough evaluation, even if only one cause may have been identified.[82]

Identification of the primary cause of shoulder pain is not always easy. Referred pain to the shoulder girdle region occurs from multiple sources other than the neck. With diaphragmatic irritation, pain is referred along the phrenic nerve to the supraclavicular region, the trapezius, and the superomedial angle of the scapula.[27] Pulmonary infarction may irritate the diaphragm. A subphrenic abscess or ruptured abdominal viscus, gallbladder, and hepatic parenchymal disease may be present with epigastric pain, as well as pain over the top of the shoulder, with concomitant tenderness and scapular pain. Gastric and pancreatic diseases may refer to the interscapular region.

The rare superior sulcus lung tumor, or Pancoast tumor, occasionally coincident with Horner's syndrome, may have shoulder pain as its initial symptom (Fig. 3-1).[90]

Prolonged vigorous aerobic and anaerobic exertions in long-distance running, causing myocardial ischemic pain, may also cause pain to radiate at the base of the neck in the clavicular region, through the shoulder, and down the ulnar border of the left arm. The transverse and descending aortic diseases classically radiate to the left shoulder, whereas those of the ascending right side of the arch radiate to the right shoulder.

Many times the cause of the referred shoulder pain cannot be established. Early on, objective findings in the shoulder are absent, whereas over time the shoulder stiffness that develops becomes a cause of pain in and of itself, with secondary ipsilateral neck and scapular muscle fatigue.

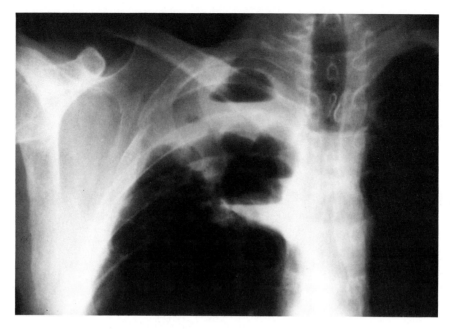

FIG. 3-1. Pancoast tumor. First symptom was shoulder pain.

Intrinsic Problems

Intrinsic causes of shoulder pain in the athlete fall into six basic groups:

1. Instability—subluxations and dislocations of the glenohumeral, acromioclavicular (AC), and sternoclavicular (SC) joints
2. Impingement lesions—rotator cuff tears and ruptures of the long head of the biceps
3. Fractures of the proximal humerus, scapula, and clavicle
4. Arthritis—SC, AC, and glenohumeral joints
5. Miscellaneous—calcific tendinitis, myositis ossificans,[95] adhesive capsulitis, tumors, and nerve or vessel injury
6. Psychologic presentations with abnormal posturing, painful subluxations, or other painful symp-

---

Intrinsic causes of shoulder pain

- Instability
- Impingement
- Fractures
- Arthritis
- Calcific tendinitis
- Myositis ossificans
- Adhesive capsulitis
- Tumors
- Neurovascular injury
- Psychologic disturbance

---

toms grossly in excess of physical findings with nonorganic or functional causes

Pain or injuries may occur in an isolated group or in combination.

MECHANISMS OF INJURY AND THEIR ROLE
Throwing Motion

Second only to running injuries, athletic injuries affecting the shoulder joint are the next most common. Throwing is the most common motion used in sports.[120] The overhead throwing motion has been extensively analyzed for the baseball pitcher.* With minor variations its biomechanics are similar to those used in football, shotput and hammer throw, all racket sports, and three of the four swimming sports, namely the freestyle, backstroke, and butterfly.[133] The throwing mechanism involves a set sequence of body motion, beginning with pelvis, upper trunk rotation, upper arm, forearm, and hand.[10] It has been divided into five stages: preparation and windup, early cocking, late cocking, forward acceleration, and follow-through with deceleration.† Skilled throwers seldom use more than 90 degrees' abduction; however, the arm rapidly moves from the extremes of external to internal rotation.[42] Preliminary EMG analysis has elucidated the shoulder and elbow function in throwing,[133,160] tennis strokes,[1,152] and swimming.[113,129,165]

These throwing motions share the common need for upper and lower body positioning and proper timing to decrease stress on the glenohumeral joint and provide power.[120] Analysis of the throwing arm angles; the mechanics of the lead shoulder, arm, and foot; the gloved arm; and the rhythm have demonstrated predictable injuries to the shoulder and elbow.[2] Poor mechanics can cause shoulder and elbow injuries.[2,56] A stiff front leg causes trunk vaulting when rotation is needed. Closing off, or getting the arm ahead of the body before significant trunk rotation, increases the load on the shoulder.

---

*References 5, 7, 80, 104, 108, 154, and 163.
†References 56, 61, 79, 81, 84, 164, and 166.

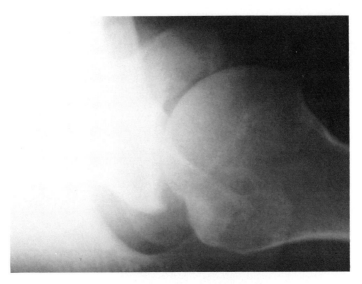

FIG. 3-2. Bennett lesion. Posterior glenoid rim fracture ossification in a 53-year-old man who pitched from age 9 until age 22, at which point pain ended his overhand throwing career.

Rushing, or opening up[77] too soon, gets the body ahead of the throwing arm, thereby increasing the stress on the anterior glenohumeral and medial elbow ligaments.[61,78,80] During the rapid change from maximal external rotation in the late cocked position to full internal rotation of the follow-through phase, the medial elbow is placed under tension with a valgus stress. The ulnar collateral ligament can be stretched or ruptured. Ulnar nerve entrapment from overuse, stretching, and fibrosis develops.[78] The lateral elbow is subjected to repeated compression.[84,94]

In the adolescent, osteochondritis dissecans of the capitellum and elbow loose bodies develop.[84,165,167] The pull of the subscapularis and longitudinal tension along the humerus serve to widen the proximal humeral epiphyseal plate that has a stress fracture.[36,65,94]

Maximal stretching in the external rotation cocking phase directly about the humeral head on the posterior glenoid rim while stretching or avulsing the anterior ligamentous and labral attachments results in recurrent anteroinferior subluxations. The force and torque pitching with the strong muscle contractions have been reported to fracture the humeral shaft.[57,85,94] The rapid deceleration in the follow-through places traction on the posterior and superior capsular and tendinous structure. Two lesions described by Bennett,[16,17] namely ossification of the triceps long head origin at the inferior glenoid and ossification at the posterior glenoid rim,[12,96] are thought to occur as a result of the traction during deceleration in pitching (Fig. 3-2). Posterior abutment of the maximally externally rotated humerus in cocking is postulated as being another cause of the posterior glenoid rim ossification and posterior humeral head defects that are separate from Hill-Sachs defects.[79] Whereas detachment of the anterior superior labrum is attributed to the pull of the long head of the biceps during the deceleration phase,[4,109] detachment of the anteroinferior labrum is one of instability from repeated stresses from extreme external rotation and abduction.

The dead arm syndrome, with transient numbness and arm weakness following a hard throw, has become a commonly accepted historical symptom indicative of shoulder subluxations.[148,151] The overuse syndromes, with subacromial impingement termed *throwers' and swimmers' shoulders* with increasing frequency, are associated with recurrent shoulder subluxations.[66,110] That glenohumeral instability can cause secondary shoulder impingement has important therapeutic implications. It explains why coracoacromial ligament release, alone or in conjunction with anterior acromioplasty,[83] often has failed to relieve the impingement symptoms, whereas treatment directed to restoring joint stability, with repair of detached ligaments or reducing the joint volume in multidirectional instability with capsular shift procedures, has been successful.[61,80,116]

Albright et al[2] reported that throwing injuries are directly related to the duration of exposure and intensity of participation. Clancy[37] recognized the role of tissue overuse in athletic shoulder injuries.

Macrotrauma

An acute forceful direct or indirect injury causing fracture-dislocation or soft-tissue disruption can be defined as macrotrauma. An acute strain or ligament tear becomes a chronic situation if an early diagnosis is not

---

Classification of injury types

- Macrotrauma
- Repetitive microtrauma
- Atraumatic injury

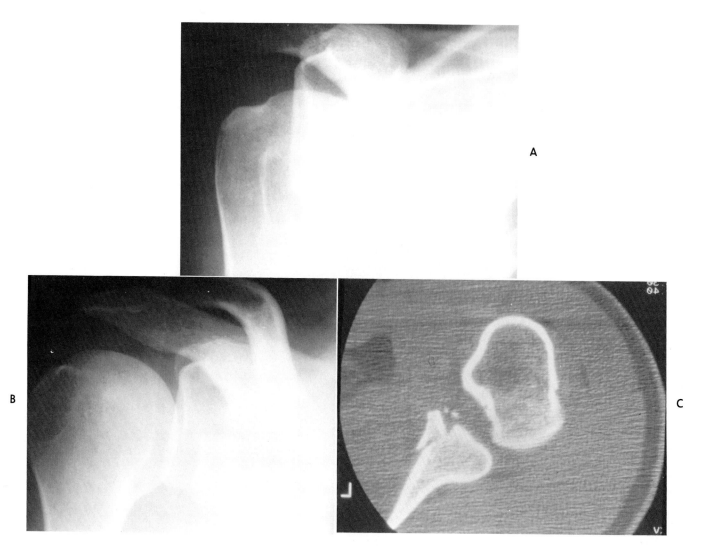

FIG. 3-3. A, Anterior humeral head dislocation from a direct blow to the posterior shoulder. **B,** Following reduction, a large anteroinferior glenoid rim fracture is evident. **C,** Computed tomography scan accurately documents the extent of glenoid involvement.

made and followed by adequate rests, splinting, repair, and reconditioning before return to the same activity.[42] Rotator cuff tears in the younger athlete are rare, but they can result from violent injuries with large avulsions. In patients over age 30 acute tears may be superimposed on more chronic degenerative impingement lesions, with or without previous cuff tearing. The initiating trauma for tearing lessens with advancing age.[107]

Repetitive Microtrauma

Chronic overuse syndromes with repetitive stretching, as in rowing, swimming, or throwing, are injuries of repetitive microtrauma. These may be associated with lack of or improper conditioning for the sport performed. Frequently there are deficiencies in one muscle group (most commonly the shoulder external rotators), lack of flexibility, or longer than normal sessions.[80,81]

Warming up is necessary for safe stretching. Without stretching for complete range of motion before beginning

competition, the muscles are more susceptible to extrinsic overload with disruption of attachments or intrinsic muscle tearing.[31] The healing sequence after tissue overload includes edema with inflammation, fibrin and granulation tissue deposition, and tissue calcification or ossification.[42] If the healing process is repeatedly interrupted, the process itself may become pathologic. The tissue then responds with different mechanical properties that decrease performance or lower threshold for new injury. An example might be the Bennett shoulder lesions with posterior glenoid calcification that eventually interferes with pitching.[16,17,96]

Atraumatic Injury

Atraumatic disorders are generally those of shoulder instability in patients with generalized ligamentous laxity or congenital hypoplasia of the glenoid. When an individual experiences pain in the absence of traumatic or overuse syndromes and with normal radiographs, the

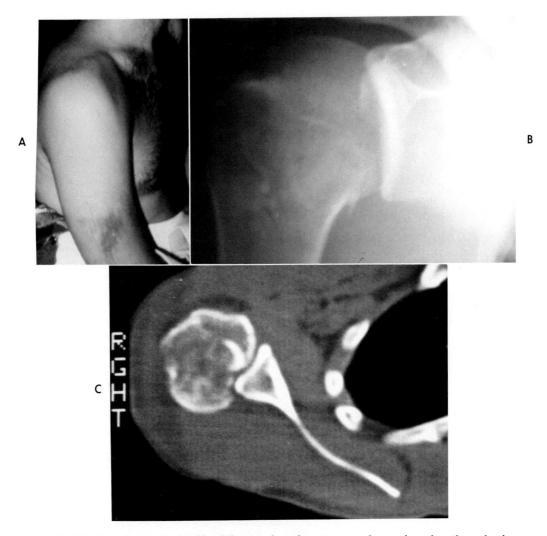

FIG. 3-4. Locked posterior shoulder dislocation from direct trauma of a tree branch striking shoulder as automobile went off the road. **A,** Long axis of the humerus is directed posteriorly proximally. The coracoid is prominent. The anterior humeral head area is depressed. A fullness is noted posteriorly. **B,** True anteroposterior view of glenohumeral joint in the scapular plane demonstrates an overlap of the head with the glenoid. **C,** Computed tomography scan demonstrates the locked posterior dislocation with an anterior humeral head impression fracture (reverse Hill-Sachs lesion).

psychologic stresses and motivation may need evaluation.*

Impact vs. Nonimpact Injuries

Whereas general mechanisms of injury may be associated with specific injuries, the condition of the athlete's tissue influences the ease with which these injuries may occur.

Impact injuries may be divided into direct and indirect trauma.[75] Nonimpact injuries occur from overuse syndromes and muscle strains, ruptures, and avulsions. In cases of direct trauma, the injury force is in direct contact with the shoulder complex. Indirect forces injuring the shoulder usually pass up through the hand, wrist, or elbow and result in a rotational or longitudinal force directed along the humerus.

Examples of direct trauma include the following:
1. Posterior dislocations of the sternoclavicular joint[174]
2. Acromioclavicular subluxations or dislocations after a fall on the posterior superior shoulder[60,138,174]
3. Direct blows to the supraclavicular brachial plexus at the base of the neck or axillary nerve as it courses under the deltoid
4. Clavicular fractures
5. Muscle contusions

Indirect trauma results in muscle, tendon, ligament, and brachial plexus stretch, strain, rupture, and bony fractures. Glenohumeral subluxations are usually from indirect forces. Anterior dislocations occur from abduc-

---

*References 14, 15, 62, 63, 147, and 150.

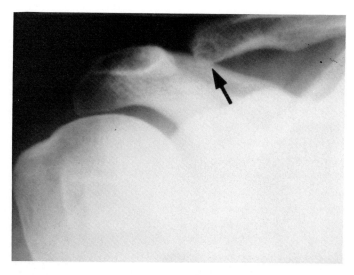

FIG. 3-5. Early osteolysis of the outer clavicle with subcortical cystic lesions in a weight lifter.

tion and external rotation of the arm, whereas traumatic posterior dislocation occurs from a forward fall on the adducted, internally rotated arm with the posterior force directed through the hand or elbow along the humeral axis. The violent muscle contractures produced by an epileptic seizure or electric shock flex, adduct, and internally rotate the humerus, forcing it posteriorly.

Although Bankart[11a] believed the prime mechanism of recurrent anterior dislocations was a direct blow to the posterior humerus, this is not common. When it does occur, the direct compression of the humeral head into the anterior glenoid rim is more likely to fracture the glenoid (Fig. 3-3). This results in an unstable joint after reduction in 80% of these fractures.[73] Similarly, a direct blow to the anterior shoulder can drive the humerus posteriorly, resulting in a locked posterior fracture-dislocation (Fig. 3-4).

Fractures of the proximal humerus occur from both direct and indirect forces. Direct blows and falls can fracture the humerus. Indirect or rotational forces with the forearm used as a lever, as in shotput[155] and wrestling,[175] can fracture the humerus. Recently, a patient was seen who fell from his bicycle, landed on his elbow, and, through this longitudinal force traveling up the humerus, sustained a midshaft clavicle fracture.

Repetitive compression or impact loading may injure the joint surface. Although this has long been associated with capitellar osteochondritis in pitchers[84,165] and osteolysis of the outer clavicle in weight lifters (Fig. 3-5),[19,33,35] it has more recently been described in the humeral head of a tennis player who hit 1000 tennis backhands a day using a ball machine.[76]

Nonimpact injuries with muscle ruptures occur when the muscle-tendon unit is forced beyond its physiologic limit. Hoyt[75] ascribed this to excessive use beyond its fatigue limits, a sudden powerful contraction against resistance initiated by the muscle antagonists, or by external force working against a muscle contraction. Exam-

ples include ruptures of the subscapularis[22] or humeral shaft from arm wrestling, rupture of the pectoralis insertion from weight lifting,[89] and extreme muscle tension resulting from hanging by the arm.[105] Wrestlers, on the other hand, are predilected to rupture at the sternocostal origin rather than at the musculotendinous junction or tendinous insertion.[44,105]

Fractures at the base of the coracoid have been reported in rugby with an unknown mechanism,[101] in trap-shooting as a stress fracture,[29] and in tennis as an avulsion fracture from the recurrent pull of the pectoralis minor.[18] An unusual example of muscle pull causing a comminuted scapular body fracture has occurred during pushups.[45] Hematoma in a scapular fracture preventing use of the supraspinatus can be confused clinically with a rotator cuff tear. Good radiographs in three right-angle planes allow differentiation of the pseudo–cuff tear.

SPECIFIC PROBLEMS
Instability

Glenohumeral instability is the most common shoulder problem in the younger athlete, yet its varied presentations can make it one of the more difficult conditions to accurately diagnose, especially because ligamentous laxity, in and of itself, may not be the cause of an athlete's shoulder pain.

Anatomic Considerations

The glenohumeral joint characteristics that make it biomechanically unique are its nearly spherical articular surfaces, a high size disparity between the humerus and glenoid, and a more extensive complex motion than any other major joint in the body.[161] Only 25% to 30% of the humeral head articulates with the glenoid at any one time. The shallow cavity is functionally deepened by the intact labral and ligamentous attachment at its perimeter. The inferior glenohumeral ligament complex is the

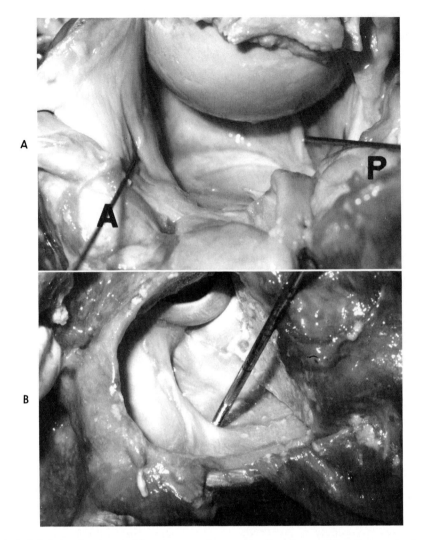

FIG. 3-6. Inferior glenohumeral ligament complex provides the prime stabilizer for anterior, inferior, and posterior stability. **A,** Thickenings of the complex form anterior *(A)* and posterior *(P)* inferior glenohumeral ligaments that pass from the humeral calcar up each side of the glenoid rim to blend with the labrum. A small inferior recess is normally between the two ligaments. **B,** The anteroinferior glenohumeral ligament as seen in a right shoulder (from behind with the humeral head removed) becomes confluent with the anterior labrum. It is the strongest glenohumeral ligament and the prime stabilizer when the arm is abducted and externally rotated.

prime static stabilizer for anterior,[168] posterior,[53,130] and inferior[116] stability (Fig. 3-6). The middle glenohumeral ligament appears to have a role secondary to the inferior glenohumeral ligament in anterior stability.[130]

The rotator cuff actively centers the humeral head in the glenoid cavity except when the arm is in extreme abduction and external rotation.[74,80] Then an obligatory posterior translation occurs. Shear forces over the articular cartilage and labral attachments occur with the forward acceleration in pitching as the humeral head glides anteriorly. Abnormal translation occurs in those with ligamentous detachments.[136,137] Once the anterior labrum has been detached, it no longer serves as a buttress to anterior subluxation or a tether to posterior instability. Increased subluxation in both directions can occur.[128,157]

The scapular rotators—namely the trapezius, rhomboids, and serratus anterior—function by positioning the glenoid for optimal stability.[79]

Classification

Shoulder instability is defined in terms of the following:

1. *Directions:* anterior, posterior, inferior, anterosuperior, and multidirectional
2. *Degree*
   a. Dislocation—humeral head escapes the glenoid cavity
   b. Subluxation—passive translation with more than 50% of the humeral head over the glenoid rim without complete dislocation[121,122,130]; ac-

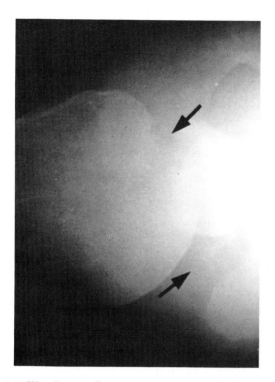

FIG. 3-7. West Point axillary view. Ectopic calcification of the anteroinferior glenoid is pathognomonic for a labral detachment and anterior instability. The posterior lateral humeral head Hill-Sachs impression fracture is the pathognomonic radiographic sign often seen in anterior dislocations after reduction.

tive translation more than 4 mm from the center of the glenoid cavity[74]

3. *Timing:* acute, recurrent, chronic, or fixed
4. *Etiologic force*
   a. Trauma—major injury
   b. Microtrauma—repetitive stretching
   c. Atraumatic—congenital ligamentous laxity
5. *Motivation*
   a. Voluntary—muscle contracture or positional with or without abnormal secondary psychologic gain
   b. Involuntary—positional or with trauma
6. *Anatomy*
   a. Bony architecture—dysplasia, hypoplasia, aplasia of glenoid or humeral head
   b. Glenoid rim fracture (Fig. 3-3)
   c. Humeral head impression fracture
   d. Anteriorly from posterior dislocation (Fig. 3-4)
   e. Posteriorly from anterior dislocation (Hill-Sachs defect) (Fig. 3-7)
   f. Ligamentous, labral, and muscle integrity, that is, labral detachment (Fig. 3-7), subscapularis avulsion, or cuff tear
   g. Neurologic status—Erb's palsy, plexus injury, or cerebrovascular accident

Anterior Instability

Anterior instability from acute trauma (as in football) or from repetitive stretching (as in pitching) occurs in

an anteroinferior direction. In up to 85% of such injuries the labrum has been detached from the anteroinferior glenoid rim.

The optimal time for postreduction immobilization for the first dislocation is thought to be between 3 and 6 weeks.[86,118] Recurrence in the athlete is probable.[42,70] The younger the athlete, the more likely is recurrence; however, it is not frequent in the nonathlete or if adequate immobilization and rehabilitation take place before the return to sports.[159]

The major diagnostic efforts are to ascertain whether the glenoid labrum and inferior glenohumeral ligaments are secure. The clinical evaluation, specialized oblique axillary radiographs (Fig. 3-7),[146] CT arthrotomography,[11,106,110,131,158] or arthroscopy[79] can provide this information. Because of the high incidence of labral detachment with first-time dislocation in the younger patient who wishes to remain active, early operative repair with confirmation of a labral detachment is becoming more popular.

Anterior dislocations require assistance with their first and often subsequent reductions. Radiographs confirm the direction and degree. Blazina and Saltzman[24] reported on recurrent anterior subluxation and advanced the understanding of more subtle forms of instability. Dislocation or subluxation of the humeral head may occur over the anteroinferior glenoid rim when the arm is in the throwing position of abduction, external rotation, and extension. With hard throwing the subluxation may manifest itself as a dead arm.[151] Transient neurologic symptoms radiate down the arm and forearm and usually to the ulnar side of the hand. For a few minutes the athlete is unable to use the arm but then recovers with residual aching. Popping, catching, and fear that the arm will slip in the provocative position are commonly reported.

Labral tearing, with subluxation manifesting as clicking, has been identified in the anteroinferior glenoid in pitching[131] and in swimming.[110] Loose bodies seen in radiographs of the shoulder are an indication of recurrent shoulder dislocations.[122]

Whereas other forms of instability are thought to be capsular in origin, anterosuperior instability is seen postoperatively after a rotator cuff or greater tuberosity dehiscence. The humeral head cannot be fixed in the glenoid cavity. It rides superiorly with the pull of the deltoid when the force couple action of the supraspinatus and long head of the biceps no longer serves as a head depressor (Fig. 3-8).

Posterior Instability

Posterior shoulder instability is classified as acute posterior dislocation, with or without a head impression fracture; chronic locked posterior dislocation (often originally missed)[68]; and recurrent posterior shoulder subluxation.

The **acute posterior dislocation** without a head impression fracture is rare, but if not reduced and immobilized in external rotation with the arm at the side, it becomes recurrent. Both the acute posterior dislocation and the posterior locked (head impression fracture) dislocation occur in sports from a fall on the elbow or out-

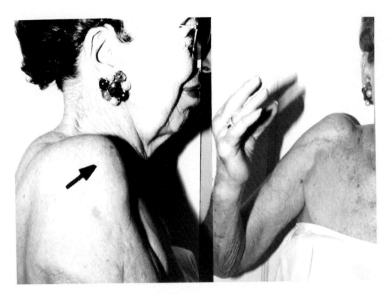

FIG. 3-8. Anterosuperior ascent of the humeral head with a large cuff tear as in this rheumatoid or tuberosity avulsion. Supraspinatus and long head of the biceps can no longer fix the humeral head in the glenoid as the deltoid attempts to elevate the arm. Following failed surgery, this is exacerbated by loss of the coracoacromial ligament as an anterior superior restraint.

stretched hand when the arm is flexed forward, adducted, and internally rotated. The same injury can occur—although not usually in sports—from electric shock, epileptic seizure, or alcoholic withdrawal seizures. Up to 80% of these are missed by the first examining physician. Although most of these result from violent muscle contractures or trauma directed along the axis of the humeral shaft, I have seen a case in which a tree limb went through a car windshield, knocking the shoulder backward with a direct blow as the car went off the road (Fig. 3-4). The history, a high index of suspicion, and an axillary radiograph or CT scan prevents missing this lesion in an individual with limitations of forward flexion, external rotation, and forearm supination (Fig. 3-4, C).

Chronic recurrent posterior subluxations are frequently demonstrable by the patient either in arm position or selected muscle contracture.[125] It may be unilateral after trauma or bilateral with pain only on one side, with or without a precipitating traumatic event. Hawkins and McCormack[69] classify four subsets as (1) voluntary habitual (emotionally disturbed), (2) voluntary, (3) not willful (muscular control), and (4) involuntary positional and involuntary unintentional (not demonstrable by patient).

The usual history is one of gradual onset in which subluxation of both shoulders can occur posteriorly either by contracture of the anterior deltoid and pectoralis (Fig. 3-9) or by arm position with the arm forward flexed (Fig. 3-10, A). Extension of the arm causes a sudden snap with a concomitant reduction (Fig. 3-10, B). If posterior shoulder subluxation occurs unintentionally with forward flexion, pain may interfere with the sport. Although it is easy to demonstrate, the athlete may not know what is happening, and the physician often does not consider

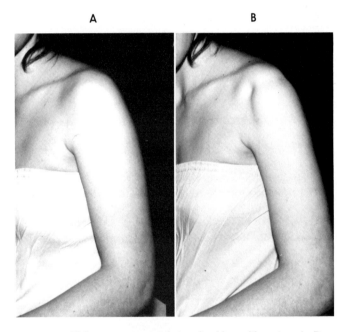

FIG. 3-9. Voluntary posterioinferior shoulder subluxation. **A,** Reduced. **B,** Subluxation and fixation by muscle contractures of the anterior deltoid and pectoralis with simultaneous relaxation of the posterior deltoid and external rotators.

it in the differential diagnosis for shoulder pain. Although apprehension is common for anterior instability, it is not reliable for posterior instability.

Athletes with recurrent posterior subluxations aggravate their shoulder problem with sports that stress the posterior capsule. In my practice these have been more common in butterfly swimmers, rowers, archers,[55] and

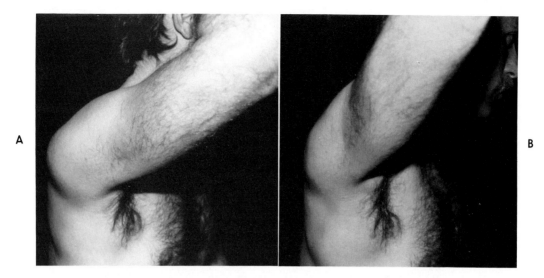

FIG. 3-10. A, Positioned posterior subluxation. **B,** Reduction with snap. This could be confused with anterior instability if the shoulder were mistakenly thought to be reduced in the first position **(A).**

weight lifters, who feel pain on bench pressing. As a result of excessive stretching, recurrent subluxations may be associated with rotator cuff tendinitis.[69] External rotational strengthening, with the arms at the side and avoidance of posterior capsular stress, have been moderately effective in alleviating patients' symptoms. For those who had a specific traumatic onset and unsuccessful conservative exercises, Fronek, Warren, and Bowen[53] report encouraging results using posterior capsular shift procedures in returning athletes to their former sports.

Multidirectional Instability

In 1980 Neer and Foster[116] identified the hallmark of multidirectional shoulder instability as abnormal inferior glenohumeral laxity in the absence of labral detachments. The typical occurrence is in an athlete with generalized ligamentous laxity without appreciable trauma. Vague aching or recurrent slipping of the shoulder with increasing disability is common in weight lifting and sports that require repetitive overhead arm movement, such as in pitching and swimming. Multidirectional subluxations might be suspected in a swimmer who reports pain in the pull-through phase in the water and recovery phase out of the water.[6] Secondary rotator cuff tendinitis may occur with normal acromial morphology in a young athlete. Transient pain and paresthesias, radiating distal to the elbow, are common with arm use, and yet neurologic evaluation is normal.

At the time of examination both shoulders can be pulled inferiorly to create a sulcus between the humeral head and acromion (Fig. 3-11, A). Shoulder subluxation also can occur anteriorly, posteriorly, or in both directions simultaneously with the aid of mild inferior traction. Radiographs, with 20-pound weights strapped to both forearms, may reveal excessive bilateral inferior laxity[122] (Fig. 3-11, B), but pain may preclude relaxation and

thereby the inferior subluxation on the symptomatic side. Correlating the patient's pain and ability to relax during the test assists in interpretation of otherwise confusing radiographs. Shoulder arthrography may demonstrate an enlarged inferior capsular pouch (Fig. 3-12, A and B); CT arthrotomography (Fig. 3-12, C) and arthroscopy reveal normal labral and ligamentous attachments.

Evaluation of other joints for laxity may demonstrate hyperextension of the elbows and knees, thumbs that can touch the forearms with wrist flexion, and ballerina-type hip laxity if the feet can be placed over the head and behind the neck (Fig. 3-13).[116,122]

Pitfalls to be avoided in the diagnosis and treatment of multidirectional instability (MDI) include the following:

1. Traumatic labral detachment allows for increased motion in all directions on examination. Repair of the labrum is sufficient; additional capsular shifting serves to overly tighten the shoulder.
2. Failure to repair labral detachments with anterior, posterior, or combined procedures may still allow for residual inferior instability and thereby mimic MDI.
3. In an athlete with MDI, overly tight anterior repairs (Putti-Platt, Magnuson-Stack, Bristow) may displace the head to the opposite side of the joint. Early arthritis with pressure necrosis of the head and glenoid results when the capsular restraints on all three sides of the joint have not been balanced, yet iatrogenically hold the head in a position of fixed subluxation (Fig. 3-14).

Matsen[103] attempted to simplify the instability considerations with two mnemonics:

TUBS   **T**raumatic etiology
       Unidirectional instability
       Bankart ligamentous detachment
       Surgical repair

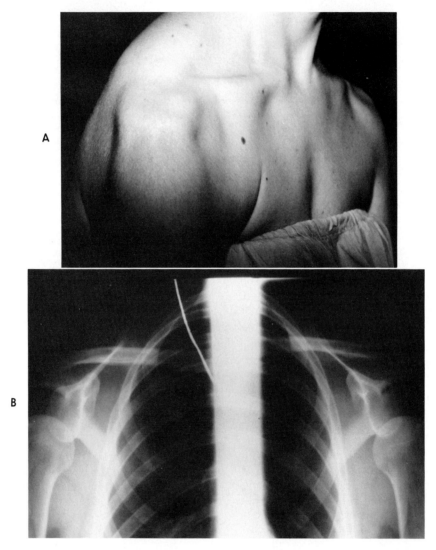

FIG. 3-11. Inferior subluxation of the glenohumeral joints. **A,** Sulcus develops between the acromion and humeral head. **B,** Radiograph demonstrating inferior capsular laxity with a 20-pound weight strapped to each forearm.

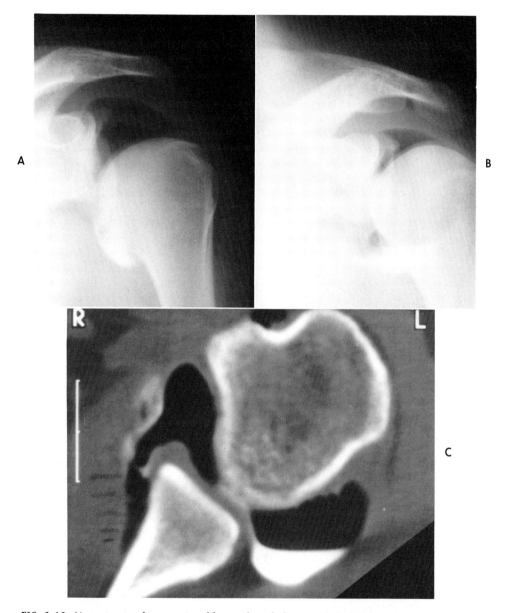

FIG. 3-12. Air-contrast arthrogram in athlete with multidirectional shoulder instability. **A,** Enlarged inferior capsular pouch. **B,** Traction obliterates inferior pouch in inferior humeral head subluxation. **C,** Computed tomography-assisted air-contrast arthrogram is normal. Dye extravasates into the subscapularis recess. Air outlines the triangular-pointed anterior labrum and more blunted posterior labrum. The margins of the labrum are intact without evidence of tearing, detachment, or abnormal straining with contrast. Positive contrast is seen in the posterior capsular pouch.

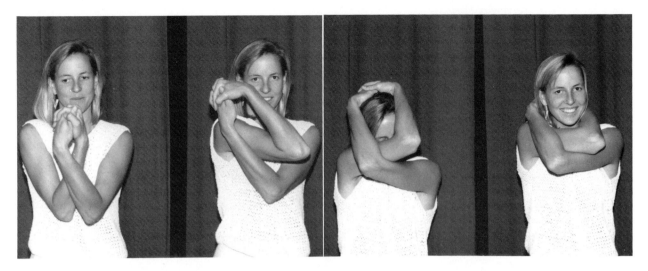

FIG. 3-13. Bilateral generalized upper extremity laxity of shoulders and wrists is required to perform this series of maneuvers. Once the symptomatic right shoulder was repaired, these maneuvers could not be repeated.

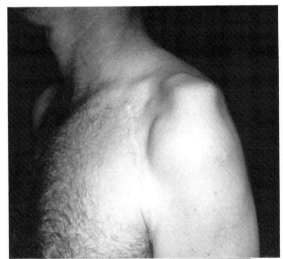

A

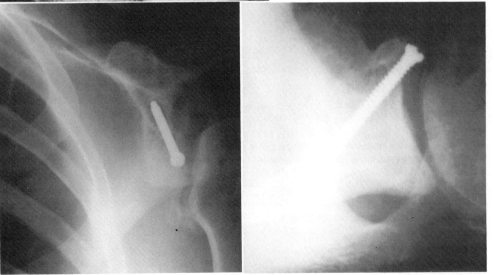

B

C

FIG. 3-14. Failed anterior instability repair. Unrepaired anterior labrum with unidirectional repair resulted in fixed posterior humeral head subluxation. Transfer of the coracoid muscles under the axillary nerve resulted in permanent paralysis even though the epineurium was intact. A prominent bony block with hardware and fixed posterior subluxation resulted in degenerative arthritis. **A,** Clinical loss of the deltoid. **B** and **C,** Hardware impingement excavates the anterior humeral head and contributes to the fixed posterior subluxation.

AMBRI **A**traumatic etiology
Multidirectional instability
Bilateral shoulders
Rehabilitation with rotational strengthening exercises as primary treatment; effective in approximately 80% of patients
Inferior capsular shift is the surgical treatment for failed exercises

Impingement

The terminology for impingement lesions has led to confusion. In 1834 Smith[160a] described rotator cuff tears as a pathologic entity. In 1934 Codman,[38] in the first book dealing with the shoulder, recognized the continuing pain and dysfunction caused by the neglected rotator cuff tear and recommended its repair. Many names and causes for this continuum have been cited, including bursitis, tendinitis, acute trauma, overuse, instability, aging, tendon degeneration, vascular deficiencies, and mechanical impingement. McLaughlin[107] noted the following:

that the rotator cuff is the only tendon situated between two bones . . . is compressed by every motion of the shoulder until it succumbs to the ravages of attrition long before most other tendons.

Neer[114] unified these concepts when he recognized the wear centered on the supraspinatus, just posterior to the long head of the biceps, as it passed underneath the anterior acromion, acromioclavicular joint, and coracoacromial ligament. Secondarily, the long head of the biceps and infraspinatus may become involved. There are four stages of impingement. Phase I, termed *edema and swelling,* is now correlated with the overuse tendinitis from sports requiring repetitive overhead arm action. Phase II, thickening and fibrosis, is correlated with incomplete thickness rotator cuff tears, as seen by ultrasonography, arthrography, and arthroscopy. Phase III comprises complete thickness tearing and bone changes consisting of sclerosis or spurring along the anterior acromion with excrescences on the greater tuberosity with subcortical cystic lesions (Fig. 3-15). Phase IV, cuff tear arthropathy,[115]

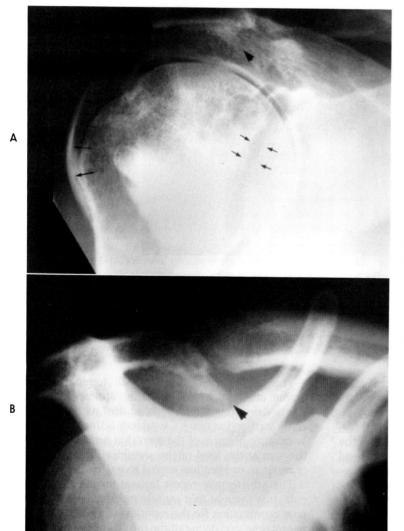

FIG. 3-15. Rotator cuff tear with Stage III impingement. **A,** The positive contrast from the shoulder arthrogram has extended beyond the normal attachment of the greater tuberosity, indicating a rotator cuff tear. The small arrows medially mark the long head of the biceps, demonstrating its integrity. If the arm was in external rotation and if dye were to extend down its sheath, the appearance should not be confused with a rotator cuff tear. Calcification extends into the coracoacromial ligament. **B,** In the lateral scapular view the supraspinatus outlet is compromised by an inferior projection of the anterior undersurface of the acromion. Calcification is seen extending into the superior portion of the coracoacromial ligament. This Type III hooked acromion (by the Bigliani-Morrison classification) is the most frequent shape associated with tearing of the rotator cuff.

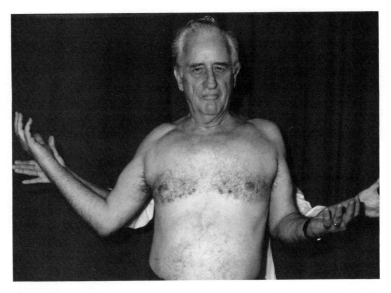

FIG. 3-19. Herniated C5-C6 disk resulting in external rotation weakness mimics rotator cuff tear of the left shoulder. Once the arms are released, the left arm falls in toward the stomach, demonstrating passive but not active external rotation.

jection of lidocaine (Xylocaine).[32,118] With incomplete thickness tears, strength returns to normal for the duration of the effects of the Xylocaine.

Ruptures of the long head of the biceps may occur at the musculotendinous area in the young athlete, but in the middle-aged or aging athlete this is usually at the top of the biceps groove and associated with an impingement lesion (Fig. 3-18).[21,90]

The differential diagnosis of rotator cuff impingement is adhesive capsulitis, nerve compression (C5-C6 disk [Fig. 3-19], suprascapular neuropathy, or other brachial plexus lesions), and shoulder instability. The provocative tests to demonstrate a positive impingement overlap with anterior apprehension in testing instability or the pain produced by stretching a partially frozen shoulder.

Calcific Tendinitis

Calcific tendinitis can occur at any age during adulthood. It has a predilection for the middle-aged athlete involved in repetitive activities. It can occur in any of the tendons of the rotator cuff, although it is more frequently seen in the supraspinatus, 1 to 2 cm from the tendon insertion in the greater tuberosity. The athlete may manifest impingement-like symptoms, with aching and pain exacerbated by activities requiring overhead arm motion. There is no correlation between the size of the deposit and the symptoms.[173] If the pain is longstanding, there is a tendency for secondary shoulder stiffness to develop in the athlete.

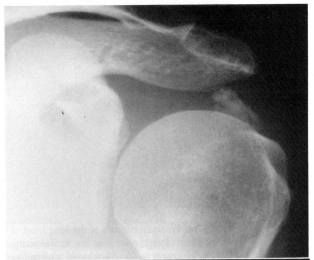

A

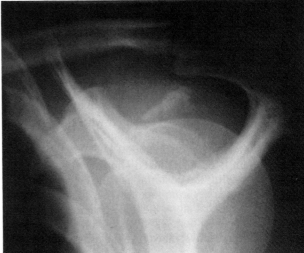

B

FIG. 3-20. Calcific tendinitis in the supraspinatus 1 cm from its insertion. **A,** External rotation view. **B,** Lateral scapula view.

AMBRI   **A**traumatic etiology
Multidirectional instability
Bilateral shoulders
Rehabilitation with rotational strengthening exercises as primary treatment; effective in approximately 80% of patients
Inferior capsular shift is the surgical treatment for failed exercises

Impingement

The terminology for impingement lesions has led to confusion. In 1834 Smith[160a] described rotator cuff tears as a pathologic entity. In 1934 Codman,[38] in the first book dealing with the shoulder, recognized the continuing pain and dysfunction caused by the neglected rotator cuff tear and recommended its repair. Many names and causes for this continuum have been cited, including bursitis, tendinitis, acute trauma, overuse, instability, aging, tendon degeneration, vascular deficiencies, and mechanical impingement. McLaughlin[107] noted the following:

that the rotator cuff is the only tendon situated between two bones . . . is compressed by every motion of the shoulder until it succumbs to the ravages of attrition long before most other tendons.

Neer[114] unified these concepts when he recognized the wear centered on the supraspinatus, just posterior to the long head of the biceps, as it passed underneath the anterior acromion, acromioclavicular joint, and coracoacromial ligament. Secondarily, the long head of the biceps and infraspinatus may become involved. There are four stages of impingement. Phase I, termed *edema and swelling,* is now correlated with the overuse tendinitis from sports requiring repetitive overhead arm action. Phase II, thickening and fibrosis, is correlated with incomplete thickness rotator cuff tears, as seen by ultrasonography, arthrography, and arthroscopy. Phase III comprises complete thickness tearing and bone changes consisting of sclerosis or spurring along the anterior acromion with excrescences on the greater tuberosity with subcortical cystic lesions (Fig. 3-15). Phase IV, cuff tear arthropathy,[115]

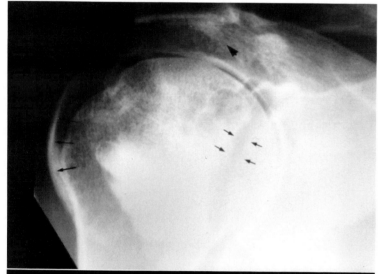

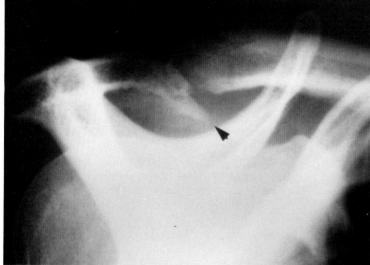

FIG. 3-15. Rotator cuff tear with Stage III impingement. **A,** The positive contrast from the shoulder arthrogram has extended beyond the normal attachment of the greater tuberosity, indicating a rotator cuff tear. The small arrows medially mark the long head of the biceps, demonstrating its integrity. If the arm was in external rotation and if dye were to extend down its sheath, the appearance should not be confused with a rotator cuff tear. Calcification extends into the coracoacromial ligament. **B,** In the lateral scapular view the supraspinatus outlet is compromised by an inferior projection of the anterior undersurface of the acromion. Calcification is seen extending into the superior portion of the coracoacromial ligament. This Type III hooked acromion (by the Bigliani-Morrison classification) is the most frequent shape associated with tearing of the rotator cuff.

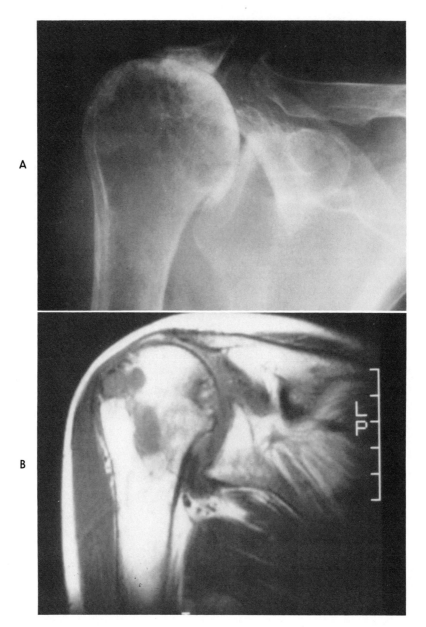

FIG. 3-16. Rotator cuff tear arthropathy with loss of supraspinatus and superior migration of the humeral head. **A,** The humeral head thins out the acromion as a new facet is formed superiorly. Humeral head can no longer be fixed within the glenoid for adequate elevation or use of the intact deltoid. **B,** An MRI in this patient following failed cuff surgery demonstrates roughening and necrosis of the subchondral bone.

may occur in a small percentage of neglected cuff tears (Fig. 3-16). Over time, humeral head subluxation occurs superiorly.[172] In some instances the combination of superior and anterior instability and loss of nutritional factors with the persistent cuff tear leads to softening of the head and rotator cuff tear arthropathy. The humeral head then erodes into the undersurface of the acromioclavicular joint in its position of superior subluxation without a stable fulcrum for the glenoid. At this advanced stage, except for sports that involve underhand throwing, like horseshoes, an athlete's career has ended.

The clinical presentations with impingement syndrome are recognized in young athletes involved in sports using repetitive overhead arm motion. They become sore, and at times a swimmer is unable to continue swimming because of the pain that accompanies use of the arm at the level of the shoulder.[66,83,134,142,143] Use of resistive paddles has served to hasten the symptoms.

The athlete may report fatigue involving the rotator cuff. It is thought that muscle imbalance contributes to poor coordination for the repetitive activities. The external rotators, consisting of the infraspinatus and teres mi-

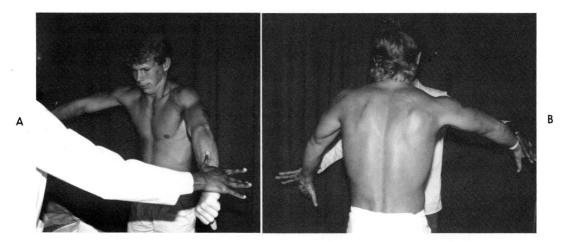

FIG. 3-17. A, Isolated testing of the supraspinatus begins with the arms in 90 degrees abduction and 30 degrees forward flexion and internal rotation with the thumbs pointing downward. **B,** This athlete is unable to resist the examiner's downward force on the left side.

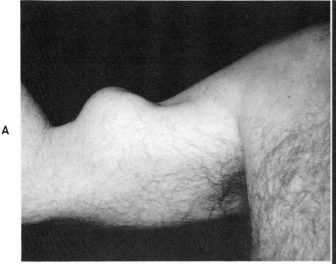

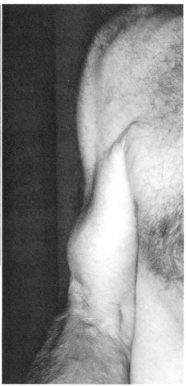

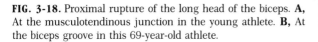

FIG. 3-18. Proximal rupture of the long head of the biceps. **A,** At the musculotendinous junction in the young athlete. **B,** At the biceps groove in this 69-year-old athlete.

nor, are much weaker as compared with the pectoralis major, latissismus dorsi, teres major, subscapularis, and anterior deltoid. Abnormal rhythm has also been implicated if there is either reduced shoulder motion with a stiffness involving the posterior capsule or, alternatively, increased joint laxity from repetitive capsular stretching. The positive clinical signs include subacromial crepitus with rotation in 90 degrees of abduction and a painful arc of motion on actively lowering the arms between 120 and 170 degrees; catching often accompanies this motion. The arm may suddenly drop or need to be supported by the other arm. Weakness of the external rotators is determined by testing the arm at the side. Isolated supraspinatus weakness may be found when the arm is tested against a downward force once placed in 90-degree abduction, 30-degree forward flexion, and full internal rotation (Fig. 3-17).

Temporary pain relief follows a 10-ml subacromial in-

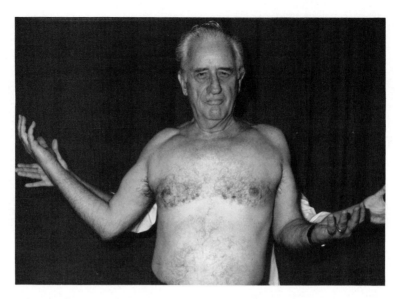

FIG. 3-19. Herniated C5-C6 disk resulting in external rotation weakness mimics rotator cuff tear of the left shoulder. Once the arms are released, the left arm falls in toward the stomach, demonstrating passive but not active external rotation.

jection of lidocaine (Xylocaine).[32,118] With incomplete thickness tears, strength returns to normal for the duration of the effects of the Xylocaine.

Ruptures of the long head of the biceps may occur at the musculotendinous area in the young athlete, but in the middle-aged or aging athlete this is usually at the top of the biceps groove and associated with an impingement lesion (Fig. 3-18).[21,90]

The differential diagnosis of rotator cuff impingement is adhesive capsulitis, nerve compression (C5-C6 disk [Fig. 3-19], suprascapular neuropathy, or other brachial plexus lesions), and shoulder instability. The provocative tests to demonstrate a positive impingement overlap with anterior apprehension in testing instability or the pain produced by stretching a partially frozen shoulder.

Calcific Tendinitis

Calcific tendinitis can occur at any age during adulthood. It has a predilection for the middle-aged athlete involved in repetitive activities. It can occur in any of the tendons of the rotator cuff, although it is more frequently seen in the supraspinatus, 1 to 2 cm from the tendon insertion in the greater tuberosity. The athlete may manifest impingement-like symptoms, with aching and pain exacerbated by activities requiring overhead arm motion. There is no correlation between the size of the deposit and the symptoms.[173] If the pain is longstanding, there is a tendency for secondary shoulder stiffness to develop in the athlete.

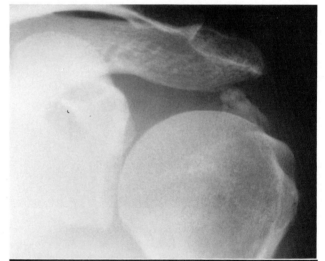

A

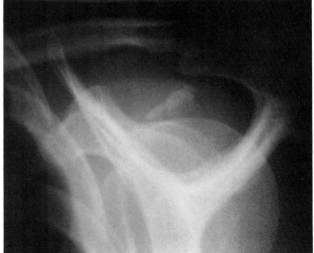

B

FIG. 3-20. Calcific tendinitis in the supraspinatus 1 cm from its insertion. **A,** External rotation view. **B,** Lateral scapula view.

The second presentation is the more severe form, with exquisite pain at rest, inability to sleep, and additional aggravation by motion. The athlete holds the arm as if it were a piece of Steuben glass. The common findings in the evaluation are point tenderness over the calcific deposit and increase in pain when the involved muscle is actively used or if the examiner stretches against the end-range stiffness. Full but guarded motion may be present. Assistance may be requested in getting the arm down to the midthoracic level on internal rotation testing.[173] It can be diagnosed with under penetrated (35% to 40%) anterior and posterior radiographic views, in internal and external rotation, and by a lateral scapular view to determine the precise location of the deposit (Fig. 3-20).

Of individuals with shoulder pain, 7% have symptomatic calcific tendinitis.[50] Approximately 3% of asymptomatic patients demonstrate calcification in the rotator cuff.[141] Of the asymptomatic individuals, 35% to 45% eventually become symptomatic.[28] Although the etiology is uncertain, Uhthoff, Sakar, and Maynard[169] proposed tissue hypoxia as the initial event leading to hydroxyapatite deposition, followed by macrophage adsorption and collagenous reconstitution.

Two types of deposits may be seen: the well-circumscribed, gritty, sandlike deposit is consistent with the chronic phase, whereas the amorphous deposit of toothpaste consistency is characteristic of the resorptive healing phase. The latter phase is associated with the exquisite pain; the former phase may be present on an incidental x-ray film without symptoms or with other chronic aching symptoms. Corticosteroid injections, and more likely the needle puncture of the deposit in the acute resorptive phase, allow the deposit to escape into the subacromial space and to resorb. Calcific deposits are seen less frequently now by the treating orthopaedic surgeon than 30 years ago. It is not clear whether this is a change in the natural history of the disease or whether the deposits are more often adequately treated by the primary care physicians.

Adhesive Capsulitis (Frozen Shoulder)

Although there are many causes of shoulder stiffness, perhaps the most perplexing is that of adhesive capsulitis resulting in a markedly restricted joint capsule.[173] There is a strong predilection for women in the menopausal and early postmenopausal age group. It is rarely associated with tearing of the rotator cuff. Its cause is unknown. Neviaser[119] reported dense adhesions in the capsule, whereas Lundberg[97] found no adhesions at surgery, with fibrosis of the deep layers on biopsy. Bland, Merritt, and Boushey[23] postulated that an autonomic dysfunction results in impaired circulation, secondary fibrosis, and stiffness. This hypothesis satisfactorily explains the lack of adhesions within the joint when the shoulder is examined arthroscopically or visualized at open surgery.

Clinically, many orthopaedists ascribe the onset to episodes of shoulder immobilization. Stiffness follows protection of the arm in adduction, internal rotation, and slight elevation of the shoulder. The precipitating cause

could be placement of the arm in a sling after a Colles' fracture, cervical radiculopathy, angina, intrinsic calcific tendinitis, or failure to mobilize the arm after a stroke. Frequently the precipitating cause is not found. The treatment goal is restoration of the inferior capsular pouch by stretching, exercises, manipulation under anesthesia, or open release. Shoulder stiffness invalidates many of the other diagnostic maneuvers for impingement and instability testing. Unfortunately, the missed posterior fracture dislocation may present as a frozen shoulder. An axillary radiograph eliminates this confusion.

Precipitating causes of adhesive capsulitis

- Forearm, wrist, and hand fractures or injuries
- Cervical radiculopathy
- Angina
- Calcific tendinitis
- After cardiovascular accident
- Unknown

Neurologic Problems

Neurologic problems occur in the amateur or young athlete more frequently than in the professional.[13] They often manifest radiating pain, burning, and numbness in the shoulder or extending down the arm, with local stunning and inability to lift the arm, forearm, or wrist. Primary shoulder injury is not associated with pain extending beyond the elbow. Spinal cord injuries and cervical spine fractures, although infrequent, still occur with spearhead football tackles or hard falls when the head and shoulder are forced apart. Common mechanisms for this include forward falls in gymnastics and skiing and being thrown over the handlebars of a speeding motorcycle or bicycle.

Paralysis of the entire limb and severe burning is a sign of nerve root avulsion; fractures of the first rib, clavicle, and coracoid are associated with severe brachial plexus stretching.[92] Those injuries caused by a hockey stick or other sharp object to the neck can result in weakness of the trapezius and a dragging, aching sensation in the shoulder.[13] The athlete may be unable to shrug the shoulder and may later report secondary impingement symptoms with attempted overhead arm extension.

Wearing a heavy backpack or falling with a backpack has been associated with **serratus anterior palsy.** Loss of the serratus anterior with traction to the long thoracic nerve of Bell has been reported in overhead weight lifters[162] and in the discus thrower, who presumably tears the scapular fixators that allow for stretching of the nerve with subsequent scapular winging.[64]

Compression or traction of the **suprascapular nerve** with pain and weakness in hitting a backhand or in serving has been seen in suprascapular nerve entrapment as well as in occult ganglions pressing the suprascapular nerve. This being the highest structure coming off the plexus, it is also susceptible to direct blows in contact sports.[13]

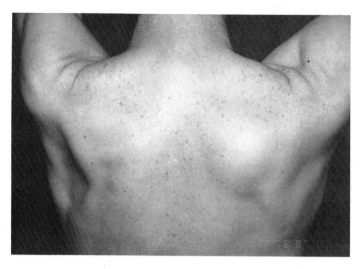

FIG. 3-21. Isolated infraspinatus atrophy of the left shoulder.

Isolated infraspinatus atrophy has occurred with traction, trauma, and ganglions (Fig. 3-21). Loss of the suprascapular nerve branch to the infraspinatus at the level of the spinoglenoid notch or distal has been reported in injuries caused by stretching.[47,51,111] The isolated infraspinatus palsy was a common finding in Italian volleyball spikers.[51] Another mechanism that caused weakness and posterior shoulder pain involved severe stretching of the infraspinatus muscle after a violent throw.[152] As seen on MRI, the infraspinatus was replaced with fatty tissue.

The relationship of the **axillary nerve** to the glenohumeral joint makes it particularly prone to injury during shoulder joint trauma.[39] The axillary nerve is susceptible to stretching with an anterior dislocation or direct contusion by a backward fall on the quadrilateral space or a blow to the deltoid.[13,40] The nerve is found to be injured in 20% to 30% of glenohumeral dislocations and humeral neck fractures when it is assessed by EMG 2 to 3 weeks after injury.[40] In those over 50 years of age, it is as high as 50%.[25,48,132] Unfortunately, sensibility testing in the axillary nerve distribution of the lateral arm has not proved reliable.[25]

The **musculocutaneous nerve** is susceptible to direct frontal blows. Athletes report numbness in the lateral forearm to the base of the thumb and have a weak to absent biceps.

Sports injuries account for 2.9% to 5.7% of all the peripheral nerve system injuries.[72,87] The radial, ulnar, peroneal, and axillary nerves are the peripheral nerves most frequently injured in sports.[72] The axillary and musculocutaneous nerves are the most likely to be injured in athletic reconstructive procedures about the shoulder (Fig. 3-14).[34,40,126]

Scapulothoracic Problems

The scapulothoracic articulation is a gliding joint between the thoracic rib cage and the scapula. It is separated by filmy bursa. Problems in this area occur from muscle paralysis, snapping scapula, and rib fractures. In

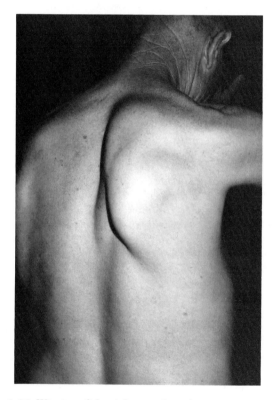

FIG. 3-22. Winging of the right scapula with serratus anterior paralysis.

the group of muscle paralyses, winging from a serratus anterior palsy and scapular ptosis or drooping from a trapezius palsy hamper the athlete because of fatigue pain and inability to adequately place the scapula under the glenoid. With a **serratus anterior palsy** the scapula cannot be fixed to the chest wall as the arm is elevated (Fig. 3-22). The winging is accentuated by contracture of the rhomboids and pectoralis minor muscles.[170] Increasing pain develops, and the athlete is unable to lift with power or push. In **trapezius palsies** impingement

is aggravated with arm abduction. The shoulder droops and is subject to easy fatigue.

Scapulothoracic crepitus, or a snapping scapula palpable at the superior medial border of the scapula, is not a well-understood entity. Rarely, an osteochondroma on the undersurface of the superior medial border of the scapula accounts for the crepitus. Alternatively, a malunion after multiple rib fractures interrupts the gliding motion of the scapula on the chest wall. More commonly, there is no known cause of the crepitation and grinding that can be produced by moving the scapula up and down against the chest wall. Snapping and pain are localized to the superior medial border as it articulates with the thorax. Modification of activities, strengthening of the subscapularis and serratus anterior, and occasionally a corticosteroid injection in the scapulothoracic bursa are sometimes successful in treatment of what can be an intermittently painful syndrome. If psychologic problems can be excluded, a subperiosteal excision of the superior medial pole through a muscle-splitting incision relieves the pain and snapping in eight of nine cases.[8] The procedure had to be repeated in one patient who was skeletally immature at the index procedure.

Arthritis

Arthritis of joints of the shoulder girdle include the sternoclavicular, acromioclavicular, and glenohumeral joints. Sporting activities that can produce arthritis include direct trauma with fractures, dislocations, and repetitive loading.

Sternoclavicular Joint Problems

Arthritis of the sternoclavicular joint may occur from direct trauma with a rare posterior dislocation or indirect trauma with the more frequent anterior subluxation and dislocations. Arthritis of this joint is rarely sports related[138] and is gradual in onset in postmenopausal women.[30] In a 27-year period Quigley[138] found few sternoclavicular joint injuries in organized college athletics at Harvard. The few severe injuries to the sternoclavicular joint are high-kinetic injuries from bicycles, motor vehicles, polo, snowskiing, and occasionally football.

Acromioclavicular Joint Problems

Weight lifters' shoulders describes a condition with repetitive loading at the acromioclavicular joint resulting in degenerative arthritis and (at times) an osteolysis of the outer clavicle.[33,35]

Glenohumeral Joint Problems

Glenohumeral osteoarthritis with eccentric wear of the posterior glenoid has been observed in weight lifting as well as in many other sports in which the strong rotator cuff muscles are intact and function well. The athlete may report aching and fatigue pain or bone-on-bone grinding noises that are accentuated with resistive muscle testing with sharp pain. The diagnosis is confirmed with radiographs. Other causes of glenohumeral arthritis to consider in the patient's history include an arthritis occurring after recurrent dislocations[122,124,125] or after fixed humeral head displacement to the opposite side

of the joint in repairs for instability that are too tight[116,117,126] or in which the humeral head abuts on metal in or near the joint.[127,176]

PSYCHOLOGIC FACTORS IN SHOULDER PAIN*

When the orthopaedic history and examination, together with any indicated special studies, are unsuccessful in clearly suggesting an anatomic diagnosis, functional causes of pain must be considered. Indeed, even when shoulder pain has an anatomic basis, psychologic factors may result in a clinical presentation which, on first regard, seems more serious than is actually the case. Although the terms **anatomic** (organic) and **functional** (nonorganic) and their variations are commonly used to describe pain, it should be understood that this dichotomy is an artificial one. Most pain—especially chronic pain—has both organic and psychologic underpinnings.

Clinicians are frequently unable to relinquish the notion that pain must always originate in peripheral receptors and nowhere else. Association pathways in the brain link peripheral pain (afferent) pathways with the limbic system, through which emotions are processed. Pain is a final common pathway that can signal disturbance in either or both the physical and the psychologic domain.

Nonorganic (or functional) causes of pain must always be included in the differential diagnosis of chronic pain. The differential diagnosis of functional pain includes depressive and anxiety spectrum disorders (including major depression, dysthymia, and generalized anxiety disorder), adjustment disorders, somatoform disorders, factitious disorders, and malingering. Sometimes chronic pain may be a manifestation of a psychotic disorder, such as schizophrenia.

Functional causes of pain

- Depression
- Anxiety disorders
- Adjustment disorders
- Somatoform disorders
- Factitious disorders
- Malingering
- Psychosis

Functional pain is not (and should never be) regarded as a diagnosis of exclusion. Certain individuals, because of events and circumstances during the formative years, are prone to pain. They are particularly vulnerable to development of chronic pain in response to events and circumstances of their adult lives that resonate (frequently at an unconscious level) with the situations in their formative years, which rendered them prone to pain in the first place. More often than not they do not understand the dynamics involved. Not realizing its origin in the psyche, they seek an organic explanation for their pain. Their conviction (which may reach delusional proportions) is that the pain is not only organic, but also (rein-

forcing the delusion) results because of a specific "target incident" or "injury." Many such injuries are red herrings that serve as a smokescreen to obscure the emotional situation responsible for and underlying the chronic pain. In the case of shoulder pain the underlying situation often has to do with *shouldering* a burden or with *shouldering* responsibility or with *bearing up* in the face of personal or financial loss.

Depressed individuals invariably have lowered tolerance of pain. They may perceive as disabling or incapacitating pain that for healthy individuals would be, at worst, an annoyance. The depressed individual uses chronic (nonorganic) pain at an unconscious level to legitimize his or her dependency (primary gain) and to secure caretaking (secondary gain) from the environment. Many young persons are driven to almost superhuman lengths to achieve athletically in an unconscious search for parental acceptance or approval. For some, the only way out without losing face is to be forced, because of a painful orthopaedic condition, to curtail their activities. Their pain bespeaks a conflict between *consciously* wanting to continue the striving for athletic achievement, on the one hand, and *unconsciously* wanting to lessen the incessant pressure to achieve, on the other. Similarly, in the individual whose emotional neediness is concealed by a façade of independence and self-sufficiency (often since a young age), a chronic pain syndrome is evidence of the conflict between consciously wanting to continue shouldering responsibility and providing, on the one hand, and unconsciously wanting passively to be taken care of and to receive the emotional nurturing denied earlier in life, on the other. In these situations the chronic pain syndrome legitimizes the curtailment of activity by the patient, who can then become passive and less dependent *without losing face*. It is this face-saving dynamic, an internal mechanism to preserve self-esteem, that is termed *primary gain*. The primary gain usually far outweighs the *secondary gain* in terms of its overall importance and should be recognized as the *raison d'etre* for the functional pain.

Pain, depression, and anxiety are frequently observed in association with one another. At times chronic pain may be an early manifestation of a depressive disorder. It is common for the patient to conclude that the chronic pain caused the depression. In most cases of functional pain it is the other way around: the pain is an early manifestation of an unrecognized or so-called masked depression that is smoldering beneath the surface.

How is the orthopaedist to recognize the patient with chronic shoulder pain in whom functional factors are of primary importance? Typically such pain has been precipitated by and reflects not physical but emotional injury. A careful history usually reveals a circumstance or event, such as separation from close ones (spouse, children, parents, siblings), material or financial loss (including job loss), or increased responsibility, in temporal proximity to the onset of functional pain. In athletes, precipitants may be particularly important athletic contests or events.

Somatization is the expression in physical terms of emotional pain. Somatists use denial and repression, and they usually externalize blame. They usually do not volunteer the precipitating psychosocial stressors that brought on their physical symptoms because they do not understand the connection. Indeed, they often resist inquiry into the important psychosocial arena with anger and the question, "What's that got to do with my shoulder pain?" It is therefore particularly important to remain mindful that individuals who, in their developmental years, have been emotionally shortchanged (by parental fighting or divorce, emotional or physical parental absence, parental alcoholism, family poverty, and the need, at an early age, to shoulder major breadwinner responsibilities, or who have been physically or sexually abused) are particularly vulnerable to somatization. It is to the benefit of the orthopaedist to spend a few minutes during the history to inquire appropriately.

The MADISON mnemonic outlines the behavioral indicators that suggest psychogenic pain.[62,63]

Multiple complaints. The patient manifests a variety of symptoms, often unrelated to the pain that brought him or her into the office. For example, a patient with shoulder pain also discusses pain in the knees, stomach pain, headaches, etc. Particularly significant is that the reports of pain are related to multiple systems in the body and are clearly unrelated to one another.

Authenticity. In this case the patient uses overkill to convince the physician of the authenticity of the pain. There may be some preamble related to other physicians who have not believed the patient. This is especially significant in those instances in which the patient attempts to "head the doctor off at the pass" to prevent the physician from forming his or her own opinion. The patient is engaged in an argument long before the doctor has arrived at that juncture.

Denial. This refers to inappropriate affect about the pain, as well as the denial of affect about other aspects of the patient's life. Doctors are attuned to the patient who complains too much, but they should also be concerned about those who deny negative effect from their injuries. The stoic or compliant patient may be easier to deal with in the office, but there is also the possibility that he or she is using the pain in some way to get a greater reward, hence the absence of negative affect about the sequelae of the injury.

Along these lines, be careful about the patient who denies any negative effect from the impact of the pain on the rest of his or her life. An essential question in an examination is, "How do you feel about your injury?"

Behavioral indicators that suggest psychogenic pain

- M—Multiple complaints
- A —Authenticity
- D —Denial
- I —Interpersonal variability
- S —Singularity
- O —Only you
- N —Nothing works

Interpersonal variability. The patient who has psychogenic pain varies his or her report of pain according to the person with whom he or is interacting, hence the office staff hears about one level of discomfort and the doctor another. It may vary in either direction, that is, the doctor getting more or less than his or her staff. Some variability is normal and appropriate. Excessive variability is indicative that there are more variables other than the organic ones that need to be considered.

Singularity. The patients report their symptoms in a manner that indicates only they have this kind or degree of pain. Any attempts to put them into a category—"people who have your kind of injury"—are met with resistance. Their request for special consideration should be heard as a warning signal.

Only you. The doctor is placed on a special level that indicates that the patient sees him or her as the only one who can help. This is particularly seductive, as it plays to the doctor's ego needs. It should serve as a warning to remember that, with many of these patients, several doctors have preceded you who have also been special, until they failed, in the patients' eyes, that is. This approach is often used as a way of engaging the doctor to behave in some way out of the ordinary, that is, extra medication, more frequent visits, or disability certification.

Nothing works. The emphasis here is on the "nothing" part of the statement. Medication, which should have some effect—however minimal—is said to be *totally* ineffective. The same is true for physical therapy and all of the other varieties of treatments. In other words the absoluteness and the uniformity of the intransigence are the issues here. Reinforcing this is an often benign indifference that the patient has toward the doctor's failure to resolve the problem. It suggests that there is some other problem that may need to be resolved before the patient is willing to allow any treatments to have an impact.

Although it is not the task of the orthopaedist to establish precise psychiatric diagnosis, it is important that functional problems not be overlooked because of failure to consider the appropriate history. It is the task of the psychiatrist and the clinical psychologist, working collaboratively, to establish the precise diagnosis. Although obtaining a Minnesota Multiphasic Personality Inventory (MMPI) with a computerized interpretation may identify *some* problems as functional, the diagnostic precision from such an approach is not great. An analogy is for the orthopaedist to rely solely on radiographic and other imaging findings out of context in diagnosing a shoulder problem. The results of the MMPI and of other diagnostic measures are best interpreted against the backdrop of a thorough history and physical and mental status examinations.

Persuading a patient to undergo psychologic evaluation can be problematic. It is almost axiomatic that the more the patient resists and the more angry he or she becomes, the more likely it is that a relevant psychiatric diagnosis is discovered. There are ways to convince the recalcitrant individual to be evaluated:

1. Some orthopaedists make such evaluation a part of their work-up in every case of chronic shoulder pain. Increasingly, physicians are including psychiatric screening of candidates for organ transplantation and for other major surgery. Such screening proves cost effective in that it can identify patients who, with special preoperative or postoperative help, will have smoother courses than they might otherwise.

2. Sometimes a patient volunteers that stress makes the pain worse. Such information can provide good reason for psychologic evaluation to understand how the individual copes with stress and to consider techniques to manage stress optimally.

3. When chronic pain is the manifested problem, it can be helpful to explain to the patient that everyone has an emotional reaction to pain and that if pain is longstanding, the emotional reaction can result in excess pain after surgery or in other postoperative morbidity. Patients should see the evaluating psychiatrist as a physician with particular understanding of chronic pain, rather than as a doctor who treats crazy persons.

However it is done, the referral should be made in a manner that reflects an acknowledgement of the validity of the patient's pain. Pain is pain and, whether of organic or functional origin or both, it hurts, and it is unpleasant. Only when the psychologic dimensions of chronic shoulder pain are understood can a rational treatment plan (with a reasonable chance of success) be devised.

PHYSICAL EXAMINATION

The shoulder evaluation begins with the patient seated. The female's gown is placed above her breasts, below the axilla, and is tied in the back. Bra straps are lowered. The male is undressed above the waist. This allows observation of the front and back, symmetry of motion, muscle atrophy, and bony prominences. By standing behind the seated patient, the examiner begins with the cervical spine. Flexion and gentle rotation are evaluated first. In the absence of rheumatoid arthritis or other significant cervical spine disease, this serves as a beginning psychologic screening test. Exaggerated reports of pain or paresthesias in nonanatomic distributions alert the examiner to possible overly anxious or hysterical responses. This provides an early basis for interpretation of subjective symptoms.

Foramenal closure maneuvers, with hyperextension and lateral bending of the neck, are used to screen for cervical radiculopathy. Mild pain in the cervical spine or radiating to the levator scapula insertion is not uncommon, whereas pain radiating to the shoulder and more distal in the upper extremity suggests that additional neurologic work-up be considered.

Sternoclavicular Joint

This joint is evaluated for sprains, anterior and posterior subluxations and dislocations, arthritis, fractures,

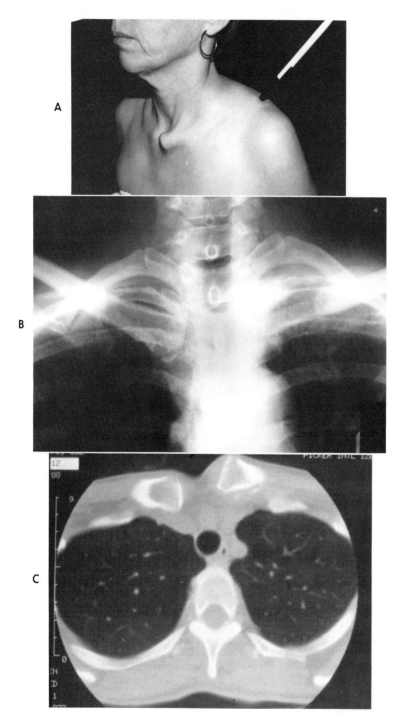

FIG. 3-23. Bipolar clavicle dislocation with anterior sternoclavicular joint dislocation and Type IV posterior acromioclavicular joint dislocation. **A,** The prominent left sternoclavicular joint is the more clinically obvious, but the posteriorly displaced distal clavicle is the more symptomatic secondary to supraspinatus impingement. **B,** Anteroposterior radiographs of the sternoclavicular joints demonstrate more high-riding left clavicle. This combined with a 15-degree cephalad tilt exaggerates the difference. **C,** Computed tomography scan documents the anterior dislocation of the left as compared with the right sternoclavicular joint.

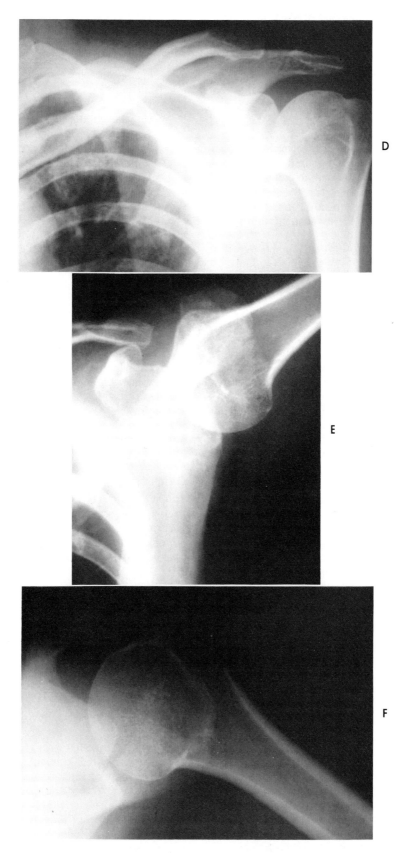

FIG. 3-23 cont'd. D, The anteroposterior radiograph of the Type IV acromioclavicular posterior dislocation shows widening at the acromioclavicular joint. **E,** Stryker notch view. **F,** Axillary view. Both of these views demonstrate the posterior displacement of the distal clavicle relative to the acromion.

and in the child, physeal injuries that may simulate a dislocation.

Observation

The patient is observed both from the front and behind for prominences, depressions, and abnormal asymmetric motion when the arms are elevated.

Palpation

The medial ends of the clavicle can be evaluated with the physician standing behind the patient. A finger can be placed in the superior sternal notch to palpate the medial clavicle above the articulation with the sternum. Direct pressure over the sternal costal articulation elicits pain if there is arthritis or a recent capsular sprain with associated swelling.

Posterior dislocations of the sternoclavicular joint are rare. Clinically they can be palpated as a depression between the sternal end of the clavicle and the manubrium. In the acute setting, pulses are palpated for a great vessel injury. The airway is assessed to ensure there is no difficulty in breathing.

Anterior subluxation or dislocation is the more common direction of instability (Fig. 3-23). The sternal end of the clavicle can be grasped between the examiner's fingers and moved cephalad or caudad. With abduction and extension of the shoulders it retracts more laterally. The subluxation may be reduced but is usually unstable. Hypertrophy and degenerative arthritis are not uncommon in postmenopausal women on the dominant arm.[26,30,145]

Provocative Tests

If the patient has reported clicking or instability, motion of the arm is encouraged to reproduce the symptoms. Grasping the sternal end of the clavicle to compress it or attempting subluxation is another means of testing the stability of the joint. Adduction of the arm across the chest can compress the involved joint. This might increase pain if there is traumatic or degenerative arthritis.

Acromioclavicular Joint

The acromioclavicular joint is a diarthrodial joint between the lateral end of the clavicle and the medial aspect of the acromion. Coracoacromial ligaments control anterior and posterior translation of the outer clavicle, whereas coracoclavicular ligaments, consisting of the trapezoid and conoid ligaments, hold the shoulder girdle up to the outer end of the clavicle. This joint is evaluated for arthritis and ligamentous disruption with instability. Allman[3] originally described three classes of acromioclavicular joint injuries. Rockwood[145] has expanded the classification to six types.

- Type I: Sprain of acromioclavicular ligaments without displacement of the joint
- Type II: Disruption of acromioclavicular ligaments, sprain of coracoclavicular ligaments, and slight upward displacement of the clavicle compared with the shoulder

- Type III: Disruption of acromioclavicular and coracoacromial ligaments with relative upward displacement of the outer clavicle and an increase of the coracoclavicular space by 25% to 100%; deltoid and trapezius muscles have been detached from the outer clavicle (Fig. 3-24)
- Type IV: Acromioclavicular ligaments disrupted, coracoclavicular ligaments partially or completely disrupted, posterior dislocation of the clavicle into the trapezius with detachment of the deltoid and trapezius from the distal clavicle (Fig. 3-23)
- Type V: Severe version of Type III with coracoclavicular interspace increased 100% to 300% compared to normal; clavicle is displaced toward the base of the neck; the deltoid and trapezius have been detached from the outer half of the clavicle
- Type VI: Acromioclavicular ligaments are disrupted, coracoclavicular ligaments may be intact or disrupted, and the clavicle is dislocated inferiorly or under the acromion or coracoid process

With this classification in mind, the acromioclavicular joint is evaluated.

Observation

The outer clavicle is viewed to determine whether it is prominent, relative to the acromion, or displaced in one of the directions consistent with an acromioclavicular joint injury. Although it is often described as upward displacement of the outer clavicle, the shoulder girdle displaces downward from the clavicle, which is normal position with coracoclavicular ligamentous disruptions.

The outer clavicle warrants careful evaluation in the presence of an obvious sternoclavicular joint dislocation. Bipolar dislocations of the clavicle are visibly noticeable at the sternal end, but clinically painful at the acromial end, with impingement on the supraspinatus when posteriorly displaced into the trapezius (Fig. 3-23).

Palpation

The acromioclavicular joint is located by palpating the base of a V formed between the spine of the scapula and the posterior clavicle as it articulates with the acromion. The anterior and posterior aspects of the acromion are then identified. The lateral acromion is palpated, and its position is confirmed by rotating the humerus when longitudinal traction is placed in the line of the humerus. Once the acromial margins can be identified, the acromioclavicular joint is palpated from posterior to anterior. Direct pressure over the acromioclavicular joint is painful in acute injuries with swelling and degenerative arthritis. Gentle ballottement confirms the joint location. Crepitus may be elicited with arthritis or instability.

The coracoid and the coracoclavicular ligaments are palpated for evidence of tenderness, indicative of a sprain, in the event that there is either no displacement of the joint seen with radiography or a tear when displacement is encountered. With Types III and V acromioclavicular joint injuries there is a prominent step-off at the outer end of the clavicle.

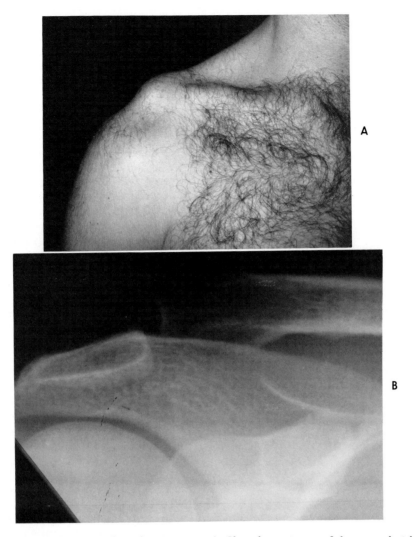

FIG. 3-24. Grade III acromioclavicular separation. **A,** Clinical prominence of the outer clavicle is demonstrated in inferior shoulder girdle subluxation. **B,** Radiographic appearance.

Provocative Tests

With pressure over the outer end of the clavicle, an upward force placed along the lines of the dependent humerus reduces suspected acromioclavicular joint subluxation or dislocation. Forward flexion of the arm with adduction across the chest accentuates a Type V acromioclavicular joint injury, tenting the skin over the outer clavicle as it comes close to tickling the ear.

Adduction of the arm across the chest also serves as a provocative compression of the intact acromioclavicular joint. This is painful with acromioclavicular arthritis or osteolysis of the outer clavicle and needs to be differentiated from posterior capsular tightness and other more severe forms of shoulder stiffness.

In a Type IV posteriorly displaced distal clavicle, the signs and tests for an impingement syndrome are positive. The outer clavicle may be more difficult to palpate because it is buried in the trapezius and supraspinatus.

Glenohumeral Joint
Observation

The muscles about the glenohumeral joint are observed for atrophy or bulges. The supraspinatus and infraspinatus are best viewed from behind and from the side. With a C5-C6 disk or with a longstanding rotator cuff tear, infraspinatus atrophy can be appreciated. Ruptures of the long head of the biceps can be viewed as a more distal enlargement of the lateral half of the biceps in the arm and later accentuated with external rotation—resistance testing or biceps muscle strength testing.

Normally the long axis of the humerus passes up through the anterior acromion. The acromion superiorly covers the posterior half of the humeral head rather than extending over it entirely. When the coracoid is prominent and there is a depression anteriorly, a posterior or locked posterior fracture dislocation must be suspected. Alternatively, psychiatrically disturbed individuals may intentionally or unintentionally hold their arm in a posi-

tion of posterior subluxation with the elbow positioned slightly forward through a strong contracture of the pectoralis and anterior deltoid (Fig. 3-9).

Inferior subluxation of the humerus with atrophy of the deltoid may be noted after a birth injury or other brachial plexus injury, a cerebral vascular accident, or a dislocation of or iatrogenic injury to the axillary nerve. A sulcus is present between the acromion and humeral head. An acute anterior dislocation of the shoulder in an athlete or a chronic fixed anterior dislocation (more commonly seen in an alcoholic) presents with a humeral head prominence anteriorly, usually in the subcoracoid region, with a depression at the upper portion of the posterior deltoid under the acromion.

Last, an anterosuperior position of the humeral head tenting the skin is noted after a massive rotator cuff tear or a cuff dehiscence after a surgical repair. Attempted forward flexion increases the proximal migration of the humeral head (Fig. 3-8).

Palpation

The bony prominences, including the coracoid, the acromioclavicular joint, and the acromion, are palpated to determine whether the humeral head is located in the glenoid cavity. The cuff insertion may be tender with calcific tendinitis or rotator cuff tears. Rotating the humerus with the finger in one position can often bring the area of the calcific deposit underneath the examining finger. The long head of the biceps tendon can be palpated in the intertubercular groove directly anteriorly when the arm is in 10 degrees of internal rotation. Firm pressure over the biceps tendon almost uniformly causes discomfort; therefore this has not been a helpful sign for evaluating tendinitis. The contour of the biceps is palpated for symmetry within each individual arm and in comparing the two arms. Ruptures of the long head of the biceps are far more common than ruptures of the medial head of the biceps. Dimpling in the upper part of the long head of the biceps and an increased girth in the lower half of the muscle on the lateral side are indicative of a proximal rupture at the musculotendinous junction in the young and through the tendon in middle-aged and older athletes (Fig. 3-18).[21]

Palpation of the supraspinatus and infraspinatus is done with the arms at the side. A hollow depression can often be appreciated in the body of the muscle if it has ruptured or if a nerve injury has occurred (Fig. 3-25). It is later palpated at the time of muscle strength testing to determine whether there are active contractions.

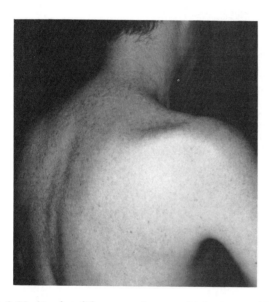

FIG. 3-25. Atrophy of the supraspinatus and infraspinatus following a difficult arthroscopic access to the glenohumeral joint and injury to the suprascapular nerve.

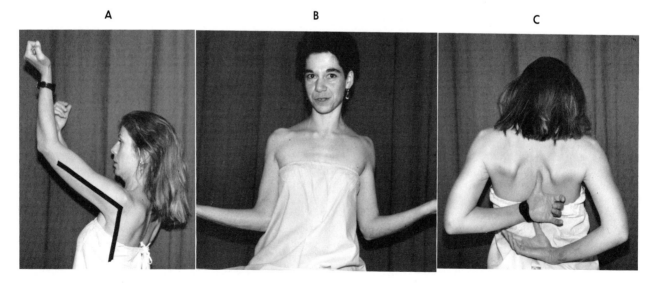

FIG. 3-26. Active range of motion. **A,** Active elevation measured in forward flexion compares the axis of the arm with that of the thorax. **B,** External rotation is measured with both arms at the side and in 90 degrees abduction. **C,** Internal rotation is measured as the patient actively brings the thumb up the midline of the spine. The nondominant arm can normally reach two vertebral levels higher. T7 to T8 correlates with the inferior pole of the scapula.

Range of Motion Testing

Active range of motion is measured with the patient sitting (Fig. 3-26). This is to avoid confusion that might otherwise occur with abnormal position through the knees or trunk. As proposed by the American Shoulder and Elbow Surgeons, total elevation is measured as the angle between the elevated arm and the thoracic rib cage (see the form on pp. 68 and 69). External rotation is measured with the elbows flexed to 90 degrees and the arms at the side, then again with the arms in 90 degrees of abduction. Active internal rotation is measured behind the back to the highest vertebral level that the patient can bring the thumb up the lumbar or thoracic spine.

Passive supine range of motion includes forward elevation with the arm close to the head, external rotation with the arms at the side, and again in 90 degrees of abduction (Fig. 3-27). With the examiner's hand placed on the scapula to prevent it from rolling forward, internal

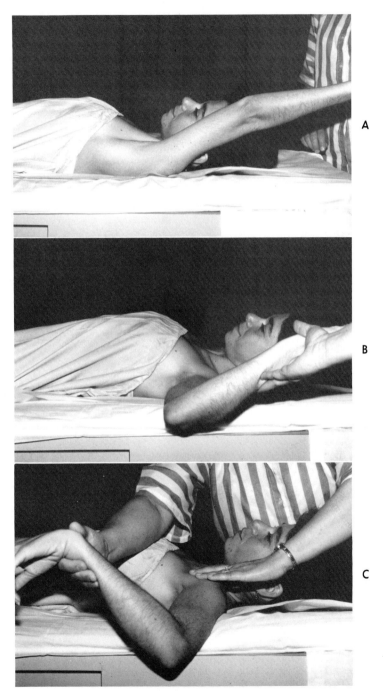

FIG. 3-27. Passive range of motion. **A,** Supine elevation. **B,** Supine external rotation in 90 degrees abduction. **C,** Internal rotation in 90 degrees abduction with a hand to stabilize the scapula from riding upward permits reproducible results. The arms are also measured for passive external rotation at the side.

AMERICAN SHOULDER AND ELBOW SURGEONS
EXAMINATION DATA FORM

Evaluation date:

Name: Chart #   Dominance:

List findings as Involved/Univnolved: (R/L)   (L/R)   Bilateral?

Diagnosis:

Previous surgery:

Number of steroid injections:

  I. Pain: / *(5 = none, 4 = slight, 3 = after unusual activity, 2 = moderate, 1 = marked, 0 = complete disability)*

 II. Shoulder Motion:
    A. Patient sitting:
      1. Active total elevation of arm: /   degrees
      2. Active external rotation with arm at side: /   degrees
      3. Active rotation - 90 degrees abduction: /   degrees
      4. Passive internal rotation (segment reached)   /   *

1 = Less than trochanter	*5 = L5*	*9 = L1*	*13 = T9*	*17 = T5*
2 = Trochanter	*6 = L4*	*10 = T12*	*14 = T8*	*18 = T4*
3 = Gluteal	*7 = L3*	*11 = T11*	*15 = T7*	*19 = T3*
4 = Sacrum	*8 = L2*	*12 = T10*	*16 = T6*	*20 = T2*

    B. Patient Supine:
      1. Passive total elevation of arm: /   degrees*
      2. Passive external rotation with arm at side: /   degrees
      3. Passive external rotation - 90 degrees abduction: /   degrees
      4. Passive internal rotation - 90 degrees abduction: /   degrees

      Total elevation of arm measured by viewing patient from side and using goniometer to determine angle between arm and thorax.

    C. Impingement:
      1. Painful arc of motion: /
      2. Relieved by subacromial xylocaine injection: /
      3. Crepitus: /

III. Strength: *(5 = normal, 4 = good, 3 = fair, 2 = poor, 1 = trace, 0 = paralysis)*
    A. Anterior deltoid: /   E. Trapezius: /
    B. Middle deltoid: /   F. Triceps: /
    C. External rotation: /   G. Biceps: /
    D. Internal rotation: /

 IV. Stability: *(5 = normal, 4 = apprehension, 3 = rare subluxation, 2 = recurrent subluxation, 1 = recurrent dislocation, 0 = fixed dislocation)*
    A. Anterior: /   C. Inferior: /
    B. Posterior: /   D. Superior: /

  V. Function: *(4 = normal, 3 = mild compromise, 2 = difficulty, 1 = with aid, 0 = unable)*

F1.	/	Use back pocket	F9.	/	Sleep on shoulder
F2.	/	Rectal hygiene	F10.	/	Pulling
F3.	/	Wash opposite underarm	F11.	/	Use hand overhead
F4.	/	Eat with utensil	F12.	/	Throwing
F5.	/	Comb hair	F13.	/	Lifting
F6.	/	Use hand/arm @ shoulder	F14.	/	Do usual work
F7.	/	Carry 10-15 lbs./arm @ side	F15.	/	Do usual sport
F8.	/	Dress			

 VI. Patient Response: / *(3 = much better, 2 = better, 1 = same, 0 = worse)*

VII.   Roentgen Assessment:
        (Circle findings, denote side)
        Plain roentgenogram_____ Fluoroscopy_____ MRI_____
        Tomography_____ CT Scan_____ Stress roentgenogram_____

A.   No abnormalities_____
B.   Arthritis: 4 = none   Glenohumeral_____
                  3 = mild   Acromioclavicular_____
                  2 = moderate   Sternoclavicular_____
                  1 = severe
     1._____ Avascular necrosis   6._____ Osteoarthritis
     2._____ Cuff tear arthropathy   7._____ Post-traumatic
     3._____ Cysplasia   8._____ Recurrent dislocations
     4._____ Metabolic   9._____ Rheumatoid
     5._____ Neuropathic   10._____ Septic

C.   Impingement:
     1. Anterior acromial spur_____ Sclerosis_____
     2. Bone reaction greater tuberosity_____
     3. Inferior spurs A-C joint_____
     4. Superior displacement humeral head: calcar/inferior glenoid
     5. Humeral head/acromion level_____ mm _____ mm
     6. Arthrogram: cuff tear: yes_____ no_____
         a. Complete thickness_____
         b. Incomplete thickness_____
     7. Sonogram: cuff tear: yes_____ no_____
         a. Complete thickness_____
         b. Incomplete thickness_____
     8. Unfused acromial epiphysis:
         pre_____ meta_____ meso_____ basi_____

D.   Instability: Anterior/Inferior/Posterior
     1. Glenohumeral dislocation
     2. Glenohumeral subluxation
     3. Inferior subluxation with weights
     4. Hill-Sachs defect
     5. Glenoid rim:
         fracture_____ bone reaction_____ anterior/posterior_____
     6. Glenoid wear: anterior_____ posterior_____
     7. Loose body

E.   Trauma/Fractures:
Proximal humerus	Scapula	Clavicle
1. Two part	1. Glenoid	1. Proximal 1/3
2. Three part	2. Other	2. Middle 1/3
3. Four part		3. Distal 1/3
4. Articular split	A-C Joint	S-C Joint
5. Humeral shaft	1. Separation	1. Separation
	Grade I II III	2. Intraarticular fracture

F.   Follow-up HHR or TSR
     1. Humeral prosthesis: (1 = no abnormalities, 2 = lucent line,
             3 = drift, 4 = loosening, 5 = fracture, 6 = ectopic cement)
     2. Glenoid prosthesis: (1 = no abnormalities, 2 = lucent line [see
             below], 3 = wear, 4 = loosening, 5 = fracture, 6 = ectopic
             cement)
             Lucent lines: complete, incomplete, loosening, progressive
     3. Position of implants: (1 = normal, 2 = subluxation, 3 = dislocation)
             (A = anterior, P = posterior, S = superior, I = inferior)
     4. Ectopic bone: (1 = none, 2 - mild, 3 = moderate, 4 = severe)

rotation in 90 degrees of abduction is measured. Testing for rotation in 90 degrees of abduction has been the most reliable method of testing glenohumeral motion as opposed to scapulothoracic motion. Thus adhesive capsulitis or a locked posterior fracture-dislocation has minimal if any motion once the scapulothoracic motion has been eliminated by bringing the arm to 90 degrees of abduction. The difference between the active and passive motion is noted. For example, a patient with a rotator cuff tear or nerve injury frequently has full passive motion but may lack active external rotation or elevation.

Muscle Strength Testing

Shoulder muscle strengths are graded on the orthopaedic grading scale: 5 is normal, 4 is good, 3 is fair, 2 is poor, 1 is trace, and 0 is paralysis. All three divisions of the deltoid, the internal rotators, the external rotators, the biceps, the triceps, the serratus anterior, and the trapezius are routinely tested.

Deltoid

The three divisions of the deltoid are tested by placing the arm in slight flexion, slight lateral abduction, and slight posterior extension, respectively (Fig. 3-28). The patient is then asked to resist the examiner's force, which

pushes the lower arm back to a neutral dependent position. Pushing at the distal humerus is preferable to pushing on the hand or wrist. This avoids the effect of active flexion or extension at the elbow that occurs when the examiner pushes on the hand or wrist.

At times there is concern that the deltoid might have ruptured from its origin, either from traumatic injury or from dehiscing after a surgical procedure in which it was detached and then repaired. To test the anterior deltoid, the arm is passively placed in 30 degrees' forward flexion, the patient's arm is supported, and he or she is asked to relax. The deltoid muscle is palpated at its acromial and clavicular origins. The patient is then asked to maintain the arm in this position. If the deltoid muscle fibers—and not an upward subluxation of the humeral head—push the fingers outward, then the integrity of the muscle and its attachments can be ensured. Another cause of weakness might be a large tear of the rotator cuff. Other divisions of the deltoid can be tested in a similar manner.

Internal Rotators

The internal rotators are tested by placing the hands in internal rotation across the abdomen (Figs. 3-29 and 3-33). The patient is asked to resist an external rotation

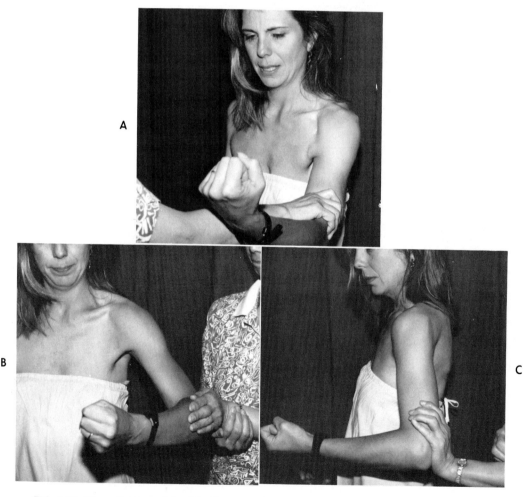

FIG. 3-28. Three divisions of the deltoid are tested for strength and appearance. **A,** Anterior. **B,** Lateral. **C,** Posterior.

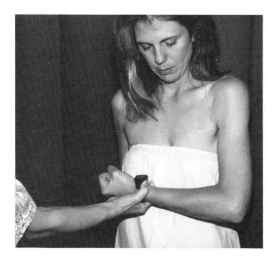

FIG. 3-29. Internal rotation strength is tested with the arm at the abdomen as the athlete resists an external rotation force.

A

B

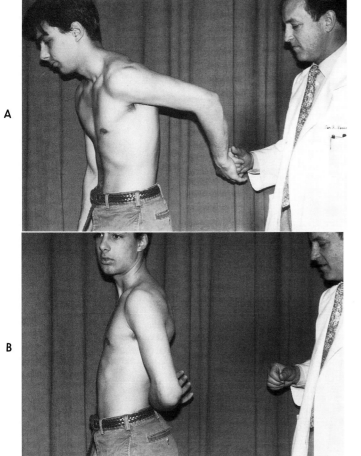

FIG. 3-30. A, Passive range of motion for internal rotation behind the back at waist level is tested. B, If the patient is unable to maintain this passive motion and the hand falls to the waist, it is likely that the subscapularis has ruptured.

force. Care is taken to ensure that the patient does not use the triceps and biceps and thereby convert a test of internal rotation muscle strength to one of the elbow flexion-extension groups. The pectoralis and latissismus dorsi muscles are tested by placing the arm in 30 degrees of abduction and asking the patient to adduct the arm against the chest wall while attempting to internally rotate it. The pectoralis is palpated over the anterior chest wall and in the anterior axillary fold for muscle contractures and possible ruptures. The latissismus dorsi is palpated over the posterior chest wall and in the posterior axillary fold for its muscle strength and integrity. The test for subscapular rupture is demonstrated in Fig. 3-30).

External Rotators

The external rotators consist of the infraspinatus and teres minor. They are tested with the arms at the side while the arms are in slight external rotation. The elbows are flexed to 90 degrees. An attempt is made by the examiner to push both hands together as the patient resists (Fig. 3-31).

If the patient cannot hold the arm in slight external rotation, then significant weakness from detachment or nerve injury is anticipated. These individuals try to comply with the test by placing the forearm on the stomach, extending the arm with the posterior deltoid, and bringing the hand to the side but not away from the body.

Supraspinatus

The supraspinatus is isolated by pushing downward on the wrists of the arms after they have been placed in 90 degrees' abduction, 30 degrees of forward flexion, and internal rotation, with the thumbs pointing downward (Fig. 3-17).

Serratus Anterior

The serratus anterior is tested by pressing forward on the thoracic spine when the individual rests both arms in front leaning on a wall with the elbows in full exten-

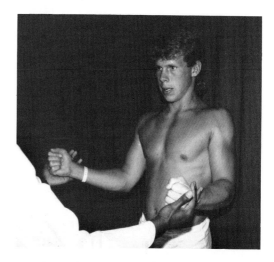

FIG. 3-31. External rotation strength testing with the arms at the side.

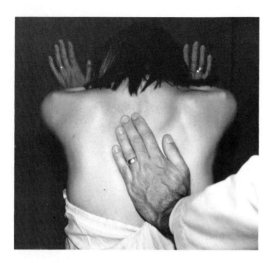

FIG. 3-32. Testing the serratus anterior to determine if winging of the scapula occurs.

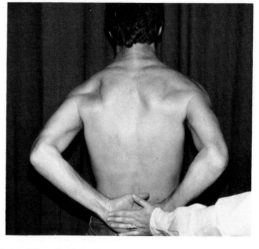

FIG. 3-33. Rhomboids and teres minor can be visualized when the athlete extends the arms behind the back against a resistance.

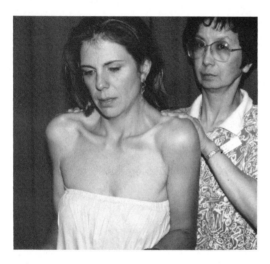

FIG. 3-34. Trapezius is tested as the individual attempts to shrug both shoulders upward.

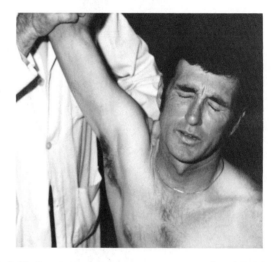

FIG. 3-35. Positive impingement sign is pain on forceful abduction of the internally rotated arm against the acromion.

sion. The muscle is intact if no significant winging occurs (Fig. 3-32).

Rhomboids and Teres Minor

Visualization and palpation of the rhomboids and the teres minor can be achieved by having the patient place both hands behind the back at the level of the buttocks and push posteriorly to extend the arms against resistance (Fig. 3-33).

Subscapularis

In Gerber and Krushell's test[58] the subscapularis is specifically tested with the arm behind the back at mid-waist level. Passive motion is determined by pulling the hand backward with the elbow bent, thereby pulling the shoulder into extension. If the patient can actively hold this position without assistance, it is likely that the subscapularis is intact. If, on release of the hand and wrist,

the patient's wrist falls back to the waist and cannot be elevated off of the waist, it is likely that the subscapularis has ruptured. Some degree of its strength or competence can be tested by asking the patient to push against the examiner's hand to maintain passive motion. In cases of partial denervation or partial rupture of the subscapularis, this active motion is weak but not absent.

Trapezius

The trapezius is tested by asking the patient to shrug both shoulders toward the ears (Fig. 3-34).

Special Tests
Impingement

The following methods are used to evaluate impingement. Subacromial crepitus can be palpated while the arm is actively or passively rotated when in 90 degrees of abduction. Painful arc of abduction, between 120 and

70 degrees, may occur as the patient gradually lowers the arm from full elevation to the side. This may be further exacerbated if the patient slightly resists a downward pressure while going through this same motion. A catch or sudden giving way of the arm at midrange reproduces Codman's drop arm test. A positive *impingement sign* occurs when the patient experiences pain on forceful abduction of the internally rotated arm against the acromion (Fig. 3-35).

The *impingement injection test* is relief of more than half of this painful arc of abduction pain after placing 10 ml of lidocaine (Xylocaine) in the subacromial space. In instances in which impingement pain may preclude a full muscle strength testing or when there is a partial thickness rotator cuff tear, the subacromial Xylocaine injection test relieves enough pain so that the patient has normal strength on the isolated supraspinatus test. For those with complete thickness rotator cuff tears, weakness is still present. The impingement sign is not a valid test in the face of a partially frozen shoulder. Even the subacromial injection of Xylocaine does not relieve the stiffness pain.

Biceps

Pathologic processes implicating the long head of the biceps include tendinitis, rupture, and instability. The pain from tendinitis or a partial thickness tearing may be exacerbated with a test of the biceps tendon gliding in its groove against resistance. This is tested by asking the patient to flex the shoulder with the elbow extended and the forearm supinated against the examiner's resistance. Production of pain in the intertubercular groove is considered a positive test.

Subluxation of the long head of the biceps may occur with large rotator cuff tears in which the transverse humeral ligament has been worn through in the impingement process, or in individuals with fractures involving the greater tuberosity that extends into the biceps groove. Recurrent subluxation of the long head of the biceps in young athletic patients has been an erroneous diagnosis in an athlete who actually has glenohumeral instability.

Instability

The patient is first asked to voluntarily reproduce subluxation of the shoulders to demonstrate their laxity (Fig. 3-9). Then provocative maneuvers to reproduce glenohumeral subluxations or dislocations can be done with the patient sitting, supine, or standing.[59,122,171] With the patient sitting, the examiner can stabilize the scapula by placing one finger on the coracoid and resting the body of the hand and forearm on the scapula. With the other hand, the index and middle fingers grasp the anterior humeral head and the thumb grasps the posterior head. Then a variation on the load shift test for knee instability is performed. A force is directed anteriorly and inferiorly (Fig. 3-36). Subluxation of the head over the anteroinferior glenoid rim is estimated as to degree. Pain may preclude this testing.

With the patient seated, abduction and external rotation of the involved arm and a force directed in an an-

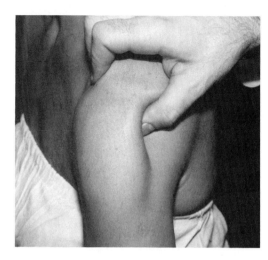

FIG. 3-36. Anteroinferior subluxation creates a void under the posterior acromion and a slight bulge below the coracoid.

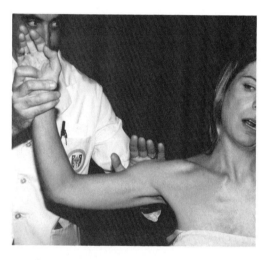

FIG. 3-37. Positive apprehension test. Attempts at anteroinferior subluxation of the abducted and externally rotated arm are exacerbated by forceful pressure on the proximal posterior humerus directed anteriorly.

teroinferior direction from behind may cause a palpable subluxation, labral crepitation, or frank dislocation (Fig. 3-37). The patient is most apprehensive and resists this maneuver when the arm is abducted to approximately 120 degrees and externally rotated. The patient's subjective apprehension that the shoulder may slip out of joint is considered a positive apprehension finding, whether or not there is actual joint subluxation. The differential diagnoses in this position are impingement and a partial frozen shoulder.

Variations of this test may be done while the patient is sitting or supine, with longitudinal traction on the arm in the axis of the slightly abducted humerus, and with a force in an anteroinferior direction from behind on the proximal humerus.[59,121,122,128]

Posterior instability testing involves static translation of the humeral head posteriorly, with the thumbs placed

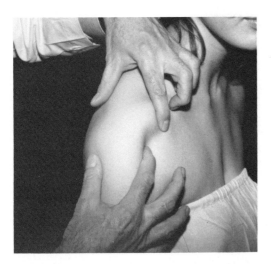

FIG. 3-38. Posterior subluxation with the scapula stabilized is considered abnormal when more than 50% of the humeral head can be translated in a posterior direction.

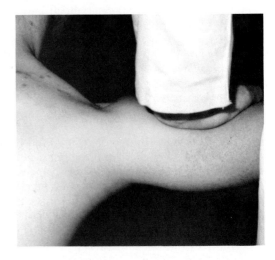

FIG. 3-40. Inferior subluxation tested in a variation of the Feagin maneuver is associated with a palpable bounce and pain.

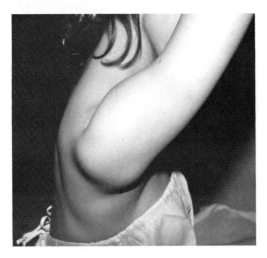

FIG. 3-39. Posterior subluxation of the humeral head is increased with a longitudinal force on the internally rotated and adducted humerus.

on the scapular spines bilaterally. Pressure over both humeral heads, from anterior in a posterior direction, may cause posterior translation (Fig. 3-38). Translation up to 50% of the humeral head diameter is considered normal.[121]

The patient may demonstrate posterior subluxation by muscular control, or either the examiner or patient may demonstrate posterior instability by positioning the arm in forward flexion, internal rotation, and directing a posterior force along the axis of the humerus (Fig. 3-39). For an individual with lax recurrent posterior subluxations, mere elevation of the arm in slight forward flexion without internal rotation may cause a subluxation. The humerus slips out posteriorly, unnoticed except as a slightly posterior bulge. The diagnosis is confirmed with extension of the arm posteriorly to the coronal plane of the scapula, which is accompanied by a quick snap

(Fig. 3-10). Reduction is more easily palpated than the subluxation. Apprehension may be present but is much less reliable than in anterior instability.

Inferior instability is tested with a downward traction of both arms at the side. A sulcus develops between the top of the humeral head and the undersurface of the acromion in lax individuals (Fig. 3-11). If this test is painful, by the time radiographs are obtained in this provocative position, some patients resist the downward pull and do not reproduce the previous clinical findings.

In the Feagin maneuver variation on the anteroinferior instability testing,[122] the examiner places the patient's arm at 90 degrees of elevation. The patient's elbow is resting on either the examiner's shoulder or on the examiner's belt. Then, with both hands over the top of the proximal humerus, the arm is pulled downward with a quick motion. Reproduction of the subluxation or palpable bounce is considered a positive finding (Fig. 3-40).

Reproduction of the pain, or fear that the shoulder is going to dislocate, is a variation of anterior apprehension. For multidirectional instability the shoulder subluxation can occur anteriorly, posteriorly, and inferiorly. All directions are tested. An estimation is recorded as to the percentage of the humeral head diameter that can be slipped over the glenoid rim. Crepitation over the labrum is common. In the absence of labral tearing, the subluxation is less painful than in traumatic anteroinferior instability lesions. Posterior apprehension is less reliable than is anterior.

Scapulothoracic Joint
Observation

Both scapulae are observed to ensure that they appear symmetric on the chest wall, both when at rest (with the arms at the sides) and through full ranges of motion. Abnormal rhythm, with greater scapular than glenohumeral motion, occurs when there is shoulder stiffness.

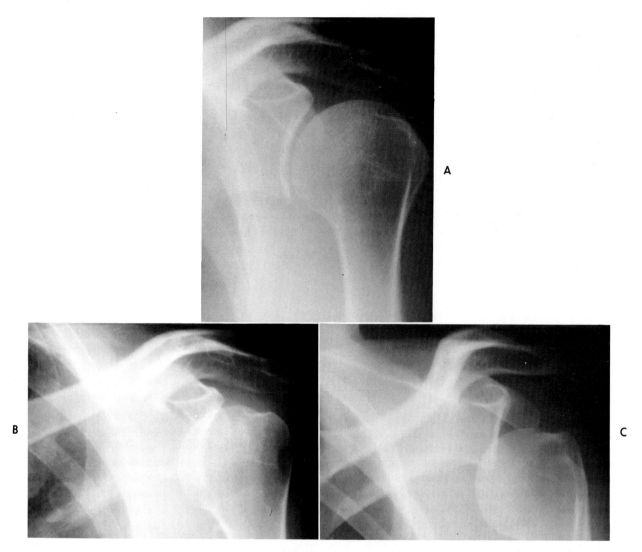

FIG. 3-41. True anteroposterior view in the plane of the scapula. **A,** Reduced glenohumeral joint with articular space visible between the head and the scapula. **B,** Posterior dislocation with overlap of the head from the glenoid in the same patient as in **A. C,** Anterior dislocation with the humeral head in a subcoracoid inferior position that slightly overlaps the glenoid.

Palpation

Muscles inserting into the scapula are palpated for tenderness or muscle spasm. Frequently the middle and posterior trapezius and the levator scapula are tight when the patient has protected the arm with adduction, internal rotation, and slight elevation of the shoulder. The common differential diagnosis is between primary cervical and painful shoulder lesions.

Range of Motion

Range of motion is evaluated in combination with the glenohumeral motion. The superior medial angle of the scapula is palpated for snapping or crepitus. The muscle strength and integrity of the rhomboids, trapezius, and serratus are evaluated. Any scar on the neck from an office node biopsy with trapezius weakness raises the suspicion of an iatrogenic spinal accessory nerve injury.

SPECIAL TESTS AND THEIR CLINICAL SIGNIFICANCE
Radiographs

Routine tests for shoulder injury begin with five screening views. The first three right-angle trauma views in the scapular plane include a true anteroposterior (AP) view of the glenohumeral joint (Fig. 3-41), a lateral scapular view (Fig. 3-42), and an axillary view.[122] The true AP view of the glenohumeral joint assesses the integrity of the cartilage, concentric reduction without the overlap of the humeral head to rule out an anterior or posterior dislocation or fracture dislocation. Loose bodies found in 10% of recurrent dislocations may be seen in the inferior capsular recess.

In the lateral scapular view the head covers the small

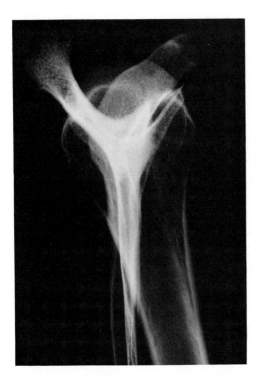

FIG. 3-42. In the normal lateral scapula view the humeral head is centered on the Y formed by the coracoid, spine of the scapula, and body of the scapula. Anterior displacement is more easily recognized than posterior displacement. Slight obliquity may exaggerate or diminish the prominence of the humeral head posteriorly in a locked posterior fracture-dislocation and thus allows the examiner to miss the diagnosis.

glenoid. It is at the center of the Y formed by the acromion, spine, and body of the scapula. Displacement of the humerus anteriorly, posteriorly, and inferiorly in respect to the scapula denotes instability or dislocation. Calcific deposits in the rotator cuff are localized as to which tendon is involved and then compared with other views. The three shapes of the acromial undersurface with a Type I flat, Type II curved, and a Type III hooked acromion require 10 to 35 degrees' caudal projection so that the medial portion of the scapula and supraspinatus fossa do not project over the acromial outline. An acromial spur or calcification extending into the coracoacromial ligament is seen in some with longstanding impingement.

The acromial morphology is further examined in the axillary view for failure of ossification of either the preacromial or mesoacromial epiphyses. The unfused acromial epiphysis has a high correlation with rotator cuff tears and long biceps ruptures after a patient is more than 30 years of age.[20,126] This is the most important view to diagnose a posterior fracture-dislocation, estimate the size of the humeral head defect, and evaluate eccentric glenoid wear (Fig. 3-43). The diagnosis, classification, and treatment recommendations for fractures of the proximal humerus are based on the above three trauma series views.

The two classic views to rule out calcific tendinitis are AP views, with the arm in internal and external rotation. Thirty-five to forty percent of underpenetrated views visualize the calcific deposits, whereas the calcium is burned out on the standard darker views.

In internal rotation the Hill-Sachs posterior lateral humeral head impression fracture after an anterior dislocation is seen as a straight line inside the most lateral portion of the head (Fig. 3-44).[71] The Stryker notch view, a supplemental view, images the defect when the patient places a hand on top of his or her head. An AP view is taken with a 10-degree cephalad tilt.

The external rotation view allows evaluation of cystic changes in the greater tuberosity, excrescences, localized osteopenia, sclerosis, and loss of the normal contour of the greater tuberosity with more advanced rotator cuff tears. The missing greater tuberosity in this view represents an avulsion. If the greater tuberosity fragment is not seen over the top of the head, it is usually hidden in the AP view behind the humeral head and glenoid but is visualized either on the lateral scapular view or axillary view (Fig. 3-45). These five views are usually sufficient for calcific tendinitis, chondrocalcinosis, degenerative arthritis, trauma, metabolic diseases, and inflammatory arthritis.[156]

Additional tests to evaluate shoulder instability include the weighted views, with 20 pounds of weight strapped to each forearm. Care is taken to have the patient not hold the weights, in an effort to avoid reduction of passive subluxation by active use of the deltoid. Bilateral inferior subluxation denotes generalized shoulder capsular laxity. Unilateral subluxation is significant on the involved side; it may represent guarding from pain, if present only on the asymptomatic side, in an otherwise lax individual.[122]

The West Point axillary view is obtained to evaluate injury of the anteroinferior glenoid rim.[146] Ectopic calcification, indicative of labral detachments, or a glenoid rim fracture in the anteroinferior quadrant is visualized on this view when often missed on the standard axillary view. This view is obtained with the patient in supine position, the arm abducted at 90 degrees on an arm board

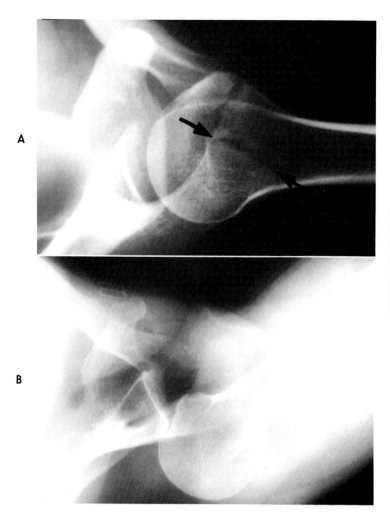

FIG. 3-43. Axillary lateral view is the third and most important view to correlate with the others to evaluate fractures of the humeral head, glenoid, unfused acromial epiphyses, cartilage wear, and coracoid stress fractures. **A,** Patient with an unfused mesoacromion has an associated rotator cuff tear. **B,** Posterior dislocation without a humeral head impression fracture in the axial plane corresponding with Fig. 3-43, *B*.

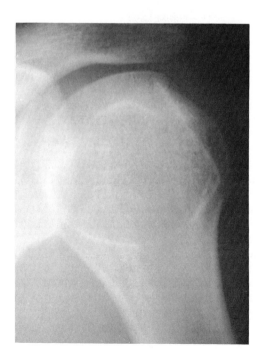

FIG. 3-44. Hill-Sachs posterolateral humeral head defect often is seen as a straight line on an internal rotation anteroposterior view.

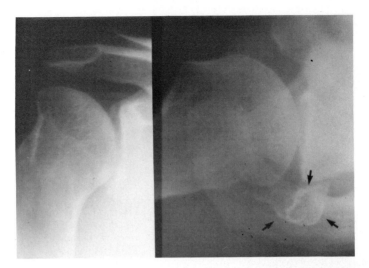

FIG. 3-45. External rotation and axillary view of a patient with a missed tuberosity avulsion. In the external rotation view, deficiency of the top portion of the humeral head is seen. In the axillary lateral view the retracted tuberosity is seen adjacent to the glenoid and no longer attached to the glenoid.

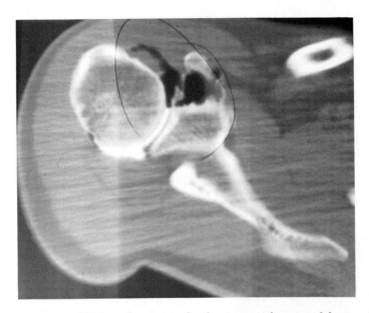

FIG. 3-46. Computed tomography arthrotomography showing partial erosion of the anterior glenoid with disruption of the anterior glenoid labrum. Positive contrast outlines the area of disruption where the anteroinferior labrum is no longer attached.

and internally rotated. The x-ray tube is placed at the hip, abducted 25 degrees, and directed downward 25 degrees from behind and above the shoulder, to pass through the coracoid.

An alternative way to visualize the anteroinferior glenoid rim is the Ciullo supine axillary view, obtained with the arm abducted and externally rotated when the tube is placed at the hip.[122]

Additional views to evaluate the degree of tearing in the rotator cuff include the Fukuda pushup views.[54] Both arms are pushed upward as the patient bears weight on the hand down at his or her side. If the

acromial-humeral interval is less than 4 mm, it is considered diagnostic of a rotator cuff tear. Cuff tears do not produce fixed superior migration early, but when the acromial humeral interval is 6 mm or less on standard non–weight-bearing views, a cuff tear is anticipated.[172]

The acromioclavicular joints are best visualized when they do not overlie the spine of the scapula. A 15-degree cephalad tilt view that is shot at approximately one-third normal exposure allows demonstration of the joint and any early osteolytic or arthritic changes.[145]

CT arthrotomography has been the most reliable technique to assess the integrity of the glenoid labrum (Fig.

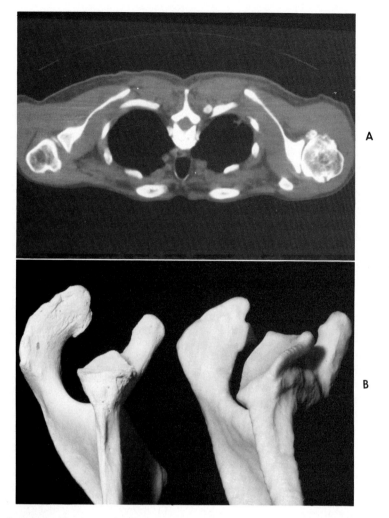

FIG. 3-47. A, Computed tomography demonstrates eccentric wear of the glenoid in this athlete with posterior erosion. **B,** Three-dimensional reconstructions of the glenoid allow the surgeon to compare a normal scapula to the amount of erosion to determine if bone grafting is necessary at the time of surgical reconstruction.

3-46).[139] Anterior detachments are best seen when the arm is scanned in internal rotation and posterior detachments when the arm is in external rotation. These positioning maneuvers relax the capsule and allow for better detail when tears are present.

Additional tests to evaluate for shoulder impingement lesions include imaging of the rotator cuff with ultrasound,[43,98] the gold standard of shoulder arthrography,[11] and, more recently, MRI.[88] For lesions with a full-thickness rotator cuff tear less than 1 cm in diameter, the ultrasound and MRI are more difficult to interpret. All three examinations have an accuracy approaching 95%. Double-contrast shoulder arthrotomography in a large series had an accuracy of 99%, with additional information as to the size of the tear.[112]

Eccentric glenoid wear and fractures are best evaluated by the CT scan. Stiffness, size, or pain often precludes adequate plain axillary views beyond establishing the lack of a dislocation. Anterior rim fractures of the glenoid (Fig. 3-3) with dislocations and eccentric posterior glenoid wear in arthritis (Fig. 3-47, A) are the two most frequently encountered conditions.

Three-dimensional plastic models, reconstructed from the uncompressed CT tape, further elucidate the amount of glenoid and humeral head distortion (Fig. 3-47, B). These reconstructions have been valuable in surgical planning, in shortening operative procedures, and for better visualization of the bony anatomy without widespread muscle detachment in shoulder arthroplasty.[123,124]

The conventional CT scan is also a valuable adjunct to radiographs in athletes with infection, osteomyelitis, foreign bodies, and soft-tissue abscesses. Increased uptake on skeletal scintigraphy may indicate neoplastic, infectious, posttraumatic, degenerative, and arthritic lesions.[156]

Early signs of osteonecrosis of the proximal humerus are most easily seen on the MRI. Later, the crescent sign is visualized on plain radiographs.

Additional testing for instability can be done with an

evaluation of the shoulder performed while the patient is under anesthesia, with [100,121,122] or without[41,121] C-arm fluoroscopy. Displacement of the humeral head greater than 50% beyond the glenoid rim denotes generalized laxity or pathologic instability. This examination is correlated with the other clinical findings.

Electrophysiologic Testing

EMG and nerve conduction studies are obtained routinely to evaluate cervical radiculopathy, brachial plexus injuries, and distal nerve entrapment lesions and also after fracture-dislocations or their treatment in which nerve deficits are anticipated.

These specialized tests confirm the clinical findings from the history and physical examination of the athlete with a painful shoulder. Only with an accurate diagnosis can meaningful comparisons of nonoperative and operative treatments be undertaken.

SUMMARY

An accurate history and thorough physical examination can yield a provisional diagnosis, subsequently confirmed by adjunctive laboratory or radiographic evaluation. The clinician well versed in the complete physical examination of the shoulder can facilitate the diagnostic work-up, avoid unnecessary tests, and provide direct, clear avenues of treatment to the athlete with a shoulder problem.

REFERENCES

1. Adelsberg A: The tennis stroke: an EMG analysis of selected muscles with rackets of increasing grip size, *Am J Sports Med* 14(2):139, 1986.
2. Albright JA et al: Clinical study of baseball pitchers: correlation of injury to the throwing arm with method of delivery, *Am J Sports Med* 6(1):15, 1978.
3. Allman FL: Fractures and ligamentous injuries of the clavicle and its articulations, *J Bone Joint Surg* 49A:774, 1967.
4. Andrews JR, Carson WG: The arthroscopic treatment of glenoid labrum tears in the throwing athlete, *Orthop Trans* 8(1):44, 1984.
5. Andrews JR, Gillogly S: Physical examination of the shoulder in throwing athletes. In Zarins B et al (eds): *Injuries to the throwing arm*, Philadelphia, 1985, WB Saunders.
6. Arendt EA: Multidirectional shoulder instability, *Orthopedics* 11(1):113, 1988.
7. Ariel G: Body mechanics. In Zarins B et al (eds): *Injuries to the throwing arm*, Philadelphia, 1985, WB Saunders.
8. Arntz CT, Matsen FR III: Disabling scapulothoracic snapping. Abstract submitted to American Shoulder and Elbow Surgeons Annual Meeting, Las Vegas, February 1989.
9. Aronoff GM, Evans WO: Evaluation and treatment of chronic pain at the Boston Pain Center, *J Clin Psychiatr* 43(8):4, 1982.
10. Atwater AE: Biomechanics of overarm throwing movements and throwing injuries, *Exerc Sport Sci Rev* 7:43, 1979.
11. Bangert BA, Pathria MN, Resnick D: Advanced imaging of the shoulder, *Surg Rounds Orthop* (June):48, 1989.
11a. Bankart ASB: Recurrent or habitual dislocation of the shoulder joint, *Br Med J* 2:1132, 1923.
12. Barnes DA, Tullos HS: An analysis of 100 symptomatic baseball players, *Am J Sports Med* 6(2):62, 1978.
13. Bateman JE: Nerve injuries about the shoulder in sports, *J Bone Joint Surg* 49(4):785, 1967.
14. Becker G: *Diagnosis: the cornerstone of treatment in chronic pain*, Paper presented at meeting of Yale Orthopaedic Association, Turtle Bay, Oahu, Hawaii, November 1986.
15. Becker G: Personal communication, June 1989.
16. Bennett GE: Shoulder and elbow lesions distinctive of baseball players, *Ann Surg* 126 (July):107, 1947.
17. Bennett GE: Elbow and shoulder lesions of baseball players, *Am J Surg* 98:484, 1959.
18. Benton J, Nelson C: Avulsion of the coracoid process in an athlete, *J Bone Joint Surg* 53A(2):356, 1971.
19. Bergfeld JA, Andrish JT, Clancy WG: Evaluation of the acromioclavicular joint following first- and second-degree sprains, *J Sports Med* 6(4):153, 1978.
20. Bigliani LU et al: The relationship between the unfused acromial epiphysis and subacromial impingement lesions, *Orthop Trans* 7(1):138, 1983.
21. Bigliani LU, Wolfe IN: Biceps tendon rupture in the athlete. In Torg JS, Welsh RP, Shephard RJ (eds): *Current therapy in sports medicine*, St Louis, 1985, Mosby.
22. Biondi J, Bear TF: Isolated rupture of the subscapularis tendon in an arm wrestler, *Orthopaedics* 11(4):647, 1988.
23. Bland JH, Merritt JA, Boushey DR: The painful shoulder, *Semin Arthritis Rheum* 7:21, 1977.
24. Blazina ME, Saltzman JS: Recurrent anterior subluxation of the shoulder in athletics—a distinct entity, *J Bone Joint Surg* 51A(5):1037, 1969.
25. Blom S, Dahlback CO: Nerve injuries in dislocations of the shoulder joint and fractures of the neck of the humerus, *Acta Chir Scand* 136:461, 1970.
26. Bonnin JG: Spontaneous subluxation of the sternoclavicular joint, *BMJ* 2:274, 1960.
27. Booth RE, Marvel JP: Differential diagnosis of shoulder pain, *Orthop Clin North Am* 6(2):353, 1975.
28. Bosworth DM: The supraspinatus syndrome: symptomatology, pathology, and repair, *JAMA* 116:2477, 1941.
29. Boyer DW: Trapshooter's shoulder: stress fracture of the coracoid process, *J Bone Joint Surg* 57A(6):862, 1975.
30. Bremner RA: Nonarticular, noninfective subacute arthritis of the sternoclavicular joint, *J Bone Joint Surg* 41B:749, 1959.
31. Brewer BJ: Athletic injuries: musculotendinous unit, *Clin Orthop* 23:30, 1962.
32. Brown JT: Early assessment of supraspinatus tears: procaine infiltration as a guise to treatment, *J Bone Joint Surg* 31B(3):423, 1949.
33. Brunet ME et al: Atraumatic osteolysis of the distal clavicle: histologic evidence of synovial pathogenesis, *Orthopedics* 9(4):557, 1986.
34. Bryan WJ, Schauder K, Tullos HS: The axillary nerve and its relationship to common sports medicine shoulder procedures, *Am J Sports Med* 14(2):113, 1986.
35. Cahill BR: Osteolysis of the distal part of the clavicle in male athletes, *J Bone Joint Surg* 64A(7):1053, 1982.
36. Cahill BR, Tullos HS, Fain RH: Little League shoulder, *J Sports Med* 2:150, 1974.
37. Clancy WG: Shoulder problems in overhead-overuse sports, *Am J Sports Med* 7(2):138, 1979.
38. Codman EA: *The shoulder*, Malabar, Fla, 1984, Robert E. Kreiger Publishing. (Reprint of Private Press 1934 Publication, Thomas Todd.)
39. Coene LN: Axillary nerve lesions and associated injuries, thesis, de Kempenaer, Oegstgeest, Holland, 1985.
40. Coene LN, Narakas AO: Surgical management of axillary nerve lesions, isolated or combined with other infraclavicular nerve lesions, *Peripheral Nerve Repair and Regeneration* 3:47, 1986.
41. Cofield RH, Irving JF: Evaluation and classification of shoulder instability, *Clin Orthop* 223:32, 1987.
42. Cofield RG, Simonet WT: The shoulder in sports, *Mayo Clin Proc* 59:157, 1984.
43. Crass JR, Craig EV: Noninvasive imaging of the rotator cuff, *Orthopedics* 11(1):57, 1988.
44. Danielsson L: Ruptur av. m. pectoralis major, en brottningsskada, *Nordisk Med* 72:1089, 1964.
45. Deltoff MN, Bressler HB: Atypical scapula fracture—a case report, *Am J Sports Med* 17(2):292, 1989.
46. Derebery UJ, Tullos WH: Low back pain exacerbated by psychological factors, *West J Med* 144:574, 1986.

47. Drez D: Suprascapular neuropathy in the differential diagnosis of rotator cuff injuries, *Am J Sports Med* 4(2):43, 1976.
48. Ebel R: Uber die Ursachen der Axillaris Parese bei Schulterluxation, *Mschr Unfallheilk* 76:445, 1973.
49. Engle G: Psychogenic pain and the pain-prone patient, *Am J Med* 26 (June):899, 1959.
50. Faure G, Daculsi G: Calcific tendinitis: a review, *Ann Rheum Dis* 42(suppl):49, 1983.
51. Ferretti A, Cerullo A, Russo G: Suprascapular neuropathy in volleyball players, *J Bone Joint Surg* 69A(2):260, 1987.
52. Ford CV: The somatizing disorders, *Psychosomatics* 27(5):327, 1986.
53. Fronek J, Warren RF, Bowen M: Posterior subluxation of the glenohumeral joint, *J Bone Joint Surg* 71A(2):205, 1989.
54. Fukuda H, Hamada K, Kobayashi Y: *"Push-up views" for the massive rotator cuff tears—a new roentgenographic projection,* Paper presented at the American Shoulder and Elbow Surgeons' Fifth Open Meeting, Las Vegas, February 12, 1989.
55. Fukuda H, Neer CS II: Archer's shoulder—recurrent posterior subluxation and dislocation of the shoulder in two archers, *Orthopedics* 11(1):171, 1988.
56. Gainor BJ et al: The throw: biomechanics and acute injury, *Am J Sports Med* 8(2):114, 1980.
57. Garth WP, Leberte MA, Cool TA: Recurrent fractures of the humerus in a baseball pitcher, *J Bone Joint Surg* 70A(2):305, 1988.
58. Gerber C, Krushell RJ: Isolated rupture of the tendon of the subscapularis muscle: clinical features in 16 cases, *J Bone Joint Surg* 73B:389, 1991.
59. Gerber C, Granz R: Clinical assessment of the shoulder, *J Bone Joint Surg* 66B:551, 1984.
60. Glick JM et al: Dislocated acromioclavicular joint: follow-up study of 35 unreduced acromioclavicular dislocations, *Am J Sports Med* 5(6):264, 1977.
61. Glousman R et al: Dynamic EMG analysis of the throwing shoulder with glenohumeral instability, *Orthop Trans* 11(2):247, 1987.
62. Goldstein R: Psychological evaluation of low back pain, *SPINE: State of the Art Reviews* 1(1):103, 1986.
63. Goldstein R: Personal communication, June 1989.
64. Gregg JR et al: Serratus anterior paralysis in the young athlete, *J Bone Joint Surg* 61A(6):825, 1979.
65. Hansen NM: Epiphyseal changes in the proximal humerus of an adolescent baseball pitcher, *Am J Sports Med* 10(6):380, 1982.
66. Hawkins RJ, Kennedy MD: Impingement syndrome in athletes, *J Sports Med* 8(3):151, 1980.
67. Hawkins RJ, Hobeika PE: Impingement syndrome in the athletic shoulder, *Clin Sports Med* 2(2):391, 1983.
68. Hawkins RJ, Neer CS II: Missed posterior dislocations of the shoulder. In Bateman JE, Welsh RP (eds): *Surgery of the shoulder,* Philadelphia, 1984, BC Decker.
69. Hawkins RJ, McCormack RG: Posterior shoulder instability, *Orthopedics* 7(1):101, 1988.
70. Henry JH, Genung JA: Natural history of glenohumeral dislocation revisited, *Am J Sports Med* 10:135, 1982.
71. Hill HA, Sachs MD: The grooved defect of the humeral head: a frequently unrecognized complication of dislocations of the shoulder joint, *Radiology* 35:690, 1940.
72. Hirasawa Y, Sakakida K: Sports and peripheral nerve injury, *Am J Sports Med* 11:420, 1983.
73. Hopkinson WJ, Ryan JB, Wheeler JH: Glenoid rim fracture and recurrent shoulder instability, *Complic Orthop* (March/April):36, 1989.
74. Howell SM et al: Normal and abnormal mechanics of the glenohumeral joint in the horizontal plane, *J Bone Joint Surg* 70A(2):227, 1988.
75. Hoyt WA: Etiology of shoulder injuries in athletes, *J Bone Joint Surg* 49:755, 1967.
76. Ishikawa H et al: Osteochondritis dissecans of the shoulder in a tennis player, *Am J Sports Med* 16(5):547, 1988.
77. Jobe FW: Shoulder problems in overhead-overuse sports, *Am J Sports Med* 7(2):139, 1979.
78. Jobe FW: Treating problem elbows in baseball pitchers, *Orthop Today,* 7:36, 1986.
79. Jobe FW: Impingement problems in the athlete. In Barr JS (ed): *Instructional course lecture 38,* Park Ridge, Ill, 1989, American Academy of Orthopaedic Surgeons.
80. Jobe FW et al: The relationship of anterior instability and rotator cuff impingement in the throwing athlete, Paper presented at the American Shoulder and Elbow Surgeons Annual Open Meeting, Las Vegas, February 12, 1989.
81. Jobe FW, Jobe CM: Painful athletic injuries of the shoulder, *Clin Orthop* 173:117, 1983.
82. Kaplan PE, Kernahan WT Jr: Rotator cuff rupture: management with suprascapular neuropathy, *Arch Phys Med Rehabil* 65:273, 1984.
83. Kennedy JC, Hawkins R, Krissoff WB: Orthopaedic manifestations of swimming, *Am J Sports Med* 6(6):309, 1978.
84. King JW, Brelsford HJ, Tullos HS: Analysis of the pitching arm of the professional baseball player, *Clin Orthop* 67:116, 1969.
85. Kircher MT, Cappuccino A, Torpey BM: Muscular violence as a cause of humeral fractures in pitchers, *Contemp Orthop* 26(5):475, 1993.
86. Kiviluoto O et al: Immobilization after primary dislocation of the shoulder, *Acta Orthop Scand* 51:915, 1980.
87. Kline DG, Lusk MD: Management of athletic brachial plexus injuries. In Schneider RC et al, eds: *Sports injuries,* Baltimore, 1984, Williams & Wilkins.
88. Kneeland JB et al: Rotator cuff tears: preliminary application of high resolution MRI with counter-rotating loop gap resonators, *Radiology* 160:695, 1986.
89. Kretzler HH, Richardson AB: Rupture of the pectoralis major muscle, *Orthop Trans* 11(1):76, 1987.
90. Leach RE, Schepsis AA: Shoulder pain, *Clin Sports Med* 2(1):123, 1983.
91. Leffert RD: *Thoracic outlet syndrome,* A correspondence newsletter to the American Society for Surgery of the Hand, December 12, 1988.
92. Leffert RD: Lesions of the brachial plexus revisited. Barr JS (ed): *Instructional course lecture 38,* Park Ridge, Ill, 1989, American Academy of Orthopaedic Surgeons.
93. Leffert RD, Gumley G: The relationship between dead arm syndrome and thoracic outlet syndrome, *Clin Orthop* 223:20, 1987.
94. Lipscomb AB: Baseball pitching injuries in growing athletes, *J Sports Med* 3(1):25, 1975.
95. Lipscomb AB, Thomas ED, Johnston RK: Treatment of myositis ossificans traumatica in athletes, *Am J Sports Med* 4(3):111, 1976.
96. Lombardo SJ et al: Posterior shoulder lesions in throwing athletes, *J Sports Med* 5(3):106, 1977.
97. Lundberg BJ: The frozen shoulder, *Acta Orthop Scand Suppl* 119:1, 1969.
98. Mack LA et al: US evaluation of the rotator cuff, *Radiology* 157:205, 1985.
99. Magni G, deBertolini C: Chronic pain as a depressive equivalent, *Postgrad Med* 73(3):79, 1983.
100. Maki NJ: Cineradiographic studies with shoulder instabilities, *Am J Sports Med* 16(4):362, 1988.
101. Mariani PP: Isolated fracture of the coracoid process in an athlete, *Am J Sports Med* 8(2):129, 1980.
102. Markey KL, DiBenedetto M, Curl WW: Upper trunk brachial plexopathy, *Am J Sports Med* 21(5):650, 1993.
103. Matsen FA: TUBS-AMBRI—mnemonics to differentiate traumatic instability from multidirectional instability, American Academy of Orthopaedic Surgeons, Summer Institute, San Diego, September 7-11, 1988.
104. McCue FC, Gieck JH, West JO: Throwing injuries to the shoulder. In Zarins B et al (eds): *Injuries to the throwing arm,* Philadelphia, 1985, WB Saunders.
105. McEntire JE, Hess WE, Coleman SS: Rupture of the pectoralis major muscle, *J Bone Joint Surg* 54A(5):1040, 1972.
106. McGlynn FJ, El-Khoury G, Albright JP: Arthrotomography of the glenoid labrum in shoulder instability, *J Bone Joint Surg* 64A:506, 1982.
107. McLaughlin HL: Rupture of the rotator cuff, *J Bone Joint Surg* 44A(5):979, 1962.

108. McLeod WD: The pitching mechanism. In Zarins B et al (eds): *Injuries to the throwing arm,* Philadelphia, 1985, WB Saunders.
109. McLeod WD, Andrews JR: Mechanisms of shoulder injuries, *Phys Ther* 66(12):1901, 1986.
110. McMaster WC: Anterior glenoid labrum damage: a painful lesion in swimmers, *Am J Sports Med* 14(5):383, 1986.
111. Mestdagh H, Drizenko A, Ghestem P: Anatomical bases of suprascapular nerve syndrome, *Anatomica Clinica* 3:67, 1981.
112. Mink JH, Harris E, Rappaport M: Rotator cuff tears: evaluation using double-contrast shoulder arthrography, *Radiology* 157:621, 1985.
113. Moynes DR et al: Electromyography and motion analysis of the upper extremity in sports, *Phys Ther* 66(12):1905, 1986.
114. Neer CS II: Anterior acromioplasty for chronic impingement syndrome in the shoulder, *J Bone Joint Surg* 54A:41, 1972.
115. Neer CS II, Craig EV, Fukuda H: Cuff tear anthropathy, *J Bone Joint Surg* 65A:1232, 1983.
116. Neer CS II, Foster CR: Inferior capsular shift for involuntary inferior and multidirectional instability of the shoulder, *J Bone Joint Surg* 62A:897, 1980.
117. Neer CS II, Watson KC, Stanton FS: Recent experience in total shoulder replacement, *J Bone Joint Surg* 64A:319, 1982.
118. Neer CS II, Welsh RP: The shoulder in sports, *Orthop Clin North Am* 8(3):583, 1977.
119. Neviaser JS: Adhesive capsulitis of the shoulder, *Med Times* 90:783, 1962.
120. Nicholas JA, Grossman RB, Hershman EB: The importance of a simplified classification of motion in sports in relation to performance, *Orthop Clin North Am* 8(3):499, 1977.
121. Norris TR: C-arm fluoroscopic evaluation under anaesthesia for glenohumeral subluxations. In Bateman J, Welsh P (eds): *Surgery of the shoulder,* Philadelphia, 1984, BC Decker.
122. Norris TR: Diagnostic technique for shoulder instability. In Stauffer ED (ed): American Academy of Orthopaedic Surgeons, *Instructional Course Lectures,* vol 34, St Louis, 1985, Mosby.
123. Norris TR: Bone grafts for glenoid deficiency in total shoulder replacements, In *Proceedings of the Third International Conference on Surgery of the Shoulder,* Tokyo, 1987, Professional Postgraduate Services.
124. Norris TR: Unconstrained prosthetic shoulder replacement. In Watson M (ed): *The shoulder,* London, 1989, Churchill Livingstone.
125. Norris TR: *Recurrent posterior subluxations: hospital medicine,* New York, 1989, Cahners Publishing.
126. Norris TR, Bigliani LU: Analysis of failed repair for shoulder instability—a preliminary report. In Bateman J, Welsh P (eds): *Surgery of the shoulder,* Philadelphia, 1984, BC Decker.
127. Norris TR, Bigliani LU: Complications following the modified Bristow procedure for shoulder instability, *J Bone Joint Surg* 11:232, 1987.
128. Norris TR et al: The unfused acromial epiphysis and its relationship to impingement syndrome, *Orthop Trans* 7(3):505, 1983.
129. Nuber GW et al: Fine wire electromyography analysis of muscles of the shoulder during swimming, *Am J Sports Med* 14(1):7, 1986.
130. O'Brien SJ et al: Capsular restraints to anterior posterior motion of the shoulder, *Orthop Trans* 12(1):143, 1988.
131. Pappas AM, Goss TP, Kleinman PK: Symptomatic shoulder instability due to lesions of the glenoid labrum, *Am J Sports Med* 11(5):279, 1983.
132. Pasila M et al: Early complication of primary shoulder dislocations, *Acta Orthop Scand* 49:260, 1978.
133. Perry J: Anatomy and biomechanics of the shoulder in throwing, swimming, gymnastics, and tennis, *Clin Sports Med* 2(2):247, 1983.
134. Pettrone FA: Shoulder problems in swimmers. In Zarins B et al (eds): *Injuries to the throwing arm,* Philadelphia, 1985, WB Saunders.
135. Poindexter DP, Johnson EW: Football shoulder and neck injury: a study of the "stinger," *Arch Phys Med Rehabil* 65:601, 1984.
136. Poppen NK, Walker PS: Normal and abnormal motion of the shoulder, *J Bone Joint Surg* 58A:195, 1976.
137. Poppen NK, Walker PS: Forces at the glenohumeral joint in abduction, *Clin Orthop* 135:165, 1978.
138. Quigley TB: Injuries to the acromioclavicular and sternoclavicular joints sustained in athletes, *Surg Clin North Am* 43(6):1551, 1963.
139. Rafii M et al: Athlete shoulder injuries: CT arthrographic findings, *Radiology* 162(2):559, 1987.
140. Reilly PJ, Torg JS: Athletic injury to the cervical nerve roots and brachial plexus, *Op Tech Sports Med* 1(3):231, 1993.
141. Resnick D: Shoulder pain, *Orthop Clin North Am* 14:81, 1983.
142. Richardson AB: Overuse syndrome in baseball, tennis, gymnastics, and swimming, *Clin Sports Med* 2(2):379, 1983.
143. Richardson AB, Jobe FE, Collins HR: The shoulder in competitive swimming, *J Sports Med* 8(3):159, 1980.
144. Robertson WC, Eichman PL, Clancy WG: Upper trunk brachial plexopathy in football players, *JAMA* 241(14):1480, 1979.
145. Rockwood CA Jr: Posterior dislocation of the shoulder. In Rockwood CA Jr, Green DP, (eds): *Fractures in adults,* Philadelphia, 1984, JB Lippincott.
146. Rokous JR, Feagin JA, Abbott HG: Modified axillary roentgenogram, *Clin Orthop* 82:84, 1972.
147. Rome HP, Harness DM: Psychological and behavioral aspects of chronic facial pain, *Otolaryngol Clin North Am* 22:6, 1989.
148. Rowe CR: Shoulder subluxation in the athlete. In Torg JS, Welsh RP, Shephard RJ (eds): *Current therapy in sports medicine,* St Louis, 1985, Mosby.
149. Rowe CF: Recurrent transient anterior subluxation of the shoulder, the "dead arm" syndrome, *Clin Orthop* 223:11, 1987.
150. Rowe CR, Pierce DS, Clark JG: Voluntary dislocation of the shoulder: a preliminary report on a clinical electromyographic and psychiatric study of 25 patients, *J Bone Joint Surg* 55A:445, 1973.
151. Rowe CR, Zarins B: Recurrent transient subluxation of the shoulder, *J Bone Joint Surg* 63A:863, 1981.
152. Ryu RKN et al: An electromyographic analysis of shoulder function in tennis players, *Am J Sports Med* 6:481, 1988.
153. Saha AK: *Theory of the shoulder mechanism: descriptive and applied,* Springfield, Ill, 1961, Charles C Thomas.
154. Sain J, Andrews JR: Proper pitching techniques. In Zarins B et al (eds): *Injuries to the throwing arm,* Philadelphia, 1985, WB Saunders.
155. Santavirta S, Kiviluoto O: Transverse fracture of the humerus in a shotputter: a case report, *Am J Sports Med* 5(3):122, 1977.
156. Sartoris DJ, Resnick D: Imaging the painful shoulder: what studies to order, *J Musculoskel Med* 5(7):21, 1988.
157. Schwartz PA, Torzilli PA, Warren RF: *Capsular restraints to anterior-posterior motion of the shoulder.* Paper presented at the 33rd Annual Meeting, Orthopaedic Research Society, San Francisco, January 19-22, 1987.
158. Shuman WP et al: Double-contrast computed tomography of the glenoid labrum, *Am J Roentgenol* 141:581, 1983.
159. Simonet WT, Cofield RH: *Prognosis in anterior dislocation.* Paper presented at American Orthopaedic Society for Sports Medicine, Anaheim, Calif, March 9-10, 1983.
160. Sisto D et al: An EMG analysis of the elbow in pitching, *Am J Sports Med* 15:260, 1987.
160a. Smith JG: Pathological appearances of seven cases of injury of the shoulder joint with remarks, *Am J Med Sci* 16:219, 1834.
161. Soslowsky LJ et al: Articular geometry of the glenohumeral joint, *Clin Orthop* 285:181, 1992.
162. Stanish WD, Lamb H: Isolated paralysis of the serratus anterior muscle: a weight training injury, *Am J Sports Med* 6(6):385, 1978.
163. Stewart MJ: The acromioclavicular joint in the throwing arm. In Zarins B et al (eds): *Injuries to the throwing arm,* Philadelphia, 1985, WB Saunders.
164. Tibone JE et al: Surgical treatment of tears of the rotator cuff in athletes, *J Bone Joint Surg* 68A(6):887, 1986.

165. Tullos HS, King JW: Lesions of the pitching arm in adolescents, *JAMA* 220(2):264, 1972.
166. Tullos HS, King JW: Throwing mechanism in sports, *Orthop Clin North Am* 4(3):709, 1973.
167. Tullos HS et al: Unusual lesions of the pitching arm, *Clin Orthop* 88:169, 1972.
168. Turkel SJ et al: Stabilizing mechanism in preventing anterior dislocation of the glenohumeral joint, *J Bone Joint Surg* 63A:1208, 1981.
169. Uhthoff HK, Sakar K, Maynard JA: Calcifying tendinitis—a new concept of the pathogenesis, *Clin Orthop* 118:164, 1978.
170. Van Nes CP, Van Nes JF: Serratus paralysis, *Arch Chir Neerl* 21(1):85, 1969.
171. Warren RF: Instability of shoulder in throwing sports. In Stauffer ED (ed): *American Academy of Orthopaedic Surgeons instructional course lectures,* vol 34, St Louis, 1985, Mosby.
172. Weiner DS, Macnab I: Superior migration of the humeral head: a radiological aid in the diagnosis of tears of the rotator cuff, *J Bone Joint Surg* 52B:524, 1970.
173. Weiss J: The painful shoulder. In Kelly WN et al (eds): *Textbook of rheumatology,* Philadelphia, 1981, WB Saunders.
174. Welsh RP: Dislocations of the shoulder: acromioclavicular and sternoclavicular joints. In Welsh RP, Shephard RJ (eds): *Current therapy in sports medicine 1985-1986,* Philadelphia, 1985, BC Decker.
175. Whitaker JH: Arm wrestling fractures—a humerus twist, *Am J Sports Med* 5(2):67, 1977.
176. Zuckerman JC, Matsen FA III: Complications about the glenohumeral joint related to the use of screws and staples, *J Bone Joint Surg* 66A(2):175, 1984.

CHAPTER 4

Diagnostic Imaging of the Shoulder

Andrew H. Turtel
Jeffrey Minkoff
Mahvash Rafii
Vincent DiStefano

There is no simple flow sheet by which diagnostic tests and treatments for the athlete with a disabled shoulder may be ordained to the satisfaction of all treating physicians. Only a few decades ago the primary weapon in the diagnostic armamentarium was the physician's examination. Third-party carriers and doubtful patients were not available in any numbers to undermine the physician's diagnosis. While the physical examination became more sophisticated throughout the 1970s and 1980s, with the common recognition of such entities as impingement and multidirectional instability, the sophistication of radiographic diagnostics has grown to a much greater extent, and arthroscopy has developed as well. Today, documentation of pathologic conditions has become a critical factor in American medicine. It satisfies the patient, the carrier, and the physician that the treatment direction is appropriate; perhaps more important, objective testing reveals whether anything serious is being overlooked, such as a tumor.

Many factors are involved in determining the extent and nature of the documentary evidence to be secured. They include the severity of manifested symptoms, the activity for which the disabled limb is to be used, expe-

diency requirements (as with professional athletes), the expertise of the physician for the limb segment being treated, the availability and effectiveness of special diagnostic tests within the community, and the variance in treatment approaches by different physicians for a given pathologic entity. These factors constitute the essence of a needed resolve between the radiologist and the sports medicine physician. The radiologist is charged with a descriptive interpretation of radiographic studies performed. The sports medicine physician, on the other hand, is charged with the ordering of such studies and, most important, the translation of their descriptive interpretations into a practical treatment plan.

The sports clinician ordinarily encounters a variety of shoulder afflictions in his or her practice. Some are sport specific and must be kept in mind. Cofield and Simonet[25] provide a partial list:

1. Weight lifters—inflammatory acromioclavicular arthritis with resorption of the distal end of the clavicle
2. Baseball pitchers—ossification of the posterior glenoid region[108]
3. Tennis serve and baseball pitching acceleration phase—impingements
4. Gymnastics—strains, impingements, and instabilities, especially attributable to the use of rings
5. Trap-shooters—fractures of the coracoid
6. Swimmers—impingement, especially on the breathing side (The parameters of swimmer's shoulder were defined by Hawkins and Kennedy [1980][78] and are associated with internal rotation and adduction and CT arthrographic findings of anterior labral detachment.[113])

This list is only a small sample of the wide array of athletically related disorders that may or may not be sport specific. Most of these conditions fall within several categories of pathology: glenohumeral instability, capsulolabral disorders, rotator cuff disease and impingement, acromioclavicular disorders, and a miscellaneous category, which includes pathologic states ranging from calcareous diseases to tumors simulating injuries. Few sports physicians would attempt to diagnose or treat any of these prospective disorders without the benefit of a radiographic assessment. Before 1970, other than for the intermittent use of arthrography, radiography consisted primarily of plain radiographs. However, there have since appeared a progression of sophisticated and high-tech radiographic techniques that have substantially enhanced the accuracy (sensitivity and specificity) of diagnosis of the above-indicated abnormalities. These techniques have included the development of specialized views, glenohumeral and bursal arthrography, arthrotomography, computed tomographic (CT) arthrography, sonography, and magnetic resonance imaging (MRI).

There is a great variance among clinicians in their capacities and confidence in the physical diagnosis of the symptomatic shoulder. No matter how confident the physician, nor how certain the apparent diagnosis, there remains an ultimate doubt, even if only with respect to the specificity or quantity of the suspected pathologic condition; certainly, there is little or no disadvantage in performing one or more of the corroborative radiographic procedures currently available. Deterrents to this pursuit might include:

1. An overconfident physician and/or undemanding patient
2. Mutual selection of an empirical or arbitrary program of conservative management—a conscious deferment of surgical considerations
3. A decision to bypass the less invasive diagnostics for an arthroscopic evaluation with the potential added benefit of a therapeutic response
4. A special expediency reasonably precluding testing delays
5. Failure of insurance to cover one or more of the proposed radiographic tests
6. Absence of facilities for the performance of these tests or expertise in their interpretation
7. Claustrophobia in regard to the MRI gantry

Regardless of any possible deterrents, there are many advantages to the performance of the specialized tests. For the patient who potentially has a surgically treatable problem, the tests may indicate in advance whether there is any reasonable benefit to be gained from surgery. Their ability to detail the pathologic condition may also help in surgical planning: open versus closed, period of expected disability (how long out of work or school), and inpatient versus outpatient treatment. For the patient without intention of surgery or with a diagnosis of a nonsurgical condition, the tests might reveal an intractable problem, treatable only by surgery (such as a bucket handle tear of the glenoid labrum). These tests rarely produce a false positive result. More often, they produce a false negative or underreading of the pathologic state. The potential consequence is that in some instances an appropriate treatment course is not pursued. In most cases, however, these tests corroborate the presence of the pathologic condition and enhance the surgeon's and patient's confidence in the treatment protocol. Objective documentation also better satisfies third-party carriers with respect to approvals, provides a mobile exhibit to facilitate second opinions, and reduces the chances of certain litigious allegations.

This chapter presents the techniques and indications for each of the radiographic techniques currently available for the diagnosis of the more common sports-related afflictions of the shoulder. The selection of tests and their relative reliability for each condition are outlined within reason at the present level of knowledge.

CONVENTIONAL (PLAIN) RADIOGRAPHY
Trauma and Instability

Most orthopaedic surgeons include conventional or plain radiography as a part of their evaluation of a shoulder disability. There is some variance, however, in defining those projections that constitute the so-called routine views of the shoulder. Is the objective to demonstrate the most evident pathologic state with the fewest number of radiographs, or is it to attempt to discover even more subtle abnormalities by ordering an expanded group of views as a routine? Thoroughness, cost, time

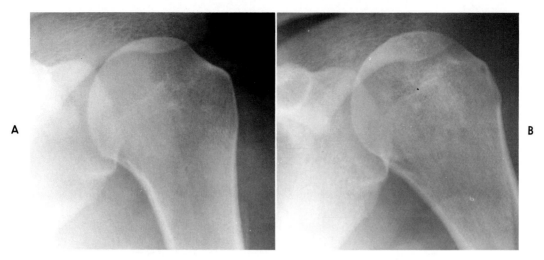

FIG. 4-1. Normal anteroposterior views of the left shoulder in external rotation (**A**) and internal rotation (**B**).

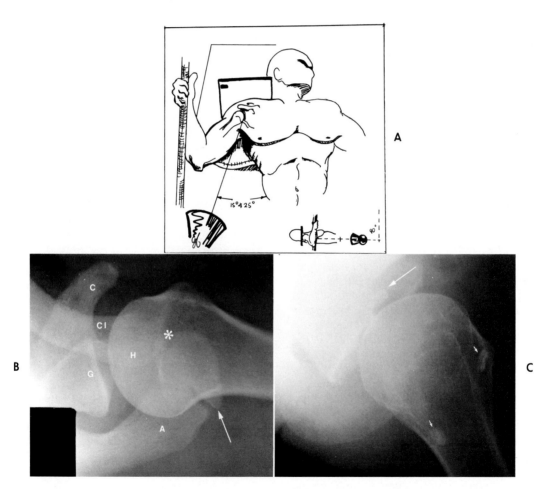

FIG. 4-2. Routine supine axillary view. Demonstrates the glenohumeral joint in craniocaudad orientation. Useful for evaluation of the glenohumeral joint alignment, the glenoid margins, and the acromion process. **A,** The patient is supine with the arm in neutral rotation and 45 degrees abduction. The film cassette is placed perpendicular to the table against the top of the shoulder. The x-ray beam is horizontal to the axilla at an angle of 15 to 25 degrees from the sagittal plane. **B,** Normal. *A,* Acromion; *C,* coracoid; *Cl,* clavicle; *G,* glenoid; *H,* humeral head. NOTE: Anterior acromion is formed by a secondary ossification center and is nonunited *(arrow)*. *Acromioclavicular joint. **C,** Anterior instability. The humeral head is subluxed anteriorly. Ossification of an existing Bankart lesion is visualized *(large arrow)*. Osteocartilaginous loose bodies are present *(small arrows)*. (**A** redrawn from Norris TR: Diagnostic techniques for shoulder instability. In AAOS: *Instructional course lectures,* vol 34, St Louis, 1985, Mosby.)

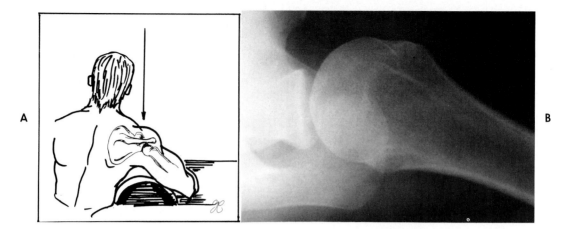

FIG. 4-3. Axillary view. Superoinferior projection. Similar to routine supine axillary view in its demonstration of the anatomic constituents of the shoulder joint. **A,** The patient is sitting with his side against the table. The arm is abducted over the curved cassette. The x-ray beam is directed in a superoinferior direction. This view may also be obtained using a regular cassette. The use of a curved cassette eliminates the excess magnification of the image because of decreased subject-film distance. **B,** Normal.

efficiency, and the suspected disorder may each be a factor shaping the routine. The suspected disorder is vital in considering the selection of one or more of the special or sports views to better delineate a particular portion of the glenoid or humeral head. In describing an approach to painful athletic injuries of the shoulder, Jobe and Jobe[87] indicate that the initial evaluation should include three views of the shoulder: anteroposterior views in internal and external rotation and a transaxillary lateral view; a West Point view may be helpful to demonstrate the anteroinferior portion of the glenoid. DeSmet[38] described an anterior oblique (**Y** view) projection (see Fig. 4-6) by which he was able to detect scapular and humeral head fractures undetected by the routine views outlined above. This scapular **Y**-view was cited by Rubin, Gray, and Green[172] as an important diagnostic aid in shoulder trauma. Pavlov and Freiberger[149] reenforce the adage that two films at right angles are important in the evaluation of all fractures. They maintain that the evaluation of the traumatized shoulder joint requires the taking of a transscapular view (**Y**-view) in conjunction with either a frontal or tangential view of the joint.

The routine views most commonly obtained for evaluating shoulder disorders always include **anteroposterior (AP) views** with internal and external rotation of the humerus (Fig. 4-1). These views provide a profile of the acromioclavicular (AC) and glenohumeral joints, the humeral head, and the tuberosities. They provide information about alignment, arthritic changes, and calcific deposits about the joint. Routine examination often also includes one of the **axillary projections** for tangential visualization of the glenohumeral joint and glenoid margins to assess alignment of the former and infractions and irregularities of the latter (Fig. 4-2). The commonly employed axillary view requires meticulous positioning with the arm in abduction (Fig. 4-3). DeSmet[39] has demonstrated its value in the nontraumatized shoulder. However, it is often poorly tolerated by patients with an acute

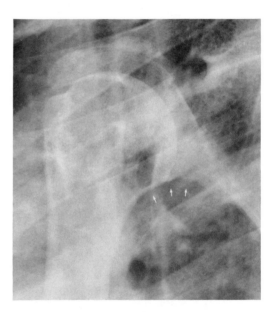

FIG. 4-4. Normal transthoracic lateral view of the shoulder. On this view the humeral shaft, the greater tuberosity, and the humeral head are clearly visualized in a true lateral projection. The coracoid process is visualized arching over the humeral head, which in turn partially overlaps the glenoid fossa. Line continuity of the lateral scapular margin and the surgical neck of the humerus, forming the scapulohumeral arch *(arrows)*, is an indicator of normal glenohumeral alignment.

shoulder injury. Hence the routine examination of patients following acute trauma, especially when fractures or dislocations are suspected, requires that the patient be positioned with minimal or no movement of the arm. The radiographic projections most often employed include an AP view without rotating the arm, and a **transthoracic lateral projection** (Fig. 4-4). These projections are usually sufficient for detecting anterior dislocations (best

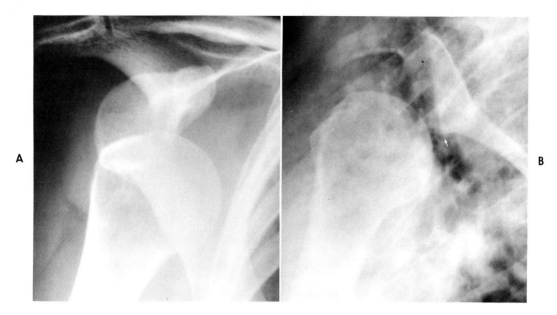

FIG. 4-5. Anterior dislocation of right shoulder. **A,** Anteroposterior view. Anterior dislocation of the humeral head is readily recognized by its marked medial displacement under the coracoid process. **B,** Transthoracic lateral view. Disruption of the scapulohumeral arch *(arrows)* is an indication of glenohumeral malalignment.

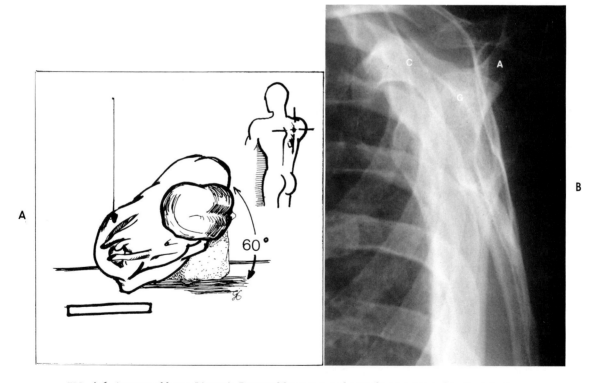

FIG. 4-6. Anterior oblique (**Y** view). Proximal humerus and scapula are projected in the lateral position. Useful for evaluating fractures and dislocations. **A,** Patient is in upright position, and the shoulder being studied is anteriorly rotated 60 degrees. The x-ray beam is in posteroanterior direction and is perpendicular to the cassette. **B,** The coracoid (C) and the acromion (A) processes and the lateral border of the scapula form the figure of **Y,** in the center of which the glenoid fossa (G) is projected en face. The humerus is in the true lateral projection and the humeral head overlaps the center of the figure **Y.**   *Continued.*

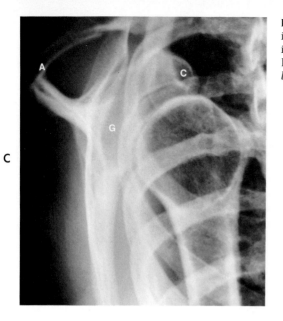

FIG. 4-6, cont'd. C, Anterior dislocation. The anteriorly displaced humeral head is demonstrated below the coracoid process in this projection. The glenoid fossa is empty, signifying the presence of a dislocation. (**A** redrawn from Norris TR: *Diagnostic techniques for shoulder instability.* In AAOS: *Instructional course lectures,* vol 34, St Louis, 1985, Mosby.)

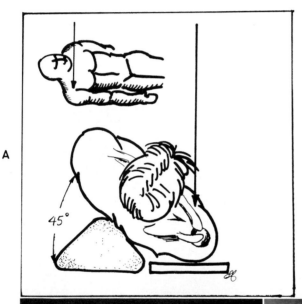

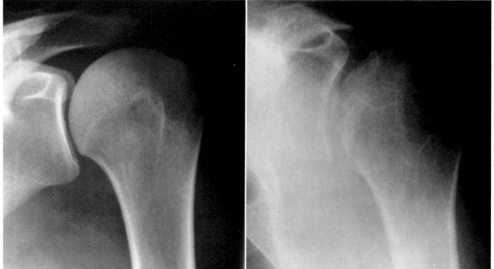

FIG. 4-7. Posterior oblique or true (tangential) AP view. The glenohumeral joint is visualized in AP orientation. Useful for evaluating humeral fractures and suspected posterior dislocation. **A,** The patient is supine or upright, and the shoulder being studied is posteriorly rotated 45 degrees. The x-ray beam is directed anteroposteriorly and perpendicular to the cassette. **B,** Normal. The glenohumeral joint space is clearly visualized. **C,** Posterior dislocation. The glenohumeral joint space is obliterated because of posterior dislocation of the humeral head, which is hinged and locked against the posterior glenoid margin. (**A** redrawn from Norris TR: Diagnostic techniques for shoulder instability. In AAOS: *Instructional course lectures,* vol 34, St Louis, 1985, Mosby.)

seen on the AP view) and for evaluating displaced fractures of the proximal end of the humerus (Fig. 4-5). They may fail to demonstrate small fractures about the joint. Contrary to common belief, the transthoracic lateral view is not particularly good for the detection of dislocations and requires painstaking scrutiny for the detection of subtle changes in scapulohumeral alignment. A **Y view** (anterior oblique projection) should be performed because of its ability to detect dislocations and fractures of the proximal end of the humerus (Fig. 4-6). Finally, a **posterior oblique view** (tangential AP) should be added for additional capability in the detection of dislocations (Fig. 4-7).

Routine views

- Anteroposterior (internal and external rotation)
- Axillary view
- Lateral in scapular plane (Y view)

Posterior dislocations are notoriously difficult to detect and may go unrecognized without employing specific views (Fig. 4-8). Vastamaki and Solonen[188] report that the diagnosis of posterior dislocation or fracture-dislocation is often delayed and that an axillary view is

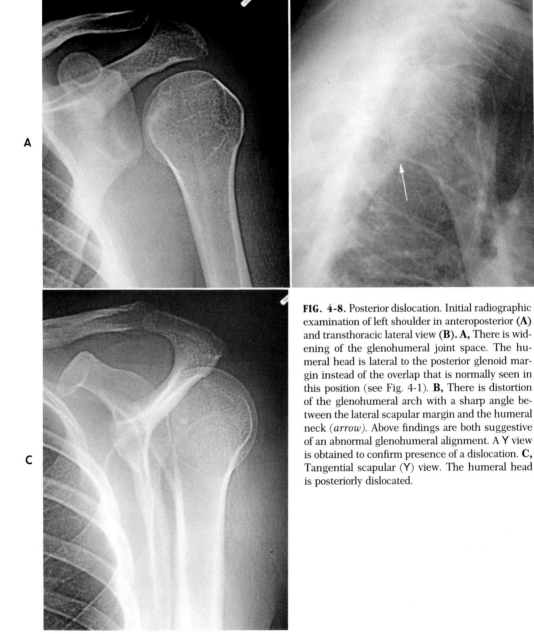

FIG. 4-8. Posterior dislocation. Initial radiographic examination of left shoulder in anteroposterior (**A**) and transthoracic lateral view (**B**). **A,** There is widening of the glenohumeral joint space. The humeral head is lateral to the posterior glenoid margin instead of the overlap that is normally seen in this position (see Fig. 4-1). **B,** There is distortion of the glenohumeral arch with a sharp angle between the lateral scapular margin and the humeral neck (*arrow*). Above findings are both suggestive of an abnormal glenohumeral alignment. A **Y** view is obtained to confirm presence of a dislocation. **C,** Tangential scapular (**Y**) view. The humeral head is posteriorly dislocated.

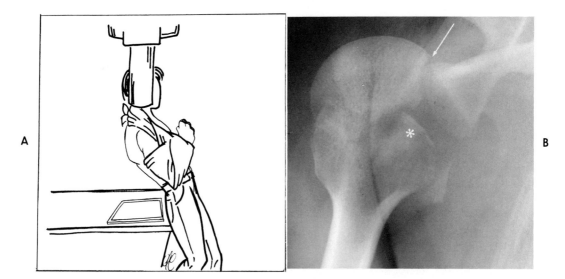

FIG. 4-9. Velpeau axillary view. A craniocaudad view of the glenohumeral joint is obtained. Useful for evaluation of the glenohumeral alignment in suspected posterior dislocation. **A,** Patient stands with back against the x-ray table. The patient arches backward over the table until the shoulder is above the cassette, which is lying on the table. The superoinferior x-ray beam is then directed through the shoulder and perpendicular to the cassette. **B,** Posterior fracture-dislocation. In addition to a comminuted fracture of the humeral neck and tuberosities, the major portion of the humeral head is posteriorly dislocated and is hinged against the posterior glenoid margin. A smaller segment of the head (*) is impacted. (**A** redrawn from Bloom MH, Obata WG: *J Bone Joint Surg* 49A(5):943, 1987.)

essential in suspected cases. Bloom and Obata[11] reinforce the diagnostic dilemma of the posterior dislocation and cite the report of Arndt and Sears,[4] which indicates that in 50% of such cases the diagnosis is tardy. Bloom and Obata sought to reconcile this dilemma of tardy diagnosis with that of attempting to position an acutely injured shoulder, and with the wisdom of Vastamaki and Solonen, by creating **Velpeau axillary** and **angle-up views.** These axillary projections can demonstrate a posterior displacement of the humeral head without a need to position the patient in a painfully compromising manner (Fig. 4-9). Horsefield and Jones[83] describe the Stripp axial view designed to evaluate the shoulder of the acutely injured patient who is unable to abduct because of pain. Another view that is useful in demonstrating glenohumeral instability and that requires no movement of the painful shoulder is the **apical oblique** projection (Fig. 4-10). In fact, Brams-Dalgaard et al[14] and Richardson et al[166] suggest that the apical oblique view was superior for providing diagnostic information when compared with other lateral views. When the apical oblique view was combined with an AP view, the authors found a great ability to establish a diagnosis compared with the transthoracic and transscapular views (see Commentary in Table 4-1).

Garth, Slappey, and Ochs[58] stated that this view, which provides a coronal profile of the glenohumeral joint, is an excellent detector of the hallmark criteria of instabilities of all ages: glenohumeral displacements, Hill-Sachs lesions, and Bankart fractures or ossifications. Nevertheless, they admitted that the West Point view of

Rokous, Feagin, and Abbott[168] was much more likely to detect Bankart lesions (Fig. 4-11).

Hill-Sachs Lesion

It is evident that the lesions of chronic or recurrent glenohumeral dislocations and subluxations are often not optimally visualized on the standard radiographic views alluded to above. The compression fracture of the posterolateral portion of the humeral head was first reported by Flower[51] in 1861, then subsequently by Eve[47] in 1880. However, it was Hill and Sachs[81] who ultimately immortalized this lesion as an accompaniment of recurrent anterior dislocation of the shoulder in a classic article in 1940. The article credits Pilz (1925) with having demonstrated that the detection of this posterolateral defect of the head is dependent on the radiographic technique employed. Although the lesion is frequently visualized on an AP internal rotation view (Fig. 4-12), it is most likely to be seen to good advantage by a **Stryker notch view** (Fig. 4-13). Pavlov et al[150] studied 83 patients with combinations of anterior shoulder subluxations and dislocations and reached the same conclusion. Danzig, Greenway, and Resnick.[35] performed cadaveric

---

Hill-Sachs lesion

- Compression fracture of the posterolateral humeral head
- Results from anterior dislocation
- Best seen on anteroposterior in internal rotation or Stryker notch view

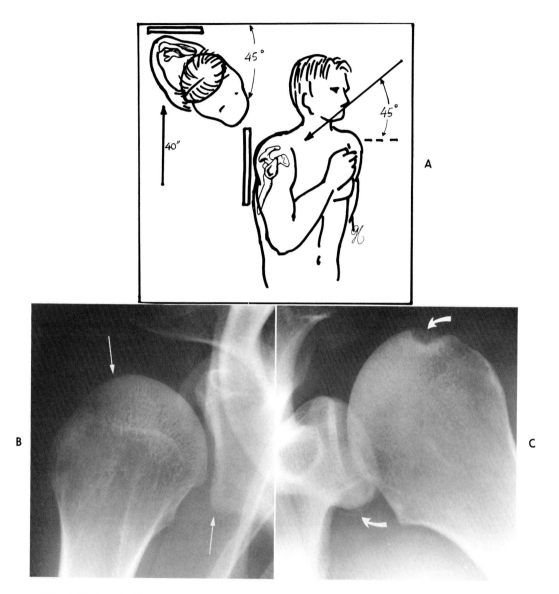

FIG. 4-10. Apical oblique or craniocaudad view. The glenohumeral joint is projected in a cranio-caudad orientation. Useful for evaluation of fracture dislocations. Specifically good for demonstra-tion of Hill-Sachs and Bankart lesions. **A,** Patient is in upright position and the shoulder being stud-ied is 45 degrees posteriorly rotated. The radiographic beam is in an anteroposterior and 45 degrees caudad direction. A variation of this view may be obtained with the patient supine. **B,** The glenohu-meral joint is tangentially visualized. Craniocaudad angulation of the x-ray beam provides a tangen-tial view of the posterosuperior aspect of the humeral head and the anteroinferior aspect of the gle-noid margins *(arrows).* **C,** Anterior instability. Hill-Sachs defect of the humeral head and ectopic ossification along the anterior glenoid margin are visualized *(arrows).* (**A** redrawn from Garth WP, Slappey CE, Ochs CW: *J Bone Joint Surg* 66A(9):1450, 1984.)

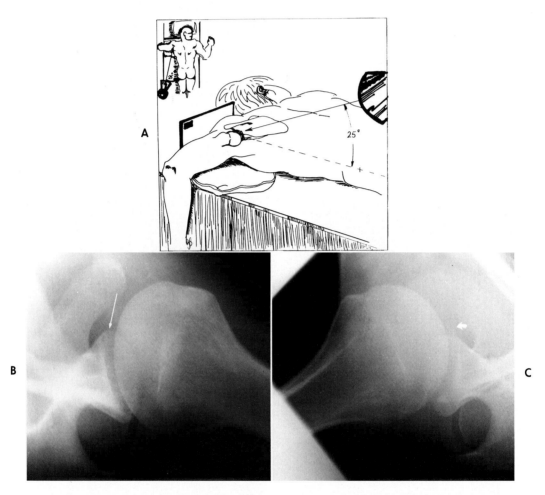

FIG. 4-11. West Point axillary view. The anteroinferior glenoid margin is visualized without structure superimposition. Specifically used for detecting osseous Bankart lesion. **A,** Patient is in prone position with shoulder propped up over a pillow. The arm is in internal rotation and hanging down from the edge of the table. The x-ray beam is angled downward 25 degrees from the horizontal plane and 25 degrees from the sagittal plane of the body. **B,** The anteroinferior glenoid margin is visualized without obstruction (*arrow*). **C,** Anterior instability. Ectopic bone formation (osseous Bankart lesion) of anterior glenoid margin is visualized (*arrow*). (**A** redrawn from Norris TR: Diagnostic techniques for shoulder instability. In AAOS: *Instructional course lectures,* vol 34, St Louis, 1985, Mosby.)

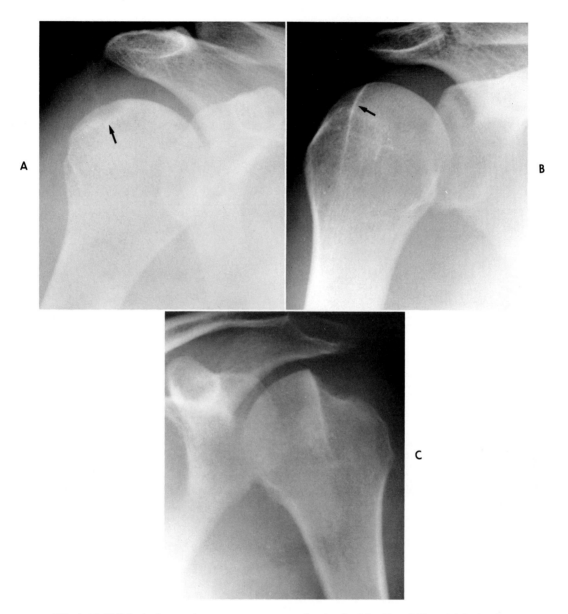

FIG. 4-12. Hill-Sachs lesion. Anterioposterior views of right shoulder (**A** and **B**) and left shoulder (**C**) in three different patients. **A,** This small Hill-Sachs defect is projected as a dense band, parallel to the posterosuperior aspect of the humeral head *(arrow)*. **B,** The posterosuperior articular surface of the humeral head is irregular and is outlined by a dense vertical band medially. This sclerotic band shows the extent of this Hill-Sachs lesion *(arrow)*. **C,** A large defect of the humeral head is visualized.

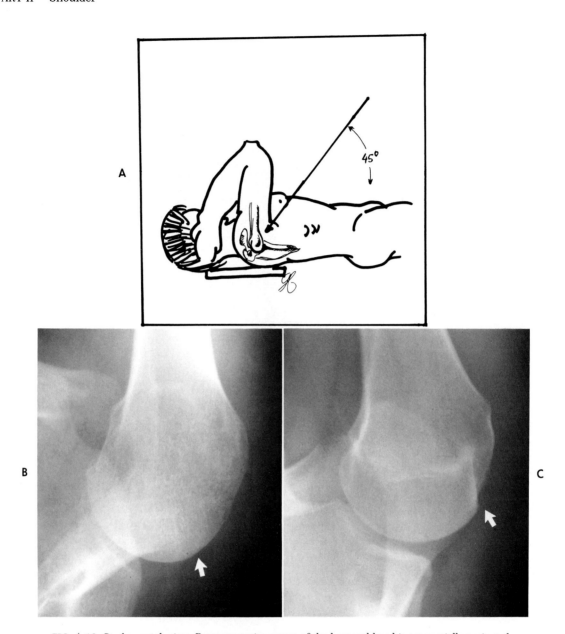

FIG. 4-13. Stryker notch view. Posterosuperior aspect of the humeral head is tangentially projected. Specifically useful for demonstrating Hills-Sachs defect. **A,** The patient is supine. The arm is elevated 90 degrees and the elbow is flexed so that the palm is on the ear or resting on the side of the head. The humerus is parallel to the sagittal plane of the body. The radiographic beam is directed to the axilla 45 degrees from the horizontal plane. A variation of the view may be obtained with a 10-degree cephalad angulation of the beam. **B,** The posterosuperior aspect of the humeral head seen in profile *(arrow)*. **C,** Anterior instability. Hill-Sachs defect is visualized *(arrow)*. (**A** redrawn from Rozing PM, deBakker HM, Obermann WR: *Acta Orthop Scand* 68:479, 1967.)

studies and clinical evaluations on a series of dislocations and concluded that the optimal means for detecting the Hill-Sachs lesion was a combination of three views: an AP view with 45 degrees of internal rotation of the humerus, a Stryker notch view, and a modified Didiee view (Fig. 4-14).[42]

In 1934 Hermodsson[80] described an axillary view performed with the patient supine (Fig. 4-15). This view was conceived to demonstrate the Hermodsson fracture (Hill-Sachs lesion) of the humeral head. In a study of 27 shoulders with recurrent anterior shoulder dislocations, Rozing, deBakker, and Obermann[171] could demonstrate the lesion in only 12 shoulders using the Hermodsson view, whereas the Stryker notch view identified the lesion in 25 of the shoulders. Warren[190] distinguishes between dislocators and subluxators and cites Pavlov et al,[150] who discovered the Hill-Sachs lesion in 80% of the former and in only 25% of the latter.

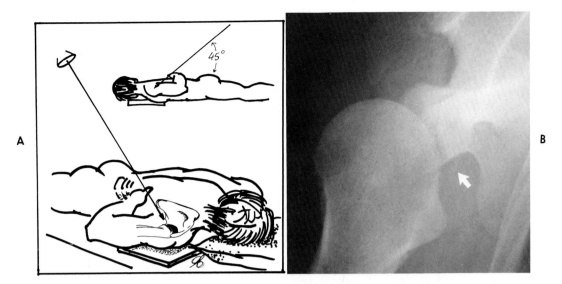

FIG. 4-14. Didiee view. Posterosuperior aspect of the humeral head and anterior glenoid margin are projected. Useful for demonstration of Hill-Sachs and Bankart lesions. **A,** Patient is in prone position. The arm is internally rotated and the dorsum of the hand rests on the iliac crest. The radiographic beam is directed to the humeral head in the plane of the humeral shaft and 45 degrees to the horizontal plane. **B,** Anterior instability. Ectopic ossification (osseous Bankart lesion) is visualized *(arrow).* (**A** redrawn from Rozing PM, deBakker HM, Oberman WR: *Acta Orthop Scand* 68:479, 1967.)

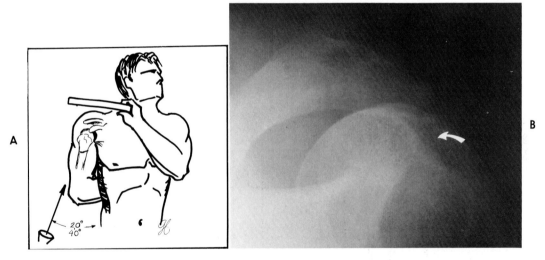

FIG. 4-15. Hermodsson view. The posterolateral aspect of the humeral head is visualized without superimpositions for evaluation of Hill-Sachs defect. **A,** The patient is upright and holds the cassette with the opposite hand against the top of shoulder. The arm is internally rotated and the hand rests against the back. The x-ray beam is directed to the back of the humeral head at an angle of approximately 30 degrees from the sagittal plane or the humeral axis. **B,** Hill-Sachs defect *(arrow).*

Bankart Lesion

In 1923 Bankart[7] contended that detachment of the glenoid labrum is the essential lesion in recurrent anterior dislocations of the glenohumeral joint. Regardless of any controversy centering about this contention, the radiologist has come to regard the presence of an osseous Bankart lesion (fracture or ectopic bone formation about the anterior glenoid rim) as pathognomonic evidence of

anterior instability.[8,13,150] In 1972 Rokous, Feagin, and Abbott[168] reported a new axillary view, now referred to as the **West Point view** (Fig. 4-11), which was conceived for the specific purpose of demonstrating the Bankart lesion.

Norris recommends assessment of the anteroinferior glenoid findings of instability by either the West Point prone axillary view or the supine external rotation

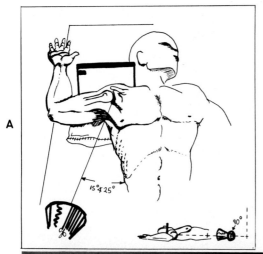

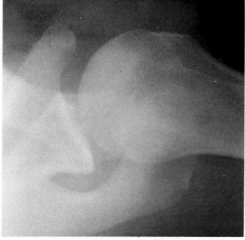

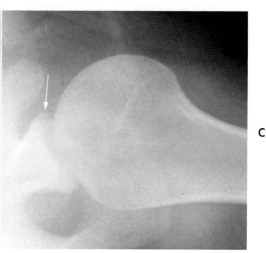

FIG. 4-16. Supine external rotation axillary view of Ciullo. For improved visualization of anteroinferior glenoid margin. Useful for Bankart lesion. **A,** The patient position is similar to that for a routine axillary view. However, the arm is abducted 90 degrees and externally rotated. **B,** Normal. **C,** Small osseous Bankart lesion is visualized (*arrow*). (**A** redrawn from Norris TR: Diagnostic techniques for shoulder instability. In AAOS: *Instructional course lectures,* vol 34, St Louis, 1985, Mosby.)

axillary view of Ciullo[22,23] (Fig. 4-16). He indicates that, although the West Point view gives better detail, the Ciullo view is less difficult to obtain for the uninitiated technician.

Pavlov et al[190] reported that the osseous Bankart lesion is best documented on the West Point and Didiee views. The latter view was described by Didiee[42] in 1930 and has value as well in the detection of the Hill-Sachs lesion, as already indicated (Fig. 4-14). The apical oblique, or craniocaudad oblique, view also has an advantage in that it can reveal both pathognomonic lesions of instability, the Hill-Sachs lesion, and the Bankart lesion (Fig. 4-10). Furthermore, it is simpler to obtain than either the West Point or the Stryker notch view. Mizuno and Hirohata,[128] using a modified West Point view, found anterior displacement of the humeral head in 11% of traumatic anterior subluxations and in 89% of involuntary multidirectional subluxations.

Posterior Instability

Consideration to chronic posterior instability must not be forsaken amidst the more voluminous information regarding anterior instabilities. The main contribution made by conventional radiography for the diagnosis of posterior instability, according to Gambrioli, Maggi, and

Randelli,[55] is the special Y view projection demonstrating the classic anterolateral lesion of the humeral head; this is the counterpart of the Hill-Sachs lesion described by McLaughlin.[112] Posterior instability counterparts of the Bankart fracture and fracture of the greater tuberosity are fractures of the posterior glenoid rim and of the lesser tuberosity. Routine supine axillary views may reveal the McLaughlin fracture as well as deformities of the glenoid margin in patients with posterior instability (Fig. 4-17). Warren[190] admonishes that both the Stryker notch and the West Point views must be carefully evaluated for posterior glenoid lesions indicative of posterior subluxation. In a study of 50 shoulders with recurrent (involuntary) posterior subluxation, Hawkins, Koppert, and Johnston[79] found no abnormalities on routine radiographs. Of these shoulders, 17 were subjected to stress radiographs and cineradiography, which demonstrated posterior instability.

Dynamic Radiography

According to Norris,[144] the conventional radiographic evaluation of inferior glenohumeral instability may be enhanced by the addition of well-padded 20-pound gauntlet forearm weights, which reveal an increased acromiohumeral interval (Fig. 4-18).

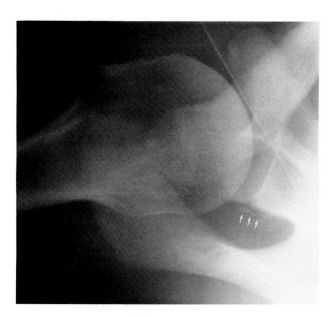

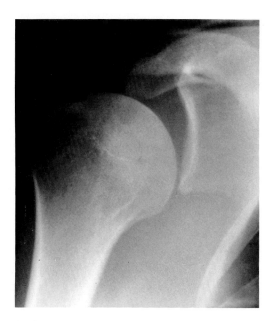

FIG. 4-17. Posterior instability, axillary view. Same patient as in Fig. 4-19. The posterior glenoid margin is irregular and ectopic ossification is present *(arrows).*

FIG. 4-18. Inferior instability. True anteroposterior view of the right shoulder with addition of 10-pound weight to the forearm. Inferior displacement of the humerus and glenohumeral malalignment is demonstrated.

Anterior and posterior drawer tests such as those described by Gerber[59] and recorded by radiographs may be performed with the patient awake or anesthetized to corroborate the presence of an instability, its direction, and its magnitude (Fig. 4-19). Confirmation and documentation of the findings in such instances are best accomplished with C-arm fluoroscopy.[144] It must be appreciated that posterior displacement of the humeral head up to 50% of its width may be within normal limits.

Discussion

In reviewing the morass of available views designed to evaluate traumatic lesions or instabilities of the glenohumeral joint, the physician finds that certain trends are evident. AP views with both internal and external rotation of the humeri are definite standards. The externally rotated view is not valuable for instability evaluation but reveals tuberosity fractures and calcifications about the rotator cuff. In acutely traumatized patients, motion of the arm may be too painful or inhibited by a dislocation. In such instances an AP view may be performed without rotation of the arm. The AP view may be further complemented by the addition of a "true" AP view (in the posterior oblique position), which permits the joint to be visualized tangentially. The transthoracic lateral view is also used in this circumstance, but as pointed out by Kornguth and Salazar[102] in their evaluation of 161 abnormal shoulders after trauma, the view has relatively poor success in detecting glenoid rim fractures, Hill-Sachs lesions, and scapular body fractures. Supine axillary views fail to reveal a number of lesions with consistency, and because positioning for these views may be too painful for many patients, other views must be considered with regularity. The Velpeau axillary, angle up, Stripp axial,

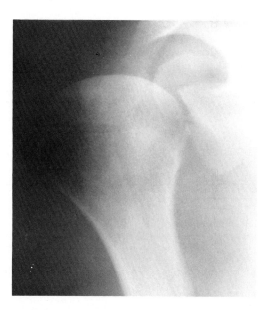

FIG. 4-19. Posterior instability. Craniocaudad (apical oblique) view of the right shoulder (same patient as in Fig. 4-17) was obtained while posterior stress was being applied. Marked posterior displacement of the humeral head is demonstrated. (Courtesy Dr. Ramesh Gidumal, NYU Medical Center.)

and anterior oblique views are helpful for patients whose arms cannot be manipulated because of pain. As noted earlier, the apical oblique, when combined with the appropriate AP examinations, may offer the best diagnostic combination with the least discomfort to the patient.[14,166]

The format and severity of instability (e.g., subluxa-

TABLE 4-1 The efficiency of various radiographic views in evaluation of shoulder abnormalities

A. Instability

1. Modified from Rozing PM, deBakker HM, Obermann WR: *Acta Orthop Scand* 68:479, 1967.
Twenty-seven shoulders, with recurrent anterior dislocation Hill-Sachs defect seen in 26; Bankart defect seen in 10.

View	Hill-Sachs	Bankart
45-degree craniocaudal	22/27	10/10
Stryker notch	25/27	1/10
Didiee	7/27	Not reported
Frontal (AP)	7/27	Not reported
Hermodsson	12/27	0/10
Axial	0/27	2/10

COMMENTARY: 45-degree craniocaudal view has high yield for both lesions. Stryker notch view excellent for Hill-Sachs.
RECOMMENDATION: Do craniocaudal view first, and if defect is not seen, do Stryker notch view. West Point and Didiee views may be added to see Bankart lesion.

2. Modified from Danzig LA, Greenway G, Resnick D: *Am J Sports Med* 8(5):328, 1980.
The Hill-Sachs Lesion in 15 patients with anterior shoulder dislocation.

View	Result
AP external rotation	1/15
AP internal rotation 45 degrees	*15/15
Axillary	7/15
AP internal rotation 20 degrees	4/15
PA external rotation 45 degrees	10/15
PA internal rotation 45 degrees	*12/15
Stryker notch	*14/15
Modified Didiee	*12/15

RECOMMENDATION: Take three views to show Hill-Sachs: AP (or PA) in 45-degree internal rotation, Stryker notch, and Didiee.
*Views that are particularly efficacious.

3. Modified from Pavlov H et al: *Clin Orthop* 194:153, 1985.
a. A study of 83 patients with unilateral anterior shoulder instability.

View	Hill-Sachs	Bankart
Internal rotation	92%	15%
External rotation	32%	65%
Axillary	44%	66%
West Point	51%	70%
Stryker notch	92%	11%
Didiee	35%	71%

COMMENTARY: Maximal yield in diagnosing the lesions of anterior instability are achieved with three combined views: AP internal rotation, Stryker notch, and either West Point or Didiee.

b. (1) Lesion %	Bankart or Hill-Sachs	Hill-Sachs and Bankart	Isolated Hill-Sachs	Isolated Bankart	Normal
	82%	16%	61%	5%	18%

(2)	Hill-Sachs	Bankart
	(with or without each other)	
Subluxations	66%	40%
Dislocations	77%	15%
Combined	87%	20%

COMMENTARY: Isolated Hill-Sachs occurs much more often than isolated Bankart. One or the other is often present, but they occur together infrequently. The type of instability bears upon defect incidence.

B. General Trauma

1. Modified from DeSmet AA: *Am J Radiol* 134:515, 1980.

Acute trauma	AP external rotation	AP external and internal rotation	Anterior oblique	AP internal rotation and anterior oblique
Anterior dislocation	0	0	0	8
Humeral head fracture	2	0	*1	4
AC separation	0	0	0	5
Clavicle fracture	0	0	0	3
Scapular fracture	0	1	3	2

NOTE: 60-degree anterior oblique = Y view.

COMMENTARY: In this series four fractures (*) would have been missed without an anterior oblique projection. It may be obtained at 45 degrees or 60 degrees and requires no movement of the humerus.

2. Modified from Kornguth PJ, Salazar AM: *Am J Radiol* 149(1):113, 1987.

Abnormality	n.	AP percent	Lateral percent	Y view percent	Apical oblique percent
Humerus fracture	56	100	70	68	93
GH dislocation	34	100	94	91	100*
Clavicle fracture	22	100	9	68	73
Glenoid rim fracture	7	39	0	11	94†
AC separation	14	100	14	21	14
Hill-Sachs lesion	5	42	8	8	100‡
Scapular fracture	9	90	30	50	50

COMMENTARY: Twenty of 161 abnormalities would have been missed in a study of 511 traumatized shoulders if an apical oblique (45-degree posterior oblique with 45-degree caudal angulation) view was not performed. It is a good view to show posterior glenohumeral dislocation (*), glenoid rim fractures (†), and Hill-Sachs lesions (‡).

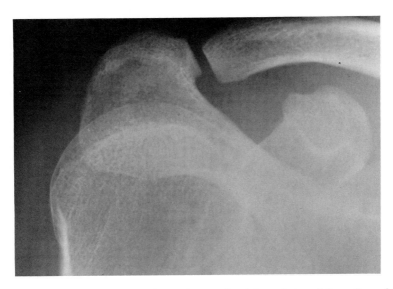

FIG. 4-20. Normal right acromioclavicular (AC) joint. Cranial angulation of the radiographic beam projects the AC joint above and clear of the acromion process.

tion vs. dislocation) may bear upon the yield of radiographic evidence for its existence on one or more of the axillary or oblique views selected for diagnosis. Garth, Slappey, and Ochs[58] suggested that the size of a Hill-Sachs lesion had no apparent relationship to the chronicity or recurrence rate of instability. Though views such as the Didiee and apical oblique are capable of revealing both Hill-Sachs and Bankart lesions, other views may be more proficient in the detection of one or the other of these lesions. Table 4-1 is a collation of studies by various authors who have attempted to compare the efficacies of different views for the detection of a variety of traumatic and instability lesions.

Acromioclavicular Joint

The AC joint is ordinarily well visualized on all AP views of the shoulder. There is, however, a technical difficulty in the radiographic examination of the acromial arch region on the AP projection. The thickness of the proximolateral aspect of the shoulder is considerably less than that of the glenohumeral and axillary regions. Therefore optimal visualization of the latter regions is often achieved at the expense of the AC joint and subacromial regions. The use of the appropriately designed filters can overcome this problem. These filters may be in the form of a graduated aluminum plate attached to the x-ray tube with its thicker end up against the top of the shoulder. They may also come in the form of a silicone rubber pad placed on the shoulder. Vezina[189] has employed a silicone absorption filter to enhance clarity of the acromioclavicular window even when performing such studies as arthrotomography in evaluating a ruptured rotator cuff. In any case, when a filter is used the beam is more attenuated by the filter's proximal end, preventing overpenetration of the proximal portion of the shoulder.

Visualization of the AC joint is also enhanced by a 15-degree cranial angulation of the x-ray beam (Fig. 4-20). This joint, however, has a variable orientation. Nevi-

aser[139] indicated that the plane of the acromioclavicular joint varies from vertical to nearly horizontal. When AC joint separation is suspected, it is common practice to examine the joint with 5 to 15 pounds of weight attached to the patient's wrists. This examination most often includes both shoulders for purposes of comparison. The apposition of the acromion to the articular end of the clavicle is evaluated, as is the coracoclavicular interval.[193] The usual coracoid to clavicle distance is 1.1 to 1.3 cm; an increase in this interval is indicative of a coracoclavicular ligamentous disruption (Fig. 4-21). With increasing severity of the grade of sprain and elevation of the lateral portion of the clavicle, there is a progressive widening of the AC joint.[150] Horizontal instability of the clavicle is not appreciated by standard radiographic techniques. Occasionally, intraarticular fractures may mimic a separation on physical inspection and/or accompany a separation (Figs. 4-22 and 4-23). Realistically, the search for fractures is perhaps more important than the evaluation for separation, since the latter is most readily discerned by physical examination. Except for the most flagrant separations, such as the subcutaneous variety of the Rockwood classification,[167] which requires a reattachment of the large extrinsic muscles, sports physicians are moving away from early operative fixations of the joint or even protracted immobilizations[30] in favor of early mobilization and strengthening.

Examination of the chronically separated joint may reveal a displaced, enlarged, and arthritic clavicular head and/or ossifications where the coracoclavicular ligaments had existed (Fig. 4-23).

In Search of the Supraspinatus Syndrome

According to Jobe and Jobe,[87] "the most common shoulder problem in sports medicine is impingement syndrome associated with bursitis, rotator cuff inflammation and tears, and bicipital tendinitis." The presence of impingement, or the supraspinatus syndrome, implies the existence of symptoms or functional disability ema-

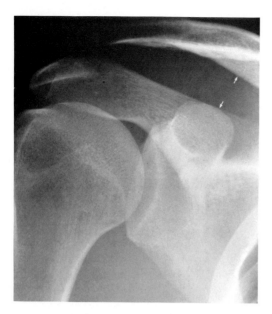

FIG. 4-21. Coracoclavicular ligament disruption. Anteroposterior view of right shoulder following acute trauma. Acromioclavicular joint separation is evident. The coracoclavicular distance *(arrows)* of 1.7 cm indicated ligamentous disruption.

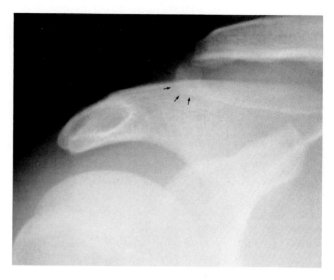

FIG. 4-22. Intraarticular fracture of the distal clavicle with acromioclavicular separation. A fracture of the distal end of the clavicle with involvement of its articular surface is demonstrated following acute trauma in this professional hockey player. The articular fracture fragment is displaced and rotated inferiorly *(arrows)*.

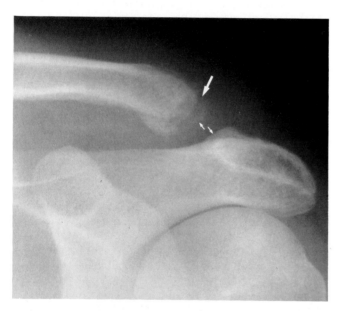

FIG. 4-23. Intraarticular fracture of the distal clavicle. A healing fracture is evident *(long arrow)*. The articular component remains properly aligned with the acromial articular surface *(small arrows)*.

nating from one or more of the tissues of which the subacromial region is comprised. Most commonly these manifestations result directly or indirectly from the inflammation or tearing of the rotator cuff or the existence of an obstruction to tissue glide within the subacromial space. The role of available diagnostic radiography for this entity and its related pathologic conditions is variable, because it is predicated on the patronage of pre-

scribing physicians whose need for quantified proof of diagnosis and prognosis is variable. The diagnosis of rotator cuff tears and impingements is based upon a spectrum of evidence that ranges from circumstantial to pathognomonic. With respect to the rotator cuff, physical examination can provide reasonably strong evidence of disruption in many cases, but pathognomonic demonstrations are accomplished only by radiography (arthrography, sonography, and MRI) and surgery. Impingement, on the other hand, is perhaps most confidently diagnosed by physical examination. Radiography merely adds credence to a strong circumstantial case. Unfortunately, there is no objective and quantitative measure of impingement. In fact, impingement is not even a single entity but a syndrome that may be multiply derived from a gamut of pathologic states. It is an eponym for a group of painful motion syndromes about the shoulder having some abnormality of glide of the subacromial structures, as a common denominator.

Preoperative radiographic evaluation must be pursued for those patients and surgeons concerned with a quantitative assessment of pathologic conditions, a measure of the difficulty of the intended surgery, an anticipation of the duration and quantity of postoperative disability, and a foreknowledge of predictive success and prognosis.

Disease of the rotator cuff tendons and dysfunction attributable to alterations of the anatomy and mechanics of the periacromial region are intimately related. These entities are also intimately related with respect to the conventional radiographic signs they produce, especially in more chronic cases.

In 1961 Golding[64] reported that cystic erosion of the anatomic neck is pathognomonic of a tear of the rotator cuff. Godsil and Linscheid[63] observed conventional radiographic alterations in 100% of patients between 36 and 76 years of age with rotator cuff tears. The duration

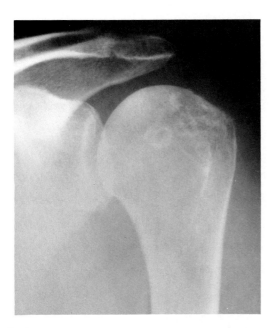

FIG. 4-24. Rotator cuff disease. Anteroposterior view of left shoulder. There are multiple cystic erosions of the anatomic neck and greater tuberosity regions. The tuberosity is flattened and the humeral head is sclerotic.

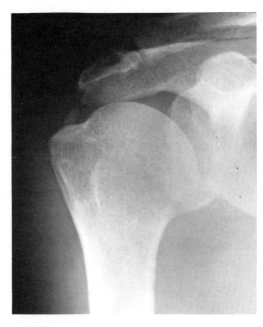

FIG. 4-25. Calcific tendonitis, right shoulder. Amorphous calcium deposition is present in the immediate vicinity of the greater tuberosity and in expected orientation of the supraspinatus tendon. The tuberosity is sclerotic and also a manifestation of impingement syndrome.

of cuff disease in the 59 patients studied was difficult to deduce. The degenerative changes observed included the following: (1) subcortical cystic erosion at the angle of cuff insertion into the greater tuberosity and (2) late sclerosis of the acromioclavicular joint and humeral head (implying their mutual articulation) (Fig. 4-24).

Both Golding[64] and Godsil and Linscheid[63] reported their observations before the renaissance of the concept of impingement. The issue is raised as to which of the radiologic observations are attributable to rotator cuff disease and which to impingement.

Impingement within or about the coracoacromial arch was an established source of shoulder disability long before Neer[132] reacquainted orthopaedists with it in 1972. According to Ciullo, Koniuch, and Teitge[23] the athletic impingement syndrome was first described in baseball pitchers (1906) by Codman. Gerber, Terrier, and Ganz[60] refer to the works of Meyer (1922) and Watson Jones (1943) as additional cornerstones in the establishment of impingement as a disabling entity for shoulders.

Conventional radiography generally reveals no evidence of impingement in its earlier stages when the soft tissues are the primary source of involvement.[25] Repetitious trauma to these tissues induces a progression of fibrin deposition, edema and inflammation, granulation formation, and tissue calcification or ossification (Fig. 4-25). Only the latter may be detected by conventional radiography. Hence, conventional radiographic evidence of impingement only becomes evident in Stage III[133] (see Chapter 8) cases when tendon degeneration or rupture has already occurred.[78] The characteristic radiographic findings of impingement thus relate more to the middle-aged groups rather than to the younger groups of patients with the syndrome.

Ellman, Hanker, and Bayer[45] operated on 50 nonath-

letic patients with shoulder pain, three quarters of whom had clinical manifestations of Neer's impingement Stages II or III.[133] Conventional radiography revealed greater tuberosity cysts in 60% and rarefaction or sclerosis in 76%. There were acromial cysts in 30% and lateral or inferior sclerosis in 74%. A concave acromial undersurface (from articulation with the humerus) was present in 36%. These findings bear more than a casual similarity to those reported by Godsil and Linscheid[63] in cases of documented rupture of the rotator cuff. Cone, Resnick, and Danzig[27] reported their findings in cases of shoulder impingement. Consistent among their findings were bony proliferation, sclerosis, and cystic changes of the greater tuberosity. These changes are more often seen in association with the presence of subacromial traction spurs, whereas a flattened, sclerotic appearance is most likely to be seen when there is an associated complete rupture of the rotator cuff. The cuff arthropathy referred to by Neer[133] obviously encompasses the changes resulting from impingement. While Neer contends that impingement precedes cuff tears and is responsible for 95% of all cuff tears, it is difficult to determine the chronology of radiographic findings attributable to each. It would certainly seem that sclerosis of the greater tuberosity, acromion, and humeral head and the concave undersurface appearance of the acromion are findings largely attributable to an associated complete rupture of the rotator cuff (Fig. 4-26). Since some of these findings imply an articulation of the humeral head with the acromion as a consequence of a reduction of tissues occupying the acromiohumeral interval, it is appropriate to interrupt the discussion of impingement in favor of a discussion of conventional radiography of the ruptured rotator cuff.

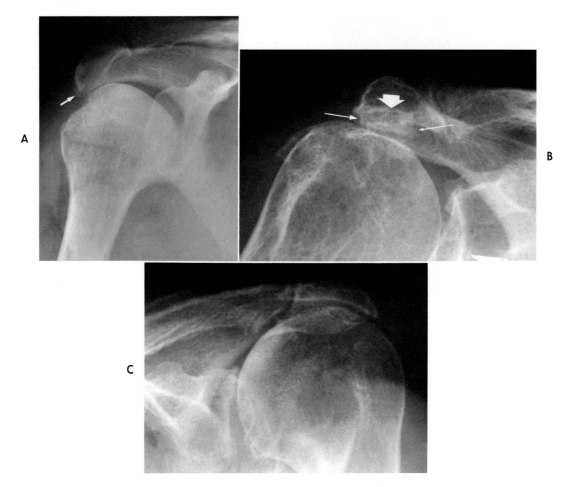

FIG. 4-26. Rotator cuff disease and impingement. **A,** Right shoulder; both the greater tuberosity and the acromion process are sclerotic. Hypertrophic changes of the peripheral margin of the acromion are also evident *(arrow)*. **B,** Right shoulder. There is bone formation *(long arrows)* along the undersurfaces of the acromion process *(large arrow)*. This occupies the subacromial space and is conformed to the humeral head contour. **C,** Left shoulder. Superior migration of the humeral head is evident. The anterior acromion process and the distal clavicle have developed a concave appearance as a result of articulation with the humeral head.

Beltran et al[9] refer to the work of Bretzke et al[17] in stating that the thickness of the supraspinatus is approximately 6 mm. Diminution of the interval between the humeral head and the acromion, which is occupied by the supraspinatus and its surrounding soft tissues, implied rupture of the rotator cuff. Petersson and Redlund-Johnell[153] studied almost 200 shoulders of almost 100 patients with neither symptoms nor degenerative changes. They measured the shortest distance between the inferior aspect of the acromion and the top of the humeral head. Remembering that the space is occupied by acromial periosteum, areolar tissue, and bursa, as well as by the supraspinatus, the measured intervals on AP radiographs were as follows:

$$\male: 9.7 \text{ mm} (\pm 1.5 \text{ mm}) \text{ to } 10.2 \text{ mm} (\pm 1.7 \text{ mm})$$
$$\female: 9.2 \text{ mm} (\pm 1.4 \text{ mm})$$

The interval diminished with age in males only. The authors stated that a space of less than 6 mm is abnormal in a middle-aged person (Fig. 4-20). Upward subluxation

of the humeral head, according to Cofield,[24] is almost always more pronounced on external than on internal rotation views (Fig. 4-26, *C*).

The acromiohumeral interval may bear prognostic as well as diagnostic import. In their study, Ellman, Hanker, and Bayer[45] found that patients whose acromiohumeral distance was less than 7 mm had larger tears and less strength and motion than others after cuff repair.

Bloom[12] and Cotty et al[29] suggest an ability to detect rotator cuff tears using an active abduction view. In the former the arm was raised against gravity, whereas the latter study used a weighted resistance. The authors noted a diminished acromiohumeral interval in some patients with rotator cuff tears later proven by arthrography.

A discussion of impingement may now be resumed with the knowledge that the most flagrant radiographic evidence of its presence is observed in association with complete ruptures of the rotator cuff.

Petersson and Gentz[152] studied 47 shoulders of pa-

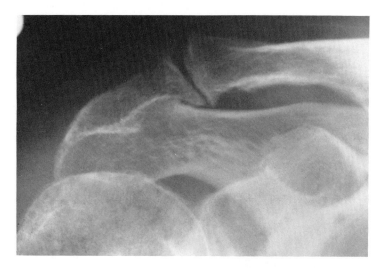

FIG. 4-27. Acromioclavicular spur. Anteroposterior view with upward angulation of the beam demonstrates inferiorly pointing osteophytes of the acromioclavicular joint.

tients with arthrographically proven supraspinatus ruptures, 50 normal shoulders, and 170 cadaveric shoulders, of which 54 had partial or complete supraspinatus rupture. Among the groups studied just over 50% of shoulders with supraspinatus ruptures had distally pointing acromioclavicular osteophytes, while less than 15% of the remaining shoulders had them (Fig. 4-27). In addition, the "ruptured" groups manifested anterior lipping of the acromion in 20% to 25% of shoulders, as described by Neer.[132] The contentions of Petersson and Gentz[152] and of Kessel and Watson,[88] who found the acromioclavicular osteophytes in one third of their supraspinatus ruptures, would point up the importance of scrutinizing the acromioclavicular joint in such cases.

Anterior acromial spurs (Fig. 4-26, *A* and *B*) and distally pointing acromioclavicular spurs have thus been identified as two important additional findings of impingement, the latter being particularly associated with ruptures of the supraspinatus. Neer[132,133] has repeatedly played up the importance of the anterior acromion in the creation of symptomatic impingements and contends that the posterior half of the acromion is not involved in the impingement process. He further asserts that individuals with a less sloped acromion and a more prominent anterior edge on its undersurface are predisposed to cuff tears secondary to impingement, and that it is therefore logical to perform acromioplasty at the time of every cuff repair. Cone, Resnick, and Danzig[27] reported some interesting observations about the relationship between subacromial spurs and other findings associated with their presence. One third of their patients evidencing such spurs also had spurs about the intertubercular sulcus, which appeared on bicipital groove views. Nearly half the patients with subacromial spurs had degenerative changes of the AC joint as opposed to only 15% of those without subacromial spurs.

Kessel and Watson,[88] who add the eponym of painful arc syndrome to those of impingement and the supraspinatus syndrome, discount the portent of the subacromial spur. However, they reassert the importance of the acromioclavicular spurs (rather than the spurs of the anterior acromion). They develop a theme that the varying manifestations (symptoms and radiographic signs) of their painful arc syndrome are in fact attributable to different subtypes of impingement.

Kessel and Watson[88] studied nearly 100 patients with painful arc syndromes. Using physical examination, local anesthetic injections, and contrast radiography to determine the sites and sources of problems, they determined that patients afflicted with the syndrome were divisible into three distinct groups of equal distribution. The third of patients with the posterior type had no visible pathologic condition, no AC joint disease, pain on internal rotation, and an excellent response to conservative management. The third with the anterior type had no visible pathologic condition, no AC joint disease, pain on external rotation, and an occasional need for surgery. The last third, with a superior type, had AC joint disease and rotator cuff degeneration. Decompressive surgery was often needed.

The findings of Cone, Resnick, and Danzig[27] are consistent with the concept of multifocal impingements and the use of impingement tests ascribable to several arcs of shoulder motion. Their fluoroarthrography studies revealed a correlation in some patients between the production of pain with elevation of the arm and the point at which the humeral tuberosities and acromion were in their closest apposition. In these cases pain was maximal during abduction of 70 to 120 degrees and 20 to 30 degrees of external rotation or during 70 to 120 degrees of elevation and more than 30 degrees of internal rotation.

Conventional radiography offers little in documenting impingement in its earlier stages. Special radiography to be presented in the ensuing sections has more to offer in this regard, particularly with respect to tears of the rotator cuff. In the advanced stages of impingement the radiographic signs discussed in the preceding paragraphs offer testimony in support of operations predicted on the concept that the acromial arch region is respon-

sible for the production of symptoms. Evidence presented in this section has derived largely from studies of nonathletic populations.

COMPUTED AXIAL TOMOGRAPHY
General Concepts

Modern CT scanners are capable of producing high-resolution images with excellent detailing of the bony architecture. Software packages are available that can selectively enhance either soft tissue or bony detail; they can enlarge focal segments of images or regions of in-

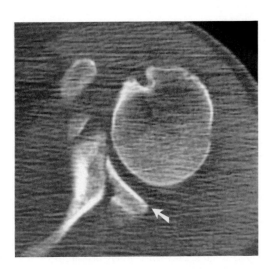

FIG. 4-28. Comminuted fracture of the left glenoid. This single computed tomography section shows that the major articular component of the glenoid as a whole is displaced posteriorly *(arrow)*. The humeral head remains in alignment with this major fragment, while a small fragment is displaced and rotated anteriorly. Superoinferior displacements are determined by viewing all axial sections.

terest as the images are being reconstructed; and they provide capability for image reformation in sagittal, coronal, or oblique planes. Additional computer hardware and software are obtainable for three-dimensional reconstruction and display.

CT of the shoulder without enhancement by contrast media is indicated when plain radiography has failed to adequately substantiate a suspected osseous or periarticular abnormality (Fig. 4-28). CT is beneficial for the evaluation of acute intraarticular fractures, such as comminuted fractures of the humeral head, as an aid to surgical planning. It is also of value in the recognition of some ossifications (Fig. 4-29) and fractures associated with glenohumeral instability. Obviously, it can document any existing degree of glenohumeral dislocations.[41] CT is indicated when there is reason to suspect the presence of osseous or soft-tissue tumors about the shoulder.

Shoulder computed tomography assets

- Intraarticular fractures
- Periarticular ossification or calcification
- Humeral head fractures
- Glenohumeral relationship

Technique

The imaging technique for the shoulder ordinarily requires patients to be placed in the supine position with the arm at the side. For patients with wide shoulder girdles, the contralateral arm must be manipulated to a position that allows the hand to cradle the back of the patient's head. In this way the formation of striking artifacts on axial images resulting from a wide shoulder girdle is avoided.

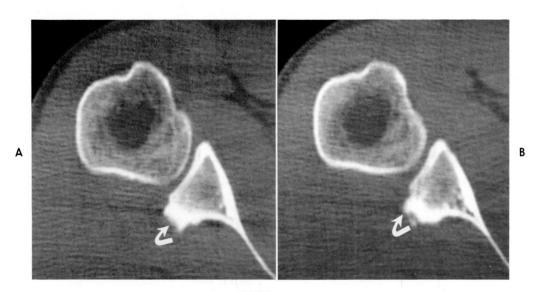

FIG. 4-29. Ossification of the posterior glenoid margin in a baseball pitcher. Consecutive computed tomography sections of the right shoulder (**A** and **B**) at approximately midglenoid level. An ossific ridge is formed along the posterior glenoid margin *(arrows)* at the site of insertion of the posterior joint capsule.

Slice thickness will vary in accordance with the pathologic entity suspected. Ordinarily, 5-mm sections provide adequate bony detail and are suitable for the evaluation of traumatic lesions of the shoulder. The slice thickness can be increased to 10 mm when larger lesions of the paraarticular structures are suspected. This is in contradistinction to the thinner, 3-mm sections commonly used in performing CT arthrography.

The hard copies are produced twice, first with wide window settings (2000/200) for bone viewing, and then with narrow window settings (500/50) for the viewing of soft tissue detail.

Scapulometry and Instability

Seltzer and Weissman[180] used CT scapulometry to evaluate certain parameters in normal patients and those with shoulder instability. The only finding of interest was the maintenance of the humeral head in the central third of the glenoid on all cuts in normal shoulders but not necessarily in those with instability. Past investigators such as Saha[173,174] have devised scapulometric techniques for the purpose of determining telltale version and torsion abnormalities of unstable shoulders. Cyprien et al[34] devised their own group of measurements and concluded that angular and torsional values vary little between normal and recurrently dislocating shoulders. Although index of contact between the humeral head and glenoid is smaller in patients with recurrent anterior dislocation than in normal patients, Cyprien et al[34] found no consistent deviations of humeral retroversion in the group of dislocators.

Norris[144] claimed that lesions and version of the glenoid and humeral head are best revealed with computed axial tomography (CAT) and may be a particular help in the planning of bony reconstructions.

Gambrioli, Maggi, and Randelli[55,162] indicated that CT scanning is valuable in the determination of three morphologic factors that Saha[174] determined to be pertinent to anterior instability:

1. *Glenoid tilt*—orientation of the glenoid articular surface in relation to the plane of the shoulder
2. *Angle of retroversion*—proximal end of the humerus
3. *Glenohumeral index*—ratio of maximal diameters (transverse) of the glenoid and humeral head

However, Gambrioli, Maggi, and Randelli[55] studied 50 normal subjects, 24 patients with anterior instability, and 9 patients with posterior instability and found no relevance of these factors to a distinction between the groups studied.

When considering operative approaches for posterior instabilities unresponsive to conservative management, Warren[190] used CT and axillary radiographs to determine the degree of glenoid version. If the version is abnormal and the angle exceeds 20 degrees, Warren considers an osteotomy of the scapular neck. It is an interesting corollary that, failing to demonstrate version alteration of the glenoid in cases of anterior instability, Gambrioli, Maggi, and Randelli[55] were able to demonstrate an increase in glenoid cavity retroversion inferiorly in chronic cases of posterior instability. Presumably this is attributable to the erosive changes of the posteroinferior portion of the glenoid over time, indenting its profile on scan cuts at inferior glenoid level.

Obviously there must be a better resolution to the controversy concerning the value of scapulometry in the formulation of surgical indications for instability. Surely the interpretation of CT requires a different and more sophisticated knowledge of anatomy. Deutsch, Resnick, and Mink[40] point out that the interpretation of shoulder pathology examined by CT is largely predicated upon a knowledge of axial anatomy. For example, the glenoid is mildly retroverted superiorly and undergoes a transition to anteversion as more caudad sections are taken.

Subcoracoid Impingement

Subcoracoid impingement was described in 1909 by Goldthwait; as with other impingement forms, radiographic evidence is limited, even on CT.[61] This form of impingement produces dull anterior shoulder pain with distal radiation, aggravated by forward flexion and internal rotation. Although the more common varieties of impingement produce pain on full forward flexion, the subcoracoid type produces maximal pain in the forward flexion arc from 80 degrees to 130 degrees and at 90 degrees of abduction with the humerus internally rotated.[60]

Gerber, Terrier, and Ganz[60] and Gerber et al[61] performed CT scapulometry to determine its relevance to the diagnosis of this syndrome. These studies revealed a narrowed coracoid-to-humeral head distance with the arm abducted and internally rotated in patients with clinically diagnosed impingement. Furthermore, patients with signs of subcoracoid impingement were 1.5 times more likely to produce a reduction of the coracohumeral space with the arm flexed and internally rotated than with the arm at the side. Recommendations for coracoacromial ligament and coracoid tip resection were made on the basis of these studies.

CONVENTIONAL SHOULDER ARTHROGRAPHY
General Concepts

Arthrography of the shoulder was initially described by Oberholzer (1933), who used air as a contrast medium to evaluate capsular distortions that occurred after dislocations. In 1939 Lindblom[106] used single contrast arthrography to document ruptures of the rotator cuff. As recently as 1968 Killoran, Marcove, and Freiberger[94] indicated that arthrography of the shoulder was not in widespread use despite its ability to demonstrate the character of the glenohumeral capsule and ruptures of the rotator cuff. Ghelman and Goldman[62] were responsible for the popularization of double contrast arthrography (1977). The diagnostic use of arthrography (with and without CT or tomography) has been expanded to include the evaluation of the glenoid labrum. On occasion distention arthrography has been used in the treatment evaluation of the frozen shoulder.

The two popular techniques used today are single and double contrast arthrography.

Technique of Single Contrast Arthrography

Routine radiographic examination of the shoulder is performed before the arthrographic procedure. Antero-

posterior, internal-external, axillary, and bicipital groove views are obtained and reviewed. The procedure is performed with the patient supine on the fluoroscopic table. Although most orthopaedic surgeons prefer to aspirate or inject a shoulder through a posterior approach, most radiologists prefer an anterior approach to the joint.

After sterile preparation of the shoulder region and the infiltration of a local anesthetic, a 20-gauge, 3.5 cm long disposable spinal needle is inserted into the glenohumeral joint using fluoroscopic guidance. If the injection

of a small amount of positive contrast material confirms an intraarticular position of the needle, 16 ml of contrast medium is injected and the needle is withdrawn. The contrast agent most often used is 60% meglumine diatrizoate.

Four views are obtained after withdrawal of the needle: AP views in internal and external rotation, an axillary view, and a bicipital groove view. Unless a complete tear of the rotator is immediately evident, the same views are repeated after the joint is exercised.

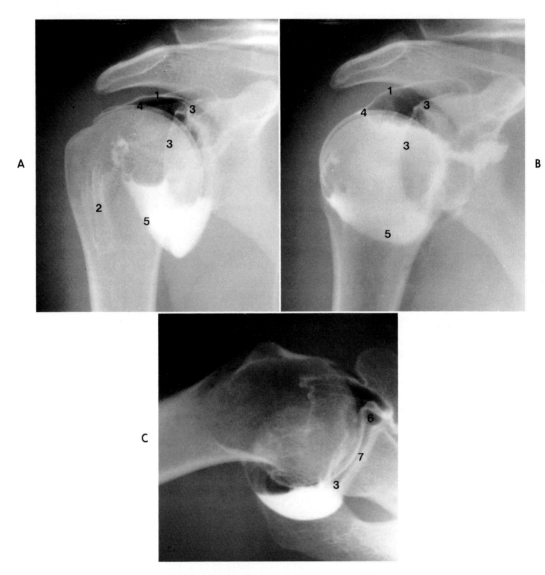

FIG. 4-30. Normal double contrast shoulder arthrogram of right shoulder. Anteroposterior views with patient standing and holding 5-pound weight, in external rotation (**A**) and internal rotation (**B**). The undersurface of the rotator cuff (*1*), the long head of the biceps tendon, (*2*) the superior and posterior glenoid labrum (*3*), the humeral articular surface (*4*), and the joint capsule (*5*) are optimally visualized. **C,** Supine axillary view. The glenohumeral articular components are visualized. The excess positive contrast is pooled in the posterior joint space and therefore the anterior glenoid labrum (*6*) is clearly visualized. A prone axillary view improves visualization of the posterior glenoid labrum (*3*), which in this view is partially obscured by pooling of contrast material. The glenoid articular cartilage (*7*) is also clearly seen.

Technique of Double Contrast Arthrography

This technique has been advocated for enhanced visualization of the rotator cuff, the joint surfaces, and the labrum (Fig. 4-30). The contrast medium used consists of 4 ml of a positive contrast agent admixed with ⅓ ml of 1:1000 epinephrine and 12 ml of room air. After the injection of contrast medium, anteroposterior views are taken with the patient in the upright position with 5-pound weights fastened to the wrists.

To enhance visualization of the rotator cuff, Garcia[56] hangs 6 to 10 pounds of weight from the patient's wrist. On AP views with 15 degrees caudal angulation of the central beam, the acromiohumeral space is increased an average of 25 to 35 mm, the tendons of the biceps and rotator cuff are well separated, and the shape of the torn segments is well visualized. An axillary view is then taken with the patient in the supine position. As with the single contrast technique, if a complete tear of the cuff is not immediately evident, the joint is exercised and the radiographic series is repeated.

Errors and Morbidity

False negative arthrographic studies are obviously a problem when rotator cuff tears are incomplete, either intratendinous or on the superior surface, or when they have been sealed by encompassing granulations. Full thickness tears are easier to detect. Nevertheless, Killoran, Marcove, and Freiberger[94] caution that errors can be made when there is inadequate distribution of contrast; a tardy arrival of contrast within the bursa may be seen on delayed films. This is the rationale for the routine taking of radiographs before and after exercise when a tear is not immediately evident. Direct and inadvertent injection into an enlarged bursa can also be misconstrued as a complete tear of the rotator cuff.

Shoulder arthrography (single or double contrast) with or without the use of epinephrine or local anesthetics as a diluting agent has, in general, been a safe procedure. Anaphylactoid reactions, chemically induced synovitis, and even infections have occurred as a consequence of arthrography, especially in its early years. Patients are most apprehensive, however, of the pain associated with the placement of a needle in the shoulder joint and of the painful aftermath reported to them by others who have undergone the procedure. Severe postprocedural pain has not been commonly reported. In our experience such pain occurs most commonly among patients with severe pain before studies are done.

Hall et al[74] could find little morbidity attributable to arthrography in a 30-year review of the English-language literature. Nevertheless, significant shoulder discomfort occurred within 48 hours of the procedure in 74% of 72 patients evaluated. The least discomfort was reported in the group subjected to double contrast arthrography. This was so despite the advocated use of epinephrine with its potentiating effects for the double contrast technique. Its use is unnecessary in single contrast arthrography, and it is rather mandatory for CT arthrography or arthropneumotomography for prolongation of the time during which an optimal tomographic study can be performed.

In a 1985 sequel study to their 1981 study,[74] Hall et al[75] found that moderate or severe delayed exacerbation of baseline discomfort after shoulder arthrography occurred in only 14% of those examined with metrizamide, an anionic medium, and in 45% of those studied with the conventional double contrast technique. Hence postprocedural pain is related to several factors, including a direct irritant effect of contrast material on the synovium and the hyperosmolar nature of these agents. The latter phenomena result in diffusion of fluids across the synovium, causing further joint distention. These effects are greater with sodium salts, rather than the meglumine salt of the contrast medium most commonly employed in arthrography. In conclusion, the double contrast arthrographic technique using the meglumine salt of the positive contrast agent without the addition of epinephrine is associated with the lowest morbidity rate. However, epinephrine must be used when arthrotomographic techniques are employed for evaluation of the glenoid labrum. Nonionic contrast agents are likely to be safer though their higher cost is a prohibitive factor.

Single Versus Double Contrast Arthrography

There is consensus that the double contrast arthrography is capable of revealing more information about the character of a cuff tear. Mink, Harris, and Rappaport[123] found double contrast arthrography to have a greater than 99% accuracy in the detection of surgically proven full-thickness tears. Pavlov and Freiberger[149] indicated that, although an accurate diagnosis of a torn rotator cuff can be made by single contrast arthrography, double contrast arthrography better delineates the size of the tear and the character of its edges (Fig. 4-31).

Goldman and Ghelman[65] reported that, although both single and double contrast techniques are accurate in diagnosing full-thickness and inferior surface tears of the rotator cuff, only double contrast arthrography can demonstrate the quality of the tendon ends and help delineate the width of a tear. Mink, Harris, and Rappaport[123] using three grades to distinguish tear size and three grades to distinguish cuff quality, found that they did not err by more than a grade as determined by surgical correlation. On the other hand, Ellman, Hanker, and Bayer[45] found that neither single nor double contrast arthrography was of consistent accuracy in quantitating the size of a tear before surgery.

Neer and Welsh[135] indicated that double contrast arthrography with or without tomography requires special experience in attempting to identify the size of identifiable tears in the rotator cuff. Cofield[24] stated that double contrast arthrography reveals more information about the synovium and articular surfaces and, when combined with tomography, may define the size of a tear. However, Cofield indicated that the single contrast arthrogram usually suffices for the diagnosis of a cuff tear and probably with fewer false negative results.

Arthrography and the Rotator Cuff

A suspected tear of the rotator cuff is the most common indication for shoulder arthrography.[65]

Incomplete tears of the rotator cuff are either of the

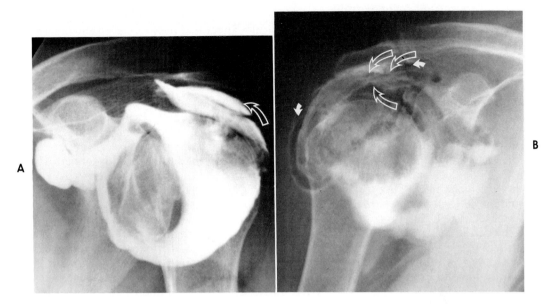

FIG. 4-31. Complete rotator cuff tear. Single and double contrast techniques. **A,** Single contrast arthrogram of left shoulder. There is opacification of the subcromion-subdeltoid bursa *(arrow)* indicating a rotator cuff tear. Although no significant degeneration of the cuff is seen, the site of the tear and the nature of torn tendinous margins cannot be determined because of pooling of contrast material. **B,** Double contrast arthrogram of right shoulder. The subacromion-subdeltoid bursa is mostly opacified by air *(solid arrows).* The rotator cuff is covered by positive contrast material. The site of tendinous tear and the quality of the tendinous margins are well demonstrated *(open arrows).*

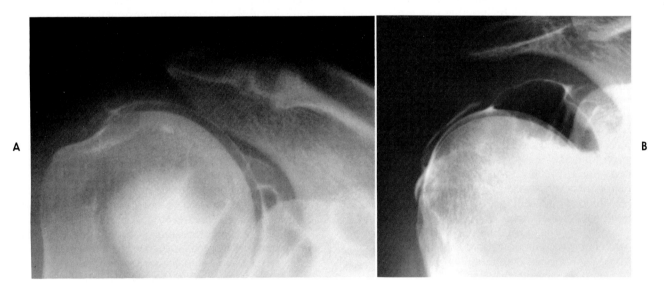

FIG. 4-32. Incomplete rotator cuff tears. **A,** Supraspinatus tear near its tuberosity insertion. A superficial fissurelike tear is visualized communicating with a longitudinal intratendinous tear. **B,** Infraspinatus tear originating at the site of posterior greater tuberosity insertion. Two tears are visualized, one forming a long intratendinous component.

intratendinous or deep surface variety and each may heal without surgery (Fig. 4-32).[142] Although tears of the undersurface of the cuff may be appreciated as an ulcerlike collection of contrast, intrasubstance tears most likely escape detection by arthrography. The import of such tears with respect to symptoms or treatment is to some extent speculative and controversial.[94] Thus Neviaser and Neviaser[142] reason that the object of an evaluation for the treatment of a cuff problem is the differentiation between complete and incomplete tears. By this hypothesis the diagnostic pursuits necessary for this distinction are of vital importance, and radiography is the most reliable pursuit; each patient with a full-thickness cuff tear should undergo surgery.

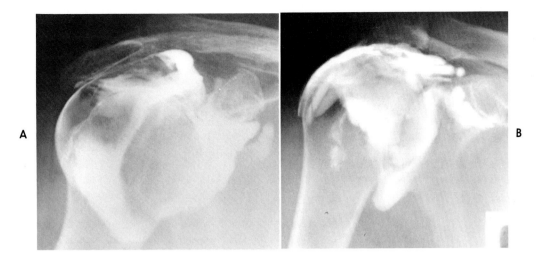

FIG. 4-33. Complete rotator cuff tear, single contrast techniques. **A,** There is opacification of the subacromion-subdeltoid bursa, indicating the presence of a rotator cuff tear. **B,** There is opacification of the subacromion-subdeltoid bursa and virtually total communication with the glenohumeral joint space because of disruption and severe degeneration of the rotator cuff tendon.

Although the authors vehemently disagree with such dogmatic formulae, and specifically with this one, investigative radiography for cuff tears must not be undervalued.

Killoran, Marcove, and Freiberger[94] indicated that the easiest diagnosis to make by arthrography is a complete rupture of the cuff because contrast extrudes blatantly into the subacromial bursa (Fig. 4-33). Neer[133] maintained that arthrography is the most reliable method of detecting a complete tear of the rotator cuff. Arthrograms, in his opinion, are indicated for patients over 40 years of age with an unresponsive impingement syndrome, sudden weakness of the shoulder after trauma, bicipital tendon rupture with persistent shoulder symptoms, and certain glenohumeral instabilities that are chronic or have occurred *de novo* in patients over 40 years of age. These recommendations were made before the advent of MRI.

Indications for arthrography (Neer)

- Unresponsive impingement syndrome (>40 years of age)
- Sudden weakness after trauma
- Bicipital tendon rupture
- Glenohumeral instability (>40 years of age)

The Neviasers[140-142] recommended five arthrographic views in the evaluation of musculotendinous injury, adding an AP view with the arm abducted to the four views reported in the sections on technique. They claim that the presence of contrast material in the subdeltoid bursa on any of the five views should be considered diagnostic of a tear.

Importance of Discovering a Cuff Tear

Among the critical diagnostic functions of the shoulder arthrogram is the determination of rotator cuff integrity. The discovery of a tear of the rotator cuff, especially a full-thickness tear, is of theoretical significance in the understanding and management of patients manifesting pain or weakness of the shoulder. Aggressive surgeons such as the Neviasers[142] suggest the repair of all full-thickness tears. Yet many patients with full-thickness tears respond well to conservative management. It is always debatable whether the manifestations of weakness and pain are particularly caused by the cuff tear, or by associated impingement, relative overuse, or rehabilitation of inadequate quantity or specificity. In this regard the study of Calvert et al[19] is of particular interest. This group studied 20 patients with double contrast arthrography after operative repair for a torn rotator cuff. Most of the patients experienced a complete remission of pain and return of shoulder elevation despite the discovery that contrast leaked into the subacromial bursa in 18 of the 20 patients studied. It is not stated, though implied, that a deimpingement was performed concurrently with the cuff repair to account for the remissions. Although Calvert et al[19] concluded that arthrography may not be helpful in the evaluation of cuff repair failures, there is another question to ponder. To what extent do leakages of contrast into the bursae of unrepaired tears implicate the cuff as the primary source of pain or motion restriction? If good operative results can be achieved despite the demonstration of leakage subsequent to repair through defects in excess of 2 cm, then the value of arthrography as an indicator for surgery may be inappropriately exaggerated.

It is noteworthy in the study of Calvert et al[19] that the only two patients with no contrast leakage were the only two patients under 50 years of age. The implications are that tear duration or the quality of surrounding tissue is important.

Detailing a Cuff Tear—Size and Character

It has already been established that among the alleged advantages of the double contrast technique (conventional or with CT or tomographic enhancement) is its ability to portray the size of a tear and the quality of the remaining tendon in which it is situated (Fig. 4-31, *A*). There is some controversy regarding the efficacy of the technique for the purpose specified.

Calvert et al[19] refer to the work of Post, Silver, and Singh,[154] which failed to demonstrate a correlation between the quantity of collected contrast in the bursa and the size of the defect. Neviaser[139,140] refuted the ability of arthrography to determine the size of the defect, whereas Goldman and Ghelman[65] and Calvert et al[19] maintained that size may be estimated using double contrast arthrography. Kilcoyne and Matsen[93] found good correlations between defect sizes estimated by arthropneumotomography and those observed at surgery.

In our opinion, there is little doubt that the double contrast techniques are superior in elucidating the tear characteristics with reasonable, though not absolute, accuracy. They are less concerned with this issue than with the more practical issue of whether such information is useful in treatment. The study of Calvert et al[65] might refute the validity of cuff-induced symptoms in many cases. Exposition of cuff tear details is nevertheless of importance to the treatment philosophies of a number of surgeons for purposes of planning an approach or for objective documentation of the nature of existing pathologic conditions for records, research, or insurance carriers.

Timing the Study

If the surgeon accepts the philosophy of Neviaser and Neviaser[142] that an acute full-thickness tear should be repaired expediently if large, then the timing of the arthrogram is of some importance. The Neviasers suggested an outside delay of 2 to 3 weeks, after which time the retraction of the edges increase the difficulty of reconstruction.

Cuff Tears and Glenohumeral Instability

The entities of glenohumeral instability and rotator cuff tear are not often considered as cohabiting pathologic states within the same shoulder. Reeves[165] has indicated that rupture of the supraspinatus is not an uncommon finding when performing arthrography on patients with acute dislocations. Other authors have been even more definitive on the subject.

In the experience of Neviaser and Neviaser[142] a tear of the rotator cuff is a more common accompaniment of an anterior dislocation than an axillary nerve palsy. Therefore, they maintain, the persistence of an inability to abduct after 1 to 2 weeks calls for an arthrogram when an axillary nerve injury has been ruled out by examination.

Although tears of the cuff occurring in conjunction with acute instability episodes may heal, there are instances when cuff injury may have existed before a dislocation or when newly acquired cuff lesions may fail to heal. In less acute circumstances, Kneisl, Sweeney, and

Paige,[100] studying patients with shoulder pain with and without instability, found rotator cuff injury in 12% of patients with instability.

Arthrography and the Unstable Shoulder

The use of arthrography for the evaluation of glenohumeral instability dates back to Lindblom.[106] Even approaching the early 1970s, when orthopaedists were reluctant to operate on a patient reporting instability without radiographic documentation, the capsular shadows perceived on arthrography were welcome corroborators of the suspected diagnosis (Fig. 4-34). Today the capsular patterns of different instabilities are reasonably well defined, and even labral and Bankart lesions are determinable without enhancement by tomography or CT.

In Kummel's study[103] of 10 unstable shoulders subjected to arthrography and surgery, three types of arthrographic defects were noted and confirmed: (1) defect of the anteroinferior capsule, filled with contrast anterior to the glenoid; (2) extravasation beyond the capsule; and (3) enlarged and irregular axillary pouch (Fig. 4-34).

Mizuno and Hirohata[128] specifically studied patients with clinical evidence of traumatic, recurrent subluxation of the shoulder. Using double contrast arthrography they determined that there is pooling of contrast material (a cap shadow) over the humeral head in looser jointed patients with inferior or multidirectional instability when traction is applied to a slightly adducted arm.

Mink, Richardson, and Grant[124] studied 12 shoulders with documented or suspected glenohumeral instability. Their technique included upright internal and external rotation, supine axillary, prone axillary, and bicipital groove views. Nine of 12 arthrograms revealed a torn labrum.

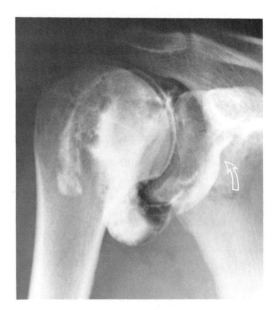

FIG. 4-34. Anterior instability. Double contrast arthrogram in a patient with history of prior dislocations. The anterior capsule is extended more medially than normal. This has resulted in almost complete obliteration of the notch normally seen between the subscapularis bursa and the joint capsule (*arrow*).

Mizuno and Hirohata[128] have described the special use of arthrography to diagnose labral tears with a relatively high positive predictive value. The presence of a Bankart lesion is demonstrable by a subscapular leakage of contrast and only when the arm is in an externally rotated position. Mizuno and Hirohata[128] observed subscapular leakage in 75% of their anterior subluxations and in only 5% of their involuntary multidirectional subluxations. They found that posterior tangential views are helpful in attempting to assess Bankart lesions. This modified West Point view demonstrates the labrum as a radiolucent shadow on the anterior and posterior portions of the glenoid, a shadow that is not observed when the labrum or glenoid cartilage has been damaged. The demonstration of a detached labrum requires a good superoinferior view. There were no false positive results among 35 patients who were operated upon. False negative outcomes could not be determined.

It is of historical and some practical interest to know that conventional arthrographic techniques can detect multiple components of glenohumeral instability. Still, the specificity and sensitivity of conventional arthrographic techniques do not begin to match those of CT arthrography and MRI, especially with respect to labral and osseous lesions.

Frozen Shoulder and Distention Arthrography

Moderate pressure is required to inject the smaller quantity of contrast material (5 to 10 ml) accepted by the tighter joint with diminutive or absent subscapularis and axillary recesses (Fig. 4-35). On very rare occasions the pressure distention needed for the study results in symp-

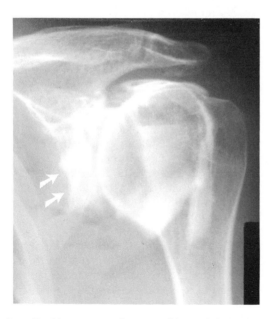

FIG. 4-35. Double contrast arthrogram of frozen left shoulder. Less than half the usual amount of contrast material could be injected. Patient experienced severe pain. The joint capsule and recesses are retracted. There is extravasation of contrast material along the anterior aspect of the capsule over the scapula (*arrows*). This occurred after forceful injection of contrast material.

tomatic relief and improved motion of the afflicted shoulder. The value of arthrography is not necessarily confined to diagnosis and surgical planning. In 1976 Older, McIntyre, and Lloyd[145] referring to Duplay's (1872) initial use of shoulder manipulation for the stiff shoulder, reported on a group of six patients they treated for stiff shoulders with distention arthrography. They distended shoulders with contrast under fluoroscopic control and obtained good results (increased motion and decreased pain) in five of the six patients. Average follow-up was nearly 2 years from the time of distention. Ten years previously (1965) Andren and Lundberg[2] had reported on a much larger series with a short follow-up. Inconsistent results were observed. These efforts are largely of historical interest now that arthroscopy accomplishes distention, fibrolysis, and visual guidance without the dangers of forcible, blind manipulation.

SPECIALIZED ARTHROGRAPHY
Subacromial Bursography

Subacromial bursography is a procedure that has been sporadically performed and studied.[27,103,186] Purposeful bursography was initially performed in the 1930s by Lindblom.[106] As remarked on in the section on conventional radiography, subacromial bursography may be accomplished inadvertently while attempting to perform a glenohumeral arthrogram.[103]

When a bursogram is performed in conjunction with an arthrogram, the thickness of the cuff is readily determined.[186] Subacromial bursography may reveal information about the superior surface of the cuff, which is not obtainable by arthrography alone. In addition, bursography can provide knowledge about impingement.[27] Its usefulness, however, may be overshadowed by the skills necessary for its performance and interpretation.

The subacromial bursa is adherent to the greater tuberosity and rotator cuff distally and to the undersurface of the acromion and the coracoacromial ligament proximally. It has a usual volume capacity of 4 to 6 ml.[103] The subacromial and subdeltoid components of the bursa are usually confluent. A subcoracoid component extending more inferiorly is not often present.[186]

In principle the technique of subacromial bursography is simple. A 20-gauge spinal needle is inserted immediately under the anterior margin of the acromion and 3 to 4 ml of contrast agent is injected. The bursa is usually opacified after slight motion of the arm. The entry of contrast material into the bursa is confirmed with an anteroposterior, internal rotation view of the shoulder.[103] Nonopacification may be seen in severe instances of bursitis.

Lie and Mast[105] were able to image a variety of disorders using bursography: degenerative rotator cuff tear, mechanical impingement, and adhesive bursitis. When a complete tear of a rotator cuff tendon is present, the contrast escapes into the glenohumeral joint. Incomplete tears of the superior cuff surface are less likely to be discovered by finding contrast-filled craters as might be found on the glenohumeral (undersurface) surface of the cuff. The implication is that subacromial bursography adds little, if anything, to the diagnosis of disorders of

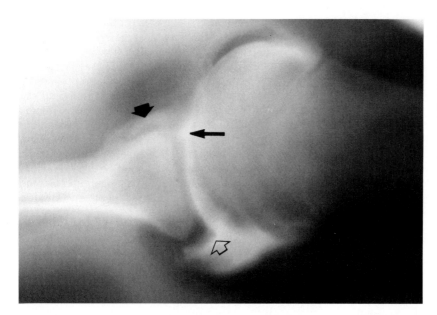

FIG. 4-36. Arthropneumotomography in anterior instability. Tomographic section of the left glenohumeral joint in the axillary position, following double-contrast arthrography. The anterior glenoid labrum is torn *(long arrow)*. There is stripping of the joint capsule; this has initiated ectopic bone formation over the scapular neck region *(short arrow)*. The posterior glenoid labrum is normal *(open arrow)*. (Courtesy Dr. Georges El-Khoury, Professor of Radiology and Orthopedics, The University of Iowa Hospitals and Clinics.)

the rotator cuff when compared to glenohumeral arthrographic techniques.

Lie and Mast[105] express a much more positive attitude with respect to the role of subacromial bursography in the diagnosis of impingement. They go so far as to say that the normal clearance of the humeral tuberosities relative to the coracoacromial arch is demonstrable only by subacromial bursography. In the presence of an intact cuff, mechanical impingement is recognized by progressive distention of the bursa as the arm is elevated into abduction. Supposedly, this distention is a consequence of the failure of the humeral head to freely clear the arch.

In a very limited series of patients subjected to bursography, Cone, Resnick, and Danzig[27] discovered rotator cuff tears and impingement evidenced by the pooling of contrast material in the subdeltoid portion of the bursa. Bursatomography was not found to enhance the observations discernible by simple bursography and fluoroscopy alone.

Strizak et al[186] studied the value of bursography in the evaluation of impingement components in 15 cadavers and 31 symptomatic patients. When the findings of bursography are normal, a diagnosis of subacromial impingement should be regarded as dubious. In fact, Strizak et al maintained that, when the bursogram is normal, deimpingement surgery has a poor prognosis in young, healthy athletes failing to respond to conservative management. Abnormal bursograms were those demonstrating an absent, small, or irregularly shaped subacromial bursa, with or without evidence of a cuff tear or thinning.

Arthropneumotomography

This technique is employed essentially for the evaluation of the glenoid labrum. Conventional, thin-section radiographic tomography is performed after double contrast arthrography has been done. Two variations of this technique have been described[16,44] based upon the manner in which the patient is positioned and the projection

in which tomographic sections are obtained. One technique uses an AP projection with a 45-degree posterior rotation of the shoulder. The images obtained with this format best demonstrate the superior and inferior portions of the labrum.[16] The middle portions of the labrum, anterior and posterior, are less well defined and are best seen by the other method, which employs an axillary projection.[44,97] The patient is positioned so that the scapula is perpendicular to the plane of the film and the arm is extended so that the patient appears to be taking a breath while swimming the crawl. This technique projects the anterior and posterior portions of the labrum in favor of the superior and inferior portions.

Double contrast arthrotomography was apparently introduced to the modern literature in 1979 when El-Khoury et al[44] described the value of the technique in the reading of labral or capsular lesions of eight patients with instability (Fig. 4-36).

Kleinman et al[97] expanded upon the report of El-Khoury et al,[44] who studied 67 arthrotomograms of patients with a variety of shoulder complaints not necessarily derived from instability per se. For the examinations performed with surgical confirmation they claimed to have had a sensitivity of 100% and a specificity of 80% for labrocapsular lesions. Braunstein and O'Connor[16] reported a small series of surgically proven labral tears predicted by arthrotomography.

Pappas, Gross, and Kleinman[148] reported no false positive or false negative results in a study of 37 labral tears confirmed by surgery using double contrast arthrotomography. They stress that axillary arthrotomography is especially useful in the detection of subtle labral lesions.

The use of arthropneumotomography for the evaluation of the labrum and capsule may have had diagnostic value in the era preceding the advent of CT arthrography.[111] Mink, Richardson, and Grant[124] contended that polytomography-augmented arthrography may be at least as accurate as double contrast arthrography in defining labral pathology but increases the dose of radia-

tion to the patient. CT arthrography and MRI are more accurate than either technique and imposes less radiation than tomography.[41]

Contrary to the arguments of such investigators as El-Khoury et al[44] that double contrast arthrotomography is a valuable screener of patients with shoulder pain and/or instability, Kneisl, Sweeney, and Paige[100] believe otherwise. Their studies revealed good reliability of the procedure for the planning of a lesion-specific operation among patients with instability. However, its low sensitivity for labral lesions and partial cuff tears leaves its value in question for painful but stable shoulders.

Arthropneumotomography has also been used in the evaluation of full-thickness rotator cuff lesions for purposes of surgical planning and prognostication. As already discussed, the premise that surgical planning is aided by a knowledge of the size of a cuff tear and the character of the surrounding tissues has been a stimulus to the "improvement" of arthrographic techniques. Kilcoyne and Matsen[93] commented about the evolution from Lindblom's single contrast method[106] to Goldman and Ghelman's double contrast technique[65] (by which cuff quality and tear size may be estimated) and compared these with their own arthropneumotomographic evaluation. This technique, culminating the 40-plus year evolution, is based on double contrast arthrography but with the addition of complex motion tomography in the upright position to better demonstrate cuff tears. Kilcoyne and Matsen[93] perform upright arthrography first and then proceed with tomography when a tear is identified by conventional radiography. A transscapular view is sometimes helpful in identifying the more elusive tears of the subscapularis, infraspinatus, and teres minor. Employing their technique in 33 shoulders that underwent subsequent surgery, they found a good correlation between predicted and actual pathologic conditions with specific reference to the size of cuff tears and the quality of the adjacent tissues. Nevertheless, the use of tomographic arthrography with its increased radiation exposure seems too heroic a technique to consider when conventional arthrography and MRI are relatively revealing.

Computed Tomography Arthrography

The evolution of CT arthrography was a natural progression after the relative successes of plain arthrotomography and CT scanning in diagnostic radiology of the shoulder. CT arthrography is able to delineate capsular redundancy, loose bodies, glenoid rim lesions, and full-thickness rotator cuff abnormalities. Its major disadvantage is its relatively poor efficacy in detailing partial rotator cuff tears and biceps/labral complex abnormalities. CT also uses ionizing radiation and poorly delineates impingement.

Technique

Following a conventional double contrast arthrogram, a CT scan of the shoulder is performed. The newer generation of scanners add approximately 15 minutes to the examination. The patient is examined in the supine position and the arm is placed at the side with the palm against the thigh (neutral position).[156-158] The neutral position of the arm is the one most commonly employed.

Deutsch et al[41] examined their patients with the arm in neutral or slight internal rotation. Singson, Feldman, and Bigliani[182] examined shoulders in neutral and occasionally in internal or external rotation. McNiesh and Callaghan[114] and DeHaven et al[36] performed examinations in neutral or in external rotation. The position of the arm plays a role in the movements of air and contrast, which may enhance or diminish visualization of a given area of study. The neutral position allows fairly uniform dispersement of contrast media. An externally rotated position may adversely prejudice interpretation of the anterior joint structures. Additional sections with the arm in external rotation can be obtained specifically to enhance visualization of the posterior portion of the glenoid labrum. Pennes et al[151] found a small increase in diagnostic yield when external rotation scans were added to those that were done initially in internal rotation. This is in accord with Deutsch et al,[40] who explain that the externally rotated position enhances posterior labral visualization by relaxing the posterior capsule and forcing air to move posteriorly. Generally, those undergoing CT scanning are not exercised, in contrast to conventional arthrographic studies. The risk of extracapsular extravasation, which interferes with the quality of the CT scan, is too great.

In the context of air-contrast dispersements, Randelli, Odella, and Gambrioli[163] indicated their experience with false positive results wherein a localized accumulation of contrast had been misconstrued as labral fragmentation. This can occur with inadvertent positioning of the needle within the labrum, especially early on in the learning curve. Adequate distention and even distribution of contrast is necessary for proper interpretation of the soft tissues. Variation in the quantities of positive contrast material or even the use of air alone has been reported.[41] The joint is scanned with 3-mm thick slices. Using special software, the computer can generate high-resolution, magnified images of the shoulder region. Wide window settings (3000/300) are used for producing hard copy images that allow various densities (bone, soft tissue, and contrast media) to be adequately resolved. Excellent visualization of the glenoid labrum, the capsular structures, including the glenohumeral ligaments and the joint surfaces, is achieved by this technique.[156] Additionally, the osseous and the periarticular structures are optimally visualized and can be evaluated for possible unexpected lesions (Fig. 4-37).

The evaluation of the extent of rotator cuff tears and degeneration by direct sagittal computed tomography (DSCT) has also been described.[9] According to Beltran et al,[9] DSCT performed with the patient seated between the gantry and the scanner table reveals greater diagnostic accuracy in the detection of rotator cuff lesions than either axial CT scanning or double contrast arthrography with plain films. Twenty-nine lesions were detected in 24 symptomatic patients: 14 by arthrogram, 19 by axial CT, and 27 by DSCT. Hence, DSCT is better for cuff injury and CAT arthrography is better for labral lesions.

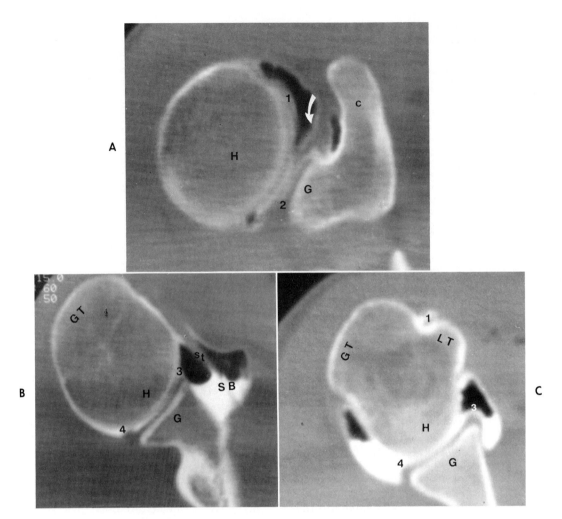

FIG. 4-37. Normal CT arthrogram of right shoulder. Representative images from proximal (**A**), middle (**B**), and distal (**C**) aspects of the glenohumeral joint. *c,* Coracoid process; *G,* glenoid; *H,* humeral head; *GT,* greater tuberosity; *LT,* lesser tuberosity; *SB,* subscapularis bursa; *st,* subscapularis tendon; *1,* long head of biceps tendon; *2,* superior glenoid labrum; *3,* anterior glenoid labrum; *4,* posterior glenoid labrum. **A,** The long head of biceps tendon and the superior glenoid labrum merge and form a common insertion onto the superior glenoid margin. The anterior aspect of the joint capsule in this vicinity forms the superior glenohumeral ligament (*arrow*). **B,** The subscapularis bursa is formed below the coracoid process as a medial extension of the synovial lining of the joint capsule along the superior free margin of the subscapularis tendon. **C,** Below the subscapularis bursa the anterior capsule extends for a distance (individually varied) medially, forms a smooth reflexion over the glenoid, and blends with the anterior glenoid labrum. The posterior capsule is intimately related to the posterior glenoid labrum. (**C** reproduced with permission from Rafii M et al: *Am J Sports Med* 16:352, 1988.)

Isolated Labrum Lesion

CT arthrography has its greatest value in the evaluation of isolated labral lesions and of labral and capsular lesions associated with glenohumeral instability. Isolated and instability lesions of the labrum are sometimes difficult to distinguish. The isolated varieties are most traditionally associated with throwing type mechanisms. Rafii et al[157,158] observe that athletes with no clinical instability had frequently demonstrable detachments of the superior labrum, the inner margin of which is weakly attached to the glenoid.[13] The second most frequent labral tear in the athlete with a stable shoulder is that of the middle anterior portion of the glenoid. Just as the supe-

rior labral detachment has been postulated by Andrews et al[3] to result from the pull of the biceps tendon during the throwing act, middle anterior lesions may be a consequence of labral impingement between the humeral head and subscapularis tendon during the act of throwing (Fig. 4-38).

According to Zarins and Matthews,[194] these labral tears occur in the anterosuperior or anterior portions of the glenoid. Vertical longitudinal or circumferential tears are seen with the greatest frequency, followed by flap tears and then complex tears. The labral lesions of instability occur more commonly, although not exclusively, about the lower hemisphere of the glenoid.

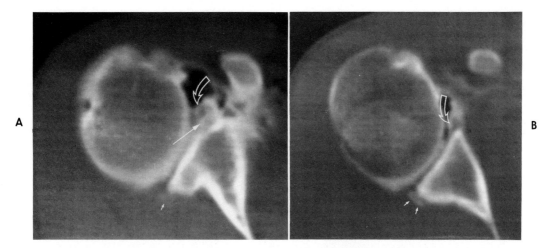

FIG. 4-38. Isolated glenoid labrum tear. Major league pitcher with right shoulder pain. **A** and **B,** Computed tomography arthrogram images from the proximal aspect of the glenohumeral joint. The anterior glenoid labrum is irregularly torn (*curved arrows*) and detached from the glenoid margin (*long arrow*). Inferior to these levels the labrum was normal. Also noted is a calcific ridge formed along the posterior capsular margin within the expected site of capsular attachment (*short arrows*).

In a study of autopsy and patient shoulders, Kohn[101] discovered a high incidence of labral pathology by gross or arthroscopic examination that could not be correlated to symptoms. He concluded that most glenoid labral lesions have little clinical relevance. DePalma's studies[37] of aging in the shoulder joint are worth mentioning at this point. They revealed a progressive degeneration of the labrum after the second decade. These changes comprise detachment of superior labrum from the glenoid (which exceeds an incidence of greater than 60% in the fifth decade) and thinning and fraying of the inferior portion of the labrum. It may be the case that many of these degenerative changes are not productive of symptoms. Nevertheless, it is evident, particularly in an athletic population, that many labral tears produce symptoms that are relieved by arthroscopic debridement. In fact, some of these tears produce not only pain and clicking, but also a sense of instability within the joint (functional instability). Pappas, Gross, and Kleinman[148] went to great lengths in creating a distinction between labrum-produced, or functional, instability treatable by excision and anatomic, or glenohumeral, instability, which may require labral repair and capsulorrhaphy. Obviously, this distinction is important in surgical planning and in patient counseling.

Shuman et al[181] studied 11 sequential patients with suspected labral pathology associated with a variety of signs and symptoms, and in each instance in which a labral tear was discovered on CT arthrography, it was confirmed at surgery. All negative studies were confirmed at surgery as well. Deutsch et al,[41] based on surgical correlation to CT arthrography, found a sensitivity for anterior labral lesions of 100%. DeHaven et al,[36] using CT arthrography to evaluate a group of patients with symptoms derived from multiple pathologic conditions, found high sensitivities for loose body detection and labral lesions; they found relatively poor sensitivities (less than 70%) in diagnosing lesions of the rotator cuff, the bicipital-labral complex, and the Hill-Sachs lesion. Although specificities were 100% for the cuff, loose body, posterior labral lesion, Hill-Sachs lesion, and bicipital-labral complex, there was less than 75% specificity and a less than 90% accuracy for anterior labral lesions. This may, in part, relate to the fact that they studied patients with the arm in an externally rotated position, which, as already indicated, is best for enhancing posterior lesions.

Labral Morphology

As pointed out in the section on the isolated labrum, the labrum can manifest a variety of tears. However, frank tears are not the only morphologic labral alterations that can be appreciated arthroscopically.[1] The labrum can appear atrophic or degenerated, loose or floppy, or even distorted in contour.[5] The significance of each of these findings is not always clear. The morphologic characteristics of the labrum as seen by CT arthrography are often different from those which may be appreciated by direct viewing using arthroscopy, lending more confusion and speculation to their significance.

McNiesh and Callaghan[114] studied 72 shoulders by double contrast CT arthrography between 1984 and 1988. They noted labra which they considered to be unusually small (though nondegenerated), some with cleavages within the normally sharply truncated shadow, and even one that was notched. They considered these to be normal variants, since subsequent arthroscopies demonstrated no apparent abnormalities in any of these labra. The corrugations that frequently develop within labra after the second decade may help to explain some of these variants.[37] They might also result from peripheral detachment or laxity as in the knee, where a normal meniscus often appears convoluted when there exists a near or distant locus of peripheral separation.

Working with a variety of co-workers, Rafii et al[156-158] noted numerous morphologic alterations in the evaluation of labra CT arthrography. Labral eversion, attenua-

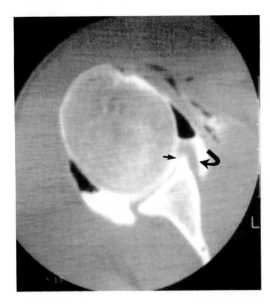

FIG. 4-39. Tear and enlargement of the glenoid labrum. (Same patient as in Fig. 4-44, *A*). An anterior labrum tear *(straight arrow)* was detected 1 week following acute trauma to the right shoulder in this professional hockey player. The torn labrum is rather enlarged and the adjacent soft tissues of the capsulolabral junction are thickened *(curved arrow)*.

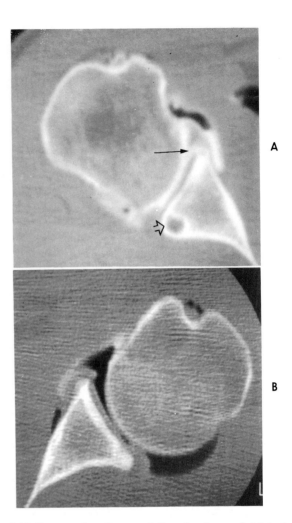

FIG. 4-40. Degenerative disease of the glenohumeral joint. **A,** Right shoulder pain in a middle-aged tennis player. The anterior and posterior glenoid labra are enlarged. The anterior labrum is also partially detached from the glenoid margin, which shows osteophyte formation *(long arrow)*. A subarticular cyst of the posterior labrum is also present *(open arrow)*. **B,** Degenerative disease in a veteran baseball player. The anterior glenoid labrum and the articular cartilage of the humeral head and glenoid are attenuated. There is an osteophyte off the anterior glenoid margin. The posterior glenoid margin is irregular.

tion, hypertrophy, and floppiness (loss of truncation) were among the findings noted. Although not even a majority of those studied eventually underwent surgery, these labral findings were considered to be abnormal and not always readily appreciated by arthroscopy. It is postulated that configurational alterations of the labrum may be more readily identifiable by the definitive geometry created by air/contrast lines than by direct gross inspection. The meaning of the morphologic variants appreciated by CT arthrography has also been speculated upon by the authors. The floppy labrum probably results from a tear with subsequent degeneration. The everted labrum is also associated with tear or detachment. The hypertrophied labrum may result from tearing with inflammation or hydrops (Fig. 4-39). DePalma's work[37] revealed that a natural progression of hypertrophy occurs within the superior portion of the labrum with aging (Fig. 4-40). DePalma ascribed this hypertrophy to the formation of synovial tabs and fringes particularly about the anterior portion of the labrum. Wilson et al,[191] in a long-term study of CT arthrography and surgical follow-up, concluded that there was a wide range of labral shapes. There was a suggestion the labra should be considered abnormal only if they are absent, markedly deformed, fragmented, or contain contrast media. For example, a small, smoothly contoured labrum with a rounded tip should be considered normal. They found a 100% sensitivity and 97% specificity while using surgery as a standard.

Whether the discovery of morphologic variants other than obvious tears relates to the isolated labral problem, to instability, or to neither, is not altogether clear. It is not yet established whether these changes have import and reliability in the planning of lesion-specific surgery.

Unstable Shoulder: Capsule and Labrum

Glenohumeral instability is most often discoverable by history and physical examination and is frequently documented by conventional radiography, as discussed on p. 100. However, when no bony lesions are present on conventional radiography, even with special views, and when there is a need for more precise evaluation of the suspected pathologic condition, special radiography such as CT arthrography becomes important.[95]

CT arthrography has value in the reaffirmation of a suspected instability, the discovery of subtle or unsuspected instability, the determination of the direction of instability, and the characterization of the type of labral lesion associated with the instability. At times, the diagnosis of the unstable shoulder can be difficult.[95] Many patients are poor at perceiving a sense of sliding and

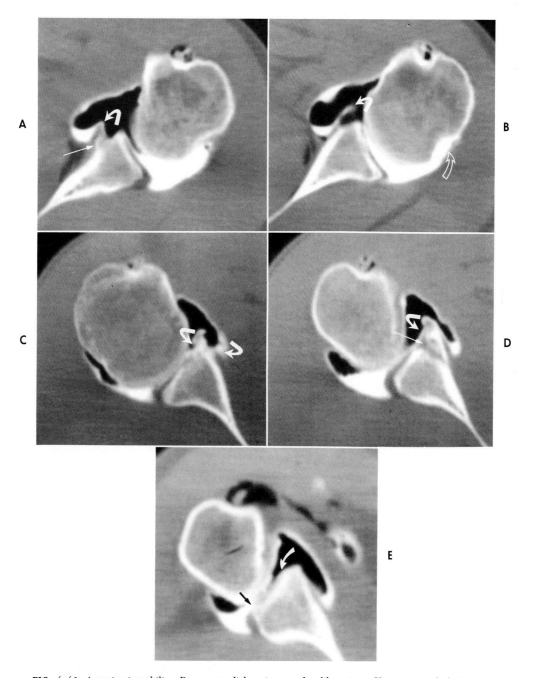

FIG. 4-41. Anterior instability. Recurrent dislocations and subluxations. Various morphologic configurations of capsulolabral lesions. **A** and **B,** Recurrent dislocation of left shoulder. The glenoid labrum *(curved arrows)* is detached and considerably attenuated. The capsulolabral junction is also detached and an enlarged anterior pouch is formed. The anterior glenoid margin is deficient and ectopic calcification is noted *(long arrow)*. A Hill-Sachs defect is also demonstrated *(hollow arrows)*. **C** and **D,** Recurrent subluxation of right shoulder. The anterior capsulolabral complex is irregularly torn in all aspects *(curved arrows)*. A fracture of anterior glenoid margin is demonstrated *(straight arrow)*. **E,** Recurrent dislocation of right shoulder. The anterior glenoid labrum is totally absent and stripping of the anterior capsule is evident. The articular cartilage of the glenoid and the osseous glenoid margin are deficient *(white arrow)*. Also, a tear of the posterior glenoid labrum is visualized *(black arrow)*.

merely experience pain as a manifestation of glenohumeral displacement. Many are too apprehensive to be adequately examined or refuse to submit to surgery or even general anesthesia for purposes of diagnosis.

In an early study, Kinnard et al[95] performed CT arthrography on 10 unstable shoulders of which seven had documented instability. All 10 were noted to have had an increase in the size of the anterior recess, which may be of no significance; seven patients had intraarticular septate adhesions; three had labral amputations; and two patients had glenoid rim fractures not discovered by routine radiography. All of the findings in this rudimentary study were substantiated by subsequent surgery.

Fifty-four shoulders, 40 with involuntary dislocations and 14 with involuntary subluxations, were studied by Singson, Feldman, and Bigliani.[182] Of the shoulders, 85% had sustained athletic trauma. Anterior labral abnormalities were present in almost 100% of cases on CT arthrography. Surgical corroboration revealed *no* false positive findings and only two false negative findings based on either an inadequate study or an inadequate prospective interpretation of positive evidence.

Randelli, Odella, and Gambrioli[163] cautioned that large capsular recesses must not automatically be assumed to represent an instability. The capsular recesses, particularly the axillary and subscapular recesses, vary considerably in size and shape among normal shoulders. Only those marked anterior capsular enlargement or detachment should be interpreted as a definite sign of instability (Fig. 4-41). This statement is corroborated by Rafii et al.[156]

Capsular recesses

- Large ones may represent normal variation
- Not a sine qua non of instability
- If detached, more likely to represent instability

Singson, Feldman, and Bigliani[182] found radiographic capsular evidence of instability in almost 80% of cases and consisted of the following: (1) medial scapular insertion; (2) glenoid stripping or detachment; and (3) capsular widening or redundant anterior recess. Morphologic description of capsular insertion made by Moseley and Overgaard[130] has been translated into radiographic description by CT arthrographic study.[156,169,196] A Type I capsule inserts near the glenoid labrum. In Types II and III, a more medial insertion is found.

The import of the location or the glenohumeral capsular insertion into the scapula was reinforced by Rothman, Marvel, and Hepenstall.[169] They indicated that the more distal capsular insertions (Types II and III) onto the neck, rather than onto the glenoid (Type I), are more likely to be associated with anterior instability. Rafii et al[158] reported that capsular findings of instability included stripping of the anterior capsule from the scapular neck; thickening or irregularity of the capsular and periosteal soft tissues about the anterior portion of the scapula; capsular tears with or without leakage; periosteal bone formation about the scapular neck; and ante-

rior or posterior capsular redundancy. One or more of these findings were present in all cases of glenohumeral instability (Fig. 4-41). Wilson et al,[191] however, believed that insertion away from the glenoid margin is such a common finding that it is probably a normal variant and is a poor predictor of shoulder abnormality. They thought that only insertions at the medial third should be considered abnormal. There was a correlation with more medial insertions and labral tears in their study.

Capsular findings associated with instability

- Stripping of anterior capsule from scapular neck
- Thickening/irregularity of capsule/periosteum
- Capsular tears
- Periosteal bone formation along scapular neck
- Capsular redundancy

Singson, Feldman, and Bigliani[182] found no essential differences in the labral lesions of recurrent subluxation and dislocation. However, capsular abnormalities were more frequent and dramatic in shoulders with recurrent dislocation. They reported that 90% of patients with a widened subscapular bursa had anterior dislocations, whereas those with only cicatricial responses within the tendon of the subscapularis tended to have only subluxations. However, it must be pointed out that subscapular cicatrix may be deduced only from circumstantial evidence.

Rafii et al[156-158] observed that all anterior instabilities were associated with lesions of the anterior portion of the labrum, which included frank tears, detachments, absences, and attenuations. In occasional cases the labrum remains intact and a frank tear is not seen (Fig. 4-42). Labral lesions on the side of the glenoid opposite the direction of instability were not uncommonly observed (Fig. 4-41, *E*). Such tears were not necessarily construed to represent a posterior instability. An instability on the side of the glenoid with a tear was most definitely accepted when there was an associated tear of the capsule, glenoid rim fracture, or peculiarity in the scapular insertion of the capsule (Fig. 4-43). This is in keeping with the findings of Singson, Feldman, and Bigliani,[182] who report that in nearly all cases in which an anterior form of instability existed an anterior labral lesion is present; all patients with posterior instability (unidirectional and multidirectional) have concomitant anterior as well as posterior labral lesions.

Labral findings associated with instability

- Tears
- Detachment
- Absence
- Alteration

Rafii et al[156-158] stressed the dilemma of diagnosing mild unidirectional or multidirectional instabilities and of distinguishing instabilities from isolated labral lesions,

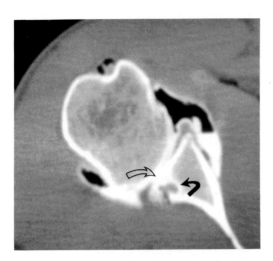

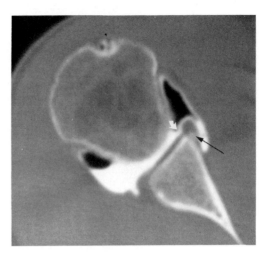

FIG. 4-42. Anterior instability. Recurrent subluxation of right shoulder. There is a small notch at the junction of the glenoid labrum and the glenoid articular cartilage (*white arrow*). The labrum is rounded in contour, but does not otherwise show a tear. Also there is small ectopic calcification adjacent to the glenoid margin (*black arrow*). A frank tear was not seen at arthroscopy.

FIG. 4-43. Posterior instability, right shoulder. The posterior glenoid labrum is torn, and there is detachment and displacement of the torn glenolabral complex (*open arrow*). The osseous glenoid margin is deficient and shows a cystic type defect (*solid arrow*). This configuration is the result of glenoid margin fracture. There is an enlarged anterior capsule with medial attachment near the scapular neck. This results from presence of large inferior subscapularis bursa in this patient. One should be alerted to the possible presence of anterior instability in this instance.

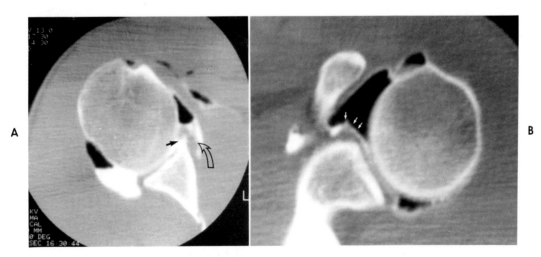

FIG. 4-44. Glenoid labrum tear resulting from acute trauma. **A,** Computed tomography (CT) arthrogram of right shoulder in a professional hockey player 3 days after acute trauma (same patient as in Fig. 4-39). The anterior labrum is shown to be torn and partially detached (*solid arrow*). There is no stripping of the capsule. However, the capsulolabral junction is swollen (*open arrow*). This finding was not considered to be a solid evidence for persistent joint instability and none was demonstrated at arthroscopy. Anterior instability became apparent at subsequent clinical examination. **B,** Professional hockey player following acute trauma to left shoulder. Representative image from proximal aspect of the joint. The anterior glenoid labrum is deformed and shows many surface irregularities (*arrows*). The entire anterior labrum showed similar abnormality. No capsular abnormality was detected. Subsequently, laxity was clinically documented. No follow-up CT arthrogram was done to evaluate any interval change. (**B** reproduced with permission from Rafii M et al: *Am J Sports Med* 16:352, 1988.)

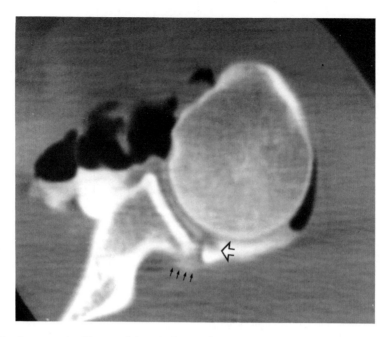

FIG. 4-45. Posterior shoulder instability. Professional hockey player following acute trauma to left shoulder. Representative computed tomography arthrogram image at the upper aspect of the joint, with a rather prominent subscapularis bursa visualized anteriorly. The posterior glenoid labrum is torn and detached, floating within the posterior aspect of the joint (*open arrow*). There is extravasation of the contrast material beyond the capsulolabral junction, indicative of capsular tear (*small arrows*). This finding was considered to be a manifestation of persistent instability.

such as those resulting from throwing activities. They further indicate the additional burden of establishing these diagnoses in the wake of a new and acute injury (Figs. 4-44 and 4-45).

Although experts in athletic medicine may be embarrassed or reluctant to admit that they are unable to discover or define all cases of instability by physical evaluation of patients in the awake or anesthetized state, the difficulty nonetheless exists in a number of instances. Even when an instability of limited magnitude is discovered, there remains the task of assigning to it a clinical (symptomatic) relevance. The concepts expressed by Pappas, Gross, and Kleinman[148] of functional instability and by Rafii et al[157] of unobtrusive laxity are not just a source of additional confusion, but are loose ends in the determination of practical treatment designs.

Rafii et al[157] specifically studied 61 shoulders with symptoms deriving from athletic trauma or performance in patients between 15 and 40 years of age. They observed that high level athletes with glenohumeral instability had fewer dramatic labral lesions and less capsular stretching than the population at large, which may relate to their youth or their resilience in achieving an elite status.[157,158]

Hill-Sachs Lesion

Among the alleged disadvantages of CT arthrography and arthrotomography is a diminished ability to detect the Hill-Sachs lesion.[36] In the series reported by Rafii et al,[157] only two Hill-Sachs lesions were identified among 14 competitive athletic patients with a known anterior instability. Using CT arthrography, a Hill-Sachs lesion was

identified in less than 40% of the 54 unstable shoulders studied by Singson, Feldman, and Bigliani.[182] Other reports, however, are more positive. Deutsch et al[41] stated that CT arthrotomography is highly sensitive in the detection of Hill-Sachs lesions and may detect these lesions when conventional radiography or arthrography fails to do so. Gambrioli, Maggi, and Randelli[55] determined that CT revealed the Hill-Sachs lesion with a similar accuracy to that of conventional radiographic views such as the Didiee, but with better definition of the extent of the lesion.

Wilson et al[191] not only demonstrated excellent detection of Hill-Sachs lesions, but also showed a correlation of this finding and bony glenoid fractures with labral tears. In any case, if the only Hill-Sachs lesions missed by CT arthrography are those that are too small to require a specific treatment for the bony defect, then the only potential loss in diagnostic confirmation of instability is the failure to detect the Hill-Sachs lesion. This is a small loss, since in virtually all but some newer cases of instability, the accurate delineations of Bankart lesions of the glenoid-labrum complex and the character of the capsular insertion onto the scapula by CT arthrography are sufficiently diagnostic of instability.

MAGNETIC RESONANCE IMAGING
General Concepts

The introduction of MRI into the armamentarium of those dealing with pathologic conditions of the shoulder has brought what amounts to a revolution in the field of diagnostic imaging. The impact on musculoskeletal im-

aging is significant because of the exquisite resolution of the various soft-tissue structures available without the use of ionizing radiation. MRI also has the capability for multiplanar imaging (including oblique orientations), which allows viewing in anatomically suitable planes, gathering information most helpful for recognition of pathologic conditions.

Advantages of magnetic resonance imaging

- High soft tissue contrast
- Multiplanar imaging capability
- Absence of bone artifacts
- No ionizing radiation
- Noninvasive

The principal advantages of MRI are summarized by Huber et al[84]: high soft-tissue contrast, multiplanar imaging capability, absence of bone artifacts, and an absence of ionizing radiation or other invasive elements.

This imaging modality has particularly affected the imaging of the hip, knee, and ankle joints. Noninvasive, and with a much greater capacity for the depiction of the ligamentous structures and the periarticular soft tissues, MRI has already eliminated the need, in most cases, for the more invasive technique of knee arthrography and even diagnostic arthroscopy. MRI is more effective than plain CT in the demonstration of shoulder joint anatomy because of its capability for multiplanar imaging and its superior resolution of soft-tissue structures.[70,84,136] Its ability to identify isolated labral abnormalities, instability patterns (labral and capsular injury), coracoacromial arch, rotator cuff, bursal, and AC injury is well documented and has largely supplanted many other invasive imaging modalities.*

The disadvantages of this powerful tool include its relative cost per study, limitations as a result of various equipment quality, reliance on expert radiologic interpretation, possible claustrophobia in the gantry, and its questionable efficacy in postoperative assessment.

Signal Generation

MRI scans are formed on the basis of signals that are received from the various tissues. The MRI signal is based on the presence, and the density of, mobile protons. Signals are produced by magnetized protons, which are then excited by a radiofrequency. The signals, or echoes, are detected and transmitted with the same or a different coil system from that which generated the original radiofrequency. The varied characteristics of signals generated, for example, short (T1, or proton density) or long (T2) ranges of listening (weighting), can determine the nature of tissue elements and therefore help in detecting pathologic processes. Anatomic detail is best seen with T1, or proton density, weighted images as compared with T2 weighting, which best outlines normal or abnormal fluid.

Cortical bone, fibrocartilage (glenoid labrum), fibrous tissue, tendons, and ligaments contain few mobile protons and produce no signal. They are depicted as black regions (signal void) in both long and short echo sequences and are identified by virtue of their anatomic location and contrast with surrounding tissues. With short echo sequences (T1, proton density) fat (subcutaneous, intramuscular, and fat planes) and bone marrow produce the highest signals appearing as bright or white areas. Water and water-containing tissue elements, such as muscles and hyaline cartilage, induce various ranges of medium signal intensity in these sequences.

In T2 sequences, fluids are depicted with high signal generation. For example, fluids such as joint effusion produce a medium signal intensity on T1 ranger and may blend with periarticular tissues when these short intervals of signal gathering are used. In long ranges of pulse sequence (T2) the intensity of signal from fluids is greatly increased. Therefore effusion is depicted as bright, providing an arthrogram effect that is distinguished from adjacent (low signal) structures during T2 sequences.

More and more the T1 sequences that were widely used in the infancy of MRI have been replaced with the improved resolution of proton density imaging and other techniques.[53,69]

Because a complete discussion of general MRI physics and the newer or weighted imaging techniques is beyond the scope of this chapter, the reader is referred to other sources for detailed information regarding this topic.[185]

Technique

The development of MRI technique for imaging of the shoulder joint has proved to be a challenging task. The shoulder is difficult to image because of the space limitations within the housing of the MRI magnet and because the shoulder cannot be positioned in the center of the magnet where the highest ranges of signal-to-noise (S/N) ratios are achieved. Seeger et al[177] explained that these problems can be overcome by combining high-resolution scanning with the use of a surface coil for the shoulder.

MRI of the peripheral joints became a clinical reality mostly after the development of high-resolution imaging techniques and the development of surface coils intended for gathering MR signals from small regions of the body. The peripheral location of the shoulder, however, necessitated further changes in imaging techniques. Ordinarily the center of the field of view is in the vicinity of the center of the magnet, where the highest S/N ratio is obtained. Although peripheral images are possible to obtain, they have poor resolution. The development of an off-center zoom technique has eliminated this problem by shifting the center of the field of view to the periphery as much as needed to produce high-resolution magnified images of the shoulder region.

The MRI examination of the shoulder is obtained with the patient supine and with the arms extended along the sides. With the palm against the thigh, the humerus is in a position midway between internal and external rotation, which is most suitable for imaging of this joint. The rotator cuff muscles and tendons also are in a relaxed state and parallel to the plane of the scapula, mak-

---

*References 46, 52, 70, 85, 92, 125, 131, 136, 159, 176, and 197-200.

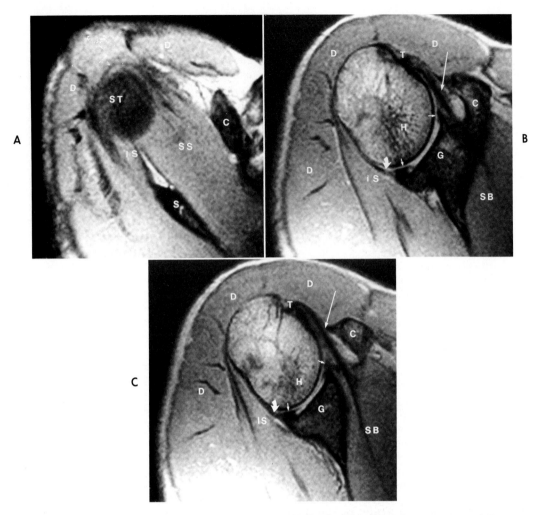

FIG. 4-46. Magnetic resonance imaging (MRI) scan of right shoulder. Normal anatomy in axial (**A** to **C**), anatomic coronal (**D** and **E**), and anatomic sagittal plane (**F** and **G**). **A,** Axial image at the level of supraspinatus fossa of the scapula. At this level the supraspinatus muscle and tendon are visualized. The plane of the coronal images is based on the orientation of this muscle in each individual. A small portion of the infraspinatus muscle is also visualized with its tendon overlapping the supraspinatus tendon. **B** and **C,** Axial images at the level of the base of the coracoid process (**B**). At this level and below the coracoid process (**C**), the glenohumeral articulation and the glenoid labrum (anterior and posterior segments) (*short arrows*) and the subscapularis, the infraspinatus, and the deltoid muscles are visualized. The anterior joint capsule and the subscapularis tendon (*long arrow*), which emerges from medioinferior margin of the coracoid process, extend laterally to the lesser tuberosity. A cross-section of the long head of the biceps tendon is seen at the top of the bicipital groove. The posterior capsule (*curved arrow*) extends from the posterior labrum along with the infraspinatus muscle and tendon to the greater tuberosity. **C,** Axial MR image below the coracoid process. The subscapularis muscle and tendon are visualized in continuity.

ing their depiction easier in the coronal plane. Seeger et al[179] performed MRI scanning with the arm in internal rotation, a position that they considered more convenient to the patient and more revealing of the pathologic state related to subacromial impingement. The imaging of the rotator cuff, the subacromial space, the AC and the glenohumeral joints are best achieved by imaging in at least two, and preferably three planes (Fig. 4-46); (1) the oblique coronal (anatomic coronal), (2) the axial, and (3) the oblique sagittal (anatomic sagittal) planes.

Scan Sequence

Because individual anatomy differs, it is important to custom tailor each study to the individual shoulder being examined. These planned scans are initiated with the coronal view. The scout coronal view is used to plan the axial cuts (Fig. 4-47). In like fashion, a scout axial view is used to plan both the oblique coronal and oblique sagittal views (Fig. 4-48). The coronal plane images are best made parallel to the course of the supraspinatus tendon and, because of its individual variability, may be best de-

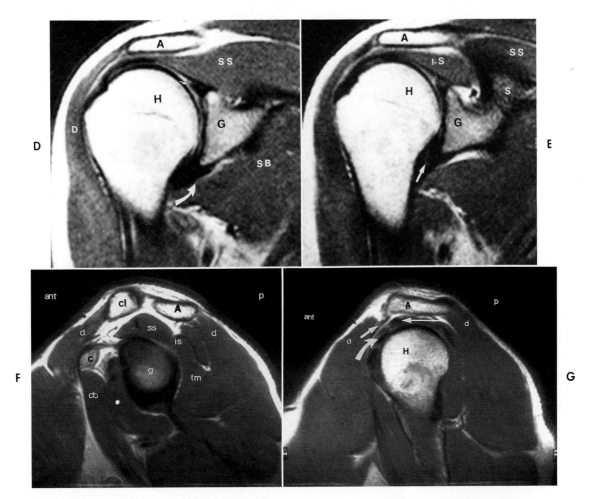

FIG. 4-46, cont'd. D, Anatomic coronal plane MRI of right shoulder oriented along the longitudinal axis of the supraspinatus muscle and tendon. The supraspinatus, the subscapularis, and the deltoid muscles are visualized extending within the subacromial space and inserting onto the greater tuberosity. The superior glenoid labrum is visualized *(short arrow).* The inferior labrum blends with the axillary pouch of the joint capsule from which it cannot be differentiated because of the normal lack of signal from both structures *(curved arrow).* **E,** Anatomic coronal plane MRI slightly posterior (lateral) to **D.** At this level the infraspinatus muscle is visualized (lateral to the scapular spine) emerging from behind the scapular spine. A portion of the supraspinatus muscle is also visualized medial (anterior) to the scapular spine. The musculotendinous junction and the tendon of the infraspinatus are visualized within the subacromial space extending toward the greater tuberosity. The inferior glenoid labrum is partially outlined on this image, probably as a result of signal arising from a small amount of joint fluid *(arrow).* **F,** Anatomic sagittal plane magnetic resonance image perpendicular to the direction of the supraspinatus, medial to humeral head. The glenoid is visualized with its circumferential labrum. The supraspinatus, infraspinatus, teres minor, and subscapularis muscles are identified. The clavicle and acromium create the roof of the subacromial space. **G,** Further laterally the humeral head is visualized with the rotator cuff assuming its narrower dimensions beneath the acromion. Coracoacromial ligament *(short arrows),* supraspinatus *(long arrows),* biceps tendon *(curved arrows); A,* acromion; *C,* coracoid process; *CB,* coracobrachialis; *CL,* clavicle; *D,* deltoid; *G,* glenoid; *H,* humeral head; *IS,* infraspinatus; *SB* subscapularis; *SS,* supraspinatus; *T,* long head of biceps tendon; *TM,* teres minor.

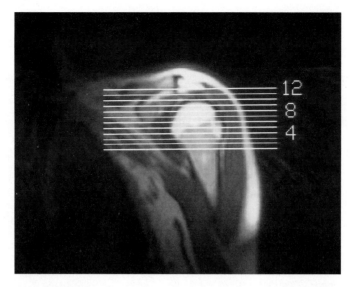

FIG. 4-47. Planned scan. Scout coronal view used for planning axial sequence. The number of cuts, cut thickness, and relation to proposed pathology can be determined. (See Fig. 4-46, *A.*)

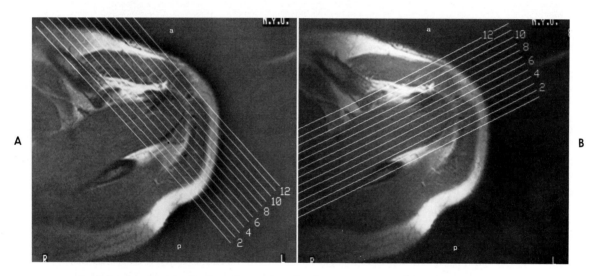

FIG. 4-48. Planned scan. Scout axial is used to plan the anatomic coronal (**A**) and anatomic sagittal (**B**) views. *a,* Anterior; *p,* posterior; *L,* lateral.

termined by a series of scout images. The sagittal images obtained are generally perpendicular to the coronal planes, parallel to the glenoid.

The oblique coronal views are most suitable for evaluation of the supraspinatus tendon, subacromial space, AC joint, glenohumeral joint, and the superior and inferior glenoid labrum. The axial images are centered on the glenohumeral joint and are most helpful for evaluation of the anterior and posterior rotator cuff, the capsule, and the labral elements. The superficial rotators and the neurovascular bundle are also well demonstrated. The oblique sagittal plane provides a cross-section of the cuff

tendons in the medial to lateral direction and describes the subacromial space from anterior to posterior.[126]

Anatomy

An historical review of pilot reports on MRI of the shoulder that addresses the structures visualized by imaging in various planes may be summarized as follows.

Huber et al,[84] in an early report on MRI of the shoulder, suggested that the rotator cuff is most usefully imaged on coronal and sagittal views.

Middleton et al[121] studied normal MRI anatomy of the shoulders of six volunteers. They found that the deltoid

was the most prominent structure, could be identified in all planes, and was easily distinguishable from the rotator cuff because of an interspace of fat in which the subdeltoid bursa and the coracoacromial ligament are identified. They detected the rotator cuff tendons most easily in the coronal and sagittal planes, as did Huber et al.[84]

Seeger et al[178] reported that the coracoclavicular ligaments, acromioclavicular joint, and superior humeral head articular cartilage are well seen in the coronal plane. They indicated that the sagittal plane reveals the horizontal axis of the acromion and its relationship to the supraspinatus tendon, whereas the oblique plane shows the supraspinatus muscle and tendon in continuity and their relationship to the acromion and acromioclavicular joint.

According to Seeger et al[177] the low signal glenoid labrum is well depicted with axial scanning, and with internal rotation the anterior labrum is larger at all levels than the posterior labrum. It is demarcated from the adjacent capsule and cuff by a thin rim of medium to high intensity produced by synovial folds within the cavity.

Kieft et al[89] devised an anatomically shaped surface coil. They indicate the most advantageous planes for viewing the various structures of the shoulder are as follows:

1. *Axial plane*—best for the biceps tendon, glenohumeral joint, articular surfaces, glenoid labrum, and neurovascular bundle
2. *Oblique plane*—(perpendicular to the glenoid) best for the rotator cuff, glenohumeral joint, and acromioclavicular joint
3. *Sagittal plane*—best for the neurovascular bundle and for staging bone tumors

Rotator Cuff Tears

Until the advent of modern techniques, surface coils, and the experience gathered over the last couple of years, detection of rotator cuff tears by MRI was fraught with problems.[92] The chief difficulty lay primarily with differentiating between small complete tears, partial tears, and tendinitis. Large tears were generally well seen. Because of the proximity of the signal void in both the cortical bone (humeral head) and closely applied tendon (rotator cuff), delineation between the two structures proved difficult. Currently the recognition of large full-thickness tears and various permutations of partial tears is well documented from the perspective of sensitivity, specificity, and accuracy.*

Present day imaging, by virtue of its excellent delineation of soft tissue anatomy, can accurately detect the basic radiologic appearance of rotator cuff tears: an interruption of tendon substance at the defect (Fig. 4-49). Under T2 sequences fluid (high signal generation) or granulation tissue (intermediate signal) is interposed in the defect created by these disruptions (Fig. 4-50). Other than directly visualizing a rotator cuff tear, there are reliable indirect telltale signs readily identified by MRI. Retraction of the musculotendinous junction of the su-

___
*References 18, 46, 49, 85, 98, 99, 129, 159, and 200.

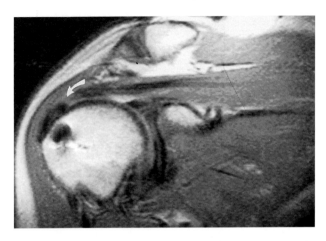

FIG. 4-49. Full-thickness rotator cuff tear. Proton density weighting. Note interruption in signal void of tendon *(arrow)*.

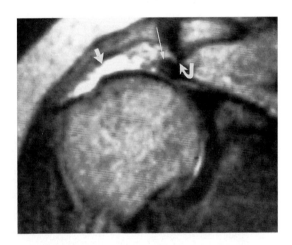

FIG. 4-50. Full-thickness rotator cuff tear (T2 weighting). The retracted supraspinatus tendon *(small arrow)* is seen under a spur from acromioclavicular joint *(curved arrow)*. High signal intensity at cuff insertion point is well delineated *(large arrow)*. The magnitude of the tear shows that a simple exploratory or decompressive procedure does not suffice. Advanced knowledge of lesion size is not possible by physical examination or arthroscopy.

praspinatus is usually seen in the case of complete tears but may be difficult to visualize in smaller tears. Atrophy of the muscle belly occurs and can be related to the chronicity of the injury. It is identified by loss of general mass and fatty infiltration into the muscle substance (Fig. 4-51). Changes in the subacromial/subdeltoid space and peribursal fat also are present. This may result in bursal fluid accumulation from the joint and diminution of fat signal secondary to scarring.

An advantage of MRI is the ability to detect size, location, and pattern of rotator cuff tears.[85] As noted earlier, the supraspinatus is best seen on the coronal views for its mediolateral dimensions and on the sagittal view for anteroposterior dimensions. This portion of the cuff is by far the most commonly involved in such tears. These

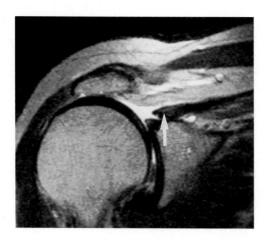

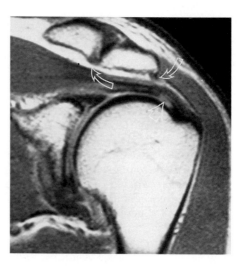

FIG. 4-51. Massive chronic rotator cuff tear. Note retraction of tendon *(arrow)*, muscle atrophy, and fatty infiltration of supraspinatus muscle belly. Compare with more acute massive tear in Fig. 4-53. There is superior migration of the humeral head with no recognizable tendinous structures seen within the markedly diminished subacromial space. The articular aspects of the acromioclavicular joint are irregular. The size and site of the cuff tear are discerned by magnetic resonance imaging, which might help in dictating ultimate treatment, including the surgical approach.

FIG. 4-52. Partial-thickness rotator cuff tear *(straight arrow)* is seen proximal to ultimate tendon insertion. Inferior osteophytes from acromioclavicular joint and acromion are seen *(curved arrows)*.

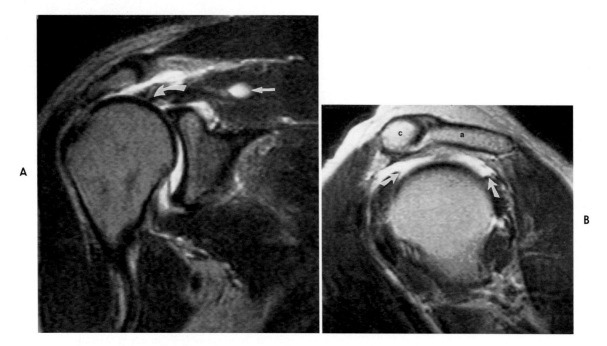

FIG. 4-53. Massive acute rotator cuff tear. **A,** Coronal view. Retracted tendon *(curved arrow)* is noted without the atrophy and fatty infiltration seen in more chronic ruptures. A small cyst is noted in the muscle belly of the supraspinatus muscle *(straight arrow)*, which might indicate earlier intrasubstance degeneration. **B,** Sagittal view. Note absence of tendinous structures between humeral head *(h)* and acromioclavicular region from arrowhead to arrowhead.

generally occur at the tendinous insertion into the greater tuberosity or the slightly more proximal critical zone, with a small portion of the tendon remaining attached to the tuberosity. These tears can extend anteriorly and include the subscapularis, but more commonly they involve the infraspinatus posteriorly.

Partial-thickness tears are generally best visualized on

T2-weighted scans (Fig. 4-52). They can manifest as a retraction of the anterior portion of the tendon from the greater tuberosity. These are often missed at arthrography due to retained fibers at either the synovial or bursal surface. Full-thickness tears are identified on T2 imaging with a high signal intensity noted at the cuff defect.

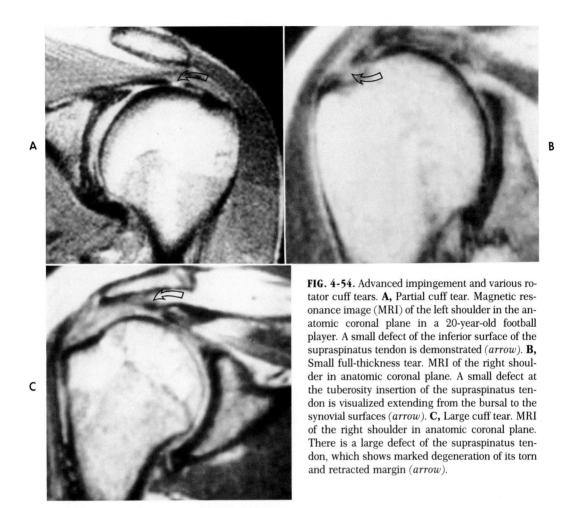

FIG. 4-54. Advanced impingement and various rotator cuff tears. **A,** Partial cuff tear. Magnetic resonance image (MRI) of the left shoulder in the anatomic coronal plane in a 20-year-old football player. A small defect of the inferior surface of the supraspinatus tendon is demonstrated (*arrow*). **B,** Small full-thickness tear. MRI of the right shoulder in anatomic coronal plane. A small defect at the tuberosity insertion of the supraspinatus tendon is visualized extending from the bursal to the synovial surfaces (*arrow*). **C,** Large cuff tear. MRI of the right shoulder in anatomic coronal plane. There is a large defect of the supraspinatus tendon, which shows marked degeneration of its torn and retracted margin (*arrow*).

Other than high or low signal generation at the tear site, morphologic changes may commonly occur. In the case of an attempted healing response, a thickened cuff edge represented by low signal (scarring) may be present. Attenuation of the tear edges may point to a more chronic condition, whereas a thickened edge with intermediate signal points to a more acute event (with bleeding and edema) (Fig. 4-53).

Evancho et al[46] used both T2 high signal intensity and morphologic identification (tendon discontinuity and irregularity) to determine rotator cuff tears. For full-thickness tears they found an 80% sensitivity, 94% specificity, and 84% accuracy in MRI performance. Overall (full-thickness and partial-thickness tears combined) there was 69% sensitivity, 94% specificity, and 84% accuracy.

Zlatkin et al,[200] using similar criteria, also included peribursal fat line abnormalities in their determinations. They found a 100% sensitivity in full-thickness and 91% sensitivity in full and partial tears combined. In conjunction with conventional arthrography, they found both a greater sensitivity and specificity for MRI in detecting full-thickness cuff tears. Burke,[18] comparing MRI, arthrography, and sonography with surgical follow-up, found a 92% sensitivity and 100% specificity of MRI

(comparable to arthrography), both of which were vastly superior to sonography.

Rafii et al[159] found a 95% sensitivity for full-thickness tears and 85% for partial tears. They determined that a high T2 signal at this site is the most common finding in cuff tears. Less commonly a low signal as a result of scarring was present.

Iannotti et al[85] with 91 patients, found that the greatest clinical value of MRI was detecting complete tears (including their size) and the muscle atrophy accompanying chronic tears. In comparing complete tears and intact rotator cuffs, they found 100% sensitivity and 95% specificity of the MRI in detecting full-thickness tears.

Impingement

Impingement and its associated disorders are the most common causes of shoulder pain. MRI can not only reveal the cuff tears that may be the final structural failure as a result of the syndrome of impingement (Fig. 4-54), but also detect rotator cuff tendinitis, subacromial bursitis, and AC joint arthritis (Fig. 4-55).

Cuff tendinitis appears on MRI scans when the normal signal void of the tendon is altered and replaced with a moderate or high signal intensity on T1-weighted images. These changes are an indication of chemical

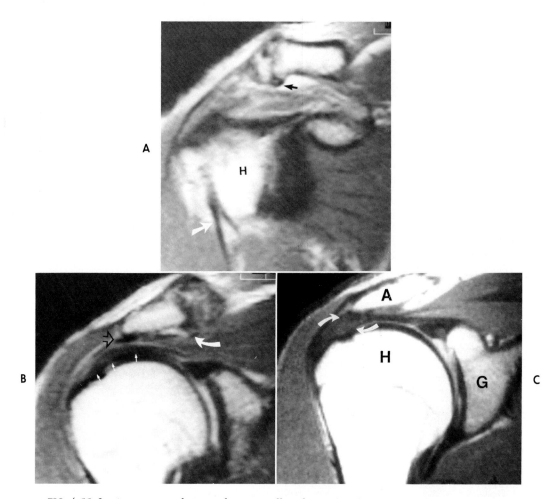

FIG. 4-55. Impingement syndrome and rotator cuff tendinitis. **A** and **B,** Magnetic resonance images (MRIs) of the right shoulder in anatomic coronal plane; **A** is anterior (medial) to **B. A,** This coronal image is at the most anterior aspect of the joint, with the humeral head *(H)* and the long head of the biceps tendon *(white arrow)* visualized. There is an inferiorly pointing osteophyte of the acromioclavicular (AC) joint *(black arrow).* **B,** This section through the supraspinatus muscle and tendon again demonstrates degenerative manifestations of the AC joint with hypertrophic changes *(curved arrow)* impinging upon the musculotendinous junction. Also an area of hypertrophic change is present at the periphery of the acromion process *(open arrow).* The supraspinatus tendon has an inhomogeneous appearance with a linear area of increased signal along its length *(small arrows).* This is indicative of tendinitis and may also indicate interstitial tendon tear. There is no complete tendon tear demonstrated. **C,** MRI of the right shoulder in the anatomic coronal plane. There is marked swelling of the distal aspect of the supraspinatus tendon (distance between *curved arrows*). Also the peribursal fat is obliterated indicating subacromial-subdeltoid bursitis. *A,* Acromion. *G,* glenoid, *H,* humeral head.

or histologic alteration within the tendon, which can reflect degenerative, inflammatory, or posttraumatic changes.[92,96,159,195] Zaslov et al[195] found histologic manifestations of degeneration in supraspinatus tendons that had high signal intensity on MRI scans. Fatty degeneration and fiber disorganization and separation were noted. They caution that MRI findings of tendinitis and interstitial tears may overlap and that these are separate stops along the line of a single pathologic process (inflammation and repair after multiple microtraumas). Seeger et al[179] studied 107 symptomatic shoulders and diagnosed impingement in 53. Three types of impinge-

ment signs were recognized: Type I—subacromial bursitis; Type IIa—supraspinatus tendinitis; and Type IIb—tendinitis with areas of tendon disruption.

As opposed to microtears, degeneration of the cuff was able to be distinguished from tendinitis in the study by Iannotti et al,[85] using surgical identification as the standard. They found a sensitivity of 82% and specificity of 85% in the differentiation of tendinitis and cuff degeneration. Also, differentiation of tendinitis and normal cuff tendons showed sensitivity of 93% and specificity of 87%.

Subacromial and subdeltoid bursitis can be detailed on

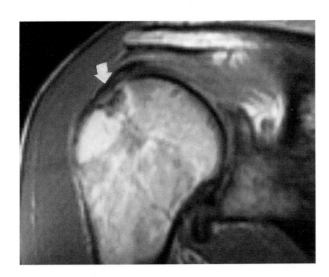

FIG. 4-56. Subcortical cystic changes *(arrow)* around greater tuberosity in subacromial impingement.

MRI scans by an alteration in the peribursal fat pattern and changes in the bursal space itself. In cases of more chronic changes, scarring or obliteration of bursal recesses and fat can be noted on T1 images. Fluid accumulation in the bursal tissue is readily noted on T2 studies and may indicate acute inflammation or fluid flow through a rotator cuff tear.

AC joint degenerative changes with both soft-tissue and osseous changes are readily noted by MRI. AC joint spurs, which may impinge on the supraspinatus tendon and musculotendinous junction, can also be demonstrated. Sclerosis and subcortical cysts (Fig. 4-56) are noted in the greater tuberosity in early stages of impingement and are readily noted by MRI.

Degenerative changes and frank rupture of the biceps tendon related to aging and acute trauma are not uncommon. In addition, tenosynovitis or subluxation of the tendon may be present secondary to trauma. MRI is particularly well suited to discern these abnormalities as changes in tendon morphology (thinning, thickening, or nonvisualization), position, or synovial surroundings are readily elicited.

Snyder et al[183] described the superior labrum anterior and posterior (SLAP) lesion regarding injuries to the biceps and its anchor at the superior labrum. Early studies[20,66,82] have documented a relative efficacy in detailing these lesions by MRI, but more work is needed in this area.

Certainly, on the basis of the clinical studies thus far available and our experience, it is evident that most osseous, bursal, and tendinous manifestations of mechanical impingement can be detected. Our experience with MRI at 1.5 T has shown a sensitivity of greater than 92% in detection of partial or complete cuff tears. At this time very few partial or small complete tears cannot be accurately differentiated from one another or from tendinitis. Also, MRI has the capability of detecting certain lesions that are usually not detectable by shoulder arthrography, such as intratendinous or bursal surface partial tears or full-thickness tears that are sealed by the synovial lining of the joint.[125]

Instability

In this era of arthroscopic labral reattachment and capsular advancement, surgeons of varied skills may hope to determine the planning of an open vs. closed procedure or attempt to predict the duration of postoperative disability on the basis of an accurate, minimally invasive diagnostic test. Kleinman et al[97] expressed many of these thoughts when contemplating the performance of CT arthrography before the advent of MRI. They stated that the need for preoperative study in the patient with documented instability "is dictated by the general approach of the orthopaedic surgeon." It is a function of what the surgeon desires to learn or to gain from the procedure, which includes the extent of labral disruption, corroboration of the direction of instability, and a diagnostic reaffirmation for the patient. In the patient without obvious instability the indications include a search for labral tears or for the discovery of an unsuspected instability. Either procedure may lead to findings that could avert an invasive procedure or help the physician avoid the selection of an inappropriate surgical approach.

Glenohumeral instability is most often discoverable by history and physical examination and is frequently documented by more conventional radiography, as discussed earlier in the chapter. However, when there is a need for more precise evaluation of the suspected pathologic condition, special studies are necessary. Until recently, only CT arthrography was able to adequately confirm these abnormalities. MRI has now stepped into the forefront to stake its claim as a powerful noninvasive implement to determine these pathologic conditions. It has value in the discovery of subtle or unsuspected instability, the determination of the direction of instability, and the characterization of the type of labral lesion associated with the instability.[57]

At times the diagnosis of the unstable shoulder can be difficult.[60] Many patients are poor at perceiving a sense of sliding and merely experience pain as a manifestation of glenohumeral displacement. Many are too apprehensive to be adequately examined or refuse to submit to surgery or anesthesia for purposes of diagnosis. MRI can be especially helpful in defining these soft tissue abnormalities in such situations.

If MRI is to be able to identify instability of the shoulder, it must be able to identify its pathologic components. Instability has many faces, each with its particular attributes. Clinically based classifications have defined instability based on direction (anterior, posterior, or multidirectional) and etiology (atraumatic [congenitally lax], macrotraumatic [an event], and microtraumatic [repetitive]).[134] Still others consider whether it is voluntary or involuntary.[170] To confuse matters, one type may be superimposed upon another within each class or cross the various classification lines.

The above descriptions do not address pathologic anatomy, which may be present. The essential anatomic lesions of anterior shoulder instability are primarily regarded to be that of capsuloglenoid/glenolabral disrup-

TABLE 4-2 Variability in anterior and posterior labral shapes in 52 asymptomatic shoulders at inferior, mild, and superior glenoid levels

Shape	Anterior Part of Labrum (%)			Posterior Part of Labrum (%)		
	Inferior	Mid	Superior	Inferior	Mid	Superior
Triangular	24 (46)	21 (40)	25 (49)	42 (81)	42 (81)	30 (58)
Rounded	8 (15)	4 (8)	17 (32)	7 (13)	7 (13)	5 (10)
Cleaved	9 (17)	13 (25)	2 (4)	0	0	0
Notched	7 (13)	6 (11)	0	0	0	0
Flat	2 (4)	6 (11)	3 (6)	3 (6)	3 (6)	4 (8)
Absent	2 (4)	2 (4)	5 (9)	0	0	13 (25)

From Neumann CH et al: *Am J Roentgenol* 157:1015, 1991.

TABLE 4-3 Variability in capsular attachment in 52 shoulders at the inferior, mid, and superior levels of the glenoid cavity

Type of Insertion	Anterior Part of Glenoid (%)			Posterior Part of Glenoid (All Levels) (%)
	Inferior	Mid	Superior	
1	17 (33)	6 (12)	50 (96)	52 (100)
2	33 (63)	42 (80)	2 (4)	0
3	2 (4)	4 (8)	0	0

From Neumann CH et al: *Am J Roentgenol* 157:1015, 1991.
NOTE: Type 1, capsular insertion on labral tip or its outer surface; Type 2, insertion immediately medial to labrum on glenoid rim; Type 3, insertion 1 cm or more medial to cartilaginous labral tip on cortical surface of glenoid neck.

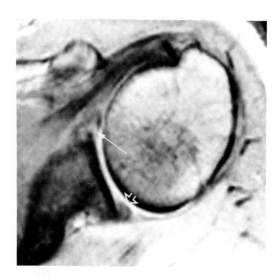

FIG. 4-57. Glenoid labrum tear. Axial magnetic resonance imaging scan of the left shoulder at the proximal aspect of the glenohumeral joint. There is an abnormal configuration of the anterior glenoid labrum, which is separated from the glenoid margin with an area of increased signal intensity (*solid arrow*). This indicates tear and detachment. The posterior labrum has a normal configuration, but demonstrates normal signal intensity (*open arrow*). This is indicative of partial tear.

tion (Bankart lesions) and frank capsular tearing.[8,77,130] In addition, Bigliani et al[10] have reintroduced the concept of capsulohumeral disruption.[143,170]

Studies comparing and detailing the efficacy of MRI and CT arthrography in the diagnosis of instability are currently available for review. Early studies by Kieft et al[90,91] noted poor visualization of capsular alterations and insertional stripping unless large effusions were present. Later studies reveal an improved accuracy in determining labral and capsular injury equal to and surpassing CT arthrography.[70,86,136,161,178] Delineation of these areas now seems to be well suited to superior soft-tissue resolution of MRIs, which may be due to better recognition of anatomic structures and technical advances (Figs. 4-57 to 4-59).*

On MRI the glenoid labrum is normally visualized as a signal void outlined by signal derived from surrounding elements (hyaline articular cartilage of the glenoid and humeral head and the small amounts of joint fluid covering the joint surfaces).[176,196,199] Neumann et al[138] performed MRI on a series of asymptomatic shoulders to ascertain labral morphology and capsular insertion patterns in theoretically normal shoulders. Their assessment of labra was based primarily upon the variations noted by McCauley et al,[110] McNiesh and Callaghan,[114]

and Rafii et al[156] seen on CT arthrography. The incidence of occurrence of labral types noted is shown in Table 4-2. The capsular attachments listed in Table 4-3 are based on the attachments described by Moseley et al.[130]

The pathologic changes of the labrum are determined mostly on the basis of its abnormal contours, relations to the glenoid margin, and areas of abnormal signal intensity. Glenoid labral lesions can be depicted as a configurational abnormality of the structure itself such as irregular outline, attenuation, and total absence. In addition, labral detachments from the glenoid or even intrasubstance tears can be depicted by abnormal signal bands, which would not ordinarily be present.[176,196,199]

The physician must be aware of normal anatomic features that might give rise to a seemingly abnormal signal.[107] McCauley et al[110] found increased signal at the bone-labrum junction in 100% of allegedly normal labra in a young population (mean age 33 years). This may be

*References 21, 68, 85, 104, 115, 131, 137, 155, 160, 175, 176, 187, 196, 197, and 199.

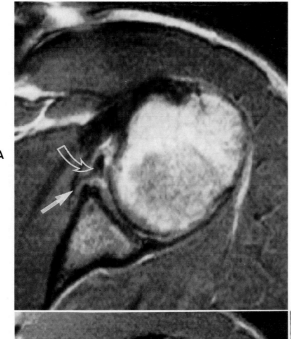

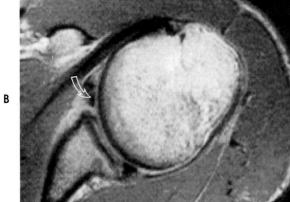

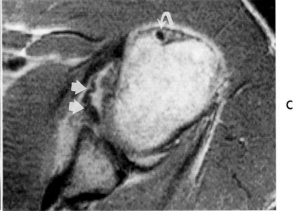

FIG. 4-58. Instability. Labral detachments in two professional hockey players after acute injuries. Note labral detachments form glenoid (*open arrows*), capsular stripping from anterior glenoid neck (*straight arrow*) in **A** and **B,** and redundant capsule (*arrowheads*) in **C.** These findings were corroborated at surgery. Resolution of biceps tendon (*curved arrow*). **B** and **C** are from the same patient at different anatomic levels.

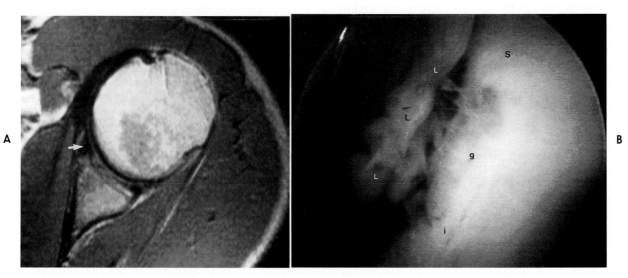

FIG. 4-59. Recurrent dislocations. Patient complained of multiple shoulder dislocations while sleeping after acute event 1 year prior (**A**). Labral detachment is seen (*straight arrow*). **B,** Intraoperative arthroscopic photo shows labral dislocation from anterior glenoid viewed from posterior portal. *g,* Glenoid; *L,* labrum; *s,* superior glenoid; *i,* inferior glenoid.

caused by a hyaline cartilage signal beneath the labrum. Although other signal abnormalities were discovered within the labra, morphologic abnormalities were essentially found only in patients with labral tears. These features, which are not recognized on CT arthrography, can be a source of error on MRI. However, they caution that morphologic changes were more predictive of labral tears vs. intralabral signal changes.

These distinctions are made even more difficult because of the varying attachments of the labral tissue into the very same glenoid at different areas. Copper et al,[28] noted different labral morphologies in relation to the superior vs. the inferior labrum. Interiorly a rounded structure firmly attached to the underlying glenoid was noted, whereas superiorly the labrum was more meniscal appearing, being more mobile and less firmly anchored.

The capsulolabral complex comprises the area of interest when dealing with the Bankart lesion. This characteristically involves the anteroinferior region of the glenohumeral ligaments with or without bony involvement of the glenoid. The labrum may be clearly torn, detached, undulating (capsular laxity), or stripped from the scapular neck. Abnormal signal intensity may also result from degenerative changes within the labrum and should not be mistaken for instability lesions.[21] The differentiation is based primarily on the characteristic location of instability lesions and the more generalized nature of degenerative changes.

In clinical studies Iannotti et al[85] noted a sensitivity of 88% and specificity of 93% when evaluating labral tears proved by subsequent surgical intervention. In defining the spectrum of labral lesions, they noted a value of MRI that could be detected neither by ultrasound nor by CT arthrogram. In 88 arthroscopically confirmed cases, Legan et al[104] noted a sensitivity and specificity of anterior labral tears of 95% and 86% and in superior labral tears 75% and 99%, respectively. The accuracy for anterior labral lesions was 92%, whereas that for superior labral lesions was 95%. Unfortunately the findings for other instability patterns were not as promising. For posterior labral abnormalities an 8% sensitivity was noted, and for the inferior labrum 40%. They noted a lesion, the glenoid labrum ovoid mass (GLOM) (Fig. 4-60), which they believed was a retraction of a torn anterior labrum. This was a dark round mass at the base of the coracoid seen best on a T2-weighted image, suggesting a retracted labral tear.

Abnormalities of the subscapularis tendon may also be noted by MRI (rupture, retraction of the musculotendinous junction, and atrophy), generally in the older population following a dislocation.[176] In addition, cartilage lesions associated with instability and Hill-Sachs deformities[192] are visualized and may be important in aiding in the diagnosis of mild instabilities.* Posterior instability manifests with lesions similar to those of its anterior counterpart, including posterior capsulolabral complex abnormalities with or without associated anterior lesions in those with multidirectional instability.[176]

The bottom line is that MRI has the lone ability to noninvasively affirm traumatic and anterior/inferior instabil-

---
*References 70, 85, 131, 136, 175, 176, 196, 197 and 199.

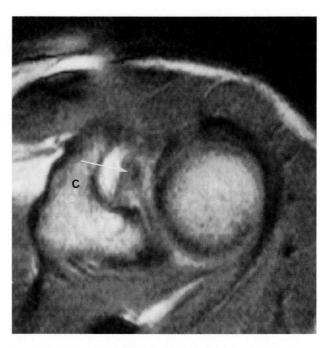

FIG. 4-60. Glenoid labrum ovoid mass (GLOM). Axial magnetic resonance imaging in same patient as Fig. 4-58, *A*. Signal void mass at base of coracoid (*c*) is thought to be retracted anterior labrum or capsule (*arrow*).

ities (macrotrauma more than microtrauma), the only ones for which there are consistent pathognomonic pathologic abnormalities. It appears that instability of the shoulder can be evaluated with MRI with a high degree of accuracy. In addition, patients who undergo MRI evaluation for capsulolabral injury are evaluated simultaneously for impingement and other forms of rotator cuff abnormalities that can develop in the unstable shoulder. With new higher resolution scanners, image clarity and interpretive confidence will continue to improve.

MRI Arthrography

Early plain MRI studies noted a high sensitivity of detection of labral injury when acute trauma was studied for instability vs. more chronic cases.[91] The presence of an effusion was very helpful in these situations because it provided an intraarticular contrast and joint distention when viewed from an MRI standpoint. Numerous authors have indicated the value of contrast imaging in assessing lesions of the labrocapsular complexes as noted above, but mostly with regard to CT scanning, not MRI.[50,156,158,161,196] The addition of contrast agents to MRI offers the potential advantages of demonstrating intraarticular anatomy, capsular ruptures, and possible enlargement of capsular pouches with greater clarity. (Fig. 4-61).[50,71,72] Enhanced injury of the labrum is noted, including biceps and SLAP lesions.[82] The potential for delineating tears of the rotator cuff is also increased. Zlatkin et al.[196] used cadaver specimens with gadolinium injections to detail the normal and abnormal cross-sectional appearance of the glenohumeral joint as a baseline for further MRI study.

Hajek et al[71,72] compared gadolinium, normal saline,

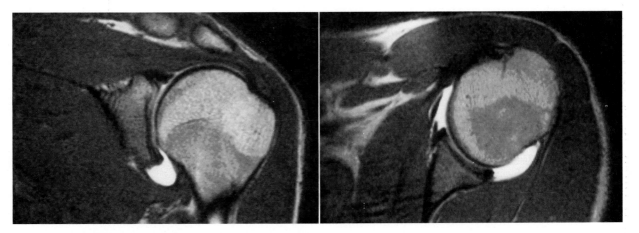

FIG. 4-61. Magnetic resonance arthrography. Intraarticular gadolinium enhances joint capsule volume. In this case no labral pathology or rotator cuff abnormalities are noted. The patient had clinical history of multidirectional instability with associated complaints of pain and weakness.

diatrizoate (Renograffin), and air as contrast agents in both shoulder and knee cadaver specimens. They found gadolinium to be a superior agent because of its high signal intensity exhibited on T1-weighted sequences. This offers excellent contrast against surrounding anatomic structures. Using the T1 sequences allows for more rapid studies and decreased chances of artifact secondary to subject motion. T2-weighted sequences were needed for use with saline and diatrizoate injections, because faster sequences did not allow adequate contrast difference between the agents and anatomic structures. Inherent in T2 weighting is its increased imaging time and lower spacial resolution. Overall, with contrast, smaller surgically created lesions were better identified than without, whereas larger lesions were noted with more confidence. In a separate study by Hajek et al[73] it was shown that gadolinium has neither macroscopic nor microscopic effects on the synovium or articular cartilage of rabbit joints; however, clinical studies are pending.

Flannigan et al[50] evaluated symptomatic shoulders by both arthrographic and nonarthrographic MRI. They reported that conventional imaging missed two thirds of the labral tears discovered at surgery, whereas MRI arthrography revealed them all (n = 9). This is disturbing considering that MRI arthrography is not an established procedure, and the lesions missed by conventional MRI were of prognostic or therapeutic import. The implications from this study are that for conventional MRI, the presence of a significant pathologic finding should be presumed valid (low percentage of false positives), whereas the absence of one (magnitude dependent) should not be presumed to be valid (potential false negatives). In other words, there is an implication that many labral tears will be missed without the use of contrast.

Although MRI contrast material has been used to evaluate various joints, several drawbacks exist. The contrast agent most commonly employed, gadolinium diethylen-etriaminepentaacetic acid (DTPA), is rather expensive. The procedure requires insertion of a needle into the joint (which needs to be proven in the fluoroscopy suite) before transferring the patient to the MRI suite. This eliminates one advantage of MRI, that is, its noninvasive nature. From the surgeon's perspective it appears that the jury is still out with regard to a strong recommendation for the routine use of contrast, except in rare instances.

Postsurgical Evaluation

Following surgical intervention reevaluation of the shoulder for persistent symptoms is occasionally necessary. With regard to both bony and soft-tissue procedures, MRI seems to be able to ascertain adequacy of the procedure performed, although, as noted previously, even undisturbed presurgical normal anatomy may be difficult to distinguish from pathologic alterations. Little has been written on the subject and, until more clinical studies are done, little can be said about the efficiency of MRI in this regard.

Owen et al[147] were able to delineate one specific use of MRI in a postoperative setting. Following surgery they were able to determine full-thickness tears with an accuracy of 90%, sensitivity of 86%, and specificity of 92% utilizing nonvisualization or a high signal on T2 studies extending through an area of the rotator cuff. They found, however, that partial tears were indistinguishable from those rotator cuffs that had been successfully repaired. With impingement their success rates of predicting this condition were relatively poor, with a sensitivity of 64%. MRI was able to exclude impingement in those thought to be free from impingement (specificity 82%), and had an overall accuracy of 74% (Fig. 4-62).

Current Status

Interpretations of MRI are best formulated after a discussion between the referring physician and radiologist in which the history, physical findings, and most particularly *the object of having ordered the imaging in the case* has been determined. An interpretation of images without the benefit of this discussion can result in more speculative interpretation as a contributing basis for treatment. Hence, the vital objective of the radiologist is to render interpretive information specifically addressed

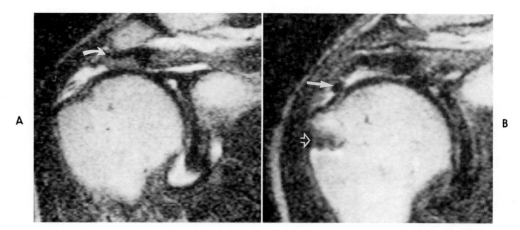

FIG. 4-62. Preoperative and postoperative magnetic resonance image (MRI). Full-thickness rotator cuff tear is seen both before (**A**) (note retracted rotator cuff tendon *[curved arrow]*), and after (**B**) open repair. After surgery patient had excellent clinical recovery including range of motion and strength and agreed to a follow-up MRI with knowledge of its academic import. Follow-up study delineates repaired tendon *(straight arrow)* and the bony trough used for reinsertion *(arrowhead)*. The tendon signal is highly irregular and does not appear to mimic a normal anatomic course. How we might use this information for clinical purposes in the case of a clinical failure after surgery is unclear at the present.

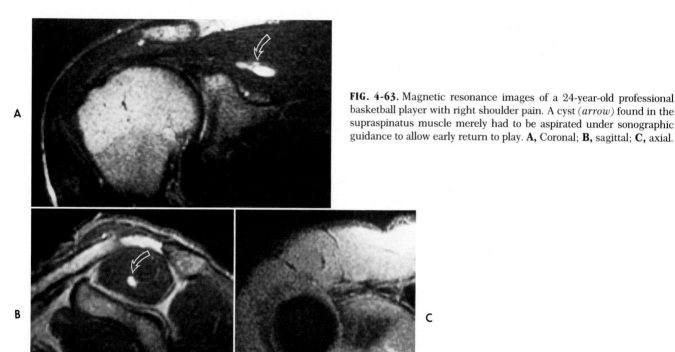

FIG. 4-63. Magnetic resonance images of a 24-year-old professional basketball player with right shoulder pain. A cyst *(arrow)* found in the supraspinatus muscle merely had to be aspirated under sonographic guidance to allow early return to play. **A**, Coronal; **B**, sagittal; **C**, axial.

to the requesting physician as opposed to any physician in general.

Some of the indications for MRI evaluation therefore include the following (after adequate history and physical examination):

1. Patient or third-party carrier requires documentation before permitting an invasive study.

2. When procedure and timing are particularly critical. A professional athlete, for example, who complains of shoulder pain that precludes effective play needs diagnostic resolution to predict length of disability and an appropriateness of treatment. Diagnostic arthroscopy or arthrogram (with or without CT) automatically costs the player days or weeks

out of the line-up, and therefore MRI is a wiser diagnostic choice. (Fig 4-63)

3. When a decision to perform an arthroscopic vs. an open procedure must be determined in advance of the surgery, or, for example, when a particular surgical facility must be decided upon (inpatient or outpatient) for open or arthroscopic procedures.

4. When the length of disability must be anticipated in advance of surgery. For example, a patient who undergoes an arthroscopic excision of a bucketed labral fragment might anticipate missing a considerably shorter period of work than would a patient who undergoes an open glenohumeral reconstruction for instability.

5. When there has been an initial subluxation or dislocation and consideration of primary repair is entertained to prevent a recurrent pattern of instability.

6. The diagnostic dilemma.

The basic advantages offered by MRI for the shoulder at this time are that it is noninvasive and provides a comprehensive, multiplanar evaluation of the joint, which can detect a moderate quantity of pathologic changes. Its most promising diagnostic advantage over other radiographic techniques is its ability to demonstrate, at once, the collective components of impingement, including rotator cuff tears and the pathologic changes found with shoulder instability. Its principal disadvantage is its high cost.

ULTRASONOGRAPHY

Ultrasonography is another technique that is noninvasive to patients.[15,76,146] It is most valuable in the evaluation of the rotator cuff.* The difficult learning curve needed for reliable interpretation has undoubtedly been a deterrent to the popularity of shoulder ultrasonography. As pointed out by Balogh et al,[6] ultrasonography, like

---

*References 48, 54, 109, 116, 122, 127, and 184.

MRI, may be studied in all planes, and the use of a real-time probe permits almost a cine-evaluation of evolving echogenicity in the study of tendon damage.

Physics of Ultrasound

Sound waves are vibrations of gases, liquids, or solids that are quantitated in terms of hertz (Hz), the international unit of frequency, equal to one cycle per second. Those in the range of 20 to 20,000 Hz are audible to the human ear. Sound vibrations below 20 Hz are termed subsonic, and those above 20,000 Hz are termed ultrasonic. Frequencies 1 to 15 million Hz or megahertz- (MHz) are used for medical diagnostic ultrasonography.

Since acoustic waves of sufficiently high frequency can be made to travel in a beam with little spreading, such a beam can explore a physical medium and detect inhomogeneities by reflection (echo). Ultrasonography is the technical procedure in which the transmitted and reflected properties of an ultrasound beam are imaged and recorded after passage through a particular area of the body. An ultrasound beam travels through tissue at a fixed rate, and thus the distance traveled by the beam and echo, when imaged, indicates the proportional distances between the structures traversed.

When an ultrasound beam is transmitted through a medium and strikes a second medium of altered density, a portion of the energy is reflected at the tissue boundary (interface) while the remaining energy penetrates the second medium. Diagnostic data are obtained by imaging the echoes at tissue boundaries. The interfaces relevant to the study of the rotator cuff are those between the differing soft tissue media of the deltoid muscle, rotator cuff, and bony humerus.

Technique

A real-time mechanic sector scanner employing a 7.5 or 10 MHz transducer is most often used (Fig. 4-64). A patient is scanned while seated with the humerus resting against the patient's side or slightly extended and in neutral or slight external rotation.

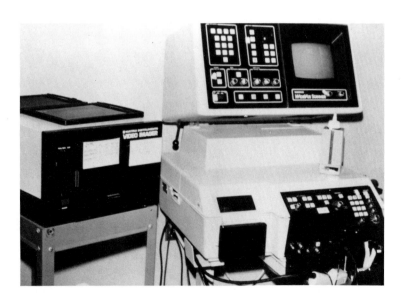

FIG. 4-64. Real-time small parts mechanical sector scanner with 10-MHz transducer.

In this position the region of insertion of the supraspinatus tendon into the greater tuberosity of the humerus lies uncovered anterior and lateral to the shadowing effect of the acromion process, exposing to the transducer the critical zone of vascularity where most rotator cuff ruptures occur.[164] The more proximal portion of the rotator cuff beneath the acromion process may be exposed by shrugging the shoulder and occasionally by simultaneously extending the humerus at the glenohumeral joint. The more lateral and posterior portions are uncovered by internal rotation of the humerus.

The bicipital groove and greater tuberosity are used as landmarks for localizing the supraspinatus tendon, which is scanned in the longitudinal (sagittal) and transverse planes (Figs. 4-65 and 4-66). Emphasis is placed on the anterior or supraspinatus portion of the cuff since most tears occur in this area, but the more posterior portions containing the tendinous insertions of the infraspi-

natus and teres minor should also be routinely scanned. Most investigators image the subscapularis only when clinical suspicion points to this area. The intraarticular and extraarticular portions of the tendon of the long head of the biceps, including the bicipital groove of the humerus, are scanned in the transverse plane (Fig. 4-67). The tendon is also imaged in the longitudinal plane along its long axis. (Fig. 4-68).[33,114,119,120]

Normal Ultrasonographic Anatomy
Rotator Cuff

The relevant anatomy of the shoulder region is easily imaged and compared with the opposite member for diagnostic purposes. The rotator cuff appears as a well-marginated band of homogenous echogenicity between the humeral head below and the deltoid muscle above. Acoustic shadowing from the acromion establishes the limit of visualization medially, while distally the aponeu-

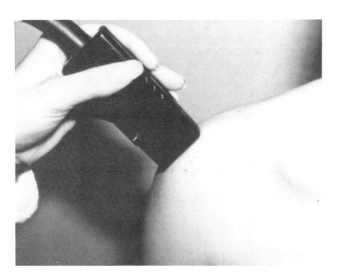

FIG. 4-65. Transducer aligned in the longitudinal (sagittal) plane of the supraspinatus tendon.

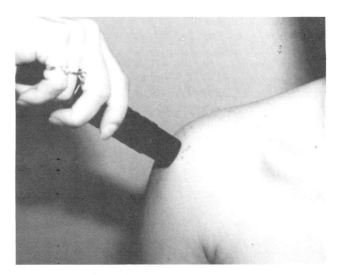

FIG. 4-66. Transducer aligned in the transverse plane of the supraspinatus tendon.

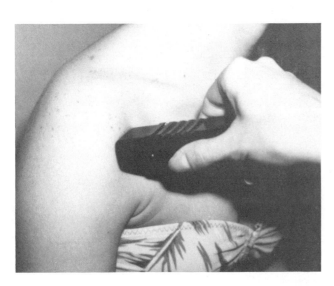

FIG. 4-67. Transducer aligned in the transverse plane of the tendon of the long head of the biceps.

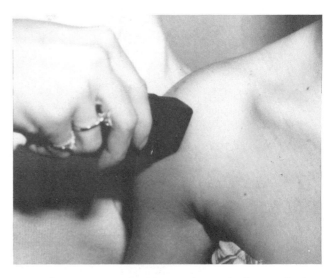

FIG. 4-68. Transducer aligned in the longitudinal (sagittal) plane of the tendon of the long head of the biceps.

rosis of the rotator cuff tapers in two directions, laterally into its bony insertion as well as posteriorly.

The rotator cuff band is bordered superiorly and inferiorly by echogenic lines of higher amplitude. The superficial line marks the interface of the deltoid muscle and rotator cuff and identifies the location of the subdeltoid bursa, which in its normal nondistended state is not resolved as a separate structure. The deep echogenic line results from reflections at the proximal humerus.

The average thickness of the anterior cuff is 6 mm and the posterior cuff 3.6 mm.[33] In most instances the rotator cuff band is thicker than the deltoid, which tends to diminish somewhat beyond the sixth decade of life. Physiologic age-related cuff thinning is represented sonographically as a homogeneous although hypoechoic band, which is symmetric with the opposite side. Increased gain settings may be used to evaluate its inter-

nal characteristics. Although focal inhomogeneities can occur in normal subjects, the echogenicity of the rotator cuff is relatively homogeneous and equal to or brighter than that of the suprajacent deltoid (Figs. 4-69 to 4-73). Comparison with the opposite side allows abnormalities to be differentiated from the physiologic reduced echogenicity seen in the elderly.

Biceps Tendon

On transverse scan the tendon of the long head of the biceps appears as an echogenic ellipse within the bicipital groove of the humerus. More proximally the tendon is found adjacent to the humeral head delineated superiorly and posteriorly by the supraspinatus and inferiorly and anteriorly by the subscapularis (Fig. 4-72). On longitudinal scans the tendon appears as a narrow band of tissue between the humerus and deep surface of the deltoid. Its echogenicity is greater than that of the deltoid muscle (Fig. 4-73).[118-121]

Abnormal Ultrasonographic Anatomy
Rotator Cuff

When the ultrasonic evaluation of the symptomatic shoulder is considered equivocal, the imaged asymptomatic side acts as a control providing a comparison with normal. Disagreement exists within the literature relative to the reliable and reproducible sonographic signs of

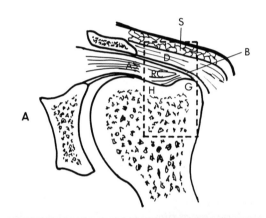

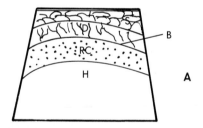

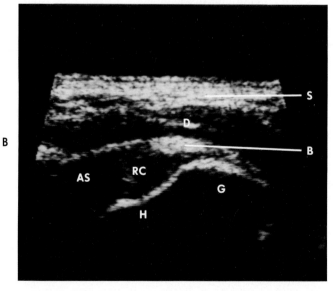

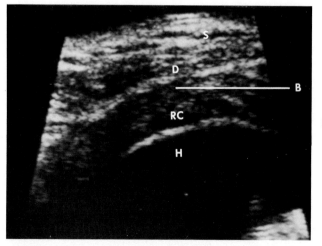

FIG. 4-69. Schematic (**A**) and sonographic (**B**) representations of the normal shoulder as seen in the longitudinal (sagittal) plane. *S*, Subcutaneous fat; *D*, deltoid muscle; *B*, echogenic line marking deltoid and rotator cuff interface and the location of the subdeltoid bursa (normally not imaged as a distinct structure); *AS*, area of acromion shadowing; *RC*, rotator cuff tendon; *H*, humerus; *G*, greater tuberosity. Note relative thickness and echogenicity of deltoid and rotator cuff images.

FIG. 4-70. Schematic (**A**) and sonographic (**B**) representations of the normal shoulder as seen in the transverse plane. *S*, Subcutaneous fat; *D*, deltoid muscle; *B*, echogenic line marking deltoid and rotator cuff interface and the location of the subdeltoid bursa (normally not imaged as a distinct structure); *RC*, rotator cuff tendon; *H*, humerus.

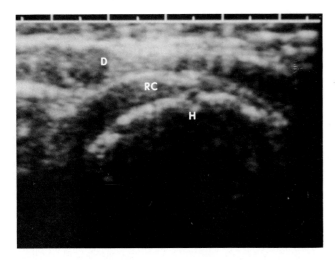

FIG. 4-71. Transverse scan in an asymptomatic subject demonstrating normal posterior thinning of rotator cuff. *D,* Deltoid; *RC,* rotator cuff; *H,* humerus.

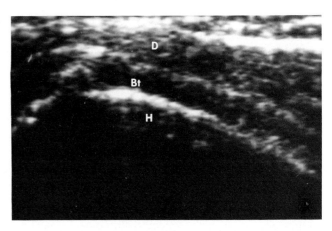

FIG. 4-73. Longitudinal scan showing tendon of the long head of the biceps between the humerus and deep surface of the deltoid. *D,* Deltoid; *Bt,* biceps tendon; *H,* humerus.

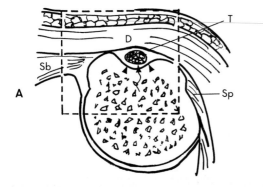

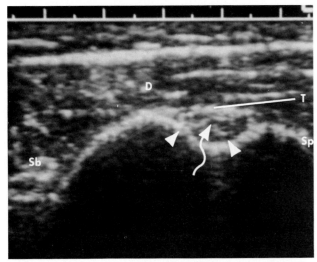

FIG. 4-72. Schematic (A) and transverse sonographic (B) representations of the normal tendon of the long head of the biceps in the bicipital groove of the humerus. *D,* Deltoid; *T,* transverse humeral ligament; *Sb,* subscapularis; *Sp,* supraspinatus. *Arrowheads,* Bicipital groove; *curved arrow,* bicipital tendon.

rotator cuff injury. Major diagnostic criteria include the following.[17,31-33,114,117-120]

Focal thinning. Focal thinning of the rotator cuff is considered a reliable sign of rupture. Although isolated tears in the posterior aspect of the rotator cuff are uncommon, suspected pathologic posterior thinning can be differentiated from normal posterior thinning by the presence of an abrupt transition between the normal and abnormal portions of the cuff. Pathologic thinning is almost always more pronounced than physiologic tapering, and symmetry is lost with the normal opposite side. Further, normal-appearing cuff tissue is not seen in an area of pathologic thinning (Figs. 4-74 and 4-75).

The intact portions of the tendons maintain the thickness of the tendon plane in smaller or incomplete tears, but the low-level echogenicity of normal tendon is replaced by high-level echoes, resulting from the many fibrous interfaces in the bursal proliferations.

An uncommon pattern of sonographic abnormality is represented as a factitious irregular thickening of the cuff with foci of increased and decreased echogenicity. The thickened appearance is caused by hypertrophied bursal elements, which are sonographically inseparable from the tendon undergoing degenerative change in the region of the tear (Fig. 4-76).

Nonvisualization. Nonvisualization of the rotator cuff is considered the most reliable criterion of rupture. In large tears in which the torn edge of the rotator cuff retracts under the acromion, the deep surface of the deltoid muscle becomes opposed to the humeral head without any intervening rotator cuff tissue. Ultrasonography demonstrates close opposition of the deep surface of the deltoid muscle to the entire humeral head (Fig. 4-77). The size of the defect that can be detected with sonography is controversial, and estimates have ranged from 1 to 3 cm.

Focal discontinuity. Small areas of discontinuity are more difficult to interpret and provide a source of false positive sonograms because of the presence of echogenic inhomogeneities seen in normal subjects (Fig. 4-78). Discontinuity occurs when rotator cuff defects fill with fluid or hyperechoic reactive tissue without opposition of

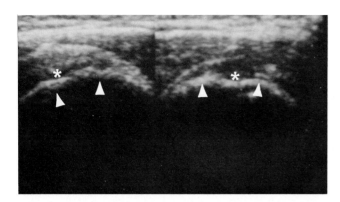

FIG. 4-74. Bilateral transverse sonograms in patient with right rotator cuff tear. Note marked thinning and absence of normal appearing cuff tissue on right. *Star,* Rotator cuff; *arrowheads,* humerus.

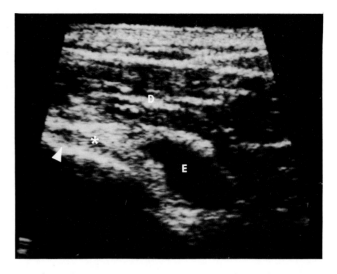

FIG. 4-75. Tranverse sonogram in a patient with complete rupture of the rotator cuff demonstrating markedly thinned and hyperechoic cuff tissue and effusion. *Star,* Thinned hyperechoic cuff tissue; *E,* effusion; *arrowheads,* humerus; *D,* deltoid.

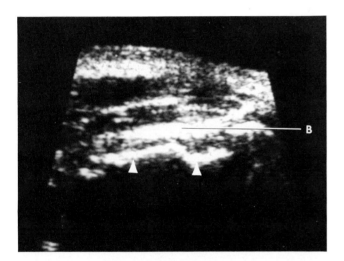

FIG. 4-76. Longitudinal scan in patient with complete rotator cuff rupture demonstrating bursal hypertrophy and marked thinning of rotator cuff. *B,* Bursal hypertrophy; *arrowheads,* humerus.

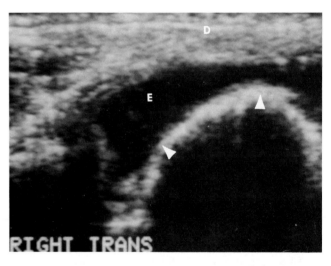

FIG. 4-77. Transverse sonogram demonstrating complete nonvisualization of rotator cuff in a patient with a large rupture that has retracted proximally. The deltoid is separated from the humeral head by a large effusion. *Arrowheads,* Humerus; *E,* effusion; *D,* deltoid.

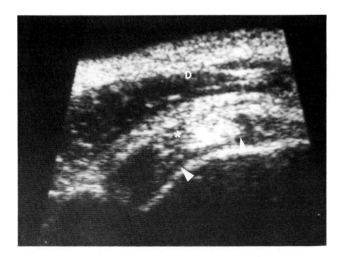

FIG. 4-78. Transverse sonogram in an asymptomatic shoulder revealing areas of echogenic inhomogeneity in the rotator cuff band. *D,* deltoid; *star,* rotator cuff; *arrowheads,* humerus.

the deltoid to the humeral head. This finding is more reliable when the discontinuity is large, well defined, and clearly asymmetric when compared with the opposite side. When the edge of the tendon is visible it may appear as a simple termination of the normal tendon or a hyperechoic and thickened border; at times it tapers toward the torn edge (Fig. 4-79).

A normal area of discontinuity is present on transverse scans between the intraarticular portion of the tendon of the long head of the biceps and the adjacent supraspinatus. This can be differentiated from a tear by first imaging the biceps tendon extraarticularly in the intertubercular groove of the humerus and following it proxi-

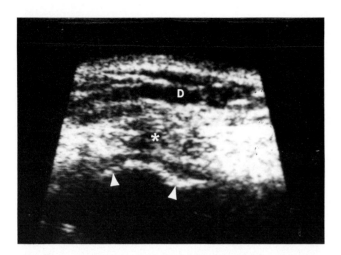

FIG. 4-79. Longitudinal sonogram demonstrating area of focal discontinuity in a patient with a moderate-sized cuff tear. *D,* deltoid; *star,* area of focal discontinuity in rotator cuff band; *arrowheads,* humerus.

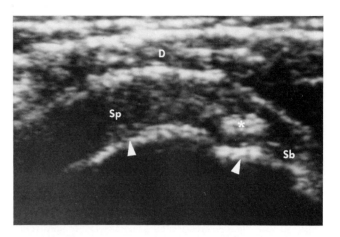

FIG. 4-80. Transverse sonogram demonstrating physiologic discontinuity surrounding intraarticular portion of biceps tendon. *D,* Deltoid; *Sp,* supraspinatus; *star,* biceps tendon; *Sb,* subscapularis; *arrowheads,* humerus.

mally over the humeral head. This strict delineation of the biceps tendon also serves to differentiate this portion of the normal shoulder anatomy from a hyperechogenic focus resulting from a cuff tear (Fig. 4-80). Discontinuity is a sign that must be interpreted on an individual basis and is generally considered a useful but not pathognomonic sign of rotator cuff tear.

Central echogenic bands. Granulation tissue and hypertrophied synovium filling the tear defect can result in the presence of a hyperechogenic band replacing the normal homogeneous echogenicity of the rotator cuff. Close comparison with the opposite side is mandatory, since echogenic bands may occur in normal shoulders (Fig. 4-81). In fact the frequency with which these bands occur in normal shoulders and the problems posed by the determination of asymmetry, the effect of technical factors, and the presence of calcification in the rotator cuff (Fig. 4-82) render it a difficult criterion to apply in most situations.

Nonspecific changes. Abnormal findings such as joint or bursal fluid, atrophy of the deltoid, and bursal hypertrophy, while not bearing a consistent association with rotator cuff tears or other shoulder lesions, do nonetheless bolster one's confidence that the shoulder has pathologic changes.

Biceps Tendon

Effusion. Effusions of the sheath of the tendon of the long head of the biceps appear on transverse scans as a penumbral area of decreased echogenicity (Fig. 4-83) and are often associated with other pathologic entities afflicting the glenohumeral joint, the most common being tears of the rotator cuff. Other lesions reported in association with effusions of the tendon sheath include adhesive capsulitis, fractures of the glenoid, osteochondral loose bodies, and subacromial fibrosis.[120]

Nonvisualization. Nonvisualization of the biceps tendon from its humeral groove suggests dislocation or rupture; tendon sheath effusion and asymmetric hyperechoic foci

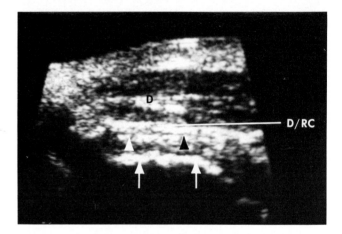

FIG. 4-81. Longitudinal sonogram in a patient with rotator cuff rupture demonstrating a central echogenic band that was not present on the opposite control. *D,* Deltoid; *arrowheads,* central echogenic band; *D/RC,* deltoid-rotator cuff interface; *arrows,* humerus.

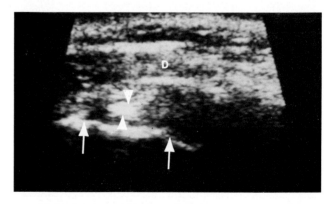

FIG. 4-82. Longitudinal scan in a patient demonstrating a hyperechogenic focus in the rotator cuff band caused by an area of calcific tendonitis. *D,* Deltoid; *arrowheads,* hyperechogenic focus (calcific deposit), *arrows,* humerus.

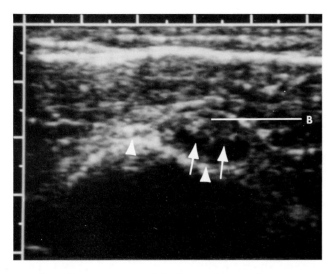

FIG. 4-83. Transverse scan of the bicipital groove demonstrating an effusion of the bicipital sheath appearing as an area of hypogenicity situated between the floor of the bicipital groove and the biceps tendon. The patient had a complete rotator cuff rupture. *B*, Biceps tendon; *arrows*, effusion; *arrowheads*, humerus.

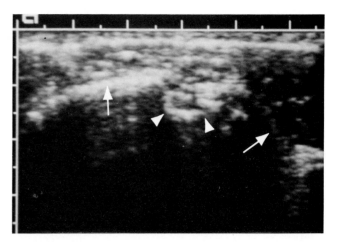

FIG. 4-84. Transverse scan of the bicipital groove in a patient with a proximal rupture of the tendon of the long head of the biceps. Scan reveals absence of the tendon from the groove, which contains echogenic fibrous tissue. *Arrowheads*, Bicipital groove; *arrows*, humerus.

within the tendon are indicative of chronic degenerative change.

Hyperechoic foci. Sonography can help delineate the site of biceps tendon rupture: visualization of the tendon within the groove places the rupture intraarticularly and allows for proper preoperative planning when surgery is anticipated (Fig. 4-84).

Loose bodies. Osteochondral loose bodies in the tendon sheath are likely to present as echogenic foci casting an acoustic shadow within a sheath effusion.

Advantages

Ultrasonography is quick, noninvasive, and painless and carries no risk of infection or allergic reaction. In most institutions its cost is only 75% or 80% that of an arthrogram and includes the routine investigation of the opposite shoulder with no morbidity.

Examination of the normal and abnormal biceps tendon is more readily and accurately accomplished with ultrasound than with contrast. Middleton et al[120] have reported considerably higher sensitivity, specificity, and accuracy values with ultrasonography when the two studies are compared.

Dynamic ultrasonographic imaging may add a new dimension to the motion study of normal and abnormal rotator cuff mechanics. These studies have shown the normal rotator cuff to glide smoothly beneath the coracoacromial arch during its excursion and suggest that the coracoacromial ligament functions as a pulley, guiding the superior rotator cuff and changing the direction and degree of the cuff indentation in abduction. Abnormal cuff mechanics have been demonstrated as a buckling or hesitancy of the cuff beneath the coracoacromial arch during motion, which corresponds with the patient's complaints of impingement pain.[26,67]

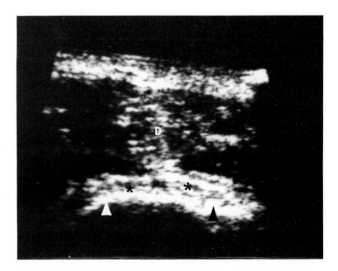

FIG. 4-85. Longitudinal scan in a patient with a recurrent rotator cuff tear. Rotator cuff band is absent and bursal elements lie opposed to the humeral head. *D*, Deltoid; *star*, bursal elements and granulation tissue; *arrowheads*, humerus.

Limitations

Ultrasonographic interpretation may be confused by altered anatomy secondary to large calcific deposits, bony deformity, or inferior subluxation of the glenohumeral joint.

In the presence of morbid obesity the transducer may not be capable of adequately penetrating to the level of the rotator cuff.

Ultrasonography of the postoperative rotator cuff is often confusing, since abnormal echogenicity resembling a tear in a patient who has not undergone surgery and distortion or absence of soft-tissue planes about the tendon persist indefinitely. As rotator cuff tears enlarge, the appearance changes from that of an echogenic area to a

gap or defect. The finding of an unequivocal defect in the rotator cuff tendon is the only reliable sign of a recurrent rotator cuff tear (Fig. 4-85).

When exaggerated anatomic variations render ultrasonographic interpretation difficult, arthrography is a more appropriate diagnostic tool.[43]

Current Status

A review of available literature uncovers a paucity of original authors and lends mute testimony to the reality that ultrasonography of the rotator cuff and biceps tendon is not in widespread use. While it appears to offer accurate data in the hands of an experienced few with a large patient population and accurate following, it remains for many an investigational procedure of unproved merit.

Diagnostic accuracy and constancy are dependent on the clinician and rely in good measure on the correct anatomic placement of the transducer, underscoring the importance of an initial interdisciplinary collaboration to include cadaveric and intraoperative study of the rotator cuff and its environs.

SUMMARY

The standard radiographic evaluation of the shoulder invariably includes anteroposterior views in internal and external rotation, and usually includes an axillary view. While these views will detect the preponderance of traumatic and nontraumatic osseous lesions, they often fail to detect posterior dislocations, certain scapular fractures, Hill-Sachs lesions, and the glenoid rim lesions of throwing and/or instability. Specialized views for the detection of these abnormalities have been reported. They include anterior (Y) and posterior oblique views, West Point and Ciullo axillary views, the Stryker notch, Hermodsson, and Didiee views. Some specialized views are of particular value for the assessment of the painful shoulder because they require no manipulation of the arm. Included among these views are the apical (craniocaudad) oblique, Velpeau, angle-up, and Stripp axial views. The anterior oblique and Didiee views both have a capability for the detection of both the Bankart and Hill-Sachs lesions of anterior instability. Conventional radiography is able to demonstrate evidence of only the intermediate or more advanced stages of subacromial impingement. To a large extent this evidence is indistinguishable from that which is ascribable to cuff arthropathy.

Simple CT has a limited role in studying the shoulder. It has value in defining some bone tumors and in the clarification of certain fractures, such as those of the humeral head with multiple parts. It can be of value in the assessment of subluxations and fractures of the clavicular articulations, especially those with the sternum. On rare occasion, CT scapulometry is used to analyze version of the scapular neck. The analysis may be useful in the planning of surgical osteotomies for posterior glenohumeral instability. Anecdotally, it should be indicated that CT scapulometry appears to have some reliability in the confirmation of subcoracoid impingement.

Simple arthrography of the shoulder remains a standard for the evaluation of full-thickness and inferior surface tears of the rotator cuff. Its use has been reported for the evaluation of capsular and even labral abnormalities of instability. However, its capacities in this regard are not comparable to those of CT arthrography and MRI. Double contrast arthrography provides more information about cuff tear morphology than does the single contrast technique. It also tends to produce less postprocedural pain. The use of subacromial bursography has been sparsely reported to have value in the diagnosis of impingement and superior surface cuff tears. The benefits of the technique for these purposes are too limited, and technical demands are too exacting to ever allow bursography to become a popular procedure.

Arthropneumotomography can effectively demonstrate lesions of the labrum, but it is a less reliable, more time-consuming procedure than CT arthrography, and it imposes a greater quantity of radiation upon the patient. CT arthrography is still an excellent radiographic procedure for demonstrating pathology of the capsulolabral osseous complexes. It demonstrates labral tears, Bankart lesions, abnormal capsular distentions and insertions, and even the directions of an instability. Yet it is relatively ineffectual in demonstrating pathologic changes of impingement other than cuff tears or degeneration. Cuff disease is probably better seen using direct sagittal rather than axial forms of CT arthrography.

Although arthrography is still a commonly used procedure in the search for rotator cuff tears, the value of arthrography is largely limited to the demonstration of full-thickness types. It is invasive by virtue of the injection of contrast media and the need for radiation. Ultrasonography, on the other hand, is a noninvasive, reliable screener of the rotator cuff. In expert hands, it offers the advantages of diagnosing partial as well as full-thickness tears without radiation or needles. The use of ultrasonography in the shoulder, however, has not become widespread; this procedure can only reveal pathologic conditions relative to the cuff; in addition, expertise in ultrasonographic interpretation of the shoulder is not rapidly developed.

MRI is the newest of the radiographic techniques. It is noninvasive and it provides images in multiple planes with equally good resolution. It can image virtually every structure and every tissue about the shoulder. It can demonstrate the labrum and the capsule, portraying abnormalities with more clarity of detail than CT arthrography. It can demonstrate most tears of the rotator cuff with good reliability. MRI can show subacromial bursitis and is a reliable diagnostic study for impingement. MRI is expected to surpass all other radiographic methods for the accurate diagnosis of any shoulder injury. Its inordinate expense has been a drawback.

In the early 1980s, arthroscopy of the shoulder was an infant procedure. Major pathologic states of the shoulder were treated by arthrotomy when surgery was indicated. By the middle 1980s, excisional arthroscopy (e.g., labral tear) and deimpingement were well established, and arthroscopically directed capsulorrhaphy for instability had been initiated. In the 1990s arthroscopy has ad-

vanced to include acute capsulolabral repair and reconstruction, even before an instability is necessarily evident and the repair of some discrete cuff tears within the avascular zone. MRI, with its detailing of cuff tears, labral disruptions, and directions of instability, has been a valued predictor and prognosticator of surgical needs. However, the sophistication of arthroscopic surgery may presently be progressing more rapidly than that of shoulder radiography. To determine whether to perform an arthroscopic procedure or to open a shoulder, whether a labrum is completely torn or simply detached, or whether an impingement is of sufficiently confined geography to be treated arthroscopically, the arthroscopist must use a radiographic procedure that is capable of spelling out the pathologic process in consummate detail.

However, it goes without saying that the value of any type of imaging to the orthopaedic surgeon is in some measure related to the confidence that he or she has in the radiologist and the equipment used. Confidence can be achieved only experientially as the surgeon learns that the technical abilities of the machinery and the interpretive skills of the radiologist are a match to the findings at surgery. If sophisticated imaging, hardware, and software are not readily available in the community, if the radiologist does not have expertise in shoulder evaluation, or if the procedures in consideration are too expensive for the patient population (insured or not), the imaging procedures will fall into disfavor with everyone involved. This is especially true when the majority of symptomatic shoulders are able to be diagnosed by simpler and time-honored evaluations.

REFERENCES

1. Altchek DW et al: Arthroscopic labral debridement, *Am J Sports Med* 20(6):702, 1992.
2. Andren L, Lundberg BJ: Treatment of rigid shoulders by joint distension during arthrography, *Acta Orthop Scand* 36(1):45, 1965.
3. Andrews JR et al: Glenoid labrum tears related to the long head of the biceps, *Am J Sports Med* 13:337, 1985.
4. Arndt JH, Sears AD: Posterior dislocation of the shoulder, *Am J Roentgenol* 94:639, 1965.
5. Baker CL et al: Arthroscopic evaluation of acute initial anterior shoulder dislocations, *Am J Sports Med* 18(1):25, 1990.
6. Balogh B et al: Sonoanatomy of the shoulder, *Acta Anat* 126:132, 1986.
7. Bankart ASB: Recurrent or habitual dislocation of the shoulder joint, *Br Med J* 2:1132, 1923.
8. Bankart ASB: The pathology and treatment of recurrent dislocation of the shoulder joint, *Br J Surg* 26:23, 1938.
9. Beltran J et al: Rotator cuff lesions of the shoulder: evaluation by direct sagittal CT arthrography, *Radiology* 160(1):161, 1986.
10. Bigliani LU et al: Tensile properties of the inferior glenohumeral ligament, *J Orthop Res* 10:187, 1992.
11. Bloom MH, Obata WG: Diagnosis of posterior dislocation of the shoulder with use of the Velpeau axillary and angle-up roentgenographic views, *J Bone Joint Surg* 49A(5):943, 1967.
12. Bloom RA: The active abduction view: a new maneuver in the diagnosis of rotator cuff tears, *Skeletal Radiol* 20:255, 1991.
13. Bost FC, Inman VT: The pathological changes in recurrent dislocation of the shoulder: a report of Bankart's operative procedure, *J Bone Joint Surg* 24:595, 1942.
14. Brams-Dalgaard E et al: Radiographic examination of the acute shoulder, *Eur J Radiol* 11:10, 1990.
15. Brandt TD et al: Rotator cuff sonography: a reassessment, *Radiology* 173:323, 1989.
16. Braunstein EM, O'Connor G: Double contrast arthrotomography of the shoulder, *J Bone Joint Surg* 64A(2):192, 1982.
17. Bretzke CA et al: Ultrasonography of the rotator cuff: normal and pathologic anatomy, *Invest Radiol* 20:311, 1985.
18. Burk DL: Rotator cuff tears: prospective comparison of MR imaging with arthrography, sonography, and surgery, *Am J Roentgenol* 153:87, 1989.
19. Calvert PT et al: Arthrography of the shoulder after operative repair of the torn rotator cuff, *J Bone Joint Surg* 68B:147, 1986.
20. Cartland JP et al: MR imaging in the evaluation of SLAP injuries of the shoulder: findings in 10 patients, *Am J Roentgenol* 159:787, 1992.
21. Chandnani V et al: MR findings in asymptomatic shoulders: a blind analysis using symptomatic shoulders as controls, *Clin Imaging* 16:25, 1992.
22. Ciullo JV: Swimmer's shoulder, *Clin Sports Med* 5(1):115, 1986.
23. Ciullo JV, Koniuch MP, Teitge RA: Axillary roentgenography in clinical orthopedic practice, *Orthop Trans* 6(3):451, 1982.
24. Cofield RH: Tears of rotator cuff, *Mayo Clin Proc* 258, 1980.
25. Cofield RH, Simonet WT: Symposium on sports medicine. II. The shoulder in sports, *Mayo Clin Proc* 59(3):157, 1984.
26. Collins RA, Gristina AG, Carter RE: Ultrasonography of the shoulder: static and dynamic imaging, *Orthop Clin North Am* 18:351, 1987.
27. Cone RO III, Resnick D, Danzig L: Shoulder impingement syndrome: radiographic evaluation, *Radiology* 150(1):29, 1984.
28. Copper DE et al: Anatomy, histology, and vascularity of the glenoid labrum: an anatomic study, *J Bone Joint Surg* 74A:46, 1992.
29. Cotty P et al: Rotator cuff tear: roentgen diagnosis, *J Radiol* 69:633, 1988.
30. Cox J: Personal communication, 1989.
31. Crass JR, Craig EV, Feinberg SB: Sonography of the postoperative rotator cuff, *Am J Radiol* 146:561, 1986.
32. Crass JR et al: Ultrasonography of the rotator cuff: surgical correlation, *J Clin Ultrasound* 12:487, 1984.
33. Crass JR et al: Ultrasonography of the rotator cuff, *Radiographics* 5:941, 1985.
34. Cyprien JM et al: Humeral retroversion and glenohumeral relationship in the normal shoulder and in recurrent anterior dislocation (scapulometry), *Clin Orthop* 175:8, 1983.
35. Danzig L, Greenway G, Resnick D: The Hill-Sachs lesion, *Am J Sports Med* 8(5):328, 1980.
36. DeHaven JP et al: *A prospective comparison study of double contrast CT arthrography and shoulder arthroscopy. Walter Reed Army Medical Center,* Paper presented at the AOSS in San Francisco, January 1987.
37. DePalma AF: *Surgery of the shoulder,* ed 3, Philadelphia, 1983, JB Lippincott.
38. DeSmet AA: Anterior oblique projection in radiography of the traumatized shoulder, *Am J Radiol* 134:515, 1980.
39. DeSmet AA: Axillary projection in radiography of the nontraumatized shoulder, *Am J Radiol* 134:511, 1980.
40. Deutsch AL, Resnick D, Mink JH: Computed tomography of the glenohumeral and sternoclavicular joints, *Orthop Clin North Am* 16(3):497, 1985.
41. Deutsch AL et al: Computed and conventional arthrotomography of the glenohumeral joint: normal anatomy and clinical experience, *Radiology* 153:603, 1984.
42. Didiee J: Le radiodiagnostic dans la luxation recidivante de l'epaule, *J Radiol Electrol* 14:209, 1930.
43. Drakeford MK et al: A comparative study of ultrasonography and arthrography in evaluation of the rotator cuff, *Clin Orthop* 253:118, 1990.
44. El-Khoury GY et al: Arthrotomography of the glenoid labrum, *Radiology* 131:333, 1979.
45. Ellman H, Hanker G, Bayer M: Repair of the rotator cuff, *J Bone Joint Surg* 68A(8):1136, 1986.
46. Evancho AM et al: MR imaging diagnosis of rotator cuff tears, *Am J Roentgenol* 151:751, 1988.
47. Eve FS: A case of subcoracoid dislocation of the humerus with

formation of an indentation on the posterior surface of the head, *Medico-Chir Trans Soc (London)* 63:317, 1880.

48. Farin PU et al: Shoulder impingement syndrome: sonographic evaluation, *Radiology* 176:845, 1990.

49. Farley TE et al: Full-thickness tears of the rotator cuff of the shoulder: diagnosis with MR imaging, *Am J Roentgenol* 158:347, 1992.

50. Flannigan B et al: MR arthrography of the shoulder: comparison with conventional MR imaging, *Am J Roentgenol* 155:829, 1990.

51. Flower WN: On the pathological changes produced in the shoulder joint by traumatic dislocation, as derived from an examination of all the specimens illustrating this injury in the museums of London, *Trans Path Soc (London)* 12:179, 1861.

52. Frittz HM et al: MR imaging of the shoulder: clinical experience and surgical correlation, *Radiology* 169:165, 1988 (abstract).

53. Fritz RC et al: Fat suppression MR arthrography of the shoulder, *Radiology* 185:(2)614, 1992 (letter).

54. Furtschegger A et al: Value of ultrasonography in preoperative diagnosis of rotator cuff tears and postoperative follow-up, *Eur J Radiol* 8(2):69, 1988.

55. Gambrioli PL, Maggi F, Randelli M: Computerized tomography in the investigation of scapulo-humeral instability, *Ital J Orthopaed Traumatol* 11(2):223, 1985.

56. Garcia JF: Arthrographic visualization of rotator cuff tears, *Radiology* 150(2):595, 1984.

57. Garneau RA et al: Glenoid labrum: evaluation with MR imaging, *Radiology* 179:519, 1991.

58. Garth WP, Slappey CE, Ochs CW: Roentgenographic demonstration of instability of the shoulder: the apical oblique projection, *J Bone Joint Surg* 66A(9):1450, 1984.

59. Gerber C: Clinical assessment of instability of the shoulder, *J Bone Joint Surg* 66B(4):551, 1984.

60. Gerber C, Terrier F, Ganz R: The role of the coracoid process in the chronic impingement syndrome, *J Bone Joint Surg* 67B(5):703, 1985.

61. Gerber C et al: The subcoracoid space, *Clin Orthop* 215:132, 1987.

62. Ghelman B, Goldman A: The double-contrast shoulder arthrogram: evaluation of rotary cuff tears, *Radiology* 124:251, 1977.

63. Godsil RD, Linscheid RL: Intratendinous defects of the rotator cuff, *Clin Orthop* 69:181, 1970.

64. Golding RC: The shoulder—the forgotten joint, *Br J Radiol* 35(411):149, 1962.

65. Goldman AB, Ghelman B: The double-contrast shoulder arthrogram, *Radiology* 127:655, 1978.

66. Grauer JD et al: Biceps tendon and superior labral injuries, *Arthroscopy* 8(4):488, 1993.

67. Gristina AG, Collins RA, Carter RE: Diagnostic ultrasound of the shoulder, *Abst Orthop Trans* 10:214, 1986.

68. Gross M et al: Magnetic resonance imaging of the glenoid labrum, *Am J Sports Med* 18:229, 1990.

69. Haacke EM et al: Fast MR imaging: techniques and clinical applications, *Am J Roentgenol* 155:951, 1990.

70. Habibian A et al: Comparison of conventional and computed arthrotomography with MR imaging in the evaluation of the shoulder, *J Comput Assist Tomogr* 13:968, 1989.

71. Hajek PC et al: MR arthrography: pathologic investigation, *Radiology* 163:141, 1987.

72. Hajek PC et al: Potential contrast agents for MR arthrography: in vitro evaluation and practical observations, *Am J Roentgenol* 149:97, 1987.

73. Hajek PC et al: The effect of intra-articular gadolinium-DPTA on synovial membrane and cartilage, *Invest Radiol* 25:179, 1990.

74. Hall FM et al: Morbidity from shoulder arthrography: etiology, incidence, and prevention, *Am J Radiol* 136:59, 1981.

75. Hall FM et al: Shoulder arthrography: comparison of morbidity after use of various contrast media, *Radiology* 154:339, 1985.

76. Harcke HT et al: Evaluation of the musculoskeletal system with sonography, *Am J Roentgenol* 150:1253, 1988.

77. Harryman DT et al: The role of the rotator interval capsule in passive motion and stability of the shoulder, *J Bone Joint Surg* 74A:53, 1992.

78. Hawkins RJ, Kennedy JC: Impingement syndrome in athletes, *Am J Sports Med* 8:151, 1980.

79. Hawkins RJ, Koppert G, Johnston G: Recurrent posterior instability (subluxation) of the shoulder, *J Bone Joint Surg* 66A(2):169, 1984.

80. Hermodsson I: Rontgenologische studien uber die traumatische und habituellen schultergelenk-verrenkungen nach vorn und nach unten, *Acta Radiol Suppl* 20:1, 1934.

81. Hill HA, Sachs MD: The grooved defect of the humeral head: a frequently unrecognized complication of dislocation of the shoulder joint, *Radiology* 35:690, 1940.

82. Hodler J et al: Injuries of the superior portion of the glenoid labrum involving the insertion of the biceps tendon: MR imaging findings in nine cases, *Am J Roentgenol* 159:565, 1992.

83. Horsefield D, Jones SM: A useful projection in radiography of the shoulder, *J Bone Joint Surg* 69B(2):338, 1987.

84. Huber DJ et al: MR imaging of the normal shoulder, *Radiology* 158:405, 1986.

85. Iannotti JP et al: Magnetic resonance imaging of the shoulder: sensitivity, specificity and predictive value, *J Bone Joint Surg* 73A:7, 1991.

86. Jahnke AH Jr et al: A prospective comparison of computerized arthrotomography and magnetic imaging of the glenohumeral joint, *Am J Sports Med* 20:(6)695, 1992.

87. Jobe FW, Jobe CM: Painful athletic injuries of the shoulder, *Clin Orthop* 173:117, 1983.

88. Kessel L, Watson M: The painful arc syndrome, *J Bone Joint Surg* 59B:166, 1977.

89. Kieft GJ et al: Normal shoulder: MR imaging, *Radiology* 159(3):741, 1986.

90. Kieft GJ et al: MR imaging of anterior dislocation of the shoulder: comparison with CT arthrography, *Am J Radiol* 150:1083, 1988.

91. Kieft GJ et al: Magnetic resonance imaging of glenohumeral joint diseases, *Skeletal Radiol* 16:285, 1987.

92. Kieft GJ et al: Rotator cuff impingement syndrome: MR imaging, *Radiology* 166:211, 1988.

93. Kilcoyne RF, Matsen FA: Rotator cuff tear measurement by arthropneumotomography, *Am J Radiol* 140:315, 1983.

94. Killoran PJ, Marcove RC, Freiberger RH: Shoulder arthrography, *Am J Radiol* 103(3):658, 1968.

95. Kinnard P et al: Assessment of the unstable shoulder by computed arthrography, *Am J Sports Med* 11(3):157, 1983.

96. Kjellin I et al: Alterations in the supraspinatus tendon at MR imaging: correlation with histopathologic findings in cadavers, *Radiology* 181:837, 1991.

97. Kleinman PK et al: Axillary arthrotomography of the glenoid labrum, *Am J Radiol* 141:993, 1984.

98. Kneeland JB et al: Rotator cuff tears: preliminary application of high-resolution MR imaging with counter rotating current loop-gap resonators, *Radiology* 160(3):695, 1986.

99. Kneeland JB et al: MR imaging of the shoulder: diagnosis of rotator cuff tears, *Am J Radiol* 149:333, 1987.

100. Kneisl JS, Sweeney HJ, Paige ML: Correlation of pathology observed in double contrast arthrotomography and arthroscopy of the shoulder, *Arthroscopy* 4(1):21, 1988.

101. Kohn D: The clinical relevance of glenoid labrum lesions, *Arthroscopy* 3(4):223, 1987.

102. Kornguth PJ, Salazar AM: The apical oblique view of the shoulder, *Am J Radiol* 149(1):113, 1987.

103. Kummel BM: Arthrography in anterior capsular derangements of the shoulder, *Clin Orthop* 83:170, 1972.

104. Legan JM et al: Tears of the glenoid labrum: MR imaging of 88 arthroscopically confirmed cases, *Radiology* 179:241, 1991.

105. Lie S, Mast WA: Subacromial bursography, *Radiology* 144:626, 1982.

106. Lindblom K: Arthrography and roentgenography in ruptures of tendons of the shoulder joint, *Acta Radiol* 20:548, 1939.

107. Liou JT et al: The normal shoulder: common variations that simulate pathologic conditions at MR imaging, *Radiology* 186:435, 1993.

108. Lombardo SJ et al: Posterior shoulder lesions in throwing athletes, *Am J Sports Med* 5(3):106, 1977.
109. Mack LA et al: Sonographic evaluation of the rotator cuff: accuracy in patients without prior surgery, *Clin Orthop* 234:21, 1988.
110. McCauley TR et al: Normal and abnormal glenoid labrum: assessment with multiplanar gradient-echo MR imaging, *Radiology* 183:35, 1992.
111. McGlynn FJ, El-Khoury G, Albright JP: Arthrotomography of the glenoid labrum in shoulder instability, *J Bone Joint Surg* 64A(4):506, 1982.
112. McLaughlin H: Posterior dislocation of the shoulder, *J Bone Joint Surg* 34A(3):584, 1952.
113. McMaster WC: Anterior glenoid labrum damage: a painful lesion in swimmers, *Am J Sports Med* 14(5):383, 1986.
114. McNiesh LM, Callaghan JJ: CT arthrography of the shoulder: variations of the glenoid labrum, *Am J Radiol* 149:963, 1987.
115. Meyer SJF et al: Magnetic resonance imaging of the shoulder, *Orthop Clin North Am* 21(3):497, 1990.
116. Middleton WD: Status of rotator cuff sonography, *Radiology* 173:307, 1989.
117. Middleton WD et al: Ultrasonography of the rotator cuff: technique and normal anatomy, *J Ultrasound Med* 3:549, 1984.
118. Middleton WD et al: Ultrasonography of the biceps tendon apparatus, *Radiology* 157:211, 1985.
119. Middleton WD et al: Pitfalls of rotator cuff sonography, *Am J Radiol* 146:555, 1986.
120. Middleton WD et al: Ultrasonographic evaluation of the rotator cuff and biceps tendon, *J Bone Joint Surg* 68A:440, 1986.
121. Middleton WD et al: High resolution MR imaging of the normal rotator cuff, *Am J Roentgenol* 148:559, 1987.
122. Miller CL et al: Limited sensitivity of ultrasound for the detection of rotator cuff tears, *Skeletal Radiol* 18(3):179, 1989.
123. Mink JH, Harris E, Rappaport M: Rotator cuff tears: evaluation using double-contrast shoulder arthrography, *Radiology* 157:621, 1985.
124. Mink JH, Richardson A, Grant TT: Evaluation of glenoid labrum by double-contrast shoulder arthrography, *Am J Radiol* 133:893, 1979.
125. Minkoff J et al: Glenohumeral instabilities and the role of MRI: the orthopedic surgeon's perspective, *MRI Clin North Am* 1(1):105, 1993.
126. Mirowitz SA: Normal rotator cuff: MR imaging with conventional and fat suppression techniques, *Radiology* 180:735, 1991.
127. Misamore GW et al: Evaluation of degenerative lesions of the rotator cuff: a comparison of arthrography and ultrasonography, *J Bone Joint Surg* 73A:704, 1991.
128. Mizuno K, Hirohata K: Diagnosis of recurrent traumatic anterior subluxation of the shoulder, *Clin Orthop* 179:160, 1983.
129. Morrison DS et al: The use of magnetic resonance imaging in the diagnosis of rotator cuff tears, *Orthopedics* 13(6):633, 1990.
130. Moseley HF et al: The anterior capsular mechanism in recurrent anterior dislocation of the shoulder: morphological and clinical studies with special references to the glenoid labrum and the glenohumeral ligaments, *J Bone Joint Surg* 44B:913, 1962.
131. Munk PL et al: Glenoid labrum: preliminary work with use of radial sequence MR imaging, *Radiology* 173:751, 1989.
132. Neer CS: Anterior acromioplasty for the chronic impingement syndrome in the shoulder: a preliminary report, *J Bone Joint Surg* 54A:41, 1972.
133. Neer CS: Impingement lesions, *Clin Orthop* 173:70, 1983.
134. Neer CS: Dislocation. In Neer CS: *Shoulder dislocation*, Philadelphia, 1990, WB Saunders.
135. Neer CS, Welsh RP: The shoulder in sports, *Orthop Clin North Am* 8(3):583, 1977.
136. Nelson MC et al: Evaluation of the painful shoulder: a prospective comparison of magnetic resonance imaging, computerized tomographic arthrography, ultrasonography and operative findings, *J Bone Joint Surg* 73A:707, 1991.
137. Neumann CH et al: MRI in the evaluation of patients with suspected instability of the shoulder joint including a comparison with CT arthrography, *Fortschr Rontgenstr* 154(6):593, 1991.
138. Neumann CH et al: MR imaging of the labral-capsular complex: normal variations, *Am J Roentgenol* 157:1015, 1991.
139. Neviaser RJ: Anatomic considerations and examination of the shoulder, *Orthop Clin North Am* 11(2):187, 1980.
140. Neviaser RJ: Arthrography of the shoulder, *Orthop Clin North Am* 11(2):205, 1980.
141. Neviaser RJ: Tears of the rotator cuff, *Orthop Clin North Am* 11(2):295, 1980.
142. Neviaser RJ, Neviaser TJ: Lesions of musculotendinous cuff of shoulder: diagnosis and management. In AAOS: *Instructional course lectures*, vol 30, St Louis, 1981, Mosby.
143. Nicola T: Anterior dislocation of the shoulder, *J Bone Joint Surg* 31A:153, 1949.
144. Norris TR: Diagnostic techniques for shoulder instability. In AAOS: *Instructional course lectures*, vol 34, St Louis, 1985, Mosby.
145. Older MWJ, McIntyre JL, Lloyd GJ: Distension arthrography of the shoulder joint, *Can J Surg* 19:203, 1976.
146. Olive RJ et al: Ultrasonography of rotator cuff tears, *Clin Orthop* 282:110, 1992.
147. Owen RS et al: Shoulder after surgery: MR imaging with surgical validation, *Radiology* 186:443, 1993.
148. Pappas AP, Gross TP, Kleinman PK: Symptomatic shoulder instability due to lesions of the glenoid labrum, *Am J Sports Med* 11:279, 1984.
149. Pavlov H, Freiberger RH: Fractures and dislocations about the shoulder, *Semin Roentgenol* 13(2): 1978.
150. Pavlov H et al: The roentgenographic evaluation of anterior shoulder instability, *Clin Orthop* 194:153, 1985.
151. Pennes DR et al: Computed arthrotomography of the shoulder: comparison of examinations made with internal and external rotation of the humerus, *Am J Roentgenol* 153:1017, 1989.
152. Petersson CJ, Gentz CF: Ruptures of the supraspinatus tendon, *Clin Orthop* 175:143, 1983.
153. Petersson CJ, Redlund-Johnell I: The subacromial space in normal shoulder radiographs, *Acta Orthop Scand* 55:57, 1984.
154. Post M, Silver R, Singh M: Rotator cuff tear, *Clin Orthop* 173:78, 1983.
155. Prendergast N et al: Magnetic resonance imaging of the shoulder joint, *Curr Opin Radiol* 4:70, 1992.
156. Rafii M et al: CT arthrography of capsular structures of the shoulder, *Am J Radiol* 146:361, 1986.
157. Rafii M et al: CT arthrography of shoulder instabilities in athletes, *Am J Sports Med* 16:352, 1988.
158. Rafii M et al: Athlete shoulder injuries: CT arthrographic findings, *Radiology* 162(2):559, 1987.
159. Rafii M et al: Rotator cuff lesions: signal patterns at MR imaging, *Radiology* 173:817, 1990.
160. Rafii M et al: High resolution glenohumeral instability lesions, *Radiology* 181(P):154, 1991.
161. Rafii M et al: Magnetic resonance imaging of glenohumeral instability, *MRI Clin North Am* 1(1):1, 1993.
162. Randelli M, Gambrioli PL: Glenohumeral osteometry by computed tomography in normal and unstable shoulders, *Clin Orthop* 208:151, 1986.
163. Randelli M, Odella F, Gambrioli PL: Clinical experience with double-contrast medium computerized tomography (arthro-CT) in instability of the shoulder, *Ital J Orthopaed Traumatol* 12(2):151, 1986.
164. Rathbun JB, McNab I: The microvascular pattern of the rotator cuff, *J Bone Joint Surg* 52B:540, 1970.
165. Reeves B: Arthrography of the shoulder, *J Bone Joint Surg* 48B(3):424, 1966.
166. Richardson JB et al: Radiographs in shoulder trauma, *J Bone Joint Surg* 70B:457, 1988.
167. Rockwood CA: Fractures and dislocations about the shoulder. II. Subluxations and dislocations about the shoulder. In Rockwood CA, Green DP (eds): *Fractures*, ed 2, Philadelphia, 1975, JB Lippincott.
168. Rokous JR, Feagin JA, Abbott HG: Modified axillary roentgenogram: a useful adjunct in the diagnosis of recurrent instability of the shoulder, *Clin Orthop* 82:84, 1972.

169. Rothman RH, Marvel JP Jr, Hepenstall RB: Anatomic considerations in the glenohumeral joint, *Orthop Clin North Am* 6:341, 1975.
170. Rowe CR: Prognosis in dislocations of the shoulder, *J Bone Joint Surg* 38A:957, 1956.
171. Rozing PM, deBakker HM, Obermann WR: Radiographic views in recurrent anterior shoulder dislocation, *Acta Orthop Scand* 57:328, 1986.
172. Rubin SA, Gray RL, Green WR: The scapular "Y" view—a diagnostic aid in shoulder trauma, *Radiology* 110:725, 1974.
173. Saha AK: Anterior recurrent dislocation of the shoulder, *Acta Orthop Scand* 68:479, 1967.
174. Saha AK: Dynamic stability of the glenohumeral joint, *Acta Orthop Scand* 42:491, 1971.
175. Seeger LL: Shoulder instability: evaluation with MR imaging, *Radiology* 168:695, 1988.
176. Seeger LL: Magnetic resonance imaging of the shoulder, *Clin Orthop* 244:48, 1989.
177. Seeger LL et al: MR imaging of the normal shoulder: anatomic correlation, *Am J Radiol* 148:83, 1987.
178. Seeger LL et al: *Shoulder MR*, Paper presented at the annual meeting of the Radiological Society of North America, Chicago, November 1987.
179. Seeger LL et al: Shoulder impingement syndrome: MR findings in 53 shoulders, *Am J Radiol* 150:343, 1988.
180. Seltzer SE, Weissman BN: CT findings in normal and dislocating shoulders, *J Can Assoc Radiol* 36(1):41, 1985.
181. Shuman WP et al: Double-contrast computed tomography of the glenoid labrum, *Am J Radiol* 141:581, 1983.
182. Singson RD, Feldman F, Bigliani L: CT arthrographic patterns in recurrent glenohumeral instability, *Am J Radiol* 149:749, 1987.
183. Snyder S et al: SLAP lesions of the shoulder, *J Arthroscopy* 6:274, 1990.
184. Sobel MG et al: Rotator cuff tear: clinical experience with sonographic detection, *Radiology* 173:319, 1989.
185. Stark DE et al: *Magnetic resonance imaging*, ed 2, St Louis, 1992, Mosby.
186. Strizak AM et al: Subacromial bursography, *J Bone Joint Surg* 64A(2):196, 1982.
187. Vahlensieck M et al: MRI of the shoulder, *Bildgebung* 59(3):123, 1992.
188. Vastamaki M, Solonen KA: Posterior dislocation and fracture-dislocation of the shoulder, *Acta Orthop Scand* 51:479, 1980.
189. Vezina JA: Compensation filter for shoulder radiography, *Radiology* 155(3):823, 1985.
190. Warren RF: Instability of shoulder in throwing sports. In Staufer ES (ed): *AAOS Instructional course lectures*, vol 34, St Louis, 1985, Mosby.
191. Wilson AJ et al: Shoulder joint: arthrographic CT and long term follow up with surgical correlation, *Radiology* 173:329, 1989.
192. Workman TL et al: Hill-Sachs lesion: comparison of detection with MRI imaging, radiography, and arthroscopy, *Radiology* 185:(3)847, 1992.
193. Zanca P: Shoulder pain: involvement of the acromioclavicular joint, *Am J Radiol* 112:493, 1971.
194. Zarins B, Matthews LS: Evaluation and treatment of glenoid labrum tears. In Jackson DW (ed): *Shoulder surgery in the athlete*, Rockville, Md, 1985, Aspen Publications.
195. Zaslov K et al: Magnetic resonance imaging of rotator cuff: anatomic and histologic correlations of alteration in signal intensity, *Orthop Trans* 14:562, 1990.
196. Zlatkin MB et al: Cross-sectional imaging of the capsular mechanism of the glenohumeral joint, *Am J Roentgenol* 150:151, 1988.
197. Zlatkin MB et al: The painful shoulder: MR imaging of the glenohumeral joint, *J Comput Assist Tomog* 12:995, 1988.
198. Zlatkin MB et al: High resolution MR imaging of the glenohumeral joint, *Top Magn Reson Imaging* 3:1, 1989.
199. Zlatkin MB et al: Magnetic resonance imaging of the shoulder, *Magn Reson Quart* 5:3, 1989.
200. Zlatkin MB et al: Rotator cuff tears, diagnostic performance of MR imaging, *Radiology* 172:223, 1989.

CHAPTER 5 Shoulder Arthroscopy

Francis X. Mendoza
C. Alexander Moskwa, Jr.

The concept of using a small telescope to visualize a joint directly was introduced by Takagi[66] in Japan in 1918. Employing a 7.3-mm cytoscope, he inspected a cadaveric knee and thereby inaugurated the field of arthroscopy. In 1931 Burman[11] reported on the arthroscopic examination of various cadaveric joints, including 25 shoulders. Using both anterior and posterior portals, he concluded that the shoulder is the easiest of all joints to visualize. Although many contemporary orthopaedic surgeons disagree with Burman's conclusion, there is no doubt that shoulder arthroscopy has significantly increased in popularity and use.

Shoulder arthroscopy has followed a development parallel to that of knee arthroscopy. Although at present it is not as universally established as knee arthroscopy, shoulder arthroscopy has grown to be the second most performed arthroscopic procedure.[36] It is beyond the stage of being predominantly an investigative or diagnostic tool, and it currently can be used for surgical treatment of certain conditions.

The advantages of shoulder arthroscopy are that it is less invasive than open surgery, permits direct visualization of intraarticular and extraarticular pathologic conditions, and allows earlier rehabilitation, with return to ac-

tivities of daily living. Prospective studies have demonstrated that an arthroscopic subacromial decompression has yielded results as good as open surgery with less operating time and faster return to premorbid functional levels.[28,35] A major disadvantage is that the physician's skill with shoulder arthroscopy is generally correlated to his or her experience. It is no surprise that those orthopaedic surgeons well trained in knee arthroscopy have found an easier transition to the art of shoulder arthroscopy than those without such previous experience.

Shoulder arthroscopy

Advantages
- Less invasive than open surgery
- Permits direct visualization
- Allows earlier rehabilitation

Disadvantages
- Skill dependent on case volume

HISTORY AND PHYSICAL EXAMINATION

A diligent history and physical examination, supplemented with plain radiographs, form the cornerstone of the appropriate diagnosis in the overwhelming majority of shoulder conditions. If necessary, additional studies, such as plain radiographs of the cervical spine, electrodiagnostic studies, and special radiographs can often be helpful after a review of the initial plain shoulder radiographs. In a comparison of magnetic resonance imaging (MRI), computed tomographic (CT) arthrography, ultrasonography, and operative findings, Nelson[49] found that MRI was the most useful modality for assessing the shoulder. In our experience, a physician cannot depend on shoulder arthroscopy to reveal the diagnosis in most situations.

SURGICAL SETUP

The patient usually receives a general anesthetic to ensure good relaxation. Recently regional anesthesia, specifically an interscalene block, has gained popularity and has been shown to provide excellent intraoperative anesthesia with good muscle relaxation.[9,60] It is critical to perform a gentle examination of the shoulder during anesthesia on all patients undergoing arthroscopy because

it affords an opportunity to assess shoulder motion and instability, if appropriate, with complete joint relaxation. When compared with operative findings, the examination of the anesthetized shoulder for instability revealed a sensitivity of 100% with specificity and predicted values of 93%.[15]

A lateral decubitus position (Fig. 5-1) is commonly used for most patients, with the involved shoulder up. The patient rests with anterior and posterior pelvic posts stabilizing the pelvis, an axillary pad under the uninvolved arm, and careful padding and positioning of all bony prominences. To enhance distention of the joint, longitudinal traction of 10 to 15 pounds is applied, with Buck's traction on the forearm directed through a commercially available shoulder suspensory device. This traction apparatus must permit changes in the degree of shoulder abduction and forward flexion (Fig. 5-2). Various authors have offered a wide range of recommendations of shoulder abduction and forward flexion to obtain maximal visualization of the joint while avoiding the neurovascular structures. Our experience indicates that approximately 60 degrees of abduction, with 5 to 10 degrees of forward flexion, allows the best glenohumeral (intraarticular) visualization, whereas 5 to 15 degrees of abduction, with zero to 10 degrees of forward flexion, maximizes visualization of the subacromial space.

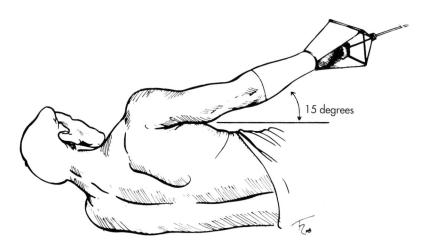

FIG. 5-1. Lateral decubitus position with longitudinal traction in 5 to 15 degrees abduction, and 0 to 10 degrees of forward flexion maximizes visualization of the subacromial space.

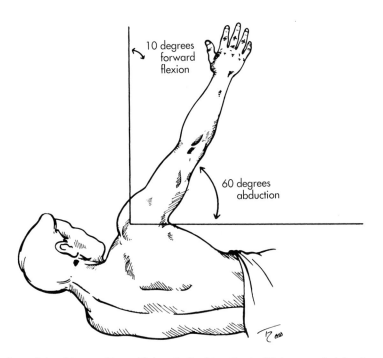

FIG. 5-2. Lateral decubitus position with longitudinal traction in 60 degrees of abduction with 5 to 10 degrees of forward flexion enhances glenohumeral intraarticular visualization.

Other methods of positioning the patient exist, such as the semirecumbent or beachchair position (see p. 187).[61] Here shoulder joint distraction is accomplished via gravity—the weight of the arm—assisted by gentle manual downward traction by the surgical assistant. Although this position is more comfortable for the surgeon, our experience reveals that it does not provide the same degree of visualization as one obtained in the lateral decubitus position, especially in muscular athletes.

EQUIPMENT

In virtually all cases the standard 30-degree angle, 4.0- or 4.5-mm arthroscope can be used in the shoulder, as in the knee. Other pieces of equipment common to knee and shoulder arthroscopy include a high-intensity fiberoptic light source; a camera; a video monitor and recorder; cannulae with sharp and semiblunt trocars; an 18-gauge spinal needle; a gravity-based irrigation system; and an assortment of arthroscopic instruments, such as probes, scissors, punches, and graspers. A power-driven rotary shaver with variable speed, suction capability, and interchangeable blades and burs is also necessary for debridement purposes. Instruments specific for shoulder arthroscopy include a cannula system with a diaphragm to prevent leakage of fluid when instruments are passed through it, a Wissinger rod to assist in creation of an anterior intraarticular portal, and an electrocautery generally used during subacromial procedures.

PORTAL SELECTION

With the patient sterilely prepared and draped, the following bony landmarks are palpated and outlined with a sterile pen: the distal clavicle, the tip of the coracoid process, and the anterolateral and posterolateral borders of the acromion. The ideal portal for joint inspection and instrumentation should meet the following criteria:
1. A relatively avascular tissue plane should be entered.
2. Adjacent neurovascular structures should be protected.
3. Tissue bulk should be minimized to ensure maximal visualization of the joint and instrument maneuverability.
4. The technique of creating the portal should be reproducible.

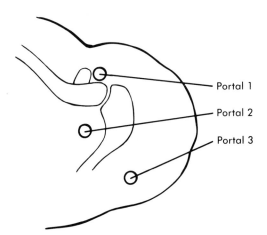

FIG. 5-3. Intraarticular portals. *Portal 1,* The anterior portal remains lateral and in line with or just superior to the tip of the coracoid process. *Portal 2,* The accessory portal for additional instrumentation or improved inflow is located superiorly just posterior to the acromioclavicular joint. *Portal 3,* The posterior portal is located in the soft spot 1 cm medial and 2 cm inferior to the posterior lateral corner of the acromion.

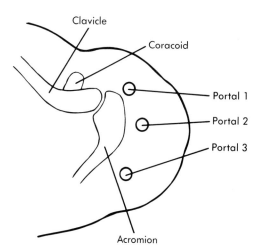

FIG. 5-4. Extraarticular subacromial portals. *Portal 1,* The instrument portal is in line with the anterior acromion and 3 cm distal to the anterolateral corner of the acromion. *Portal 2,* The arthroscopic portal is located 1.5 to 2 cm anterior to the posterior corner of the acromion and 1.5 cm distal to the lateral acromion. *Portal 3,* The posterior inflow portal is located 2 cm distal to the posterior acromion and angled toward the anterior acromion.

Portal site selection

- Through a relatively avascular plane
- Avoid or protect adjacent neurovascular structure
- Minimize tissue bulk
- Technique is reproducible

Many portals have been successfully used for shoulder arthroscopy. Nonetheless, procedures involving the glenohumeral joint (intraarticular) (Fig. 5-3) necessitate different portals than those procedures performed in the subacromial space (extraarticular) (Fig. 5-4).

Intraarticular Portals

The **posterior portal** has been accepted as the standard for the initial entry into the shoulder joint. In a cadaveric study using 51 shoulders, Rojvanit[58] found that the posterior approach had a wider field of view as compared to the anterior and superior approaches, and better anatomic orientation was obtained.

The posterior intraarticular portal is located approximately 1 cm medially and 2 cm inferiorly to the posterolateral corner of the acromion. The location corresponds to the palpable posterior soft spot of the shoulder, which represents the interval between the infraspinatus and teres minor muscles. With the middle finger palpating the coracoid process and the thumb on the posterior soft spot, the surgeon inserts an 18-gauge spinal needle through the soft spot directed at the coracoid process. Approximately 30 cc of sterile saline are injected through the spinal needle to distend the shoulder joint and to demonstrate free backflow, thereby confirming joint entry. The spinal needle is then withdrawn, and a small incision is made through the skin. The arthroscopic sheath with its semisharp trocar is used to penetrate the soft tissues into the shoulder. A blunt trocar should be inserted before any further manipulation within the shoulder joint. Adequate joint distention is maintained with a continuous gravity inflow of saline from elevated saline fluid bags.

An **anterior intraarticular portal** is then made by advancing the arthroscope to the anterior capsule, where the intraarticular triangle, consisting of the humeral head, glenoid, and biceps tendon, is visualized as described by Matthews et al (Plate 1).[37] The authors confirm through anatomic studies that instruments passing through the area cause little risk to adjacent neurovascular structures. Further safety is ensured if the anterior portal remains in the area lateral and adjacent or just superior to the coracoid process.

Two common techniques exist for the safe and reproducible method used to create an anterior intraarticular portal. The arthroscopic sheath may be advanced anteriorly to abut against the anterior capsule bounded between the superior and middle glenohumeral ligaments and the subscapularis tendon (Plate 2). The arthroscope is then exchanged for a Wissinger rod, which is advanced through the arthroscopic sheath to rest at the previously determined point on the anterior capsule and just

lateral to the coracoid process. An anterior skin incision is made over the tip of the Wissinger rod, and a cannula is placed over the anteriorly existing rod and advanced in a retrograde fashion into the joint. The rod is then removed, and the accessory anterior portal is ready to accept instruments or an arthroscope.

An alternate method for the creation of an anterior intraarticular portal is described by Matthews et al,[37] who employed a 22-gauge spinal needle entering through the intraarticular triangle under arthroscopic visualization. The needle is placed superior to the middle glenohumeral ligament but inferior to the biceps tendon. After satisfactory placement is confirmed, a small skin incision is made and a semisharp trocar and cannula are inserted following the previously defined angle to create the anterior portal (Plate 3).

A third **accessory intraarticular portal** may at times be necessary for improved fluid inflow or additional instruments. This portal may be created adjacent to the initial anterior portal, using the previously described techniques. Care must be taken to remain somewhat more superior and lateral to the coracoid process to avoid jeopardizing the musculocutaneous nerve. An alternative site for this accessory portal is located superiorly on the shoulder just posterior to the acromioclavicular joint (Plate 4). From that point, an 18-gauge spinal needle is aimed toward the center of the axilla and monitored arthroscopically as it enters the joint through the superior posterior capsule just posterior to the posterior glenoid rim. The needle is then withdrawn, and a cannula with a semisharp trocar is inserted through the previously defined track establishing the **superior portal**.[51] Only the muscular portions of the trapezius and supraspinatus are traversed in creating this portal. However, rigorous technique must be employed to avoid violating the tendinous portion of the supraspinatus.

Extraarticular Portals

The technique for performing subacromial endoscopic procedures demands that different portals be used.[51] The arthroscope is inserted into the subacromial space through a posterolateral subacromial portal located approximately 1.5 to 2.0 cm anterior to the posterior lateral corner of the acromion and 1.5 cm distal to the lateral acromion. A posterior subacromial portal used for inflow is placed 2 cm distal to the posterior acromion and angled toward the anterior edge of the acromion. An instrument portal is generally selected in line with the anterior edge of the acromion and lies approximately 3 cm distal to the anterolateral edge.

ARTHROSCOPIC ANATOMY

A detailed knowledge of normal anatomy and its variants is absolutely essential for arthroscopic surgery. All anatomic structures and viewing orientation can be related to four anatomic landmarks (Plate 1): (1) articular surface of the humeral head; (2) articular surface of the glenoid; (3) tendon of the long head of the biceps; and (4) tendon of the subscapularis.

The humeral head and glenoid face opposite one an-

A   B

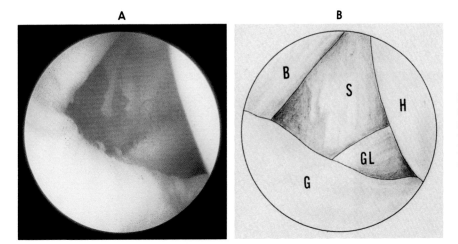

PLATE 1. **A,** Intraarticular reference landmarks are visualized. **B,** Glenoid (*G*), humeral head (*H*), long head of biceps tendon (*B*), subscapularis tendon coursing vertically from behind humeral head (*S*), and glenohumeral ligaments oriented obliquely to glenoid (*GL*).

A   B

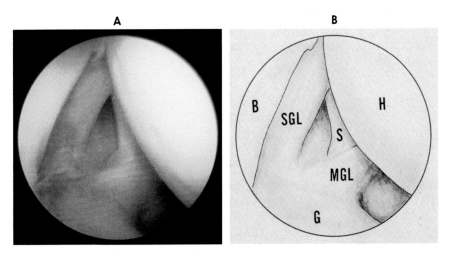

PLATE 2. **A,** Anterior portal capsule visualized. **B,** Capsule bordered by superior glenohumeral ligament (*SGL*), superior edge of subscapularis tendon (*S*), and middle glenohumeral ligament (*MGL*). Long head of biceps tendon (*B*), humeral head (*H*), glenoid (*G*).

A   B

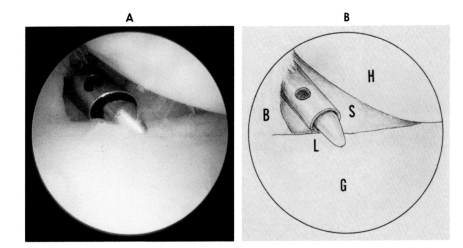

PLATE 3. **A,** Obturator and cannula enter joint anteriorly through intraarticular triangle. **B,** Obturator rests on anterior labrum (*L*) and glenoid (*G*). Long head of biceps (*B*), superior edge of subscapularis tendon (*S*), humeral head (*H*).

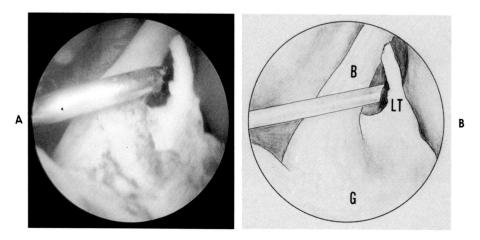

PLATE 4. A, Spinal needle enters joint through accessory superior portal. **B,** Portal provides a posterior superior view of long head of biceps tendon origin *(B)*, anterior superior labral tear *(LT)*, and superior glenoid *(G)*.

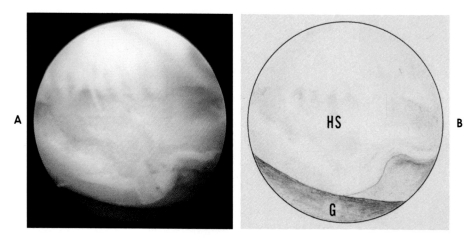

PLATE 5. A, Hill-Sachs lesion. A pathologic denuding of the posterior humeral head cartilage secondary to anterior glenohumeral instability. **B,** Hill-Sachs lesion *(HS)*, glenoid *(G)*.

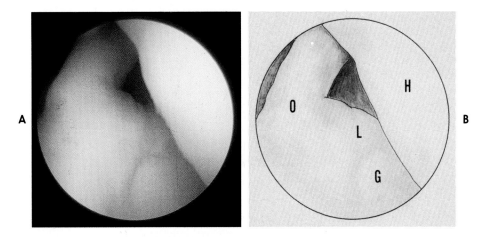

PLATE 6. A, The origin of the long head of biceps tendon from the supraglenoid tubercule and superior labrum. **B,** Origin biceps tendon *(O)*, superior labrum *(L)*, glenoid *(G)*, humeral head *(H)*.

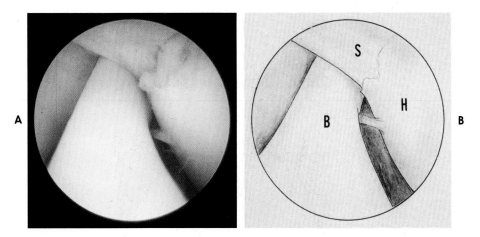

PLATE 7. A, Long head of biceps tendon is seen just before entering into the bicipital groove. The tendon traversing anterior to the biceps is the supraspinatus. **B,** Humeral head *(H)*, biceps tendon *(B)*, supraspinatus tendon *(S)*.

PLATE 8. A, Insertion of the oblique broad band of ligamentous tissue consisting of the middle and inferior glenohumeral ligaments is identified with a spinal needle. **B,** Middle and inferior glenohumeral ligaments (*GL*), subscapularis tendon (*S*), glenoid (*G*), humeral head (*H*).

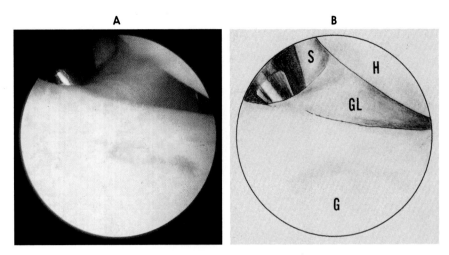

PLATE 9. A, Identified are the long head of biceps tendon; the superior, middle, and inferior glenohumeral ligaments. The subscapularis tendon edge is visualized in the background. **B,** Biceps tendon (*B*), superior glenohumeral ligament (*SGL*), middle and inferior glenohumeral ligaments (*MGL*), subscapularis tendon courses vertically behind (MGL). Humeral head (*H*), glenoid (*G*).

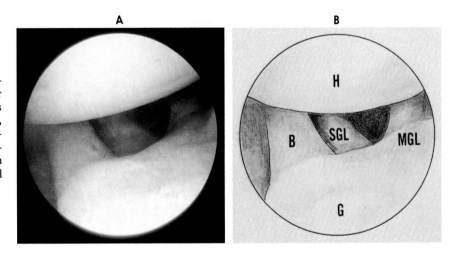

PLATE 10. A, Detached anterior labrum consistent with recurrent anterior glenohumeral subluxations. **B,** Detached labrum (*L*), humeral head (*H*), glenoid (*G*).

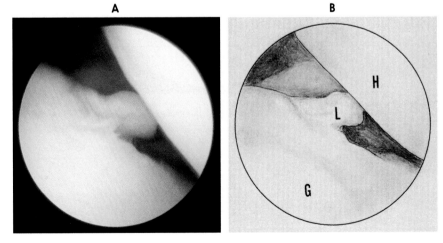

other and contain smooth articular cartilage covering their surfaces. A normal sulcus exists circumferentially on the humeral head, which represents an area of bare bone between the insertion of the capsule and the edge of the humeral articular cartilage.[16] An increase in size of this bare area posteriorly should not be considered pathologic because it is thought to be part of the normal aging process. Clinically, the physician must be careful not to confuse this normal bare area of posterior humeral head with a Hill-Sachs lesion, which represents a pathologic denuding of the posterior humeral cartilage secondary to anterior glenohumeral instability (Plate 5).

The glenoid is surrounded by a wedge-shaped labrum and is intimately related to the capsule and ligaments. It is important to note that not all detachments of the labrum are pathologic. DePalma[16] noted that superior labral detachments frequently occur with advancing age. Our experience suggests that symptoms from anterior superior labral tears do occur but are uncommon.

The tendons of the long head of the biceps and of the subscapularis are both prominent structures within the glenohumeral joint. The biceps tendon can be followed arthroscopically from its insertion at the supraglenoid tubercle and superior labrum (Plates 6 and 7) to its exit at the opening of the bicipital groove. Two rare variants of the biceps tendon should be noted: double-headed biceps and intracapsular biceps,[16] which may lead to initial confusion during arthroscopy. Located at approximately 90 degrees to the glenoid, the biceps tendon forms the anterior border of the insertion of the supraspinatus before entering the bicipital groove (Plate 7). Thus the biceps tendon is helpful in locating the rotator cuff, where the supraspinatus tendon is seen just superior to it. The infraspinatus and teres minor tendons can also be seen by directing the arthroscope farther posteriorly and superiorly.

The superior edge of the subscapularis tendon is also an intraarticular structure and can be seen against the anterior capsule (Plate 8). It, too, courses at approximately 90 degrees to the glenoid, and it is roughly parallel in orientation to the biceps tendon. The subscapularis tendon is helpful in locating the capsular ligaments. Of the three capsular ligaments, the inferior glenohumeral ligament is usually the largest, and its superior

band can be seen crossing the superior edge of the subscapularis tendon at about 90 degrees near its attachment to the glenoid (Plate 9). The middle glenohumeral ligament crosses the superior edge of the subscapularis at approximately 60 degrees (Plate 9), and it is slightly anterior to the superior band of the inferior glenohumeral ligament. The smallest capsular ligament, the superior glenohumeral ligament, is usually obscured from view by the biceps tendon. It can, however, be seen by switching to an anterior or superior portal.

With an intimate familiarity with the four anatomic landmarks of the articular surfaces of the humerus and glenoid, the long head of the biceps tendon, and the subscapularis tendon, the physician can view nearly the entire glenohumeral joint in an orderly fashion. A standardized viewing sequence is important so that no accessible area is overlooked. Many different regimens for systematically viewing the glenohumeral joint have been proposed, and the selection of a particular regimen is at the discretion of the arthroscopist.

Our approach is to access the aforementioned orienting landmarks completely at the start. We then proceed anteriorly to view the anterior capsule, glenohumeral ligaments, and subscapularis recess and its opening. The examination then goes to the superior portion of the glenohumeral joint, followed by the inferior and posterior portions, where the rotator cuff and capsule are inspected. With this approach the entire joint has been inspected, and all critical structures are noted.

INDICATIONS

The indications for shoulder arthroscopy have yet to be definitely outlined and substantiated by long-term prospective studies. Diagnostic shoulder arthroscopy should be limited to the occasional patient in which the history, physical examination, plain radiographs, and other less invasive special radiographs failed to reveal the diagnosis.

Subacromial Impingement and Rotator Cuff Tears

The use of arthroscopic surgery in the subacromial space has been shown to be effective in the appropriate patient. As defined by Neer,[47,48] the impingement syndrome is a mechanical compression of the rotator cuff by the subacromial arch. The diagnosis continues to be a clinical one, and the treatment depends on the stage of impingement. Stage 1 impingement consists of a mechanical bursitis and inflammation of the rotator cuff tendons, which is reversible and thus responsive to conservative treatment. Stage 2 impingement consists of a bursitis, tendinitis, and fibrosis within the soft tissues, which compromise the subacromial space. Nonoperative treatment is generally successful, with avoidance of overhead activities, the use of oral inflammatory medication, the prudent use of one or two cortisone injections, and strengthening exercises for the rotator cuff musculature. If symptoms persist for greater than 6 to 9 months, these patients may be candidates for a decompressive procedure.

An arthroscopic subacromial decompression is recom-

mended by many physicians for those Stage 2 patients without acromioclavicular joint involvement. This technique was introduced by Ellman in 1985.[20] Numerous studies have reported good to excellent results in 80% to 90% of cases with appropriate patient selection and surgical techniques.*

An open surgical procedure continues to be the preferred method of decompressing Stage 2 shoulders with concomitant acromioclavicular joint involvement. The efficacy of accomplishing this more complex decompression arthroscopically is under investigation, but results are still pending.

Stage 3 subacromial impingement consists of advanced Stage 2 pathologic findings, with an additional rotator cuff tear. The use of surgical arthroscopy is limited with respect to treatment of Stage 3 disease. There is little scientific evidence that debridement of a partial rotator cuff tear leads to an increased healing response, although clinical improvements have been noted. Andrews, Broussard, and Carson[3] reported that 85% of competitive athletes with partial tears of the supraspinatus portion of the rotator cuff had good to excellent results after an arthroscopic debridement of the tear. Gartsman[25] reported that 83% of patients who underwent an acromioplasty with debridement of partial rotator cuff tears had major improvements in ratings for pain, activities of daily living, work, and sports; but debridement of full-thickness tears was not as successful, with only 56% being satisfied with the results. Ellman, Kay, and Wirth[22] have found that older individuals involved in nonstrenuous activities with massive irreparable tears rated their results as satisfactory in nearly 90% of their cases after an arthroscopic decompression and debridement.

A more intriguing application of arthroscopy is to identify the rotator cuff tear and to repair it via a limited deltoid splitting approach or with arthroscopic suture fixation. Levy, Uribe, and Delaney[33] evaluated 25 patients with a 1-year follow-up after an arthroscopic subacromial decompression with a mini open repair of the cuff tears; 100% of the patients with small to moderate tears had a satisfactory rating. Long-term results following arthroscopic suture fixation of small tears or mini open rotator cuff repairs for full-thickness tears found at arthroscopy are still pending.

Our experience is that arthroscopy is helpful in identifying small to incomplete tears of the rotator cuff that are not identified by an arthrogram and that judicious debridement may be of some value at the time of an arthroscopic subacromial decompression. In complete tears, however, arthroscopic debridement in the athlete, despite decompression, is of little value because symptoms attributable to weakness and discomfort commensurate with the size of the tear manifest themselves during attempts at high-performance use of the shoulder. Furthermore, this may worsen the athlete's condition, with possible extension of the tear and an exacerbation of the overall condition. Some of the more demanding open rotator cuff repairs that we have encountered have been failures after an arthroscopic debridement, where loss of tendon substance has been thought to compromise the open repair directly.

Instability

The term *shoulder instability* encompasses the entire spectrum, from unidirectional to multidirectional and from subluxation to frank dislocation. Current thinking reflects that glenohumeral instability depends on an interrelationship between the capsule, labrum, glenohumeral ligaments, and rotator cuff tendons, as well as the humeral head and bony glenoid.

Use of shoulder arthroscopy to treat instability is still in its developmental stages (see p. 191). In recent years Johnson has popularized a technique of an arthroscopic staple capsulorrhaphy. After scarification of the anterior scapular neck, the glenohumeral ligaments were grasped with a tine of a staple and advanced and fixed into the newly created bony bed. Nottage, Duge, and Fields[52] reported that double contrast computed arthrotomography is useful in helping to select patients for staple capsulorrhaphy by identifying large labral lesions with sufficient tissue suitable for the procedure.

Other arthroscopic procedures include suture anchors, screw fixation[69] of the advanced capsule or placing sutures[44] through the anterior scapular neck, tying them posteriorly to obtain fixation of the anterior capsulorrhaphy. Duncan and Savoie[19] reported that an arthroscopic capsular shift procedure with suture fixation demonstrated satisfactory results in 10 patients in their preliminary report after a 1- to 3-year follow-up. McIntyre and Caspari,[40] using a suture technique, reported a 4% recurrence rate with an average follow-up of 33 months, whereas Wolf[70] employed a suture anchor to perform an anterior capsulolabral repair with favorable results.[1] Although early results with all of these techniques are encouraging, Johnson[56] reported a 21% recurrence rate of instability after the arthroscopic staple capsulorrhaphy in 106 shoulders with a minimal 2-year follow-up, and Lane, Sachs, and Riehl[30] reported a 33% recurrence rate with an average follow-up of 39 months. These results, as of yet, do not compare favorably with currently accepted open surgical repair failure rates of 3%.[57] Furthermore, the placement of metallic devices into the scapular neck has been replete with problems in open surgical procedures,[72] and their use arthroscopically must be weighed accordingly. Perhaps the development of biodegradable staples may eliminate some of the problems associated with metallic devices.

The diagnosis of shoulder instability is still primarily based on the history and clinical findings. It is uncommon when shoulder arthroscopy is needed for the diagnosis. Cofield[14] found that approximately 90% of arthroscopy was either optional or unnecessary in diagnosing or altering the treatment of cases of shoulder instability. In difficult cases of recurrent subluxations a careful evaluation of the shoulder with the patient under anesthesia, supplemented with image intensification and perhaps an arthroscopic evaluation, may be effective in yielding the diagnosis.[17]

Zarins[71] has found that the direction of abnormal sub-

---

*References 1, 12, 24, 28, 42, 46, 55, 59, 64, and 65.

luxations can be inferred by the location of the labral injury present at the time of arthroscopy (Plate 10). Other arthroscopic findings that may be supportive of recurrent glenohumeral subluxations include attenuation of the inferior glenohumeral ligament, a peripheral erosion of the glenoid cartilage, loose bodies, and a humeral head Hill-Sachs lesion (Plate 5).[13,23,39,43]

Arthroscopic findings in subluxation

- Labral tears
- Inferior glenohumeral ligament attentuation
- Glenoid cartilage erosion
- Loose bodies
- Humeral head Hill-Sachs lesion

Labral Tears

Labral injury continues to be an area of much interest. Labral fraying and tears are known to occur with instability, as well as degenerative conditions.[16] Mechanical symptoms arising from labral tears unassociated with clinical glenohumeral instability (functional tears) have been described. More recently, we have identified tears of a nonfunctional nature associated with chronic subacromial impingement.

Pappas, Goss, and Kleinman[54] divided labral lesions into those occurring with instability and those that are functional and cause painful clicking in the stable shoulder. Treatment in the former group must be directed primarily at the clinical instability. On the other hand, open debridement of functional tears leads to improvement.

Andrews, Carson, and McLead[4] found that functional anterosuperior labral tears are also seen in throwing athletes who complain of pain or popping during the throwing motion, and that, after an arthroscopic debridement of these tears, many athletes had excellent or good results and returned to pitching. Glasgow et al[26] reported 91% good or excellent results in overhead throwing athletes after labral debridement in stable shoulders with a minimum of 2 years' follow-up. However, Altchek et al[2] noted that arthroscopic debridement was not an effective long-term solution for the overhead athlete, with only 7% of athletes having relief of symptoms with a minimum of 2 years' follow-up. However, 40% of his patients had unstable shoulders upon initial examinations.

Snyder et al[63] have described another type of superior labral tear caused by a compression loading of the shoulder. The superior labrum anterior and posterior (SLAP) lesion of the shoulder extends from posterior to anterior within the superior glenoid labrum but stops before the midglenoid notch and includes the anchor of the biceps tendon to the labrum. Four separate types have been described, which can be treated arthroscopically, thereby eliminating the complaints of painful catching and clicking with overhead activities.

Mendoza, Nicholas, and Reilly[41] have found that anterosuperior glenoid labral tears without true detachments occur more commonly than previously believed but are not necessarily symptomatic. These tears gener-

ally extend from the long head of the biceps tendon distally, but they are confined to the anterosuperior quadrant of the glenoid and do not cross the equator into the inferior quadrant. This configuration of tear is frequently found in shoulders of athletes suffering from Stage 2 subacromial impingement, and successful results continue to be obtained by a subacromial decompression without debridement of the labral tear, further supporting the nonfunctional nature of this type of tear. Much more uncommon is the throwing shoulder with symptoms suggestive of recurrent anteroinferior subluxations, which cannot be shown to be clinically unstable. This latter group of shoulders with an additional concomitant anterosuperior labral tear has improved, with return to throwing, after an arthroscopic debridement of the labral tear. This supports the functional nature of the tear. Labral tears associated with anteroinferior glenohumeral instability have been shown to extend from the anterosuperior quadrant of the glenoid to the inferior quadrant, or they remain confined in the inferior quadrant.[41] Arthroscopic debridement of these lesions as a sole treatment is contraindicated, and a repair against the instability continues to be the most effective treatment. Nonetheless, Neviaser[50] has reported a type of superficial anterior inferior labral tear associated with an adjacent glenoid articular cartilage injury without evidence for anterior instability. Simple debridement of these lesions relieved the symptoms of anterior shoulder pain.

Bicipital Tendinitis

Intraarticular fraying and synovitis of the biceps tendon are often seen in overhead throwers, as well as in older individuals in conjunction with degenerative arthritis.[16] These pathologic implications remain unclear. Nonetheless, some authors arthroscopically debride the tendon and enlarge the entrance into the bicipital groove.[53] Partial and complete tears of the biceps tendon are more often noted as part of the impingement syndrome, and therapeutic intervention should be directed there. Mechanical symptoms resulting from a ruptured intraarticular biceps tendon stump are uncommon but may be eliminated by an arthroscopic debridement of the stump.

Glenohumeral Arthritis

The role of arthroscopy in this entity depends on the severity of the disease.[53] In mild osteoarthritis, Ogilvie-Harris and Wiley[53] obtained successful results with debridement of chondral debris and synovium in about two thirds of cases. In severe osteoarthritis only one third of patients had favorable results. Early rheumatoid arthritis without radiographic evidence of disease had improvement after arthroscopic synovectomy with approximately 1-year follow-up. Long-term results are still pending.

Adhesive Capsulitis

After arthroscopy of 24 patients with adhesive capsulitis, Ha'eri and Maitland[27] found a decreased glenohumeral joint volume in 60% and synovitis in 21% of patients. In a similar study Uitvlugt et al[68] found varying degrees of capsular contracture and synovitis in all 21

shoulders reported. Although a more rapid recovery from this condition has been reported after arthroscopy, presumably by stretching soft-tissue contractures,[53] we have found that improvement is short term, and an intensive course of physical therapy is overall a more effective and predictable method of treatment without the attendant risk of surgery.

Loose Bodies

Loose bodies of the glenohumeral joint are a telltale sign and can occur in association with conditions such as instability, arthritis, chondromatosis, and an osteochondral fracture. Although retrieval of loose bodies can be accomplished arthroscopically in the shoulder without resorting to open techniques,[38] emphasis should be placed on treatment of the primary condition rather than only on the loose bodies.

Calcific Tendinitis

A large single calcific deposit may be amenable to arthroscopic needling and curettage after failure of conservative methods.[21] Ark et al[6] have reported 91% good and satisfactory results after arthroscopic calcium removal and subacromial bursectomy. However, if multiple or small deposits exist, the technical difficulties encountered in locating the tendinous deposits and their boundaries within the surrounding chemical bursitis may be such that an open procedure is necessary for proper treatment.

Other Conditions

Shoulder arthroscopy has been successfully used for irrigation and debridement of septic shoulders, biopsy of tissue in polymyalgia rheumatica,[18] treatment of pigmented villonodular synovitis, debridement of hemodialysis-related shoulder arthropathy,[67] and removal of painful and loose hardware from previous open shoulder procedures.[7] Also of interest, a successful arthroscopically assisted glenohumeral arthrodesis has been reported with fusion at 6 weeks.[45]

COMPLICATIONS

In his reported series of 439 surgical shoulder arthroscopies, Ogilvie-Harris and Wiley[53] reported a complication rate of 3%, all of which were without residual sequelae. These complications included massive leakage of fluid from the shoulder, abrasion of the articular cartilage, sepsis, and musculocutaneous nerve palsy.

Fluid leakage into the surrounding soft tissues poses a theoretical complication of neurovascular compromise, but the fluid usually begins to resorb within the first 12 hours.[34] Nonetheless, there are case reports of pneumomediastinum secondary to severe subcutaneous emphysema following shoulder arthroscopy.[31,32] Early diagnosis and appropriate treatment can be lifesaving.

Neurologic injury is a potential serious complication that can be minimized with careful arthroscopic technique. In anatomic studies Bryan, Schauder, and Tullos[10] demonstrated the potential for direct nerve injury because the standard posterior portal of entry passes only

from 0.5 to 2.5 cm superior to the main trunk of the axillary nerve. Transient neurologic compromise ranging from paresthesias to palsies has been reported, with an incidence of 10% to 30%.[29] The commonly affected nerves are the musculocutaneous and ulnar.[5] Positioning of the upper extremity and the degree of applied traction have been found to be contributing factors. The positions of least strain on the brachial plexus that allow maximal visualization are 45 degrees of forward flexion and 90 degrees of abduction, or 45 degrees of forward flexion and 0 degrees of abduction.[29]

In a survey on arthroscopy of the knee and other joints, the Arthroscopic Association of North America reported that anterior staple capsulorrhaphy for shoulder instability had a complication rate of 5.3%—the highest rate of any joint arthroscopic procedure. Subacromial decompression had a rate of only 0.76%.[62] Similarly, in a more recent review, Bigliani, Flatow, and Deliz[8] noted that the highest complication rate of 3.2% was associated with staple capsulorrhaphy. Subacromial decompression had a complication rate of less than 1% with infection rates in the range of 0.04% to 3.4%. Thus the technique of anterior staple capsulorrhaphy continues to need further refinement.

SUMMARY

Shoulder arthroscopy has, without a doubt, increased our knowledge of anatomy as well as pathology. Although its role as a diagnostic tool in the shoulder is currently minimal, its effectiveness as a surgical tool is ever increasing. Its continued success can only be further enhanced by a sound understanding of the appropriate preoperative diagnosis. Long-term results of surgical arthroscopy are still pending in many areas, but the future of this minimally invasive alternative to open surgery is encouraging.

REFERENCES

1. Altchek DW et al: Arthroscopic acromioplasty technique and results, *J Bone Joint Surg* 72:1198, 1990.
2. Altchek DW et al: Arthroscopic labral debridement: a three-year follow-up study, *Am J Sports Med* 20:702, 1992.
3. Andrews JR, Broussard TS, Carson WG: Arthroscopy of the shoulder in the management of partial tears of the rotator cuff: a preliminary report, *J Arthroscopy* 1:117, 1985.
4. Andrews JR, Carson WG, McLeod WD: Glenoid labrum tears related to the long head of the biceps, *Am J Sports Med* 13:337, 1985.
5. Andrews JR, Carson WG, Ortega K: Arthroscopy of the shoulder: technique and normal anatomy, *Am J Sports Med* 12:1, 1984.
6. Ark JW et al: Arthroscopic treatment of calcific tendinitis of the shoulder, *Arthroscopy* 8:183, 1992.
7. Bach BR Jr: Arthroscopic removal of painful Bristow hardware, *Arthroscopy* 6:324, 1990.
8. Bigliani LU, Flatow EL, Deliz ED: Complications of shoulder arthroscopy, *Orthop Rev* 20:743, 1991.
9. Brown AR et al: Interscalene block for shoulder arthroscopy: comparison with general anesthesia, *Arthroscopy* 9:295, 1993.
10. Bryan WJ, Schauder K, Tullos H: The axillary nerve and its relationship to common sports medicine shoulder procedures, *Am J Sports Med* 14:113, 1986.
11. Burman MS: Arthroscopy or the direct visualization of joints: an experimental cadaver study, *J Bone Joint Surg* 13:669, 1931.

12. Burns TP, Turba JE: Arthroscopic treatment of shoulder impingement in athletes, *Am J Sports Med* 20:13, 1992.
13. Caspari RB: Shoulder arthroscopy: a review of the present state of the art, *Contemp Orthop* 4:523, 1982.
14. Cofield RH: Arthroscopy of the shoulder, *Mayo Clin Proc* 58:501, 1983.
15. Cofield RH, Nessler JP, Weinstabl R: Diagnosis of shoulder instability by examination under anesthesia, *Clin Orthop* 291:45, 1993.
16. DePalma AF: *Surgery of the shoulder,* ed 3, Philadelphia, 1983, JB Lippincott.
17. Dolk T, Gremark O: Arthroscopy and stability testing of the shoulder joint, *Arthroscopy* 2:35, 1986.
18. Douglas WAC, Martin EA, Moms JH: Polymyalgia rheumatica: an arthroscopic study of the shoulder joint, *Ann Rheum Dis* 42:311, 1983.
19. Duncan R, Savoie FH III: Arthroscopic inferior capsular shift for multi-directional instability of the shoulder: a preliminary report, *Arthroscopy* 9:24, 1993.
20. Ellman H: Arthroscopic subacromial decompression, *Orthop Trans* 9:48, 1985.
21. Ellman H: Arthroscopic subacromial decompression: analysis of one- to three-year results, *Arthroscopy* 3:173, 1987.
22. Ellman H, Kay SP, Wirth M: Arthroscopic treatment of full thickness rotator cuff tears: 2- to 7-year follow-up study, *Arthroscopy* 9:195, 1993.
23. Garth WP, Allman FL, Armstrong WS: Occult anterior subluxations of the shoulder in noncontact sports, *Am J Sports Med* 15:579, 1987.
24. Gartsman GM: Arthroscopic treatment of stage 11 subacromial impingement, *Orthop Trans* 12:731, 1988.
25. Gartsman GM: Arthroscopic acromioplasty for lesions of the rotator cuff, *J Bone Joint Surg* 72:169, 1990.
26. Glasgow SG et al: Arthroscopic resection of glenoid labral tears in the athlete: a report of 29 cases, *Arthroscopy* 8:48, 1992.
27. Ha'eri GB, Maitland A: Arthroscopic findings in the frozen shoulder, *J Rheumatol* 8:149, 1981.
28. Holsbeeck EV et al: Subacromial impingement: open versus arthroscopic decompression, *Arthroscopy* 8:173, 1992.
29. Klein AH et al: Measurement of brachial plexus strain in arthroscopy of the shoulder, *Arthroscopy* 3:45, 1987.
30. Lane JG, Sachs RA, Riehl B: Arthroscopic staple capsulorrhaphy: a long-term follow-up, *Arthroscopy* 9:190, 1993.
31. Lau KY: Pneumomediastinum caused by subcutaneous emphysema in the shoulder, *Chest* 103:1606, 1993.
32. Lee HC, Dewan N, Crosby L: Subcutaneous emphysema, pneumomediastinum, and potentially life threatening tension pneumothorax: pulmonary complications from arthroscopic shoulder decompression, *Chest* 101:1265, 1992.
33. Levy HJ, Uribe JW, Delaney LG: Arthroscopic assisted rotator cuff repair: preliminary results, *Arthroscopy* 6:55, 1990.
34. Lilleby H: Shoulder arthroscopy, *Acta Orthop Scand* 55:561, 1984.
35. Lindh M, Norlin R: Arthroscopic subacromial decompression versus open acromioplasty, *Clin Orthop* 290:174, 1993.
36. Lombardo SJ: Arthroscopy of the shoulder, *Clin Sports Med* 2:309, 1983.
37. Matthews LS et al: Anterior portal selection for shoulder arthroscopy, *J Arthroscopy* 1:33, 1985.
38. McGinty JB: Arthroscopic removal of loose bodies, *Orthop Clin North Am* 13:313, 1982.
39. McGlynn FJ, Caspari RB: Arthroscopic findings in the subluxating shoulder, *Clin Orthop* 183:173, 1984.
40. McIntyre LF, Caspari RB: The rationale and technique for arthroscopic reconstruction of anterior shoulder instability using multiple sutures, *Orthop Clin North Am* 24:55, 1993.
41. Mendoza FX, Nicholas JA, Reilly J: Anatomic patterns of anterior glenoid labrum tears, *Orthop Trans* 11:246, 1987.
42. Mendoza FX, Nicholas JA, Rubinstein MP: The arthroscopic treatment of subacromial impingement, *Clin Sports Med* 6:573, 1987.
43. Mizuno K, Hirohata K: Diagnosis of recurrent traumatic anterior subluxation of the shoulder, *Clin Orthop* 179:160, 1983.
44. Morgan CD, Bodenstab AB: Arthroscopic Bankart suture repair: technique and early results, *Arthroscopy* 3:111, 1987.
45. Morgan CD, Casscells CD: Arthroscopic assisted glenohumeral arthrodesis, *Arthroscopy* 8:262, 1992.
46. Morrison DS: Correlation of acromial morphology and the results of arthroscopic subacromial decompression, *Orthop Trans* 12:731, 1988.
47. Neer CS II: Anterior acromioplasty for the chronic impingement syndrome in the shoulder: a preliminary report, *J Bone Joint Surg* 54A:41, 1972.
48. Neer CS II: Impingement lesions, *Clin Orthop* 173:70, 1983.
49. Nelson MC et al: Evaluation of the painful shoulder: prospective comparison of magnetic resonance imaging, computerized tomographic arthrography, ultrasonography, and operative findings, *J Bone Joint Surg* 73:707, 1991.
50. Neviaser TJ: The GLAD lesion, *Arthroscopy* 9:22, 1993.
51. Nottage WM: Shoulder arthroscopy: portals and surgical techniques, *Tech Orthop* 3:23, 1988.
52. Nottage WM, Duge WD, Fields WA: Computed arthrotomography of the glenohumeral joint to evaluate anterior instability: correlation with arthroscopic findings, *Arthroscopy* 3:273, 1987.
53. Ogilvie-Harris DJ, Wiley AM: Arthroscopic surgery of the shoulder: a general appraisal, *J Bone Joint Surg* 68B:201, 1986.
54. Pappas AM, Goss TP, Kleinman PK: Symptomatic shoulder instability due to lesions of the glenoid labrum, *Am J Sports Med* 11:279, 1983.
55. Paulos LE, Franklin JL: Arthroscopic shoulder decompression development and application: a five-year experience, *Am J Sports Med* 18:235, 1990.
56. Rockwood CA Jr: Shoulder arthroscopy, *J Bone Joint Surg* 70A:639, 1988 (editorial).
57. Rockwood CA Jr, Green DP, Bucholz RW: *Fractures in adults,* ed 3, Philadelphia, 1991, JB Lippincott.
58. Rojvanit F: Arthroscopy of the shoulder joint: a cadaver and clinical study, vol 1, Cadaver study, *J Jpn Orthop Assoc* 58:1035, 1984.
59. Ryu RKN: Arthroscopic subacromial decompression: a clinical review, *Arthroscopy* 8:141, 1992.
60. Sandin R: Interscalene plexus block for arthroscopy of the humeral-scapular joint, *Acta Anesthesiol Scand* 36:493, 1992.
61. Skyhar MJ, Altcheck DW, Warren RF: Shoulder arthroscopy in the seated position, *Orthop Rev* 10:1033, 1988.
62. Small NC: Complications in arthroscopy: the knee and other joints, *Arthroscopy* 2:253, 1986.
63. Snyder SJ et al: SLAP lesions of the shoulder, *Arthroscopy* 6:274, 1990.
64. Snyder SJ et al: Partial thickness rotator cuff tears: results of arthroscopic treatment, *Arthroscopy* 7:1, 1991.
65. Speer KP, Lohnes J, Garrett WE: Arthroscopic subacromial decompression: results in advanced impingement syndrome, *Arthroscopy* 7:291, 1991.
66. Takagi K: Practical experiences using Takagi's arthroscope, *J Jpn Orthop Assoc* 8:132, 1933.
67. Takenaka R et al: Surgical treatment of hemodialysis-related shoulder arthropathy, *Clin Nephrol* 38:224, 1992.
68. Uitvlugt G et al: Arthroscopic observations before and after manipulation of frozen shoulder, *Arthroscopy* 9:181, 1993.
69. Wolf EM: Arthroscopic anterior shoulder capsulorrhaphy, *Tech Orthop* 3:67, 1988.
70. Wolf EM: Arthroscopic capsulolabral repair using suture anchors, *Orthop Clin North Am* 24:59, 1993.
71. Zarins B: Current concepts in the diagnosis and treatment of shoulder instability in athletes, *Med Sci Sports Exerc* 16:444, 1984.
72. Zuckerman JD, Masten FA: Complications about the glenohumeral joint related to the use of screws and staples, *J Bone Joint Surg* 66A:175, 1984.

12. Burns TP, Turba JE: Arthroscopic treatment of shoulder impingement in athletes, *Am J Sports Med* 20:13, 1992.
13. Caspari RB: Shoulder arthroscopy: a review of the present state of the art, *Contemp Orthop* 4:523, 1982.
14. Cofield RH: Arthroscopy of the shoulder, *Mayo Clin Proc* 58:501, 1983.
15. Cofield RH, Nessler JP, Weinstabl R: Diagnosis of shoulder instability by examination under anesthesia, *Clin Orthop* 291:45, 1993.
16. DePalma AF: *Surgery of the shoulder,* ed 3, Philadelphia, 1983, JB Lippincott.
17. Dolk T, Gremark O: Arthroscopy and stability testing of the shoulder joint, *Arthroscopy* 2:35, 1986.
18. Douglas WAC, Martin EA, Moms JH: Polymyalgia rheumatica: an arthroscopic study of the shoulder joint, *Ann Rheum Dis* 42:311, 1983.
19. Duncan R, Savoie FH III: Arthroscopic inferior capsular shift for multi-directional instability of the shoulder: a preliminary report, *Arthroscopy* 9:24, 1993.
20. Ellman H: Arthroscopic subacromial decompression, *Orthop Trans* 9:48, 1985.
21. Ellman H: Arthroscopic subacromial decompression: analysis of one- to three-year results, *Arthroscopy* 3:173, 1987.
22. Ellman H, Kay SP, Wirth M: Arthroscopic treatment of full thickness rotator cuff tears: 2- to 7-year follow-up study, *Arthroscopy* 9:195, 1993.
23. Garth WP, Allman FL, Armstrong WS: Occult anterior subluxations of the shoulder in noncontact sports, *Am J Sports Med* 15:579, 1987.
24. Gartsman GM: Arthroscopic treatment of stage 11 subacromial impingement, *Orthop Trans* 12:731, 1988.
25. Gartsman GM: Arthroscopic acromioplasty for lesions of the rotator cuff, *J Bone Joint Surg* 72:169, 1990.
26. Glasgow SG et al: Arthroscopic resection of glenoid labral tears in the athlete: a report of 29 cases, *Arthroscopy* 8:48, 1992.
27. Ha'eri GB, Maitland A: Arthroscopic findings in the frozen shoulder, *J Rheumatol* 8:149, 1981.
28. Holsbeeck EV et al: Subacromial impingement: open versus arthroscopic decompression, *Arthroscopy* 8:173, 1992.
29. Klein AH et al: Measurement of brachial plexus strain in arthroscopy of the shoulder, *Arthroscopy* 3:45, 1987.
30. Lane JG, Sachs RA, Riehl B: Arthroscopic staple capsulorrhaphy: a long-term follow-up, *Arthroscopy* 9:190, 1993.
31. Lau KY: Pneumomediastinum caused by subcutaneous emphysema in the shoulder, *Chest* 103:1606, 1993.
32. Lee HC, Dewan N, Crosby L: Subcutaneous emphysema, pneumomediastinum, and potentially life threatening tension pneumothorax: pulmonary complications from arthroscopic shoulder decompression, *Chest* 101:1265, 1992.
33. Levy HJ, Uribe JW, Delaney LG: Arthroscopic assisted rotator cuff repair: preliminary results, *Arthroscopy* 6:55, 1990.
34. Lilleby H: Shoulder arthroscopy, *Acta Orthop Scand* 55:561, 1984.
35. Lindh M, Norlin R: Arthroscopic subacromial decompression versus open acromioplasty, *Clin Orthop* 290:174, 1993.
36. Lombardo SJ: Arthroscopy of the shoulder, *Clin Sports Med* 2:309, 1983.
37. Matthews LS et al: Anterior portal selection for shoulder arthroscopy, *J Arthroscopy* 1:33, 1985.
38. McGinty JB: Arthroscopic removal of loose bodies, *Orthop Clin North Am* 13:313, 1982.
39. McGlynn FJ, Caspari RB: Arthroscopic findings in the subluxating shoulder, *Clin Orthop* 183:173, 1984.
40. McIntyre LF, Caspari RB: The rationale and technique for arthroscopic reconstruction of anterior shoulder instability using multiple sutures, *Orthop Clin North Am* 24:55, 1993.
41. Mendoza FX, Nicholas JA, Reilly J: Anatomic patterns of anterior glenoid labrum tears, *Orthop Trans* 11:246, 1987.
42. Mendoza FX, Nicholas JA, Rubinstein MP: The arthroscopic treatment of subacromial impingement, *Clin Sports Med* 6:573, 1987.
43. Mizuno K, Hirohata K: Diagnosis of recurrent traumatic anterior subluxation of the shoulder, *Clin Orthop* 179:160, 1983.
44. Morgan CD, Bodenstab AB: Arthroscopic Bankart suture repair: technique and early results, *Arthroscopy* 3:111, 1987.
45. Morgan CD, Casscells CD: Arthroscopic assisted glenohumeral arthrodesis, *Arthroscopy* 8:262, 1992.
46. Morrison DS: Correlation of acromial morphology and the results of arthroscopic subacromial decompression, *Orthop Trans* 12:731, 1988.
47. Neer CS II: Anterior acromioplasty for the chronic impingement syndrome in the shoulder: a preliminary report, *J Bone Joint Surg* 54A:41, 1972.
48. Neer CS II: Impingement lesions, *Clin Orthop* 173:70, 1983.
49. Nelson MC et al: Evaluation of the painful shoulder: prospective comparison of magnetic resonance imaging, computerized tomographic arthrography, ultrasonography, and operative findings, *J Bone Joint Surg* 73:707, 1991.
50. Neviaser TJ: The GLAD lesion, *Arthroscopy* 9:22, 1993.
51. Nottage WM: Shoulder arthroscopy: portals and surgical techniques, *Tech Orthop* 3:23, 1988.
52. Nottage WM, Duge WD, Fields WA: Computed arthrotomography of the glenohumeral joint to evaluate anterior instability: correlation with arthroscopic findings, *Arthroscopy* 3:273, 1987.
53. Ogilvie-Harris DJ, Wiley AM: Arthroscopic surgery of the shoulder: a general appraisal, *J Bone Joint Surg* 68B:201, 1986.
54. Pappas AM, Goss TP, Kleinman PK: Symptomatic shoulder instability due to lesions of the glenoid labrum, *Am J Sports Med* 11:279, 1983.
55. Paulos LE, Franklin JL: Arthroscopic shoulder decompression development and application: a five-year experience, *Am J Sports Med* 18:235, 1990.
56. Rockwood CA Jr: Shoulder arthroscopy, *J Bone Joint Surg* 70A:639, 1988 (editorial).
57. Rockwood CA Jr, Green DP, Bucholz RW: *Fractures in adults,* ed 3, Philadelphia, 1991, JB Lippincott.
58. Rojvanit F: Arthroscopy of the shoulder joint: a cadaver and clinical study, vol 1, Cadaver study, *J Jpn Orthop Assoc* 58:1035, 1984.
59. Ryu RKN: Arthroscopic subacromial decompression: a clinical review, *Arthroscopy* 8:141, 1992.
60. Sandin R: Interscalene plexus block for arthroscopy of the humeral-scapular joint, *Acta Anesthesiol Scand* 36:493, 1992.
61. Skyhar MJ, Altcheck DW, Warren RF: Shoulder arthroscopy in the seated position, *Orthop Rev* 10:1033, 1988.
62. Small NC: Complications in arthroscopy: the knee and other joints, *Arthroscopy* 2:253, 1986.
63. Snyder SJ et al: SLAP lesions of the shoulder, *Arthroscopy* 6:274, 1990.
64. Snyder SJ et al: Partial thickness rotator cuff tears: results of arthroscopic treatment, *Arthroscopy* 7:1, 1991.
65. Speer KP, Lohnes J, Garrett WE: Arthroscopic subacromial decompression: results in advanced impingement syndrome, *Arthroscopy* 7:291, 1991.
66. Takagi K: Practical experiences using Takagi's arthroscope, *J Jpn Orthop Assoc* 8:132, 1933.
67. Takenaka R et al: Surgical treatment of hemodialysis-related shoulder arthropathy, *Clin Nephrol* 38:224, 1992.
68. Uitvlugt G et al: Arthroscopic observations before and after manipulation of frozen shoulder, *Arthroscopy* 9:181, 1993.
69. Wolf EM: Arthroscopic anterior shoulder capsulorrhaphy, *Tech Orthop* 3:67, 1988.
70. Wolf EM: Arthroscopic capsulolabral repair using suture anchors, *Orthop Clin North Am* 24:59, 1993.
71. Zarins B: Current concepts in the diagnosis and treatment of shoulder instability in athletes, *Med Sci Sports Exerc* 16:444, 1984.
72. Zuckerman JD, Masten FA: Complications about the glenohumeral joint related to the use of screws and staples, *J Bone Joint Surg* 66A:175, 1984.

CHAPTER 6 Acromioclavicular Complex

John A. Bergfeld
Richard D. Parker

Injuries to the acromiocoracoclavicular ligament complex are a common problem in athletics.

MECHANISMS OF INJURY

A knowledge of the pertinent anatomy is important in understanding the rationales for intervention (Fig. 6-1). The box below summarizes the acromioclavicular complex components.

The acromioclavicular (AC)-coracoclavicular (CC) complex is usually injured by a fall in which the athlete lands on the tip of the acromion, forcing the scapula caudally (Fig. 6-2).[2,21] If the clavicle does not break, the AC and CC ligaments may be sprained. Other mechanisms of injury include a direct lateral blow on the shoulder (crushed in a pile-up) or a posterior blow to the scapula.

An indirect injury may result from a fall on the outstretched arm or elbow. These are rare mechanisms by far. The fall in which the outer edge of the shoulder (tip of the acromion) is landed on is the most common mechanism. Injury to the AC-CC complex is common in football, rugby, ice hockey, skiing, wrestling, horseback riding, and, to a lesser extent, basketball, tumbling, and soccer.

CLASSIFICATION OF INJURIES

The prioritization of injuries developed by Rockwood allows us to effectively group the injuries for diagnosis, treatment, and prognosis (Fig. 6-3).[21] Grade I injuries represent a mild sprain of the AC-CC ligaments, with no anatomic disruption of either the AC joint or the CC ligaments.[2] Grade II represents a partial displacement of the AC joint, less than the width of the clavicle, representing a second-degree sprain of both the AC and CC ligaments. Grade III represents complete loss of the integrity of the AC and CC ligaments. Grade IV is a posterior dislocation of the clavicle on the acromion, with complete disruption of the AC joint and ligaments, although the CC ligaments may remain intact. Grade V represents complete loss of the AC joint and ligaments and CC ligaments as well as the trapezius and deltoid muscle attachment to the clavicle and acromion. Often the acromion buttonholes through the muscle. Grade VI represents the clavicle being displaced inferiorly to the coracoid. This is a rare injury in athletics, and usually occurs only with massive trauma, such as that sustained in a motorcycle or motor vehicle accident.

GRADE I INJURIES

Grade I is the most common injury but often goes unnoticed until the day after the injury and sometimes until the late sequela of posttraumatic arthritis causes dis-

---

Acromioclavicular-coracoclavicular complex

- Acromioclavicular joint—acromioclavicular ligaments
- Coracoclavicular interval—coracoclavicular ligaments
(conoid and trapezoid)

Grade I injury

- Point tenderness on acromioclavicular joint
- No instability of joint
- Minimal or no loss of shoulder motion
- Normal radiograph

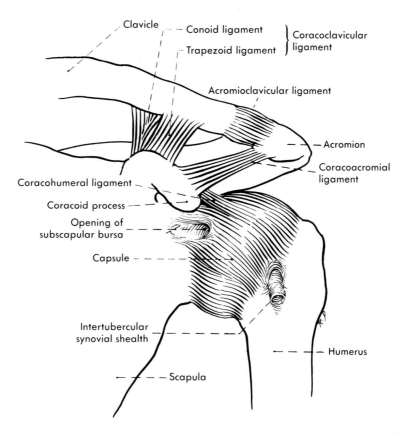

FIG. 6-1. Ligaments of the acromial end of the clavicle and the anterior aspect of the shoulder joint.

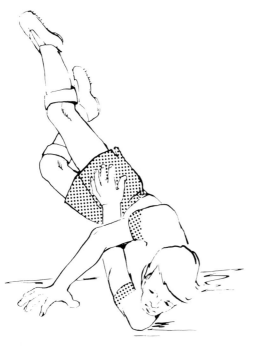

FIG. 6-2. Most common mechanism of injury is a direct force that occurs from a fall on the point of the shoulder. (From Rockwood CA, Jr, Williams GR, Young DC: Injuries to the acromioclavicular joint. In Rockwood CA, Jr, Green DP, Bucholz RW (eds): *Rockwood and Green's fractures in adults*, ed 3, Philadelphia, 1991, JB Lippincott.)

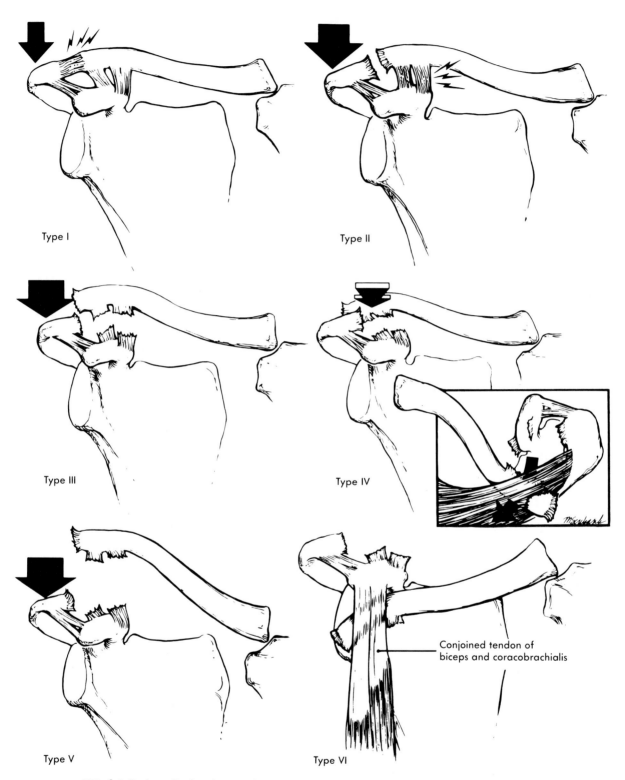

Type I

Type II

Type III

Type IV

Type V

Type VI

Conjoined tendon of
biceps and coracobrachialis

FIG. 6-3. Rockwood's classification of injuries to the acromiocoracoclavicular complex. (From Rockwood CA, Jr, Williams GR, Young DC: Injuries to the acromioclavicular joint. In Rockwood CA, Jr, Green DP, Bucholz RW (eds): *Rockwood and Green's fractures in adults*, ed 3, Philadelphia, 1991, JB Lippincott.)

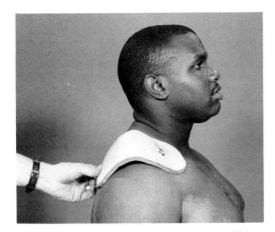

FIG. 6-4. Following Grade I injury the shoulder is padded to allow return to competition.

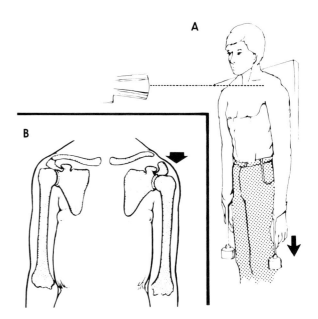

FIG. 6-5. Technique of obtaining stress radiographs of the acromioclavicular (AC) joint. **A,** Anteroposterior radiographs are made of both AC joints with 10 to 15 lbs of weight hanging from the wrists. **B,** The distance between the superior aspect of the coracoid and the undersurface of the clavicle is measured to determine whether the coracoclavicular ligaments have been disrupted. One large horizontal-positioned 14 × 17-inch radiograph cassette can be used in small patients to visualize both shoulders on the same film. In large patients it is better to use two horizontal-placed smaller cassettes and take two separate radiographs for the measurements. (From Rockwood CA, Jr, Williams GR, Young DC: Injuries to the acromioclavicular joint. In Rockwood CA, Jr, Green DP, Bucholz RW (eds): *Rockwood and Green's fractures in adults,* ed 3, Philadelphia, 1991, JB Lippincott.)

comfort in the shoulder. Physical examination is characterized by point tenderness directly over the AC joint, a good diagnostic point to differentiate this injury from the shoulder pointer (contusion on the acromion), or strain of the rotator cuff. The joint is stable, and often there is no loss of motion of the shoulder joint; the athlete reports only mild discomfort at the extremes of motion, especially abduction. Radiographs are negative. A good physical examination should preclude the need for stress radiographs to rule out further injury.

Treatment

Treatment of the acute Grade I injury is symptomatic. These measures include ice, antiinflammatory medication, and padding of the shoulder to prevent direct pressure over the joint (Fig. 6-4). Often the athlete is able to return to competition immediately, and certainly within 2 days to 2 weeks, depending on the sport.

Stress views

- Specific views must be taken of the acromioclavicular joint
- Proper exposure and angulation of the beam is essential
- Stress radiographs require passive stretching of the joint, with weights suspended from both the injured arm and the contralateral arm
- Often the patient is mistakenly asked to hold the weights in the hands, with the resulting muscle contraction negating the displacement of the joint

---

GRADE II INJURIES

The athlete is usually aware of a Grade II injury because of the pain and functional disability. Physical examination reveals mild laxity of the AC joint and a step-off that may be felt between the clavicle and the acromion. There is limitation of abduction and adduction of the shoulder. Radiographs without stress show the classic appearance of the acromion being depressed less than

the width of the clavicle. Occasionally the radiographs are normal, and stress radiographs are necessary (Fig. 6-5). We find the need for stress a rare situation. After some experience, the physician should be able to tell if there is instability of the AC-CC complex on a physical examination.

Grade II injury

- Moderate discomfort
- Palpable (mild) acromioclavicular joint step off
- Limitation of abduction and adduction

Treatment

Treatment of a Grade II injury is again symptomatic, but now the physician must be more aggressive in supporting the joint. Usually a sling is sufficient, but we often use a modified Kinney-Howard sling to get proper support of the joint (Fig. 6-6). The length of treatment depends on the symptoms and the level of competition in all but a few sports that produce unusual stress across the AC joint (e.g., parallel bar). The athlete may return to sports usually as soon as he or she is free from pain;

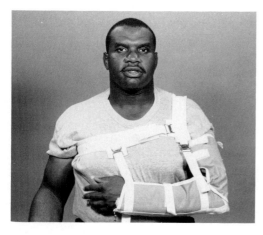

FIG. 6-6. Modified Kinney-Howard sling for proper support of the acromioclavicular joint.

this requires anywhere from 1 to 4 weeks. The deformity that is initially present with the joint remains a permanent deformity.

LONG-TERM SEQUELAE
Grades I and II Injuries

Often little concern is given to the sequelae of Grade I and II injuries in the textbooks for general orthopaedics. These injuries may cause significant problems for the athlete in the future. A follow-up study of midshipmen carried out at the U.S. Naval Academy by Bergfeld et al[4] in 1973 and a similar study, repeated by Cox[11] at the U.S. Naval Academy, revealed a surprisingly large number of persistent positive physical findings and radiographic changes, and significant symptoms (Table 6-1).

The positive physical findings consist of thickening and prominence of the AC joint. Abnormal radiographic findings include posttraumatic changes about the AC joint, loss of the joint space, bony spurring, and soft-tissue calcification. A minor radiographic finding commonly linked to the first-degree AC separation is **osteolysis of the lateral clavicle.** This was an identical finding in both studies and did not correlate with symptoms. Many authors postulate that this osteolysis is caused by avascular necrosis of the lateral clavicle secondary to undecompressed pressure from intraarticular hematoma in a first-degree injury.[9,16] We have seen an osteolytic clavicle recalcify, and we have also noted avascular necrosis in a resected lateral clavicle that had been symptomatic after Grade I AC injuries.

The significant aftersymptoms in athletes with Grade I injuries include pain with heavy activity, such as dips between parallel bars, bench pressing heavy weights, and overhand serving in tennis, as well as throwing a ball. The cause of these symptoms is usually the incongruity of the AC joint as the result of tearing of the meniscus between the clavicle and the acromion or simply posttraumatic arthritis with loss of the articular surface and spur formation.

TABLE 6-1 Long-term findings in Grades I and II acromioclavicular injuries

	Grade I	Grade II
Positive physical examination	43%	71%
Abnormal radiograph	29%	48%
Support system	3.5%*	13%*
	9%†	23%†

*Data from Cox JS: *Am J Sports Med* 5:258, 1977.
†Data from Bergfeld JA et al: *Am J Sports Med* 6:153, 1978.

Treatment of Chronic Symptoms

Treatment of chronically symptomatic Grade I or II injury is to first ensure that there is full strength and endurance of the shoulder musculature. If not, rehabilitation is initiated with particular attention placed on strengthening of the periscapular muscles (especially the serratus anterior) as well as the rotator cuff, deltoid, trapezius, and pectoralis minor and major.

It is imperative that the physician be sure he or she is dealing with AC joint injury alone and not subacromial impingement syndrome as well. This is particularly important in athletes or ex-athletes in the 40+ age group. AC joint symptoms and impingement syndrome symptoms can be differentiated by history, physical examination, radiographs, and injection tests. Athletes with AC joint injury alone complain of pain with the following:
1. Pressure over the joint
2. Bench press
3. Adduction and forward flexion or extension

On the other hand, athletes with impingement syndrome complain of pain:
1. Along the anterior acromion and laterally along the deltoid
2. At night
3. With above-head activities

Physical examination of the athlete with AC joint symptoms alone creates pain primarily with the following:
1. Palpation on the AC joint and distal clavicle
2. Adduction, forward flexion, or extension of the shoulder

Athletes with impingement syndrome as well have pain with the following:
1. Impingement sign (internal rotation/forward flexion)
2. Weakness of the rotator cuff
3. Palpation of the anterior acromion

Radiographic evaluation should consist of an anteroposterior (AP) view, axillary view, supraspinatus outlet view, and AC joint view without weights. Radiographic evidence of AC joint arthritis (Fig. 6-7) and evaluation of the morphologic appearance of the anterior acromion on the supraspinatus outlet view should be emphasized. Further evidence of AC joint arthritis can be provided by a bone scan, especially if surgical excision is contemplated (Fig. 6-8). Rarely if ever is magnetic resonance imaging (MRI) indicated because it is expensive and oversensitive.

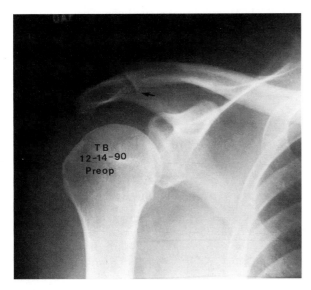

FIG. 6-7. Anteroposterior radiograph of the right shoulder in a 20-year-old athlete after a Grade I acromioclavicular (AC) joint sprain with radiographic evidence of posttraumatic arthritis. Notice the thickening, sclerosis, and joint space narrowing present at the AC joint.

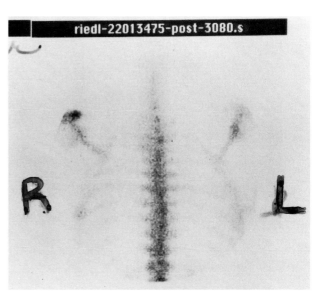

FIG. 6-8. Technetium bone scan of the right shoulder showing increased radiopharmaceutical uptake in the area of the acromioclavicular joint, indicative of posttraumatic arthritis.

Injection tests can help differentiate pain secondary to impingement syndrome and AC joint injury. Injection of 3 ml of 2% lidocaine into the AC joint followed by repeat physical examination helps both the examiner and patient understand the source of the pain. If this injection eliminates the pain completely, both the patient and physician can be assured that the AC joint is the sole locus of symptoms. If incomplete relief is accomplished by the AC joint injection, then 10 ml of 1% lidocaine can be injected subacromially followed by repeat physical examination. If this eliminates the remaining pain, the physician should suspect associated subacromial impingement syndrome.

Nonoperative treatment is the mainstay of treatment of AC joint arthritis and consists of a 3-week course of a nonsteroidal antiinflammatory drug (NSAID). If NSAID medication is unsuccessful, an injection of a soluble corticosteroid into the AC joint is indicated. If impingement syndrome is also present, subacromial bursal corticosteroid injection can also be performed. Injections can be repeated one or two times if there is persistent discomfort, but no more than three injections should be given over a 1-year period. If either the NSAID or corticosteroid injection is successful in decreasing inflammation and pain, rehabilitation is stressed. Rarely do local modalities such as electric stimulation, diathermy, or ultrasound provide lasting relief, although ice and phonophoresis with cortisone cream may be successful because the AC joint is superficial. Another form of treatment is modification of activities such as overhead throwing, bench press, or any activity that seems to aggravate the symptomatic AC joint. Adequate time should be given to allow symptoms to decrease. A minimum of 6 months of nonoperative treatment is recommended before additional treatment is contemplated. Fortunately the nonoperative treatment just discussed achieves satisfactory improvement in most athletes' symptoms.[12,13,20]

Operative treatment is reserved for those athletes with chronic symptoms that have not responded to nonoperative treatment. To have a successful surgical outcome, it is imperative that the physician be absolutely sure of the etiology of the patient's symptoms. If the patient's symptoms are secondary to AC joint arthritis alone, the AC joint excision is sufficient. However, if impingement syndrome is also present, a subacromial decompression as well as an AC joint excision should be performed. In the majority of young athletes with impingement syndrome, decompression of the subacromial space by resecting the subacromial bursa suffices, whereas anterior acromioplasty should be reserved for older athletes or young athletes with acromial spurs or hooks.

AC joint excision with or without subacromial decompression can be performed via an open or arthroscopic technique.[12,13,20] **Open excision of the AC** joint is performed through a longitudinal incision over the distal end of the clavicle. Before incision of the skin, the AC joint and deep tissues are injected with 20 ml of 0.25% bupivacaine (Marcaine) with 1:100,000 epinephrine to decrease bleeding as well as pain during and after the surgical procedure (preemptive anesthesia). The incision is approximately 3 cm in length. The periosteum over the distal clavicle, AC joint, and medial superior acromion is incised horizontally and reflected such that the deltoid anteriorly and the trapezius posteriorly are attached to the reflected periosteum (Fig. 6-9). Small Bennett retractors are placed anteriorly and posteriorly, thus exposing and defining the distal clavicle. An oscillating power saw is then used to resect the distal 1.5 cm of the distal (lat-

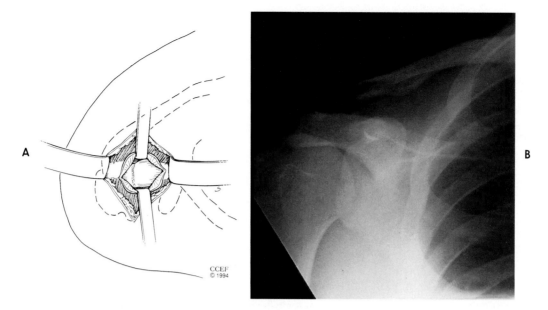

FIG. 6-9. A, Vertical 3-cm incision is placed over the acromioclavicular joint for open excision of the distal 1.5 cm of the clavicle. Note that the periosteum overlying the joint is horizontally incised so as to be able to reflect the trapezius and periosteal sleeve posteriorly and the deltoid and periosteal sleeve anteriorly. This allows for a more stable closure and thus earlier rehabilitation. It is imperative that the posterior and anterior aspects of the distal clavicle are visualized so that adequate bone resection is carried out. **B,** Postoperative anteroposterior radiograph revealing adequate distal clavicle excision (1.5 cm).

eral) clavicle. A rongeur is then used to resect the degenerative meniscus and capsular fibrotic tissue as well as any osteophytes along the medial acromion. Following excision of the distal clavicle the surgeon's index finger is placed in the defect created, and the operative arm is then taken through a range of motion, especially cross-body adduction. If the surgeon's finger is pinched, more distal clavicle should be excised. If no pinching occurs, then adequate resection has been accomplished. If a subacromial decompression is required, the incision can be enlarged, the bursae and coracoacromial ligament excised, and, if indicated, an anterior acromioplasty performed through the defect created by the distal clavicle resection. From 1 to 1½ cm of deltoid may need to be detached from the acromion to gain exposure but does not alter the postoperative rehabilitation. Once adequate bone resection has been performed, the edges are smoothed and wounds are irrigated. The periosteum is then closed with a long-lasting absorbable suture followed by subcuticular skin closure to enhance cosmesis.

Arthroscopic excision of the distal clavicle can be performed by one of two different techniques.[12,13,20] One technique results in excision of the distal clavicle from underneath the AC joint through the subacromial space (Fig. 6-10). The other technique excises the distal clavicle from above the joint through a transcutaneous approach (Fig. 6-11). An advantage of the arthroscopic approach over the open approach is that it allows for complete inspection of the glenohumeral joint, subacromial space, and rotator cuff. One of the many pitfalls of the

arthroscopic approach is incomplete resection (Fig. 6-12), which unfortunately can happen early on the learning curve. Therefore we recommend that the surgeon wishing to learn this arthroscopic approach perform the procedure arthroscopically on cadaveric specimens and then open the AC joint to assess the degree of resection. Once the surgeon has mastered the arthroscopic technique on cadaveric specimens, he or she should then feel comfortable performing this procedure on his or her patients. This ensures a good outcome while still learning a new technique.

We find the open approach to be easier and more reproducible than the arthroscopic approach. Both procedures may be performed as an outpatient procedure. The arthroscopic approach may be a triumph of technology over reason because it is harder to perform, is less reliable, and requires more operative time.

Postoperative management is the same for the arthroscopic and open approaches to distal clavicle excision. A sling is worn for 3 or 4 days, and the athlete begins exercises on the first postoperative day. Pendulum exercises are advised as a gentle warm-up. Active and passive elevation and external rotation movements are performed, and after 10 to 14 days the athlete is encouraged to use the arm as normally as possible. Patients begin a program of isometric and functional strengthening 1 to 2 weeks postoperatively and are permitted to resume sports when they are having no pain or discomfort and have regained functional strength adequate for the sport. A stretching program is stressed after 3 weeks to regain internal rotation and cross-body adduction, thus dimin-

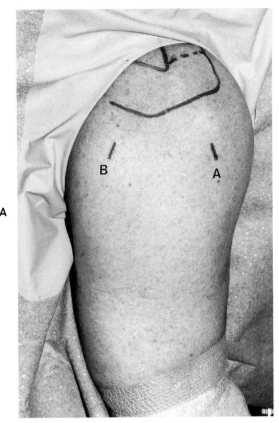

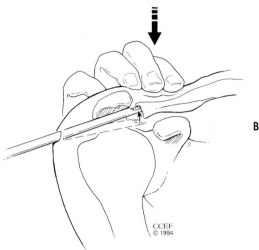

FIG. 6-10. A, Operative photograph of a right shoulder in a beach chair position marking the lateral (A) and posterior (B) portals for subacromial excision of the acromioclavicular joint. The lateral portal is used for the high-powered bur and the posterior portal for arthroscope placement. **B,** Subacromial excision of the distal clavicle. Note how manual pressure from above facilitates adequate resection and visualization.

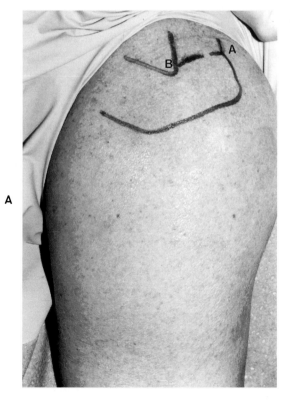

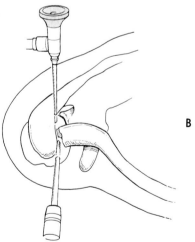

FIG. 6-11. A, Operative photograph with the anterior and posterior excisions marked for transcutaneous approach to the excision of the distal clavicle. The arthroscope can be placed in either the anterior (A) or posterior (B) portal and the bur and synovial receptor in the opposite portal to allow for a systematic excision of the distal clavicle. **B,** Arthroscope and power bur in their respective portals. These instruments can be switched back and forth until adequate excision of the distal clavicle has occurred.

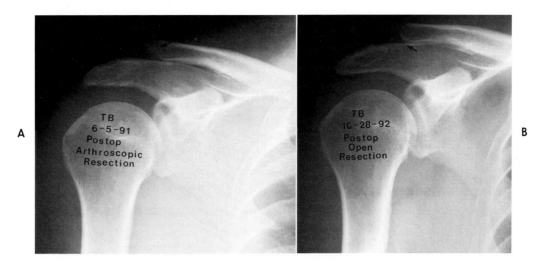

FIG. 6-12. A, Anteroposterior radiograph of a 30-year-old patient who has undergone arthroscopic subacromial excision of the distal clavicle, which failed to resolve the patient's symptoms. **B,** Upon open excision it was discovered that incomplete posterosuperior resection of the distal clavicle had been carried out arthroscopically. This is a common pitfall of the arthroscopic approach.

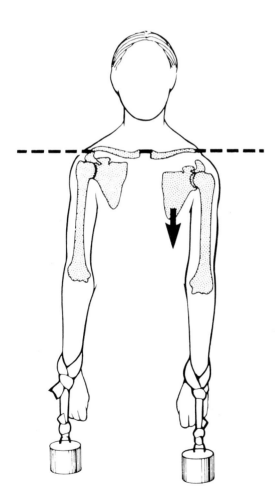

FIG. 6-13. Complete Grade III acromioclavicular dislocation. The major deformity seen in this injury is a downward displacement of the scapula and upper extremity and *not* an upward elevation of the clavicle.

ishing posterior capsular tightness and increasing rotator cuff flexibility.

GRADE III INJURIES

Grade III injury is more severe, and the injured athlete experiences immediate pain, limitation of motion, and possible disability. Often the athlete comes out of athletic participation supporting the shoulder with the opposite arm. Inspection of the shoulder reveals the downward displacement of the acromion, and often the physician hears that the clavicle is riding high (Fig. 6-13). This is an illusion because the clavicle remains at the same level as its counterpart; it is the scapula that is driven caudally. The clavicle is freely movable, and there is complete loss of integrity of the AC joint and CC ligaments. An occasional patient may have a posterior subluxation or dislocation of the clavicle in relation to the acromion (Rockwood Grade IV).

Grade III injury

- Severe pain
- Marked limitation of motion
- Downward acromion displacement

In mild Grade IV injury the CC ligaments remain intact. In Grade III injury, although there is complete loss of the ligamentous stability, the trapezius and deltoid muscles are only partially torn from the clavicle. As with any injury, especially involving the shoulder, careful neurologic examination should be carried out. It is interesting to note that it is rare to see a brachial plexus

injury associated with a Grade III AC sprain in the athlete. We believe the dissipation of the energy through rupturing of the AC and CC ligaments relieves the abnormal stress on the brachial plexus. It may also be that the blow to the shoulder that causes the brachial plexus injury is more toward the top of the shoulder and closer to the spine, such as might occur in making a tackle in American football (see Chapter 31).

Treatment

Treatment of Grade III injury has changed in the past 15 years. In 1974 a poll of Chairmen of the Teaching Programs revealed that 95% of those who responded believe this injury requires surgery to restore the normal anatomy, although a similar recent survey by Cox[11] found that only 40% of the respondents believe surgery is necessary. An informal poll of orthopaedists who treat athletes exclusively raises the percentage of those advocating nonoperative treatment to approximately 90%. This is not to say that nonoperative treatment may return the anatomy to normal, but, as Hippocrates said, "No impediment, small or great, will result from such an injury [Grade III AC separation]; however there would be [malposition] or deformity, for the bone cannot be properly restored to its rational situation."[1]

Before proceeding further, let us say that Grade V injury (complete loss of the attachment of the trapezius and deltoid muscles) should be repaired surgically because this is a severe loss of muscle and ligamentous integrity of the AC joint. Resultant deformity is such that functional use of the shoulder is severely compromised. Fortunately, this is a rare injury in all sports, except motorcycling.

Several considerations must go into the treatment of the common Grade III injury. There are problems and complications in both open and closed methods.

Common problems (open and closed treatment) in Grade III injury

- Posttraumatic arthritis
- Deformity vs. scar
- Calcification of soft tissues
- Pain and disability with sports activity

Overall, a 5% to 10% incidence of significant problems can be anticipated with a Grade III AC injury, no matter whether it is treated by closed or open means.

A review of the literature reveals a multiplicity of surgical procedures designed for AC separations.* At present there appear to be three basic procedures commonly performed: (1) AC joint fixation with wires,[6] (2) circumferential Dacron or wire immobilization of the coracoid and clavicle,[18,22] and (3) screw fixation of the clav-

---

*References 3, 8, 10, 19, 23, and 24.

Complications or problems in treating Grade III injury

Closed method
- Deformity
- Patient intolerance
- Failure to obtain reduction
- Failure to maintain reduction
- Postimmobilization joint stiffness
- Compression neuropathy

Open method
- Anesthesia
- Infection
- Cosmetic scar
- Fixation device failure
    - a. Breaks become loose
    - b. Migrate
    - c. Erode through bone
    - d. Second operation to remove
- Expense
- Time loss from competition
- Longer than nonoperative treatment

---

icle to the coracoid.[7] After personally treating many of these injuries, using all of the above methods at one time or another, we have elected to now treat these injuries by closed method. The closed method falls into two categories—symptomatic and aggressive (Table 6-2).[5,15,25,26]

Closed Symptomatic Treatment

Closed symptomatic treatment might be called, by some, skillful neglect. This is because any method requires attention to the details of splint adjustment and rehabilitation. The closed symptomatic treatment has many advantages, including earlier return to competition.[5,17] One hundred percent have some residual deformity of the AC joint. Approximately 5% to 10% of the individuals find the cosmetic appearance disturbing. However, little correlation is found between the final radiograph, the clinical appearance,[14] and the incidence of significant pain and disability. Like other methods the closed symptomatic treatment yields a 5% to 10% incidence of later problems requiring medical attention.

Closed Aggressive Treatment

The closed aggressive treatment has other advantages for certain situations. An attempt is made to restore normal anatomy; therefore the resultant deformity is not as severe as with the closed symptomatic treatment. These techniques are difficult to carry out, however, if patient compliance is poor, and particularly after 3 weeks from the initial injury. The closed aggressive treatment has the same incidence of persistent significant pain and disability as other methods.

Techniques of Treatment

If seen at the site of injury, a Grade III AC joint sprain can often be easily reduced and held with a modified

TABLE 6-2 Closed treatment

Symptomatic	Aggressive
Immobilization for comfort	Reduce with a splint
Begin rehabilitation when tolerated	Attempt to maintain reduction
	Begin rehabilitation when tolerated

Kinney-Howard sling. Once the AC joint is reduced, the athlete is given pain medication and instructions to keep the shoulder quiet, not to remove the sling unless there is severe pain, and report for daily adjustment of the sling. If symptomatic treatment is elected, the AC sling is discontinued when symptoms allow, usually after 7 to 10 days. While the patient is in the sling, isometric exercises are begun; the sling is loosened for range of motion exercises and these are performed through the range of motion with the athlete or the therapist supporting the AC joint. Progressive resistance exercises are begun as soon as they can be tolerated by the athlete.

If aggressive treatment is elected, an attempt is made to keep the joint reduced for 6 full weeks, during which time isometric exercises are instituted and periodic checks of sling position are made. Experience shows that patent compliance drops off after approximately 3 weeks, and the sling is found to be worn only in the doctor's office or the training room.

More commonly, the athlete is seen several hours after the injury and moderate to severe swelling as well as pain is present. An attempt to reduce the joint and support it with the AC sling is a difficult, uncomfortable experience for the athlete and is frustrating for the physician, therapist, or trainer. If a sling is applied and tightened only for pain reduction, this is also often unsuccessful. An injection into the area with local anesthetic can assist in obtaining a good reduction, essentially a hematoma block, much like treatment of a Colles fracture. The joint is fixed in the sling. This often requires admission to the hospital, where pain medication and attention to the sling at frequent intervals can be carried out. With both symptomatic and aggressive treatment, once the sling is discontinued the athlete is allowed to return to competition when he or she can demonstrate a full range of motion and reasonable strength in the shoulder. A recent report by Walsh et al[27] showed that there was no decrease in strength compared with the normal shoulder in the third-degree AC separations treated by nonoperative means, as opposed to a 19.8% deficit in those shoulders treated surgically. This report tends to give support to nonsurgical treatment of this problem, especially in the athlete or worker who requires good strength in his or her shoulder.

In certain Grade III injuries closed treatment may not be satisfactory. This might be a body builder or fashion model who, for cosmetic reasons, absolutely needs to restore normal anatomy. In the question of a throwing athlete, the need to restore anatomy also may arise, although a majority of the team orthopaedic surgeons treating throwing athletes often resort to closed method of treatment. A preferable surgical technique is the method de-

scribed by Bosworth[7] and popularized by Neer and Rockwood.[21] The AC joint is debrided and the CC ligaments are repaired as best as possible. The AC joint, now reduced, is held with a lag screw (or, in some instances, a Dacron tape is used).

Braided polydioxanone suture (PDS) suture can be used in place of a Dacron tape. This material loses its strength and dissolves within the body after 8 to 10 weeks, thereby negating the need to go back and cut the tape or remove the lag screw. At the time of surgery, all muscles are repaired.

Long-Term Sequelae

For the athlete who has the residuum of a third-degree AC separation with significant pain and disability, we prefer a modification of the procedure described by Weaver and Dunn.[28] This consists of resection of the lateral clavicle, reconstruction of the CC ligaments using the coracoacromial ligament, and stabilization of the coracoid to the clavicle using a lag screw or Dacron tape (or PDS suture) (Fig. 6-14). With this technique the screw must be removed and the tape cut at 8 to 10 weeks postoperatively.

Often there is a severe calcification and scarring in the area of the CC ligaments, making any reduction of the space between the clavicle and the coracoid difficult. In this situation a simple resection and contouring of the lateral clavicle is appropriate.

POSTERIOR DISLOCATION

The clinician should look closely for the third-degree posterior dislocated clavicle because this injury tends to have an increased incidence of chronic functional disability. Acutely, there may be difficulty reducing this separation with a sling, necessitating an open reduction. Most often the examiner can determine by physical examination that the clavicle is posterior to the acromion. If the examiner is unable to determine this, a hint that there is a posterior subluxation of the clavicle on the acromion is indicated by the clavicle and acromion being at the same level, although there is a widened space between the acromion and the clavicle. If there is any question that there is a posterior dislocation of the clavicle, a computed tomography (CT) scan with comparison to the opposite shoulder is often helpful.

In our clinic we have treated one young patient who sustained an interesting posterior subluxation of the clavicle, having split through its periosteum. The athlete then began to regenerate a second clavicle in its initial position, necessitating resection of the distal portion of the initial clavicle, which was ruptured posteriorly. Posterior subluxation of the clavicle tends to occur, in our experience, in the younger athlete and most commonly in wrestlers. It is not a common injury in the person who is fully skeletally mature.

REHABILITATION

As with all athletic injuries, rehabilitation should begin as soon as possible to avoid the deleterious effects of

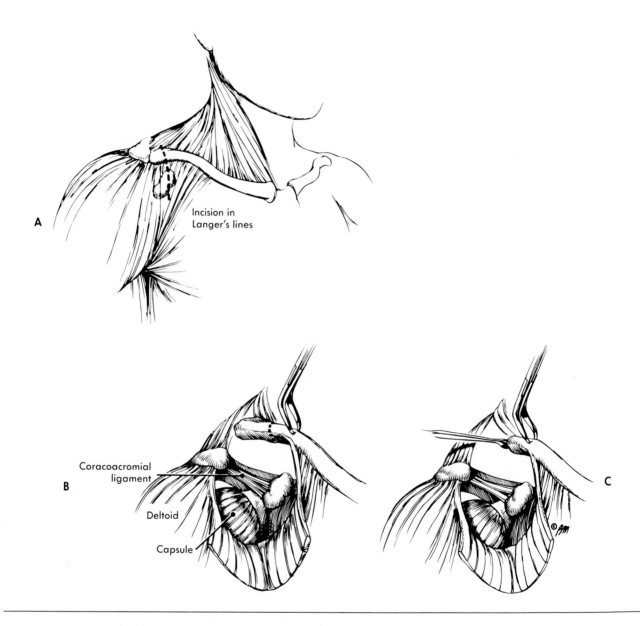

A
Incision in
Langer's lines

B
Coracoacromial
ligament

Deltoid

Capsule

C

FIG. 6-14. A through **H,** Authors' method to reconstruct a Type III acromioclavicular (AC) dislocation. See text for description. Preoperative **G** and postoperative **H** x rays of a chronic Type III AC
dislocation treated with an AC reconstruction. There are degenerative changes in the AC joint that
were causing pain in this man who is a manual worker. The coracoacromial ligament will be used to
reconstruct the coracoclavicular (CC) ligaments. Following removal of the distal 1¼ inches of the
clavicle, the coracoacromial ligament, which was detached from the acromion, was transferred into
the medullary canal of the distal clavicle. The CC lag screw holds the clavicle in position for 8 to 12
weeks until there is secure fixation of the ligament to the clavicle. (From Rockwood CA, Jr,
Williams GR, Young DC: Injuries to the acromioclavicular joint. In Rockwood CA, Jr, Green DP,
Bucholz RW (eds): *Rockwood and Green's fractures in adults,* ed 3, Philadelphia, 1991, JB Lippincott.)

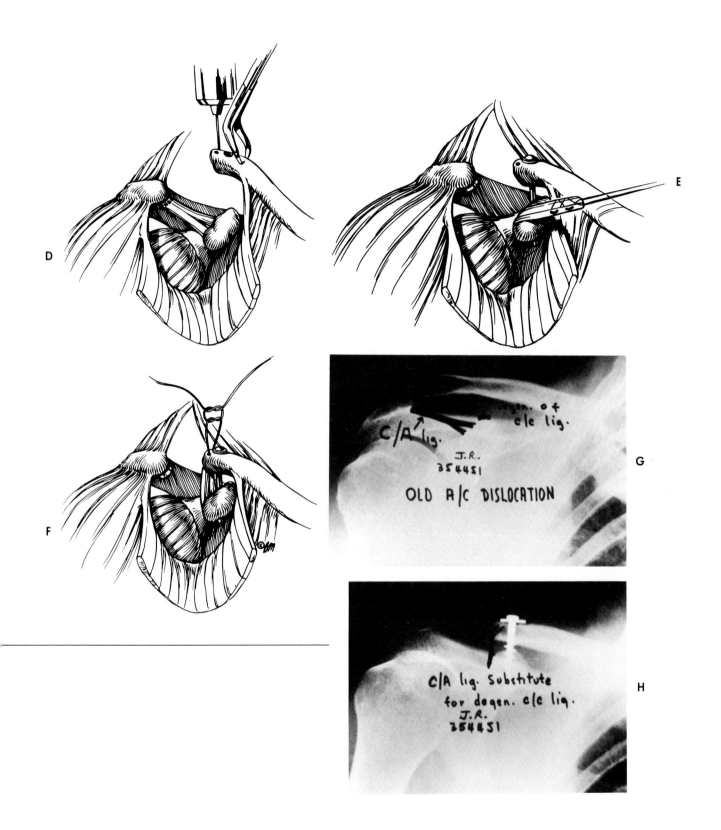

D

E

F

G

OLD A/C DISLOCATION

H

immobilization. As soon as the shoulder is stabilized, by sling or surgically, isometric contraction of the shoulder musculature should be instituted. After surgical treatment, a gentle, full range of motion of the joint can be started when shoulders are pain free. Light resistive exercises can be begun at 3 weeks and weight lifting at 8 to 10 weeks.

With closed treatment, range of motion can be started after 2 weeks, with an assistant stabilizing the AC joint. Eventually the athlete is able to stabilize his or her own AC joint with the opposite hand. Modified resistive exercise can be started immediately, progressing to full progressive resistance exercise at 8 to 10 weeks after injury. Returning to sports activity must be individualized, depending on the athlete and the sport.

REFERENCES

1. Adams FL: *The genuine work of Hippocrates,* vols 1 and 2, New York, 1986, William Wood.
2. Allman FL Jr: Fractures and ligamentous injuries of the clavicle and its articulation, *J Bone Joint Surg* 9A:774, 1967.
3. Bailey RW: A dynamic repair for complete acromioclavicular joint dislocation, *J Bone Joint Surg* 47A:858, 1985.
4. Bergfeld JA et al: Evaluation of the acromioclavicular joint following first and second degree sprains, *Am J Sports Med* 6:153, 1978.
5. Bjerneld H et al: Acromioclavicular separations treated conservatively, *Acta Orthop Scand* 54:743, 1983.
6. Bloom FA: Wire fixation in acromioclavicular dislocation, *J Bone Joint Surg* 27:273, 1945.
7. Bosworth BM: Acromioclavicular separation—a new method of repair, *Surg Gynecol Obstet* 73:866, 1941.
8. Browne J et al: Acromioclavicular joint dislocations—comparative results following operative treatment with and without primary distal clavisectomy, *Am J Sports Med* 5:258, 1977.
9. Cahill BR: Osteolysis of the distal part of the clavicle in male athletes, *J Bone Joint Surg* 64A:1053, 1982.
10. Cook FF et al: The Mumford procedure in athletes: an objective analysis of function, *Am J Sports Med* 16(2):97, 1988.
11. Cox JS: The fate of the acromioclavicular joint in athletic injuries, *Am J Sports Med* 5:258, 1977.
12. Gartsman GM et al: Arthroscopic acromioclavicular joint resection: an anatomical study, *Am J Sports Med* 19(1):2, 1991.
13. Gartsman GM: Extra-articular uses of the arthroscope—acromioclavicular arthroplasty, *Clin Sports Med* 12(1):111, 1993.
14. Glick JM et al: Dislocated acromioclavicular joint follow-up study of 35 unreduced acromioclavicular dislocations, *Am J Sports Med* 5:264, 1977.
15. Imatani RJ et al: Acute complete acromioclavicular separations, *J Bone Joint Surg* 57A:328, 1975.
16. Jacobs P: Post-traumatic osteolysis of the outer end of the clavicle, *J Bone Joint Surg* 46B:705, 1964.
17. McDonald PB et al: Comprehensive functional analysis of shoulders following complete acromioclavicular separation, *Am J Sports Med* 16(5):475, 1988.
18. Monem MS, Balduini FC: Coracoid fractures as a complication of surgical treatment by coracoclavicular tap fixation, *Clin Orthop* 168:133, 1982.
19. Mumford EB: Acromioclavicular dislocation, *J Bone Joint Surg* 23:799, 1941.
20. Myers JF: Arthroscopic debridement of the acromioclavicular joint and distal clavicle resection. In McGinty JB et al (eds): *Operative arthroscopy,* New York, 1991, Raven Press.
21. Neer CS, Rockwood CA: Fractures and dislocations of the shoulder. In Rockwood CA, Green DP (eds): *Fractures in adults,* ed 3, vol 1, Philadelphia, 1991, JB Lippincott.
22. Nelson CL: Repair of acromioclavicular separations with knitted dacron graft, *Clin Orthop* 143:289, 1979.
23. Park JP et al: Treatment of acromioclavicular separation, *Am J Sports Med* 7:65, 1979.
24. Powers JA, Bach PJ: Acromioclavicular separation—closed or open treatment, *Clin Orthop* 104:213, 1974.
25. Smith MJ, Stewart MJ: Acute acromioclavicular separation, *Am J Sports Med* 7:65, 1979.
26. Stewart MJ: The acromioclavicular joint in the throwing arm. In Zarins B et al (eds): *Injuries to the throwing arm.* Philadelphia, 1985, WB Saunders.
27. Walsh WM et al: Shoulder strength following acromioclavicular injury, *Am J Sports Med* 13:153, 1985.
28. Weaver JK, Dunn HK: Treatment of acromioclavicular injuries, especially complete acromioclavicular separation, *J Bone Joint Surg* 54A:1187, 1972.

CHAPTER 7 Instability of the Shoulder

Michael J. Pagnani
Russell F. Warren

Shoulder instability is common in the athletic population. The large forces directed on the shoulder in contact sports are a frequent cause of injury, and the repetitive loads generated at the glenohumeral joint in throwing, swimming, and racquet sports often lead to pathologic changes in the athletes who perform these activities.

No single essential lesion is responsible for all cases of glenohumeral instability. Injury varies with the degree and type of instability, and different anatomic structures play stabilizing roles as the position of the shoulder changes. Attempts at treatment should specifically address the pathologic condition encountered in a particu-

lar case, and stability should not be obtained at the expense of function.

STABILIZERS OF THE SHOULDER

Instability of the shoulder may be defined as a clinical situation in which there is excessive translation of the humeral head on the glenoid fossa. Because there is variation in the amount of normal glenohumeral translation for a given individual, relative laxity of the shoulder may exist without the accompanying symptoms of instability. Indeed, Harryman et al,[38] in an in vivo assessment of glenohumeral translation in normal subjects, noted wide variations in anterior, posterior, and inferior translations among individuals. Although laxity is not synonymous with instability, an abnormal increase in translation that results in the development of symptoms is the hallmark of shoulder instability.

To permit freedom of movement, the shoulder has evolved with minimal bony constraint. As a result, the surrounding soft-tissue envelope is the primary contributor to the stability of the normal glenohumeral joint (Fig. 7-1). Generally, this stability is attributed to both the static effect of ligaments and tendons and to dynamic mechanisms associated with muscular contraction.

The shoulder capsule is large, loose, and redundant to allow for the large range of shoulder motion. The capsule contains discrete thickenings or capsular ligaments that are important in understanding the pathomechanics of shoulder instability. Three anterior glenohumeral ligaments have been described: the **superior glenohumeral ligament (SGHL)**, the **middle glenohumeral ligament (MGHL)**, and the **inferior glenohumeral ligament complex (IGHLC)** (Fig. 7-2).[27,89] The role of the shoulder capsule and the anterior glenohumeral ligaments in preventing instability is complex and varies with shoulder position and with the direction of the translating force. Discrete anatomic deficiencies in these capsular structures appear to be responsible for the vast majority of unstable shoulders.

Selective cutting studies of the capsule have helped define the relative importance of static restraints in various shoulder positions.[14,88,121,127,129] The inferior capsular structures are preeminent in stabilizing the shoulder near full elevation, and the superior capsular structures gain in importance as the arm is adducted. The IGHLC

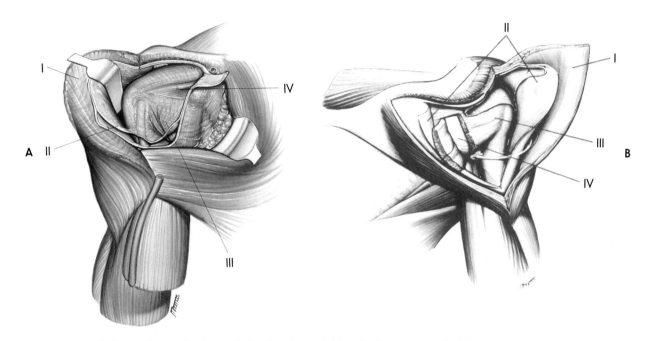

FIG. 7-1. Supporting layers of the glenohumeral joint. **A,** Anterior view: *I,* deltopectoral musculature; *II,* clavipectoral fascia; *III,* rotator cuff muscles and tendons; *IV,* shoulder capsule; **B,** Posterior view: *I,* deltopectoral musculature; *II,* posterior scapular fascia; *III,* rotator cuff muscles and tendons; *IV,* shoulder capsule. (From Cooper DE et al: *Clin Orthop* 289:144, 1993.)

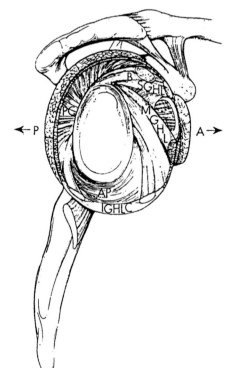

FIG. 7-2. Section of the glenohumeral articulation through the plane of the joint demonstrating the capsular ligaments. *B,* Biceps tendon; *SGHL,* superior glenohumeral ligament; *MGHL,* middle glenohumeral ligament; *AB,* anterior band of inferior glenohumeral ligament complex; *AP,* axillary pouch of inferior glenohumeral ligament complex; *PB,* posterior band of inferior glenohumeral ligament complex; *IGHLC,* inferior glenohumeral ligament complex; *PC,* posterior capsule; *A,* anterior; *P,* posterior. (From O'Brien SJ et al: *Am J Sports Med* 18:449, 1990.)

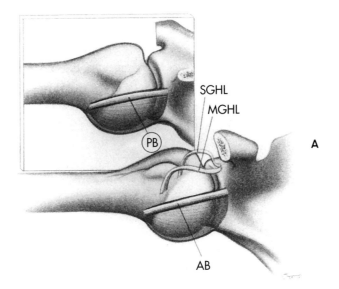

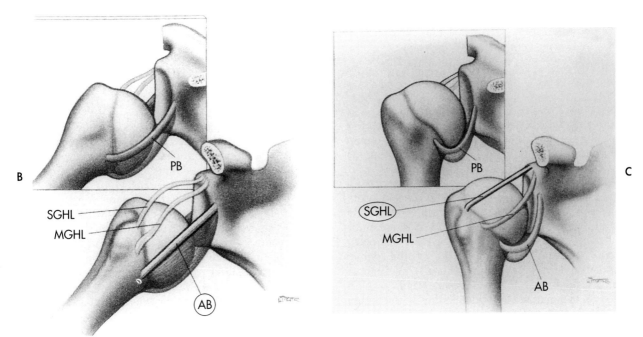

FIG. 7-3. Roles of the capsular ligaments in varying arm positions. **A,** Capsular ligaments with the humerus in 90 degrees of abduction and neutral rotation. *Bottom,* Glenohumeral joint from the anterior aspect. *Top,* Mirror view showing the posterior aspect of the joint. In this position the inferior glenohumeral ligament complex is the primary static restraint against anterior, posterior, and inferior translation. Note that the anterior and posterior bands are taut in this position. *PB,* Posterior band of inferior glenohumeral ligament complex; *AB,* anterior band of glenohumeral ligament complex; *SGHL,* superior glenohumeral ligament; *MGHL,* middle glenohumeral ligament. **B,** Capsular ligaments with the humerus in 45 degrees of abduction and neutral rotation. *Bottom,* Glenohumeral joint from the anterior aspect. *Top,* Mirror view showing the posterior aspect of the joint. In this position the inferior glenohumeral ligament complex remains the primary static restraint against inferior translation. The superior and middle glenohumeral ligaments appear to act as secondary restraints if the inferior glenohumeral ligament complex is disrupted. **C,** Capsular ligaments with the humerus in zero degrees of abduction and neutral rotation. *Bottom,* Glenohumeral joint from the anterior aspect. *Top,* Mirror view showing the posterior aspect of the joint. In this position the superior glenohumeral ligament is the primary static restraint against inferior translation. The middle glenohumeral ligament and the inferior glenohumeral ligament complex appear to act as secondary restraints if the superior glenohumeral ligament is disrupted. (From Warner JJP et al: *Am J Sports Med* 20:675, 1992.)

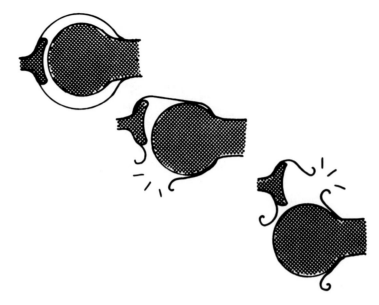

FIG. 7-4. Circle concept of the capsular contribution to shoulder stability. Complete dislocation requires capsular deformation on both the same side and on the opposite side of the joint.

is the primary static restraint against anterior, posterior, and inferior translation between 45 and 90 degrees of glenohumeral elevation (Fig. 7-3, *A*). In the midrange of elevation the MGHL and subscapularis appear to assist the IGHLC in resisting anterior translation, whereas the teres minor and infraspinatus may help prevent posterior translation (Fig. 7-3, *B*). With the arm adducted, the SGHL and the MGHL stabilize against anterior movement, the posterior capsule and the SGHL resist posterior motion, and the SGHL and IGHLC are the primary restraints against inferior translation (Fig. 7-3, *C*).

Rupture or deformation of the capsule would result in specific translational increases, depending on the portion of the capsule involved.

The classic Bankart lesion (capsular-periosteal separation at the anteroinferior glenoid neck) causes dysfunction of the important IGHLC.[77] However, it appears that capsular stripping must be accompanied by plastic deformation of the capsule to allow complete dislocation.[115] This deformation may involve both sides of the capsule.

The circle concept of shoulder instability has been formulated to describe this phenomenon.[129] In essense this concept states that abnormal glenohumeral translation in one direction requires capsular damage on both the same side and on the opposite side of the joint (Fig. 7-4). Recent data suggest a role for the circle concept in the pathomechanics of anterior instability as well as posterior instability. Blaiser, Guldberg, and Rothman[13] and Terry et al[117] have supported the circle concept in that both the anterior and the posterior capsule were noted to be important in controlling anterior translation of the humeral head on the glenoid.

Insufficiency of the capsule may also result from abnormal laxity without capsular detachment or periosteal

stripping. This laxity may occur on a genetic basis or may be caused by plastic deformation from extrinsic forces.

The space between the superior border of the subscapularis and the anterior margin of the supraspinatus has been termed the *rotator interval* (Fig. 7-5).[81] The SGHL is located in this region of the capsule. A relatively large interval has been associated clinically with inferior instability[86] as well as anterior instability.[103,105] Harryman et al[39] recently found that this portion of the capsule plays a significant role in preventing inferior subluxation of the adducted shoulder and acts as a secondary restraint against posterior translation. Enlargement of the rotator interval appears to result in abnormal inferior translation and may also be related to increases in anteroposterior (AP) motion.

The glenoid labrum is a fibrous structure that is intimately attached to the circumference of the glenoid rim.[24,79] Mobility of the labrum above the transverse equator of the glenoid is normal and not necessarily pathologic; in contrast, inferior mobility is abnormal (Fig. 7-6). The tendon of the long head of the biceps, the SGHL, and the MGHL insert in association with the superior labrum; the IGHLC blends into the inferior labrum. Labral detachment may reduce the restraining effect of these capsular structures. The labrum deepens the glenoid socket and may predispose to instability when it is damaged or inherently small.[49,113,116]

The rotator cuff, biceps, and scapular rotator muscles also play an important role in the stability of the glenohumeral joint. Contraction of the cuff and biceps is believed to compress the humeral head into the glenoid fossa, increasing the load needed to translate the humeral head.[64,69,70] Selective contraction of the individual muscles may adjust tension within the capsuloligamen-

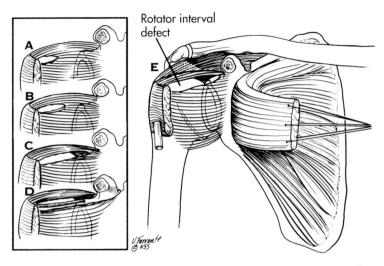

FIG. 7-5. Rotator interval. The interval may be variable in size (**A** to **D**). In some cases the superior genohumeral ligament will be seen crossing through the defect (**D**).

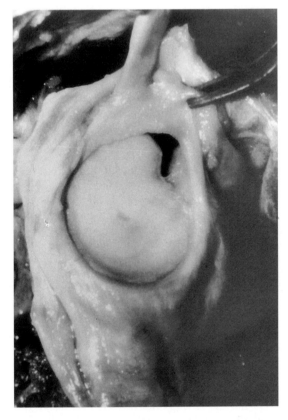

FIG. 7-6. Glenoid labrum of a right shoulder. Note that the superior portion of the labrum is loose while the inferior portion is relatively immobile. The opening at the anterosuperior portion of the glenoid is a normal variant, which should not be confused with a pathologic lesion. (From Cooper DE et al: *J Bone Joint Surg* 74A:46, 1992.)

tous structures.[117] Muscular forces may be particularly important in the midrange of glenohumeral motion, where the capsular system is relatively lax.[64]

The stabilizing effect of the glenohumeral musculature may involve more than simple joint compressive forces. The effects of these periarticular muscles appear to depend on joint position.[73,74,91] A change in position alters the line of action of a particular muscle and, as a result, alters its ability to stabilize against a given translation. For instance, in lower ranges of elevation the subscapularis tendon lies anterior to the joint where its contraction appears to be effective in limiting anterior translation. When the shoulder is fully elevated, the line of action of the subscapularis moves superior to the joint. In this position it seems unlikely that the subscapularis would be an effective restraint against anterior translation. This theory could explain why muscular forces are insufficient to control translation in the face of extensive capsular injury.[22]

Another group of muscles affects glenohumeral stability. The scapular rotators (trapezius, rhomboids, latissimus dorsi, serratus anterior, and levator scapulae) position the scapula to provide a stable platform beneath the humeral head. This allows the glenoid to adjust to changes in arm position. Itoi et al[53] found that the scapular inclination angle had a significant effect in preventing inferior translation of the adducted shoulder. Dysfunction of the scapular rotators may contribute to or result from instability. We have observed that winging of the scapula is associated with both anterior and posterior instability.

Warner et al[126] found that axioscapular muscle dysfunction is common in patients with anteroinferior instability. It remains to be determined whether this represents a primary or secondary phenomenon. These authors believed that periscapular dysfunction could prevent the coracoacromial arch from avoiding the advancing greater tuberosity during forward flexion.

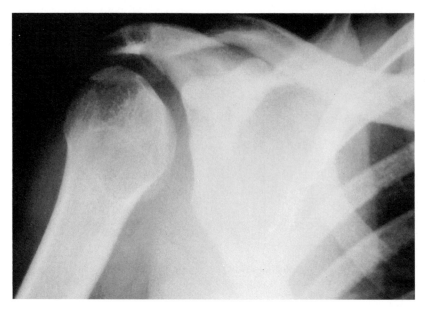

FIG. 7-7. Bony dysplasia of the humeral neck and glenoid in a patient with Erb's palsy.

This could help explain concomitant impingement in patients with instability.

The scapula must rotate upward (horizontally protract) in synchrony with arm elevation. Dysfunction of the serratus anterior, which is primarily responsible for this motion, may predispose to increased stress and subsequent injury.

The complex function of the shoulder in athletic activities requires a coordinated, synchronous interaction of all of these muscles. Muscular dysfunction may predispose to instability, and, conversely, instability may result in a musculotendinous pathologic condition as secondary mechanisms of restraint become overwhelmed.

Abnormalities in bony anatomy may be related to some cases of instability. The articular portion of the glenoid has a small surface area that is incapable of covering the larger humeral head. The surface area of the humeral head is two to four times that of the glenoid,[113] and the diameter of the head is nearly twice that of the glenoid when measured in the transverse plane.[14,67,107] This lack of articular contact contributes to the inherent instability of the glenohumeral joint. Instability is not attributable to a lack of congruence between those portions of the articular surfaces that are in contact. The corresponding articular surfaces of the humeral head and glenoid are nearly congruous in the normal situation.[52,114]

Patients with a relatively shallow glenoid fossa or with an abnormal size or tilt may be at increased risk for instability. This situation could be most applicable to cases in which a developmental anomaly (e.g., Erb's palsy) leads to bony dysplasia (Fig. 7-7). Abnormal glenoid version angles have been associated with instability, particularly of the posterior type.[18,50] However, a wide range of version angles have been recorded in both normal controls and in patients with instability.[50] We have found that measurement of glenoid version and humeral tor-

sion using plain radiographs or computed tomography (CT) are often unreliable and inconsistent. In a study using the posterior border of the acromion as the reference axis for glenoid version, Galinat, Howell, and Kraft[31] found no association between version and anterior or posterior instability. Theories that attribute instability to abnormal humeral torsion also remain questionable.[60]

The glenohumeral joint is normally bathed in less than 1 ml of free synovial fluid. This joint fluid aids in holding the articular surfaces together with viscous and intermolecular forces.[70] Additionally, the normal intraarticular pressure is negative, creating a relative vacuum that resists translation.[20,33,62] If these properties are disrupted by venting the capsule with a needle and introducing air or fluid, subluxation tends to occur.[33,62]

Gibb et al[33] found that venting the capsule reduced the force necessary to the translate the humeral head. Habermeyer, Schuller, and Wiedemann[36] noted that traction on the arm caused an increase in negative pressure in normal shoulders but that no increase occurred in unstable shoulders with a Bankart lesion, suggesting that the vacuum effect is somehow lost in the unstable shoulder (Fig. 7-8). These authors compared the glenohumeral joint with a piston (the humeral head) surrounded by a valve. In their view the glenoid labrum acts as a valve block, sealing the joint from atmospheric pressure. In theory, a labral tear eliminates this seal.

CLASSIFICATION OF SHOULDER INSTABILITY

Shoulder instability may be classified on the basis of frequency, acuity, direction, degree, etiology, and volition. The condition may be described as acute, recurrent, or chronic. Instability may occur anteriorly, posteriorly, inferiorly, or it may be multidirectional. The articular surfaces may become completely separated (dislocation), or

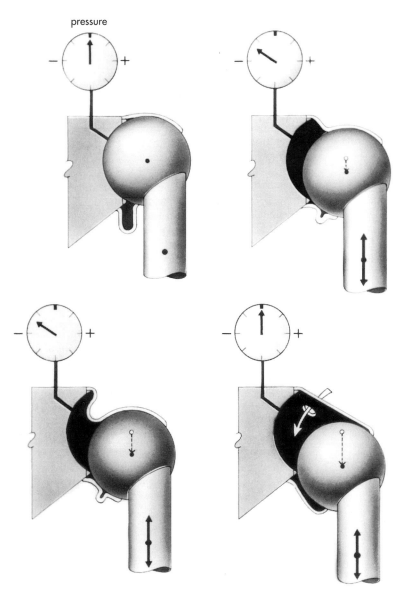

pressure

FIG. 7-8. Effect of negative intraarticular pressure on joint stability. *Left,* In the normal situation, traction on the arm causes an increase in negative intraarticular pressure. *Right,* If the capsule is vented with a needle and air or fluid is introduced into the joint, traction on the arm no longer affects intraarticular pressure.

symptoms may occur from abnormal translation without complete separation (subluxation).

Instability classification factors

- Frequency
- Acuity
- Direction
- Degree
- Etiology
- Volition

A specific traumatic episode is a common inciting event with anterior dislocation but is less common in patients with posterior or multidirectional instability. A mi-

crotraumatic etiology associated with repetitive use is common in anterior subluxation as well as in the posterior and multidirectional groups, especially in throwers and swimmers. Some patients are unable to relate the onset of their symptoms to either trauma or repetitive use; this atraumatic subgroup is more commonly of the multidirectional type.

Some patients are able to voluntarily display instability. A certain number of these patients are psychologically disturbed. Although the traditional approach has been to avoid operation in all patients with voluntary instability,[101] there is recent evidence of a subgroup of patients who can voluntarily demonstrate their instability but who do not have underlying psychiatric disease. Generally, these patients have a positional type of instability in which the head slides posteriorly with flexion, adduction, and internal rotation of the arm.[30]

PHYSICAL EXAMINATION OF THE UNSTABLE SHOULDER

A careful history and a physical examination remain the cornerstone of diagnosis in shoulder instability. Examination of the glenohumeral joint is generally performed in two parts: first with the patient standing, and subsequently with the patient in the supine position.

A **visual inspection** is made for deformity, asymmetry, and atrophy. A routine **neurovascular assessment** should be made. The shoulder region is **palpated** for evidence of local tenderness. Passive and active **arcs of motion** in each shoulder are determined. **Muscular strength,** particularly in abduction and external rotation of the shoulder, is evaluated. Tests that more specifically address the issue of instability are then performed.

Drawer tests are designed to assess translation of the humeral head on the glenoid. The degree of translation is noted in anterior, posterior, and inferior directions. Normally translation is equal anteriorly and posteriorly and is greatest in neutral flexion-extension and neutral rotation. These tests are best performed with the patient in both the supine and the standing positions. The arm is generally examined in 0 and 90 degrees of abduction and in neutral rotation. Other positions of abduction and rotation may also be examined in an attempt to correlate the pathologic condition with the existing basic science data presented earlier. Translation is graded as 1+ if there is increased translation compared with the opposite shoulder but if subluxation or dislocation does not occur. If head subluxation is over the glenoid rim but then spontaneously reduces, translation is graded as 2+. Frank dislocation without spontaneous reduction constitutes 3+ translation.[2] It is essential that the opposite shoulder be tested for comparison.

Grading of the sulcus sign is based on the distance between the inferior margin of the lateral acromion and the humeral head when a downward traction force is applied to the adducted arm (Fig. 7-9, *A*). Less than 1 cm of distance represents a 1+ sulcus, 1 to 2 cm indicates a 2+ sulcus, and more than 2 cm is a 3+.[2] A 3+ sulcus sign reflects laxity of the SGHL and IGHLC and is indicative of inferior instability. It is pathognomonic of multidirectional instability. Assessment of inferior translation with the arm abducted more than 45 degrees more accurately reflects tension on the inferior capsule.[14,127] Helmig et al,[47] in a cadaveric study, noted that maximal inferior humeral migration occurred with the arm in 20 degrees of abduction and neutral rotation. We generally assess inferior stability at 0 and 90 degrees of abduction with the arm in neutral rotation.

Apprehension tests are designed to induce anxiety and protect muscular contraction as the shoulder is brought to a position associated with instability. The anterior apprehension test is performed with the arm abducted and externally rotated. The examiner progressively increases the degree of external rotation and notes the development of patient apprehension. The posterior stress test (Fig. 7-9, *B*) is performed with the arm inter-

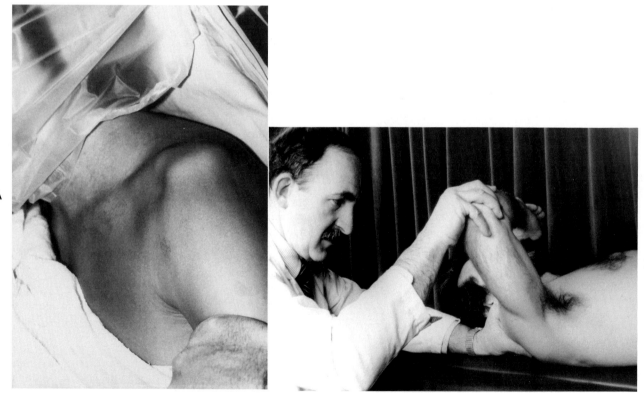

FIG. 7-9. Physical examination for shoulder instability. **A,** Sulcus sign. An extremely large sulcus is indicative of multidirectional instability. **B,** Posterior stress test.

nally rotated and forward flexed to 90 degrees. Apprehension is unusual in this position, but pain or a palpable jump may be noted as the humerus is loaded in an anteroposterior direction and progressively adducted across the chest.

The **relocation test** is also helpful in evaluating anterior instability.[54] The examiner's hand is placed over the anterior shoulder of the supine patient. A posteriorly directed force is applied with the hand to prevent anterior translation of the head. The shoulder is then abducted and externally rotated in a manner similar to the anterior apprehension test. A positive relocation test is obtained when this anterior pressure allows increased external rotation and diminishes associated pain and apprehension. The relocation test appears to be sensitive in the detection of anterior instability, but the test may lack specificity.[115]

Ligamentous laxity is commonly associated with shoulder instability and can be measured objectively on physical examination. The degree of thumb hyperabduction with the wrist volar flexed can be noted by the distance between the thumb and volar forearm. If the thumb reaches the forearm, the test is considered positive. An assessment is also made for index metacarpophalangeal hyperextension in excess of 90 degrees, elbow hyperextension, and knee hyperextension (Fig. 7-10).

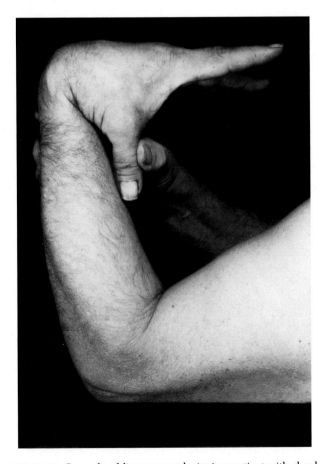

FIG. 7-10. Generalized ligamentous laxity in a patient with shoulder instability.

Assessment of ligamentous laxity
■ Thumb hyperabduction with wrist palmar flexion
■ Index metacarpophalangeal hyperextension
■ Elbow hyperextension
■ Knee recurvatum

Examination under anesthesia is a valuable tool because the awake patient often guards against vigorous attempts to evaluate translation. With the patient under anesthesia the shoulder is stressed inferiorly at 0 and 90 degrees of elevation with the arm in neutral rotation. To assess AP laxity at 90 degrees of elevation, one of the examiner's hands is used to deliver a translational load to the humerus. The opposite hand is used to sense the degree of translation and the presence of crepitation. By placing the arm in neutral rotation, translation is maximized. The examiner must be careful in interpreting translation in the anesthetized patient: normal posterior translation may be as much as 50% of the glenoid diameter.[43] During the examination the head may displace to the posterior edge of the glenoid, and a jump may be noted. Although a similar degree of *anterior* translation is normally present,[88] the examiner usually perceives anterior translation to be less than posterior translation. The reason for this perception is unclear.

RADIOGRAPHY

Routine radiographic examination of the acutely injured shoulder includes an AP view (deviated 30 to 45 degrees from the sagittal plane of the body to parallel the plane of the glenohumeral joint) and a transscapular (**Y**) lateral. The axillary view is extremely valuable in the assessment of glenoid version, in the demonstration of humeral head impression fractures, and in revealing the position of the humeral head relative to the glenoid. These three views constitute the *trauma series*.

In the assessment of recurrent shoulder instability, additional views are helpful in the determination of bony anatomy and pathology. The West Point view[98] often reveals the presence of a fracture or ectopic bone production at the anterior glenoid rim, which may not be visualized in other projections. This projection is obtained by placing the patient prone with the arm in 90 degrees of abduction and neutral rotation. The cassette is placed at the superior aspect of the shoulder. The radiographic beam is projected cephalad at an angle of 25 degrees from the horizontal and medially at an angle of 25 degrees. The beam is centered inferomedially to the acromioclavicular joint. The Stryker notch view[37] is especially helpful in demonstrating the Hill-Sachs lesion (the notch in the posterolateral humeral head) (Fig. 7-11). In this radiographic technique the patient lies supine with the palm of the hand placed on top of the head. The cassette is placed posterior to the shoulder. The arm is aligned in slightly more than 90 degrees of forward flexion, slight internal rotation, and neutral abduction. The

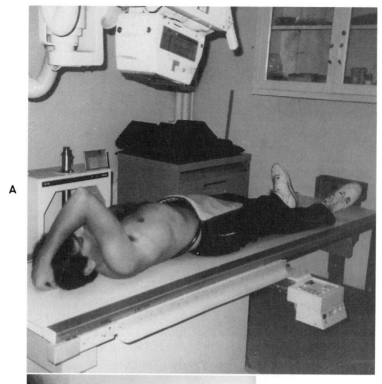

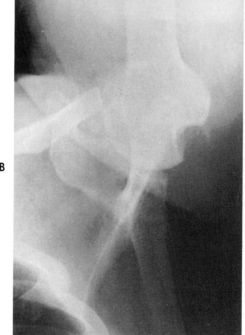

FIG. 7-11. Stryker notch view. **A,** Patient positioning for the Stryker notch view. **B,** Stryker notch view demonstrating a Hills-Sachs lesion in a patient with anterior instability.

beam is then centered on the coracoid and is tilted 10 degrees from the vertical.

The apical oblique projection described by Garth, Slappey, and Ochs[32] may be helpful in detecting Hill-Sachs and glenoid fractures, especially if the shoulder is acutely injured, because positioning for the West Point or Stryker notch views may be painful in these patients. This is essentially a true AP view (in the plane of the joint) modified by aiming the beam from above downward.

An arthrogram may be considered after dislocation in patients older than 45 years of age, especially if the patient seems to be slow to recover after dislocation. Magnetic resonance imaging (MRI) and computed arthrotomography have been reported to be sensitive in the detection of labral abnormalities.[35,51,83] MRI may be par-

ticularly helpful when performed shortly after a dislocation when the attendant joint effusion permits better visualization of these structures.[123] In the absence of an effusion, intraarticular injection of gadolinium may improve the resolution of these tissues. MRI is also a valuable aid when significant cuff injury is associated with instability.

ANTERIOR INSTABILITY
Acute Anterior Dislocation

Anterior instability of the glenohumeral joint is the most common type of shoulder instability. In Rowe's series of 500 shoulder dislocations,[99] 98% occurred in the anterior direction. Indirect forces that are applied to the upper extremity are the most common cause of anterior dislocation. These forces generally place the shoulder in a position of extreme external rotation, which is combined with abduction or hyperextension.[65] In shoulders of patients with inherent soft-tissue laxity, dislocation can occur with little or no injury. In Rowe's series,[99] 4.4% of the dislocations were of this atraumatic subtype.

Forces associated with anterior dislocation

- Abduction
- External rotation
- Extension

The diagnosis of an anterior dislocation is usually readily apparent on physical examination. The arm is held in a slightly abducted and externally rotated position. Internal rotation and full abduction are not possible. The humeral head may be palpable anteriorly, and the distal acromion may be more prominent than usual. The posterior aspect of the joint appears hollow.

The first step in management is to obtain a brief history to determine the mechanism of injury and the direction of dislocation as well as any previous evidence of instability. Although an anterior dislocation is by far the most common type, the caretaker should beware of the possibility of a posterior dislocation. A careful evaluation of the neurovascular status of the involved extremity is important before any attempt at reduction is made. After the diagnosis has been made, the shoulder should be reduced as quickly and as gently as possible. In older or debilitated patients radiographs should be obtained before attempts at relocation are made to rule out concomitant fracture. However, if an anterior dislocation is encountered in a healthy, young athlete by a knowledgeable individual who is skilled in methods of reduction, an immediate reduction maneuver may be performed on the playing field before the onset of muscular spasm. We generally prefer manipulation in forward flexion and gentle internal rotation in reducing an anterior dislocation.

If this maneuver is unsuccessful, the patient should be taken to the locker room where radiographs should be taken if the facilities are available. If no x-ray facili-

ties are present, it is prudent to transfer the patient to an emergency room for these studies. The standard trauma series consists of AP, transscapular (Y) lateral, and axillary views of the shoulder.

As the radiographs are being obtained, pain relief should be provided. If narcotics or benzodiazepines are to be administered, an intravenous line should be placed. An alternative method of reduction may be attempted at this point.[4] The patient is placed prone with the arm hanging free, and weight is attached to the upper extremity. The scapula is then manipulated by lifting its vertebral border to unlock the anterior aspect of the joint so that the glenoid in placed beneath the dislocated humeral head.

If the shoulder remains unreduced after an attempt at scapular rotation, alternative methods of analgesia such as the injection of local anesthetic into the joint or an interscalene nerve block can facilitate reduction. Adequate muscular relaxation is extremely important in these difficult cases. The final reduction maneuver is modified from that described by Kocher.[59] The patient is positioned supine, and one sheet is tied around the patient's chest and axilla. This sheet is then tied to the table or held by an assistant to provide countertraction. A second sheet is then wrapped around the physician's waist as he or she stands in the axillary region. The patient's elbow is flexed to 90 degrees, and the sheet is applied to the forearm just distal to the antecubital fossa. Traction is then applied to the upper extremity by the backward lean of the physician with the arm held in slight abduction. The arm is then gently moved in external and internal rotation until the shoulder reduces. The modified Kocher maneuver carries a risk of iatrogenic damage to bony and neurovascular structures.

Radiographs of the injured shoulder should always be obtained after reduction. Evidence of bony damage to the humeral head or glenoid should be noted. Hovelius et al[48] noted Hill-Sachs lesions in 55% of primary dislocators, whereas Rowe[99] found this defect in 38%. Greater tuberosity fractures occur in approximately 15% of anterior shoulder dislocations.[99]

A neurovascular examination should be performed before and after reduction. The axillary nerve is the most frequently damaged neurologic structure after an anterior dislocation. Sensory testing of the lateral shoulder may be unreliable in the assessment of axillary nerve function, since the motor component of the nerve appears to be more vulnerable to traction injury.

Several factors may influence the rate of recurrence after an anterior dislocation. In patients whose injuries recur, the majority sustain an additional dislocation within the first 2 years after the primary event. The age of the patient at the time of initial dislocation has been shown to have a major effect on the incidence of recurrence. Rowe and Sakellarides[102] noted a 94% recurrence rate in those patients under 20 years of age at primary dislocation but found that only 14% of those patients over 40 years of age had a recurrence. In addition, Rowe[99] noted increased recurrence in those patients who sustained an atraumatic dislocation when compared to traumatic dislocators. Simonet and Cofield[111] noted that ath-

letes tended to have injuries recur more commonly than did nonathletes. Concomitant greater tuberosity fractures greatly reduce the risk of recurrence.[48,99] The effect of a Hill-Sachs lesion on recurrence rates is controversial. Rowe[99] found that the presence of a Hill-Sachs lesion was related to higher recurrence rate. In contrast, Hovelius et al[48] did not find that the risk of recurrence was increased in the presence of a head defect.

The effect of immobilization and rehabilitation on recurrence rates is also somewhat controversial. Yoneda, Welsh, and MacIntosh[135] reported that only 17% of young males developed recurrent instability after a 5-week period of sling and swathe immobilization. Aronen and Regan[8] reported that a supervised rehabilitation program reduced the incidence of recurrence in U.S. Naval Academy midshipmen. In contrast, Simonet and Cofield[111] reported that immobilization had no effect on recurrence, and Wheeler et al[131] believed that rehabilitation did not reduce recurrence in U.S. Military Academy cadets after a primary dislocation.

We generally immobilize young patients who suffer a traumatic anterior dislocation for 4 to 6 weeks. The available basic science data suggest that, for optimal capsular healing to occur, immobilization of this duration is required. This period is followed by a rehabilitative regimen that employs rotator cuff and scapular rotator strengthening. External rotator strengthening receives particular emphasis. Positions of extreme abduction and external rotation are avoided for 3 months after removal of the sling. A full range of motion, complete return of strength, and the absence of pain are prerequisites to the return to sports and overhead activities. When the patient returns to athletic activities, a harness that limits abduction may provide additional security against recurrent damage.

In older patients, especially those over 40 years of age, immobilization is continued only until pain subsides; 7 to 10 days in a sling are usually required. Because of the diminished risk of recurrence and the difficulty in regaining motion in this age group, the rehabilitation program is started earlier.

If progress with therapy seems slow, an arthrogram or MRI should be obtained to rule out a rotator cuff injury, particularly in the older age group. The posterior mechanism of dislocation with an associated cuff tear is common in this population.[84] Evidence of deltoid weakness suggests the need for electromyographic studies to evaluate the axillary nerve.

Open reduction of acute anterior shoulder dislocations is necessary in those rare cases which are irreducible by closed methods and in dislocations which are more than 6 weeks old at the time of presentation. Displaced fractures of the greater tuberosity and large fractures of the glenoid rim may also require surgical treatment in the acute setting.

The role of operative **stabilization of acute dislocations** in young, scholastic athletes is controversial. These patients appear to be at extremely high risk for recurrence. The acute dislocation often curtails sports activity for the current year, and the development of recurrent instability results in an extended period away

from athletics and other activities. This may be particularly problematic in throwing and overhead athletes. For some patients this long absence from their sport may be extremely undesirable.

Arciero et al[7] reported a dramatic decrease in the recurrence rate in army cadets after arthroscopic Bankart repairs for initial anterior dislocations. About 80% of cadets treated with 4 weeks of immobilization followed by 4 months of rehabilitation developed recurrent instability. In contrast, only 14% of the operatively treated patients suffered recurrence.

The treatment of these patients should be individualized on a case-by-case basis. The risk of recurrence should be explained as well as the potential risks of a surgical procedure. In some young athletes engaged in throwing sports, early restoration of the disrupted anatomy appears to provide the best opportunity to continue in their sport without losing a significant period of the following season. In contact sports, operative stabilization can be performed at the end of the season.

In summary, the management of an initial dislocation depends on the age, activity, and goals of the patient. Those dislocations encountered at an athletic event in the presence of an experienced physician may be reduced promptly. If any difficulty is encountered in achieving reduction, radiographs are obtained. If the patient is first seen in an emergency room, a radiographic trauma series is routinely obtained both before and after reduction. The period of postinjury protection varies with age and goals. Early surgery, either following the acute event or at the end of the season, may be considered in selected patients with a high probability of recurrence or when recurrence could compromise the ability to compete in athletics.

Recurrent Anterior Dislocation

The diagnosis of recurrent anterior dislocation is usually made without difficulty. The patient typically gives a history of a specific initial injury in which the shoulder "popped out" followed by multiple similar episodes that tended to occur with a lesser amount of trauma and were more easily reduced. In some patients recurrent dislocation occurs without a history of significant trauma.

Recurrent anterior instability classification

- Traumatic vs. atraumatic
- Voluntary vs. involuntary
- Subluxation vs. dislocation

Upon physical examination, patients with recurrent anterior dislocation demonstrate increased anterior translation of the humeral head on the glenoid. The apprehension and relocation tests are positive.

Patients who develop recurrence should have a complete radiographic evaluation for evidence of bony injury. Both Pavlov et al[94] and Rowe et al[99] noted Hill-Sachs lesions in 77% of recurrent anterior dislocators. Pavlov and

associates[94] also noted ectopic bone production or fracture of the anterior glenoid in 15% of these patients.

Rowe, Patel, and Southmayd[100] noted the Bankart lesion in 85% of the cases that came to operation. Those patients who did not demonstrate a Bankart lesion frequently had an atraumatic etiology. In Rowe's experience the great majority of dislocations were intracapsular, with only 6% demonstrating perforation of the capsule by the humeral head. Reeves[96] thought that capsular-periosteal disruption was common in younger patients but that capsular rupture was the primary mode of failure in the older age group. On occasion lateral capsular disruption from the humeral neck may occur.[9,85] This detachment is usually secondary to trauma and should be searched for in traumatic dislocators in whom no Bankart lesion is found.

Recurrent Anterior Subluxation

The signs and symptoms of recurrent anterior subluxation are often more subtle. The patient with recurrent subluxation is usually unaware that the shoulder has popped out. The chief complaint may be vague, such as a sense of movement, pain, or clicking with certain activities. The pain is often localized posteriorly because of strain on the posterior capsule and tendons in resisting anterior translation. Rowe and Zarins[103] have described the dead arm syndrome in patients with anterior subluxation. In this situation the patient experiences sharp pain when the arm is placed in extreme external rotation. The patient loses control of the extremity and drops any object that is held in the hand. After the acute episode the severe pain usually subsides quickly, but the shoulder may remain sore and weak.

In throwers, pain is often associated with the cocking or acceleration phases, but it may occasionally occur during follow-through. Swimmers commonly experience pain with the backstroke or during turns. Racquet sports, volleyball, and water polo are also commonly associated with recurrent anterior subluxation.

A traumatic event may be related to the onset of symptoms. Often the inciting episode involves extreme external rotation of the arm combined with either abduction or hyperextension. Tackling in football and diving back to a base in baseball may result in this positioning. Anterior dislocations can lead to recurrent anterior subluxation.

In other patients there is no history of macrotrauma. Instead, repetitive low loading appears to result in microtraumatic changes associated with overuse.

The findings on physical examination are also often subtle. Tenderness may be noted over the posterior shoulder. In throwers a 10- to 15-degree loss of internal rotation and a similar gain in external rotation may represent normal physiologic changes and are not necessarily pathologic. The anterior apprehension test usually causes pain to a greater degree than it causes apprehension. This pain is relieved upon performance of the relocation test.

In addition to the physical findings mentioned above, examination may reveal the presence of impingement and rotator cuff signs. Jobe and Kvitne[55] have identified two groups of throwing or overhead athletes with concomitant impingement and instability, based on clinical and operative findings. In one group instability was thought to occur because of chronic labral microtrauma with impingement occurring secondarily. These patients were noted to have damage to the labrum and attenuation of the IGHLC. In the second group instability was thought to occur as a result of hyperlaxity. These patients had an intact labrum and demonstrated laxity of the glenohumeral ligaments. The physical findings in the two groups were similar with the exception that the hyperlax patients were noted to have generalized laxity of other joints. In these patients MRI may be helpful in evaluation of the rotator cuff.

Humeral hypertrophy[128] is another normal physiologic response to throwing that may be noted radiographically. Hill-Sachs lesions are seen in 25% of patients with recurrent anterior subluxation. Calcification of the antero-inferior glenoid margin is found in approximately 50%.[87,94]

Nonoperative Treatment of Recurrent Anterior Instability

The treatment of recurrent anterior instability begins with a period of rest. After an acute event an arm sling is worn for a few days for comfort. Nonsteroidal antiinflammatory medication is administered during this time. In those individuals in whom the instability becomes recurrent, the likelihood of soft-tissue healing with subsequent immobilization becomes less likely. Therefore prolonged immobilization after the second dislocation is of no apparent value.

A rehabilitation program that emphasizes rotator cuff and periscapular muscle strengthening is then employed.[125] Early rehabilitation is directed at reduction of pain and restoration of motion. Subsequently, an aggressive strengthening program is instituted. This regimen is generally started at 2 weeks in throwers and overhead athletes. Stretching exercises are incorporated in an attempt to regain full motion. In recurrent posttraumatic anterior instability, losses of external rotation at 0 and 90 degrees of abduction are common. Even if the shoulder is no longer unstable, these individuals often present with pain because of abnormal shoulder mechanics due to the contractures. One goal of rehabilitation should be restoration of a normal range of motion with special attention given to external rotation loss in the functional position of abduction.

Range of motion exercises that are performed in a therapeutic pool may be helpful; the buoyancy of water and the warmer water temperature appear to facilitate motion.

Attention should also be directed at proper conditioning of scapular musculature. There is some evidence to suggest that scapular position is altered in patients with recurrent instability. Again, whether this is a primary or a secondary phenomenon is unknown. The scapular rotators are conditioned by a combination of shoulder shrugs, horizontal adduction exercises, seated rows, pulldowns, chest presses, and serratus anterior presses. Initially, these exercises are performed in an isotonic mode.

Deltoid isometrics for each of the three divisions are also employed. Good deltoid and scapular rotator function should be evident before commencing with rotator cuff strengthening.

Strengthening exercises should include both concentric and eccentric modalities. Isokinetic testing can help identify specific muscular weakness and can provide a baseline for comparison during the rehabilitative process.[55] Selective weakness in a particular muscle suggests the need for strengthening.

Rotator strengthening may be performed with elastic resistance bands, an isotonic machine, or an isokinetic dynamometer. Stabilization of the scapula is facilitated by positioning the patient supine on an exercise bench. Slow angular velocities allow the patient to relax while the shoulder is moved through a range of motion. In the early phase of therapy, especially in patients with concomitant impingement, these activities should be performed with the arm at the side or in the lower ranges of elevation to protect the rotator cuff. Later, these exercises may be performed in higher degrees of elevation as well. Muscular endurance should be emphasized in addition to strengthening.

Recently, Townsend et al[120] have described four specific exercises that, based on electromyographic data, provide specific strengthening to the glenohumeral muscles.

1. Elevation of the arm in the scapular plane with the arm internally rotated and the thumbs down
2. Elevation of the arm in the sagittal plane
3. Horizontal adduction from the prone position with the arm externally rotated
4. The press-up: in a seated position, the hands are placed upon the seat and the body is lifted from the chair by extension of the upper extremities

The first of these four exercises may aggravate rotator cuff symptoms and should be avoided if rotator cuff pathology is present.

The final phase of rehabilitation involves the restoration of functional activity. Proprioceptive neuromuscular facilitation (PNF) patterns are instituted within a specific range of motion using manual resistance, isokinetic machines, or pulley systems. Later, more aggressive measures are implemented for overhead athletes. Plyometrics involve quick movements in which muscles are stretched before a rapid, reflex contraction. Theoretically, prestretch of a muscle increases its potential energy and allows it to generate more force. Thus the goals of plyometric exercise are increases in force and speed through activity-related rehabilitation. A medicine ball two-hand overhead throw is one example of such an activity. A medium weight ball is used initially with both pure overhead and diagonal patterns. Sport-specific drills are introduced as motion and strength return to normal.

Throwing is not allowed until strength and motion are normal. Throwing is slowly progressed in distance, velocity, frequency, and duration. The patient's pitching mechanics should be adjusted to provide efficient energy transfer from the lower extremities and thorax to the shoulder. Specific activities that seemed to incite pain before the institution of therapy are withheld for a longer time.

In sports that do not require overhead activity, an abduction harness may be worn to prevent elevation above 90 degrees. This device is especially useful for selected positions in football (see Fig. 12-6).

A rehabilitative program often succeeds in patients with atraumatic instability. In these patients instability may exist on the basis of inherent soft-tissue laxity about the shoulder. These individuals commonly start to develop symptoms when the joint is stressed in specific positions during sports participation. Traumatic dislocators appear to respond less favorably to a rehabilitative program. Burkhead and Rockwood[22] reported that an exercise program led to a good or excellent result in 80% of shoulders with atraumatic subluxation but in only 16% of shoulders with traumatic subluxation.

Operative Treatment of Recurrent Anterior Instability

The indications for surgical treatment of recurrent anterior shoulder instability are highly subjective and include recurrence, pain, or activity limitation after a thorough trial of nonoperative management. Some surgeons believe that the presence of a Bankart lesion on arthroscopic evaluation is another indication for a stabilization procedure because conservative methods may be likely to fail in the face of this type of pathologic condition. As discussed earlier, the treatment of acute instability in young athletes is controversial.

Patients with voluntary anterior instability are often poor operative candidates and require psychologic testing and a rigorous attempt at rehabilitation.[101]

Patients with concomitant instability and impingement who fail conservative treatment should have surgical intervention to provide stability. Subacromial decompression is not recommended as a primary procedure in these patients. Occasionally, anterior acromioplasty may be required as a secondary part of treatment.[45]

In general, the surgeon should have a clinical sense of the direction and degree of instability from the office evaluation, and this impression should be confirmed by the examination under anesthesia. On occasion the findings may be equivocal, and the arthroscope may add objective data to the evaluation.

Arthroscopy

Although arthroscopy of the shoulder does not usually play a major diagnostic role in evaluation of shoulder instability, it is highly useful in some cases. Throwers with concomitant instability and rotator cuff symptoms are particularly good candidates for arthroscopy. Arthroscopy is also of value in those patients in whom the direction or degree of instability is in doubt. The arthroscopic examination may help in identifying intraarticular injury and in the detailed planning of an open or an arthroscopic stabilization procedure. However, the tendency to overemphasize minor changes that are noted arthroscopically should be avoided.[6] Degenerative lesions of the labrum are common in patients older than 40 years of age.[5,27]

Our basic approach is to perform an arthroscopic examination in all traumatic types of anterior instability,

since the likelihood of capsular-periosteal disruption of the anterior glenoid is high in these patients. In patients with an atraumatic etiology, an open technique is generally used.

Technique. We perform shoulder arthroscopy in the modified beach-chair position.[1] The patient's back is placed at an angle of approximately 75 degrees from the floor, the hips are flexed to 90 degrees, and the knees are set in 30 degrees of flexion. The thorax is rotated slightly toward the nonoperative shoulder to expose the medial border of the scapula on the operative side. The position is fixed by molding a beanbag to the body and then deflating the beanbag to make it firm (Fig. 7-12).

We believe that there are several advantages to the beach-chair position. We perform the vast majority of our shoulder procedures under interscalene block anesthesia. The patients are more comfortable in the semisitting position than in the lateral decubitus position and are able to observe the procedure on the arthroscopic monitor. The beach-chair position allows the surgeon to examine the shoulder in various positions of abduction and rotation because there is no traction on the arm. There is also a lower risk of neurapraxia[58] from traction, and the anterior structures are not placed in a stretched, nonanatomic orientation. The beach-chair position allows easier access to the anterior shoulder during an arthroscopic stabilization. In addition, an arthroscopic procedure can be simply converted to an open procedure without the need for extensive repositioning and redraping. The beanbag is simply deflated, and the head of the operating table is lowered to the appropriate level.

The posterior arthroscopic portal is placed 3 cm inferior and 2 cm medial to the posterolateral corner of the acromion. The anterior portal is situated lateral to the coracoid. Placement of the anterior portal in a position that is medial to the coracoid risks neurovascular injury.[71] The anterior cannula enters the joint in the triangular area bounded by the biceps tendon, the subscapularis tendon, and the anterosuperior glenoid.

Arthroscopic examination of the shoulder should be performed in a standard, systematic fashion in which all significant anatomic structures are viewed in turn. The first step in our routine is to examine the biceps tendon throughout its intraarticular course. The anterior labrum is then probed for evidence of detachment or tearing. The presence of a labral sulcus near the 2 o'clock position is a normal variant and should not be confused with a pathologic change.[24] The presence and qualities of the SGHL, the MGHL, the subscapularis tendon, and the anterior band of the IGHLC are ascertained. Next, the axillary pouch is inspected to assess excess volume and to search for loose bodies. Internal and external rotation of the arm will reveal whether the normal mechanism of reciprocal tightening of the IGHLC components is functional.

The articular surfaces of the glenoid and humeral head are checked for damage. The undersurface of the rotator cuff is evaluated, including its insertion on the greater tuberosity. The presence or absence of a defect in the posterolateral head is noted.

Translational forces may be delivered in both anterior and posterior directions to assess the relationship between the head and the glenoid.

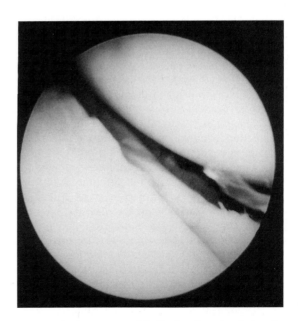
FIG. 7-13. Arthroscopic view of the Bankart lesion with detachment of the anteroinferior labrum and capsule from the glenoid neck.

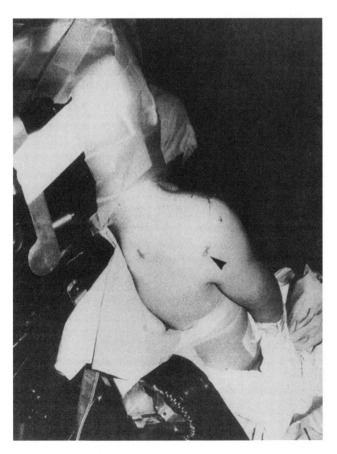
FIG. 7-12. Beach chair position for shoulder arthroscopy.

Pathologic findings. Pathologic findings during the arthroscopic examination include detachment of the anteroinferior capsulolabral structures (Fig. 7-13), stretching of the IGHLC, and fraying or tearing of the anteroinferior labrum. Laxity of the pouch is present when the arthroscope is easily passed into the anteroinferior joint cavity without the normal restraint of the capsular tissues. This phenomenon is referred to as the drive-through sign.

SLAP lesions. Recently Snyder, Karzel, and Del Pizzo[112] have coined the term *SLAP lesion* to describe "an injury to the superior aspect of the labrum which begins posteriorly and extends anteriorly . . . including the 'anchor' of the biceps tendon to the glenoid."

The arthroscopist must be careful not to mistake the normal mobility of the superior portion of the labrum or the labral sulcus for the SLAP lesion.[24] Snyder, Karzel, and Del Pizzo[112] classified the lesion into four types based on arthroscopic findings:

Type I: Fraying of the superior labrum, but firm attachment of the labrum to the glenoid

Type II: Stripping of the superior labrum and biceps tendon off the underlying glenoid, resulting in instability of the labral-biceps anchor

Type III: Bucket-handle tear of the labrum with an intact biceps insertion

Type IV: Bucket-handle tear of the labrum that extends into the biceps tendon

In the Snyder series the SLAP lesion was most commonly caused by a fall onto the outstretched arm with the shoulder in abduction and slight forward flexion. Traction injuries were also associated with this lesion. Andrews, Carson, and McLeod[5] noted that lesions of the superior labrum are frequently found in throwers. Patients in the Snyder series had a high incidence of associated pathology including anterior instability and rotator cuff disease. Increased biceps activity has been noted in throwers with anterior instability and was felt to represent a possible mechanism of secondary restraint in the unstable shoulder.[34] Tension on the tendon of the long head of the biceps as it resists humeral head translation may be related to the pathogenesis of superior labral lesions.[91,92] In our experience these lesions are not usually associated with overt instability, but the affected patient may have a sense of looseness in the shoulder. In a recent biomechanical investigation we noted moderate multidirectional increases in glenohumeral translation after creation of a Type II lesion in a cadaveric model.[92]

Symptoms include pain, which worsened with overhead activity, and a sensation of catching or popping in the shoulder. Andrews, Kupferman, and Dillman[6] described the *clunk test* to aid in the diagnosis of these lesions. With the patient in the supine position, one of the examiner's hands is placed posterior to humeral head and used to apply an anteriorly directed force to the humerus while the opposite hand rests on the humeral condyles and is used to rotate the humerus. A clunk or grind noted with the arm in the full overhead abducted position is suggestive of a labral tear. These subtle clinical findings and changes in the superior labrum on MRI may suggest the diagnosis of a superior labral lesion.

We have had successful results in a series of 21 patients with unstable lesions of the superior labrum who were treated with arthroscopic fixation of the lesion to the superior glenoid. Of these patients, 19 were able to return to their premorbid levels of function. A biodegradable tack was used to fix the labrum in the vast majority of these cases. Debridement of the unstable superior labral lesions has not been highly successful in our experience.[3] Debridement alone may be considered in isolated lesions of the anterosuperior labrum that do not involve the biceps insertion.

Labral flaps. Anteroinferior labral flaps are often associated with instability. Large labral flaps that appear nonfunctional can be debrided, but the surgeon must not destabilize the IGHLC. Altchek et al[3] recently reported that arthroscopic debridement of labral flaps provided temporary pain relief, but symptoms generally recurred upon resumption of normal activities and sports. Patients with evidence of labral detachment and instability did especially poorly. We do not recommend debridement of anteroinferior labral insufficiency as an isolated treatment.

Open Stabilization Procedures

Procedural options. Many operative procedures have been described for the treatment of anterior shoulder instability. The Putti-Platt[90] and Magnuson-Stack[66] procedures stabilize the shoulder by limiting external rotation. Such functional restraint severely limits the patient in an unnecessary manner. The Putti-Platt procedure, in particular, may cause degenerative arthritis when the subscapularis is shortened excessively.[42,108]

Isolated bone block procedures, such as the Bristow, also fail to address anteroinferior capsulolabral insufficiency.[46] The concept of an anterior bony buttress (upon which these procedures are based) may be invalid, particularly in patients with subluxation.[109] Only 16% of throwing athletes were able to return to preinjury level of performance after a modified Bristow procedure.[119] This functional deficit was attributed to weakness with extreme rotation of the arm. When metal hardware is used to fix the bone block, there is a high risk of complications from penetration of the joint or loosening.[138] A revision stabilization procedure is especially difficult after a Bristow procedure because of extensive scarring of the anterior capsule and subscapularis tendon.[136]

Regan et al[97] noted limitation and weakness of external rotation in all patients after Bristow, Magnuson-Stack, and Putti-Platt procedures. Of these three procedures the Putti-Platt affected external rotation to the greatest degree. Surprisingly, external rotation was better in patients who had undergone a Magnuson-Stack than in patients who had been treated with a Bristow. None of these three procedures addresses excess capsular laxity.

The concept of repairing the capsular-periosteal separation at the anterior glenoid neck was first proposed by Perthes[95] and later expounded upon by Bankart.[10,11] This technique attacks the pathologic condition at its most common site and is directed at reconstitution of the primary static stabilizer of the shoulder, the IGHLC. If

abnormal capsular laxity is encountered, the procedure is easily modified to account for this pathologic factor as well. In a long-term review of 50 patients treated by Bankart and his colleagues between 1925 and 1954, recurrence occurred in only two patients.[29] Rowe et al[100] noted a 3.5% recurrence rate in 145 patients after a Bankart procedure. When properly performed, the procedure results in a superior functional outcome compared to the previously discussed operations. In the series of Rowe et al[100] 69% of the patients regained full range of motion. Jobe et al[56] using a modification of Bankart's technique, reported that more than two thirds of elite throwing athletes were able to return to their previous levels of competition for at least 1 year.

Our basic procedure for the open surgical treatment of recurrent anterior glenohumeral instability is a modification of the Bankart procedure. Bone blocks are considered only in those rare cases in which there is a severe deficiency (greater than 40%) of the anterior glenoid and, even then, the bone block is used in conjunction with a repair of the capsulolabral system. Procedures that are designed to limit external rotation are not a part of our armamentarium in the initial surgical treatment of anterior instability.

Operative technique. The patient is positioned supine with the head of the operating table raised 30 degrees and the arm abducted 45 degrees on an armboard. A folded towel is placed between the scapulae to rotate the scapula on the involved side laterally.

The skin incision is started just lateral to the coracoid and extended approximately 6 cm distally along Langer's lines. (In some cases where cosmesis is a special concern, the shoulder can be approached from low in the axilla.[63] The axillary approach requires a considerable subcutaneous dissection and offers a limited view when dealing with capsular laxity.) The deltopectoral interval is identified. The cephalic vein is retracted laterally because there are fewer branches on the medial side. The surgeon must take care not to damage the vein as it crosses the superior aspect of the wound.

After dissection through the deltopectoral interval, the coracoid process and the clavipectoral fascia are identified. The fascia is incised lateral to the muscle belly of the short head of the biceps. To facilitate exposure in some cases a partial, oblique incision is made in the conjoined tendon just distal to the coracoid. Avoid the musculocutaneous nerve, which may enter the tendon as close as 1 cm distal to the coracoid. We do not recommend coracoid osteotomy or complete detachment of the tendon.

The arm is then externally rotated, and the insertion of the subscapularis tendon is revealed. Three small branches of the anterior circumflex vessels (the three sisters) lie near the inferior edge of the tendon and may require ligation. A small transverse incision (3 to 4 mm in length) is made at the inferior border of the tendon at the musculotendinous junction. The anterior capsule is visualized through this incision. A Kelly clamp or a periosteal elevator is then passed from inferomedial to superolateral in the interval between the anterior capsule and the tendon. The medial portion of the tendon is tagged with heavy, nonabsorbable sutures. The tendon is then incised obliquely over this clamp (Fig. 7-14, A). The medial portion of the tendon is dissected from the capsule with a periosteal elevator.

Because the ability to throw commonly diminishes after operative treatment for shoulder instability, Jobe et al[56] have developed an approach in which the subscap-

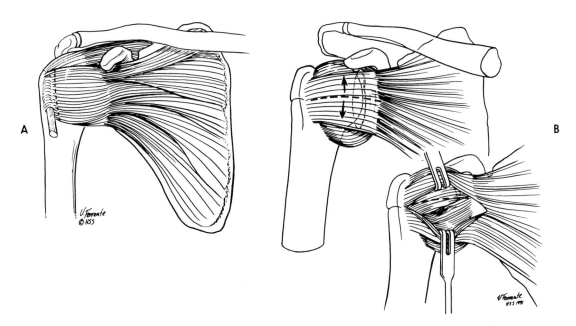

FIG. 7-14. Division of the subscapularis tendon for exposure of the anterior capsule. **A,** Tendon is generally divided medial to its insertion on the lesser tuberosity. **B,** In throwers with mild degrees of instability, exposure of the anterior capsule may be obtained through a longitudinal split in the subscapularis tendon.

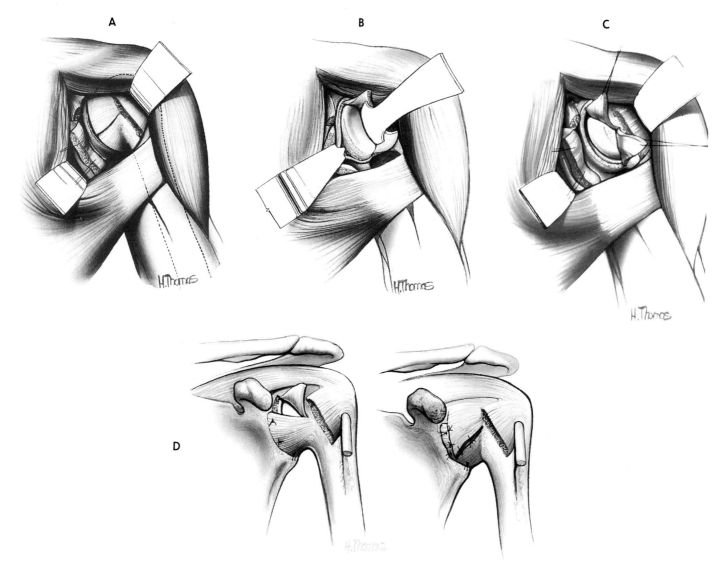

FIG. 7-15. Modified Bankart repair in a patient with a Bankart lesion and mild capsular laxity. **A,** Capsule is incised obliquely to view the joint. **B,** Humeral head retractor is placed, and the presence of a Bankart lesion is noted. **C,** Vertical limb is then created at the glenoid margin. **D,** Inferior limb of the capsular incision is advanced superomedially to eliminate capsular laxity and the Bankart lesion is obliterated. The superior limb is then brought inferomedially to reinforce the repair. The arm is placed in 40 to 50 degrees of abduction and 30 degrees of external rotation during the capsular repair. The sutures are tied, demonstrating the end result of a medial capsular repair.

ularis tendon is split longitudinally rather than divided (Fig. 7-14, *B*). We recommend this method in throwers and overhead athletes with minimal microinstability. A variation of this approach may be used in patients with a greater degree of instability; however, it is difficult to detect and correctly apply tension to an enlarged rotator interval with this method.

The laxity and quality of the capsule are assessed. If trauma played a significant role in the development of instability, a small transverse capsulotomy is performed (Fig. 7-15, *A*), and the joint is explored for evidence of damage to the anteroinferior labrum or to the bony glenoid. The joint is irrigated to remove any loose bodies.

If there is no evidence of capsulolabral separation from the glenoid neck, the shoulder should be reassessed for evidence of multidirectional instability. If there is no abnormal inferior translation in the absence of a Bankart lesion, superior advancement of the capsule may be all that is required.

If there is evidence of capsular-periosteal separation, a vertical capsulotomy is created at the glenoid margin. The capsular separation is extended medially to allow for placement of a retractor along the glenoid neck. A humeral head retractor is then carefully placed within the joint (Fig. 7-15, *B*). The glenoid neck is prepared with an osteotome to provide a bleeding surface of bone. Prep-

aration of the glenoid neck is an important step. Zarins, Rowe, and Stone[137] and Rowe, Zarins, and Ciullo[105] have implicated inadequate attention to this point in the etiology of failed reconstructions.

If the labrum is well attached, the capsule may be sutured to it. If the labrum is detached or attenuated, a dental drill is used to place three or four holes at the edge of the glenoid. The holes are then prepared with an awl, and nonabsorbable sutures are passed through the holes. Recently we have used suture anchors (Acufex Microsurgical Inc., Mansfield, MA) rather than drill holes to place these sutures. If suture anchors are used, they must be placed at the edge of the glenoid and not along its neck. The capsule is then reattached but not overly tightened. The lateral flap is advanced slightly medially and superiorly with the arm in 45 to 60 degrees of external rotation. Each suture is passed through the capsule, and the sutures are tied over the capsule. The labrum may also be reattached to the glenoid if the labrum is not degenerated. The goal is not to reduce external rotation but to obliterate excess capsular volume and to reattach the IGHLC to the glenoid.

If there is evidence of capsular laxity, the T-plasty modification is used to shift the capsule (Fig. 7-15, C, and D). The small transverse capsulotomy is enlarged, and the capsulotomy is converted to a T shape by the addition of a vertical limb. If a Bankart lesion is present in addition to capsular laxity, this vertical limb should be placed medially at the glenoid margin. The axillary nerve is protected when this limb is created. The capsule is then shifted to correct abnormal anterior or inferior laxity. Specifically, the inferior flap can be taken superiorly and medially to eliminate an abnormally large axillary recess. The same sutures may then be passed through the superior flap for reinforcement and additional tensioning. Again, tension on the capsule should be adjusted with the arm in at least 45 degrees of external rotation to prevent overtightening.

If no Bankart lesion is noted in cases with capsular redundancy, the vertical limb of the T-shaped capsulotomy may be placed either medially or laterally. The capsular shift may be technically easier when this limb is placed laterally. An arthroscopic examination before the open procedure may help in the planning of the type of capsulorraphy to be performed.

The presence of an enlarged rotator interval is important to note during the assessment of the capsule. If present, an enlarged interval must be closed to create adequate tension in the capsular system. Closure of the interval may be performed before the creation of a formal capsulotomy, or it may be done after the capsular tissue has been reattached to the glenoid.

After the capsule has been satisfactorily addressed, the subscapularis tendon is reapproximated but not tightened. If the conjoined tendon was partially released, it is repaired. A subcutaneous drain is placed, and the wound is closed.

After an open anterior stabilization, pendulum exercises are instituted after 1 or 2 days. Passive motion using a pulley system for forward flexion may also be instituted. Active range of motion at the wrist and elbow is encouraged. Active rotation, abduction, and flexion of the

shoulder are allowed after 3 weeks with resistance gradually increased in each subsequent week. The anterior capsule is protected during the early phase (first 6 weeks) by limiting external rotation and horizontal abduction.

Weight training is not allowed in the early healing period. At 6 weeks aggressive measures are used to increase range of motion. External rotation must be carefully monitored. The exercises outlined in the section on nonoperative treatment are also applicable to postoperative therapy. Generally, external rotation exercises are performed with the arm at the side for the initial 10 weeks. Later these activities are performed at higher elevation angles. The continuous passive motion (CPM) mode found on active isokinetic systems is a safe and useful means for increasing rotation.

Postoperative rehabilitation is more aggressive in throwers. In this group the goal is to restore full range of motion by 6 weeks postoperatively. Heavy lifting, contact sports, and throwing are avoided for 6 months after operation.

Arthroscopic Stabilization Procedures

Until recently the only available methods of surgical stabilization of the shoulder required an extensive anatomic dissection to address the pathologic process. These open techniques result in a significant amount of perioperative pain and morbidity and require inpatient hospitalization. In addition, overhead athletes and throwers are often unable to return to their premorbid level of function after such a procedure.[100]

Arthroscopic shoulder stabilization procedures were developed in the early 1980s. These arthroscopic techniques can be performed on an outpatient basis and offer the advantage of reduced perioperative pain and morbidity. Because of minimal surgical trauma, there is hope that these techniques will better maintain function in overhead athletes.

Techniques of arthroscopic stabilization are still in their infancy. Several early reports revealed postoperative recurrence rates of 15% to 20%.[40,72,133,134] At present, these procedures should be performed only by experienced arthroscopists in selected patients. A well-performed open stabilization is certainly preferable to a failed arthroscopic procedure.

Arthroscopic techniques allow reattachment of the anterior capsule and labrum in those patients who have a demonstrated Bankart lesion. Patients with capsular laxity, atraumatic dislocations, or enlargement of the rotator interval frequently do not have a Bankart lesion. Arthroscopic stabilization techniques do not appear to be appropriate for these patients at the present time. Multidirectional instability and voluntary instability are absolute contraindications to an arthroscopic stabilization procedure. The finding of a poorly formed IGHLC or the lack of a Bankart lesion on arthroscopic examination is also a contraindication. Some surgeons believe that an arthroscopic method should not be used in the presence of a large Hill-Sachs lesion. Morgan[76] recommended against using an arthroscopic technique in collision athletes.

We have experience with two forms of arthroscopic

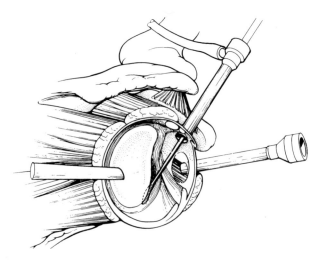

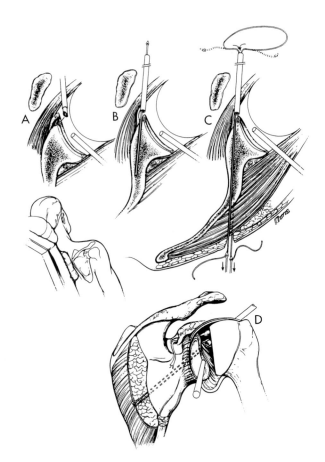

FIG. 7-16. Arthroscopic stabilization using transglenoid suture technique. *A,* Preparation of a bleeding bed on the anterior glenoid neck using a rasp. *B,* Labrum and anteroinferior capsule are repositioned on the glenoid neck. A pin is then drilled from the anterior glenoid neck and through the bony glenoid. *C,* The pin and one end of the sutures are recovered as they exit the skin posteriorly. The anterior halves of the sutures are paired together and tied. *D,* Tension is then placed on the posterior halves of the sutures to pull the capsulolabral structures to the glenoid neck. The posterior halves of the sutures are then tied over a fascial bridge.

stabilization procedures. The first type of stabilization employs sutures that are passed through drill holes in the glenoid neck and are tied posteriorly. The second technique involves the use of an absorbable tack. We have recently begun to experiment with the arthroscopic use of suture anchors. We do not recommend the routine use of metal hardware around the shoulder.

Operative technique—sutures. This method of arthroscopic stabilization was derived from the pull-out suture techniques described for open Bankart repair by Luckey[65] and by Viek and Bell.[124] A standard arthroscopic examination is performed. The glenoid labrum and anteroinferior portion of the shoulder capsule (including the anterior band of the IGHLC) are carefully assessed to determine the quality of these tissues.

If the quality of the capsulolabral tissues is felt to be sufficient to allow the performance of an arthroscopic stabilization, the anterior glenoid neck is carefully debrided to bleeding bone using a bone rasp or a motorized arthroscopic bur (Fig. 7-16, *A*).

An arthroscopic grasping instrument is used to advance the capsulolabral tissue in a medial and superior direction. When the labrum is detached, it is grasped from the anterior portal and an observation is made to assess the tension within the system. If the labrum is absent, the anterior band of the inferior glenohumeral ligament is advanced with the grasping instrument. In some cases electrocautery is used to extend the separation from the anterior glenoid neck to allow sufficient ad-

vancement of the capsulolabral system. If the glenoid attachments of both the labrum and anteroinferior capsule are noted to be intact, an open procedure is performed.

A specially designed pin (Biomet, Warsaw, IN) with a drill point at one end and small holes at the blunt, opposite end has been developed to facilitate the procedure (Fig. 7-16, *B*). The sharp end of the pin is used to spear a robust portion of the capsulolabral tissue, and the pin is placed on the glenoid neck. The pin is then drilled in a posterior direction at an angle that is approximately 45 degrees medial to the sagittal plane of the anterior glenoid and 25 degrees inferior to its transverse plane. The entry point of the pin is 2 to 3 mm medial to the edge of the glenoid articular surface. The pin is drilled through the posterior cortex of the glenoid and was recovered after exiting from the posterior skin.

A 5-mm incision is made at the posterior exit point. The drill is detached from the tail of the pin, and two zero-gauge sutures are passed through the eyelet of the pin. One end of each suture was held anteriorly as the pin is advanced completely out of the posterior shoulder. The posterior halves of the sutures are tagged, and the anterior halves are brought out of an anterior portal.

The process is then repeated so that at least one additional pair of sutures are placed at a more inferior site along the glenoid margin.

The anterior halves of the sutures can then be paired together so that each suture is coupled with a suture from the other drill hole. The sutures are then tied to-

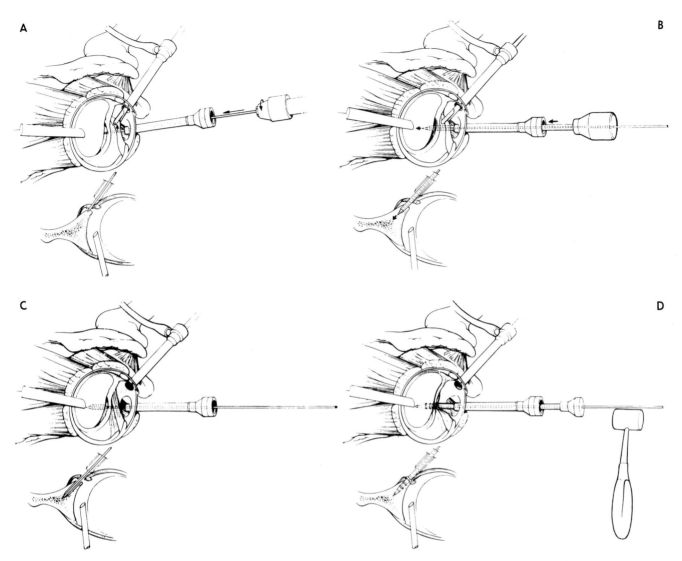

FIG. 7-17. Arthroscopic stabilization using biodegradable tacks. **A,** Cannulated drill bit and guide wire are used to advance the capsular tissues to the glenoid neck. **B,** Hole is drilled in the anterior glenoid neck. **C,** Drill bit is removed and the guide wire is left in place. **D,** Biodegradable tack is then placed over the guide wire and impacted into place with a cannulated pusher.

gether anteriorly to form a loop. Alternatively, multiple mulberry knots may be placed in the anterior ends of the sutures; these knots prevent the sutures from being pulled through the mobilized tissue.

Tension is then applied to the posterior halves of the sutures to bring the capsulolabral structures into position on the neck. A subcutaneous tunnel is created posteriorly from one group of sutures to the exit point of the other group. The posterior halves of the sutures are tied together in a subcutaneous location.

After the sutures have been tied, there should be good tension in the anterior capsulolabral system, and the drive-through sign should be eliminated.

Operative technique—biodegradable tack. In an effort to avoid the problems associated with tying sutures over a fascial bridge in proximity to the suprascapular nerve as well as the technical difficulty of transglenoid drilling, we

have recently used an absorbable tack (Acufex Microsurgical Inc., Norwood, MA) as a fixation device for arthroscopic stabilizations. The tack is cannulated and is made of polyglyconate. Its strength diminishes over 4 weeks. Ribs on the shaft of the tack increase its pullout strength to approximately 100 N. The tack's broad, flat head allows it to capture soft tissue.

The same basic arthroscopic technique is used with the tack as was described for the suture technique. The glenoid neck is prepared, and an accessory portal is created to grasp and tension the capsulolabral tissue. A cannulated drill bit that contains a guide wire is placed through the anterior portal. The wire is locked so that it protrudes a few millimeters from the end of the drill bit. The wire is used to pierce the capsulolabral tissue, and the tissue is then brought to the 2 o'clock position on the glenoid neck (Fig. 7-17, *A*). The drill bit is advanced to

a depth of approximately 12 mm into the bony glenoid (Fig. 7-17, *B*). The wire is then unlocked from the drill bit and gently tapped to free it from the drill bit. The drill bit is removed, leaving the wire in place (Fig. 7-17, *C*). A tack is then placed over the wire and impacted into place using a cannulated pusher (Fig. 7-17, *D*). We generally attempt to place a second tack at the 4 o'clock position.

In some patients a combination of the two techniques may be needed for optimal tensioning of the tissue. In this situation sutures are used superiorly to put tension on the tissues, and then a tack is placed at the 4 o'clock position to close the defect.

After an arthroscopic stabilization, a longer period of immobilization may be required to avoid postoperative instability.[40] Patients are maintained in internal rotation in a shoulder immobilizer for 4 weeks postoperatively. Shoulder pendulum and elbow range of motion exercises are encouraged during this period. Shoulder motion is increased at 4 weeks using active-assisted and passive techniques. When approximately 160 degrees of forward flexion and 30 degrees of external rotation have been obtained, resistance exercises are instituted. At 4 months the patient may resume light throwing and underhand racquet sports. Contact sports and unrestricted activity are permitted after 6 months.

At the present time the risk of recurrence after arthroscopic anterior stabilization is higher than that after an open procedure. Early reports revealed recurrence rates of between 15% and 20% after arthroscopic stabilization procedures.[40,72,133,134] The use of metal staples has consistently been associated with a high incidence of postoperative instability as well as frequent problems related to staple loosening.[23,26,40] Recently Morgan[76] reported a recurrence rate of only 5% after a 1- to 7-year follow-up of 175 patients who had undergone an anterior stabilization using a transglenoid suture technique. Suture anchors (which are drilled into the anterior glenoid neck) and biodegradable tacks appear to offer promising alternatives to the transglenoid suture technique. However, the results of these techniques of stabilization are preliminary.

There is a great hope that arthroscopic techniques will increase postoperative range of motion and will improve the results of the operative treatment of instability in throwers. In the series of Rowe et al,[100] 69% of those patients treated by an open Bankart procedure regained full motion. Morgan[76] reported recovery of full range of motion in 87% of the first 55 patients that he had treated arthroscopically. Coughlin et al[26] noted disappointing results (less than 50% success rate) in returning overhead athletes to their premorbid level of function after metal staple capsulorraphy. We have noted a better outcome in overhead athletes after transglenoid suture stabilization.[93] Of these 12 individuals, 8 were able to return to their premorbid function.

Consistently poor outcomes in terms of postoperative instability have been noted in patients with capsular laxity, absence of a Bankart lesion, or poorly defined glenohumeral ligaments, and in patients involved in contact sports.* The results of open capsular repairs in contact athletes have not been investigated. Although the results of arthroscopic stabilization procedures in such patients may be less encouraging than those in a more sedentary population, it is unclear if a matched population would fare better with an open procedure.

POSTERIOR INSTABILITY
Acute Posterior Dislocation

Posterior dislocations constitute only 2% to 4% of all shoulder dislocations. The largest series, 37 patients, was reported by Malgaigne[68] in 1855. Probably because of the relative infrequency of posterior dislocation, the diagnosis is initially missed in 50% to 80% of cases.[15,104]

Indirect forces are common causative factors. The classic examples are those associated with electrical shocks and with seizures. In these situations the powerful internal rotators (latissimus dorsi, pectoralis major, and subscapularis) are thought to overcome the weaker external rotators and force the humeral head posteriorly.[70] A less common mechanism of an indirect force that can cause posterior dislocation is a fall on an outstretched hand with the arm in a relatively adducted position. Atraumatic posterior dislocations may occur in patients with congenital laxity.

The patient who presents with an acute posterior dislocation will have an internal rotation deformity and limited external rotation of the arm (Fig. 7-18). The arm will also be adducted with abduction usually limited to less than 90 degrees. In thin patients posterior prominence of the shoulder and anterior prominence of the coracoid may be noted.[75] The patient will be unable to fully supinate the forearm with the arm forward flexed.[104] After reduction of the shoulder only increased posterior translation and posterior apprehension may be evident.

Several radiographic signs have been described to aid in the detection of posterior dislocation on an anteroposterior view; this view is rarely diagnostic, however. The axillary view is generally the most helpful view if one suspects a posterior dislocation. The presence and assistance of a physician may be required to obtain an adequate study.

Posterior dislocations may be associated with disruption of the posterior labrum or capsule[130]; however, Warren et al[129] have shown that detachment of the entire posterior capsule does not cause posterior dislocation unless it is accompanied by disruption of the anterosuperior capsule as well.

Lesser tuberosity fractures are commonly associated with posterior dislocations, and the presence of such a fracture should alert the clinician to rule out a posterior dislocation. Neurovascular injuries and rotator cuff tears are less common after posterior dislocation when compared with anterior dislocations. Recurrence is also more infrequent after a traumatic posterior dislocation than after a traumatic anterior dislocation.[70]

---

*References 23, 26, 28, 40, 77, 93, 106, and 125.

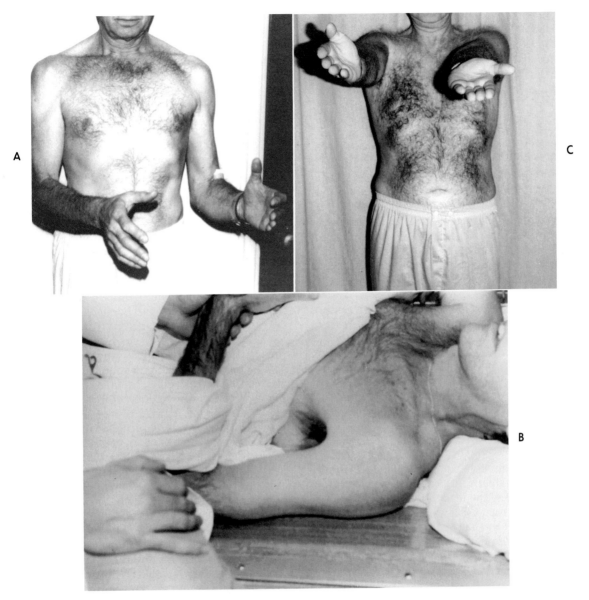

FIG. 7-18. Posterior shoulder dislocation. **A,** Patient with a posterior dislocation is unable to externally rotate the arm. **B,** Acute posterior dislocation. Note prominence of coracoid process. **C,** Rowe sign. Inability to fully supinate the forearm in a patient with a posterior dislocation.

Treatment of the acute posterior dislocation usually begins with an attempt at closed reduction if no fracture lines are seen in the humeral head.[110] Any associated fracture may extend and result in displacement of the head fragment during reduction. If an attempt at closed reduction is believed to be safe, the patient should be suitably sedated with an intravenous benzodiazepine and a narcotic. Some patients may require general anesthesia. The patient is positioned supine. Lateral traction is applied to the arm, and gentle *internal* rotation is used to unlock the impaction fracture from the glenoid. Use of an excessive *external* rotation force at this point may displace the head fragment. Posterior pressure is then applied to the head, and a longitudinal traction force is placed on the adducted arm. The head is gently lifted back into the glenoid as the arm is externally rotated.

If the reduction is stable, the arm is immobilized in 0 degrees of abduction and in slight extension. When the shoulder is unstable after reduction, the arm is externally rotated to 20 degrees in a splint or brace. Young patients are immobilized for 4 to 6 weeks and then are started on an aggressive physical therapy program that emphasizes external rotator strengthening. Older patients are immobilized for only 2 to 3 weeks.

Operative treatment with open reduction is indicated if closed reduction fails, if there is a significant risk of further damage to the head with closed reduction, and in cases where there is major displacement of a head or

glenoid fragment. A posterior approach to the shoulder is preferred, since damage to the posterior capsule can be addressed via this approach.

Postoperatively the arm is splinted in neutral rotation, slight abduction, and extension for 6 weeks. Rehabilitation is instituted after 6 weeks and initially consists of passive and active-assisted range of motion exercises. Muscle strengthening is begun after the patient has achieved a nearly normal range of motion.

Recurrent Posterior Dislocation

Recurrent posterior dislocation, as mentioned earlier, is unusual. Voluntary posterior dislocation has been reported.[21,101] Boyd and Sisk[16] noted posterior Bankart lesions in four of nine shoulders that were operated on for recurrent posterior dislocation. Rowe[99] found posterior labral or capsular detachment in three of eight cases that were operated upon. Rowe also noted an anteromedial head defect in three of ten patients who had this condition.

Neer[82] reported a series of 23 patients with recurrent posterior dislocation in which no additional recurrences were noted after a posterior capsular shift procedure was performed. Patients with recurrent posterior subluxation may have been included in this series. Operative intervention should be considered if more than one recurrence is noted in a traumatic dislocator. We recommend a posterior capsulorraphy procedure as described in the following section.

Recurrent Posterior Subluxation

Recurrent posterior subluxation is the most common form of posterior instability. Although this is increasingly recognized in athletes, the diagnosis is often missed or delayed. In a recent report diagnosis was made, on average, 14 months after the onset of symptoms.[15]

These patients often have a history of overuse rather than of macrotrauma. They usually present because of pain, which may be localized anteriorly or posteriorly. Symptoms do not usually limit the activities of daily living or work, but they may interfere with athletic performance. Symptoms tend to worsen when the arm is flexed, adducted, and internally rotated. The follow-through phase of overhead sports and the pull-through phase of swimming are commonly associated with pain. Symptoms may also increase during the bench press in weightlifters and are not uncommon in baseball batters and during pass-blocking drills performed by offensive linemen in football.

Instability is usually a secondary complaint. Instability symptoms tend to increase with time, however, and they appear to be more common in patients who have had a distinct episode of trauma.

Physical examination typically reveals pain or symptoms of instability with the arm flexed, adducted, and internally rotated. Examination should be performed with the patient supine and the arm abducted 90 degrees and in neutral rotation. A posterior force is exerted while a gentle axial load is provided to the elbow. Posterior subluxation of the head on the glenoid may be noted with the arm in this position. The examiner should note pos-

terior translation with a click. Painful or marked instability will be rare. These patients should be carefully evaluated for concomitant inferior instability to rule out multidirectional instability. Increased ligamentous laxity is not uncommon in recurrent posterior subluxation.

Many patients with recurrent posterior subluxation learn to voluntarily subluxate their shoulder.[15,30,41,43,82] In most of these patients it is their involuntary instability which leads them to seek treatment. Two types of voluntary instability have been described.[30] In the *positional* type the head subluxates posteriorly as the arm is forward flexed and internally rotated. The head then reduces with extension of the arm. The majority of patients who can voluntarily display positional posterior subluxation have no underlying psychiatric disease. The second group incorporates selective activation of the internal rotators to cause posterior subluxation. This *muscular* type of voluntary instability is believed to be indicative of a poor response to surgical management.

The pathoanatomy of recurrent posterior subluxation is often subtle. A reverse Bankart lesion is not usually present although clefts may be found in the posterior labrum.[43] Articular cartilage degeneration may also be noted. Radiographic studies are rarely diagnostic. About 20% of affected patients exhibit calcification of the posterior glenoid rim and capsule. Another 20% have been found to have some erosion of the posterior glenoid.[15]

Most patients with recurrent posterior subluxation, especially those with atraumatic or microtraumatic etiologies, respond well to an aggressive rehabilitation program that emphasizes rotator cuff strengthening. Patients with complaints of instability and those with a history of macrotrauma appear to do less well after a trial of physical therapy.[15,30]

Operative treatment is indicated in patients with pain or unintentional instability despite rehabilitation, in those with pain during the activities of daily living, and in competitive athletes who develop symptoms during strenuous activity.[30] The early published results of operative treatment for recurrent posterior subluxation were not encouraging. Hawkins et al[43] noted a 50% failure rate after a variety of stabilization procedures including glenoid osteotomy, biceps transfer, and capsulorraphy. There is a substantial risk of glenohumeral arthritis after posterior glenoid osteotomy.[57] Tibone and Ting[118] reported a 30% failure rate following open posterior staple capsulorraphy. More recently, Bowen et al[15] reported a more favorable outcome (with a 12% recurrence rate) after posterior T-plasty capsular shift.

Operative Technique

The technique of posterior T-plasty capsular shift is as follows. The patient is placed in either the lateral decubitus or, more recently, the modified beach-chair position. Initially, a horizontal skin incision was used. The horizontal incision is placed 1 cm inferior to the scapular spine and allows the surgeon to obtain a bone graft from the scapular spine if indicated. A vertical incision is used in most patients (Fig. 7-19, *A*).[19] The vertical alternative is made midway between the lateral border of the acromion and the posterior axillary crease. The su-

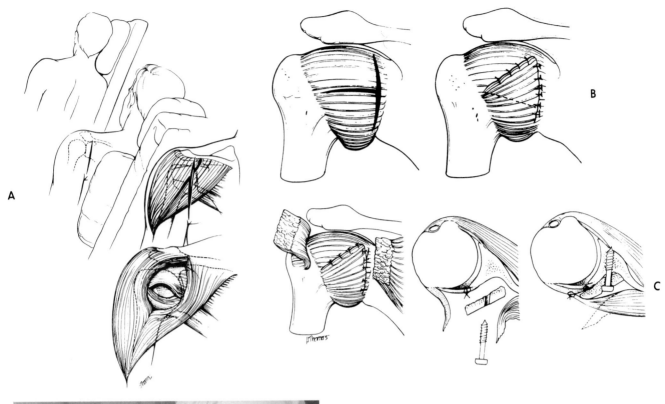

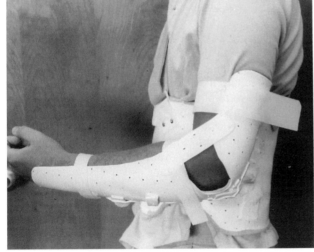

FIG. 7-19. Posterior capsular repair for recurrent posterior instability. **A,** Glenohumeral joint may be approached with the patient in the modified beach chair position. A longitudinal skin incision is used. The deltoid is split in the direction of its fibers. An interval is then created within the infraspinatus tendon to expose the joint. If the capsule is of poor quality, the infraspinatus may be tenotomized and used to reinforce the capsular repair. **B,** Posterior laxity may be eliminated and a posterior Bankart lesion obliterated by performing a T-plasty capsular incision and shifting the capsule. **C,** In rare cases a bone block may be required when the posterior glenoid has eroded. **D,** Immobilization in an Orthoplast splint.

perficial deltoid fascia is identified, and the deltoid is split to expose the infraspinatus and teres minor tendons. Division of the deltoid begins at the scapular spine and proceeds inferiorly.

Next the infraspinatus tendon is incised vertically with a large portion of the tendon remaining laterally. (In throwers the capsule may be exposed by developing an interval within the infraspinatus tendon without division of the tendon. This option is especially useful if the tissue is of good quality. If tissue quality is suboptimal, the approach may be converted by obliquely incising the tendon.) The surgeon should be mindful of the axillary nerve and the posterior circumflex humeral vessels, which exit the quadrilateral space immediately inferior to the teres minor.

A T-shaped capsular incision is then made. The vertical limb of the incision is placed medially, near the glenoid (Fig. 7-19, *B*). An incision of this type allows easier Bankart repair if a Bankart lesion is present. The horizontal limb of the capsular incision is extended laterally from the vertical component. With the arm in neutral rotation and 30 to 40 degrees of abduction, the capsule is reattached to the glenoid through drill holes or using suture anchors. Before reattachment the inferior limb of

the capsule is advanced medially and superiorly to eliminate laxity in the posteroinferior capsule. If marked capsular laxity is noted with the arm in a position of abduction despite the medial T-plication, a second vertical capsular incision is placed laterally to create an H-plasty. The inferior portion of the capsule can be advanced further by this method. Inferior laxity with the arm in adduction may indicate that the superior structures need additional tensioning. Tensioning of the superior structures may be technically difficult from a posterior approach. This difficulty has led some surgeons to consider an anterior approach in selected cases.[17]

The capsular repair may be reinforced with the infraspinatus tendon if local tissue is thought to be insufficient. If a large posterior defect is found on the glenoid, consideration can be given to obtaining a tricortical bone block from the scapular spine to compensate for the bony deficiency. When it is used, the graft is placed at the posteroinferior quadrant of the glenoid to increase the articulating surface of the glenoid at a point which is contiguous with its curvature (Fig. 7-19, C). The humeral head should not be allowed to impinge on the bone graft. The bone block technique has been used infrequently in the past 5 years.

The patient is maintained in an orthoplast splint with the arm in external rotation for the first 6 weeks after operation (Fig. 7-19, D). In throwers, early passive motion may be instituted with rotation from neutral to full external rotation. Full internal rotation should be avoided. Flexion is best avoided for 6 weeks, but elevation in the plane of the scapula allows healing to occur without undue stress to the repair.

The anterosuperior capsule has been shown to be an important stabilizer against posterior translation of the humeral head.[129] In our experience it has not been necessary to specifically address the anterior structures at the time of reconstruction; however, the surgeon may have to consider the role of the anterosuperior capsule in posterior instability. Additional tensioning of this area may be especially applicable to cases with an atraumatic etiology.

The role of arthroscopic Bankart repair in the treatment of recurrent posterior subluxation remains undefined. Arthroscopic findings include attenuation, capsular-periosteal separation of the posterior capsule, tearing or detachment of the posterior labrum, and the reverse Hill-Sachs lesion. We have used an absorbable tack for arthroscopic stabilization of recurrent posterior subluxation in a small group of patients with labral detachment.[118]

Possible indications for posterior glenoid osteotomy in the treatment of recurrent posterior subluxation include glenoid retroversion in excess of 20 degrees and congenital hypoplasia of the glenoid.[70] In our opinion this procedure is rarely indicated.

MULTIDIRECTIONAL INSTABILITY

Multidirectional instability is increasingly recognized as an important subtype of shoulder disability in the athletic population. The signs and symptoms associated with multidirectional instability are often subtle, and the results of treatment have often been less than satisfactory. Recent advances involving the recognition and pathoanatomy of the multidirectionally unstable shoulder have led to an improved outlook with regard to the treatment of this condition.

It is generally believed that the basic lesion in multidirectional instability is excessive joint volume with laxity of the capsular ligaments. In the athlete this laxity may be an inherent condition that becomes more pronounced with the superimposed trauma of sport. In addition, multidirectional instability may occur as a result of extensive capsulolabral trauma in patients who do not appear to have laxity of other joints.

The pathologic condition of the multidirectionally unstable shoulder of the *atraumatic* type usually consists of a large inferior capsular pouch that extends both posteriorly and anteriorly.[80] Anterior capsulolabral detachment is generally not associated with this capsular redundancy. In contrast a *traumatic* type of multidirectional instability exists and can be seen to a varying degree depending on the physician's patient population. In loose-jointed athletes, particularly, a traumatic event may result in a shoulder with both multidirectional instability and a Bankart lesion of varying size.

Although the shoulder capsule normally contains numerous synovial recesses, *abnormal* capsular redundancy is an important factor in the pathogenesis of multidirectional instability.[80] Gradual stretching of the capsule may occur with repetitive microtrauma, which is a common etiologic factor in multidirectional instability. On the other hand capsular laxity most commonly is caused by inherent soft-tissue laxity. These patients may have a mild form of a generalized connective tissue disorder. Belle and Hawkins[12] cultured fibroblasts from the skin of patients with multidirectional instability and discovered a significant increase in the relative amount of collagen produced in the multidirectional group.

Uhthoff and Piscopo[122] have suggested that a congenitally abnormal insertion of the capsule into the glenoid neck may predispose to capsular redundancy. This theory is based on anatomic dissections of fetal and embryonic shoulders.

Enlargement of the rotator interval appears to result in abnormal inferior translation and may also be related to increases in anteroposterior motion.[39,86,103,105] Assessment of the presence and size of the rotator interval is extremely important during operative repair for multidirectional instability. Closure of the interval often significantly diminishes excess capsular laxity.

Three basic types of multidirectional instability can be differentiated on the basis of the direction and degree of abnormal translation. We have recently noted a fourth type. Type I comprises patients who have global instability and dislocate in all three directions. Type II patients demonstrate anterior and inferior dislocation as well as mild posteroinferior subluxation. Patients with posterior and inferior dislocation and mild anteroinferior laxity are classified as Type III. In rare cases (Type IV), there are patients who appear to have abnormal anterior and posterior translation, both to the point of dislocation, with-

out significant inferior translation. These cases, although uncommon, present a difficult management problem as the inferior component of instability is absent at both 0 and 45 degrees of abduction.

Multidirectional instability

Type I
- Global instability
- Dislocation in all three directions

Type II
- Anterior and inferior dislocation
- Posteroinferior subluxation

Type III
- Posterior and inferior dislocation
- Mild anteroinferior laxity

Type IV
- Abnormal anterior and posterior translation
- No abnormal inferior translation

Most athletes with multidirectional instability present with a sense of looseness and associated discomfort of the shoulder. Symptoms tend to occur with overhead and contact activities. Those patients with an atraumatic history or a loose capsule usually are able to reduce their shoulders spontaneously without assistance. Repetitive use injury (often throwing) commonly results in symptoms consistent with subluxation. In the traumatic setting or with repeated injury, complete dislocation may occur.

Pain is an uncommon complaint except when associated with an acute event. However, the occasional patient has pain while carrying a bag or with overhead activity. We have noted that patients with multidirectional instability often have a history of paresthesia in the involved upper extremity. Symptoms of thoracic outlet syndrome are frequently associated with multidirectional instability and may result from traction on the brachial plexus associated with increased inferior translation of the shoulder.

These patients often present with bilateral complaints. Morrey and Janes[78] reported an increased failure rate after standard anterior stabilization in patients with bilateral instability and in those with a family history of instability. These groups of patients may have generalized ligamentous laxity and require a careful evaluation for evidence of multidirectional instability.

The patient with multidirectional instability usually exhibits symptomatic inferior instability in addition to anterior or posterior instability. The sulcus sign is therefore positive in these patients. The presence of inferior instability has been considered to be a requirement for the diagnosis of multidirectional instability.[82] However, we have noted a select group of patients who demonstrate marked anterior and posterior translation without significant inferior laxity.

Physical examination of the athlete with *atraumatic* multidirectional instability usually reveals little or no pain or apprehension in any direction. Those with a *trau-matic* etiology and anterior subluxation are more likely to have positive apprehension signs and associated pain.

Approximately 50% of patients with multidirectional instability have evidence of generalized ligamentous laxity. Concomitant findings of impingement occur in approximately 20% of patients with multidirectional instability.[2]

In the athlete with atraumatic multidirectional instability it is unusual to see a bony abnormality. If trauma is an etiologic factor, the development of radiographic abnormalities is more likely. We have not found stress or traction films[82] to be necessary in delineating inferior instability. Whereas weighted views may reveal inferior subluxation when the glenohumeral muscles are relaxed, clinical examination with simple inferior traction is sufficient to demonstrate a sulcus sign.

Nonoperative Treatment of Multidirectional Instability

To paraphrase Neer,[82] "Not all loose shoulders are painful and not all require treatment." Symptomatic patients with multidirectional instability should be given a thorough trial of internal and external rotator strengthening. Patients with atraumatic multidirectional instability often respond to nonoperative therapy.

A rehabilitation program that emphasizes rotator cuff and periscapular muscle strengthening is then employed. Kronberg, Brostrom, and Nemeth,[61] in an electromyographic study of patients with generalized ligamentous laxity, have noted decreased activity of the anterior and middle deltoid with abduction and flexion of the shoulder as well as increased activity of the subscapularis during internal rotation. Isokinetic testing can help identify specific muscular weakness and can provide a baseline for comparison during the rehabilitative process.[55,120] Rotator cuff strengthening begins with rubber tubing exercises, progresses to spring exercises, and then advances to Nautilus or isokinetic exercises. We also emphasize elevation with weights in the scapular plane and seated push-ups in which the body is lifted from a chair by extension of the upper extremities with the hands placed on the seat. Weights should be held so that they do not create an inferior traction force on the shoulder. If there is a positional component to the instability, then that position should be avoided.

In the early phase of therapy, especially in patients with concomitant impingement, these activities should be performed with the arm adducted or in the lower ranges of abduction to protect the rotator cuff.[137] Later, these exercises may be performed in 90 degrees of elevation in the scapular plane as well. Muscular endurance should be emphasized in addition to strengthening. The scapular rotators are conditioned by a combination of shoulder shrugs, horizontal adduction exercises, pull-downs, chin-ups, and push-ups with the elbows kept at the sides.[55]

Throwing is not allowed until strength and motion are normal. Throwing is slowly progressed in distance, velocity, frequency, and duration. The patient's pitching mechanics should be adjusted to provide efficient energy transfer from the lower extremities and thorax to the

shoulder. Specific activities that seemed to incite pain before the institution of therapy are withheld for longer periods.

A rehabilitative program often succeeds in patients with atraumatic instability. Traumatic dislocators appear to respond less favorably. Recently, Burkhead and Rockwood[22] reported that an exercise program led to a good or excellent result in 80% of shoulders with atraumatic subluxation, but in only 16% of shoulders with traumatic subluxation.

Operative Treatment of Multidirectional Instability

Candidates for surgical stabilization of multidirectional instability should be well motivated, since adherence to the postoperative rehabilitative program is extremely important to achieving a successful result. Atraumatic types of multidirectional instability appear to have higher postoperative recurrence rates than traumatic types.

In cases with a traumatic etiology, whether superimposed upon generalized laxity or not, our impression is that exercises are less helpful. These patients will note a specific event that produced their symptoms. As was mentioned earlier, traumatic conditions are more frequently associated with capsulolabral disruption (the Bankart lesion), which may be extensive enough to result in multidirectional instability. These patients frequently note a significant degree of pain and apprehension.

Arthroscopy currently plays a small role in the treatment of multidirectional instability, particularly of the atraumatic type. In general, if there is a significant component of inferior instability or subluxation, arthroscopy is avoided and an open procedure is performed. In our opinion there is no current role for an arthroscopic stabilization procedure in the treatment of multidirectional instability. Current techniques of arthroscopic stabilization do not permit sufficient mobilization of capsular laxity, do not address the rotator interval, and thus are associated with a high failure rate in the treatment of multidirectional instability.[2,7,8]

The type of operative approach for multidirectional instability should be determined by the patient's history and physical findings. Generally, the approach should be made on the side associated with the greatest amount of clinical instability. In general, we prefer to approach the shoulder anteriorly because the soft tissues are of better quality, the capsular shift is more easily performed, and an enlarged rotator interval can be identified and addressed. However, in dealing with traumatic types of instability, a posterior approach is used if the clinical evaluation reveals that the principal direction of instability is posteroinferior with only mild anterior subluxation. In patients with primarily posterior instability with an atraumatic etiology, the surgeon may consider closure of the rotator interval through a small anterosuperior incision after a posterior capsulorrhaphy has been performed.

Patients with inferior laxity may fail standard operative procedures designed for unidirectional instability. In some cases these procedures may cause excessive tightness on one side of the hypermobile shoulder. Subluxa-

tion or dislocation then occurs in the opposite direction, and glenohumeral arthritis may ensue.

Anterior Approach

After exposure of the anterior capsule by division of the subscapularis tendon the exact type of repair is determined by the size of the rotator interval, the degree of capsular laxity, and the presence or absence of a Bankart lesion. Excess capsular laxity may be dealt with on the medial side of the joint, the lateral side of the joint, or on both sides of the joint. If a Bankart lesion is present, we prefer a medial T-plasty capsulorrhaphy to allow correction of both the Bankart lesion and the capsular laxity. If only capsular laxity is found, it is technically easier to perform a lateral capsular shift as described by Neer and Foster.[80]

A search is made for the presence of a rotator interval. The rotator interval is, in essence, a hiatus for passage of the oblique head of the subscapularis tendon toward its insertion on the lesser tuberosity. Generally, the interval is small, but if it extends to the coracoid process, the superior capsule is left open with no attachment to the superior aspect of the glenoid. An enlarged rotator interval will allow abnormal anteroinferior or posteroinferior translation of the humeral head. If present, an enlarged interval must be closed to create adequate tension in the capsular system. Otherwise, a repair that advances tissue superiorly may stretch out. At times, closure of the interval alone may be sufficient to control excessive translation. In many cases, however, additional tensioning of the capsule is required. The interval may be closed before the creation of a formal capsulotomy, or the joint may be inspected through the interval if the interval is sufficiently large (Fig. 7-20, *A*). When closure of the interval alone is insufficient to control translation and the joint has been inspected via the rotator interval, the interval can be incorporated into the capsulotomy by creating vertical capsular incisions on the medial and/or lateral sides of the interval and then advancing the capsule proximally (Fig. 7-20, *B* to *D*). In this method the interval forms the transverse base for the capsular repair. Closure of the interval is accomplished with multiple nonabsorbable No. 1 sutures running from the base of the coracoid laterally to the humeral head.

If the rotator interval is not used to inspect the joint, the labrum is viewed via an oblique capsulotomy, which is created proximal to the IGHLC (Fig. 7-21, *A*). This nearly transverse incision can then be extended either medially or laterally, depending on the presence or absence of a Bankart lesion. If a Bankart lesion is noted, the capsulotomy is converted to a T by creating a vertical limb at the glenoid margin, which extends back to the posterior capsule (Fig. 7-21, *B*). The axillary nerve is vulnerable during this portion of the procedure and must be protected. The anterior glenoid margin is exposed and is roughened to a bleeding surface with a small osteotome or burr (Fig. 7-21, *C*). Drill holes are created at the glenoid margin for the passage of heavy nonabsorbable sutures. The inferior flap is then advanced superiorly to eliminate inferior laxity and medially while the arm is held in 30 to 45 degrees of external rotation and

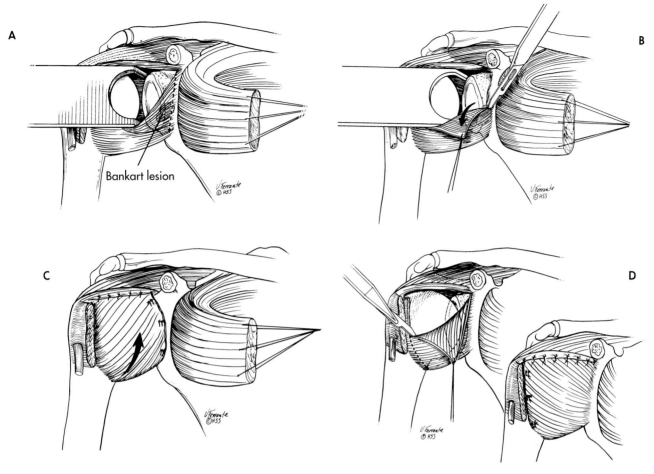

FIG. 7-20. Capsular exposure through an enlarged rotator interval. **A,** When the rotator interval is large, it can be used to examine the joint for the presence or absence of a Bankart lesion. **B,** If a Bankart lesion is encountered in a patient with multidirectional instability, the rotator interval can be connected to a medial capsular incision to eliminate both the Bankart lesion and the abnormal capsular laxity. **C,** After creation of the medial limb of the capsular incision, the capsule is shifted superomedially and the rotator interval is closed with nonabsorbable sutures. **D,** In cases with a large rotator interval in which no Bankart lesion is found, the interval may be incorporated into a lateral capsular shift. In this case the capsule is shifted superolaterally.

40 to 50 degrees of abduction (Fig. 7-21, *E*). In a thrower or swimmer the maximum degree of external rotation that maintains stability of the shoulder is preferable. The sutures are passed through the inferior limb and are tied. Next, the superior flap is advanced distally, and the sutures are passed a second time (Fig. 7-21, *F*). The goal is not to overtighten the capsule medially but to tension it superiorly.

Recently we have used suture anchors (Acufex Microsurgical Inc., Mansfield, MA) to allow direct suture placement and to obviate the need for drill holes (Fig. 7-21, *D*). If suture anchors are used, they must be prestressed by pulling on the sutures before passage through the capsule. The anchors should be placed at the glenoid margin and not medially along the glenoid neck.

If no Bankart lesion is found, the vertical limb of the **T** is placed laterally near the humeral neck (Fig. 7-22).

The lateral limb allows easier and safer access to the posterior capsule and is preferable if there is no evidence of capsulolabral stripping from the anterior glenoid. The lateral incision is made directly on the bone if the humeral attachment of the capsule is attenuated or if there is stripping of the capsule from the humeral neck. In this situation drill holes in the proximal humerus may be used for suture placement, but these are difficult to position, particularly inferiorly. Suture anchors are an excellent alternative, but the quality of the bone must be assessed following their placement, particularly in the superior portion of the humeral head. If the capsule is stripped from the humeral neck, its attachment should be moved proximally to decrease the volume of the axillary recess.

In some cases with extreme inferior laxity an anterior **H**-plasty may be necessary to allow sufficient mobilization of the capsule. This is accomplished by creating both

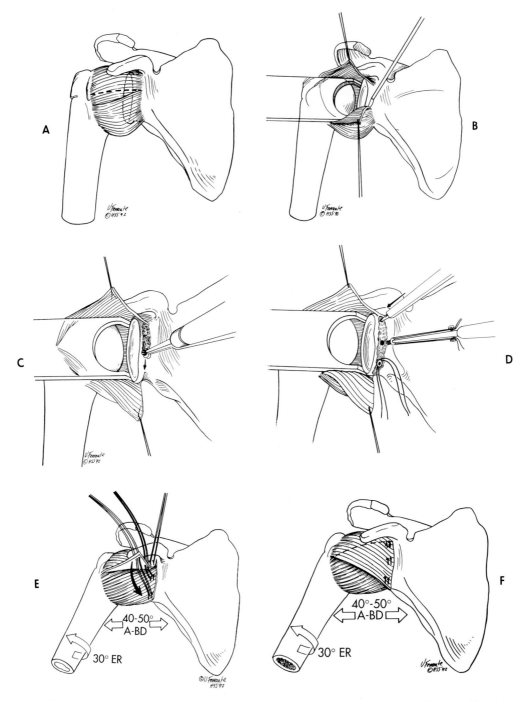

FIG. 7-21. T-plasty modification of the Bankart procedure for multidirectional instability. **A,** Oblique (almost transverse) capsular incision is made to view the joint. **B,** If a Bankart lesion is encountered, the capsule is stripped medially from the glenoid neck. **C,** Motorized burr is used to create a bleeding bed of bone. **D,** Suture anchors are placed at the glenoid margin. **E,** Inferior capsular limb is shifted superomedially. **F,** Superior capsular limb is shifted inferomedially, and the sutures are tied.

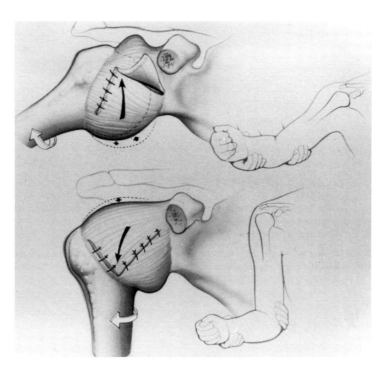

FIG. 7-22. Lateral capsular shift. In cases where no Bankart lesion is present, it is less technically demanding to shift the capsule on the lateral side of the joint.

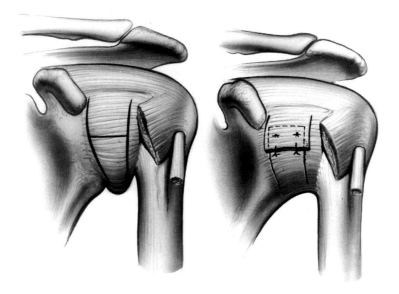

FIG. 7-23. Anterior H-plasty.

medial and lateral vertical limbs in the capsulotomy and then advancing the inferior flap superiorly (Fig. 7-23).

After an anterior capsulorrhaphy for multidirectional instability, the patient is placed in a shoulder immobilizer, and the arm is kept in adduction and internal rotation for 6 weeks. We formerly placed these patients in an orthoplast splint in slight abduction and internal rotation, but we have found that this is not necessary if the inferior instability has been eliminated when the repair is tested in the operating room. Pendulum exercises are ini-

tiated soon after surgery. Gentle passive flexion exercises to 90 degrees are instituted after 3 weeks. At 6 weeks active-assisted range of motion exercises are begun. When full range of motion is obtained, active resistance exercises are started to strengthen the internal and external rotators and the deltoid.

In individuals in whom there was a component of inferior instability, care must be taken in the early rehabilitative phase not to create high loads in a downward direction on the repaired structures. A common scenario

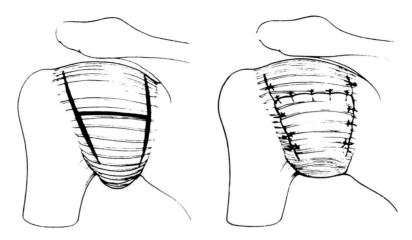

FIG. 7-24. Posterior H-plasty. This type of capsular repair is frequently required in patients with multidirectional instability and a predominant posterior component.

is the use of free weights with the arms held at the sides. When muscle fatigue occurs, the weights can generate downward stress on the repaired tissue. In this setting isokinetic machines may be preferred. If only free weights are available, the therapist should have the patient lift the weights from a waist-high platform and then replace the weights to the platform after the exercise. This maneuver allows the weight to be held only when the muscle is contracting and prevents the downward pull when the muscle is fatigued.

Light throwing and sidearm racquet sports are permitted after 6 months. At 6 to 9 months patients with a traumatic etiology may return to contact sports, hard throwing, and overhead racquet sports. Patients of the atraumatic type are protected from these activities for 9 to 12 months.

Posterior Approach

Although some surgeons prefer an anterior approach for all types of multidirectional instability, we believe that a posterior approach should be used when the predominant clinical direction of instability is posterior. This is particularly true for patients in whom trauma played an etiologic role. In patients with no history of trauma a combined anterior and posterior approach may be preferable.

The posterior approach for posttraumatic multidirectional instability is similar to the posterior T-plasty capsular shift that was described for the treatment of recurrent posterior subluxation. In the patient with multidirectional instability, conversion of the capsulotomy to an H-plasty is often necessary to eliminate inferior redundancy by advancing the inferior capsule superiorly (Fig. 7-24). It is important to dissect inferiorly to a degree that is sufficient to allow advancement of the posterior band of the IGHLC. The inferior capsule is then brought superiorly so that posterior laxity is eliminated with the arm in neutral rotation. The capsular repair may be reinforced with the infraspinatus tendon if local tissue is thought to be insufficient.

The anterosuperior capsule has been shown to be an important stabilizer against posterior translation of the humeral head.[129] In our experience it has not been necessary to specifically address the anterior structures at the time of reconstruction; however, the surgeon may have to consider the role of the anterosuperior capsule in posterior instability. Additional tensioning of this area may be especially applicable to cases with an atraumatic etiology. Inferior laxity with the arm in adduction may indicate that the superior structures need additional tensioning. Tensioning of the superior structures is technically difficult from a posterior approach. This difficulty has led some surgeons to consider an anterior approach in selected cases.

After a posterior capsular repair for multidirectional instability, the patient is maintained in an orthoplast splint with the arm in extension and neutral rotation for the first 6 weeks after operation. In throwers, early passive motion may be instituted with rotation from neutral to full external rotation. Full internal rotation should be avoided. Flexion is best avoided for 6 weeks, but elevation in the plane of the scapula allows healing to occur without undue stress to the repair.

Combined Approaches

Both anterior and posterior approaches may be required on some occasions.[82] Patients with atraumatic multidirectional instability with a predominant posterior component tend to have high postoperative recurrence rates. In this group one should consider performing a posterior repair followed by closure of the rotator interval via a small anterosuperior approach.

The combined approaches may also be indicated when significant anterior labral detachment is noted during a posterior approach, when there is doubt concerning the adequacy of stabilization after capsular repair of the first side, or when prior surgery has resulted in a contracture on the opposite side of the joint and release is required before a capsular shift can be performed.

Clinical Results

The results of the surgical treatment of shoulder instability in the face of capsular laxity have historically been less successful than those for unidirectional anterior instability. Results have improved with current techniques, however.

Neer and Foster,[80] in their classic 1980 article describing the inferior capsular shift procedure, reported a successful outcome in 36 of 37 shoulders with multidirectional instability. Neer[82] has subsequently written that he has performed more than 100 additional inferior capsular shifts "with similar satisfactory results."

Altchek et al[2] noted four recurrences in 40 patients (42 shoulders) and a 95% patient satisfaction rate at 2-year minimum follow-up after T-plasty repair for anterior and inferior (Type II) multidirectional instability. One of the patients had a single postoperative episode of anterior subluxation, and three patients developed signs of posterior instability. In one of these three a subsequent posterior stabilization was required. No patient lost more than 5 degrees of abduction, forward flexion, or internal rotation. Approximately half of the patients regained external rotation to a degree that was equal to the opposite side. The vast majority of patients who lost motion were noted to have diminished motion preoperatively. No patient lost more than 20 degrees of external rotation; 33 of the patients reported full return to sports.

Cooper and Brems[25] described a series of 38 patients (43 shoulders) who were followed for a minimum of 2 years after inferior capsular shift through an anterior approach. The majority of these patients had generalized ligamentous laxity. Seven shoulders demonstrated a Bankart lesion. Postoperatively 91% functioned well without instability. Only four patients were not satisfied with the procedure. None of these patients had been elite athletes; 28 patients were recreational athletes. Sixteen of these were able to return to the same sport, although some returned at a reduced level of activity.

Hawkins et al[44] reported on 31 patients followed 2 to 5 years after an inferior capsular shift. Nineteen patients had a satisfactory result, only two of whom had significant posterior instability. Twelve patients had unsatisfactory outcomes. Of these 12, 7 had significant posterior instability, 10 had undergone a previous attempt at surgical stabilization, and 6 had osteoarthritic changes in the shoulder. The authors concluded that patients with primarily posterior instability fared more poorly, particularly if they had undergone previous surgery. It should be noted that, in contrast to the series of Altchek et al,[2] most of the patients in Hawkins's series had the more classic findings of an atraumatic etiology and no Bankart lesion. This population tends to produce excessive collagen which may have poorer strength characteristics.

SUMMARY

Glenohumeral instability is a common cause of disability in the athletic population. The shoulder joint is extremely mobile, and bony stability has been sacrificed to allow for this motion. Glenohumeral stability is primarily dependent upon the soft tissues surrounding the joint. These soft-tissue stabilizers operate in a complex pattern that varies with shoulder position and activity. If a primary stabilizer is damaged, there appear to be secondary restraints to abnormal translation. The high loads incurred at the shoulder during athletic activity can overwhelm both primary and secondary mechanisms of stability.

Posterior and multidirectional instabilities of the glenohumeral joint are important causes of shoulder disability. Although there is an increased recognition of these types of instability, diagnosis is commonly missed or delayed due to the relative infrequency of presentation and the subtlety of the associated physical findings.

A thorough understanding of the pathomechanics of shoulder instability is required for the proper treatment of these lesions. Nonoperative treatment and rehabilitation are based on the principle of secondary mechanisms of restraint. If operative intervention is employed, the surgeon should carefully define the problem and address the pathologic anatomy accordingly. The operative treatment of anterior instability should attend to damage to the anterior capsulolabral system and to excess capsular laxity. Standard procedures for unidirectional anterior instability are likely to fail in the treatment of posterior or multidirectional instability and may, in fact, worsen the problem. A specific, selective capsulolabral repair should be the mainstay of operative treatment. The goal is the restoration of normal capsular anatomy to prevent instability while retaining maximal function.

REFERENCES

1. Altchek DW, Skyhar MJ, Warren RF: Shoulder arthroscopy for shoulder instability In Barr J (ed): *American Academy of Orthopedic Surgeons instructional course lectures*, vol 38, Park Ridge, Ill, 1989, AAOS.
2. Altchek DW et al: T-plasty modification of the Bankart procedure for multidirectional instability of the anterior and inferior types, *J Bone Joint Surg* 73A:105, 1991.
3. Altchek DW et al: Arthroscopic labral debridement: a three-year follow-up study, *Am J Sports Med* 20:702, 1992.
4. Anderson D, Zuirbulis R, Ciullo J: Scapular manipulation for reduction of anterior shoulder dislocation, *Clin Orthop* 164:181, 1982.
5. Andrews JR, Carson WG, McLeod WD: Glenoid labrum tears related to the long head of the biceps, *Am J Sports Med* 13:337, 1985.
6. Andrews JR, Kupferman SP, Dillman CJ: Labral tears in throwing and racquet sports, *Clin Sports Med* 10(4):901, 1991.
7. Arciero RA et al: *Arthroscopic Bankart repair for acute, initial anterior shoulder dislocations*, Paper presented at Annual Meeting of the American Academy of Orthopaedic Surgeons, San Francisco, 1993.
8. Aronen JG, Regan K: Decreasing the incidence of recurrence of first time anterior shoulder dislocations with rehabilitation, *Am J Sports Med* 12:283, 1984.
9. Bach BR, Warren RF, Fronek J: Disruption of the lateral capsule of the shoulder: a cause of recurrent dislocation, *J Bone Joint Surg* 70B:274, 1988.
10. Bankart ASB: Recurrent or habitual dislocation of the shoulder-joint, *Br Med J* 2:1132, 1923.
11. Bankart ASB: The pathology and treatment of recurrent dislocation of the shoulder-joint, *Br J Surg* 26:23, 1938.
12. Belle RM, Hawkins RJ: Collagen typing and production in multidirectional instability of the shoulder, *Orthop Trans* 15:188, 1991.
13. Blasier RB, Guldberg RE, Rothman ED: Anterior shoulder stability: contributions of rotator cuff forces and the capsular lig-

aments in a cadaver model, *J Shoulder Elbow Surg* 1:140, 1992.

14. Bowen MK, Warren RF: Ligamentous control of shoulder stability based on selective cutting and static translation experiments, *Clin Sports Med* 10(4):757, 1991.
15. Bowen MK et al: Posterior subluxation of the glenohumeral joint treated by posterior stabilization, *Orthop Trans* 15(3):764, 1991.
16. Boyd HB, Sisk TD: Recurrent posterior dislocation of the shoulder, *J Bone Joint Surg* 54A:779, 1972.
17. Brems JJ: Anterior approach to posterior instability, *J Shoulder Elbow Surg* 2(suppl):S26, 1993.
18. Brewer BJ, Wubben RG, Carrera GF: Excessive retroversion of the glenoid cavity, *J Bone Joint Surg* 68A:724, 1986.
19. Brodsky JW, Tullos HW, Gartsman GM: Simplified posterior approach to the shoulder joint, *J Bone Joint Surg* 69A:773, 1987.
20. Browne AO et al: The influence of atmospheric pressure on shoulder stability, *Orthop Trans* 14:259, 1990.
21. Budd FW: Voluntary bilateral posterior dislocation of the shoulder joint, *Clin Orthop* 63:181, 1969.
22. Burkhead WZ, Rockwood CA: Treatment of instability of the shoulder with an exercise program, *J Bone Joint Surg* 74A:890, 1992.
23. Cook M, Richardson AB: Arthroscopic staple capsulorraphy for treatment of anterior shoulder instability, *Orthop Trans* 15:1, 1991.
24. Cooper DE et al: Anatomy, histology, and vascularity of the glenoid labrum: an anatomical study, *J Bone Joint Surg* 74A:46, 1992.
25. Cooper R, Brems J: The inferior capsular shift procedure for multidirectional instability of the shoulder, *J Bone Joint Surg* 74A:1516, 1992.
26. Coughlin L et al: Arthroscopic staple capsulorraphy for anterior shoulder instability, *Am J Sports Med* 20:253, 1992.
27. DePalma AF, Callery G, Bennett GA: Variational anatomy and degenerative lesions of the shoulder joint. In Blount W, Banks S (eds): *The American Academy of Orthopaedic Surgeons Instructional Course Lectures,* Ann Arbor, Mich, 1949, JW Edwards.
28. Detrisac DA: Arthroscopic shoulder staple capsulorraphy for traumatic anterior instability. In McGinty J (ed): *Operative arthroscopy,* New York, 1991, Raven Press.
29. Dickson JW, Devas MB: Bankart's operation for recurrent dislocation of the shoulder, *J Bone Joint Surg* 39B:114, 1957.
30. Fronek J, Warren RF, Bowen M: Posterior subluxation of the glenohumeral joint, *J Bone Joint Surg* 71A:205, 1989.
31. Galinat BJ, Howell SM, Kraft TA: The glenoid-posterior acromion angle: an accurate method of evaluating glenoid version, *Orthop Trans* 12:727, 1988.
32. Garth WP, Slappey CE, Ochs CW: Roentgenographic demonstration of the shoulder: the apical oblique projection: a technical note, *J Bone Joint Surg* 66A:1450, 1984.
33. Gibb TD et al: The effect of capsular venting on glenohumeral laxity, *Clin Orthop* 268:120, 1991.
34. Glousman R et al: Dynamic electromyographic analysis of the throwing shoulder with glenohumeral instability, *J Bone Joint Surg* 70A:220, 1988.
35. Gross ML et al: Magnetic resonance imaging of the glenoid labrum, *Am J Sports Med* 18:229, 1990.
36. Habermeyer P, Schuller U, Wiedemann E: The intra-articular pressure of the shoulder: an experimental study on the role of the glenoid labrum in stabilizing the joint, *Arthroscopy* 8:166, 1992.
37. Hall RH, Isaac F, Booth CR: Dislocations of the shoulder with special reference to accompanying small fractures, *J Bone Joint Surg* 41A:489, 1959.
38. Harryman DT II et al: Laxity of the normal glenohumeral joint: a qualitative in vivo assessment, *J Shoulder Elbow Surg* 1:66, 1992.
39. Harryman DT II et al: Role of the rotator interval capsule in passive motion and stability of the shoulder, *J Bone Joint Surg* 74A:53, 1992.
40. Hawkins RB: Arthroscopic stapling repair for shoulder instability: a retrospective study of 50 cases, *Arthroscopy* 5:122, 1989.

41. Hawkins RJ, Belle RM: Posterior instability of the shoulder. In Barr J (ed): *American Academy of Orthopaedic Surgeons Instructional Course Lectures,* vol 38, Park Ridge, Ill, 1989, AAOS.
42. Hawkins RB, Hawkins RJ: Failed anterior reconstruction in shoulder instability, *J Bone Joint Surg* 67B:709, 1985.
43. Hawkins RJ, Koppert G, Johnston G: Recurrent posterior instability (subluxation) of the shoulder, *J Bone Joint Surg* 66A:169, 1984.
44. Hawkins RJ, Kunkel SS, Nayak NK: Inferior capsular shift for multidirectional instability of the shoulder: 2-5 year follow-up, *Orthop Trans* 15:765, 1991.
45. Hawkins RJ, Mohtadi NGH: Controversy in anterior shoulder instability, *Clin Orthop* 272:152, 1991.
46. Helfet AJ: Coracoid transplantation for recurring dislocation of the shoulder, *J Bone Joint Surg* 40B:198, 1958.
47. Helmig P et al: Distal humeral migration as a component of multidirectional shoulder instability: an anatomical study in autopsy specimens, *Clin Orthop* 252:1990, 1990.
48. Hovelius L et al: Recurrences after initial dislocation of the shoulder: results of a prospective study of treatment, *J Bone Joint Surg* 65A:343, 1983.
49. Howell SM, Galinat BJ: The glenoid-labral socket: a constrained articular surface, *Clin Orthop* 243:122, 1989.
50. Hurley JA et al: Posterior shoulder instability: surgical versus conservative results with evaluation of glenoid version, *Am J Sports Med* 20:396, 1992.
51. Iannotti JP et al: Magnetic resonance imaging of the shoulder: sensitivity, specificity, and predictive value, *J Bone Joint Surg* 73A:17, 1991.
52. Iannotti JP et al: The normal glenohumeral relationships: an anatomical study of one hundred and forty shoulders, *J Bone Joint Surg* 74A:491, 1992.
53. Itoi E et al: Scapular inclination and inferior stability of the shoulder, *J Shoulder Elbow Surg* 1:131, 1992.
54. Jobe FW: Impingement problems in athletes. In Barr J (ed): *American Academy of Orthopaedic Surgeons Instructional Course Lectures,* vol 38, Park Ridge, Ill, 1989, AAOS.
55. Jobe FW, Kvitne RS: Shoulder pain in the overhead athlete: the relationship of anterior instability and rotator cuff impingement, *Orthop Rev* 18:963, 1989.
56. Jobe FW et al: Anterior capsulolabral reconstruction of the shoulder in athletes in overhead sports, *Am J Sports Med* 19:428, 1991.
57. Johnston HH et al: A complication of posterior glenoid osteotomy for recurrent posterior shoulder instability, *Clin Orthop* 187:147, 1984.
58. Klein AH, France JC: Measurement of brachial plexus strain in arthroscopy of the shoulder, *Arthroscopy* 3:45, 1983.
59. Kocher ET: Eine neue reduction methode fur schulterverrenkung, *Berl Klin Wochenschr* 7:101, 1870.
60. Kronberg M, Brostrom L-A: Humeral head retroversion in patients with unstable humeroscapular joints, *Clin Orthop* 260:207, 1990.
61. Kronberg M, Brostrom L-A, Nemeth G: Differences in shoulder muscle activity between patients with generalized joint laxity and normal controls, *Clin Orthop* 269:181, 1991.
62. Kumar VP, Balasubramianium P: The role of atmospheric pressure in stabilizing the shoulder: an experimental study, *J Bone Joint Surg* 67B:719, 1985.
63. Leslie JT, Ryan TJ: Anterior axillary approach to the shoulder joint, *J Bone Joint Surg* 44A:1193, 1962.
64. Lippitt SB et al: Glenohumeral stability from concavity-compression: a quantitative analysis, *J Shoulder Elbow Surg* 2:27, 1993.
65. Luckey CA: Recurrent dislocation of the shoulder: modification of the Bankart capsulorraphy, *Am J Surg* 77:220, 1949.
66. Magnuson PB, Stack JK: Recurrent dislocation of the shoulder, *JAMA* 123:889, 1943.
67. Maki S, Gruen T: Anthropometric studies of the glenohumeral joint, *Trans Orthop Res Soc* 1:173, 1976.
68. Malgaigne JF: *Traite des fractures et des luxations,* Paris, 1855, JB Bulliere.
69. Matsen FA, Harryman DT, Sidles JA: Mechanics of glenohumeral instability, *Clin Sports Med* 10(4):783, 1991.

70. Matsen FA, Thomas SC, Rockwood CA: Anterior glenohumeral instability. In Rockwood C, Matsen F (eds): *The shoulder,* Philadelphia, 1990, WB Saunders.
71. Matthews LS et al: Anterior portal selection for shoulder arthroscopy, *Arthroscopy* 1:33, 1985.
72. Matthews LS et al: Arthroscopic staple capsulorraphy for recurrent anterior shoulder instability, *Arthroscopy* 4:106, 1988.
73. McKernan DJ et al: *Significance of a partial and full Bankart lesion: a biomechanical study,* Paper presented at Annual Meeting of the Orthopaedic Research Society, Las Vegas, 1989.
74. McKernan DJ et al: The characterization of rotator cuff muscle forces and their effect on glenohumeral joint stability: a biomechanical study, *Orthop Trans* 14:237, 1990.
75. McLaughlin HL: Posterior dislocations of the shoulder, *J Bone Joint Surg* 34A:584, 1952.
76. Morgan CD: Arthroscopic transglenoid Bankart suture repair, *Oper Techn Orthop* 1:171, 1991.
77. Morgan CD, Bodenstab AB: Arthroscopic Bankart suture repair: technique and early results, *Arthroscopy* 3:111, 1987.
78. Morrey BF, Janes JM: Anterior dislocation of the shoulder: long-term follow-up of the Putti-Platt and Bankart procedures, *J Bone Joint Surg* 58A:252, 1976.
79. Moseley HJ, Overgaard B: The anterior capsular mechanism in recurrent dislocation of the shoulder: morphological and clinical studies with special reference to the glenoid labrum and glenohumeral ligaments, *J Bone Joint Surg* 44B:913, 1962.
80. Neer CS, Foster CR: Inferior capsular shift for involuntary inferior and multidirectional instability of the shoulder: a preliminary report, *J Bone Joint Surg* 62A:897, 1980.
81. Neer CS II: Displaced proximal humeral fractures. Part II. Treatment of three-part and four-part displacement, *J Bone Joint Surg* 52A:1077, 1970.
82. Neer CS II: *Shoulder reconstruction,* Philadelphia, 1990, WB Saunders.
83. Nelson MC et al: Evaluation of the painful shoulder: a prospective comparison of magnetic resonance imaging, computerized tomographic arthrography, ultrasonography, and operative findings, *J Bone Joint Surg* 73A:707, 1991.
84. Neviaser RJ, Neviaser TJ, Neviaser JS: Concurrent rupture of the rotator cuff and anterior dislocation of the shoulder in the older patient, *J Bone Joint Surg* 70A:1308, 1988.
85. Nicola T: Anterior dislocation of the shoulder: the role of the anterior capsule, *J Bone Joint Surg* 24:614, 1942.
86. Nobuhara K, Ikeda H: *Rotator cuff interval lesion, Clin Orthop* 223:44, 1987.
87. O'Brien SJ, Warren RF, Schwartz E: Anterior shoulder instability, *Orthop Clin North Am* 18:395, 1987.
88. O'Brien SJ et al: Capsular restraints to anterior/posterior motion of the shoulder, *Orthop Trans* 12:143, 1988.
89. O'Brien SJ et al: The anatomy and histology of the inferior glenohumeral ligament complex of the shoulder, *Am J Sports Med* 18:449, 1990.
90. Osmond-Clarke H: Habitual dislocation of the shoulder: the Putti-Platt operation, *J Bone Joint Surg* 30B:19, 1948.
91. Pagnani MJ et al: *Effect of the long head of the biceps brachii on glenohumeral translation,* Paper presented at The Hospital for Special Surgery Fellows' Research Symposium, New York, 1993.
92. Pagnani MJ et al: *Effect of superior labral lesions on glenohumeral translation,* Paper presented at The Hospital for Special Surgery Fellows' Research Symposium, New York, 1993.
93. Pagnani MJ et al: *Arthroscopic shoulder stabilization using transglenoid sutures: an end-result study,* Paper presented at the Annual Meeting of the American Academy of Orthopaedic Surgeons, Orlando, 1995.
94. Pavlov H et al: The roentgenographic evaluation of anterior shoulder instability, *Clin Orthop* 194:153, 1985.
95. Perthes G: Ueber operationen der habituellen schulterluxation, *Deutsche Ztschr Chir* 85:199, 1906.
96. Reeves B: Experiments on the tensile strength of the anterior capsular structures in man, *J Bone Joint Surg* 50B:858, 1968.
97. Regan WD et al: Comparative functional analysis of the Bristow, Magnuson-Stack, and Putti-Platt procedures for recurrent dislocation of the shoulder, *Am J Sports Med* 17:42, 1989.
98. Roukos JR, Feagin JA, Abbott HG: Modified axillary roentgenogram: a useful adjunct in the diagnosis of recurrent instability of the shoulder, *Clin Orthop* 82:84, 1972.
99. Rowe CR: Prognosis in dislocations of the shoulder, *J Bone Joint Surg* 38A:957, 1956.
100. Rowe CR, Patel D, Southmayd WW: The Bankart procedure: a long-term end-result study, *J Bone Joint Surg* 60A:1, 1978.
101. Rowe CR, Pierce DS, Clark JS: Voluntary dislocation of the shoulder: a preliminary report on a clinical, electromyographic, and psychiatric study of twenty-six patients, *J Bone Joint Surg* 55A:445, 1973.
102. Rowe CR, Sakellarides HT: Factors related to recurrences of anterior dislocations of the shoulder, *Clin Orthop* 20:40, 1961.
103. Rowe CR, Zarins B: Recurrent transient subluxation of the shoulder, *J Bone Joint Surg* 63A:863, 1981.
104. Rowe CR, Zarins B: Chronic unreduced dislocations of the shoulder, *J Bone Joint Surg* 64A:494, 1982.
105. Rowe CR, Zarins B, Ciullo JV: Recurrent anterior dislocation of the shoulder after surgical repair, *J Bone Joint Surg* 66A:159, 1984.
106. Sachs RA, Lane JG, Riehl B: *Arthroscopic staple capsulorraphy: a long-term follow-up,* Paper presented at Annual Meeting of American Academy of Orthopaedic Surgeons, Washington, DC, 1992.
107. Saha AK: Dynamic stability of the glenohumeral joint, *Acta Orthop Scand* 42:491, 1971.
108. Samilson RL, Prieto V: Dislocation arthropathy of the shoulder, *J Bone Joint Surg* 65A:456, 1983.
109. Schauder KS, Tullos HS: Role of the coracoid bone block in the modified Bristow procedure, *Am J Sports Med* 20:31, 1992.
110. Schwartz E et al: Posterior shoulder instability, *Orthop Clin North Am* 18(3):409, 1987.
111. Simonet WT, Cofield RA: Prognosis in anterior shoulder dislocation, *Am J Sports Med* 12:19, 1984.
112. Snyder SJ, Karzel RP, Del Pizzo W: SLAP lesions of the shoulder, *Arthroscopy* 6:274, 1990.
113. Soslowsky LJ et al: Articular geometry of the glenohumeral joint, *Clin Orthop* 285:181, 1992.
114. Soslowsky LJ et al: Quantitation of in situ contact areas at the glenohumeral joint: a biomechanical study, *J Orthop Res* 10:524, 1992.
115. Speer KP, Hannafin JA, Warren RF: *An evaluation of the relocation test,* Paper presented at Annual Meeting of American Shoulder and Elbow Surgeons, San Francisco, 1993.
116. Speer KP et al: A biomechanical evaluation of the Bankart lesion, *J Bone Joint Surg* (in press).
117. Terry GC et al: The stabilizing function of passive shoulder restraints, *Am J Sports Med* 19:26, 1991.
118. Tibone JT, Ting A: Capsulorraphy with a staple for recurrent posterior dislocation of the shoulder, *J Bone Joint Surg* 72A:999, 1990.
119. Torg JS et al: A modified Bristow-Helfet-May procedure for recurrent dislocation of the shoulder: report of two hundred and twelve cases, *J Bone Joint Surg* 69A:904, 1987.
120. Townsend H et al: Electromyographic analysis of the glenohumeral muscles during a baseball rehabilitation program, *Am J Sports Med* 19:264, 1991.
121. Turkel SJ et al: Stabilizing mechanisms preventing anterior dislocation of the glenohumeral joint, *J Bone Joint Surg* 63A:1208, 1981.
122. Uhthoff HK, Piscopo M: Anterior capsular redundancy of the shoulder: congenital or traumatic? an embryological study, *J Bone Joint Surg* 67B:363, 1985.
123. Vellet AD, Munk PL, Marks P: Imaging techniques of the shoulder, *Clin Sports Med* 10(4):712, 1991.
124. Viek P, Bell BT: The Bankart shoulder reconstruction: the use of pull-out wires and other practical details, *J Bone Joint Surg* 41A:236, 1959.
125. Warner JJP et al: Arthroscopic Bankart repair with an absorbable, cannulated fixation device, *Orthop Trans* 15:761, 1991.
126. Warner JJP et al: Scapulothoracic motion in normal shoulders and shoulders with glenohumeral instability and impingement syndrome: a study using moire topographic analysis, *Clin Orthop* 285:191, 1992.

127. Warner JJP et al: Static capsuloligamentous constraints to superior-inferior translation of the glenohumeral joint, *Am J Sports Med* 20:675, 1992.

128. Warren RF: Instability of the shoulder in throwing athletes. In Murray J (ed): *American Academy of Orthopaedic Surgeons instructional course lectures,* vol 34, St Louis, 1985, Mosby.

129. Warren RF, Kornblatt IB, Marchand R: Static factors affecting posterior shoulder stability, *Orthop Trans* 8:89, 1984.

130. Weber SC, Caspari RB: A biomechanical evaluation of restraints to posterior shoulder dislocation, *Arthroscopy* 5:115, 1989.

131. Wheeler JH et al: Arthroscopic versus nonoperative treatment of acute shoulder dislocations in young athletes, *Arthroscopy* 5:213, 1989.

132. Wickiewicz TL, Pagnani MJ, Kennedy K: Rehabilitation of the unstable shoulder, *Sports Med Arthroscopy Rev* 1:227, 1993.

133. Wiley AM: Arthroscopy for shoulder instability and a technique for arthroscopic repair, *Arthroscopy* 4:25, 1988.

134. Yahiro MA, Matthews LA: Arthroscopic stabilization procedures for recurrent anterior shoulder instability, *Orthop Rev* 11:1161, 1989.

135. Yoneda B, Welsh RP, MacIntosh DL: Conservative treatment of shoulder dislocation in young males, *J Bone Joint Surg* 64B:254, 1982.

136. Young CA, Rockwood CA: Complications of a failed Bristow procedure and their management, *J Bone Joint Surg* 73A:969, 1991.

137. Zarins B, Rowe CR, Stone JW: Shoulder instability: management of failed reconstructions. In Barr J (ed): *American Academy of Orthopaedic Surgeons Instructional Course Lectures,* vol 38, Park Ridge, Ill, 1989, AAOS.

138. Zuckerman JD, Matsen FA III: Complications about the glenohumeral joint related to the use of screws and staples, *J Bone Joint Surg* 66A:175, 1984.

CHAPTER 8 Impingement and Rotator Cuff Lesions

Keith Watson

The impingement syndrome is one, if not the most, common cause of pain and dysfunction in the athlete's shoulder.[2,3,10] The pathomechanics of this syndrome implicate activities that repetitively place the arm in overhead positions. The majority of athletes who manifest this condition participate in baseball, swimming, and tennis, but it is by no means confined to these sports. The importance of its recognition is that impingement is often a progressive condition that, if recognized and treated early, can have a more favorable outcome. Delay in recognition and treatment can allow secondary changes to occur, with resultant limitations in treatment options and expectations.

PATHOPHYSIOLOGY

In response to the demands placed on it, the shoulder has evolved from a massive appendage supporting the weight of the trunk to a lightweight, fully suspended structure that allows the greatest range of motion of any joint in the body. To accomplish this, the anatomic arrangement demands a precise balance among the bony and soft tissues. As in a finely tuned machine, the tolerances are quite precise. Specifically, the rotator cuff functions essentially to maintain a force-couple with the deltoid that secures the humeral head in the glenoid. When this arrangement is compromised, the pull of the deltoid forces the humeral head proximally and the rotator cuff can be compressed (impinged) beneath the unyielding coracoacromial arch.[9] Neer[6] proposed a progressive staging of this condition that helps define treatment options as well. According to this scheme an initial injury produces acute changes in the rotator cuff, such as edema and hemorrhage. These changes, which are transient and fully reversible, are considered Stage 1. In response to repeated irritation over time, fibrosis and chronic tendinitis may develop—a subacute condition considered Stage 2. Finally, in response to persistent impingement over time, there are both adaptive and degenerative structural changes in the rotator cuff, bursa, acromial arch, and even the greater tuberosity. Once irreversible structural alterations have occurred, the process is then considered Stage 3.

Because the demands an athlete places on the shoulder may exceed those of the average person, the degree and progression of the impingement process are accelerated. Because bone reacts and adapts more slowly than soft tissues, there may be an accelerated rate of wear to the soft tissues that is not reflected by changes in the bony structures. Therefore when dealing with the athlete, some have found it convenient to modify these stages. Stage 3 represents relatively small rotator cuff defects, whereas an additional Stage 4 subclassification represents tears larger than 1 cm.[5] In essence the condition is not necessarily different in athletes, but the body's response is more limited.

What is not clear is who develops progressive impingement and why. Certainly not everyone who experiences injury to the shoulder or who participates in activities that require overhead arm movement acquires impingement, just as nerve root compression will not develop in everyone who experiences a ruptured disk. Current work suggests there are predisposing anatomic variations that affect the response of the body to injury or activity.[1]

Variations in the shape and slope of the acromion have been implicated. The concept of the **supraspinatus outlet** has been proposed to describe this confined space through which the supraspinatus is exposed to impingement.[7] The presence of bony intrusions (e.g., subacromial spurs, inferior acromioclavicular osteophytes, even the presence of an unfused acromial epiphysis) into a supraspinatus outlet is associated with a high probability of impingement (Fig. 8-1). Therefore it can be postulated that an injury (either microtraumatic or macrotraumatic) may occur with resultant reaction in the rotator cuff.

FIG. 8-1. Usual cause of subacromial impingement is narrowing of the supraspinatus outlet or variation in the shape or slope of the acromion. **A,** Anterior acromial spur formation. **B,** Prominence of the distal end of the clavicle or the inferior edge of the acromioclavicular joint. **C,** Flattening of the slope of the acromion. **D,** Nonunion or malunion of the acromion is a less common cause. (From Poppen NK: Soft-tissue lesions of the shoulder. In Chapman MW, ed: *Operative orthopaedics*, Philadelphia, 1988, JB Lippincott.)

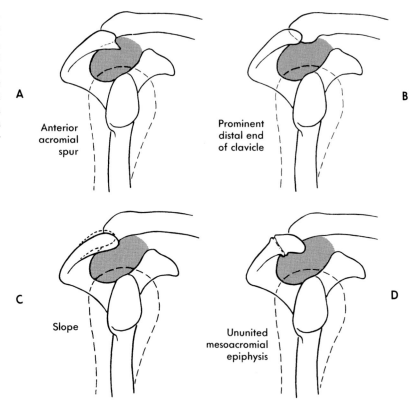

However, in individuals who are predisposed by a compromised supraspinatus outlet the condition does not resolve but becomes one of a viscious cycle, with further use causing further irritation. This concept can explain the predilection for supraspinatus involvement, as well as the variations in presentation with regard to acute injury versus overuse. The concept of impingement can also explain the relationships among bursitis, tendinitis, and rotator cuff tears.

Factors contributing to impingement syndrome

- Shape and slope of acromion
- Subacromial spurs
- Inferior acromioclavicular osteophytes
- Unfused acromial epiphysis

CLINICAL EVALUATION

Diagnosing the cause of shoulder pain in the athlete is difficult because it is almost exclusively a clinical diagnosis. This is especially true for impingement and instability, which are the two most common pathologic conditions.

History

A history of recurrent episodes of pain associated with a particular activity is usually what causes the athlete to seek the treatment of a physician. Often the athlete has been told by the trainer that it is strained or it is bursitis. The usual local remedies—heat, ice, salves, and rest—have not been effective. Quite likely there is no pain unless the athlete is involved in play. Sometimes there is a dull background ache when the athlete is at rest. Most athletes have a history of some earlier injury but often are not sure which shoulder was involved. Specific questions regarding fatigue and feelings of looseness may help in directing the examination to rule out instability. It is not unusual for patients with impingement to notice easy fatigability rather than sensations of slipping.

Inspection

Initial examination of the patient should include a visual scan from behind. Specific attention should be paid to identify atrophy of muscle groups, prominence of the acromioclavicular joint, and asymmetry of posture. Active elevation and abduction of both arms should reveal any disturbance of the normal scapulohumeral rhythm and the presence of any winging. Palpation can then elicit any areas of sensitivity. Tenderness is not specific for impingement but would be consistent at the anterior acromion, along the coracoacromial ligament, and at the greater tuberosity. It is particularly important to assess the acromioclavicular joint in this way. The coracoid process is generally tender whenever there is any shoulder problem and is therefore not necessarily a helpful sign. Tenderness at the biceps groove is also consistent with suspected impingement because most episodes of bicipital tendinitis are thought to be secondary to impingement.

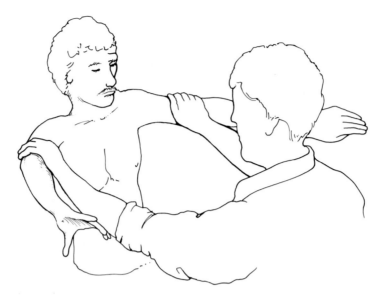

FIG. 8-2. Supraspinatus test. Patient upright, shoulder 90 degrees of abduction, 30 degrees of horizontal adduction, and full internal rotation. Patient maintains position against downward resistance. (From Jobe FW, Jobe CM: *Clin Orthop* 173:117, 1983.)

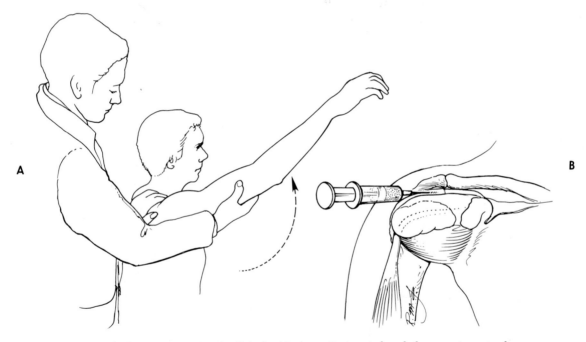

FIG. 8-3. A, Impingement sign is elicited with the patient seated and the examiner standing. Scapular rotation is prevented with one hand while the other hand raises the arm in forced forward elevation. This maneuver produces pain in patients with impingement lesions. **B,** Impingement injection test is useful in separating impingement lesions of all stages from other causes. (From Neer CS II: *Clin Orthop* 173:70, 1983.)

Arc of Motion Evaluation

The presence of a painful arc of motion is a significant finding. As the arm is lowered from 120 degrees to 70 degrees, maximum tension is developed in the rotator cuff. If this produces pain, it is suggestive of tendinitis. Jobe and Jobe[5] have further defined this part of the examination to better isolate the supraspinatus. With the shoulder at 90 degrees of abduction the arm is then brought forward 30 degrees, in line with the spine of the scapula (i.e., the scapular plane), and then internally rotated so the thumb then points to the floor (Fig. 8-2). Muscle testing against resistance is more likely to elicit discomfort in patients whose symptoms occur only with strenuous effort.

Impingement Sign

An impingement sign should also be sought (i.e., the production of pain when the arm is forcibly elevated in

the forward plane while the scapula is stabilized) (Fig. 8-3, *A*). This actually compresses the irritated tissues and is frequently positive in impingement. If this sign is absent, the diagnosis of impingement should be suspected. A full passive range of motion is necessary for the accuracy of the clinical examination. If stiffness is present, it should be addressed vigorously with stretching exercises and the patient reevaluated. Stiffness can occur as a result of impingement but also from other causes.

Strength Evaluation

Muscle testing should be undertaken with close attention to the external rotators. The majority of external rotation power comes from the infraspinatus and teres minor. Involvement of the rotator cuff can cause dysfunction either through direct injury or pain. The identification of external rotation weakness indicates a more involved condition.

Injection Test

Finally, if a painful arc, a positive impingement sign, weakness of external rotation—any or all—is identified, then a subacromial injection with a local anesthetic agent—the injection test—is recommended to support the diagnosis (Fig. 8-3, *B*). In the absence of any additional contributing factors (e.g., acromioclavicular joint stiffness, radiculitis) the injection should significantly reduce the sensitivity of the subacromial space, usually eliminating painful arc and the impingement sign and restoring external rotation power.

DIAGNOSTIC STUDIES
Radiographs

Although subacromial impingement is basically a clinical diagnosis in the later stages of the condition, there can be some diagnostic findings that are corroborative. Bony changes are necessarily slow to develop and are less likely to be of help in the athlete. Changes that are typically seen in the more advanced impingement stages include the development of an anterior acromial spur (an actual morphologic change in the origin of the coracoacromial ligament in response to increased tension in the ligament, much as the heel spur develops in the plantar fascia). Reciprocal changes are seen on the greater tuberosity with the cortical fragmentation and irregularity. Finally, with large defects in the rotator cuff, there may be a decrease of the acromiohumeral interval as the humeral head buttonholes through the defect.

For most athletes, however, these changes are not found because the dysfunction represented by such changes would have prevented participation much earlier.[10] However, there are some abnormalities detectable on plain radiographs that would support a predisposition to the development of impingement in an athlete. These areas should be closely examined and require three different radiographic projections, in addition to routine views. A good examination of the acromioclavicular joint is important. It is one of the joints to demonstrate earliest degenerative change, and identification of osteophytic proliferation is important because it can compro-

mise the supraspinatus outlet. Routine views of the shoulder, however, are often overpenetrated, and frequently there is overlapping of bone that prevents a fair assessment of this joint. It is recommended that a **10- to 15-degree cephalad projection** be obtained with less penetration. Second, evaluation of the supraspinatus outlet and the profile of the acromion can be of benefit. The identification of a Type III acromion would support a clincal diagnosis of impingement. The **outlet view** is obtained by shooting along the spine of the scapula (as is done in the lateral scapular view of the trauma series) and angling the tube caudad 0 to 10 degrees, depending on the contour of the patient. Third, an **axillary view** is recommended to rule out the presence of an unfused acromial epiphysis with an increased incidence of impingement.

Radiographic signs of impingement

- Anterior acromial spur
- Subchondral sclerosis/cysts of greater tuberosity

Ancillary Tests

Additional diagnostic studies may be of benefit to pin down the diagnosis or better assess the condition of the soft tissues. **Ultrasound** has been recently popularized as an inexpensive and noninvasive technique to evaluate the rotator cuff. For full-thickness tears more than 1 cm in size, it has achieved some success. There is disagreement, however, about its usefulness and accuracy with small tears (less than 1 cm) and partial or incomplete tears of the rotator cuff. In addition, there is some degree of operator dependency with a significant learning curve, which may preclude its usefulness in the general setting. Similarly, **magnetic resonance imaging (MRI)** is an excellent noninvasive technique, but it also has shortcomings, similar to those of ultrasound, in addition to requiring unusual and sophisticated equipment and being relatively expensive (see Chapter 4).

The importance of **arthrography** in evaluating the condition of the rotator cuff is well recognized, but unless there is a full-thickness tear, arthrography is not likely to be helpful. In the athletic population arthrography should be reserved for situations in which there is significant weakness, a major acute injury, or a failure to respond to conservative treatment. Other invasive testing, such as **computed tomography (CT) arthrography** and **bursography,** have not produced refinements in the diagnosis of subacromial impingement.

Once again, the diagnosis of subacromial impingement may be made solely on clinical grounds and, especially in the athletic population, diagnostic tests may be negative.

TREATMENT

Once the diagnosis of subacromial impingement has been made, treatment decisions must be undertaken.

The desire of the athlete to remain competitive makes this process more difficult. Although this desire is beneficial when it comes to applying oneself to a rehabilitative regimen, it can conflict with the dictates of physiology regarding healing and recovery times. Whether athletic or not, almost all patients want to consider themselves quick healers, and the athlete more than anyone must confront this time barrier.

Initial treatment must be directed at resting the irritated shoulder. This does not necessarily mean complete inactivity, and certainly not bracing or immobilization, but rather discontinuance of the activity that precipitated the condition. At the same time it is important to maintain mobility with stretching techniques and muscle tone with isometric and isokinetic exercises that are below the range of sensitivity. In addition, a short course of a non-steroidal antiinflammatory medication may be helpful in decreasing sensitivity and promoting rapid recovery.

A subacromial injection performed to clarify the diagnosis (injection test) can often be combined with a cortisone derivative to decrease the irritation in the subacromial bursa. (Such injections are made into the bursal space only and never within the tendon tissues). Such injections, although they can provide significant alleviation in symptoms, must be used quite sparingly and only in the acute phase of the condition. Once the acute phase has subsided and the athlete is pain free with full mobility, then the activity may be pursued, but with attention to correcting poor mechanics or techniques that may have initiated the process. It is helpful for the athlete (as well as coaches and trainers) to understand the possible causes of the condition to help identify any easily correctable component. It is important to detect this condition in the early stages, when treatment can be most effective, and to stress the importance of gradual resumption of play, with proper conditioning ahead of time.

Once stiffness and sensitivity have been overcome, then attention should be directed toward recovering tone and strength (see Chapter 11). This is accomplished with a series of exercises performed within the comfort range and not in the impingement arc. Allowance of sufficient time for tissue recovery is essential before the athlete returns to the sport. One of the most common mistakes made is the athlete's attempt to return to the sport too early. The only contraindication to at least 9 months of conservative treatment is the presence of a full-thickness defect in the rotator cuff. (Operative treatment may then be indicated to prevent further progression.)

Conservative treatment must be pursued for an extended period because it is the best chance the athlete has to return to his or her sport. The result of operative decompression for high-level athletes has not been adequate to present this as a reliable option.

If conservative measures are inadequate, the athlete faces a difficult choice. He or she must be counseled that more aggressive treatment has proved effective for decreasing pain, but return to preinjury level of competition is not as predictable. The goal of further treatment is, of course, to remove the impingement. Unfortunately, this requires resection of the anterior acromion and coracoacromial ligament.[8] The anatomic sites of impingement have been well identified over the last 2 decades, and the importance of the anterior acromion and coracoacromial ligament has been emphasized.

Since the work of Neer[6] in the early 1970s, the anterior acromioplasty has taken the forefront in the treatment of advanced subacromial impingement. Attempts to treat early stages of the condition with coracracromial ligament division alone have not withstood the test of time. Certainly, in this younger population it would be attractive to accomplish adequate results using a soft-tissue procedure that would necessarily have a shorter period of rehabilitation. Arthroscopy has been shown to be able to remove adequate amounts of the anterior acromion and, although early reports are encouraging, the long-term results are unknown. The open procedure described by Neer results in a significant surface of exposed bone, which necessitates a vigorous and prolonged period of rehabilitation. This, along with the unpredictability of the functional outcome, means this procedure should be approached as a final option in the high-level athlete. Obviously this is not as serious a concern to the recreational athlete.

The presence of a full-thickness tear of the rotator cuff as diagnosed by arthrography or arthroscopy dictates decompression and repair or discontinuance. The pathophysiology of the condition precludes healing, and continued participation in the sport would exacerbate the situation. In this situation the athlete is usually caught between the proverbial rock and a hard place.

DISCUSSION

The majority of the work regarding subacromial impingement has been developed working with the older patient (over 40 years of age) in whom this entity is much more likely to occur. Extrapolation of the theories and treatment options into the younger population may not be valid. Certainly, younger individuals do develop rotator cuff tears, and excessive demands placed on an athlete's shoulder may accelerate the pathologic process so that these advanced changes are seen at a younger age. However, a complicated spectrum of shoulder pathology has been implicated in the development of rotator cuff lesions in some young high-level athletes (18 to 35 years of age).[4] This concept identifies a select group of very high–performance throwing athletes who are at risk for developing anterior instability secondary to repetitive microtrauma. The inefficiency of the rotator cuff allows excessive migration of the humeral head, producing subacromial impingement and (secondarily) damage to the rotator cuff, which from all outward appearances seems to be typical of impingement. The problem, however, is not adequately addressed by treatment for impingement (either conservative or surgical). Treatment of these unique individuals must be directed toward improving the stability of the shoulder and efficiency of the rotator cuff. If conservative measures are inadequate, then it is recommended that stabilization be carried out surgically, but not decompression (see Chapters 7 and 33). It must be pointed out, though, that this is a special subset of athletes involved at a very high intensity, and most ath-

letes with signs and symptoms of impingement have the classic form.

SUMMARY

The athlete's shoulder is a challenging problem for the sports medicine physician. Many of these patients manifest problems of attrition and degeneration not expected or anticipated at their age. Because they must often function at the limits of their capabilities, the chance of a successful result is markedly diminished. The range of shoulder problems attributable to subacromial impingement (bursitis, tendinitis, rotator cuff tears, frozen shoulder, bicipital tendinitis) makes the shoulder a likely candidate for many athletes' difficulties.

By far, the majority of impingement problems, if identified and treated early, can be resolved with conservative measures. The key is awareness. There is a recognized difference in the impact of the impingement syndrome on the high-level athlete as opposed to the recreational athlete. There is necessarily a greater flexibility in the treatment of the recreational athlete with regard to time and expectations. Unfortunately, the high-level athlete who has the greatest need for a gradual and prolonged recovery period is not in a position to accept this approach.

The emphasis must be on rehabilitation and conservative treatment for the high-level athlete. Operative decompression should be considered when there is a full-thickness defect of unsuccessful conservative treatment for 9 to 12 months. The athlete must understand that operative decompression is effective in the reduction of pain but not predictable in regard to return of function.

REFERENCES

1. Bigliani LU et al: Morphology of the acromion and its relationship to rotator cuff tears, *Orthop Trans* 10:228, 1986.
2. Hawkins RJ, Kennedy JC: Impingement syndrome in athletes, *Am J Sports Med* 8:151, 1980.
3. Jackson PW: Chronic rotator cuff impingement in the throwing athlete, *Am J Sports Med* 4:231, 1976.
4. Jobe FW: Impingement problems in the athlete. In AAOS: *Instructional course lectures,* vol 35, St Louis, 1989, Mosby.
5. Jobe FW, Jobe CM: Painful athletic injuries of the shoulder, *Clin Orthop* 173:117, 1983.
6. Neer CS II: Impingement lesions, *Clin Orthop* 173:70, 1983.
7. Neer CS II, Poppen NK: The supraspinatus outlet, *Orthop Trans* 11:234, 1982.
8. Penny JW, Welsh RP: Shoulder impingement syndrome in athletes and their surgical management, *Am J Sports Med* 9:11, 1981.
9. Post M, Cohen J: Impingement syndrome: a review of late stage II and early stage III lesions, *Clin Orthop* 207:126, 1986.
10. Tibone JE et al: Surgical treatment of tears of the rotator cuff in athletes *J Bone Joint Surg* 68A:887, 1986.

CHAPTER 9

Overview of Soft-Tissue Injuries of the Shoulder

Allen B. Richardson

The diagnosis and treatment of athletic injuries to the upper extremity involve the soft tissues, including muscles, tendons, ligaments, bursae, and fibrous (capsular) structures. Primary bony injuries are much less common.

The shoulder joint is unique in that the articular surface of the humeral head is large in relation to the glenoid fossa, resulting in an inherently unstable joint. This permits a global motion of the shoulder joint, which allows the performance of many sports activities. It also results in a joint that must be stabilized and mobilized by the surrounding soft tissues. In simple terms, the capsule and its ligaments hold the humeral head and glenoid together; the labra expand the effective size of the glenoid while maintaining flexibility of the rim of the shoulder socket; and the surrounding muscles provide the motor units to carry the shoulder through a global range of motion. A description and discussion of dysfunc-

tion of these three soft-tissue groups in the athletic population are the subject of this chapter.

ADHESIVE CAPSULITIS

Commonly known as frozen shoulder,[67] this disease process is characterized by rapidly progressive limitation of shoulder motion, with increasing pain diffusely about the shoulder. It is often preceded by a relatively minor trauma, which usually is not expected to cause an inflammatory or fibrous reaction but does engender the short period of immobility common to patients with this disorder. This condition is unique to the shoulder joint; although adhesions and lack of range of motion occur in other joints such as the knee and elbow, they always follow a significant injury or surgical procedure in those joints.

Although adhesive capsulitis is uncommon in patients under 40 years of age, it certainly should remain in the differential diagnosis of the stiff shoulder. Other associated disease processes such as cervical disk disease, hyperthyroidism, pulmonary disorders, and diabetes mellitus should be considered as antecedent causes.

The diagnosis is usually easily made on the basis of a typical history and examination of the shoulder. Radiographs should be obtained to rule out other entities (degenerative arthritis). Computed tomography (CT) and magnetic resonance imaging (MRI) scans are not productive or helpful. An arthrogram shows decreased capacity of the shoulder capsule but is not usually necessary to make the diagnosis.

The pathologic condition of adhesive capsulitis seems to lie with inflammation of the glenohumeral joint, followed by capsular adhesions. Arthroscopy of the shoulder joint[92,96] with adhesive capsulitis reveals patchy, matted, vascular granulation tissue. The most constant location of these changes is the area surrounding the entrance to the subscapularis bursa anteriorly, including the area of attachment of the long head of biceps brachii and the superior glenoid labrum. The infraglenoid recess is not involved or obliterated, and there are usually no intraarticular adhesions.

The goal of treatment is to restore shoulder range of motion. Most surgeons first recommend a course of vigorous range of motion exercises. If this is unsuccessful

over a specified period (usually 4 to 6 weeks), a manipulation of the shoulder under anesthesia greatly increases range of motion. An alternative to this method, especially in severe cases, is to proceed with manipulation immediately followed by range of motion exercises. Arthroscopy has not been shown to enhance the long-term results of simple manipulation and therefore is not recommended. The efficacy of injectable, intraarticular corticosteroids is a subject of controversy.

Once shoulder range of motion is achieved, the patient should be advised to continue a series of home exercises designed to maintain that range of motion. Recurrence of adhesive capsulitis is rare.

IMPINGEMENT SYNDROME

Commonly known as bursitis, cuffitis, and supraspinatus syndrome,[18,19] impingement syndrome is the most common soft-tissue injury of the shoulder for which an athlete seeks treatment. The work of Neer[62] has provided great enlightenment to all surgeons in this area.

Anatomy

The rotator cuff (made up of the subscapularis, supraspinatus, infraspinatus, and teres minor muscles) inserts like a cowl onto the humeral head. The overlying acromion serves as the bony attachment for the deltoid muscle; it also protects the rotator cuff from direct blows. The coracoacromial ligament is simply a nonossified extension of the acromion anteriorly, spanning a gap between two parts of the same bone (the acromion and the coracoid process). As a soft-tissue structure it allows for full forward flexion of the upper extremity, while still acting as a roof to the humeral head, preventing unrestricted forward elevation of the arm.

The origins of the rotator cuff muscles on the scapula are slightly caudad to their insertions on the humerus, and all tend to depress and rotate the humeral head in relation to the glenoid (Fig. 9-1). This depressive function normally helps prevent the humeral head from migrating upward and impinging the overlying acromion and coracoacromial ligament. Indeed, in older patients one of the radiographic signs of a nonfunctioning rotator cuff is elevation of the humeral head relative to the glenoid (Fig. 9-2).[94]

Rathbun and MacNab[74] have demonstrated a tenuous vascular supply to the anterior rotator cuff, specifically the area of insertion of the supraspinatus and the long biceps tendon. Both structures come into contact with the overlying coracoacromial ligament with forward flexion of the shoulder during overhead activities.

Bigliani, Morrison, and April[17] have described three anatomic configurations of the acromion. A Type I acromion is characterized by a flat or convex undersurface (17.1%); a Type II acromion has a curved undersurface (42.9%); and a Type III acromion has an anterior hook (39.3%). Their clinical studies conclude that anterior im-

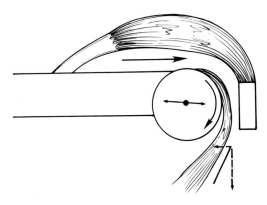

FIG. 9-1. Mechanics of humeral head motion. With the arm fully adducted, contraction of the deltoid muscle leads to superior migration of the humeral head.

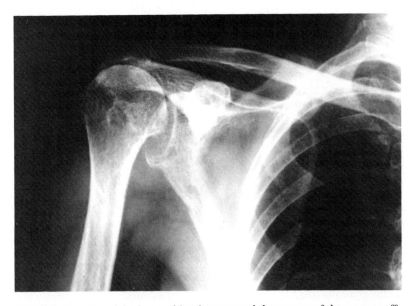

FIG. 9-2. Elevation of the humeral head occurs with large tears of the rotator cuff.

pingement and rotator cuff tears are related to the shape of the bony acromion. A modification of these conclusions, which should have more bearing on rotator cuff damage, focuses primarily on the relationship of the acromion to the humeral head on the routine outlet view. Therefore, regardless of the shape of the acromion, a Type I subacromial space implies anterior divergence of the undersurface of the acromion and humeral head (Fig. 9-3); a Type II subacromial space implies anterior congruence of the undersurface of the acromion and the humeral head; and a Type III subacromial space indicates anterior convergence of the anterior acromion and the humeral head.

Biomechanics

In nearly all sports involving the shoulder (e.g., throwing and racquet sports and competitive swimming) emphasis is placed on the power (pull-through) phase, or that phase requiring forced, rapid, internal rotation and adduction of the humerus.[77,89] Most weight-training programs and apparatus designed for athletic muscle-strengthening programs concentrate on strengthening the internal rotators of the shoulder. Emphasis is commonly placed on development of the pectoralis major and latissimus dorsi muscles. Relatively few programs emphasize the external rotator muscle groups, which are the muscles of cocking and recovery. External rotation is a function of the posterior cuff musculature—infraspinatus and teres minor.

Because of this relative imbalance between the internal and external rotator muscles of the shoulder, the rotator cuff (the primary external rotator of the shoulder) is unable to prevent the humeral head and the attachments of the rotator cuff muscles from migrating proximally and impinging the undersurface of the acromion. Full abduction of the humeral head places the area of attachment of the rotator cuff muscles well under the acromion (Fig. 9-4). With repeated abrasion of this area the

subacromial bursa becomes inflamed, edematous, and scarified, resulting in less effective space between the acromion and the rotator cuff and therefore more impingement.

Most athletes begin sports participation when they are relatively young. By adolescence, many have already experienced symptoms.[88] The average competitive swim-

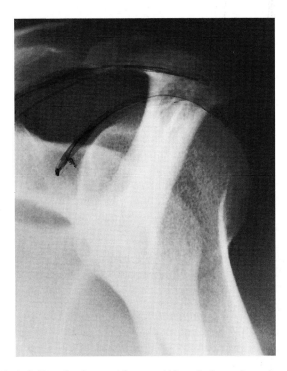

FIG. 9-3. Type I subacromial space. Although the undersurface of the acromion is concave (curved), the subacromial outlet is divergent.

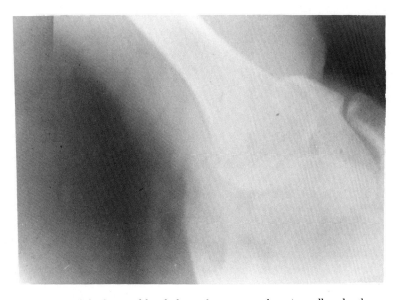

FIG. 9-4. Abduction of the humeral head places the greater tuberosity well under the acromion.

mer puts each arm through some 1.5 million strokes per year over a career that may last 8 to 15 years; baseball pitchers might throw as many as 15,000 pitches per year, most of those at high speeds. It is little wonder that these shoulders eventually wear out and become painful.

Diagnosis

The diagnosis of impingement syndrome is usually not difficult. The patient complains of pain about the acromion, often described as deep within the shoulder under the acromion. The pain is diffuse and, depending on which part of the cuff is inflamed, can occur anteriorly about the coracoacromial ligaments, laterally at the insertion of the infraspinatus, or posteriorly at the insertion of the teres minor muscle.

The pain may be aggravated by direct palpation of the insertion of the rotator cuff under the acromion. The so-called **impingement sign,** which attempts to reproduce the compression of the rotator cuff between the acromion and humeral head, is performed by forcibly forward-flexing the humerus against a fixed acromion.

Neer[62] has also described the painful arc of active elevation from 70 to 120 degrees of forward flexion. This is the range of motion during which the area of insertion of the supraspinatus into the greater tuberosity is passing under the anterior acromion and coracoacromial ligament.

Hawkins and Kennedy[35] have described three stages of clinical symptoms that are helpful in classifying patients with impingement syndrome: (1) minimal pain with activity, no weakness, and no restriction of motion; (2) marked reactive tendinitis with significant pain and a diminished range of motion; and (3) pain with significant weakness (rotator cuff tear). The level of treatment, including restriction from sport, can then be related to these three functional stages of impingement syndrome.

Differential Diagnosis

The long biceps tendon is intimately involved with the rotator cuff, interposed between the subscapularis and supraspinatus muscles and attaching to the superior glenoid labrum. As expected, **tears of the long biceps tendon** can occur in conjunction with subacromial impingement.[63] Intraarticular ruptures of the biceps tendon may cause pain about the shoulder indistinguishable from impingement syndrome. An arthrogram may yield negative results and, if the tendon does not slide in the bicipital groove, may not produce the familiar deformity of contracture of the biceps muscle of the arm. The only means of diagnosis may be MRI or arthroscopic examination (Fig. 9-5).

Extraarticular tears of the long biceps tendon almost always occur in or near the bicipital groove between the tuberosities of the humeral head. The etiology of this rupture is, once again, impingement of the tendon on the undersurface of the anterior acromion. Contracture of the biceps leads to a characteristic prominence of the muscle belly (Fig. 9-6). In the great majority of older patients little disability results from this injury. However, there is some measurable loss of flexion and supination power. In the young active athlete persistent weakness and pain can result. Treatment in this latter group of patients is exploration and tenodesis of the ruptured long biceps tendon. Simultaneous arthroscopic examination of the shoulder eliminates the missed intraarticular fragment of the tendon and perhaps a tear of the superior glenoid labrum.

McMaster[57] has described tears and abrasion of the glenoid labra as causes of shoulder pain in competitive

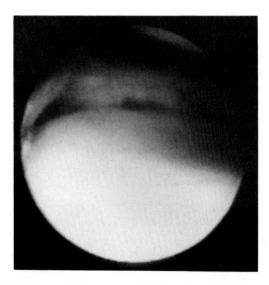

FIG. 9-5. Intraarticular rupture of the biceps tendon. This patient did not demonstrate contracture of the biceps muscle belly.

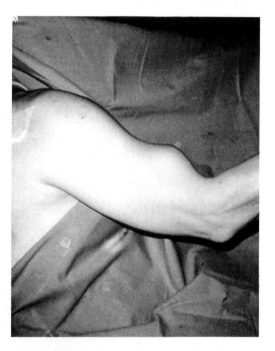

FIG. 9-6. Prominence of the biceps muscle belly following rupture of the long biceps tendon.

swimmers. Although the usual pain of swimmer's shoulder represents a variation of the impingement syndrome, the physician should always keep in mind that overuse can lead to several distinct but related injuries.

Actual tears of the rotator cuff, except in professional throwers, are uncommon in athletes under 40 years old unless there is a distinct history of direct trauma to the shoulder. Suspicion of a rotator cuff tear is increased if external rotation strength is impaired and if pain awakens the patient from sleep. An anteroposterior radiograph of the shoulder does not usually reveal the upward migration of the humeral head seen in larger, global tears.[94]

Diagnostic Imaging

It should be remembered that the diagnosis of impingement syndrome is one largely determined by a careful physical examination. In most cases diagnostic imaging only confirms an established diagnosis and rules out other less common entities. In this era of escalating health care costs, the physician should carefully weigh the need for expensive diagnostic tests vs. the likelihood that the tests will dictate any change in treatment.

Plain radiographs (internal and external rotation anteroposterior films, an outlet view, and an axillary view) should always be obtained in any patient who complains of shoulder pain for any prolonged period of time. They are, however, usually unremarkable and show no bony damage. An outlet view,[93] demonstrating the anatomic configuration of the acromion and its relation to the humeral head, should be a part of every routine radiographic examination of the shoulder joint (Fig. 9-7). Other views (e.g., West Point, true AP) may be obtained as clinical findings dictate. Particular attention should be directed to inspection of the acromioclavicular joint because pain resulting from degeneration of this joint can produce symptoms similar to subacromial impingement syndrome.

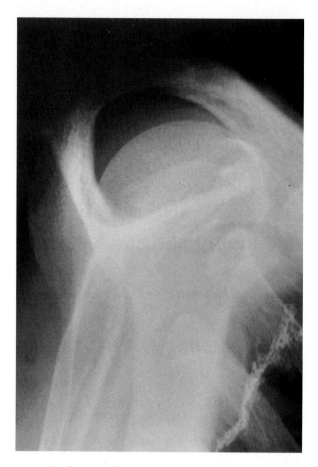

FIG. 9-7. Outlet view showing the relationship of the acromion to the humeral head.

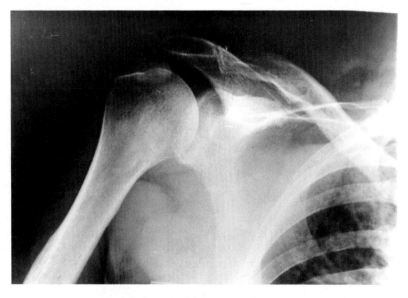

FIG. 9-8. Calcification of the insertion of the rotator cuff.

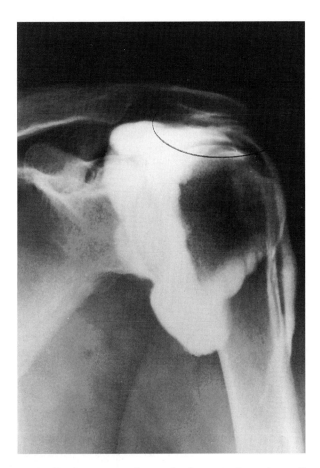

FIG. 9-9. Single contrast arthrography demonstrating extravasation of dye into the subacromial space through a rupture of the rotator cuff.

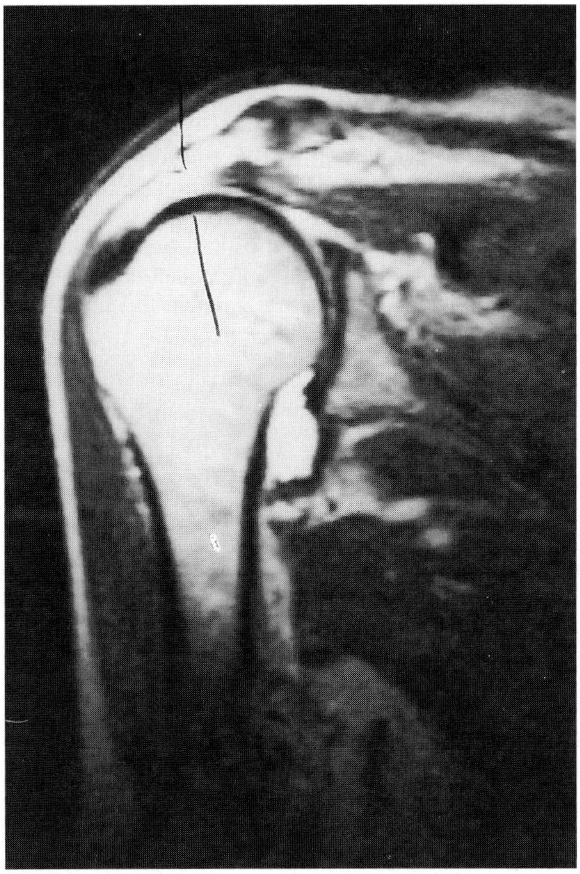

FIG. 9-10. Magnetic resonance imaging examination of a shoulder with a tear of the rotator cuff.

Calcific tendinitis, or calcification of the insertion of the rotator cuff, is occasionally seen on plain radiographs (Fig. 9-8). Microscopic tears of rotator cuff fibers result in inflammation, scarification, and calcification. Although it is conceivable that these calcific crystals are a physical cause of pain, it is the partial tear of the rotator cuff that causes the symptoms of pain with overhead activities. Single contrast arthrography of the shoulder is still a helpful procedure in ruling out tears of the rotator cuff structures (Fig. 9-9). Although the area of abrasion and impingement is on the upper surface of the rotator cuff muscles, most partial tears of the cuff muscles are on the articular side of the cuff and are therefore demonstrable by arthrography.

MRI is commonly used for the evaluation of shoulder rotator cuff problems. Several authors* have reported an accuracy rate of up to 90% in identifying full-thickness tears of the rotator cuff (Fig. 9-10). Partial cuff tears are indistinguishable from repaired tendons, and there is a 74% accuracy in diagnosing impingement. Focal signal intensity in the distal rotator cuff tendon as well as edema in the subacromial bursa are common findings of impingement syndrome in symptomatic patients. The

primary advantage to MRI examination is that the physician can evaluate the integrity of the entire Rotator Cuff,[75] which is difficult to do by any other means; although this may be of help in planning a surgical approach to the older patient with a large rotator cuff tear, most athletic patients have only localized damage to their cuff tissues.

Treatment

Nonoperative Treatment

Impingement syndrome is a problem of inflammation of the subacromial bursa and the surrounding structures (the rotator cuff) as a result of a relative lack of sufficient space for movement of the humeral head under the coracoacromial arch. The goals of treatment, therefore, are to decrease the inflammatory response to this constant abrasion and to increase the effective space between the acromion and the rotator cuff. Decreasing the inflammation by itself increases the effective subacromial space.

Ice therapy remains the most practical treatment for impingement syndrome of the shoulder. McMaster, Liddle, and Waugh[58] have demonstrated in the laboratory that ice is effective in decreasing inflammation, producing analgesia, and decreasing muscle spasm. The ice-cup massage is perhaps the easiest and most effective

---

*References 20, 28, 29, 32, 38, 44, 48, 65, and 69.

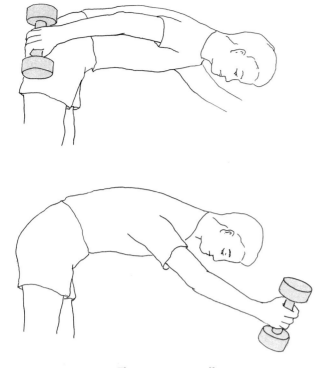

FIG. 9-11. Fly-away rotator cuff exercises.

means of applying cold to the inflamed rotator cuff. Commonly available ice-cube packs, ice gels, and packs of frozen vegetables are reasonable alternatives.

If available, physical therapy modalities such as electrogalvanic stimulation (EGS) and ultrasound can be helpful. Ultrasound should be used with some caution because it is actually a form of deep heat and can sometimes aggravate the pain of impingement syndrome.

Once the acute pain has resolved, a regular exercise program should be instituted to prevent recurrence of impingement syndrome. Simply, all such programs are directed at strengthening the rotator cuff muscles (or the muscles of deceleration, recovery, and cocking).

Fly-away shoulder exercises are done with the body forward flexed 90 degrees and supported with the non-involved arm on a table (Fig. 9-11). The involved arm is then taken through a series of fly-away exercises at 45, 90, and 135 degrees of abduction to strengthen the muscles of the rotator cuff. By bending forward, most deltoid function is eliminated. It should be emphasized that these exercises are prophylactic rather than therapeutic.

Injections of corticosteroids remain controversial. Although there is little question that these agents effectively decrease inflammation, there is also ample evidence to indicate that, by inhibiting this inflammatory process, tissue will not heal as well following injury. Under certain circumstances, however, there is little choice when dealing with chronic and persistent impingement syndrome; the physician either attempts a course of no more than four dilute corticosteroid injections or proceeds to a surgical approach to the problem.

The physician, coach, and athlete should study the athlete's biomechanics and workout schedule. Certain simple changes in the athlete's movements might lead to less pain and better efficiency for the particular sport. For example, the competitive swimmer might increase body roll while swimming freestyle or backstroke, decreasing swimmer's shoulder pain and increasing stroke efficiency.[77] Likewise, if a baseball pitcher is "opening up" too soon (turning the body toward home plate well ahead of the throwing shoulder), correction should lead to less shoulder pain and better accuracy and power during the pitching motion.

Certain exercise techniques should be eliminated. For the competitive swimmer, hand paddles (which act to increase resistance for the swimmer underwater) produce, increase, and aggravate shoulder pain. There is evidence to indicate that excessive overhead weight training (e.g., bench pressing and military presses) can result in shoulder pain. These should be modified so that stress on the subacromial bursa area is decreased.

Selective rest should be instituted for athletes with shoulder pain. Complete rest from their sport is often unnecessary. There is usually some type of related activity in which the athlete can participate that can be used to strengthen parts of the athlete's performance. For example, the baseball pitcher who is recovering from a shoulder problem might work on forearm and grip strength, which certainly helps the pitcher's return to throwing.

Exercises that may increase impingement in swimmers

- Use of hand paddles
- Overhead weight training

Operative Treatment

The goal of any surgical approach to impingement syndrome of the shoulder is direct: to increase the subacromial space. Neer[62] has provided the clearest direction in the approach to subacromial decompression. The undersurface of the acromion is excised along with the coracoacromial ligament, and the subdeltoid bursa is removed. The classic approach is through a small anterior shoulder incision and, as described, involves detachment of a small part of the deltoid muscle.

The advent of arthroscopy has added a dimension to decompression of the subacromial space. Arthroscopic visualization of the subacromial space, with excision of the undersurface of the acromion and coracoacromial ligament, is the standard approach to the problem of impingement syndrome by orthopaedic surgeons. Not only has this become an outpatient procedure, but also insult to the deltoid muscle is considerably less, allowing more rapid rehabilitation to overhead (throwing and swimming) activities.

Arthroscopy also allows the surgeon to inspect the superior and inferior surfaces of the rotator cuff for partial tears. Calcific deposits can be directly removed. Other

causes of periacromial pain can be evaluated (e.g., occult rupture of the long tendon of the biceps muscle).

Postoperatively the patient can begin passive range of motion exercises on the day following surgery and continue this through the first 10 days (see Chapter 11). Active range of motion may then start and continue through the next 2 weeks. It is not unusual to begin easy throwing maneuvers at 3 weeks after surgery and slowly increase these activities until a full return has been achieved.

Bateman[11] and Jobe and Jobe[39] have described operative treatment of tears of the rotator cuff in athletes (see Chapter 33). These injuries, as previously mentioned, are unusual in the average recreational athlete. Rehabilitation after surgical repair is prolonged, averaging 13 to 18 months. The athlete with a torn rotator cuff must understand that return to full throwing activities might prove extremely difficult.

OVERUSE SYNDROMES

Although the impingement syndrome is fundamentally a problem of friction and abrasion of bony parts (with the rotator cuff being caught between), overuse syndromes imply an overload of activity on a muscle, tendon, ligament, or joint capsule, resulting in inability of that structure to perform its normal duties. The syndrome usually develops in the absence of a specific injury and is an injury of attrition.

Most of these injuries can be categorized depending on whether they occur in the cocking (recovery) phase, the acceleration phase, or the follow-through (deceleration) phase of the throwing (or overhead) motion.

Cocking Phase

The cocking (recovery) phase is that part of the throwing motion in which the arm is brought into a position of preparation for the power (acceleration) phase. The most common problems develop from eccentric muscle loading as a musculotendinous unit is undergoing elongation during contraction. An excellent example[3] occurs when a thrower begins forward shoulder motion too early, resulting in **tendinitis of the anterior shoulder muscle tendons.** In this case the tendon of the pectoralis major, latissimus dorsi, or anterior shoulder capsule is affected. Barnes and Tullos[10] described anterior shoulder pain in 29 of 56 baseball players, in which five had tendinitis of the insertion of either the pectoralis major or the latissimus dorsi.

Hyperflexibility, which so often leads to improved ability to perform in many sports, may be a liability in some cases because the joint, tendons, and ligaments pass well beyond the optimal length of the musculotendinous unit that must control that joint. Repeated stretching of the surrounding capsule can lead to a persistent inflammation of the anterior capsular structures.

Acceleration Phase

The acceleration phase leads most commonly to fatigue injuries about the shoulder. Muscles, bones, ligaments, and tendons hypertrophy when subjected to a gradually increasing load. If, however, the resistive load is more than the surrounding structures can withstand, a fatigue injury occurs.

An example of this is cited by Fulton, Albright, and El-Khoury,[30] who interviewed and examined 16 male gymnasts. Eight of these athletes demonstrated a **hypertrophic cortical lesion of the upper humerus** at the site of insertion of the pectoralis major and the latissimus dorsi. These muscles, in particular, are important to and repeatedly stressed by the male gymnast who must often develop power to hold positions (such as in the ring event) and achieve extreme flexibility.

Tullos and King[88] and Tullos et al[90] have described the **spontaneous ball-throwing fracture of the humerus,** which has all the characteristics of a stress fracture. After a study of throwing mechanics, Gainor et al[31] noted that the torque developed during the power phase is "considerably larger than the fracture torques of the humerus." Finally, Adams[1] described **osteochondrosis of the proximal humeral epiphysis** in which the force of throwing results in widening, demineralization, and fragmentation of the proximal humeral epiphysis.

Follow-Through Phase

Posterior shoulder pain is characteristic of injuries resulting from the follow-through phase of throwing sports. Most of these injuries are seen in sports requiring a hard forward motion of the upper extremity, such as tennis, baseball pitching, volleyball spiking, and javelin throwing. Jobe et al,[40,41] in two reports of electromyographic (EMG) analysis of the throwing motion, concluded that, immediately after the ball (or javelin) is released, the posterior muscles of the shoulder and the posterior capsule must decelerate the arm. As might be expected, most strengthening and exercise programs are directed toward the anterior (power) muscles and little emphasis is given to the muscles that must decelerate the upper extremity following the acceleration phase.

This follow-through phase is characterized by large eccentric loads placed on the posterior structures of the shoulder. Barnes and Tullos[10] described this as **posterior capsule syndrome.** Lombardo et al[50] found posterior shoulder pain in four athletes and related the pain to the cocking and follow-through phases of the throwing arm. Bennett[13-15] described an exostosis of the posteroinferior glenoid that results from repeated traction of the inferior capsular structures.

The end stage of this repeated stress on the posterior capsular structures is posterior subluxation of the shoulder. Many athletes, in a variety of sports, may develop posterior subluxation of the shoulder. It is not nearly as rare a lesion as reflected in the literature. For most athletes the condition remains asymptomatic; however, if the athlete is vigorous with overhead, throwing-motion activities, treatment is extremely difficult. Symptoms of posterior shoulder pain and a feeling of instability with throwing are characteristic of the condition (see Chapter 7).

Another injury that usually develops in the follow-through phase is a painful scapula, or **snapping scapula.** Normally there is a small bursa located beneath the

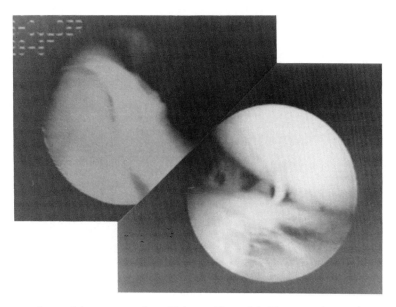

FIG. 9-12. Avulsion of the superior glenoid labrum. *Upper left,* Tear extends into the proximal biceps tendon.

medial border of the scapula. It serves to lubricate the motion of the scapula against the thoracic wall. Unfortunately, because of the large amount of motion between the scapula and the chest wall, bursitis can develop, resulting in pain and occasionally a snapping sensation as the swollen tissues impinge the underlying rib cage. Diagnosis is straightforward; however, treatment is often difficult and consists of antiinflammatory measures. There is no widely accepted surgical treatment of this condition, although Sisto and Jobe[84] have described excision of the inflamed bursa in professional pitchers.

The diagnosis of injuries of the follow-through phase is almost entirely clinical. Palpation of the tender structures posteriorly usually allows the physician to identify the pain as emanating from the posterior glenoid and the capsule or from the teres minor or major muscles. Manual manipulation of the shoulder usually demonstrates posterior subluxation of the shoulder as it is present. The physician should be particularly careful to examine the shoulder for all types of instability because multidirectional instability is always a potential problem and changes the treatment plan drastically.

The double-contrast arthrogram[59] is useful in outlining the glenoid labrum, both anteriorly and posteriorly. MRI and perhaps the magnetic resonance arthrogram (MRA) described by Flannigan et al[29] may be helpful in defining the pathologic lesion in the posterior shoulder.[21] The interpretation of the MRI (or MRA) depends, however, on the experience of the radiologist or orthopaedic surgeon with a wide array of shoulder MRI images.[66]

The arthroscope is, of course, most accurate in identifying intraarticular pathologic conditions.[24,37,54] Andrews and Carson[5] and Andrews, Carson, and Ortega,[7] in describing arthroscopic techniques for the shoulder, advocated simple excision of tears of the glenoid labrum. Although this may eliminate some of the immediate

symptoms of shoulder catching and locking,[4] all tears of the labrum indicate some degree of instability of the shoulder, and this instability often becomes symptomatic at a later date. Therefore, if a labral tear is excised, the surgeon should be aware that this "cure" may only be temporary.

Finally, Andrews, Carson, and McLeod[6] have described avulsion of the superior glenoid labrum by the long biceps tendon (Fig. 9-12). They believe this develops because of marked contraction of the biceps muscle, which is decelerating the elbow joint during the follow-through phase. Snyder et al[85] have termed this the **superior labrum anterior-posterior (SLAP) tear.** Four types have been described: Type I is labral fraying at the insertion of the biceps tendon; Type II is fraying and stripping of the superior glenoid labrum; Type III is a bucket-handle tear of the superior glenoid labrum in the region of the biceps tendon; and Type IV is a bucket-handle tear of the superior labrum with extension into the biceps tendon itself.

Surgical treatment currently consists of excision of the torn superior labrum. Reattachment of the long biceps tendon is only necessary for Type IV lesions, and in these cases tenodesis to the humeral head is the most efficient and successful approach.

TRACTION INJURIES
Avulsion of the Pectoralis Major

Avulsion of the pectoralis major was first described by Patissier[72] in 1822; by 1972 only 44 additional cases had been reported.[*] The most common site of rupture is at or near the bone-tendon junction. Ruptures occur when the muscle is at full tension and an additional force is

---

*References 8, 16, 45, 53, 56, 71, 73, and 98.

added. The most common sources of this additional force are the bench press and breaking a fall by catching one's weight with one arm.

Diagnosis is, again, relatively straightforward. Most patients experience pain and swelling over the anterior aspect of the shoulder joint and relate that "something ripped." Mild to moderate ecchymosis indicates that bleeding has taken place deep within the shoulder joint. Physical examination may not demonstrate a defect in the muscle tendon; however, if the patient forcefully claps the hands together, the defect is usually obvious. Although Gudmundsson[33] advocated nonoperative treatment, several authors noted that muscle power is markedly decreased in flexion and internal rotation. Therefore it is my opinion that operative repair of the ruptured tendon offers the patient the best possible result.[45] This advice applies even to chronic tears of the pectoralis major.

Lateral Acromion Apophysitis

In the adolescent athlete repeated traction on the lateral acromion by the deltoid muscle can lead to a painful apophysitis of this area. This apophysis usually closes at approximately 16 to 19 years of age, which coincides with the usual age when the athlete is achieving his or her greatest growth and maturity. Time usually allows resolution of this problem, and at present I am unaware of an instance in which the lateral acromion required excision with reattachment of the deltoid to the remaining acromion.

PROBLEMS OF INSTABILITY

When the capsular and labral structures about the shoulder joint become deficient either because of acute or chronic trauma or because of congenital deficiencies, instability of the glenohumeral joint occurs. The direction of this dissociation of the humeral head in relation to the glenoid fossa depends on the specific location of the capsulolabral deficiency. The specific location of the capsulolabral deficiency, then, dictates the shoulder motions that reproduce this instability.

Once the capsule and labrum are compromised, the resulting instability is chronic and recurrent. Tsai et al.[87] document the well-known natural history of shoulder function in patients with known anterior instability.

Anterior Instability

Anterior instability of the glenohumeral joint is perhaps the most common traumatic soft-tissue injury about the shoulder in athletes. Its diagnosis and treatment have been described at length in the literature. The essential lesion is believed to be the torn anterior glenoid labrum (Fig. 9-13).[9,70] This labrum is a thick, fibrous expansion of the anterior shoulder capsule.[61] Attached to the labrum are thickened bands of capsule known as the superior, middle, and inferior glenohumeral ligaments, which provide support to the anterior joint during abduction and external rotation (Fig. 9-14). If repeated humeral head subluxation or dislocation from the glenoid occurs, a compression fracture of the posterior humeral

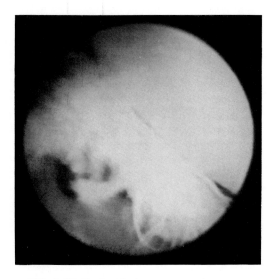

FIG. 9-13. Bankart lesion seen at arthroscopy.

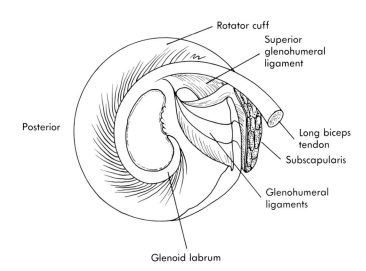

FIG. 9-14. Anterior glenohumeral ligaments.

head, commonly known as a Hill-Sachs lesion, may develop.

Diagnosis is, again, primarily clinical. The history of the shoulder coming out when the arm is in an overhead, externally rotated position is common and classic. Patients often describe waking with the shoulder either completely or partially dislocated. The dead arm syndrome can result from transient anterior subluxations of the shoulder joint.[81,82] This usually occurs with abduction and extreme external rotation; however, the athlete may not give a clear history of this maneuver. The examiner can usually demonstrate laxity of the shoulder capsule by grasping the scapula in one hand and the humeral head in the other and moving them apart (see Chapter 3).

Radiographs, although usually unremarkable, occasionally reveal two findings:

1. Hill-Sachs lesion: this is a compression fracture of the posterior humeral head that can often be seen

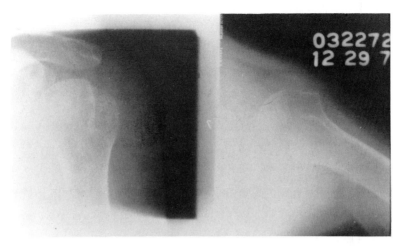

FIG. 9-15. Hill-Sachs lesion.

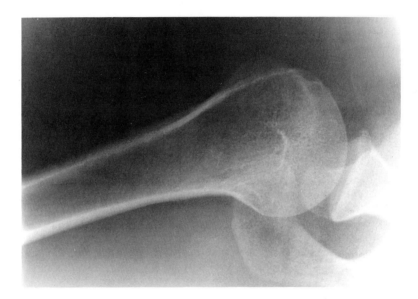

FIG. 9-16. Osteophyte formation on the anterior glenoid neck resulting from recurrent dislocations of the shoulder.

on the anteroposterior radiograph with the arm internally rotated (Fig. 9-15).

2. Osteophyte of the anterior glenoid: this represents calcification of the defect in the anterior glenoid labrum (Fig. 9-16). A modified axillary radiograph, as described by Rokous, Feagin, and Abbot,[79] can be helpful in delineating this small osteophyte.

Double contrast arthrography, as described by Mink, Richardson, and Grant,[59] may also shed light on the diagnosis by showing the torn labrum. CT arthrography and MRI have both been used to make a definite diagnosis of instability.[34] The MRI is more accurate in evaluating labral lesions (88% accuracy); however, neither test can accurately assess the capsular structures. Once again, a careful clinical examination can usually easily define instability of the shoulder, and the various techniques currently available play only a confirmatory role.

Most accurate of all diagnostic modalities of the shoulder is arthroscopy. Not only can the internal structures of the shoulder be directly visualized, but also the shoulder can be examined under anesthesia.

Almost all of the recorded procedures to prevent anterior instability of the shoulder are designed to eliminate the laxity of the anterior soft-tissue structures that stabilize the shoulder.[91] Therefore a part of their purpose must be to limit abducted external rotation. Early range of motion exercises may allow return to most activities[80]; however, Lombardo and Kerlan[49] have noted that the Bristow procedure does not readily allow the active baseball pitcher to return to his or her sport. Regan et al,[76] in comparing the Bristow, Magnuson-Stack, and Putti-Platt procedures, found that functional return to sports

TABLE 9-1 Average recurrence rate following surgical repair of the shoulder for anterior dislocation

Procedure	Recurrence
Putti-Platt	3.0%
Magnuson-Stack	4.1%
Bankart	3.3%
Bristow	1.7%

From Rockwood CA, Green DP: *Fractures,* Philadelphia, 1984, JB Lippincott.

favored the Bristow repair. Because flexibility, especially with abducted external rotation, is necessary for hard throwers such as pitchers and javelin throwers, the mere presence of anterior instability of the shoulder in these types of athletes may signal the end of their career as a high-speed and power thrower, regardless of the type of surgery performed.

Of the more common repairs done in the United States, the Bankart repair most recreates the normal anatomy by reattaching a shortened anterior glenoid labrum to the anterior glenoid rim.[9] The Putti-Platt repair[68] attempts to shorten the various anterior structures by sewing the capsule and subscapularis tendon in overlapping fashion in separate layers. The Bristow repair[36] not only places a bone block anteriorly, but also slings the conjoined tendon of the short biceps tendon and the coracobrachialis across the humeral head to prevent anterior motion of the head. The Magnuson-Stack procedure[51] reattaches the subscapularis further laterally on the humeral head in the hope that this will result in a dynamic tightening across the humeral head. Jobe et al[42] report on the anterior capsulolabral reconstruction (ACLR) procedure, citing good to excellent results in 92%; they believe that this procedure reproduces the normal anatomy better than a Bankart repair because the anterior capsule and the anterior labrum are reconstructed.

The efficacy of all these procedures in preventing future anterior instability of the shoulder is excellent (Table 9-1),[78] and most surgeons determine their choice of procedure by their experience in both training and practice.

Where there is recurrence of the instability after surgical repair, a repeat procedure usually leads to encouraging results.[82] Failure of the initial procedure, however, should prompt the clinician to evaluate the athlete for a multidirectional instability pattern.

Arthroscopic repair of the anterior structures is a relatively new procedure that has the advantages of no hospital stay, a shortened rehabilitation period, and much smaller scars. Johnson[43] popularized the technique of using barbed staples placed under direct vision to fix the anterior glenoid labrum and capsule to the bony glenoid. DuToit[25] described a similar technique done through an arthrotomy. Long-term results[23,26,52,55] to date, however, have not supported the efficacy of this procedure, and it is now done infrequently. Caspari,[22] Landsiedl,[46] Morgan and Bodenstab,[60] Benedetto and Glotzer,[12] and Wolf[97] have introduced other methods of arthroscopic repair of the lax anterior

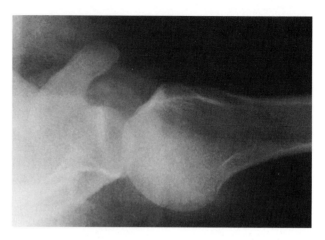

FIG. 9-17. Posterior axillary stress view of the shoulder.

capsule and labrum. All of these methods require placing intraarticular sutures through a variety of means to fix the anterior capsule and labrum to the glenoid neck. Wiley[95] has described a method employing a rivet that is removed at a future date. Although early experience with these techniques is encouraging, larger patient populations and longer follow-up are necessary.

Because open repairs can be done through relatively small incisions, hospital stay is often unnecessary, and rehabilitation time is about the same, the surgeon must question whether an arthroscopic repair offers any, other than cosmetic, advantages over an open technique. Certainly, the inexperienced surgeon should not undertake an arthroscopic repair without appropriate prior training.

Posterior Instability

Posterior instability is distinctly less common than anterior instability; however, it is not so rare among athletes as it is among the general population.[2,27] Athletes require a certain degree of instability of the shoulder to perform their activities to maximal advantage. Posterior instability (subluxation) occurs in competitive swimmers, volleyball players, throwers, and weight lifters, among others. Voluntary posterior subluxation is not readily treatable; all surgical attempts at repair are probably doomed to failure.

Stress axillary views (Fig. 9-17) are helpful in defining this entity. Comparative stress axillary views are also helpful in ruling out a bilateral condition.

In many cases this condition remains asymptomatic; unfortunately, in the patient who complains of posterior instability of the shoulder, surgical stabilization may be difficult to attain. Samilson and Prietto[83] reported good results with tenodesis of the long head of the biceps to the posterior scapular neck. Most authors have realized equivocal results with posterior stabilization procedures.[34,86] I believe that posterior instability should be considered as a multidirectional instability and treated as described in the following section.

Multidirectional Instability

In 1980 Neer and Foster[64] reported on the inferior capsular shift procedure as treatment for multidirectional in-

stability of the shoulder. Until that time the concept of instability of the shoulder occurring simultaneously in several directions was not clearly defined. Since that time this difficult entity has been recognized with increasing frequency.

Complaints of instability and pain at the extremes of motion, particularly forward horizontal flexion, are common. Examination of the athlete in the supine position demonstrates posterior instability to posterior manual stress, with the typical relocation of the humeral head into the glenoid fossa. Anterior and posterior stress axillary view radiographs are, once again, helpful in delineating this condition.

Unfortunately, muscular rehabilitation and exercises are not routinely helpful in preventing instability in the active athlete, and surgical intervention is often necessary. Procedures aimed at stabilization of either the anterior or posterior structures alone are likely to fail. The essential lesion appears to be laxity of the posteroinferior capsule. The inferior capsular shift procedure, described by Neer and Foster,[64] simply detaches the lax portion of the inferior and posterior capsule from the anterior, inferior, and posterior humeral head and advances it anteriorly and superiorly, thereby eliminating the redundancy of the capsule both inferiorly and posteriorly.

SUMMARY

The approach to the athlete with shoulder pain involves a careful clinical assessment and appropriate radiographic studies to arrive at an exact anatomic diagnosis. Secondary imaging techniques may be used to confirm diagnoses. The differential diagnosis of most shoulder problems includes adhesive capsulitis, impingement syndrome and rotator cuff injuries, overuse injuries, traction injuries, and instability. Accurate diagnosis is essential to implementation of appropriate therapy. With proper treatment most athletes can return to competitive or recreational athletics as they desire.

"There is a very fine line between pitching the batter out and injuring the shoulder."

Frank Jobe, 1979

REFERENCES

1. Adams JE: Little League shoulder: osteochondrosis of the proximal humeral epiphysis in boy baseball pitchers, *Calif Med* 105:22, 1966.
2. Ahlgren S, Hedlung T, Nistor L: Idiopathic posterior instability of the shoulder joint, *Acta Orthop Scand* 49:600, 1978.
3. Albright JA et al: Clinical study of baseball pitchers: correlation of injury to the throwing arm with method of delivery, *Am J Sports Med* 6:15, 1978.
4. Altchek DW et al: Arthroscopic labral debridement, *Am J Sports Med* 20:702, 1992.
5. Andrews JR, Carson WG: The arthroscopic treatment of glenoid labrum tears in the throwing athlete, *Orthop Trans* 8:44, 1984.
6. Andrews JR, Carson WG, McLeod WD: Glenoid labrum tears related to the long head of the biceps, *Am J Sports Med* 13:337, 1985.
7. Andrews JR, Carson WG, Ortega K: Arthroscopy of the shoulder: technique and normal anatomy, *Am J Sports Med* 12:1, 1984.
8. Bakalim G: Rupture of the pectoralis major muscle, *Acta Orthop Scand* 36:274, 1965.
9. Bankart ASB: Recurrent or habitual dislocation of the shoulder-joint, *Br Med J* 2:1132, 1923.
10. Barnes DA, Tullos HS: An analysis of 100 symptomatic baseball pitchers, *Am J Sports Med* 6:62, 1978.
11. Bateman JE: Cuff tears in athletes, *Orthop Clin North Am* 4:721, 1973.
12. Benedetto KP, Glotzer W: Arthroscopic Bankart procedure by suture technique: indications, technique, and results, *Arthroscopy* 8:111, 1992.
13. Bennett GE: Shoulder and elbow lesions of professional baseball pitcher, *JAMA* 117:510, 1941.
14. Bennett GE: Shoulder and elbow lesions distinctive of baseball players, *Ann Surg* 126:107, 1947.
15. Bennett GE: Elbow and shoulder lesions of baseball players, *Am J Surg* 98:484, 1959.
16. Berson B: Surgical repair of pectoralis major rupture in an athlete, *Am J Sports Med* 7:348, 1979.
17. Bigliani LU, Morrison DS, April EW: The morphology of the acromion in its relation to rotator cuff tears, *Orthop Trans* 10:228, 1986.
18. Bosworth DM: An analysis of twenty-eight consecutive cases of incapacitating shoulder lesions, radically explored and repaired, *J Bone Joint Surg* 22:369, 1940.
19. Bosworth DM: Supraspinatus syndrome: symptomatology, pathology, and repair, *JAMA* 117:422, 1941.
20. Burk DL et al: MR imaging of the shoulder: correlation with plain radiography, *Am J Roentgenol* 154:549, 1990.
21. Burk DL et al: MR imaging of shoulder injuries in professional baseball players, *Magn Reson Imaging* 1:385, 1991.
22. Caspari RB: *Suture techniques for arthroscopic stabilization of shoulder instability,* Paper presented at the Tenth International Seminar on Operative Arthroscopy, UCLA Extension, Kauai, Hawaii, Oct, 1988.
23. Coughlin L et al: Arthroscopic staple capsulorrhaphy for anterior shoulder instability, *Am J Sports Med* 20:253, 1992.
24. Dolk T, Gremark O: Arthroscopy and stability testing of the shoulder joint, *Arthroscopy* 2:35, 1986.
25. DuToit JG: Recurrent dislocation of the shoulder: a 24-year study of the Johannesburg stapling operation, *J Bone Joint Surg* 38A:1, 1956.
26. Eckert RR, Richardson AB, Dericks GH: Arthroscopic shoulder stapling for instability: a review of 57 cases followed up to 2 years. In Post M, Morrey BF, Hawkins RJ (eds): *Surgery of the shoulder,* St Louis, 1990, Mosby.
27. English E, MacNab I: Idiopathic posterior instability of the shoulder, *Can J Surg* 17:147, 1974.
28. Farley TE et al: Full-thickness tears of the rotator cuff of the shoulder: diagnosis with MR imaging, *Am J Roentgenol* 158:347, 1992.
29. Flannigan B et al: MR arthrography of the shoulder: comparison with conventional MR imaging, *Am J Roentgenol* 155:829, 1990.
30. Fulton MN, Albright JP, El-Khoury GY: Cortical desmoidlike lesion of the proximal humerus and its occurrence in gymnasts (Ringman's shoulder lesion), *Am J Sports Med* 7:57, 1979.
31. Gainor BM et al: The throw: biomechanics and acute injury, *Am J Sports Med* 8:114, 1980.
32. Gross ML et al: Magnetic resonance imaging of the glenoid labrum, *Am J Sports Med* 18:229, 1990.
33. Gudmundsson B: A case of agenesis and a case of rupture of the pectoralis major muscle, *Acta Orthop Scand* 44:213, 1973.
34. Hawkins RJ: *Posterior dislocations of the shoulder:* instructional course lectures, American Academy of Orthopaedic Surgeons Annual Meeting, New Orleans, January 1972.
35. Hawkins RJ, Kennedy JC: Impingement syndrome in athletes, *Am J Sports Med* 8:57, 1980.
36. Helfet AJ: Coracoid transplantation for recurring dislocation of the shoulder, *J Bone Joint Surg* 40B:198, 1958.
37. Hurley JA, Anderson TE: Shoulder arthroscopy: its role in evaluating shoulder disorders in the athlete, *Am J Sports Med* 18:480, 1990.
38. Jahnke AH et al: A prospective comparison of computerized arthrotomography and magnetic resonance imaging of the glenohumeral joint, *Am J Sports Med* 20:695, 1992.
39. Jobe FW, Jobe CM: Painful athletic injuries of the shoulder, *Clin Orthop* 173:117, 1983.

40. Jobe FW et al: An EMG analysis of the shoulder in throwing and pitching: a preliminary report, *Am J Sports Med* 11:3, 1983.

41. Jobe FW et al: An EMG analysis of the shoulder in pitching: a second report, *Am J Sports Med* 12:218, 1984.

42. Jobe FW et al: Anterior capsulolabral reconstruction of the shoulder in athletes in overhead sports, *Am J Sports Med* 19:428, 1991.

43. Johnson LL: *Arthroscopic reconstruction of the unstable shoulder—indications, techniques, and results with a one- to five-year follow-up,* Paper presented at the Ninth International Seminar on Operative Arthroscopy, UCLA Extension, Maui, Hawaii, Oct, 1987.

44. Kaplan PA et al: MR imaging of the normal shoulder: variants and pitfalls, *Radiology* 184:519, 1992.

45. Kretzler HH, Richardson AB: Rupture of the pectoralis major muscle, *Am J Sports Med* 17:453, 1989.

46. Landsiedl F: Arthroscopic therapy of recurrent anterior luxation of the shoulder by capsular repair, *Arthroscopy* 8:293, 1992.

47. Lindenbaum BL: Delayed repair of the ruptured pectoralis muscle, *Clin Orthop* 109:120, 1975.

48. Liou JT et al: The normal shoulder: common variations that simulate pathologic conditions at MR imaging, *Radiology* 186:435, 1993.

49. Lombardo SJ, Kerlan RK: The modified Bristow procedure for recurrent dislocation of the shoulder, *J Bone Joint Surg* 58A:256, 1976.

50. Lombardo SJ et al: Posterior shoulder lesions in throwing athletes, *Am J Sports Med* 5:106, 1977.

51. Magnuson PB, Stack JK: Recurrent dislocation of the shoulder, *JAMA* 123:889, 1943.

52. Maki NJ: Arthroscopic stabilization for recurrent shoulder instability. In Post M, Morrey BF, Hawkins RJ (eds): *Surgery of the shoulder,* St Louis, 1990, Mosby.

53. Marmor L et al: Pectoralis major muscle: function of sternal position and mechanism of rupture of normal muscle: case reports, *J Bone Joint Surg* 43A:81, 1961.

54. Matthews LS, Terry G, Vetter WL: Shoulder anatomy for the arthroscopist, *Arthroscopy* 1:83, 1985.

55. Matthews LS et al: Arthroscopic staple capsulorrhaphy for recurrent anterior shoulder instability, *Arthroscopy* 4:106, 1988.

56. McEntire JE et al: Rupture of the pectoralis major muscle, *J Bone Joint Surg* 54A:1040, 1972.

57. McMaster WC: Anterior glenoid labrum damage: a painful lesion in swimmers, *Am J Sports Med* 14:383, 1986.

58. McMaster WC, Liddle S, Waugh TR: Laboratory evaluation of various cold therapy modalities, *Am J Sports Med* 6:291, 1978.

59. Mink JH, Richardson AB, Grant TT: Evaluation of glenoid labrum by double-contrast shoulder arthrography, *Am J Roentgenol* 133:833, 1979.

60. Morgan CD, Bodenstab AB: Arthroscopic Bankart suture repair: technique and early results, *Arthroscopy* 3:111, 1987.

61. Moseley HF, Overgaard B: The anterior capsule mechanism in recurrent anterior dislocation of the shoulder: morphological and clinical studies with special reference to the glenoid labrum and the glenohumeral ligaments, *J Bone Joint Surg* 44B:913, 1962.

62. Neer CS: Anterior acromioplasty for the chronic impingement syndrome in the shoulder, *J Bone Joint Surg* 54A:41, 1972.

63. Neer CS, Bigliani LW, Hawkins RJ: Rupture of the long head of the biceps tendon related to subacromial impingement syndrome, *Orthop Trans* 1:111, 1977.

64. Neer CS, Foster CR: Inferior capsular shift for voluntary inferior and multidirectional instability of the shoulder: a preliminary report, *J Bone Joint Surg* 62A:897, 1980.

65. Neumann CH et al: MRI in the evaluation of patients with suspected instability of the shoulder joint including a comparison with CT-arthrography, *ROFO Fortschr Geb Rontgenstr Nuklearmed* 154:593, 1991.

66. Neumann CH et al: MR imaging of the shoulder: appearance of the supraspinatus tendon in asymptomatic volunteers, *Am J Roentgenol* 158:1281, 1992.

67. Neviaser RJ: Adhesive capsulitis of the shoulder, *J Bone Joint Surg* 27:211, 1945.

68. Osmond-Clarke H: Habitual dislocation of the shoulder: the Putti-Platt operation, *J Bone Joint Surg* 30B:19, 1948.

69. Owen RS et al: Shoulder after surgery: MR imaging with surgical validation, *Radiology* 186:443, 1993.

70. Pappas AM, Goss TP, Kleinman PK: Symptomatic shoulder instability due to lesions of the glenoid labrum, *Am J Sports Med* 11:279, 1983.

71. Park JY, Espinella JL: Rupture of pectoralis major muscle, *J Bone Joint Surg* 52A:577, 1970.

72. Reference deleted in proofs.

73. Pulaski EJ, Chandler BH: Ruptures of the pectoralis major muscle, *Surgery* 10:309, 1941.

74. Rathbun JB, MacNab I: The microvascular pattern of the rotator cuff, *J Bone Joint Surg* 52B:540, 1970.

75. Recht MP, Resnick D: Magnetic resonance-imaging studies of the shoulder, *J Bone Joint Surg* 75A:1244, 1993.

76. Regan WD et al: Comparative functional analysis of the Bristow, Magnuson-Stack, and Putti-Platt procedures for recurrent dislocation of the shoulder, *Am J Sports Med* 17:42, 1989.

77. Richardson AB, Jobe FW, Collins HR: The shoulder in competitive swimming, *Am J Sports Med* 8:151, 1980.

78. Rockwood CA, Green GP: *Fractures,* Philadelphia, 1984, JB Lippincott.

79. Rokous JR, Feagin JA, Abbot HG: Modified axillary roentgenogram: a useful adjunct in the diagnosis of recurrent instability of the shoulder, *Clin Orthop* 82:84, 1972.

80. Rowe CR, Patel D, Southmayd WW: The Bankart procedure: a long-term end-result study, *J Bone Joint Surg* 60A:1, 1978.

81. Rowe CR, Zarins B: Recurrent transient subluxation of the shoulder, *J Bone Joint Surg* 63A:863, 1981.

82. Rowe CR, Zarins B, Ciullo JV: Recurrent anterior dislocation of the shoulder after surgical repair, *J Bone Joint Surg* 66A:159, 1984.

83. Samilson RL, Prietto V: Posterior dislocation of the shoulder in athletes, *Clin Sports Med* 2:369, 1983.

84. Sisto DJ, Jobe FW: The operative treatment of scapulothoracic bursitis in professional pitchers, *Am J Sports Med* 14:192, 1986.

85. Snyder SJ et al: SLAP lesions of the shoulder, *Arthroscopy* 6:274, 1990.

86. Tibone JE et al: Staple capsulorrhaphy for recurrent posterior shoulder dislocations, *Am J Sports Med* 9:135, 1981.

87. Tsai L et al: Shoulder function in patients with unoperated anterior shoulder instability, *Am J Sports Med* 19:469, 1991.

88. Tullos HS, King JW: Lesions of the pitching arm in adolescents, *JAMA* 220:264, 1972.

89. Tullos HS, King JW: Throwing mechanism in sports, *Orthop Clin North Am* 4:809, 1973.

90. Tullos HS et al: Unusual lesions of the pitching arm, *Clin Orthop* 88:169, 1972.

91. Turkel SJ et al: Stabilizing mechanisms preventing anterior dislocation of the glenohumeral joint, *J Bone Joint Surg* 63A:1208, 1981.

92. Uitvlugt G et al: Arthroscopic observations before and after manipulation of frozen shoulder, *Arthroscopy* 9:181, 1993.

93. Watkins GL, Moore TF: *Atypical orthopedic radiographic procedures,* St Louis, 1993, Mosby.

94. Weiner DS, MacNab I: Superior migration of the humeral head, *J Bone Joint Surg* 52B:514, 1970.

95. Wiley AM: Arthroscopy for shoulder instability and a technique for arthroscopic repair, *Arthroscopy* 4:25, 1988.

96. Wiley AM: Arthroscopic appearance of frozen shoulder, *Arthroscopy* 7:138, 1991.

97. Wolf EM: *Arthroscopic capsulo-labral reconstruction using suture anchors,* unpublished material presented at 14th International Seminar on Operative Arthroscopy (UCLA Extension), Maui, Hawaii, Oct, 1992.

98. Zeman SC et al: Tears of the pectoralis major muscle, *Am J Sports Med* 7:343, 1979.

CHAPTER 10

Degenerative Joint Disease of the Shoulder

John J. Brems

In discussing degenerative joint disease in the athlete, the physician must first define it as a clinicopathologic condition and second, which is considerably more difficult, one must define an athlete.

For purposes of discussion in this chapter degenerative joint disease of the shoulder is defined as a pathologic process caused by a mechanical aberration of joint function that results in joint incongruity. This, of course, excludes certain types of degenerative diseases. Rheumatoid arthritis and crystalline and septic processes are purposely excluded from the following discussion. Furthermore, vascular causes of degenerative disease such as osteonecrosis are not addressed.

Having now defined the condition, I must set about the more difficult task of defining an athlete. Whereas just 10 to 15 years ago an athlete could be defined merely by age, an ever-increasing awareness of the benefits of physical activity has given the term *athlete* a wider domain. It is only fair to consider the 7-year-old gymnast as much an athlete as the senior citizen who plays two games of tennis a week.

Perhaps it is too difficult to adequately define the study group from this perspective; nevertheless, the following discussion is a pragmatic approach to and discussion of degenerative conditions of the shoulder and elbow that are commonly associated with competitive and noncompetitive sports activities.

The moving shoulder actually consists of four articulations: the sternoclavicular joint, the scapulothoracic joint, the acromioclavicular joint, and the glenohumeral joint. Because degenerative joint disease of the sternoclavicular and scapulothoracic joint is exceedingly rare, it is not considered here. However, acromioclavicular and glenohumeral degenerative joint disease is common in athletes and is therefore discussed in detail.

DEGENERATIVE DISEASE OF THE ACROMIOCLAVICULAR JOINT

Isolated arthritic conditions of the acromioclavicular joint have significant impact on the function of the throwing shoulder. With full elevation of the arm, 20 degrees of axial rotation motion alone occurs at the acromioclavicular joint. Depalma,[7] in a classic study in 1957, examined 223 sets of human acromioclavicular and sternoclavicular joints from infancy to age 94 years. Significant changes in the anatomy and composition of the meniscus were directly correlated with degenerative changes. Because the acromioclavicular joint is so superficial, it is subject to frequent trauma. Furthermore, the joint's small size and incongruence of its mating surfaces lead to high sheer stresses and increase the likelihood of degenerative changes.

The treatment of acute injuries is not the subject of this discussion, but the reader is referred to a pertinent synopsis.[9]

History

Patients with degenerative disease of the acromioclavicular joint may be of any age. Most younger patients clearly have a history of trauma within 12 to 24 months of their presentation. At the other extreme are patients who present typically over age 40 who rarely have a history of any antecedent trauma. Furthermore, in my experience, patients who present in middle age with acromioclavicular arthritis have associated subacromial impingement and rotator cuff injury in the majority of circumstances. The most common symptoms are pain with overhead activity and particularly with activities that require use of the arm across the midline. With the arm

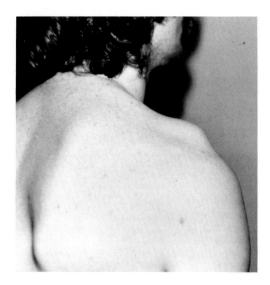

FIG. 10-1. This 40-year-old javelin thrower demonstrates the marked prominence of an arthritic acromioclavicular (AC) joint. There has been no history of AC joint separation and the prominence is caused solely by the hypertrophic spurring on both the clavicular and acromial sides of the AC joint. Also note the marked atrophy of the supraspinatus and infraspinatus fossae.

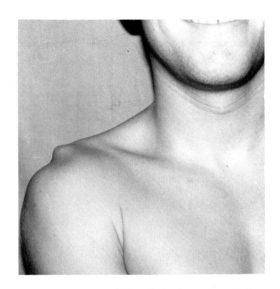

FIG. 10-2. This 30-year-old baseball player sustained an acute trauma by falling on the point of his left shoulder. He demonstrates the clinical findings of an acute third-degree acromioclavicular (AC) joint separation. A physician would expect no muscular atrophy in an acute situation. Furthermore, palpation of the acromial side of the AC joint indicates osteophytes if a chronic degenerative process is present.

adducted, compression of the acromioclavicular joint occurs. Because of this, patients frequently complain of pain at night when they roll over on their affected shoulder.

Physical Examination

The physical examination of any part of the shoulder begins by inspection. Often prominence of the acromioclavicular joint is seen together with significant muscular atrophy about the involved shoulder (Fig. 10-1). The physician should not mistake the prominence of a remote second- or third-degree acromioclavicular joint separation with degenerative changes (Fig. 10-2). True arthritis of the joint has osteophytic changes on both the clavicular and acromial side of the joint. When the examining physician then palpates the joint, there is tenderness directly over the acromioclavicular region. There may or may not be observable instability, especially if there is pain, but the physician should assess superior-inferior and anterior-posterior stability.

The passive and active ranges of motion are then examined. Characteristic changes include pain with elevation but minimal if any pain with external rotation because this latter maneuver results in only minimal motion at the acromioclavicular joint. As noted previously, passive or active motion with the arm moving in front of the body characteristically produces pain (Fig. 10-3).

The throwing athlete may find it difficult to differentiate the pain of subacromial origin from that of acromioclavicular joint origin. Here the injection test is most valuable. An injection of 10 ml of 1% lidocaine without epinephrine is given in the subacromial bursa (Fig. 10-4), and the shoulder is reexamined. With the subacro-

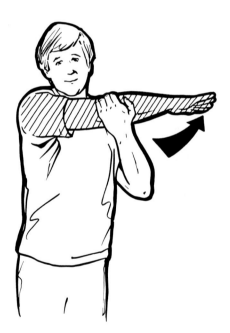

FIG. 10-3. Position that most characteristically reproduces the pain of acromioclavicular (AC) joint pathologic conditions. Forcing the arm across the chest in this adducted position compresses the AC joint and is likely to reproduce symptoms.

mial mechanism now anesthetized, the pain of impingement and cuff tear should be eliminated. If the patient's symptoms abate following the injection, the injury is *not* at the acromioclavicular joint. If the patient's symptoms persist and are still referable to the acromioclavicular joint, a further injection of 6 ml of 1% lidocaine is given

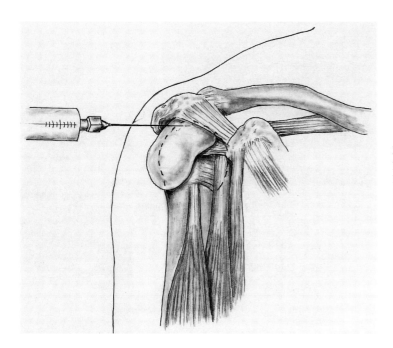

FIG. 10-4. As described, the injection test is performed by placing lidocaine initially in the subacromial bursa. If the pain persists following the subacromial injection, the lidocaine is then brought in from above and placed directly in the acromioclavicular joint.

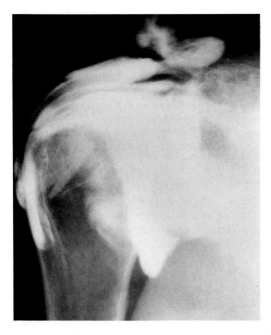

FIG. 10-5. This arthrogram shows an incompetent acromioclavicular (AC) joint capsule. The contrast can readily be seen entering the AC joint from its undersurface. The contrast agent was initially placed in the inferior aspect of the true glenohumeral joint. When there is a large rotator cuff tear, as demonstrated here, there frequently is destruction of the AC joint and repair of the rotator cuff requires concomitant excision of the distal clavicle.

into the acromioclavicular joint. The patient is once again examined, and the pain associated with acromioclavicular joint injury should now improve. I have found the diagnostic value of this test increased while performing the injections in the order described. If the physician's clinical suspicion is so directed to the acromiocla-

vicular joint, the injection could be given initially in that joint. In my experience an injection into the acromioclavicular joint can also diminish the pain of subacromial impingement. However, the converse is not true unless there is incompetence of the inferior capsule, allowing the lidocaine to enter from the underlying subacromial bursa. In severe degenerative joint disease of the acromioclavicular joint the inferior capsule is not present, as evidenced by the geyser sign seen on arthrography (Fig. 10-5).[6]

Radiographic Evaluation of the Acromioclavicular Joint

The most appropriate views to obtain when visualizing the acromioclavicular joint are the true anteroposterior (AP) view of the shoulder and the modified West Point view obtained as shown (Figs. 10-6 and 10-7). As in other joint evaluations, the physician should never accept anything less than two orthogonal views. The radiographic findings include irregularity of the joint surfaces, calcification in and about the acromioclavicular joint capsule, calcification of the coracoclavicular ligaments, and resorption of the lateral end of the clavicle to varying degrees (Figs. 10-8 and 10-9). As mentioned previously, hy-

---

Radiographic findings of acromioclavicular degenerative joint disease

- Joint surface irregularity
- Calcification of the acromioclavicular joint capsule
- Calcification of the coracoclavicular ligament
- Hypertrophic spurring
- Cyst formation
- Osteolysis of lateral clavicle (variable)

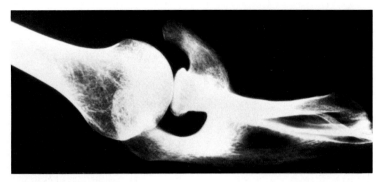

FIG. 10-6. Radiographic appearance of this modified West Point view. This provides excellent projection of the glenohumeral and acromioclavicular joints.

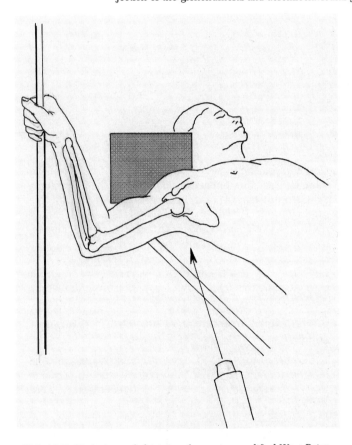

FIG. 10-7. Technique of obtaining the supine modified West Point view. With the patient laying supine and holding on to an IV pole, the x-ray tube is angled 20 degrees upward from the floor and 20 degrees away from the long axis of the patient's body. This effectively provides the lateral view of the shoulder and the acromioclavicular joint.

pertrophic spurring is usually seen on both the acromial and clavicular side of the joint. Cyst formation in the medial acromion or lateral clavicle is also significant evidence for osteoarthritic degenerative changes.

Treatment

Treatment of any condition must rely on an understanding of the natural history of the pathologic process. However, in the case of the acromioclavicular joint, the

TABLE 10-1 Chemical classes of nonsteroidal antiinflammatory agents

Chemical Class	Medication
Oxicams	Piroxicam (Feldene)
Salicylates	Aspirin
	Salsalate (Disalcid)
	Choline magnesium trisalicylate (Trilisate)
	Ascriptin
Acetic acids	Indomethacin (Indocin)
	Sulindac (Clinoril)
	Tolmetin sodium (Tolectin)
Propionic acids	Ibuprofen (Advil, Motrin)
	Naproxen (Naprosyn)
	Fenoprofen calcium (Nalfon)
	Ketoprofen (Orudis)
	Flurbiprofen (Ansaid)
Fenamates	Meclofenamate sodium (Meclomen)
Pyrazolines	Phenylbutazone (Butazolidin)
Phenylacetic acids	Diclofenac (Voltaren)

natural history and the rate of progression of the arthritis appear to be activity related. Also, it must be remembered that, as in most musculoskeletal conditions, the treating physician never treats the x-ray study. Asymptomatic patients with marked degenerative changes radiographically need no treatment. Conversely, patients with minimal radiographic findings can have severe disabling pain with recreational and nonrecreational activities.

Nonoperative Management

Nonoperative management of painful, degenerative joint disease involving the acromioclavicular joint begins with modification of activity. Daily stretching and oral nonsteroidal antiinflammatory agents (NSAIAs) are important adjuncts. Once symptoms abate, a muscle-strengthening program involving the trapezius and the remainder of the shoulder girdle muscles is initiated. Multiple nonsteroidal antiinflammatory drugs (NSAIDs) are available; my preference is one that provides the fewest doses, which (ideally) increases patient compliance. The patient must take the medication 2 to 3 weeks before evaluating its efficacy. If the initial antiinflammatory agent is not of significant benefit, at least two others of a different chemical class should be tried (Ta-

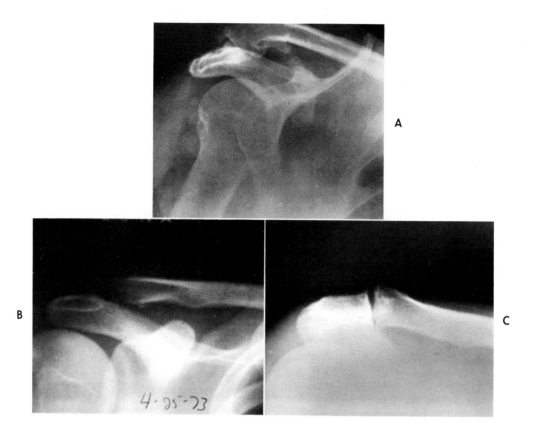

FIG. 10-8. A, Severe arthritis of the acromioclavicular (AC) joint. Note the calcification of the conoid and trapezoid ligament complex, the marked narrowing of the AC joint with irregularity of the joint surfaces, and the osteophyte process involving both the distal clavicle and medial aspect of the acromion. B, This radiograph of degenerative disease of the AC joint shows significant resorption of the lateral clavicle, cyst formation, and some early calcification of the conoid and trapezoid ligament complex. C, Note the AC joint arthritis manifested by joint space narrowing, particularly at the posteroinferior corner of the joint with cyst formation on both sides of the joint and prominence on the acromial and clavicular portions.

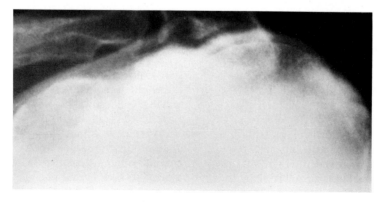

FIG. 10-9. Typical findings of arthritis of the acromioclavicular (AC) joint are seen with significant changes on the acromial side. Taken as part of an arthrogram study, absence of contrast in the AC joint can be seen, indicating integrity of the joint capsule.

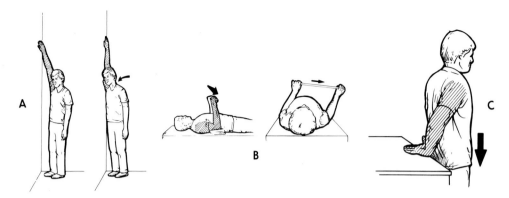

FIG. 10-10. Stretching exercises are an important part in the rehabilitating process of pathologic shoulder conditions. Cardinal motions are demonstrated here. **A,** Passive elevation is performed with the patient standing in the corner and elevating the arm in the plane of the scapula. The patient then leans against the wall trying to approximate the axilla to the wall itself, as shown. **B,** Supine external rotation is performed using a stick as shown. It is important to keep the elbow off the table so that the humerus remains parallel with the ground. **C,** Internal rotation is performed by having the patient force the thumb along the dorsal spine. This may be done by using the other arm to pull the affected arm up the back or may be performed as demonstrated.

ble 10-1). In most patients I reserve intraarticular steroids until two or three NSAIAs have been unsuccessful. If a patient is not responsive to the oral medications or has other contraindications to them, intraarticular corticosteroids may be given. If the oral agent is beneficial, it should be continued for 8 to 12 weeks after symptoms diminish to minimize the rapid return of symptoms. In addition to medication, it is equally important for the patient to modify activities. As previously mentioned, the use of the arm across the chest compresses the joint and should therefore not be allowed. Repetitive activity with the arm above the shoulder should also be kept to a minimum for the first 4 weeks of treatment. After the first month, patients may be allowed nonrepetitive use of the involved arm. Loss of motion, stiffness, and crepitus are common sequelae when treatment consists solely of limiting activity. Therefore daily stretching is also an important component of the nonoperative management of this condition. The patient must stretch in external rotation, internal rotation, and elevation at least once a day and at most twice a day during this recovery period (Fig. 10-10).

Operative Management

If nonoperative management fails to alleviate the patient's symptoms, surgical excision of the lateral clavicle may be indicated. This procedure was first described by Mumford[12] and Gurd[8] in 1941. Details of the technique are readily found in the standard texts,[16] but a few points should be emphasized. For this procedure to be successful, the coracoclavicular ligaments must be intact. If these ligaments are incompetent, significant instability of the medial clavicle remnant usually results in pain and marked weakness of elevation and forward throwing motions.

When performing the osteotomy of the clavicle, an osteotome should be used instead of a reciprocating saw. The saw creates bone dust and debris, which may result

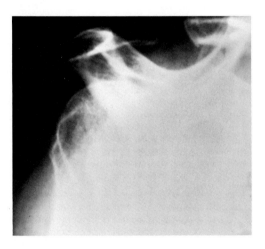

FIG. 10-11. Radiographic view after resection of the distal clavicle. Angular relationships are important to prevent impingement with motion following surgery. The lateral aspect of the clavicle is seen with slightly more bone removed inferiorly than superiorly, and the joint remains nearly parallel in appearance when comparing the lateral clavicle and medial acromion in this projection.

in myositis ossificans of the deltoid muscle. Furthermore, it has much more potential to cause soft-tissue injury involving especially the deltoid and trapezius muscles. Careful consideration must be given to the direction of the osteotomy. The AP and West Point views of the joint should provide a guide as to the angulation required for the clavicular osteotomy. When the osteotomy is complete, the new lateral end of the clavicle should represent a near parallelogram that is parallel to the plane of the medial acromion as seen in the diagram (Fig. 10-11).

In the usual case the physician resects slightly more bone posteriorly than anteriorly and slightly more bone inferiorly than superiorly. The surgeon must also remember the skeletal anatomy about the acromioclavicular joint. The trapezius inserts along the posterior distal clav-

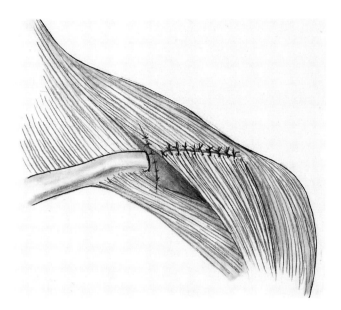

FIG. 10-12. Following clavicular resection it is imperative to reattach the deltoid muscle to the trapezius muscle directly. The deltoid takes its origin from this lateral clavicle; failure to reattach this securely results in weakness of elevation, and the athlete has difficulty in racquet and throwing sports.

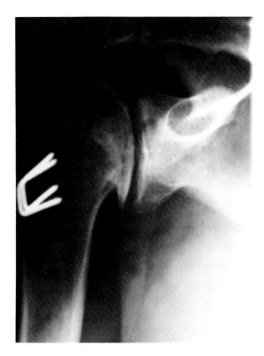

FIG. 10-13. Shoulder of a 21-year-old college football player who sustained multiple dislocations. Because he was thought to have anterior instability, repair was with a Magnuson-Stack procedure. However, because of the unrecognized inferior component, he developed the classic arthritis of recurrent dislocation. Loss of sphericity of the humeral head with degenerative changes at the glenohumeral joint can be seen. The most characteristic findings are inferior glenoid osteophytes with the osteophyte on the inferior aspect of the humerus. This osteophyte is not only present inferiorly. The more anterior portion of the osteophyte is superimposed on the anatomic neck of the humerus and cannot be visualized in this projection.

icle, and the deltoid originates on the anterior distal clavicle. As shown in Fig. 10-12, it is most important to reattach the deltoid origin to the trapezius insertion. Simply repairing the clavicular periosteum is not sufficient, and if this suture line fails, the anterior deltoid becomes markedly weak.

The aftercare of lateral clavicular resection consists of early passive motion in all planes, but active use of the arm must be restricted for 4 weeks. This permits satisfactory healing of the deltoid to the trapezius muscle. Strengthening programs are begun 1 month following surgery, and the athlete is allowed to return to activity any time thereafter without restriction. Within 3 to 4 months following surgery the athlete has nearly full range of motion and nearly symmetric strength with the contralateral arm.

DEGENERATIVE DISEASE OF THE GLENOHUMERAL JOINT

This discussion is concerned with the diagnosis and treatment of glenohumeral joint destruction. Although primary idiopathic glenohumeral arthritis is not usually seen until the fifth or sixth decade, a sizable number of patients, usually athletes, have a condition called *arthritis of dislocation*. This diagnosis was first used by Neer, Watson, and Stanton[14] when they reviewed their total shoulder experiences. In the cohort of patients who had arthritis of dislocation, the average age at the time of total joint arthroplasty for severe degenerative joint disease was 37 years old. Whether those athletes who use their arms in their chosen sport are at risk for primary glenohumeral arthritis is unknown. The association seems dubious outside the spectrum of minor and major instabilities. On the other hand, patients who undergo joint replacement for degenerative disease of the shoulder are not only allowed, but also encouraged to return to noncontact sports such as tennis, golf, and swimming.[13]

Because instability is a common problem in the athlete, some discussion of this condition seems appropriate. To begin, the physician must ask, "What is the natural history of instability?" Untreated, the natural history of the unstable shoulder does not seem to be degenerative joint disease. Clearly, a few patients with severe degenerative disease of their shoulder who seek an orthopaedist in the fifth decade and beyond give a history of untreated instability. Arthritis of dislocation appears to be an iatrogenic condition.

A review of 500 patients who had a degenerative disease of the glenohumeral joint yielded 103 patients who had a history of instability.[1] Of these 103 patients, 97 had prior surgery for their instability. Only six patients had a history of untreated instability and developed arthritis in this series. Although this series may not represent a true cross section of the population with instability, it is hard to ignore the findings. In careful studying of these patients, several potential etiologic factors come to light. The most common cause identified was the surgeon's failure to recognize the scope of the instability. Anterior instability is thought to be the most common type in the

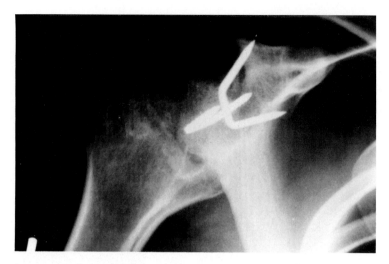

FIG. 10-14. A 19-year-old man following a failed Boyd staple capsulorrhaphy. The staples have become loosened and migrated, and the shoulder is now in a fixed, subluxation position with severe degenerative changes.

athletic population; hence the popularity of the Bristow, Boyd, Putti-Platt, and Magnuson procedures. Newer concepts of the unstable shoulder include simultaneous components of anterior, inferior, and posterior laxity to varying degrees. When an unrecognized multidirectional instability is repaired with the standard anterior procedures, the humeral head subluxation continues into the areas of untreated laxity (Fig. 10-13). This incongruity becomes exaggerated as the patient returns to activity, and degeneration of the joint then proceeds. In the reported series, 50 of the 103 patients required either total joint or humeral head replacement, and the average age was only 37 years. The second most common cause of arthritis of dislocation was related to the use of metal around the shoulder. It must be recognized that well-placed screws and staples at the time of surgery may become loose and migrate or they may fracture. If these metallic remnants find their way into the glenohumeral joint, severe destructive arthritis rapidly ensues. The literature has numerous reports on the complications of metal about the shoulder (Fig. 10-14).[10,17]

History

The active athletic patient usually has a chief complaint relating to loss of motion, stiffness, and pain in varying proportions. A history of acute trauma is usually absent. If there is a history of instability, the injury has, more often than not, been surgically treated. Night pain is not as characteristic as with subacromial impingement and rotator cuff injury. Pain is usually activity related and relieved by rest. Characteristically the pain is described as dull, aching, and poorly localizable. Because loss of external rotation is usually seen early in the degenerative process, patients complain of an inability to get the hand behind the head, especially in racquet and throwing sports. Initially patients get relief from over-the-counter antiinflammatory medications and analgesics.

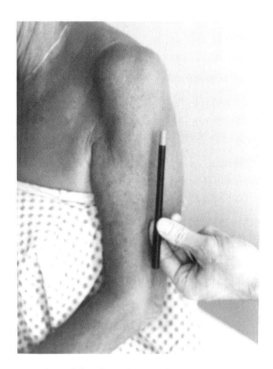

FIG. 10-15. One of the characteristic changes in arthritis of recurrent dislocation and generalized osteoarthritis of the shoulder is posterior migration of the humerus on the glenoid. When observing the patient from the lateral aspect, the more posterior position of the arm with respect to the shoulder becomes evident.

Physical Examination

In all patients who are being evaluated for shoulder injury a physical examination must begin at the cervical spine. The fact that both idiopathic cervical degenerative disease and glenohumeral degenerative dis-

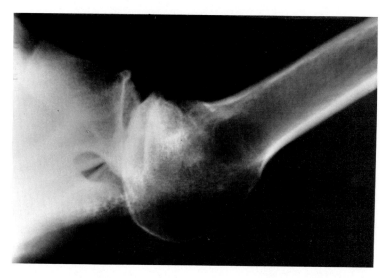

FIG. 10-16. Modified West Point view shows the marked posterior subluxation and migration in this 37-year-old baseball player. Patient had undergone a Putti-Platt procedure because he was thought to have isolated anterior instability. When his anterior capsule was made tight in the presence of some posterior laxity, the head was forced out the back, causing severe degenerative changes.

ease occur in the same age group makes these conditions difficult, yet mandatory for differentiation. Therefore a well-performed neck examination is critical. The patient is seated, both shoulders simultaneously exposed, and the neck is examined. Range of motion and degree of extension, flexion, rotation, and lateral bend are noted. Especially important is the combined maneuver of extension and lateral bend, which may close the neuroforamen and reproduce the patient's shoulder symptoms. Any limitation of cervical motion warrants a radiographic examination in the AP, lateral, and oblique planes at the least.

The shoulders are then visually inspected, noting atrophy, symmetry, and centering (Fig. 10-15). Degenerative joint disease of the glenohumeral joint characteristically causes posterior glenoid wear. As seen in Fig. 10-16, when viewed from a lateral side the humerus tends to lie more posterior than on the uninvolved side.

Clinical findings in glenohumeral degenerative joint disease

- Posterior position of humerus (axis)
- Supraspinatus/intraspinatus atrophy
- External rotation weakness
- Internal rotation contracture
- Loss of elevation

There is usually marked atrophy of the supraspinatus and infraspinatus muscles. Because loss of external rotation is so characteristic, the infraspinatus (the only true external rotator of the shoulder) is usually markedly affected. To a lesser degree clinically are the supraspinatus and deltoid visibly affected, but a Cybex evaluation

usually demonstrates clear differences between the involved and uninvolved sides.

The shoulder is then palpated, and it is imperative to examine the acromioclavicular joint. Forces that led to the glenohumeral degenerative disease were also present in some magnitude at the acromioclavicular joint. Concomitant acromioclavicular arthritis requiring surgical attention at the time of glenohumeral arthroplasty is present nearly 20% of the time in my experience. Only rarely is a true lateral clavicular resection (Mumford procedure) necessary. More commonly, an inferior claviculoplasty is performed. The sternoclavicular joint should also be examined and palpated at this time.

The patient is positioned supine, and passive range of motion is measured and recorded in both arms. When compared with the normal extremity, there is considerable loss of elevation in the scapular plane. Pain and crepitus are also frequently associated findings during this maneuver. While the patient remains supine, external rotation is measured. This characteristically has the greatest percentage loss when compared with the normal arm (Fig. 10-17). Often not only is the joint incongruity impeding motion, but also pain in itself limits motion.

The patient is once again placed in the sitting position, and internal rotation and active elevation are measured and recorded. A basic strength examination is performed by assessing the rotator cuff and deltoid. The examiner must recall that strength is modified by pain and therefore all weakness does not portend a cuff tear or nerve injury. Clinical assessment of rotator cuff integrity is best determined by evaluating the strength of external rotation. The patient positions the arms against the side with the elbows flexed 90 degrees. While the elbows are held at the sides, both arms are externally rotated

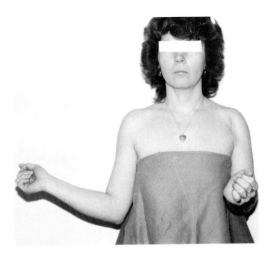

FIG. 10-17. This 27-year-old woman has severe arthritis of recurrent dislocation. She is demonstrating her maximal external rotation of the left shoulder. Careful observation shows several findings of the arthritis of dislocation. There is evidence of previous surgery with an anterior scar and marked atrophy of the anterior deltoid. The loss of external rotation and the posterior position of the humerus on the shoulder both are clinical signs of this condition.

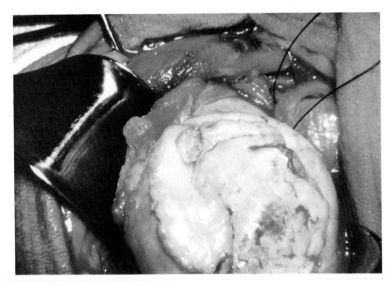

FIG. 10-18. This intraoperative view shows the circumferential nature of the osteophytes on the humeral head. On the anterior projection of this shoulder only the inferior osteophytes are seen. The more anterior and posterior osteophytes are not seen because they are projected over the anatomic neck of the humerus.

against the resistance of the examiner. Symmetric resistance implies cuff integrity, whereas weakness of external rotation may indicate rotator cuff injury. It should be understood that a careful neurologic examination documenting the integrity of the suprascapular and axillary nerve along with the remaining brachial plexus is required.

Radiographic Examination

As was noted previously, the most important films to obtain are the true AP and the modified West Point views (Figs. 10-6 and 10-7). Both of these projections provide an excellent view of a glenohumeral joint. The physician is able to appreciate the characteristic posterior glenoid wear (Fig. 10-16). The glenoid bone stock available for a glenoid replacement is seen only on the modified West Point view. Furthermore, the acromioclavicular joint can be radiographically evaluated and correlated with the

physical examination. The AP view should include the proximal two thirds of the humeral shaft so that the physician can safely estimate the appropriate humeral component diameter. On the AP view only inferior osteophytes are seen, but in fact these osteophytes are present circumferentially about the anatomic neck of the humerus (Fig. 10-18). Because they are superimposed on the anatomic neck at the periarticular margin (Fig. 10-19), they are seen only in their inferior projection. When clinically indicated, the radiographic examination of the shoulder must include a cervical spine series, as previously discussed.

Treatment
Nonoperative Management

Once again, the natural history of degenerative joint disease involving the glenohumeral joint must be considered. Whereas the natural history of untreated arthri-

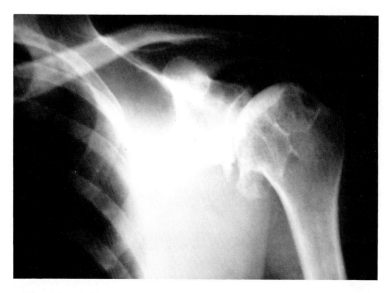

FIG. 10-19. This 40-year-old avid golfer complains of loss of motion. Four years before this radiograph, the patient had a Bankart type repair to correct recurrent and anterior instability. Once again the characteristic inferior glenoid osteophyte is seen with loss of sphericity of the humeral head. Only the inferior osteophyte is seen, but if the physician looks carefully at the anatomic neck region of the humerus, the anterior and posterior extent of the osteophyte is appreciated.

tis of the shoulder typically results in progressive loss of motion and increasing pain, the time course over which it occurs is remarkable for its unpredictability. In that context, treatment of degenerative joint disease of the shoulder by any means is always elective and based on patient symptoms. With both increased activity among patients well into the sixth and seventh decades and the near normal return of function and strength with shoulder replacement, an increasing role is played in surgical management of the athlete with degenerative joint disease of the shoulder.

Nonoperative management should consist of oral NSAIAs, a very occasional intraarticular corticosteroid, physical therapy primarily for isometric strengthening, and range of motion exercises only to the point of pain. There is little to gain in trying to increase the range of motion in a noncongruent arthritic joint. However, when performing isometric exercises, strength may be maintained in the face of a poorly moving joint. Periods of rest for the joint, the use of oral antiinflammatory agents, and isometric strengthening of the infraspinatus muscle often afford months of subjective relief in the face of clinical and radiographic severe shoulder arthritis.

Operative Management

Most surgeons consider it inappropriate to discuss the use of any joint replacements in young, active athletic people. Even in 1980 in a standard orthopaedic text, shoulder replacement was considered experimental.[15] Nevertheless, it has been recognized that a large proportion of the indications for surgical management (shoulder replacement) are in young, active athletic people. Other procedures, including cheilectomy, synovectomy, and joint lavage, should be avoided because they have

not been shown to increase motion or alter the natural history of the condition.

Those procedures, however, do result in scarring of the muscles, which leads to a poor outcome from subsequent arthroplasty. On the other hand, shoulder replacement, regardless of age, when performed properly has the potential in these young active patients to provide near normal motion and strength. Shoulder arthrodesis and joint resections make it impossible to use muscles effectively, and for this reason those procedures should be considered more radical than shoulder replacement even in the young active age groups.

In Neer, Watson, and Stanton's review of 500 shoulder replacements,[14] 95 (19%) had primary idiopathic osteoarthritis. These patients were generally young and engaged in activities such as tennis, golf, and swimming. Of those 500, 32 had arthritis of recurrent dislocation. This entity is extremely important in a sports medicine patient. The patients were athletically active, and the majority had had previous surgery. Most significant is that the average patient age was only 37 years. There was no good alternative to shoulder replacement; arthrodesis would have laid to waste good functional muscle. The patient seen in Fig. 10-20 was only 27 years old and had four procedures for instability with resultant severe osteoarthritis. Postoperatively the patient was engaged in activities that included butterfly swimming.

Principles in shoulder replacement

- Remove minimal bone.
- Preserve intact muscles.
- Restore muscles to anatomic lengths.
- Release adhesions.

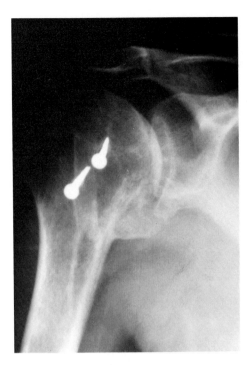

FIG. 10-20. This 27-year-old man has had four previous operations for anterior instability. The radiograph shows evidence of a previous Nicola procedure and a Magnuson-Stack type procedure as evidenced by the nails. Additionally, a Bankart type procedure was performed with anterior bone block. Now this patient has severe arthritis of dislocation, markedly limited motion, and severe pain. The only reasonable option in this young patient is shoulder replacement. In the absence of sepsis or paralysis arthrodesis would not be performed, since it would waste potentially good functioning muscle.

Surgical Technique

As with acromioclavicular joint procedures, literature on the technique of shoulder replacement is available,[3] and in this discussion only additional principles are presented. The principle in all shoulder procedures is to restore normal anatomy and, above all, consider shoulder replacement a soft-tissue procedure. The physician must remove only minimal bone, preserve intact muscles, and restore them to their anatomic lengths and release adhesions.

My preference is to perform shoulder replacements under regional interscalene block anesthesia, which offers several advantages over the general anesthetics. There is significantly less blood loss, minimal postoperative nausea, and patients are able to ambulate within 2 to 3 hours of their surgical procedure. Analgesia lasts as long as 8 hours and only gradually wears off. The most significant benefit is that the patient is able to observe their range of motion following surgery; with the patient sitting on the operating table, I place the arm through a range of motion for him or her to see.

The patient is placed in the beach-chair position, and a long deltopectoral incision is made from the clavicle to the deltoid insertion. The deltoid is not removed from its origin on the clavicle and acromion; rather, a portion of its insertion is released if necessary for increased expo-

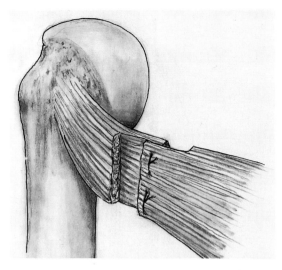

FIG. 10-21. Technique of lengthening the subscapularis capsule complex. Functional success of shoulder replacement depends on adequate external rotation. Because the arthritic process usually results in marked loss of external rotation preoperatively, the surgeon must nearly always lengthen this structure as the shoulder is approached surgically. Despite the previous history of instability, following shoulder replacement for arthritis the stability of the joint depends on the version of the components and does not depend on a tight anterior subscapularis or capsule complex. When the operative procedure is complete and the shoulder closed, the arm should be able to reach nearly 45 to 50 degrees of external rotation with no tension on the new suture line.

sure. The superior one third of the pectoralis major is released from the humeral shaft, taking care not to injure the tendinous portion of the long head of the biceps muscle. Remembering that 60 to 70 degrees of external rotation is paramount for return to most athletic activities, the surgeon must now assess the external rotation. The subscapularis capsule complex must be lengthened (Fig. 10-21) so that following anterior rotator cuff repair the arm can reach 45 to 50 degrees of external rotation with no tension on the new suture line. Care must be taken to balance soft tissues to minimize postoperative instability of the arthroplasty.[11]

When the humeral osteotomy is performed, great care must be taken to ensure that the axis of the head of the component is above the tip of the greater tuberosity (Fig. 10-22). In doing this, the deltoid and rotator cuff muscle lengths are maintained and strength recovery is more predictable. The myofascial sleeve of the upper arm must remain taut following replacement to allow full active elevation.

The use of cement in joint arthroplasty has a long, stormy history. However, in shoulder replacements there has never been more than an occasional case report of clinical loosening of either the humeral or glenoid components.[2] In one series[4] glenoid lucency rate was nearly 70% at 5-year follow-up, but none was clinically loose or required revision. More significant was the fact that 68% of the lucent lines were present within 1 week of the operative procedure, and less than 7% progressed over the 5-year follow-up period. It is my opinion that cement

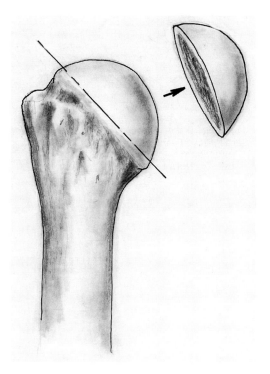

FIG. 10-22. Appropriate location for the humeral osteotomy. The axis of the component must lie above the tip of the greater tuberosity as seen.

should be routinely used for the glenoid at present with prior meticulous bone preparation. New glenoid components that are becoming available allow for bone ingrowth.[5] Anatomically, however, there appears to be so little bone available for ingrowth that the physician should be careful of jumping into a new technology when the past has offered so few problems. In considering cement for the humeral component, the key is immediate axial and rotational stability. The most important consideration must be early shoulder motion and rehabilitation. If a component cannot be seated firmly, it should be cemented without regard to patient age. With careful technique, however, nearly all humeral components can be placed adequately without the use of methyl methacrylate in the young active athletic patient with primary degenerative joint disease.

Aftercare and Rehabilitation

The physician must be intimately involved in the management of the physical therapy program after shoulder replacement. Only the surgeon is aware of the quality of the soft tissues and rotator cuff. Handing the patient a prescription and sending him or her to the local physical therapist for rehabilitation is an invitation to failure. All therapy must begin and continue as surgeon directed and surgeon modified.

Passive range of motion, including elevation and external rotation, are begun the morning following surgery. By the fourth or fifth day internal rotation stretching is begun. Because the deltoid was not detached, active elevation may begin as soon as 2 to 3 days following surgery if passive motion allows. Patients with osteoarthri-

tis and arthritis of recurrent dislocations should elevate near 150 to 160 degrees within 7 days. External rotation should reach at least 45 degrees also within a week if appropriate measures were undertaken to lengthen the anterior subscapularis capsule complex at the time of arthroplasty. The physician must encourage and reassure the patient that recovery continues well into 9 to 12 months following surgery.

With a properly implanted prosthesis and with proper physician-directed rehabilitation, patients have been allowed to return to nearly all noncontact recreational activities. Football, wrestling, and downhill skiing are not allowed, but most patients engage in activities including tennis, swimming, golf, and basketball. Bowling and other racquet sports are also permitted. Strengthening exercises below the horizontal are begun with rubber tubing, progressing to springs, and eventually free weights to a limit of 50 pounds. Push-ups are allowed, but pull-ups, chin-ups, and overhead exercises with Nautilus equipment are discouraged.

Athletic activity following shoulder replacement

Permitted (noncontact, recreational)
- Tennis
- Swimming
- Golf
- Basketball
- Bowling

Forbidden
- Football
- Wrestling
- Downhill skiing
- Pull-ups
- Chin-ups

For the young, active athletic patient who has developed degenerative joint disease of the shoulder, shoulder replacement provides predictable relief of pain and, when performed according to previously described surgical principles, patients may return to nearly all activities without restrictions.

REFERENCES
1. Brems JJ: *Arthritis of recurrent dislocations,* Paper presented at Annual New York Orthopaedic Hospital Alumni Meeting, New York, 1984.
2. Brems JJ: The glenoid component in total shoulder arthroplasty, *J Shoulder Elbow Surg* 1(5):47, 1992.
3. Brems JJ, Neer CS: Technique of shoulder replacement, *Sound Slide Library,* Cleveland, 1985, AAOS.
4. Brems JJ, Wilde AH: Glenoid lucent lines. In *Transactions of the Annual Meeting of American Shoulder and Elbow Surgeons,* New Orleans, 1986, The Academy.
5. Cofield RH, Daly PJ: Total shoulder arthroplasty with tissue ingrowth glenoid component, *J Shoulder Elbow Surg,* 1(2):77, 1992.
6. Craig EV: The geyser sign and torn rotator cuff—clinical significance and pathomechanics, *Clin Orthop* 191, 1984.
7. Depalma AF: *Surgery of the shoulder,* Philadelphia, 1983, JB Lippincott.

8. Gurd FB: The treatment of complete dislocation of the outer end of the clavicle—A hitherto undescribed operation, *Ann Surg* 113:1041, 1941.

9. Harres TJ, Cox JS: Acromioclavicular injuries and surgical treatment. In Jackson DW (ed): *Shoulder surgery in the athlete,* Gaithersburg, Md, 1985, Aspen Press.

10. Lower RF, McNeish LM, Callaghan JJ: Computed tomographic documentation of intraarticular penetration of a screw after operations on the shoulder, *J Bone Joint Surg* 67A:1120, 1985.

11. Moeckel BH et al: Instability of the shoulder after arthroplasty, *J Bone Joint Surg* 75A:492, 1993.

12. Mumford EB: Acromioclavicular dislocations, *J Bone Joint Surg* 23:799, 1941.

13. Neer CS, Brems JJ: Shoulder replacement in the active and athletic patient. In Jackson DW (ed): *Shoulder surgery in the athlete,* Gaithersburg, Md, 1985, Aspen Press.

14. Neer CS, Watson KC, Stanton FJ: Recent experiences in total shoulder replacement, *J Bone Joint Surg* 64:319, 1982.

15. Sisk DT, Wright PE: Arthroplasty of the shoulder and elbow. In Crenshaw AH (ed): *Campbell's operative orthopaedics,* ed 8, St Louis, 1992, Mosby.

16. Lavelle DG: Acute dislocations. In Crenshaw AH (ed): *Campbell's operative orthopaedics,* ed 8, St Louis, 1992, Mosby.

17. Zuckerman JD, Matsen FA: Complications about the glenohumeral joint related to the use of screws and staples, *J Bone Joint Surg* 66A:175, 1984.

CHAPTER 11 — Principles of Shoulder Rehabilitation in the Athlete

Francis X. Mendoza
Andrew K. Sands

The shoulder is the most mobile joint in humans, and, as such, it is frequently injured during athletic activities. This is especially true with modern sports, which tend to overemphasize use of the upper extremity and eye-hand coordination, as well as physical contact.

Shoulder injuries can result from either macrotrauma or microtrauma.[13] Macrotraumatic injuries occur as a result of an explosive force, such as during a tackle in a football game or a fall during a gymnastic maneuver. Microtraumatic injuries, on the other hand, occur from repetitive motions that result in overuse of the shoulder.[11] In this case the muscle activity and force generated are not necessarily maximal, but the number of times the shoulder is repetitively cycled leads to injury.

All injuries of the athlete's shoulder must be rehabilitated to allow painless range of motion with flexibility and strength. This encourages participation without further injury. The rehabilitation program can be divided into three phases. Phase I emphasizes diminishing the inflammation and discomfort that result from the acute injury or surgical repair. Phase II directs treatment toward achieving and maintaining full, painless range of motion. Phase III concentrates on increasing strength and endurance in all planes of shoulder motion.

The physician and the therapist must communicate during the different phases of rehabilitation to tailor specific aspects of the treatment to the individual athlete and allow safe and expedient recovery.

It must be remembered that, through the musculoskeletal *linkage system,* the shoulder is intimately related to the cervical spine, as are the elbow and distal arm. To treat the athlete successfully, the shoulder rehabilitation program must incorporate these additional regions.[26] Similarly, it is imperative to continue overall body conditioning during the shoulder rehabilitation program, to facilitate full return of the athlete on completion of treatment.

EVALUATION

Before initiation of treatment after a shoulder injury, a thorough history and physical examination enable the physician and the therapist to create a treatment program. This allows different aspects within the three phases of rehabilitation to be effectively tailored to the individual athlete.

History

The patient's age, arm dominance, sport, and level of competition, as well as any previous injury, should be ascertained.

A detailed description of the current injury, including the position of the shoulder and arm at the time of injury, is necessary to determine whether the injury was predominantly the result of macrotrauma (such as an acute dislocation), or microtrauma (as is often the case with atraumatic subluxations). Knowledge of any previous shoulder injury should include a diagnosis, the type and duration of immobilization, the number of steroid injections, the type of therapy used, the type of surgical repair and findings at the time of surgery, and the athlete's overall response to treatment. Furthermore, a history of injury to the uninvolved shoulder and the treatment for the injury may be useful.

Physical Examination

Examination commences with observation of the patient's use of the upper extremity while removing outer

garments, such as sweaters and coats. Generally, the uninvolved shoulder should be used as a standard of comparison with the injured shoulder. Asymmetry and atrophy are more easily appreciated when both shoulders are observed from behind. The range of motion, both passive and active, should be recorded in degrees for total elevation (Fig. 11-1), for external rotation with the arm at the side (Fig. 11-2), and for external rotation with the arm at 90 degrees of abduction. Internal rotation can be recorded using the vertebrae as landmarks (Fig. 11-3).

The presence of swelling, discrete areas of tenderness, and joint laxity should be noted. Additionally, if appropriate, the presence of an impingement sign and an apprehension sign in the anterior, inferior, or posterior directions should be recorded. Neurologic and vascular examinations of both upper extremities should routinely be performed, noting any restrictions of cervical spine motion and discomfort, as well as any differences in the peripheral pulses. Abnormalities in the degree of elbow, wrist, and hand motion and strength should also be recorded.

Manual muscle testing can be accomplished in different functional planes of motion, comparing both shoulders. Quantification of strength can be achieved using a Cybex isokinetic dynamometer or a NISMAT manual tester, although discomfort of the injured shoulder invariably has an adverse effect on the reliability of the results.

BASIC SHOULDER REHABILITATION PROGRAM

The cornerstone to successful shoulder rehabilitation is implementation of a basic three-phase program that guides the therapist and enables assessment of the athlete's progress as each phase is completed. Although the

---

General shoulder rehabilitation

- Phase I—Diminish inflammation and discomfort
- Phase II—Achieve full range of motion
- Phase III—Develop strength and endurance

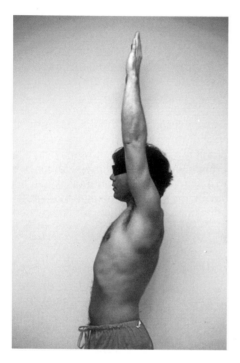

FIG. 11-1. Total elevation is measured from 0 degrees with the arm at the side to 180 degrees.

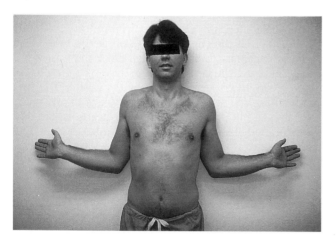

FIG. 11-2. External rotation is measured from 0 to 90 degrees with the proximal arm at the side and the elbow flexed to 90 degrees.

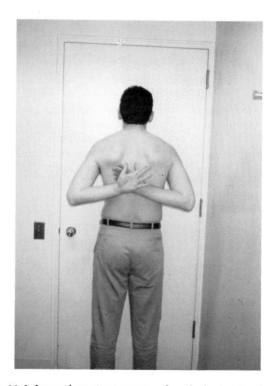

FIG. 11-3. Internal rotation is measured up the back using the vertebrae.

professional athlete can generally be treated with supervision on a daily basis, the usual frequency of treatment for nonprofessionals is 2 to 3 times a week, with close monitoring of a home exercise program.

Phase I

The primary goal of Phase I treatment is to diminish pain and inflammation during acute and subacute phases of the injury. The type of injury sustained or surgical repair performed determines the amount of shoulder motion allowed during this period of treatment. For instance, an athletic shoulder injury that results in an acute hemorrhagic bursitis may benefit from 3 to 5 days of sling immobilization. This helps control swelling and discomfort before initiation of range of motion exercises.[25] On the other hand, a shoulder surgically repaired to prevent anterior instability generally requires 2 to 6 weeks of immobilization, depending on the procedure used, to encourage healing and decrease discomfort before initiation of range of motion exercises. Thus during Phase I a variable amount of immobilization is generally necessary.

In the acute period, the first 24 to 48 hours after injury, application of ice (cryotherapy) to the area of injury for 10-minute intervals assists in the control of swelling and pain. Discomfort can be further reduced with the use of analgesics, oral nonsteroidal antiinflammatory drugs (NSAID), and transcutaneous electric nerve stimulation (TENS).[28] As the athlete progresses into the subacute period, application of heat for 10- to 15-minute intervals, alone or alternated with ice treatments, is beneficial (contrast therapy).[20]

Throughout the Phase I period of rehabilitation isometric contractions of 5-second duration followed by 2- to 3-second relaxations are instituted for the elbow, wrist, and hand. When the specific injury allows, gentle isometrics are introduced for the shoulder. These exercises can be performed using the uninvolved arm to resist the contraction of the shoulder, elbow, or wrist of the injured extremity while a soft rubber ball or putty is squeezed for hand exercises.

As soon as the acute shoulder discomfort is effectively controlled, overall aerobic and anaerobic fitness of the athlete is maintained. Although immobilization of the injured arm may still be required, a stationary bicycle, in conjunction with strengthening and flexibility exercises of both lower extremities, the trunk, and the uninvolved upper extremity, is used.

Phase I

- Immobilization
- Cryotherapy
- Analgesics
- Nonsteroidal antiinflammatory drugs
- Transcutaneous electric nerve stimulation
- Contrast therapy
- Isometrics
- Maintenance of fitness level

The amount of time necessary to complete Phase I depends on the degree of swelling and discomfort and the length of time immobilization is needed for healing of soft tissue and bone. This phase of rehabilitation generally takes 2 to 3 weeks to complete but may require up to 6 weeks.

Phase II

Phase II of the shoulder program concentrates on obtaining full, painless range of motion. During this phase of rehabilitation the therapist works closely with the athlete, using passive-assisted stretching (the therapist or the patient's uninvolved arm passively stretches the injured shoulder) range of motion techniques (Figs. 11-4

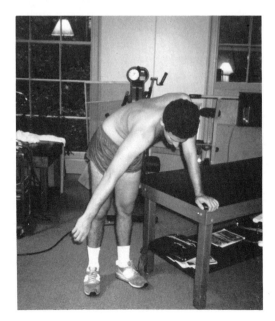

FIG. 11-4. Gentle pendulums can be used as warm-up exercises. They are performed clockwise, counterclockwise, forward and backward, and in an abduction to adduction direction.

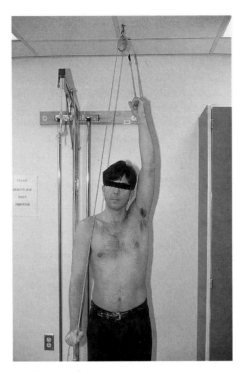

FIG. 11-5. Pulley powered by the uninvolved left arm stretches the right shoulder in total elevation.

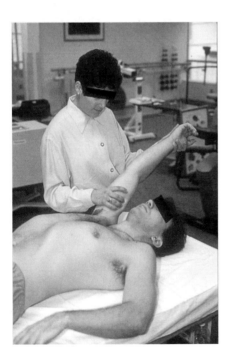

FIG. 11-6. Total elevation stretching assisted by a therapist.

to 11-7). This removes any residual shoulder stiffness that resulted from the injury or immobilization.

Any anticipated limitations of motion after a particular injury or surgical procedure should be understood. Aggressive attempts to overcome these limitations may not be appropriate and could cause undue discomfort

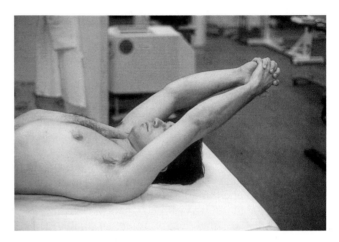

FIG. 11-7. Supine forward elevation stretching of the right shoulder provided by the left, uninvolved, arm.

during rehabilitation. Electromyographic evidence indicates that early stretching in the supine position rather than the erect position may be advantageous to ensure minimal muscle activity.[17]

The athlete must be aware that, unlike other aspects of physical therapy, passive-assisted stretching causes some discomfort. Tolerance varies with each individual. To encourage patient participation and minimize discomfort, heat is applied to the shoulder for 10 to 15 minutes before the stretching sessions. Additionally, TENS and neuromuscular electric stimulation techniques[2] have been reported to assist in relaxing the patient during maximal soft-tissue stretches. Toward the end of a stretching session, heat is applied to the shoulder girdle for 10 minutes; this is followed by the passive stretch being manually sustained during the cooling period to ensure that the motion gained during treatment is not lost.[27] Also, brief, frequent stretching sessions rather than prolonged periods are emphasized. If progress is slower than expected, the use of hydrotherapy early in this phase has been found to be useful.[33]

Because the range of shoulder motion is so extensive, the therapist must regain motion in an orderly manner. Predictably good results continue to be obtained with warm-up pendulum range of motion exercises, followed by passive-assisted stretching in the cardinal planes of total elevation, external rotation with the arm at the side, and internal rotation (Figs. 11-8 to 11-11).[24] Any later stiffness at the extremes of adduction must be eliminated (Fig. 11-12), as well as any residual stiffness that restricts full external rotation at 90 degrees of abduction (Fig. 11-13).

Throughout Phase II of the shoulder program the therapist can use the motion of the uninvolved shoulder as a standard of comparison for the gains achieved after therapy. For optimal function, *the goal of rehabilitation should be to achieve nearly symmetric range of motion in all planes of the shoulder*. Nonetheless, with knowledge of the athlete's specific shoulder injury or surgical procedure, it may be desirable to limit a particular shoul-

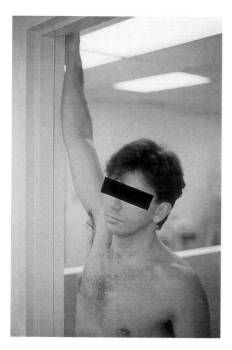

FIG. 11-8. Advanced total elevation stretching by leaning against a door edge.

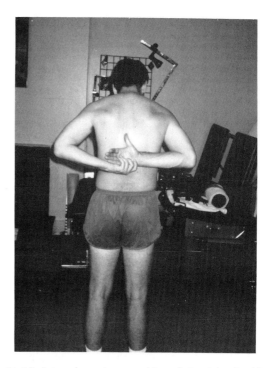

FIG. 11-10. Internal rotation stretching of the right shoulder assisted by the uninvolved left arm.

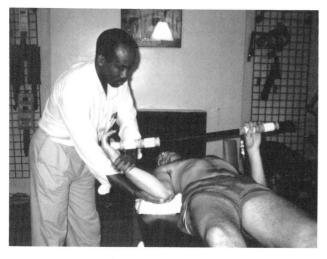

FIG. 11-9. Supine external rotation stretching of the right shoulder with a stick powered by the uninvolved arm or a therapist. A small pillow under the elbow maintains the humerus in the mid-coronal plane.

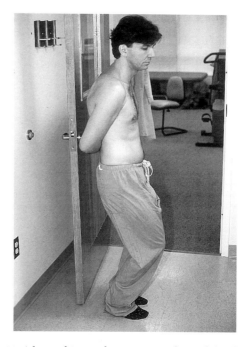

FIG. 11-11. Advanced internal rotation stretching of the shoulder performed by holding a doorknob along the center line of the back and then squatting.

der motion. For example, after an anterior dislocation, imposing a mild (10-degree) restriction of motion at the extreme of external rotation may discourage recurrent instability. Similarly, it must be recognized that many athletes involved in sports that require throwing have excessive external rotation of the dominant shoulder with a concomitant loss of internal rotation. This asymmetry may not be pathologic.

During Phase II—as recovery allows—progressive isometric exercises are instituted for the internal rotators and adductors, external rotators, abductors, anterior and posterior deltoid muscles, biceps and triceps brachii muscles, and the scapula-stabilizing muscles of the shoulder. This group of exercises is usually performed 10 to 20 times, each with a 5-second contraction and a 2- to 3-second relaxation. The uninvolved extremity or a wall

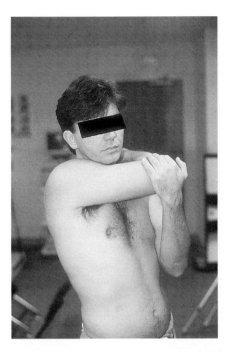

FIG. 11-12. Stretching the posterior right shoulder soft tissues in adduction with a hugging motion powered by the uninvolved left arm.

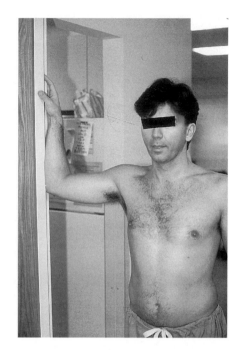

FIG. 11-13. Terminal stretching in 90 degrees of abduction and external rotation can be achieved by leaning in a doorway. This exercise must be used cautiously because it can encourage instability.

is used to resist the contraction. The entire group of shoulder isometrics can generally be performed three times a day.

On completion of Phase II stretching the athlete enters Phase III of the program, which is directed at progressive strengthening.

Phase II

- Passive-assisted range of motion
- Heat
- Transcutaneous electric nerve stimulation
- Neuromuscular stimulation
- Isometrics

Phase III

Phase III initially emphasizes strengthening against resistance (isometric), followed by advanced (isotonic and isokinetic) strengthening. Each muscle of the rotator cuff should be individually strengthened[14] to facilitate optimal recovery. During Phase III the athlete must perform a gentle daily shoulder stretch in the previously noted cardinal planes of motion to ensure that the range of motion is maintained.

When the athlete's performance with the isometric contractions improves, the patient then progresses to isotonic strengthening exercises using surgical tubing or free weights (Figs. 11-14 to 11-19). These exercises are generally most effective if performed slowly and, initially, in the underhorizontal shoulder planes. To promote

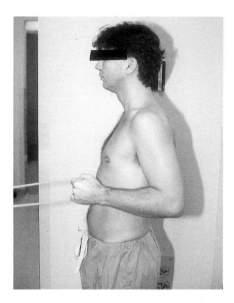

FIG. 11-14. Internal rotators are strengthened using elastic tubing on a doorknob.

rhythmic scapula motion and avoid substitution maneuvers, the patient is closely observed during each eccentric and concentric contraction. Short-term discomfort caused by muscle fatigue is acceptable and can be used as a guide to determine the number and frequency of exercise repetitions to be performed. Prolonged discomfort, precipitated by excessive repetitions of exercises or by a particular exercise, should be avoided.

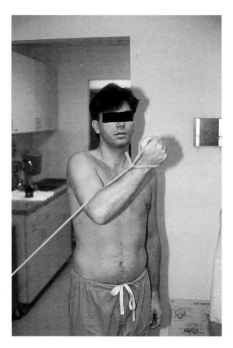

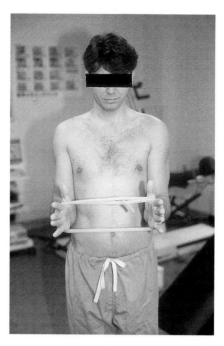

FIG. 11-15. Adductors and internal rotators are strengthened by pulling the elastic tubing across the chest toward the opposite arm.

FIG. 11-16. External rotators and abductors are strengthened using elastic tubing.

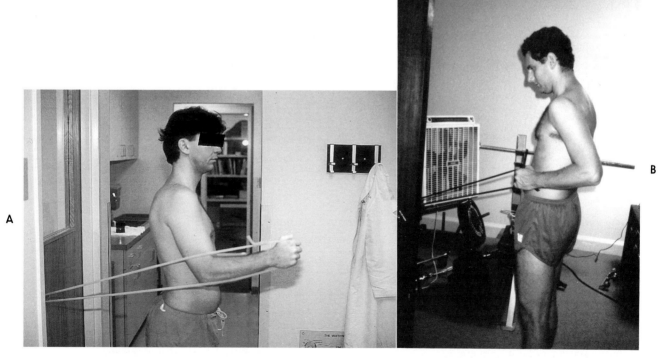

FIG. 11-17. Anterior and posterior deltoid muscles are strengthened by pushing (**A**) or pulling (**B**) the elastic tubing, which is anchored on a doorknob.

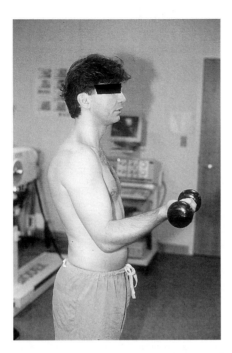

FIG. 11-18. Biceps brachii strengthening can be accomplished with a free weight.

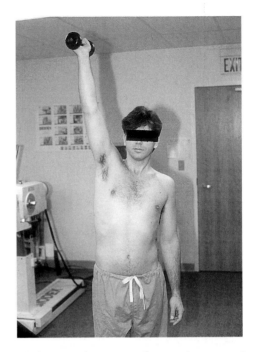

FIG. 11-19. As strength improves, free weights are used in over-horizontal planes.

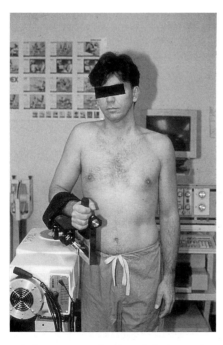

FIG. 11-20. Isokinetic strengthening of the internal rotator muscles.

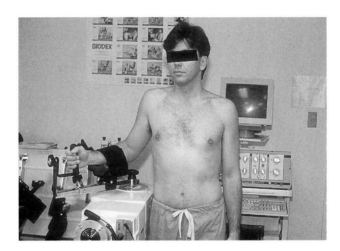

FIG. 11-21. Isokinetic strengthening of the external rotator muscles.

As performance increases with isotonic strengthening, the therapist introduces **isokinetic training,** which permits limb exercise at both slow and fast velocities. Slow speeds focus on residual strength deficits, whereas high-speed training enhances power and endurance (Figs. 11-20 to 11-22).[16,39] The therapist begins with the underhorizontal planes of motion, then progresses into the cardinal and diagonal planes. The diagonal motions are in functional planes and closely simulate patterns that are necessary for everyday activities (Fig. 11-23).[6,35]

Throughout the isokinetic strengthening period, but on alternate days, the athlete continues more advanced isotonic training in similar planes with free weights or with a Nautilus-type machine. During the advanced strengthening program, continued close supervision is warranted to further encourage normal, rhythmic scapular motions. As isometric and isokinetic strengthening nears completion, the athlete involved with repetitive motions of the shoulder may benefit from a plyometric strengthening program.[4,38] Here the therapist employs different size medicine balls to simulate the sport-

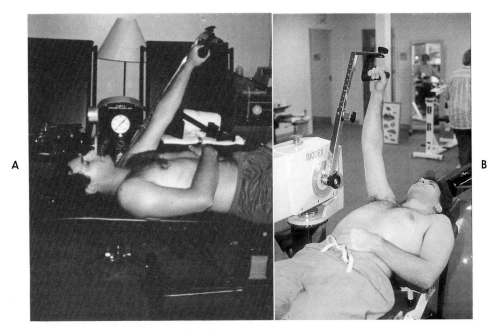

FIG. 11-22. Isokinetic strengthening in forward flexion (**A**) and total elevation (**B**).

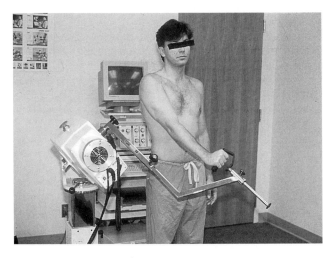

FIG. 11-23. Isokinetic strengthening in diagonal planes of function.

specific motion performed by the athlete to further enhance strength. For example, the throwing athlete performs a gradual eccentric contraction of the internal rotators (cocking phase) followed by a more rapid concentric contraction of the internal rotators (acceleration phase).

Generally during this period the athlete's strength is sufficient to allow limited participation in sports activities. The athlete's return to sports is monitored and adjusted as progress allows. When clinical examination and strength testing indicate excellent strength has been achieved, the athlete is allowed to return to full activity and continues preinjury conditioning and strength maintenance program.

Phase III

- Maintenance of range of motion with daily stretching
- Isometric exercises
- Isotonic and isokinetic exercises
- Plyometric sport-specific exercises
- Monitoring of progressive return to sports

REHABILITATION OF COMMON SHOULDER INJURIES
Anterior Shoulder Instability
Nonoperative Program

After an anteroinferior dislocation is reduced or following a traumatic subluxation, assuming no earlier history of instability, rehabilitation should be instituted. Recognizing that the glenohumeral ligaments, capsule, and surrounding musculature have been stretched by the trauma, Phase I of the treatment emphasizes immobilization with a sling and swathe. Application of ice and the use of other modalities decrease tissue edema and hemorrhage, and gentle isometric exercises are begun for the elbow, wrist, and hand. When discomfort allows, gentle Phase I isometrics are initiated while the shoulder is still immobilized.

The period of immobilization after glenohumeral dislocations is a topic of considerable debate, and reports range from 0 to 6 weeks.* Additionally, there is evidence that the age of the patient at the time of the first dislocation considerably influences the overall recurrance

---

*References 10, 12, 25, 29, 30, and 32.

Conservative management after acute anterior dislocation

Phase I
- Sling
- Ice
  Isometrics for the elbow, wrist, and hand
  Isometrics for shoulder (when comfortable)
- Aerobic work

Phase III
- Early
  Isotonic strengthening under horizontal plane
  Emphasis on internal rotators
- Middle
  Addition of external rotators and shoulder girdle to isotonic strength program
  Initiation of isokinetic work in cardinal planes of motion
- Late
  Isokinetic strengthening in diagonal planes
  Plyometric sport-specific program
  Monitored progressive return to sports

---

rate of instability, with rates reported as high as 85% to 90% for patients less than 20 years of age.[31] A well-planned rehabilitation program, however, can decrease the recurrance rate to as low as 17%.[1,40] In our experience, for best results the athlete's shoulder should be immobilized from 4 to 6 weeks, depending on his or her age, the sport to which he or she must return, the degree to which the injured shoulder is involved in the sport, and the amount of clinical laxity of the uninvolved shoulder.

During the period of immobilization and when the discomfort allows, isometric contractions of the shoulder musculature are initiated within the patient's tolerance. Throughout this period the athlete is instructed to maintain the axis of the arm anterior to the midcoronal plane of the body so as not to encourage anterior instability. On completion of the immobilization period, Phase II is initiated, with concentration on gentle, passive, assisted stretching exercises to regain the range of motion.

During Phase II, emphasis is placed on the gentle nature of the stretching exercises because these shoulders tend to regain motion rapidly. Progress is enhanced when stretching exercises are supplemented with other soft-tissue treatment modalities, such as ice, heat, and TENS. The goals of phase II should be to provide the athlete with painless, full total elevation, full internal rotation, and ideally a mild (10-degree) limitation of external rotation with the arm at the side.

The athlete then enters Phase III. Isotonic strengthening exercises should begin from the underhorizontal position. This encourages stability and diminishes mechanical irritation from the injured capsule and ligaments.[23] The internal rotators are emphasized because these are the most effective dynamic restraints against anterior instability in the middle to lower ranges of abduction.[5,34] As progress is made, strengthening proceeds to include the external rotators and remaining shoulder musculature. Isotonic strengthening is progressed in the cardinal planes of motion and then advanced isokineti-

cally to the cardinal and diagonal planes of motion. If appropriate, plyometric sport-specific exercises are then implemented.

Before initiation of full, unprotected activity of the arm, the range of motion of the shoulder must be painless, with good strength and endurance as compared with the uninvolved arm. Furthermore, sufficient external rotation strength at 90 degrees of abduction (the position at which the shoulder is generally most vulnerable to anterior instability) should be obtained without apprehension to allow comfortable participation in the athlete's particular sport. The period of recovery through phases II and III can vary from 6 weeks to 4 months.

Postoperative Program

The principles of rehabilitation of the surgically repaired shoulder against anterior instability are similar to those for the nonsurgically treated shoulder. Modifications depend on the type of procedure used, the time necessary for maturation of the repair, and any imposed motion limitations that are innate to the procedure. As previously noted, progression through all phases can vary and full rehabilitation is generally obtained within 6 months to 1 year.

In our experience[18] the modified Neer inferior capsular shift repair for anterior instability, supplemented with repair of a detached labrum if present, and bone grafting of a significant glenoid deficiency, has been used in treatment of athletes and yields a high degree of success. The shoulder is generally immobilized in a sling for 6 weeks. Isometric exercises for the elbow, wrist, and hand are used during this period. Thereafter, immobilization by sling is discontinued, and the rehabilitation progresses as previously discussed for the nonsurgically treated athlete after an anterior dislocation. Full, unrestricted use of the arm is generally allowed 9 months after surgery. The average athlete, before resumption of full activity, has regained full total elevation, full internal rotation, and generally lacks 10 degrees of external rotation with the arm at the side. Shoulder strength and endurance are regained without apprehension.

Criteria for return to play following an anterior dislocation

- Painless range of motion
- Strength and endurance parity
- Sufficient external rotation at 90-degree abduction without apprehension

---

Impingement Syndromes

The impingement syndrome has been characterized as a mechanical compression of the rotator cuff tendons beneath the subacromial arch.[21] In our experience this syndrome occurs in athletes[3,9,19,25] and can result in a progression of stages, from an acute hemorrhagic, engorged bursitis and tendinitis (Stage 1), to a recurrent fibrotic bursitis and tendinitis (Stage 2), and finally, to a rotator cuff tear (Stage 3).[22] The etiologic cause in most athletes

is attributed to microtrauma from activities involving repetitive movement of the arms above the head. Less frequently, macrotraumatic shoulder injuries resulting in recurrent bursitis or in an actual rotator cuff tear have been recognized.

Stages 1 and 2

Nonsurgical treatment of Stages 1 and 2 impingement syndromes is generally successful and is based on decreasing rotator cuff inflammation and increasing the strength of the shoulder musculature. As the soft-tissue inflammation of the bursa and tendons decreases, their volume effectively decreases, thus encouraging excursion without impingement. Similarly, by strengthening the rotator cuff muscles and the scapula-stabilizing muscles, a dynamic depressor effect on the humeral head is achieved. This maximizes the size of the subacromial space and further enhances function without impingement.

Phase I rehabilitation for either Stage 1 (acute) or Stage 2 (recurrent) impingement is essentially the same. To discourage reinjury, the athlete is advised to use the involved arm for only light underhorizontal activities. Shoulder isometric exercises are initiated shortly thereafter. In the more extreme case, immobilization by sling may be necessary for a brief period of 3 to 4 days until soft-tissue inflammation diminishes sufficiently to allow light active underhorizontal use of the arm. NSAIDs, ice, TENS, and ultrasound treatments have all been used successfully to expedite the diminishment of inflammation of the bursa and rotator cuff tendons.[9]

Within 10 to 14 days progress usually permits initiation of Phase II rehabilitation, primarily aimed at a gentle daily stretch in the cardinal planes of motion. This prevents shoulder stiffness at the extremes, whereas the lack of repetitive overhorizontal exercises discourages the impingement syndrome. Shoulder isometrics are progressed in the underhorizontal, nonpainful planes. On occasion the prudent use of a steroid injection into the subacromial space may be warranted to enhance progress through Phase I or II. Nevertheless, this latter adjunct should be used with extreme discretion; the potential hazards of steroid injections are well known.[15]

When progress through Phase II allows, Phase III is introduced, with isotonic strengthening exercises in the underhorizontal planes for the internal and external rotators, the scapular stabilizers, and the biceps brachii muscle (a humeral head depressor). As strength improves and range of motion is maintained, the patient is advanced to isotonic strengthening exercises in the overhorizontal nonpainful planes of motion.

Finally, the therapist begins isokinetic strengthening exercises using a Cybex isokinetic dynamometer with progressive advancement into the cardinal and diagonal (overhorizontal) planes. Strength may be further enhanced with a plyometric program. When satisfactory strength and endurance are achieved with full painless range of shoulder motion and there is no clinical evidence of impingement, rehabilitation is complete. Full recovery may require up to 4 months.[37]

On occasion, Phase II impingement may be refractory to nonsurgical treatment and an operative decompression of the subacromial space is necessary. Traditionally, this type of surgery has been performed in an open manner.[21] In recent years Stage 2 impingement with and without acromioclavicular joint involvement has been successfully treated by an arthroscopic decompression,[7,8,19] which does not disturb the origin of the deltoid muscle and allows a more rapid return to competitive athletics.

After an arthroscopic decompression, sling immobilization during Phase I is brief. The next morning, use of the sling is discontinued and Phase II is begun with pendulum range of motion exercises and passive-assistive stretching in total elevation, external rotation, and internal rotation. Each exercise is performed 20 times, and the entire group is repeated five times daily. Light activities of the arm in all planes are encouraged.

Two weeks after arthroscopic surgery the Phase II program is advanced to include stretching in any areas of residual stiffness. Phase III is introduced, with elastic tubing underhorizontal strengthening exercises for the internal and external rotators.

Six weeks after arthroscopy Phase III strengthening is advanced as tolerated. Although complete rehabilitation may require up to 6 months for the higher level athlete, throughout this period progressive participation in sports that involve repetitive, overhead arm movement is well tolerated.

Stage 3

The conservative treatment of Stage 3 subacromial impingement parallels Stage 1 and Stage 2. If this approach is unsuccessful, a surgical, open decompression and repair of the rotator cuff tear is recommended.[9,36]

Postoperatively, after sling and swathe immobilization (Phase I) for approximately 24 to 48 hours. Phase II is begun with pendulum exercises. As patient tolerance allows, passive-assistive total elevation with a pulley, supine external rotation stretching with a stick, and internal rotation stretching exercises are implemented. All four exercises are performed 20 times each, with four to five sessions daily. Throughout this period of Phase II the use of analgesics and the application of heat to the shoulder for 10-minute intervals before and after exercising improve overall patient compliance and performance. The patient is instructed to wear a sling between exercise sessions and while sleeping. Isometrics are used for the elbow, wrist, and hand.

Six weeks postoperatively Phase II passive-assistive stretching exercises are advanced to include supine elevation with and without abduction and more aggressive internal rotation stretching. The goal of phase II should be to obtain full passive motion in all planes by 3 months. This allows the rotator cuff and deltoid muscle repairs to adequately mature before initiation of active exercises.

Three months after surgery use of the sling is discontinued and Phase III exercises are introduced with shoulder isometrics. The patient is encouraged to use the arm actively in overhead planes for natural activities of daily living, without the use of weights. Four and a half months after repair, progress generally allows isotonic

strengthening, followed by an isokinetic program as patient tolerance permits.

If the rotator cuff tear was a particularly large one, the rehabilitation program is initially modified by placing the patient in an abduction brace immediately after surgery. Within 48 hours pulley exercises are begun with the brace in place. Six weeks after repair the brace is removed and Phase II is progressed as previously outlined to include pendulum, external rotation with the stick, and internal rotation stretching exercises. The use of the abduction brace in this manner delays the overall program by 6 weeks. Complete rehabilitation after a Stage 3 surgical repair generally takes 9 to 12 months.

SUMMARY

Perhaps because of the emphasis in our society on sports that involve the upper extremities, the shoulder continues to be susceptible to injury. A carefully organized and thorough rehabilitation program can often lead to a more expedient return to athletics and perhaps extend the athlete's career.

The rehabilitation process can be divided into three phases. Phase I deals with the immediate postinjury period in which immobilization allows for the reduction of inflammation and discomfort and isometrics are used to maintain muscle tone. The athlete then enters Phase II, which focuses primarily on regaining passive range of motion. Finally, Phase III emphasizes progressive strengthening by use of isotonic, isokinetic, and plyometric techniques.

Once full range of motion and normal strength have been achieved, the athlete can return to competition without restrictions. A premature return can lead to reinjury or injury of another area as the athlete changes form in an attempt to compensate.

REFERENCES

1. Aronen JG, Regan K: Decreasing the incident of recurrence of first time anterior shoulder dislocations with rehabilitation, *Am J Sports Med* 12:283, 1984.
2. Baker LL, Parker K: Neuromuscular electrical stimulation of the muscles surrounding the shoulder, *Phys Ther* 66:1930, 1986.
3. Ciullo JV: Swimmers shoulder, *Clin Sports Med* 5(1):15, 1986.
4. Davies GJ, Dickoff-Hoffman S: Neuromuscular testing and rehabilitation of the shoulder complex, *J Orthop Sports Phys Ther* 18:449, 1993.
5. Derscheid G: Rehabilitation of common orthopedic problems, *Nurs Clin North Am* 16:709, 1981.
6. Einhorn AR, Jackson DW: *Rehabilitation of the shoulder in shoulder surgery in the athlete*, Baltimore, 1985, University Park Press.
7. Ellman H: Arthroscopic subacromial decompression: analysis of one to three year results, *Arthroscopy* 3(1):73, 1987.
8. Gartsman GM: *Arthroscopic subacromial decompression: a clinical study*, Paper presented at the American Academy of Orthopaedic Surgeons meeting, Atlanta, Feb 7, 1988.
9. Hawkins RJ, Kennedy JC: Impingement syndrome in athletes, *Am J Sports Med* 8:151, 1980.
10. Henry JH, Genung JA: Natural history of glenohumeral dislocation—revisited, *Am J Sport Med* 10:135, 1982.
11. Hill JA: Epidemiologic perspective on shoulder injuries, *Clin Sports Med* 2:241, 1983.
12. Hovelius L et al: Recurrence after initial dislocation of the shoulder, *J Bone Joint Surg* 65A:343, 1983.
13. Jobe FW, Jobe CM: Painful athletic injuries of the shoulder, *Clin Orthop* 173:117, 1983.
14. Jobe FW, Moynes DR: Delineation of diagnostic criteria and a rehabilitation program for rotator cuff injuries, *Am J Sports Med* 10:336, 1982.
15. Kennedy JC, Willis RB: The effects of local steroid injections on tendons: a biomechanical and microscopic corrective study, *Am J Sports Med* 4:11, 1976.
16. Leffert RD, Harris BA: The role of physical therapy in rehabilitation of the shoulder. In Rowe CR (ed): *The shoulder*, New York, 1988, Churchill Livingstone.
17. McCann PD et al: A kinematic and electromyographic study of shoulder rehabilitation exercises, *Clin Orthop* 288:179, 1993.
18. Mendoza FX, Nicholas JA, Reilly JP: Neer inferior capsular shift repair for anterior glenohumeral instability, *Orthop Trans* 10:221, 1986.
19. Mendoza FX, Rubinstein M: The arthroscopic treatment of subacromial impingement, *Clin Sports Med* 6:573, 1987.
20. Moynes DR: Prevention of injury to the shoulder through exercise and therapy, *Clin Sports Med* 2:413, 1983.
21. Neer CS: Anterior acromioplasty for the chronic impingement syndrome in the shoulder: a preliminary report, *J Bone Joint Surg* 54A:41, 1972.
22. Neer CS: Impingement lesions, *Clin Orthop* 173:70, 1983.
23. Neer CS, Foster CR: Inferior capsular shift for involuntary inferior and multidirectional instability of the shoulder, *J Bone Joint Surg* 62A:897, 1980.
24. Neer CS, Hughes M: Glenohumeral joint replacement and post operative rehabilitation, *Phys Ther* 55:850, 1975.
25. Neer CS, Welsh RP: The shoulder in sports, *Orthop Clin North Am* 8:583, 1977.
26. Nicholas JA et al: The importance of a simplified classification of motion in sports in relation to performance, *Orthop Clin North Am* 8:499, 1977.
27. Nitz AJ: Physical therapy management of the shoulder, *Phys Ther* 66:1912, 1986.
28. Roeser WM et al: The use of transcutaneous nerve stimulation for pain control in athletic medicine: a preliminary report, *Am J Sports Med* 4:210, 1976.
29. Rowe CR: Prognosis in dislocations of the shoulder, *J Bone Joint Surg* 380A:957, 1956.
30. Rowe CR: Acute and recurrent anterior dislocation of the shoulder, *Orthop Clin North Am* 11:253, 1980.
31. Rowe CR, Sakellarides HT: Factors related to recurrence of anterior dislocations of the shoulder, *Clin Orthop* 20:40, 1961.
32. Simonet WT, Cofield RH: Prognosis in anterior shoulder dislocations, *Am J Sports Med* 12:19, 1984.
33. Speer KP et al: A role for hydrotherapy in shoulder rehabilitation, *Am J Sports Med* 21:850, 1993.
34. Turkel SJ et al: Stabilizing mechanisms preventing anterior dislocation of the glenohumeral joint, *J Bone Joint Surg* 63A:1208, 1981.
35. Voss DE et al: *Proprioceptive neuromuscular facilitation: patterns and techniques*, ed 3, Philadelphia, 1985, Harper & Row.
36. Warren RF: *Surgical considerations for rotator cuff tears in athletes*, Baltimore, 1985, University Park Press.
37. Wilk KE, Andrews JR: Rehabilitation following arthroscopic decompression, *Orthopedics* 16:349, 1993.
38. Wilk KE, Arrigo C: Current concepts in the rehabilitation of the athletic shoulder, *J Orthop Sports Phys Ther* 18:365, 1993.
39. Wooden MJ: Isokinetic evaluation and treatment of the shoulder. In Donatelli R (ed): *Physical therapy of the shoulder*, New York, 1987, Churchill Livingstone.
40. Yoneda B et al: Conservative treatment of shoulder dislocation in young males. (Proceedings of The Canadian Orthopedic Association), *J Bone Joint Surg* 64B:254, 1982.

CHAPTER 12 Shoulder Equipment

Robert C. Reese, Jr.
T. Pepper Burruss
Joseph Patten

Shoulder pads
Upper arm padding
Shoulder harness

SHOULDER PADS

The shoulder region is often a point of contact in sports. Contact can occur between an athlete's shoulder and another athlete or an object, such as a piece of equipment or a playing surface.

Shoulder pads are among the most common pieces of protective equipment used in contact sports. They are designed to protect the shoulder by covering the middle and lateral portions of the clavicle, the acromion, scapular body, and proximal humerus. The area protected depends greatly on the style and trim of the specific pads used (Fig. 12-1).

There is a variety of configurations and sizes in shoulder padding. Pads are generally sport specific, but even within sports, shoulder pads can vary by player position and individual requirements. By far the sports that most commonly use shoulder pads are football, hockey, and lacrosse.

In football the largest pads are often worn by linebackers, who require protection to the shoulder region because of their role as tacklers. They contact opposing players with the shoulder as the point of impact, and the shoulder pads, if appropriate in size and configuration, can protect the region from most contusions and other direct-contact injuries. In contrast, quarterbacks and wide receivers require mobility in the shoulder and arm and often wear shoulder pads with little bulk that allow extensive mobility.

Proper fitting is essential for shoulder protection, while full range of motion of the shoulders, arms, and neck remains unobstructed. Shoulder pads that are too small can allow portions of the region to go unprotected. Conversely, shoulder pads that are too large do not permit normal shoulder mobility, and this restriction can lead to injury. Care must be taken at all times to fit the shoulder pad in relation to the helmet. Interference can occur between the helmet and shoulder pads if the shoulder pads do not allow room for proper helmet fit and head and neck motion.

Additional padding can be used beneath shoulder pads. These are designed to add further impact protection to the region and are generally one of two types: foam or air (Fig. 12-2). These pads are either applied to the shoulder before the shoulder pads are put on or fastened directly to the pads themselves.

Custom padding can also be created for use with shoulder pads. Customizing techniques are most often used when an injured area requires additional protection. For example, strips of foam can be secured to the underside of a shoulder pad just anteroposterior to the acromioclavicular joint. These strips provide relief to the joint and can permit the athlete to return to competition with additional protective padding. An alternative to the strips of foam is a high-density foam donut. This can be applied directly over the acromioclavicular joint, either by using adhesive elastic tape or an elastic bandage. Hard shells fabricated from Orthoplast or other thermomoldable plastics can be made for the same purpose and taped directly to the shoulder (Fig. 12-3).

UPPER ARM PADDING

In general, shoulder pads provide sufficient protection for the upper arm. Areas that can sustain injury are the distal deltoid and the proximal and middle thirds of the biceps or triceps. Contusions can occur at the edge of the standard shoulder pads and, if repeated extensive muscle contusion continues, myositis ossificans can result. These areas of ossification can be quite tender and require additional protective padding. Often, firm areas called *blocker's nodes* develop at the site of injury, usually in the lateral aspect of the upper arm.

If additional protection is required at the deltoid insertion, an extension can be added to the standard shoulder pads (Fig. 12-4). It is difficult to protect the anterior or posterior portion of the arm with a hard shell. If padding is required in these regions, an elastic knee pad can prove invaluable. These pads can be slipped up the arm and placed over the injured region (Fig. 12-5). Their flexibility permits continued unrestricted motion in the area.

SHOULDER HARNESS

Chronic anterior shoulder instability can, at times, be managed nonoperatively. One of the cornerstones of this treatment is aggressive internal rotator muscle strength-

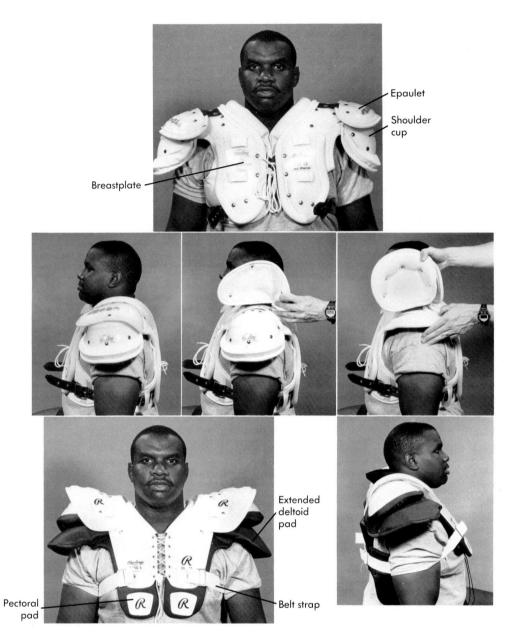

FIG. 12-1. Shoulder pads.

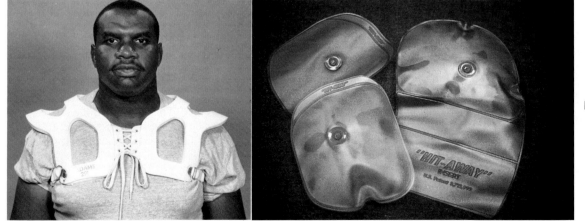

FIG. 12-2. Supplemental pads. These go beneath shoulder pads to provide additional protection to the shoulder region. **A,** Foam. **B,** Air.

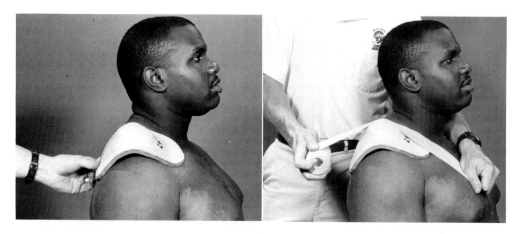

FIG. 12-3. Customized pads made from foam and orthoplast thermoldable plastic are placed on the underside of the shoulder pad to provide additional protection.

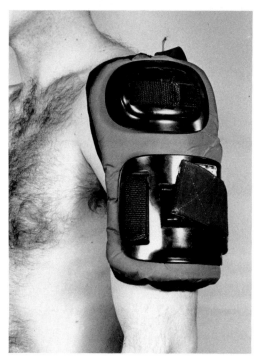

FIG. 12-4. Deltoid pad provides additional protection to the lateral arm.

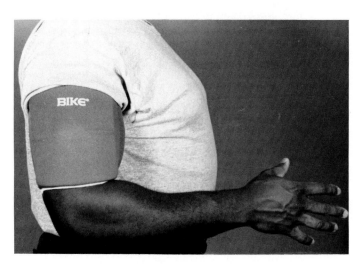

FIG. 12-5. Elastic knee pad can provide extra padding to the anterior or posterior arm.

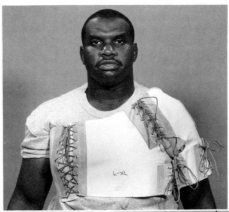
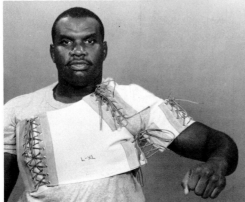
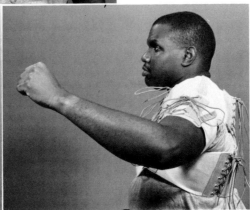

FIG. 12-6. Shoulder harness.

ening to assist in maintaining shoulder stability. In contact sports, however, abduction and external rotation forces that exceed the strength of the muscular and capsular restraints can occur at the shoulder. The shoulder harness is a piece of equipment that can be used as an adjunct in the treatment of anterior shoulder instability.

The basic principle of the shoulder harness is that shoulder instability can be controlled by avoiding abduction and external rotation of the shoulder. The design of the harness includes a chest vest, a shoulder cap, and a biceps cuff.

One commercially available harness is the C.D. Denison–Duke Wyre shoulder vest (Fig. 12-6). The brace was developed in the mid-1950s by the late Duke Wyre, former head athletic trainer at the University of Maryland, in conjunction with the late Cedric Denison, former president and chief orthotist of C.D. Denison. At that time, each brace was fabricated to custom-fit the individual athlete. In 1961 standard sizes and designs of the vest were developed and the brace was marketed throughout the United States. The design has remained

constant through the years, the only change being the replacement of rawhide laces with nylon nonstretch laces.

The main controlling feature of the harness is the lacing that connects the chest vest to the biceps cuff. This lacing is a direct restraint to shoulder abduction. The degree of limitation can be adjusted by varying the tension of the laces running from the chest to the biceps cuff. In addition, the shoulder cap also is laced to the chest vest, adding limitation to abduction and extension range of motion.

These vests come in a variety of standard sizes based on chest and biceps circumference. Right, left, or bilateral models are available. The harness is fitted to the individual; the laces are used to adjust the biceps cuff and the shoulder cap to the chest vest. The degrees of control can be varied by tightening or loosening the various laces. To prevent skin irritation from the vest, the athlete should consider wearing a well-fitted cotton T-shirt beneath the vest.

PART III   Elbow

CHAPTER 13 Anatomy and Physical Examination of the Elbow

Thomas E. Anderson

ANATOMY
Surface Anatomy

The superficial anatomy about the elbow is dominated by the bony prominences and the shape of the predominant musculature. The bony prominences include the readily palpable medial and lateral epicondyle as well as the olecranon tip. In the midportion of the arm the lateral and medial margins of the humeral shaft can be palpated. As the examiner nears the elbow, the humerus wings out, with the epicondyles becoming much more distinct to palpation. The palpable muscles (Figs. 13-1 and 13-2) include the biceps anteriorly and the biceps tendon and its aponeurosis (lacertus fibrosus) extending medially. The aponeurosis can be followed distally and medially as it blends with the medial fascia of the forearm, often forming an indentation in the flexor-pronator muscle group. Anteriorly the brachialis muscle is not readily palpable because of its deep location beneath the biceps muscle and tendon.

Laterally and slightly distal is the extensor muscle group of the forearm. This group, or mobile wad as it is sometimes called,[2,5] is readily palpable as a group of muscles originating from the lateral distal humerus and epicondyle. The group includes the brachioradialis, extensor carpi radialis longus, and extensor carpi radialis brevis. Just distal to the epicondyle is the tendinous portion of the extensor carpi radialis longus and brevis musculature and the extensor digitorum musculature. The

> **Mobile wad extensors**
> - Brachioradialis
> - Extensor carpi radialis longus
> - Extensor carpi radialis brevis

transition between the muscle and tendinous portion is not palpable.

Medially the flexor-pronator muscle group coming from the medial epicondyle is also readily palpable. This group includes the pronator teres, flexor carpi radialis, palmaris longus, and flexor carpi ulnaris. Proximally the pronator teres originates with a muscular attachment on the medial humeral bony wing. This origin also blends in with a common tendinous attachment to the medial epicondyle for the rest of this muscle group. The palmaris longus is absent in 14% of limbs. It may also present in one forearm and be absent in the contralateral forearm.[4]

> **Flexor-pronator muscle group**
> - Pronator teres
> - Flexor carpi radialis
> - Palmaris longus
> - Flexor carpi ulnaris

Posteriorly the triceps muscle is the dominant structure with its tendinous margins palpable distally as it inserts onto the olecranon. The margin of the triceps tendon can be palpated laterally and can be used in locating portals for elbow arthroscopy. The medial border is also readily palpable, and adjacent to this lies the ulnar nerve. The ulnar nerve is the only nerve about the elbow that is readily palpable in the superficial anatomy. In the distal aspect of the arm the ulnar nerve runs along the medial border of the triceps tendon and in the ulnar groove before disappearing underneath the flexor carpi ulnaris muscles distal to the medial epicondyle.

Superficial or cutaneous nerves of the forearm are not readily palpable because they are so small. Along the lat-

261

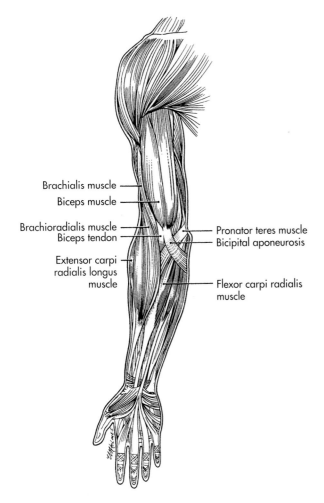

Brachialis muscle

Biceps muscle

Brachioradialis muscle
Biceps tendon

Extensor carpi
radialis longus
muscle

Pronator teres muscle
Bicipital aponeurosis

Flexor carpi radialis
muscle

FIG. 13-1. The superficial muscles of the anterior aspect of the elbow.

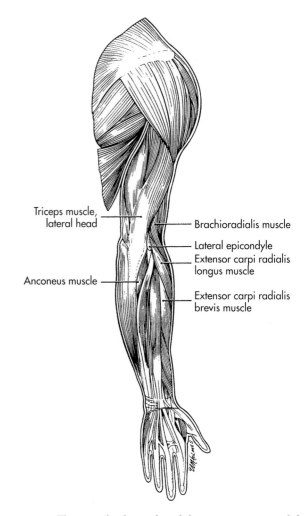

Triceps muscle,
lateral head

Anconeus muscle

Brachioradialis muscle

Lateral epicondyle
Extensor carpi radialis
longus muscle

Extensor carpi radialis
brevis muscle

FIG. 13-2. The superficial muscles of the posterior aspect of the elbow.

eral aspect of the elbow they run primarily longitudinally and are not a significant problem with lateral surgical approaches to the elbow. Medially, however, they tend to extend from the volar surface to the dorsal surface. These branches of the medial cutaneous nerve of the forearm often cross proposed incisions for exposure of the ulnar nerve or medial epicondyle. Care in avoiding injury to these cutaneous nerves during the exposure lessens the likelihood of any painful neuroma formation postoperatively. They may, however, be numerous enough and small enough that they are impossible to avoid during the exposure.

At the elbow, just medial to the biceps tendon, the brachial artery is palpable. Just distal to the elbow it divides into the radial and ulnar arteries, the division of which is not usually readily palpable. The palpable venous anatomy is the superficial cephalic vein and the basilic vein. The cephalic vein is located medially in the antecubital area. There are often intercommunication veins between the two primary veins, and these are given various names, such as the *median cephalic vein* or *median basilic vein,* depending on the individual pattern.

Deep Soft-Tissue Anatomy

Once the skin surface and subcutaneous tissue have been removed, the intervals between the muscles can be visualized. Laterally and anteriorly the lateral margin of the biceps and brachialis is readily distinguishable from the brachioradialis (Fig. 13-1). In this interval and just deep to the brachioradialis lies the radial nerve. Proximal to the elbow joint the radial nerve divides into a deep and a superficial branch. The deep branch of the radial nerve dives deep between the heads of the supinator muscle. This branch wraps around the posterolateral aspect of the radial neck and emerges as the posterior interosseous nerve. The supinator is the base of this interval and occupies the distal portion. The superficial branch of the radial nerve continues distally along the undersurface of the brachioradialis. Adjacent to the deep branch of the radial nerve lies the recurrent radial artery. It has come off the radial artery, just distal to the biceps tendon, and courses proximally, essentially wrapping around the biceps tendon.[3] This recurrent radial artery needs to be identified when performing an exposure in the area, for example, repair of a ruptured distal biceps

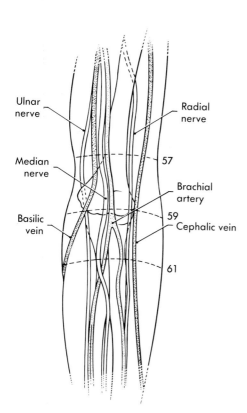

Ulnar
nerve

Radial
nerve

Median
nerve

Brachial
artery

57

59
Cephalic vein

Basilic
vein

61

FIG. 13-3. Anterior view of the relationship of the neurovascular structures about the left elbow.

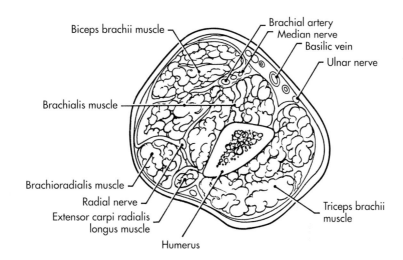

Biceps brachii muscle

Brachial artery
Median nerve
Basilic vein
Ulnar nerve

Brachialis muscle

Brachioradialis muscle

Radial nerve

Extensor carpi radialis
longus muscle

Triceps brachii
muscle

Humerus

FIG. 13-4. Cross-sectional anatomy correlating with level 57 on Fig. 13-3, looking from proximal to distal.

tendon or when exploring the deep radial nerve for entrapment (Figs. 13-3 to 13-6).

An interval is formed medial to the biceps tendon by the tendon and the flexor-pronator muscle group. This group consists of, from lateral to medial, the pronator teres, the flexor carpi radialis, the variable palmaris longus, and finally the flexor carpi ulnaris. In the interval on the medial side of the biceps tendon lies the brachial

artery and median nerve. These course distally, deep to the bicipital aponeurosis. The median nerve sends off several muscular branches before diving deep into pronator teres musculature.

Deep to the pronator teres muscle the median nerve continues to the flexor digitorum superficialis muscle. The flexor digitorum takes its origin from the medial epicondyle, medial coronoid process of the ulna, and proxi-

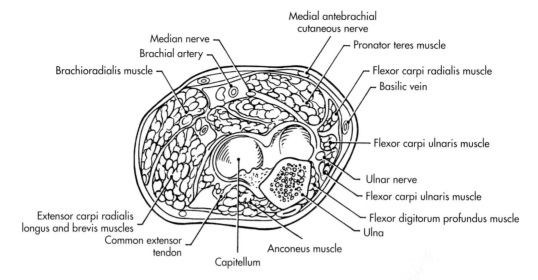

FIG. 13-5. Cross-sectional anatomy correlating with level 59 on Fig. 13-3, looking from proximal to distal.

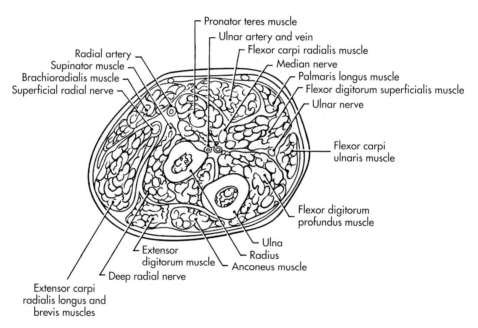

FIG. 13-6. Cross-sectional anatomy correlating with level 61 on Fig. 13-3, looking from proximal to distal.

mal radius. The brachial artery divides, as it nears the attachment site of the biceps tendon, into the radial and ulnar arteries. The ulnar artery further divides and sends off a recurrent ulnar artery and the common interosseous artery as well. The ulnar artery continues distally, diving deep to the sublimis (or flexor digitorum superficialis) to run between it and the flexor digitorum profundus. It then continues in this plane to the wrist. In approximately 3% of elbows the ulnar artery follows an anomalous course, descending superficially to the flexor muscles.[4]

Deep volar musculature

- Flexor pollicis longus
- Flexor digitorum profundus
- Pronator quadratus

The deepest layer of muscle in the anterior aspect of the forearm is composed of three muscles. Laterally is the flexor pollicis longus, which comes off the volar shaft of the radius and interosseous membrane. More medially the flexor digitorum profundus comes off the upper volar and medial ulna, as well as the medial coronoid process and interosseous membrane. The third muscle is the pronator quadratus muscle, although this is quite distal in the forearm.

The median nerve, after dividing the pronator teres heads, dives deep to the flexor digitorum superficialis and then lies superficial to the flexor digitorum profundus musculature as it courses distally to the wrist. It finally passes through the carpal tunnel, deep to the transverse carpal ligament and ulnar to the palmaris longus tendon (if present). The ulnar nerve, after diving posterior to the medial epicondyle, passes between the flexor carpi ulnaris and the flexor digitorum profundus muscles. Distal in the forearm the nerve lies adjacent to the ulnar artery, coursing with it toward Guyon's canal at the wrist.

The ulnar artery gives off the common interosseous branch before lying adjacent to the ulnar nerve. The anterior interosseous artery comes off the common interosseous artery and courses distally superficial to the flexor pollicis longus and the profundus muscles. The anterior interosseous artery courses deep to the pronator quadratus just proximal to the wrist. The posterior interosseous artery goes deep to the profundus through the interosseous membrane and is adjacent to the posterior interosseous nerve as the nerve exits the supinator.

The radial artery, after giving off the recurrent radial branch, courses in the interval with a superficial branch of the radial nerve deep to the brachioradialis muscle. As the brachioradialis attaches to the distal radius, the radial artery courses along the superficial palmar aspect of the radius to the level of the wrist. The superficial branch of the radial nerve runs underneath the brachioradialis muscle, coursing distally to the radial and dorsal aspect of the wrist.

Looking at the posterior aspect of the elbow, the most dominant muscle is the triceps, which extends onto the olecranon. Also prominent is the brachioradialis coming off the lateral aspect of the humerus. Just distal to this and lateral is the extensor carpi radialis longus and the extensor carpi radialis brevis musculature. Originating more inferior and somewhat more distal is the extensor digitorum communis musculature and the extensor digiti minimi muscle. Finally, the extensor carpi ulnaris muscle is noted lying on the lateral aspect of the ulna with the flexor carpi ulnaris muscle lying on the medial aspect. Portions of the extensor digitorum communis and extensor carpi ulnaris muscles cover the anconeus, which extends from the lateral epicondyle to the border of the ulna.

Deep to the brachioradialis and extensor carpi radialis longus brevis musculature on the anterior aspect lies the supinator muscle. Portions of the supinator originate from the lateral epicondyle, the radial collateral and annular ligaments, and the ulnar shaft below the radial notch. It inserts onto the radius distal to the bicipital tu-

berosity and along its lateral aspect. Extending down the forearm, the abductor pollicis longus muscle and extensor pollicis brevis muscle originate from the lateral dorsal ulna, the interosseous membrane, and the dorsal radius.

Just ulnar at this level lie the extensor pollicis longus and extensor indicis proprius, both originating from the dorsal surface of the ulna and the interosseous membrane. These two muscles are believed to have developed later in the phylogenic history and may be variable in their development at birth.[16] The neural structure in this area is primarily the posterior interosseous (or deep radial) nerve that dives through the supinator. It then courses along to the abductor pollicis longus and extensor pollicis brevis musculature, giving off musculature branches. It finally innervates the extensor pollicis longus and the extensor indicis. These distal nerve branches appear in a fanlike fashion along the area just superficial to the deep muscle group (composed of the abductor pollicis longus, extensor pollicis brevis, extensor pollicis longs, and extensor indicis proprius).

Osteology
Distal Humerus

The distal humerus is composed of two condyles forming the articular surfaces of the trochlea and capitellum (Figs. 13-7 and 13-8). It develops from a number of separate epiphyses about the distal humerus. These coalesce at varying ages, and all close at skeletal maturity. Medially (or ulnarly) the epicondyle is prominent and serves as a source of attachment for the ulnar collateral ligament and the flexor pronator muscle group. *The size of the prominence of the medial epicondyle provides a mechanical advantage for the ligament and muscle groups that attach there.* Just distal to the epicondyle is the condylar articular surface of the trochlea.

The lateral epicondyle is much less prominent and is located just proximal to the capitellum. This provides less

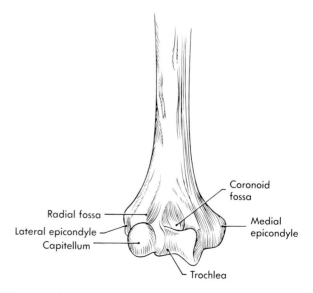

FIG. 13-7. Anterior view of the distal humerus. Unless noted otherwise, all views represent the right elbow.

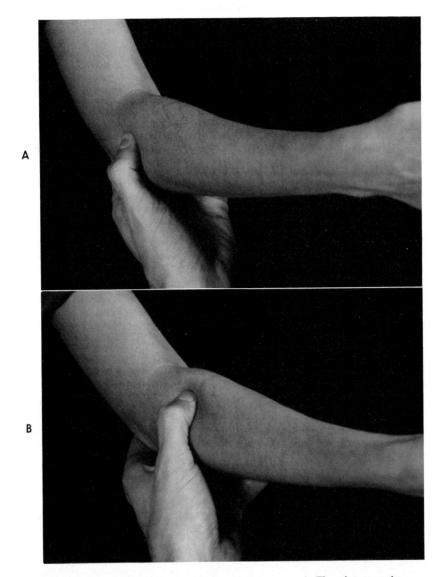

FIG. 13-19. Exact location of the most tender area is important. **A,** Thumb is over the common extensor tendon and radial head. **B,** Thumb is over the supinator and radial nerve. This small difference in location is important on the differential diagnosis.

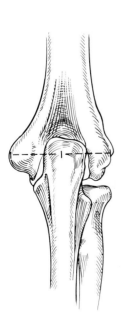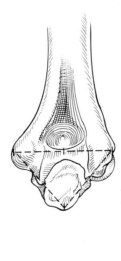

FIG. 13-20. Relationship of the palpable landmarks of the medial and lateral epicondyles of the humerus and the olecranon tip of the ulna. This is demonstrated on full extension and at 90 degrees of flexion of the elbow.

The deepest layer of muscle in the anterior aspect of the forearm is composed of three muscles. Laterally is the flexor pollicis longus, which comes off the volar shaft of the radius and interosseous membrane. More medially the flexor digitorum profundus comes off the upper volar and medial ulna, as well as the medial coronoid process and interosseous membrane. The third muscle is the pronator quadratus muscle, although this is quite distal in the forearm.

The median nerve, after dividing the pronator teres heads, dives deep to the flexor digitorum superficialis and then lies superficial to the flexor digitorum profundus musculature as it courses distally to the wrist. It finally passes through the carpal tunnel, deep to the transverse carpal ligament and ulnar to the palmaris longus tendon (if present). The ulnar nerve, after diving posterior to the medial epicondyle, passes between the flexor carpi ulnaris and the flexor digitorum profundus muscles. Distal in the forearm the nerve lies adjacent to the ulnar artery, coursing with it toward Guyon's canal at the wrist.

The ulnar artery gives off the common interosseous branch before lying adjacent to the ulnar nerve. The anterior interosseous artery comes off the common interosseous artery and courses distally superficial to the flexor pollicis longus and the profundus muscles. The anterior interosseous artery courses deep to the pronator quadratus just proximal to the wrist. The posterior interosseous artery goes deep to the profundus through the interosseous membrane and is adjacent to the posterior interosseous nerve as the nerve exits the supinator.

The radial artery, after giving off the recurrent radial branch, courses in the interval with a superficial branch of the radial nerve deep to the brachioradialis muscle. As the brachioradialis attaches to the distal radius, the radial artery courses along the superficial palmar aspect of the radius to the level of the wrist. The superficial branch of the radial nerve runs underneath the brachioradialis muscle, coursing distally to the radial and dorsal aspect of the wrist.

Looking at the posterior aspect of the elbow, the most dominant muscle is the triceps, which extends onto the olecranon. Also prominent is the brachioradialis coming off the lateral aspect of the humerus. Just distal to this and lateral is the extensor carpi radialis longus and the extensor carpi radialis brevis musculature. Originating more inferior and somewhat more distal is the extensor digitorum communis musculature and the extensor digiti minimi muscle. Finally, the extensor carpi ulnaris muscle is noted lying on the lateral aspect of the ulna with the flexor carpi ulnaris muscle lying on the medial aspect. Portions of the extensor digitorum communis and extensor carpi ulnaris muscles cover the anconeus, which extends from the lateral epicondyle to the border of the ulna.

Deep to the brachioradialis and extensor carpi radialis longus brevis musculature on the anterior aspect lies the supinator muscle. Portions of the supinator originate from the lateral epicondyle, the radial collateral and annular ligaments, and the ulnar shaft below the radial notch. It inserts onto the radius distal to the bicipital tu-

berosity and along its lateral aspect. Extending down the forearm, the abductor pollicis longus muscle and extensor pollicis brevis muscle originate from the lateral dorsal ulna, the interosseous membrane, and the dorsal radius.

Just ulnar at this level lie the extensor pollicis longus and extensor indicis proprius, both originating from the dorsal surface of the ulna and the interosseous membrane. These two muscles are believed to have developed later in the phylogenic history and may be variable in their development at birth.[16] The neural structure in this area is primarily the posterior interosseous (or deep radial) nerve that dives through the supinator. It then courses along to the abductor pollicis longus and extensor pollicis brevis musculature, giving off musculature branches. It finally innervates the extensor pollicis longus and the extensor indicis. These distal nerve branches appear in a fanlike fashion along the area just superficial to the deep muscle group (composed of the abductor pollicis longus, extensor pollicis brevis, extensor pollicis longs, and extensor indicis proprius).

Osteology
Distal Humerus

The distal humerus is composed of two condyles forming the articular surfaces of the trochlea and capitellum (Figs. 13-7 and 13-8). It develops from a number of separate epiphyses about the distal humerus. These coalesce at varying ages, and all close at skeletal maturity. Medially (or ulnarly) the epicondyle is prominent and serves as a source of attachment for the ulnar collateral ligament and the flexor pronator muscle group. *The size of the prominence of the medial epicondyle provides a mechanical advantage for the ligament and muscle groups that attach there.* Just distal to the epicondyle is the condylar articular surface of the trochlea.

The lateral epicondyle is much less prominent and is located just proximal to the capitellum. This provides less

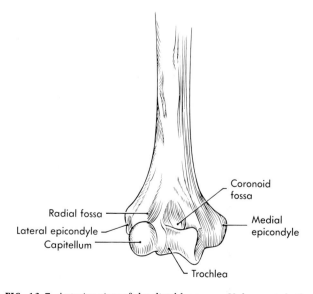

FIG. 13-7. Anterior view of the distal humerus. Unless noted otherwise, all views represent the right elbow.

Coronoid fossa

Radial fossa

Medial epicondyle

Lateral epicondyle

Capitellum

Trochlea

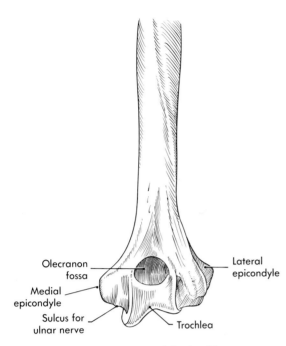

FIG. 13-8. Posterior view of the distal humerus.

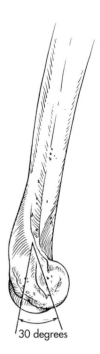

FIG. 13-9. Lateral view of the distal humerus demonstrating the anterior orientation of the articular surfaces.

of a mechanical advantage to the attachment of the extensor muscle group as well as the radial collateral ligament. Anterior and proximal to the articular surface are two indentations, or fossae. Laterally the indentation just proximal to the capitellum accommodates the radial head when the elbow is in full flexion and is referred to as the radial fossa. Just medial to the radial fossa is a deeper fossa that accommodates the coronoid process of the ulna (Fig. 13-11). The coronoid process gives the fossa its name, the coronoid fossa, which is just proximal to the trochlea. Posteriorly the olecranon fits into a deep olecranon fossa in the humerus, allowing full extension of the elbow as well as flexion to approximately 145 to 150 degrees. These bony prominences of the ulna and radius fit closely into their respective fossae.

The primary structural integrity of the distal humerus comes from medial and lateral supracondylar columns. The medial column is slightly smaller than the lateral column. The posterior aspect of the epicondyles is relatively flat, and the anterior portions are curved forward. This places the articular surfaces anteriorly and oriented approximately 30 degrees anterior to the long axis of the humerus (Fig. 13-9). The capitellum is spherical over the surface it presents to the radial head. It extends from the radial fossa distally to the distal end of the humerus (Fig. 13-10). It does not continue posteriorly in a circumferential pattern as the trochlea does. The axis of the elbow is directed through the trochlea and the capitellum in approximately 6 degrees of valgus as compared with the axis of the epicondyles. Thus the medial trochlea is somewhat longer and projects more distal (Figs. 13-7 and 13-8).

The trochlea itself is covered with articular cartilage from the coronoid fossa anteriorly to the olecranon fossa posteriorly. This presents a continuous surface of articular cartilage covering the anterior, distal, and posterior aspects of the distal humerus and forms an arc of 300 to 330 degrees.[7] This allows for only a small area of bone to exist between the coronoid fossa and the olecranon fossa. Indeed, in some individuals only a membrane is present. Occasionally this area appears to be filled with what radiographically looks like a loose body. This, however, is an anatomic variant. The trochlea itself is not symmetric because the medial lip is larger and projects more distal. A small groove that appears in the interval between the capitellum and the trochlea is covered with hyaline cartilage and articulates with the radial head when the elbow is appropriately loaded. This allows for rotation of the radial head when abutting the humerus. In the axial view the distal humerus has approximately 5 degrees of internal rotation of the articular surface in relation to the epicondylar axis (Fig. 13-10). Medially in the interval between the epicondyle and trochlea is a groove through which the ulnar nerve courses (Fig. 13-8). More proximally and medially along the area of the intermuscular septum a supracondylar process may be observed in approximately 1% to 3% of individuals.[4] From this process a fibrous band may attach to the medial epicondyle. This band and bony prominence may form an anomalous insertion of the coracobrachialis muscle or origin of the pronator teres. Additionally, it may be involved with aberrant routes of the median and ulnar nerves. The fibrous portion of this complex is the ligament of Strothers.

Proximal Radius

The shape of the proximal radius in cross section is almost cylindrical and becomes more elliptical as one

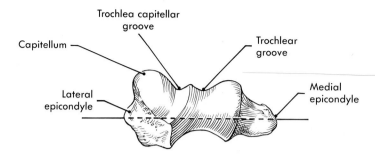

FIG. 13-10. Distal view of the distal humerus. Note medial rotation of the articular surfaces compared to the axis of the epicondyles.

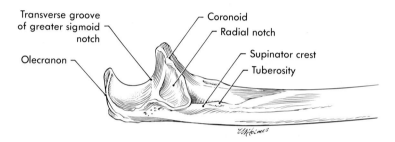

FIG. 13-11. Lateral view of the proximal ulna.

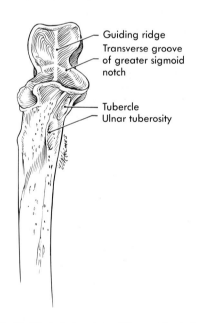

FIG. 13-12. Anterior view of the proximal ulna.

goes distal into the forearm. The proximal portion is also termed the *radial head,* and it articulates with the capitellum.[2] It presents a concave surface to accommodate the capitellum within the cylindrical outline of the radial head. Hyaline cartilage covers the proximal radial head as well as the sides of the radial head. This outer surface of the radial head is covered for approximately 240 degrees.[7] The anterior lateral third of the circumference of the radial head is void of cartilage. This area is not involved in articulation. Because it is not normally stressed, it is slightly weaker and is prone to fracture when stressed, as in a fall. Distal to the radial head the bone tapers to the radial neck. Somewhat distal to the radial neck is a prominence of the radial tuberosity on which the biceps tendon attaches (Fig. 13-17). Often adjacent to the attachment of the biceps tendon is a small bursa to protect the biceps tendon when in full pronation. In addition, the radial head and neck are not colinear with the long axis of the radius. They also form an angle of approximately 15 degrees with the shaft. This is oriented opposite the direction of the radial tuberosity.

Proximal Ulna

The proximal ulna essentially grasps the distal humerus and is responsible for the majority of the bony stability at the elbow. Distal to the elbow the ulna tapers rapidly to assume first a triangular and then a cylindrical shape. Proximally the ulna forms the greater sigmoid notch, which articulates with the trochlea of the humerus. The proximal and distal portions of this notch are composed of the olecranon tip and the coronoid process, respectively. Additionally, the coronoid process serves as an insertion site to the brachialis muscle with the olecranon serving as the attachment of the triceps. Along the lateral aspect of the coronoid process there is a small semilunar notch or radial notch into which the radial head fits that is roughly perpendicular to the long access of the bone. The circular margin of the radial head articulates and is stabilized within the radial notch (Figs. 13-11, 13-12, and 13-17). Just distal to the radial notch is a

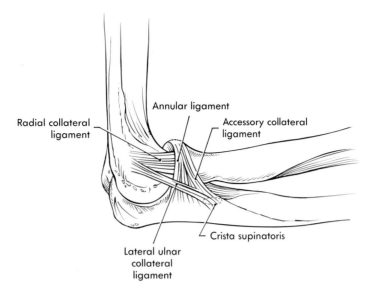

FIG. 13-13. Lateral view of the lateral collateral and annular ligaments.

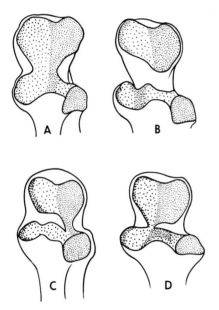

FIG. 13-14. Various configurations of the articular surfaces of the proximal left ulna. Pattern **B** is the most common, representing 63% of cases studied. Patterns **A, C,** and **D** represent 3%, 32%, and 2%, respectively.[6,7,10]

crest of bone that is the site of the ulnar origin of the supinator muscle. Additionally, on this crest, also called the *crista supinatorus*, is the insertion of the accessory lateral collateral ligament (Fig. 13-13). This ligament serves a twofold purpose: to tether the annular ligament and to supplement the radial collateral ligament. This is also important to prevent ulnohumeral rotation and posterolateral rotatory instability of the elbow.[1,8,9]

The medial aspect of the coronoid process serves the site of attachment of the anterior portion of the medial collateral ligament (Figs. 13-12 and 13-16).

The greater sigmoid notch is not covered continuously with hyaline cartilage; indeed, in the majority of cases there is a transverse portion composed of fatty tissue and not hyaline cartilage (Fig. 13-14). With the anterior and posterior portions of the sigmoid notch being composed of articular cartilage, there is normally a depression in the sigmoid notch in the central region. This depression, however, is not apparent on radiographs nor is it apparent on skeletal bone samples because it is devoid of articular cartilage and produces a prominence rather than an additional depression of subchondral bone. There is also a longitudinal ridge in the greater sigmoid notch producing a medial and lateral surface (Figs. 13-12 and 13-14). The sigmoid notch forms an arc of approximately 180 degrees and is angled approximately 30 degrees to the long axis of the ulna. This, coupled with the 300 to 330 degrees of articular surface of the trochlea, allows for between 120 and 150 degrees of flexion of the elbow. Along the lateral aspect of the proximal ulna is a lesser sigmoid notch or radial notch. This depression has an arc of approximately 60 to 70 degrees and articulates with the radial head. This articulation of 60 to 70 degrees, coupled with the radial head surface being covered for 240 degrees of its outside circumference, allows for pronation and supination of 170 to 180 degrees. The greater sigmoid notch is also not completely perpendicular to the longitudinal axis of the ulna. It is in slight valgus angulation with respect to the shaft, representing approximately 4 degrees. This valgus, coupled with the 6 degrees of the distal humerus, creates the **carrying angle,** the angle between the shaft of the humerus and the shaft of the ulna. The carrying angle may normally vary from 10 to 18 degrees with any particular angle being normal only when compared with the contralateral elbow.

The capsule of the elbow joint is covered anteriorly by the brachialis and posteriorly by the triceps. The fibrous portion of the capsule is attached to the humerus ante-

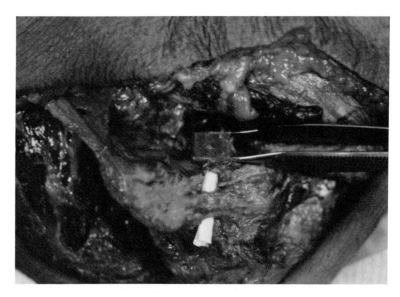

FIG. 13-15. Cadaver dissection of a left elbow. The forceps is beneath the capsule, which can be quite thin. The white marker has been passed deep to the anterior bundle of the ulnar collateral ligament.

riorly above the radial and coronoid fossa and posteriorly above the olecranon fossa.[6] Distally the capsule attaches to the anterior margin of the coronoid medially and to the annular ligament laterally. Posteriorly and distally the attachment is along the medial and lateral articular margins of the sigmoid notch. Laterally it attaches along the lateral aspect of the sigmoid notch and blends with the annular ligament.[7] This capsule is normally thin and transparent (Fig. 13-15). Studies by Morrey[7] reveal that the anterior capsule provides a significant portion of varus and valgus stability when the elbow is extended. This appears to be the result of transverse and oblique fiber bands within the capsule itself. The greatest capacity of the capsule is in approximately 60 degrees of flexion and is therefore the most comfortable position when a tense effusion is present.

The synovial membrane courses just deep to the capsule with the exception of the radial and coronoid fossa anteriorly and the olecranon fossa posteriorly. Here the synovial membrane first turns down over pads of fat in the fossa to reach the edges of the articular surfaces; thus the synovial membrane runs over the bone only a short distance to reach the articular cartilage. Most structures within the capsule of the elbow joint either are covered with fat and synovial membrane or are articular cartilage.[6] The fat pads play a significant role in evaluation of effusions of the elbow joint when they are observed in a lateral radiographic view of the elbow.

Ligaments

The ligaments about the elbow represent distinct thickening of the capsule of the elbow. These ligaments are located primarily in the medial and lateral aspects of the elbow.

Medial Collateral Ligament Complex

The medial collateral ligament of the elbow is the most important ligament for stability of the elbow joint. It is

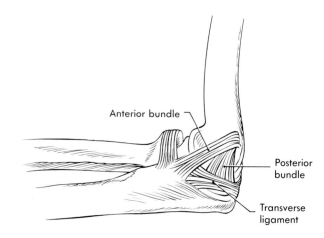

FIG. 13-16. Medial view of the medial collateral ligament bundles.

frequently divided into three bundles denoted by their anatomic location—anterior, posterior, and transverse (Fig. 13-16).[13] The posterior bundle appears to provide some support when the elbow is flexed 90 degrees or greater. The transverse ligament has little to do with elbow stability. The origin of the medial collateral ligament is from the medial epicondyle along its distal portion.[7] It inserts along the medial aspect of the coronoid process (Fig. 13-15). This insertion of the anterior bundle is firmly attached to the ulna at the margin of the articular cartilage. There is no cavity or open area under this anterior bundle at its ulnar insertion. A small potential space exists at the origin between the attachment site and the joint line.[11] The mean length of the anterior component of the complex is about 27 mm. The width of the anterior bundles is approximately 4 to 5 mm.[7] There is a slight ridge along the medial side of the olecranon to which the ligament attaches.

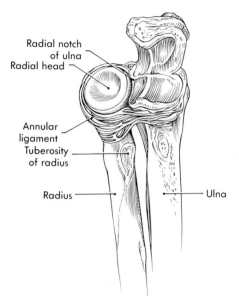

Radial notch
of ulna
Radial head

Annular
ligament
Tuberosity
of radius

Radius

Ulna

FIG. 13-17. Anterior view of the proximal radioulnar complex. Note the congruency of the radial head, annular ligament, and radial notch of the ulna.

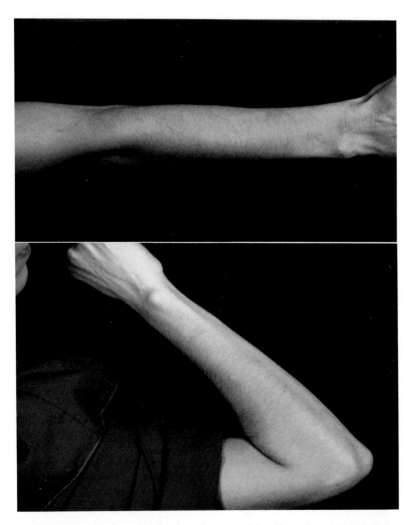

FIG. 13-18. Demonstration of a normal range of motion of the elbow. Symptoms of ulnar nerve entrapment at the elbow may be reproduced when the patient demonstrates range of motion.

Lateral Collateral Ligament Complex

The lateral ligament complex is formed by the radial collateral ligament, the annular ligament, the lateral ulnar collateral ligament, and the accessory collateral ligament.[7] The radial collateral ligament originates from the lateral epicondyle and terminates along the course of the annular ligament (Fig. 13-13). A posterior portion of this ligament extends distally onto the crista supinatorus, which is a small prominence of the lateral ulna just distal to the lesser sigmoid notch. This separate portion is termed the *lateral ulnar collateral ligament*. Additionally, a band of the annular ligament also joins it at its attachment to the crista supinatorus and is termed the *accessory collateral ligament*. The annular ligament itself forms the remaining portion of the circle (the initial portion formed by the lesser sigmoid or radial notch) and is attached at the margins of the radial notch of the ulna. This annular ligament fits tightly around the head and upper portion of the neck (Fig. 13-17) and does not allow distal migration of the radius to occur in the adult; however, in the young child or infant this may occur and result in a "pulled elbow." This ligamentous complex, combined with the radial notch of the ulna, forms a structure with the radial head that is built to close biomechanical tolerances. Any disruption of this area often results in a loss of pronation and supination. If any of these structures loses its symmetry, congruous surfaces may no longer be present. This loss of congruity, limiting pronation and supination, is a frequent occurrence following radial head fractures. The origin of the radial collateral ligament appears to be in the anatomic center of rotation.[7]

Bursa

Although there are several bursae noted about the elbow, the most clinically relevant is the olecranon bursa between the olecranon and the skin surface. This is a clinical entity when it has been enlarged because of hematoma, chronic irritation, or rheumatoid synovitis. Occasionally it may need to be surgically excised for relief of symptoms.

PHYSICAL EXAMINATION

An integral part of any evaluation of the elbow is the history and physical examination.[12] The most important question to ask the individual about the elbow is "What bothers you the most about your elbow?" This type of question elicits the chief complaint and may also aid in getting through some extraneous information as well. Next, allow the patient to point to the location where he or she senses the problem is located and ask if there is any radiation of pain or paresthesias from this area. Next the examiner should ask about the date of onset or reinjury that initiated this problem. Finally, the examiner needs to ask the "how" questions: "How does this bother you now? How have you treated this? How do you make it worse? How do you make it better? How has your training program changed over this time period?"

The actual examination begins initially with **inspection.** The examiner should be able to completely visualize both elbows during the examination. Differences may be noted related to muscle hypertrophy or atrophy, swelling, and also previous surgical incisions. **Motions** should be recorded from full extension (approximately 0 degrees) to full flexion (approximately 150 degrees) (Fig. 13-18). Record supination and pronation with the elbow at a right angle. When going through this range of motion, the examiner should note if there is any discomfort noted and have the individual point to the area of this discomfort. A locking or lack of full motion may indicate loose body formation, articular surface defect, or muscle tightness secondary to a muscle strain. Localization of the tenderness by **palpation** is helpful. I often palpate areas of possible tendinitis or nerve entrapment that do not fit the patient's chief complaint and use these for comparison later when the more painful areas are palpated (Fig. 13-19). The location of the most tender area needs to be noted. The underlying structures that pressure has been applied to in Fig. 13-19, *A,* differ from the structures in Fig. 13-19, *B.* A change in location of the most tender area changes the proposed differential diagnosis.

In acute injury the pain experienced by the patient may be too great to evaluate the range of motion. A helpful examination after an acute injury is to palpate the epicondyles and the tip of the olecranon. The line formed by the epicondyles should be perpendicular to the shaft of the humerus. If it is not, a humeral fracture should be suspected. If the position of the elbow is at 0 degrees of flexion, the epicondyles and the olecranon should form a straight line. With the elbow flexed to 90 degrees these palpable prominences should form a triangle with the sides adjacent to the olecranon being equal.[15] Should this not be the case, either a fracture, a dislocation, or both should be suspected (Fig. 13-20).

Following initial palpation the physician then begins the **stress examination** of the elbow. Because of the amount of rotation that occurs at the shoulder, it is difficult to adequately apply varus or valgus stress to the elbow. This needs to be performed at multiple angles from full extension to full flexion at every 20-degree interval.[14] The distal humerus should be grasped with one hand while the stress is applied to the distal forearm with the other (Fig. 13-21). Any toggle or play in motion, as well as elicitation of pain, is significant, especially when compared with the motion of the opposite elbow. The elbow needs to be flexed to 30 degrees to unlock the olecranon from the olecranon fossa when stressing the medial or ulnar collateral ligament. Testing for posterolateral rotatory instability also relies on reproduction of symptoms because actual instability often is not appreciated clinically. With the patient in the supine position the shoulder is flexed and externally rotated (this aids with patient relaxation and limits further external rotation of the humerus). The forearm is fully supinated while the elbow is in full extension. The elbow is then flexed slowly. Full supination and valgus stress dislocate the radiohumeral joint posterolaterally. Maximum subluxation (dislocation) occurs around 40 degrees with further flexion producing a sudden palpable reduction. Extension may reproduce the subluxation.[8,9] The angle at

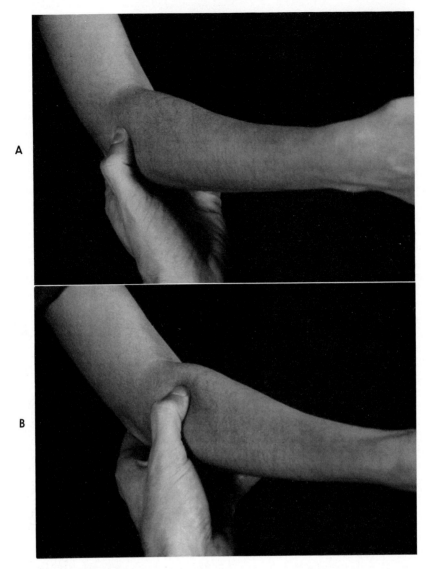

FIG. 13-19. Exact location of the most tender area is important. **A,** Thumb is over the common extensor tendon and radial head. **B,** Thumb is over the supinator and radial nerve. This small difference in location is important on the differential diagnosis.

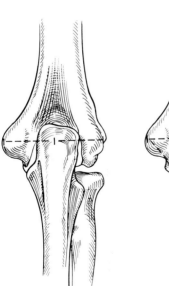
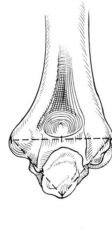

FIG. 13-20. Relationship of the palpable landmarks of the medial and lateral epicondyles of the humerus and the olecranon tip of the ulna. This is demonstrated on full extension and at 90 degrees of flexion of the elbow.

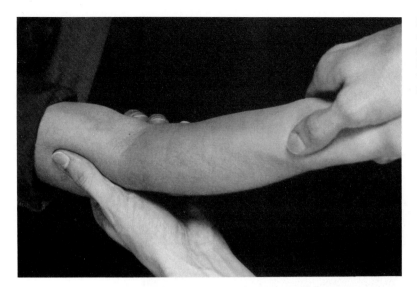

FIG. 13-21. During varus and valgus stress testing applied to the elbow, one needs to palpate the amount of rotation of the humerus as well. Laxity is best detected at approximately 30 degrees of flexion, which unlocks the olecranon tip from the olecranon fossa and releases the anterior capsule.

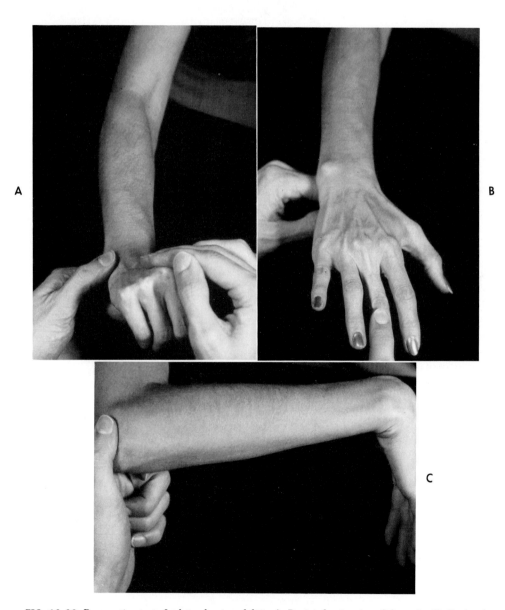

A

B

C

FIG. 13-22. Provocative tests for lateral epicondylitis. **A,** Resisted extension of the wrist. **B,** Resisted extension of the third digit, stressing the extensor digitorum muscle and tendon. **C,** The wrist palmar flexed and the forearm fully pronated. Extension of the elbow will stretch the common extensor tendon and reproduce symptoms if tendinitis is present.

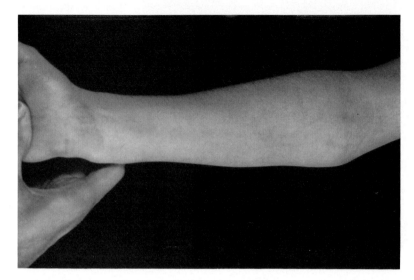

FIG. 13-23. Provocative test for flexor tendinitis is resisted wrist palmar flexion.

which symptoms are reproduced may vary with the sport. Baseball players are more apt to have their symptoms reproduced at 60 to 80 degrees of flexion. Volleyball and underhand throwers are more likely to have their symptoms at 30 to 40 degrees of flexion, indicative of the position of the elbow when the most stress from that motion is experienced.

A number of **provocative tests** can be applied for specific problems. The discomfort of lateral tendinitis can be reproduced if the extensor carpi radialis longus and brevis muscles or the extensor digitorum communis is stressed with the wrist extended (Fig. 13-22). Additionally, discomfort may be reproduced with palmar flexion of the wrist, pronation, and gradual extension of the elbow, thus stretching the extensor tendon (Fig. 13-22, *C*). Tightness along the flexor pronator muscle mass or tendinitis may also be elicited with extension of the elbow and dorsiflexion of the wrist (Fig. 13-23).

Palpation of areas that are suspected of being involved by the history obtained should then be performed. The exact location of their tenderness, whether in the proximal, middle, or distal portion, is important. At this time the patient should also be asked to demonstrate any type of motion that recreates the symptoms most completely. If there is an area of tenderness, the examiner must recall the structures beneath this area and try to determine the origin of the pain. This may be accomplished by applying stress to various structures without stressing all of them. At this time the examiner needs to correlate the history with the findings on physical examination and the radiographic evaluation. From this the physician should have at least a good differential diagnosis of the problem if not the diagnosis. Further diagnostic or therapeutic procedures are then appropriately planned.

REFERENCES

1. Angelo RL, Soffer SR: Elbow anatomy relative to arthroscopy. In Andrews JR, Soffer SR (eds): *Elbow arthroscopy*, St Louis, 1994, Mosby.
2. Bogumill GP: Functional anatomy of the shoulder and elbow. In Pettrone FA (ed): *Upper extremity injuries in athletes*, St Louis, 1987, Mosby.
3. Crenshaw AH: Surgical approaches. In Edmondson AS, Crenshaw AH (eds): *Campbell's operative orthopaedics*, ed 6, St Louis, 1980, Mosby.
4. Grant JC, Boileau JCB: *An atlas of anatomy*, ed 6, Baltimore, 1972, Williams & Wilkins.
5. Henry AK: *Extensile exposure applied to limb surgery*, Baltimore, 1945, Williams & Wilkins.
6. Hollinshead WH: *Textbook of anatomy*, ed 2, New York, 1967, Harper & Row.
7. Morrey BF: Anatomy of the elbow joint. In Morrey BF (ed): *The elbow and its disorders*, Philadelphia, 1985, WB Saunders.
8. Nestor BJ, O'Driscoll SW, Morrey BF: Ligamentous reconstruction for posterolateral rotatory instability of the elbow, *J Bone Joint Surg* 74A:1235, 1992.
9. O'Driscoll SW, Ball DF, Morrey BF: Posterolateral rotatory instability of the elbow, *J Bone Joint Surg* 73A:440, 1991.
10. Tillman B: *A contribution to the functional morphology of articular surfaces*, Stuttgart, 1978, Georg Thieme.
11. Timmerman LA, Andrews JR: Undersurface tear of the ulnar collateral ligament in baseball players, *Am J Sports Med* 22:33, 1994.
12. Tullos HS, Byron WJ: Examination of the throwing elbow. In Zarins B, Andrews JR, Carson WG Jr (eds): *Injuries to the throwing arm*, Philadelphia, 1985, WB Saunders.
13. Tullos HS, Byron WJ: Functional anatomy of the elbow. In Zarins B, Andrews JR, Carson WG Jr (eds): *Injuries to the throwing arm*, Philadelphia, 1985, WB Saunders.
14. Tullos HS et al: Factors influencing elbow instability. In Murray DG (ed): *AAOS instructional course lectures*, vol 30, St Louis, 1981, Mosby.
15. Wadsworth TG: Introduction. In Wadsworth TG (ed): *The elbow*, New York, 1982, Churchill-Livingstone.
16. Wood VE: Thumb-clutched hand, congenital hand deformities. In Green DP (ed): *Operative hand surgery*, New York, 1982, Churchill-Livingstone.

CHAPTER 14 Radiographic Evaluation of the Elbow

George H. Belhobek

STANDARD RADIOGRAPHIC PROJECTIONS

The anteroposterior (AP), lateral, and external and internal oblique projections are the radiographs most commonly ordered to evaluate the elbow joint. These views offer valuable information about the integrity of the bony structures and the elbow joint, the presence of loose bodies, and the periarticular soft-tissue calcifications.

Anteroposterior Projection

The **AP projection** is produced with the elbow placed on the x-ray cassette in the extended position and the hand positioned in full supination to prevent overlapping of the forearm bones. The anterior surface of the elbow is parallel to the cassette surface. The central x-ray beam is centered perpendicular to the elbow joint. The correct projection is obtained when the radial head, neck, and biceps tuberosities are slightly superimposed over the proximal ulna. The distal humerus, the proximal radius and ulna, and the elbow joint space are well seen in this projection (Fig. 14-1).[1,6]

Lateral Projection

A **lateral projection** is obtained by placing the 90-degree flexed elbow on the x-ray cassette in the lateral position. The hand is placed in the lateral position, and the humeral condyles are perpendicular to the x-ray film. The central x-ray beam is directed perpendicular to the elbow joint. Positioning of the elbow in 90 degrees of flexion is important for proper visualization of the olecranon process and for proper projection of the elbow fat pads. The lateral projection of the elbow provides a lateral view of the distal humerus and the proximal forearm and provides a clear view of the olecranon process (Fig. 14-2).[1,6]

Oblique Projection

Medial and lateral oblique projections are useful in the evaluation of the traumatized elbow. The **lateral oblique view** is made with the elbow extended and the hand rotated laterally to place the posterior surface of the elbow at an angle of 40 degrees to the x-ray cassette. The central x-ray beam is directed vertically to the midpoint of the joint. The correct projection should demonstrate the radial head, neck, and tuberosity free from overlap of the ulna. The external oblique projection optimizes visualization of the radial head and neck area (Fig. 14-3).[1,6]

The **medial oblique view** is made with the elbow extended and the hand pronated, with the elbow adjusted so that its anterior surface is at an angle of 40 to 45 de-

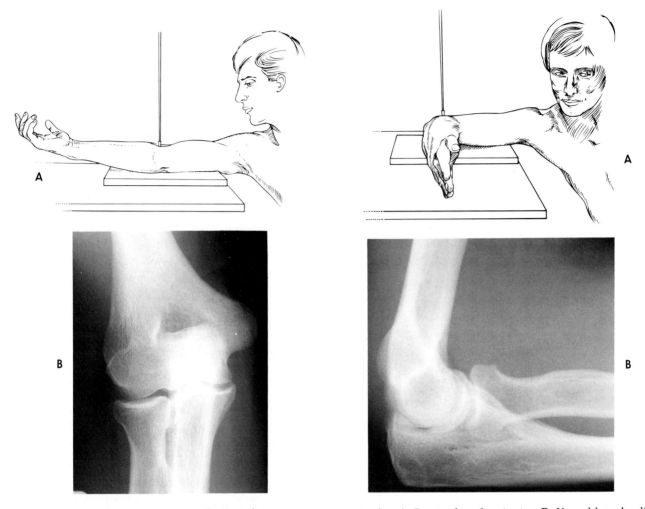

FIG. 14-1. **A,** Anteroposterior projection. **B,** Normal anteroposterior radiograph.

FIG. 14-2. **A,** Routine lateral projection. **B,** Normal lateral radiograph.

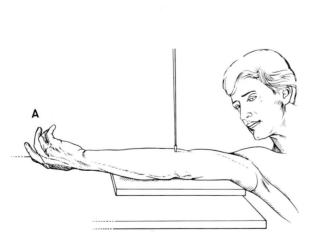

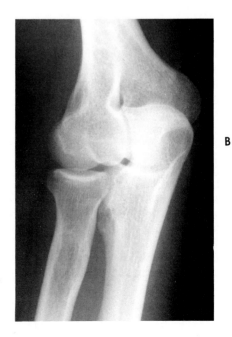

FIG. 14-3. **A,** Lateral oblique projection. **B,** Properly projected lateral oblique radiograph.

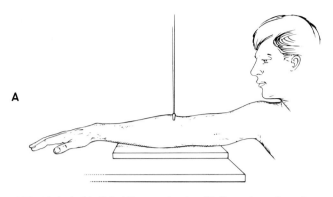

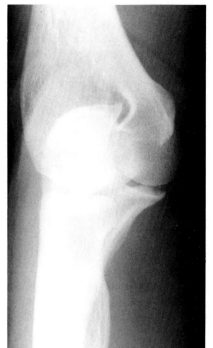

FIG. 14-4. A, Medial oblique projection. **B,** Properly projected medial oblique radiograph.

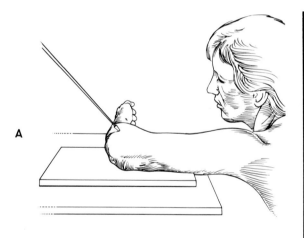

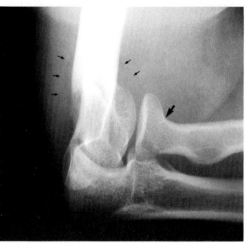

FIG. 14-5. A, Radial head—capitellum view. **B,** Radial head—capitellum view may be helpful in demonstrating subtle fractures of the radial head, the capitellum, and the coronoid process of the ulna. This radiograph demonstrates a slightly impacted fracture at the base of the radial head *(large arrow).* Notice the positive fat pad signs, indicating the presence of an elbow joint effusion *(small arrows).*

grees to the x-ray cassette. This should project the coronoid process in profile. The radial head and neck are superimposed on the ulna. The internal oblique projection optimizes visualization of the coronoid process of the ulna (Fig. 14-4).[1,6]

ADDITIONAL RADIOGRAPHIC PROJECTIONS

Subtle bony and soft-tissue pathologic conditions cannot always be defined by routine radiographs. A number of specialized projections are available to visualize selected areas of the elbow joint.

Special elbow radiographs

- Radial head projection
- Radial head–capitellum view
- Axial view
- Cubital tunnel view

Radial Head Projection

The radial head can sustain occult fractures that may be difficult to document on standard radiographs of the elbow. In the face of a high clinical suspicion for radial head fracture and nondiagnostic standard radiographs, several alternative radiographic procedures may be employed to enhance visualization.

Radiographs of the radial head in various degrees of rotation improve visualization of this structure. These can be made as spot images obtained under fluoroscopic control or as overhead radiographs made during various degrees of rotation of the radius. These procedures project the various surfaces of the radial head in profile, which improves the chances of demonstrating subtle radial head fractures. Optimal fluoroscopic spot images are obtained with fluoroscopic spot film devices employing small focal spot x-ray tubes (0.3 mm or less).

Radial Head–Capitellum View

The radial head–capitellum view is useful in evaluating patients with elbow joint injuries. This radiograph is made with the elbow placed on the x-ray cassette in the lateral position and in 90 degrees of flexion. The thumb is pointed upward, and the humeral condyles are perpendicular to the cassette. The central x-ray beam is angled 45 degrees to the forearm and passes through the radial head dorsoventrally.[21] This projection eliminates the overlap at the humeroradial and humeroulnar articulations and projects the radial head anterior to the coronoid process (Fig. 14-5).

The radial head–capitellum view is particularly useful in demonstrating fractures of the posterior aspect of the radial head (those obscured by the overlapping ulna on a conventional lateral view), fractures of the coronoid process, and fractures of the capitellum. Subtle osteochondritis dissecans lesions in the capitellum may be more clearly visualized with the radial head–capitellum view than by standard radiographs.[22,23] This view should be employed as an additional radiograph when clinical findings strongly suggest an elbow fracture and standard radiographs fail to visualize the abnormality.[26]

Axial View

The axial view of the elbow is made by placing the 45-degree flexed elbow on the x-ray cassette and making an x-ray exposure that is perpendicular to the humerus. This view images the olecranon process in an axial projection, whereas the lateral and medial epicondyles are seen in profile (Fig. 14-6).[1,6] The sulcus between the olecranon process and the capitellum, a potential space for small loose bodies, is demonstrated. Osteophytes arising at the medial and lateral aspects of the olecranon-trochlear joint are best seen in this projection (Fig. 14-7). The soft tissues adjacent to the olecranon process and the medial and lateral epicondyles are also demonstrated for evaluation of postinflammatory or posttraumatic calcification.

Cubital Tunnel View

A radiograph to profile the cubital tunnel is made by placing the maximally flexed and 15 degrees externally rotated elbow on the x-ray cassette. This position causes a vertical x-ray beam to project the cubital tunnel in profile (Fig. 14-8).[53]

The cubital tunnel, the fibroosseous passageway adjacent to the medial aspect of the elbow through which the

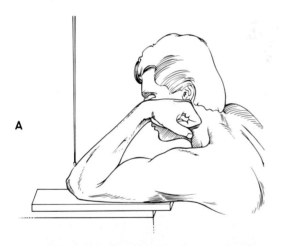

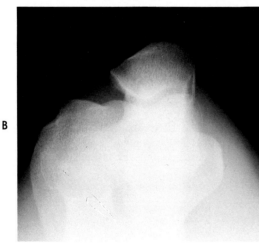

FIG. 14-6. **A,** Axial projection of elbow. **B,** Axial view of normal elbow.

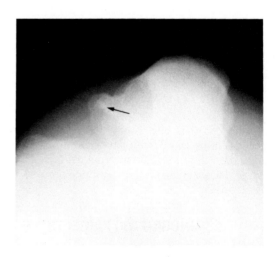

FIG. 14-7. Prominent osteophyte projecting from the lateral aspect of the olecranon process *(arrow).*

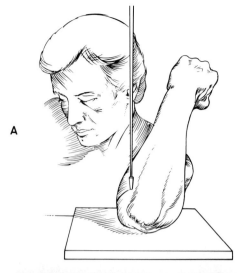

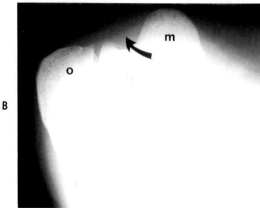

FIG. 14-8. A, Cubital tunnel view. **B,** Cubital tunnel radiograph of normal elbow. *Curved arrow,* Cubital tunnel; *M,* medial epicondyle; *O,* olecranon process.

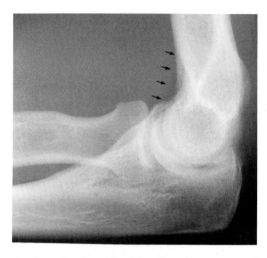

FIG. 14-9. Lateral radiograph of the elbow demonstrating the normal appearance of the anterior fat pad *(arrows).* The posterior fat pad is normally obscured by the humeral condyles.

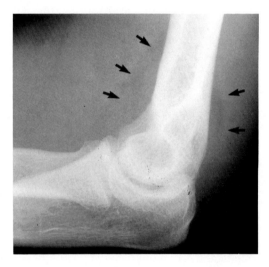

FIG. 14-10. Lateral radiograph of the elbow demonstrating positive anterior and posterior fat pad signs *(arrows).*

ulnar nerve courses, was first described by Feindel and Stratford in 1958.[17] The tunnel roof is formed by an aponeurotic arch (the arcuate ligament) that bridges the two heads of the flexor carpi ulnaris muscle. The floor of the tunnel is composed of the medial ligament of the elbow joint. Ulnar entrapment neuropathy, often referred to as cubital tunnel syndrome, can result from medial trochlear osteophytes that elevate the medial ligaments from the floor of the tunnel, resulting in diminished space for the nerve in the tunnel.[53] Lateral shift of the olecranon process during elbow flexion can result in a medial incongruity of the olecranon-trochlear joint space. A medial incongruity of greater than 5 mm is said to be a potential cause of ulnar nerve compression.[53]

ELBOW FAT PADS

Norell,[40] in 1954, was the first to suggest that displacement of the posterior fat pad of the elbow was commonly seen in patients with elbow fractures. Bledsoe and Izenstark[5] in 1959 pointed out that displacement of the fat pads anterior to the elbow joint was also seen following elbow trauma.

The radiographically visible fat pad anterior to the elbow joint is a summation of the fat collections located in the radial and coronoid fossae. When viewed on the lateral radiograph of a normal elbow, these fat collections are superimposed on each other and appear as a radiolucent triangle along the anterior aspect of the distal humerus (Fig. 14-9).

The posterior fat pad at the elbow joint is located in the olecranon fossa. On the lateral view this posterior fat collection is normally hidden from view by the humeral condyles. The anterior and posterior fat pads are positioned between the flexible joint capsule and the synovium layer of the elbow joint.[39,52]

Any intracapsular collection of fluid (transudate, exudate, or hemorrhage) or tissue leading to capsular distention causes the anterior fat pad to be displaced anteriorly and the posterior fat pad to be displaced posteriorly. As a result, the anterior fat pad assumes a convex shape on the lateral radiograph (ship's sail configura-

tion), whereas the posterior fat pad is visualized posterior to the humeral condyles (Fig. 14-10).[39] In acute elbow trauma, positive fat pad signs are the result of intracapsular bleeding secondary to intraarticular fracture.

The radiographic projection of the elbow necessary for proper fat pad evaluation is a true lateral view made with 90 degrees of flexion.[24] A slight obliquity of the projection may be enough to obscure the sign.[39] A true positive fat pad sign following acute elbow trauma is an excellent indicator of an intraarticular fracture. Examinations of the elbow that demonstrate even slight displacement of the fat pads following trauma are likely to reveal fractures if the examiner persists in seeking a positive skeletal finding by using anteroposterior, lateral, oblique, and special radiographic views as necessary. Clear radiographic evidence of a joint effusion following acute trauma is considered by many as an indication for conservative treatment and radiologic reexamination in 5 to 7 days if initial radiographs do not demonstrate a fracture.[7,52]

A false negative anterior fat pad sign can occur with poor patient positioning, extracapsular fracture, and capsular rupture.[31] According to Murphy and Siegel,[39] a false positive posterior fat pad sign may occur when the elbow is filmed in extension. A paradoxical positive posterior fat pad sign may occur when the periosteum is stripped from the humerus just proximal to the olecranon fossa, such as with hemorrhage from a supracondylar fracture or subperiosteal neoplasm.[39]

PLAIN RADIOGRAPHIC DIAGNOSIS
Stress Injuries

The elbow is the focus for excessive forces in a number of today's popular sports activities. The elbow is particularly prone to injury in throwing sports such as baseball and javelin and in racquet sports such as tennis and racquetball. The plain radiographic examination can demonstrate and document many of these stress-related injuries to the elbow joint.

Slocum[51] was the first to suggest categories of elbow injury based on precipitating stress. A number of authors have elaborated further on this subject.[13,25,32,48,56] Gore et al[20] defined five categories of stress-related elbow injuries: diffuse generalized stress, rotational humeral shaft stress, medial tension stress, lateral compression stress, and extension stress. Stresses encountered during the act of pitching are representative of these injury-producing stresses. Effects of these pressures on the elbow joint and the upper extremity are different in the adult and adolescent athlete because of structural differences between the mature and immature skeleton.

Osseous changes about the elbow joint can develop from conditioning of an extremity for throwing or stroking. Conditioning in the mature athlete results in cortical and trabecular hypertrophy and narrowing of the medullary canal of the throwing extremity (Fig. 14-11).[30] The bony hypertrophy is thought to be the result of hyperemia, which leads to accelerated bony remodeling.[20] In the adolescent athlete diffuse upper extremity stress produces hypertrophy and hypermaturity of the epiphyses and apophyses of the elbow joint.[20,25,32]

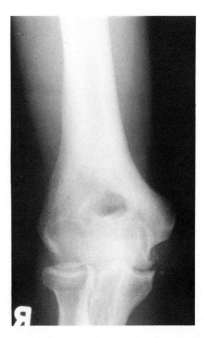

FIG. 14-11. Anteroposterior view of the distal humerus and elbow joint demonstrating cortical and trabecular hypertrophy of the distal humerus in a 28-year-old professional pitcher. This is the result of years of conditioning.

The stresses responsible for most elbow injuries from pitching occur during the acceleration phase. The forearm is forced into a valgus attitude with respect to the distal humerus during this phase, which results in distraction forces at the medial aspect of the elbow joint (medial tension stress) and impaction forces at the radial-capitellar articulation (lateral compression stress). In the adult, where the ulnar collateral ligament is the primary medial stabilizer of the elbow, most medial tension injuries result from chronic strain of the ulnar collateral ligament at its attachment on the coronoid tubercle. In the adolescent the ulnar collateral ligament is relatively lax, and the flexor-pronator muscle group becomes the primary medial support for the valgus strain of throwing. Excessive medial tension stresses on the immature skeleton, therefore, result in injury to the medial epicondylar apophysis, the point of attachment of the flexor-pronator muscles.[20,25,32,51]

The most common radiographic manifestation of medial tension stress in the throwing adult athlete is a traction spur arising from the medial aspect of the coronoid tubercle (Fig. 14-12). Gore et al[20] reported that 75% of the 16 professional baseball players they studied for radiographic manifestations of elbow stress demonstrated these spurs.

Unusually excessive strain on the ulnar collateral ligament may lead to a cortical avulsion fracture of the medial epicondyle or a rupture of the medial collateral ligament itself. An examination of the elbow under fluoroscopy may be necessary to adequately assess the degree of joint instability following a medial collateral ligament tear. Findings in the injured joint should always be compared with those found during a similar examination of the patient's uninjured elbow.

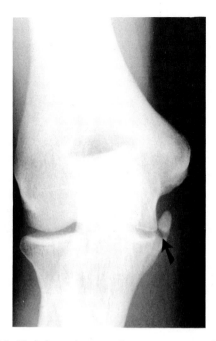

FIG. 14-12. Medial traction spur is a common manifestation of chronic elbow stress in the throwing athlete. In this case a remote fracture of this spur has healed with a fibrous union *(arrows)*.

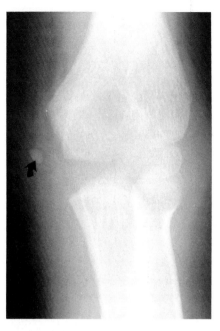

FIG. 14-13. Occasionally a complete avulsion of the medial epicondylar apophysis *(arrows)* can occur from a single stress event. The avulsion fracture illustrated followed a particular violent throw by this young athlete.

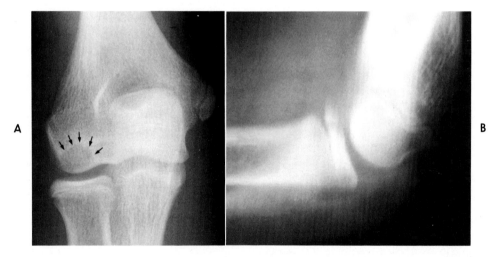

FIG. 14-14. A, Cyst outlined *(arrows)* in the capitellum of this 13-year-old gymnast is compatible with either posttraumatic osteochondrosis or an osteochondral fracture. **B,** Traumatic osteochondrosis of the radial head demonstrated on this lateral tomogram of a 14-year-old pitcher is an unusual manifestation of chronic lateral elbow stress.

Posttraumatic changes in the medial epicondylar physis and apophysis may be seen in the juvenile pitcher. This injury has become known as **little leaguer's elbow.**[8] The injury is caused by excessive pull of the flexor-pronator muscle group at its insertion on the medial epicondylar apophysis. The radiographic changes seen with little leaguer's elbow include fragmentation, irregularity, enlargement, and mild separation of the apophysis. These are the result of chronic valgus stress. Occasionally frank avulsion of the apophysis results from a single traumatic event (Fig. 14-13).[8,32,48]

While strong tension forces are applied to the medial aspect of the elbow during the acceleration phase of throwing, equally strong compression forces occur laterally, causing impaction of the radial head on the capitellum. In the adult thrower Gore et al[20] found that lateral compression forces could occasionally result in an acute osteochondral fracture of the lateral margin of the capitellum. Chronic lateral compartment compression can lead to articular cartilage shaving, which results in degenerative joint disease and loose body formation. Adolescent athletes are more likely to develop lateral com-

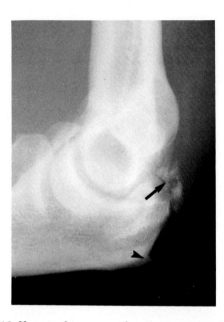

FIG. 14-15. Hypertrophic spurs at the posterior aspect of the olecranon process *(arrowhead)* commonly develop because of violent traction forces that are applied by the triceps tendon during the release and follow-through phases of the pitching motion. Notice the bony excrescences at the posterior tip of the olecranon process *(straight arrow)*.

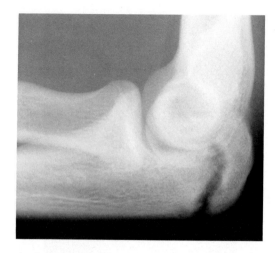

FIG. 14-16. Lateral radiograph demonstrates widening of the olecranon apophyseal plate in an adolescent pitcher. The fracture went on to heal with conservative treatment.

pression injuries because they lack the protective cubitus valgus present in adult throwers and because they exhibit a relative laxity of medial joint support.[20] Repeated lateral compression forces in the young thrower can result in osteochondral fractures or traumatic osteochondrosis of the capitellum. Traumatic osteochondrosis of the radial head is an uncommon manifestation of chronic lateral stress.[20,25,32] Subchondral bone deformity, cystic changes, and scattered areas of bone sclerosis are the radiographic hallmarks of these injuries (Fig. 14-14).

During the release and follow-through phases of pitching, the elbow goes from a position of acute flexion to complete extension with the application of a violent force. This force places severe traction on the triceps at its attachment on the olecranon process. In the adult the repeated pull of the triceps muscle results in formation of traction spurs on the posterior aspect of the olecranon process. Stress or avulsion fractures of the olecranon process may occasionally occur.[20,51,56] Loose body formation is a chronic manifestation of posterior stress (Fig. 14-15). Fractures of the olecranon apophysis have been reported in the adolescent throwing athlete (Fig. 14-16).[42,55]

Loose Body Formation

In the adult, loose body formation may be the result of shaving of the cartilaginous joint surfaces by chronic trauma or the result of fracture of an osteophyte about the elbow joint. Gore et al[20] suggest that the joint incongruity that follows the bony hypertrophy of skeletal conditioning applies pathologic stresses to the synovium, resulting in synovial shredding and metaplasia that leads to loose body exfoliation. In the adolescent, loose bodies

may be the result of osteochondral fractures or posttraumatic osteochondroses.[2] The plain radiographic projections of the elbow are useful in demonstrating periarticular calcifications and ossifications that are potential loose bodies. Fluoroscopy may be useful in the demonstration and localization of loose bodies. Intraarticular loose bodies move freely with flexion and extension. Extraarticular bodies or those wedged in the joint or fixed to the synovium move little if at all. Confirmation of a free intraarticular location, however, requires an arthrographic examination.

CONVENTIONAL TOMOGRAPHY

The complexity of the elbow anatomy results in superimposition of the osseous structures on plain radiographs. Thin-section tomographic images may occasionally be helpful in better defining subtle bony injury. The projection and slice thickness should be tailored to demonstrate areas in question. Fluoroscopy may be useful in determining the optimal tomographic projection.

COMPUTED TOMOGRAPHY

Computed tomography (CT) is another imaging modality that has proven to be a successful adjunct to plain radiography in demonstrating subtle elbow injury. State-of-the-art CT scanners provide high-resolution, thin-section images primarily in the axial plane.[18] CT data can be reconstructed to provide images in the coronal and sagittal planes. CT studies are particularly helpful in demonstrating occult fractures and osteochondral injuries as well as in localizing loose bodies and osteophytes located out of the plane of conventional radiographs. CT scans can also be useful in clarifying joint deformities resulting from significantly angled elbow fractures (Fig. 14-17).

The elbow joint and the upper extremity distal to it can be examined by positioning the arms above the patient's head with the elbows extended or flexed and positioned

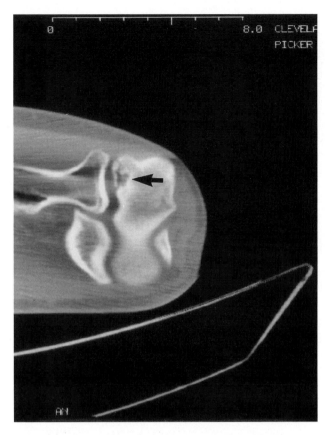

FIG. 14-17. Computed tomography scan made through the joint line of the elbow demonstrates osteochondritis dissecans in the subchondral bone of the capitellum.

at the level of the scanning gantry. Scans are usually made in a high-resolution algorithm. Patel, Barton, and Green[41] have discussed a modified patient position that may be used when clinical conditions do not allow the patient to be positioned in the scanner in the traditional way. The anatomy and mobility of the proximal radioulnar articulation can also be studied with CT.[10]

RADIONUCLIDE IMAGING

Conventional radiographs, particularly in multiple projections, are useful diagnostic tools for demonstrating traumatic injuries of the elbow joint. These examinations are hampered, however, by limited spatial resolution and by the inability of the various radiographic projections to visualize all of the complex anatomy of the elbow adequately. Although conventional tomography and CT improve the ability to demonstrate subtle pathologic conditions of the elbow, occult fractures may go undetected unless the appropriate imaging procedure is directed to the location of injury. In addition, several weeks of symptoms precede any radiographic evidence of a stress fracture (e.g., periosteal reaction, endosteal callus, focal bone sclerosis, and ultimately a fracture line).

The radionuclide bone scan, by virtue of its ability to demonstrate physiologic changes in bone, can image the abnormal physiologic changes of a stress injury or an oc-

cult fracture considerably earlier than radiographic methods can image anatomic evidence of the injury. Early diagnosis of these osseous lesions and their differentiation from soft-tissue pathologic states is of primary importance to the competitive athlete who wants to continue training unless significant injury can be documented.[28]

Three-Phase Scanning

Three-phase radionuclide imaging following bolus intravenous injection of 20 mCi (740 mEq) of ^{99m}Tc-labeled methylene diphosphonate (^{99m}Tc MDP) is the bone-imaging protocol favored by most nuclear medicine specialists.[46]

The three-phase technique consists of (1) rapid-sequence radionuclide images obtained during the first pass of tracer through the body (vascular phase), (2) blood pool images obtained about 10 minutes after injection (blood pool image), and (3) delayed images obtained 2 to 3 hours after injection (delayed image). The three-phase bone scan, therefore, demonstrates the perfusion of a lesion (phase 1), the relative vascularity of a lesion (phase 2), and the relative bone turnover of a lesion (phase 3).[35]

Three-phase bone scan

- Phase 1—Vascular phase
- Phase 2—Blood pool images
- Phase 3—Delayed images

Stress Fractures

The radionuclide bone scan has been shown by numerous authors* to be highly sensitive in detecting bone stress injuries when conventional radiographs are normal. All three phases of the scan are positive in a patient with an acute stress fracture. Fractures are imaged as focally intense areas of tracer accumulation involving 50% or more of the bone cortex.[34] A positive bone scan can be expected considerably before the 2 to 3 weeks necessary for documentation of a stress injury with conventional radiographs. Conventional tomography or CT scans of the positive area can be helpful in confirming the fracture and in differentiating it from other pathologic conditions that can cause positive three-phase bone scans (e.g., osteoid osteoma or Brodie's abscess [Fig. 14-18]).

Wilcox, Moniot, and Green[58] suggested that the pain associated with a stress fracture may not be present before the radionuclide scan becomes positive. The sensitivity of radionuclide scanning in demonstrating active stress injuries is such that, when a scan is negative, a stress fracture is unlikely.[34,45]

The radionuclide angiogram and blood pool images have been found to be helpful in assessing healing of bone stress injuries. As healing occurs, first the radio-

---

*References 11, 19, 28, 34, 35, and 45.

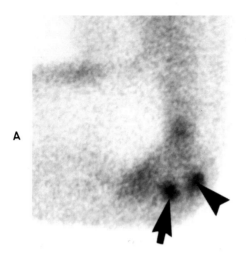
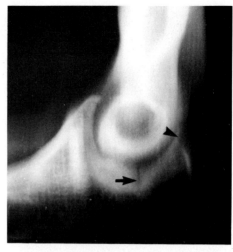

FIG. 14-18. **A,** This delayed image from a three-phase ⁹⁹ᵐTc MDP bone scan was obtained on a 26-year-old professional pitcher with unexplained chronic elbow pain. The scan demonstrates two focal areas of increased radionuclide activity representing foci of abnormal bone metabolism in the olecranon process *(short arrow* and *arrowhead)*. **B,** Lateral tomogram of this elbow demonstrates that the more anterior focus of activity corresponds to a stress fracture through the subarticular region of the olecranon process *(short arrow)*. The more posterior focus of activity *(arrowhead)* relates to a posttraumatic osteophyte.

nuclide angiogram and then the blood pool images become normal. The intensity of radionuclide uptake on delayed images decreases over 3 to 6 weeks but can still be increased for 8 to 10 months after injury.[46] Simple periosteal reaction is differentiated from a true stress fracture by its superficial and linear scintigraphic appearance compared with the fusiform configuration of a stress fracture.

Occult Fractures

The radionuclide bone scan can also be helpful in documenting and localizing occult posttraumatic fractures when standard radiographs are negative. According to Matin,[34] almost all fractures are detected by bone scintigraphy within 1 day of injury and certainly within 3 days of the trauma. Conventional tomographic or CT images made through the area of the positive scan help document the fracture.

ELBOW ARTHROGRAPHY

Radiographic techniques, including conventional tomography and CT, have only limited value in evaluating the soft tissues and cartilaginous structures of the elbow joint. Radiographic imaging following the intraarticular injection of radiographic contrast material provides information about the articular surfaces of the joint, the synovial lining of the joint, and the relationship of periarticular calcifications and masses to the joint cavity.

Elbow arthrography was first described by Lindblom in 1952.[33] In 1962 Del Buono and Solarino[14] supported the use of double contrast elbow arthrography in the diagnosis of chondromatosis, osteochondritis dissecans, detached osseous fragments, and posttraumatic calcifications and fibrosis. Since these early reports the proce-

dure has undergone significant refinement, including the application of conventional tomography[16] and CT.[50]

Techniques

Elbow arthrography can be carried out using either single or double contrast techniques. Scout radiographs of the elbow in at least AP, lateral, and both oblique projections should precede the arthrographic procedure. Arthrocentesis is generally carried out under fluoroscopic control using a lateral approach to the joint. A 1- or 1½-inch (2.5 or 3.8 cm) hypodermic needle is adequate for this purpose. A posterior approach to the elbow joint has been noted to be helpful in patients who have undergone resection of the radial head.[29]

Standard Arthrography

Single contrast arthrograms are produced by injecting the volume of water-soluble iodinated contrast material necessary to mildly distend the joint capsule (Fig. 14-19). The contrast material may be diluted with sterile water or saline to decrease its density. This allows better visualization of intraarticular loose bodies.[4,37] **Double contrast arthrography** is carried out with 0.5 ml of iodinated contrast material followed by the injection of 6 to 12 cc of room air.

With single contrast arthrography standard radiography in the AP, lateral, and both oblique projections are obtained following contrast material injection. Follow-up fluoroscopy of the joint has been noted to be useful.[4,29] Similar radiographs are obtained during the double contrast technique.

Arthrotomography

The complexity of the anatomy of the elbow makes it difficult to demonstrate all of the articular surfaces in

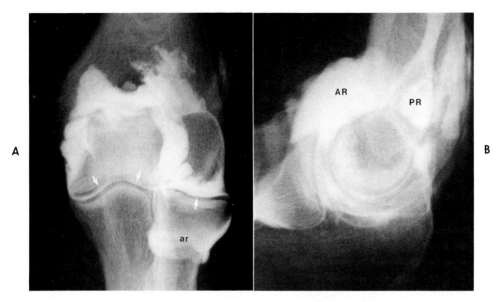

FIG. 14-19. AP **(A)** and lateral **(B)** radiographs of the elbow made during a single contrast elbow arthrogram demonstrate the articular cartilage *(arrows)* with normal filling of the anterior recess *(AR)*, the posterior recess *(PR)*, and the annular recess *(ar)*.

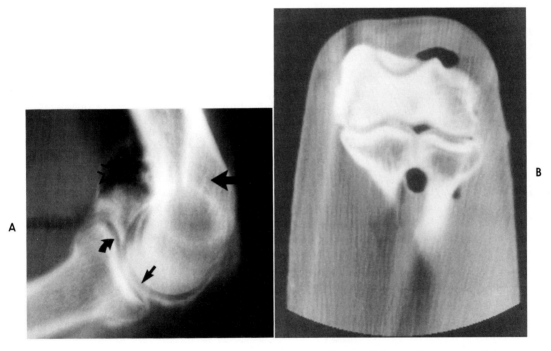

FIG. 14-20. A, This double contrast arthrotomogram through the radial capitellum portion of the elbow joint defines the normal articular cartilage of the radius *(curved arrow)* and capitellum *(straight arrow)*. The anterior recess *(open arrowhead)* and posterior recess *(closed arrowhead)* are also demonstrated. **B,** Normal elbow double contrast CT arthrotomogram demonstrates intact articular cartilage.

profile on standard radiographic projections obtained during elbow arthrography. The coupling of conventional tomography with elbow arthrography has been shown to provide additional information over conventional arthrographic techniques.[16,29,57] Arthrotomography is particularly useful in localizing articular cartilage defects and

in demonstrating small intraarticular loose bodies. Arthrotomography is particularly effective when coupled with the double contrast arthrographic technique. Scout tomograms at about 3-mm intervals in the AP and lateral projections are obtained preceding the arthrogram. Identical sections are then made after the introduction

of contrast medium. Tomography is followed by a fluoroscopic examination.

Currently CT scanning is the preferred imaging method in the arthrotomographic technique. Thin, high-resolution CT scans (2- to 3-mm thickness) of the elbow's contrast-enhanced anatomy can be reconstructed in multiplanar images following scanning in a single plane (Fig. 14-20).[50]

Loose Bodies

Elbow arthrography or arthrotomography is most commonly employed for the demonstration and localization of intraarticular loose bodies (Fig. 14-21). Arthrography can determine which paraarticular calcific densities seen

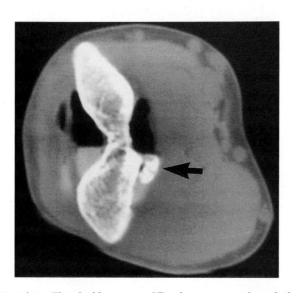

FIG. 14-21. This double contrast CT arthrotomogram through the supracondylar region of the distal humerus demonstrates a loose body in the anterior joint compartment of the elbow (arrow).

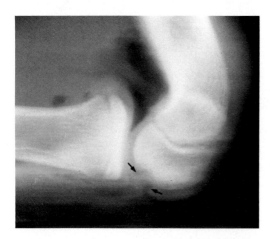

FIG. 14-22. Lateral arthrotomogram through the radial-capitellar portion of the elbow of a 12-year-old pitcher with unexplained elbow symptoms. The arthrotomogram demonstrates an articular cartilage defect that could not be diagnosed on plain radiographs and plain tomograms.

on plain radiographs lie within the joint cavity and which are embedded in the soft tissues. Occasionally arthrotomography demonstrates a cartilaginous loose body that has not been suspected on the basis of a plain radiographic examination. Intraarticular loose bodies are diagnosed when they are shown to be completely surrounded by air or contrast material and are demonstrated to move freely within the joint during the postarthrography fluoroscopic examination. Calcifications that are fixed in the periarticular soft tissues may move, but they do so less freely than loose bodies. They do not repeatedly roll over, and they do not fall into dependent portions of the joint.[29] Decreased joint motion resulting from impingement by thickened synovium or bony prominences can also be documented during arthrotomography and fluoroscopy.

Articular Cartilage

Arthrography may also be helpful in assessing the articular surfaces of patients with osteochondritis dissecans or osteochondral fractures. The plain radiographic examination often suggests subchondral bone irregularity in these patients. Occasionally, however, the only diagnostic information to be obtained is an articular cartilage defect demonstrated by arthrotomography (Fig. 14-22).

MAGNETIC RESONANCE IMAGING

Magnetic resonance imaging (MRI) is an exciting computerized imaging technology that continues to grow in importance as a method of demonstrating musculoskeletal injuries. The unique ability of MRI to provide superior soft-tissue contrast and its ability to image the bone marrow provides physicians with the capability of documenting soft-tissue injury including muscle, nerve, ligament, and articular cartilage injuries, to localizing loose bodies, and to imaging osteochondral and osseous injury.[12,38] Recent advances in MRI technology, such as off-axis imaging capability, the development of surface coils, and multiplanar reconstruction capabilities, have greatly enhanced its ability to image joints such as the elbow.

Technical Considerations

MRI is based on the principle of nuclear magnetic resonance, where tomographic images similar to those of x-ray CT are produced without the use of ionizing radiation.

The MR image is created from the interaction between radio waves and hydrogen protons of tissues. It is composed of picture elements (pixels) generated by a computer similar to the mechanism of image production with CT.

The intensity of the MR signal is determined by the density of the resonating protons and by two chemical parameters called relaxation times: T1 and T2.[43,49] Both normal and abnormal tissues can be characterized by their T1 and T2 values. When tissues are altered by disease or trauma, their T1 and T2 values may be altered, so pathologic tissues can be distinguished from normal

tissues on MR images. Scan techniques (pulse sequences) can be operator selected to enhance tissue T1 and T2 differences, thereby improving image contrast between normal and abnormal tissues. Images made with techniques that emphasize T1 tissue characteristics (T1-weighted images) generally show excellent spatial resolution producing good demonstrations of anatomy. MR images made with techniques that emphasize T2 characteristics (T2-weighted images) generally provide decreased spatial resolution, but maximize differences in contrast.

Spin-echo imaging techniques are the most widely employed pulse sequences to demonstrate musculoskeletal injury.[27] Pathologic tissues generally have increased free water, which causes lengthening of their T1 and T2 values. These abnormal tissues generally demonstrate an isointense or decreased MR signal (darker) on T1-weighted images, whereas these tissues demonstrate increased MR signal (bright) on T2-weighted images. Fluid, such as joint effusion, is uniformly bright on T2-

weighted images.[3] Fatty tissue and yellow bone marrow, because of short T1 values, have a bright signal on T1-weighted images (Table 14-1).[43] Subacute hematomas and tissues with high protein content have a relatively bright MR signal on T1- and T2-weighted images.[15,54]

Several additional pulse sequences that have been developed serve as adjuncts to standard T1- and T2-weighted spin-echo techniques. Three-dimensional gradient-echo techniques provide thin-section images that can be reconstructed in nonorthogonal planes. This technique can be helpful in demonstrating articular cartilage injury and in documenting intraarticular loose bodies. Fat saturation techniques also produce images that improve the ability to evaluate articular cartilage abnormalities.[27]

In extremity imaging, including the elbow, a dedicated extremity coil or surface coil is necessary to obtain high-resolution images. Optimal images are obtained on MR imagers that have off-access imaging capabilities. This allows the examination to proceed with the arm positioned at the patient's side. On equipment where off-axis imaging is not available, the arm must be raised above the head to center the elbow in the main magnetic field of the scanner. The elbow may be extended or flexed depending on the patient's ability to cooperate.[47]

Practical Applications

Considerable experience is now available in regard to the MRI evaluation of large joints such as the knee, hip, and shoulder. Advances in MR technology have led to improved image quality with smaller joints; because of this, enthusiasm for imaging the elbow is growing.

Publications by Middleton et al[36] and Bunnell et al[9] describe the normal MR anatomy of the elbow (Fig. 14-

TABLE 14-1 Magnetic resonance imaging gray scale: normal anatomy—T1-weighted spin-echo technique

Anatomic Structure	Signal Intensity	Gray Scale
Areolar tissue	High	White
Yellow bone marrow	High	White
Muscle	Intermediate	Gray
Articular cartilage	Intermediate	Gray
Tendons and ligaments	Low	Gray-black
Flowing blood	Low	Black
Fibrocartilage	Low	Black
Cortical bone	Low	Black

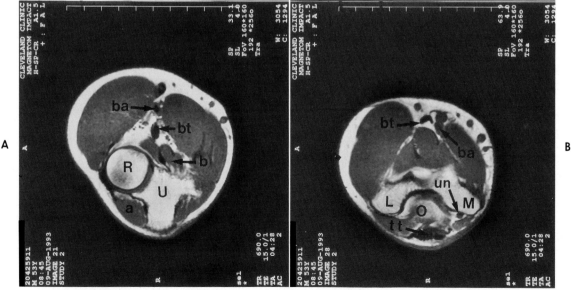

FIG. 14-23. These T_1-weighted spin-echo images of a normal elbow (**A,** level of radioulnar articulation; **B,** level of intercondylar region) demonstrate the signal intensities of normal tissues. *r,* Radial head; *u,* ulna; *a,* anconeus muscle; *b,* brachialis muscle; *bt,* biceps tendon; *ba,* brachial artery; *l,* lateral epicondyle; *m,* medial epicondyle; *o,* olecranon process; *tt,* triceps tendon; *un,* ulnar nerve.

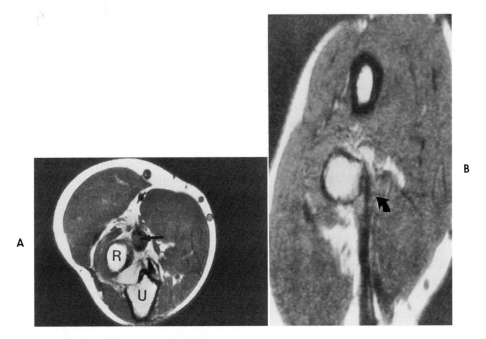

FIG. 14-24. A, This axial T₁-weighted spin-echo image at the level of the radius-biceps tubercle demonstrates increased MR signal in the distal biceps tendon near its bony attachment *(arrow).* This would suggest tendinopathy or partial tearing of the tendon. **B,** Three-dimensional gradient-echo image of the same patient reconstructed to demonstrate the attachment of the biceps tendon on the radius *(arrow).* Notice the thinning and frayed appearance of the tendon, documenting a partial tendon tear.

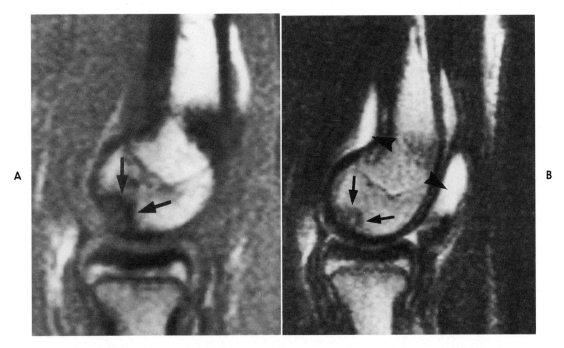

FIG. 14-25. T₁-weighted **(A)** and T₂-weighted **(B)** spin-echo images of a 12-year-old gymnast document the clinically suspected diagnosis of osteochondritis dissecans. Arrows point out the lesion in the subchondral bone of the capitellum. Articular cartilage associated with the lesion is intact. Arrowheads in image **B** (T₂ weight) point out high-signal joint fluid.

23). Recent publications by Murphy[38] and Ho and Sartoris[27] outline specific elbow injuries that can be evaluated with MRI (Fig. 14-24). The articular cartilage can be directly imaged for surface irregularities and focal defects, and osteochondral injuries can be documented (Fig. 14-25). The presence of joint fluid facilitates the evaluation of joint cartilage and loose bodies based on the bright MR signal (arthrographic effect) seen with fluid on T2-weighted spin-echo and gradient-echo images. However, the evaluation of loose bodies with MRI can be difficult even in the presence of joint fluid; on this basis double contrast CT arthrography may be more useful in this regard.[27]

Muscle tears and acute hemorrhage demonstrate bright MR signal on T2-weighted spin-echo images, whereas subacute hematomas show increased signal on both T1- and T2- weighted sequences. Rosenberg et al[44] pointed out the value of MRI in the evaluation of nerve entrapment syndromes and neuropathies at the elbow joint. Periarticular soft-tissue masses are best evaluated with MRI.

SUMMARY

Conventional radiographs in standard projections should remain the primary imaging examination for the evaluation of the injured elbow. Specialized radiographic projections may provide additional information if they are obtained in appropriate circumstances. Fluoroscopy may provide a cost-effective method of imaging subtle posttraumatic changes.

The use of more sophisticated and costly procedures should be reserved for those cases where appropriate information cannot be obtained with simpler technology. CT, by virtue of its improved contrast resolution over conventional radiographs and its ability to provide images in the axial plane, has proved to be an effective method of documenting injuries in complex anatomic structures such as the elbow. The three-phase technetium radionuclide bone scan is an efficient method of localizing subtle bone pathologic conditions, providing a road map for further analysis with additional imaging techniques.

Arthrography and arthrotomography provide information about the intraarticular and paraarticular structures of the elbow. MRI has proved to be an excellent method of imaging soft tissues such as muscle, tendons, ligaments, and articular cartilage and most certainly will play an increasingly important role in the evaluation of intraarticular and extraarticular injuries to the elbow joint.

The effective use of all of these imaging techniques is predicated on an understanding of their usefulness in providing information about a suspected clinical problem. They should be ordered only after a thorough clinical evaluation has been performed, and the imaging procedure should always be tailored to fit the need of the individual patient.

REFERENCES

1. Ballinger PW: *Merrill's atlas of radiographic positions and radiologic procedures*, ed 6, St Louis, 1986, Mosby.
2. Bassett LW et al: Posttraumatic osteochondral "loose body" of the olecranon fossa, *Radiology* 141:635, 1981.
3. Beltran J et al: Joint effusions: MR imaging, *Radiology* 158:133, 1986.
4. Blane CE et al: Arthrography in the posttraumatic elbow in children, *Am J Roentgenol* 143:17, 1984.
5. Bledsoe RC, Izenstark JL: Displacement of fat pads in disease and injury of the elbow: a new radiographic sign, *Radiology* 73:717, 1959.
6. Bontrager KL, Anthony BT: *Textbook of radiographic positioning and related anatomy*, ed 2, St Louis, 1987, Mosby.
7. Brodeur AE et al: The basic tenets for appropriate evaluation of the elbow in pediatrics, *Curr Probl Diagn Radiol* 12(5):1, 1983.
8. Brogdon BG, Crow NE: Little leaguer's elbow, *Am J Roentgenol* 83:671, 1960.
9. Bunnell DH et al: Elbow joint: normal anatomy on MR images, *Radiology* 165:527, 1987.
10. Cone RO et al: Computed tomography of the normal radioulnar joints, *Invest Radiol* 18(6):541, 1983.
11. Dakins DR: Differential diagnosis key to sports injury evaluation, *Diagn Imag* 9:146, 1987.
12. Dalinka MK et al: Modern diagnostic imaging in joint disease, *Am J Roentgenol* 152:229, 1989.
13. Dehaven KE, Evarts CM: Throwing injuries of the elbow in athletes, *Orthop Clin North Am* 4(3):801, 1973.
14. Del Buono MS, Solarino GB: Arthrography of the elbow with double contrast media, *Ital Clin Orthop* 14:223, 1962.
15. Ehman RL, Berquist TH: Magnetic resonance imaging of musculoskeletal trauma, *Radiol Clin North Am* 24(2):291, 1986.
16. Eto RT, Anderson PW, Harley JD: Elbow arthrography with the application of tomography, *Radiology* 115:283, 1975.
17. Feindel W, Stratford J: The role of the cubital tunnel in tardy ulnar palsy, *Can J Surg* 1:287, 1958.
18. Genant HK: Computed tomography. In Resnick D, Niwayama G (eds): *Diagnosis of bone and joint disorders with emphasis on articular abnormalities*, Philadelphia, 1981, WB Saunders.
19. Geslien GE et al: Early detection of stress fractures using technetium 99m-polyphosphate, *Radiology* 121:683, 1976.
20. Gore RM et al: Osseous manifestations of elbow stress associated with sports activities, *Am J Roentgenol* 134:971, 1980.
21. Greenspan A, Norman A: The radial head–capitellum view: useful technique in elbow trauma, *Am J Roentgenol* 139:1186, 1982.
22. Greenspan A, Norman A: Radial head–capitellum view: an expanded imaging approach to elbow injury, *Radiology* 164:272, 1987.
23. Greenspan A, Norman A, Rosen H: Radial head–capitellum view in elbow trauma: clinical application in radiographic-anatomic correlation, *Am J Roentgenol* 143:355, 1984.
24. Griswold R: Elbow fat pads: a radiography perspective, *Radiol Technol* 53:303, 1982.
25. Gugenheim JJ et al: Little League survey: the Houston study, *Am J Sports Med* 4(5):189, 1976.
26. Hall-Craggs MA, Shorvon PJ, Chapman M: Assessment of the radial head–capitellum view and the dorsal fat pad sign in acute elbow trauma, *Am J Roentgenol* 145:607, 1985.
27. Ho CP, Sartoris DJ: Magnetic resonance imaging of the elbow, *Rheum Dis Clin North Am* 17(3):705, 1991.
28. Holder LE: Radionuclide bone imaging in the evaluation of bone pain, *J Bone Joint Surg* 64A:1391, 1982.
29. Hudson TM: Elbow arthrography, *Radiol Clin North Am* 19:227, 1981.
30. Jones HH et al: Humeral hypertrophy in response to exercise, *J Bone Joint Surg* 59A(2):204, 1977.
31. Kohn AM: Soft tissue alterations in elbow trauma, *Am J Roentgenol* 82:867, 1959.
32. Larson RL et al: Little League survey: the Eugene study, *Am J Sports Med* 4(5):201, 1976.
33. Lindblom K: Arthrography, *J Fac Radiol* 3:151, 1952.
34. Matin P: Bone scintigraphy in the diagnosis and management of traumatic injury, *Semin Nucl Med* 13:104, 1983.
35. Maurer AH et al: Three-phase radionuclide scintigraphy of the hand, *Radiology* 146:761, 1983.
36. Middleton WD et al: MR imaging of the normal elbow: anatomic correlation, *Am J Roentgenol* 149:543, 1987.

37. Mink JH, Eckardt JJ, Grant TT: Arthrography in recurrent dislocation of the elbow, *Am J Roentgenol* 136:1242, 1981.
38. Murphy BJ: MR imaging of the elbow, *Radiology* 184:525, 1992.
39. Murphy WA, Siegel MJ: Elbow fat pads with new signs and extended differential diagnosis, *Radiology* 124:659, 1977.
40. Norell HG: Roentgenologic visualization of the extracapsular fat: its importance in the diagnosis of traumatic injuries of the elbow, *Acta Radiol* 42:205, 1954.
41. Patel RB, Barton P, Green L: CT of isolated elbow in evaluation of trauma: a modified technique, *Comput Radiol* 8(1):1, 1984.
42. Pavlov H, Torg JS, Jacobs B: Non-union of olecranon epiphysis: two cases in adolescent baseball pitchers, *Am J Roentgenol* 136:819, 1981.
43. Richardson ML: Optimizing pulse sequences for magnetic resonance imaging of the musculoskeletal system, *Radiol Clin North Am* 24(2):137, 1986.
44. Rosenberg ZS et al: The elbow: MR features of nerve disorders, *Radiology* 188:235, 1993.
45. Roub LW et al: Bone stress: a radionuclide imaging perspective, *Radiology* 132:431, 1979.
46. Rupani HD et al: Three-phase radionuclide bone imaging in sports medicine, *Radiology* 156:187, 1985.
47. Sauser DD, Thordorson SH, Fahr LM: Imaging of the elbow, *Radiol Clin North Am* 28(5):923, 1990.
48. Schwab GH et al: Biomechanics of elbow instability: the role of the medial collateral ligament, *Clin Orthop* 146:42, 1980.
49. Sims RE, Genant HK: Magnetic resonance imaging of joint disease, *Radiol Clin North Am* 24(2):179, 1986.
50. Singson RD, Feldman F, Rosenberg ZS: Elbow joint: assessment with double contrast CT arthrography, *Radiology* 160:167, 1986.
51. Slocum DB: Classification of elbow injuries from baseball pitching, *Tex Med* 64:48, 1968.
52. Smith DN, Lee JR: The radiological diagnosis of post-traumatic effusion of the elbow joint and its clinical significance: the displaced fat pad sign, *Injury* 10:115, 1978.
53. St. John JN, Palmaz JC: The cubital tunnel in ulnar entrapment neuropathy, *Radiology* 158:119, 1986.
54. Swensen SJ et al: Magnetic resonance imaging of hemorrhage, *Am J Roentgenol* 145:921, 1985.
55. Torg JS, Moyer RA: Non-union of a stress fracture through the olecranon epiphyseal plate observed in an adolescent baseball pitcher: a case report, *J Bone Joint Surg* 59A:264, 1977.
56. Tullos HS et al: Unusual lesions of the pitching arm, *Clin Orthop* 88:169, 1972.
57. Ward WL, Belhobek GH, Anderson TE: Arthroscopic elbow findings: correlation with preoperative radiographic studies, *Arthroscopy* 8(4):498, 1992.
58. Wilcox JR, Moniot AL, Green JP: Bone scanning in the evaluation of exercise-related stress injuries, *Radiology* 123:699, 1977.

CHAPTER 15 Arthroscopy of the Elbow

Howard J. Sweeney

Arthroscopy is a useful procedure in the armamentarium for therapy of various problems of the elbow joint. The elbow is potentially the most dangerous joint in terms of possible complications experienced in arthroscopic surgery. It is essential that during arthroscopy the elbow be held in a 90-degree flexed position and maximally inflated with liquid before insertion of the arthroscope. These two points are emphasized a number of times in this chapter because they are key issues in protection against neurovascular damage.[15]

INDICATIONS

The most common indication for arthroscopy of the elbow is the removal of anterior and posterior loose bodies.[3-5,16,24] Synovectomy for rheumatoid arthritis and partial debridement for degenerative joint disease are also valuable procedures. Various bony spurs can be removed from the joint (anteriorly and posteriorly) in an attempt to increase motion. Osteophytes have been removed from the distal humerus, the coronoid process, and the olecranon to reduce pain and to attempt to increase range of motion. Procedures have also been performed to debride osteochondritis dissecans of the capitellum and on occasion to internally fixate the piece. It is also to be noted that arthroscopic surgery can be per-

---

Indications for elbow arthroscopy

- Removal of loose bodies
- Synovectomy
- Debridement of osteophytes
- Debridement or fixation of osteochondritis dissecans
- Olecranon bursectomy
- Diagnostic problems

---

formed on the olecranon bursa, debriding through two or three portals to avoid a large incision.

TECHNIQUE
Initial Setup: Supine Position

Initial setup for arthroscopy of the elbow includes the following steps:

1. The arm is shaved from the middle upper area to midforearm and is scrubbed for 10 minutes with soap and water.
2. The patient is given general anesthesia while lying supine and remains in the supine position.
3. The patient's body is moved to the edge of the table on the side of the affected elbow (Fig. 15-1).
4. A tourniquet is applied to the upper arm and is elevated to 250 mm Hg pressure, subsequent to wrapping the entire arm with an Esmark bandage for exsanguination.
5. The forearm is suspended, with elbow flexed 90 degrees, using Zim-Foam material, an elastic wrap, a traction spreader, rope, an overhead pulley, and 3 to 4 pounds of weight. The elastic bandage should be tight enough around the forearm to stop slippage of the suspension setup (Fig. 15-2).
6. The entire arm is also supported with the standard thigh holder used for knee surgery. This is applied over the arm tourniquet and snugged down loosely. The holder restricts side-to-side motion of the elbow. The superior aspect of the holder is left open, so the surgeon may lift the entire arm superiorly to approach the posterior aspect of the elbow as needed (Fig. 15-3). This same system could be accomplished with two posts, one on either side of the upper arm.
7. The arm is then painted with Betadine, and sterile draping is carried out.

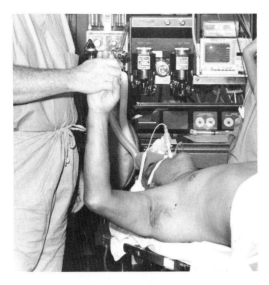

FIG. 15-1. Patient shifted to edge of table, in supine position, with general endotracheal anesthesia.

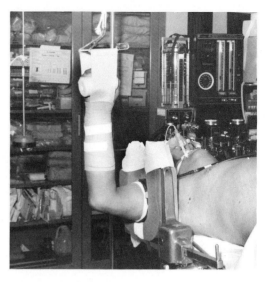

FIG. 15-2. Arm is suspended with elbow at the 90-degree position. Leg holder stabilizes arm. Elbow is easily accessible.

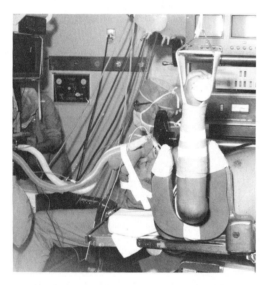

FIG. 15-3. Upper portion of leg holder is kept open to lift arm up and allow elbow extension.

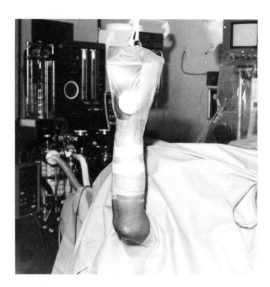

FIG. 15-4. Sterile wrap is applied to suspensory apparatus near operative field.

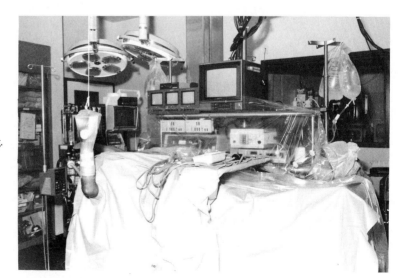

FIG. 15-5. Final preparation and draping.

8. The forearm suspension system is covered with sterile plastic draping material (Fig. 15-4).
9. The television monitor, camera, motorized system, and light source are all placed on the opposite side of the operating table directly across from the surgeon for good, straight-ahead viewing.
10. All the equipment listed in step 9 is covered with a sterile, see-through plastic drape, for ease of adjustment by the sterile scrub nurse (Fig. 15-5).

Arthroscopic Portals

A variety of portals can be used to visualize the different compartments of the elbow.[7,8,11] Portals most commonly used include inferior posterolateral inflow portal, anteromedial, anterolateral, inferior posterolateral, superior posterolateral, and posterior. Establishment of these portals is discussed in the following sections.

Portals

- Inferior posterolateral inflow portal
- Anteromedial
- Anterolateral
- Inferior posterolateral
- Superior posterolateral
- Posterior

Inferior Posterolateral Inflow Portal

The initial approach to the elbow for arthroscopy involves inflation of the joint through a posterolateral approach with either saline or Ringer's lactate solution.[10] An 18-gauge spinal needle is placed posterolaterally in the soft spot between the radial head and the olecranon. Using a syringe and extension tubing 40 ml of fluid is passed into the elbow joint (Fig. 15-6). One can feel the joint expand anteriorly, and, if the tubing is removed from the needle, there is adequate flow return from the needle. The initial distention fluid is a combination of Ringer's lactate and epinephrine. Place 1 ampule of epinephrine into 1 L of Ringer's lactate and use 40 ml of

---

Initial distention solution

- Ringer's lactate
- Epinephrine

---

this to expand the joint. We never use more than 1 L of this solution.

This same location is used later as a viewing portal. This location is also the surgeon's standard approach for aspiration of any elbow fluid.

Anteromedial Portal

With the joint well expanded and with the elbow flexed 90 degrees the initial scope portal is made anteromedially. This portal is placed 2 cm distal and 2 cm anterior to the medial epicondyle of the humerus (Fig. 15-7). An 18-gauge spinal needle is placed into the joint at that point, and good flow should be obtained before making the definitive arthroscope portal (Fig. 15-8). Poehling et al[20] use a more proximal location for this approach.

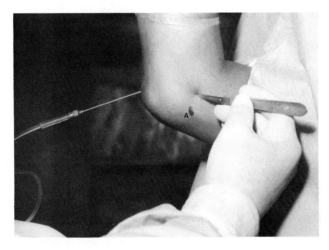

FIG. 15-7. Medial aspect of right elbow. *A,* Medial epicondyle.

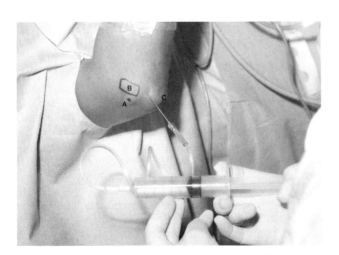

FIG. 15-6. Lateral aspect of right elbow. *A,* Lateral epicondyle; *B,* radial head; *C,* tip of olecranon.

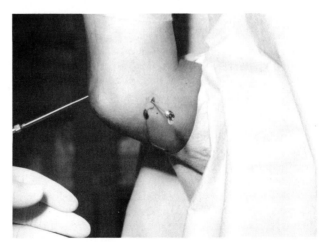

FIG. 15-8. Spinal needle inserted to identify anteromedial portal site.

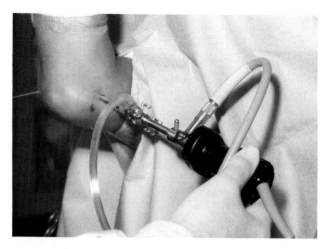

FIG. 15-9. Arthroscope in anteromedial portal.

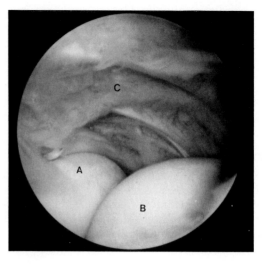

FIG. 15-10. Arthroscopic view from anteromedial portal. *A,* Radial head; *B,* capitellum; *C,* anterolateral synovium.

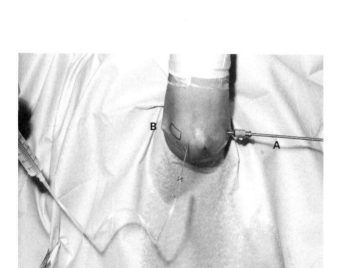

FIG. 15-11. *A,* Wissinger rod; *B,* rod tenting skin anterolaterally deep to radial nerve.

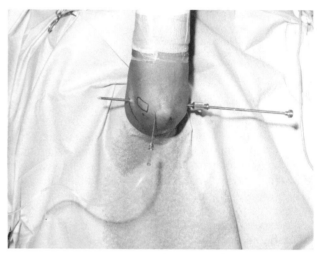

FIG. 15-12. Wissinger rod passed through joint from medial to lateral side.

The skin is incised with a No. 11 scalpel blade, taking care not to pass the blade too deeply under the skin.

The arthroscopic sheath is then passed into the joint by angling posteriorly toward the joint and aiming at the center of the joint, piercing the joint capsule. One must not pass the scope sheath directly across the elbow because the joint will be missed. Angle directly at the bone and feel the way along the bone. When the trocar is removed, fluid exudes from the joint. As the arthroscopist tries to puncture the joint capsule, the assistant should maximally inflate the joint through the 18-gauge posterolateral spinal inflow needle (Fig. 15-9).

The arthroscope is placed into the sheath, and the joint is inspected. Once again, inflate the joint with the needle placed posterolaterally. One can view across the joint in this position and very adequately see the radial head, capitellum, portions of the trochlea, the coronoid process, and the anterior recesses of the joint superiorly (Fig. 15-10).

Before making this portal ensure that the patient has not had a previous ulnar nerve transposition.

Anterolateral Portal

To establish an anterolateral portal, the arthroscope is then passed transversely to the opposite side of the joint, just anterior to the radial head and capitellum. Firmly holding the arthroscope sheath in this position, pass a Wissinger rod through the sheath, puncturing the capsule so it will appear under the skin anterolaterally (Fig. 15-11). Incise skin over the rod and complete passage of rod. In this position the surgeon is deep to the radial nerve. This technique adds a great measure of safety to the establishment of this portal (Fig. 15-12).

One now has made anteromedial and anterolateral portals into the joint at this point. With the use of switching sticks, one can move the scope from anteromedial to anterolateral. Either portal can then be used for viewing, probing, and cutting, with inflow through the scope or

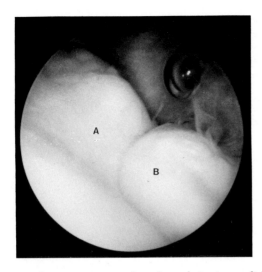

FIG. 15-13. Scope now in anterolateral portal viewing medially. *A,* Trochlea; *B,* coronoid process.

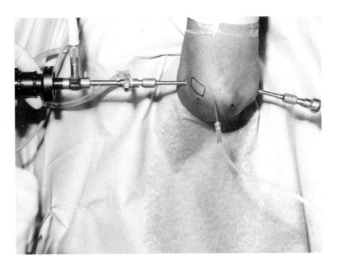

FIG. 15-14. Scope and inflow in anterolateral portal. Synovial resector will be placed in anteromedial portal. Eighteen-gauge spinal needle is shown posterolaterally and is not being used at the moment.

posterolaterally (Figs. 15-13 and 15-14). These two portals solve most of the problems anteriorly. Smith[23] has pointed out the usefulness of 70-degree, 90-degree, and 120-degree scopes in the elbow joint to view either side of the joint.

The anterolateral portal can also be established in fashion similar to the anteromedial portal, if one wishes to make a direct approach from outside at this point. Locate the lateral epicondyle and establish a point 3 cm distal and 1 cm anterior to the epicondyle. Make a small 5-mm skin incision at this point, taking care not to penetrate deeply.

Once again, penetrate with the arthroscope sheath and trocar through the skin portal and angle toward the bone so the joint is entered directly, thus avoiding the radial nerve, which will be anterior to the scope sheath. If this anterolateral portal is used initially, the scope can be passed across to the opposite side of the joint anteromedially and then the Wissinger rod can be used to establish an anteromedial portal.

There is no agreement about whether it is safer to start anterolateral or anteromedial with the initial portal.[26] I believe they are of equal danger in terms of the relationship of the brachial artery, median nerve, and radial nerve to the distended joint capsule in the 90-degree flexed position. Lindenfeld[13] demonstrated greater safety medially in cadaver dissections.

Lynch et al[14] demonstrated that flexion of the elbow to 90 degrees and distention of the joint greatly increase the distance between the scope sheath and various nerves. They found the mean distance between the scope sheath in the anterolateral portal and the radial nerve was 4 mm before and 11 mm after maximal distention.

Techniques to avoid nerve injury

- Flex elbow to 90 degrees
- Distend joint maximally

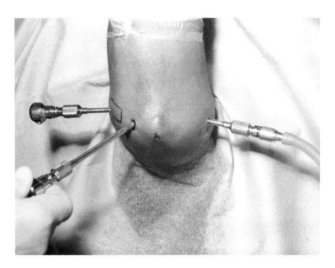

FIG. 15-15. Direct inferior posterolateral portal into soft spot. Inflow anteromedially. Cannula with blunt trocar left in place anterolaterally to stop outflow through this portal and help maintain joint distention.

Using the same technique, they found "the median nerve was a mean distance of 4 mm anterior to the sheath without distention and 14 mm anterior with 35 to 40 ml of distention."

Inferior Posterolateral Portal

The inferior posterolateral portal is placed in the soft spot on the lateral side of the elbow between the radial head and the olecranon. The surgeon already has had the inflow needle in this spot; the same portal should be used for putting the scope in posterolaterally. The joint is inflated through one of the anterior portals using a syringe to produce as much distention as possible for posterolateral scope penetration. A 4-mm or 2.7-mm scope can be used (Fig. 15-15). (I prefer a 2.7-mm scope.) This portal

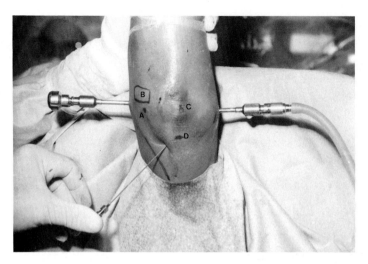

FIG. 15-16. Superior posterolateral portal. *A,* Lateral epicondyle; *B,* radial head; *C,* olecranon; *D,* proximal tip olecranon—needle being inserted posterolaterally.

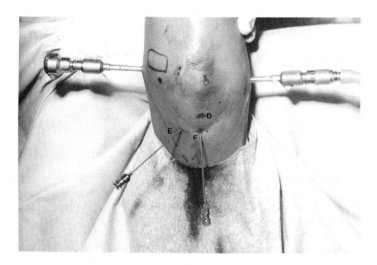

FIG. 15-17. Straight posterior portal through triceps. *D,* Proximal tip of olecranon; *E,* posterolateral portal; *F,* straight posterior portal.

shows the radial head, the lateral side of the olecranon, and a portion of the capitellum. By moving the elbow back and forth the arthroscopist can see these areas quite well. Then the arthroscope is directed along the lateral side of the olecranon toward the posterior aspect of the elbow to visualize osteophytes along the lateral surface of the olecranon.

Superior Posterolateral Portal

A portal can be placed posterolaterally 3 cm proximal to the olecranon tip and 2 to 3 cm lateral from that point, aiming directly into the olecranon fossa. This portal is located near the lateral edge of the triceps and posterior to the lateral epicondyle of the humerus (Fig. 15-16).

Direct Posterior Portal

A portal can be made directly into the olecranon fossa by measuring 3 cm proximal to the tip of the olecranon, passing through the triceps tendon directly into the olec-

ranon fossa for triangulation purposes (Fig. 15-17). When establishing posterior portals, distend the elbow fully through an anterior portal to distend the posterior area as much as possible. Reducing the elbow flexion to 20 or 30 degrees also contributes to successful posterior capsular entry.

Initial Setup: Lateral Decubitus Position

The lateral decubitus position is preferable and is now used routinely (Figs. 15-18 to 15-20). The patient is positioned with the injured arm flexed 90 degrees at the shoulder and elbow. After elevating the tourniquet on the upper arm to 250 mg Hg, place the arm on a bolster supported on a rod. The hand is in a dependent position. All portals are the same as those used in the supine position. The advantage is an easier approach to the posterior compartment and much easier use of instruments posteriorly. Prone position can be used, but it is more cumbersome.[6]

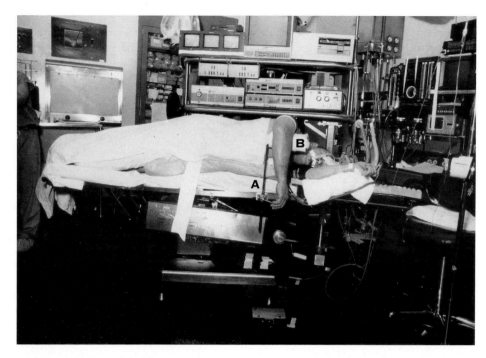

FIG. 15-18. Lateral decubitus position. *A*, Vertical arm support; *B*, bolster under upper arm.

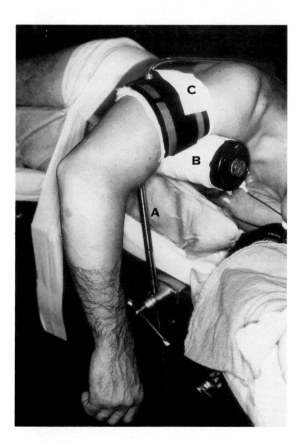

FIG. 15-19. *A*, Vertical arm support; *B*, bolster under arm; *C*, tourniquet.

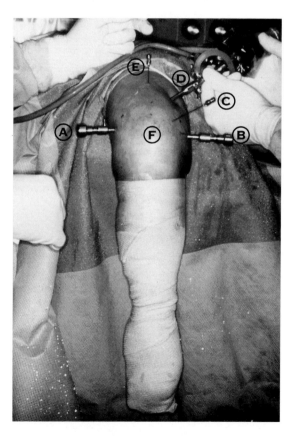

FIG. 15-20. *A*, Anteromedial portal; *B*, anterolateral portal; *C*, inferior posterolateral portal; *D*, superior posterolateral portal; *E*, straight posterior portal; *F*, tip of olecranon.

Completion of Procedure

To complete arthroscopy of the elbow, take these steps:

1. Flush the joint well with Ringer's lactate solution.
2. Bupivacaine HCl (Marcaine) 0.25% may be instilled into the joint to reduce postoperative pain. I prefer not to use this because of possible dissection of Marcaine into anterior elbow structures, producing confusing neurologic pictures postoperatively.
3. Suture all portals with subcuticular 5-0 Vicryl sutures. I believe this reduces changes of retrograde infection (for knee arthroscopy no sutures are used).
4. Remove drapes, arm-holding devices, and tourniquet. Check distal circulation for adequacy.
5. Apply sterile 4-inch by 4-inch dressings, wrap well from metacarpophalangeal joints to middle upper arm with elastic bandage, and place in a sling with 90-degree elbow flexion.
6. Elevate the elbow on two pillows in the recovery room.
7. Discharge the patient the same day after again checking neurovascular status.
8. Check the patient in the office within 2 to 3 days of surgery.

POSTOPERATIVE CARE

Dressings can be replaced with plastic Band-Aid bandages in 48 hours. Motion is started as soon as possible, and a sling is used only for a day or 2 postoperatively. Patients are advised to avoid getting the elbow wet for at least 48 hours, and total immersion in water is prohibited for 10 days.[9]

COMPLICATIONS

The 1986 Report from the Arthroscopic Association of North America Complications Committee was based on 1569 elbow arthroscopies out of a total of 395,566 arthroscopies reported. Small[22] reported the "average responding surgeon doing elbow arthroscopy was doing 0.74 cases per month." One radial nerve injury was reported.

Thomas[25] and Papilion[19] each reported single cases of radial nerve injury. Andrews[1,2] reported a transient median nerve palsy secondary to extravasation of local anaesthetic used during the procedure. O'Driscoll and Morrey[17,18] reported 10% of 70 patients had complications, including three transient radial nerve palsies, four pa-

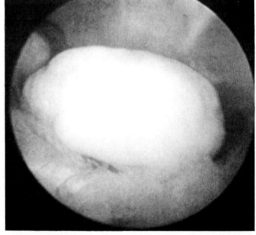

FIG. 15-21. Large, loose body lying anterolaterally in elbow joint.

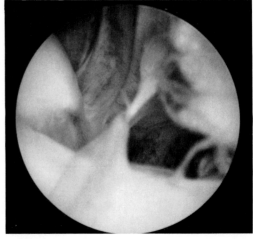

FIG. 15-22. Synovitis. Nonspecific anterior elbow compartment.

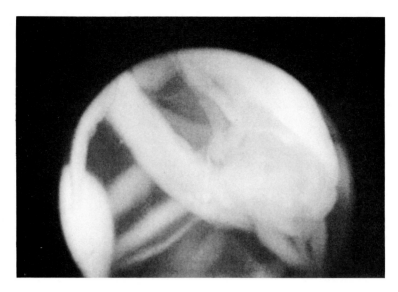

FIG. 15-23. Interior view, olecranon bursa.

tients with persistent drainage and negative cultures, and one patient with mild loss of range of motion.

The potential for serious nerve damage is evident, based on anatomy, and must be guarded against.

SUMMARY

Thus far the indications for elbow arthroscopy are not completely developed. However, the following list represents our present views on the subject:

1. Loose bodies, or suspicion of loose bodies, is the primary indication. Anterior loose bodies are the easiest to remove (Fig. 15-21).
2. Various types of chronic synovitis (e.g., rheumatoid arthritis, pigmented villonodular) may be helped by arthroscopic synovectomy (Fig. 15-22).
3. Bands of scar, located intraarticularly, that restrict motion may be excised.
4. Osteochondritis dissecans of the capitellum can be debrided.[21] Johnson[12] has reported intraarticular fixation of fragments with cannulated screws followed by successful healing.
5. Resection of intraarticular spurs of olecranon, coronoid, and humerus can be done. Twenty-four month follow-up reported by Ward[27] in 1993 demonstrated an improvement of 9 degrees of flexion and 6 degrees of extension. Longer term results will be more illuminating.
6. The "diagnostic problem" can be handled. When a patient complains of pain or swelling but no answer has appeared from the work-up, elbow arthroscopy becomes a valuable diagnostic tool.
7. Olecranon bursitis can be debrided arthroscopically, avoiding wound sloughs and possible ulnar nerve damage from open bursal resections (Fig. 15-23).

Keeping these indications in mind, the sports medicine physician can now use arthroscopy of the elbow as a potent tool in the diagnosis and treatment of a variety of elbow conditions. Attention to detail is important to avoid potential complications during the procedure.[28]

REFERENCES

1. Andrews JR: Arthroscopy of the elbow, *Arthroscopy* 1920:97, 1985.
2. Andrews JR: Bony injuries about the elbow in the throwing athlete, *Instruct Course Lect* 34:323, 1985.
3. Andrews JR: Arthroscopy of the elbow, *Clin Sports Med* 5(4):653, 1986.
4. Andrews JR, Soffer SR: *Elbow arthroscopy,* St Louis, 1994, Mosby.
5. Angelo RL: Advances in elbow arthroscopy, *Orthopedics* 16(9):1037, 1993 (review).
6. Baker CL Jr, Shalvoy RM: The prone position for elbow arthroscopy, *Clin Sports Med* 10(3):623, 1991 (review).
7. Boe S: Arthroscopy of the elbow, *Acta Orthop Scand* 57:52, 1986.
8. Carson WG Jr: Arthroscopy of the elbow, *Instruct Course Lect* 37:195, 1988 (review).
9. Dutka M: Elbow and wrist arthroscopy: perioperative nursing care, *Orthop Nurs* 5(5):5, 1986.
10. Ericksson E: Arthroscopy and arthroscopic surgery in a gas versus a fluid medium, *Orthop Clin North Am* 13(2):293, 1982.
11. Guhl JF: Arthroscopy and arthroscopic surgery of the elbow, *Orthopedics* 8(10):1290, 1985.
12. Johnson L: Elbow arthroscopy. In Johnson L (ed): *Arthroscopic surgery,* ed 2, St Louis, 1986, Mosby.
13. Lindenfeld TN: Medial approach in elbow arthroscopy, *Am J Sports Med* 18(4):413, 1990.
14. Lynch GJ et al: Neurovascular anatomy and elbow arthroscopy: inherent risks, *Arthroscopy* 2(3):191, 1986.
15. Marshall PD et al: Avoiding nerve damage during elbow arthroscopy, *J Bone Joint Surg* 75B(1):129, 1993.
16. McGinty JB: Arthroscopic removal of loose bodies, *Orthop Clin North Am* 13(2):313, 1982.
17. Morrey BF: Arthroscopy of the elbow, *Instruct Course Lect* 35:102, 1986.
18. O'Driscoll SW, Morrey BF: Arthroscopy of the elbow: diagnostic and therapeutic benefits and hazards, *J Bone Joint Surg* 74(1):84, 1992.
19. Papilion JD, Neff RS, Shall LM: Compression neuropathy of the radial nerve as a complication of elbow arthroscopy, *Arthroscopy* 4(4):284, 1988.
20. Poehling GG et al: Elbow arthroscopy: a new technique, *Arthroscopy* 5(3):222, 1989.

21. Ruch DS, Poehling GG: Arthroscopic treatment of Panner's disease, *Clin Sports Med* 10(3):629, 1991 (review).
22. Small NC: Complications in arthroscopy: the knee and other joints, *Arthroscopy* 2(4):253, 1986.
23. Smith JB: Personal communication.
24. Tedder JL, Andrews JR: Elbow arthroscopy, *Orthop Rev* 21(9):1047, 1992 (Review).
25. Thomas M: Radial nerve damage as a complication of elbow arthroscopy, *Clin Orthop* 215:130, 1987.
26. Verhaar J, van Mameren H, Brandsma A: Risks of neurovascular injury in elbow arthroscopy: starting anteromedially or anterolaterally? *Arthroscopy* 7(3):287, 1991.
27. Ward WG, Anderson TE: Elbow arthroscopy in a mostly athletic population, *J Hand Surg* 18A(2):220, 1993.
28. Woods GW: Elbow arthroscopy, *Clin Sports Med* 6(3):557, 1987 (Review).

CHAPTER 16   Acute Injuries to the Elbow

James B. Bennett

Acute injuries to the elbow in athletes are common. Diagnosis is not always easy. Factors that can aid accurate diagnosis include the location of pain about the elbow joint, the patient's age, and the sports activity involved. The examining physician must understand both the structural anatomy of the elbow and the biomechanics of the elbow joint as it relates to the specific activity. With this understanding, complaints of pain with activity may be better localized and the specific injury treated.[4,28]

ANATOMIC CONSIDERATIONS
Osseous Structures

Anatomically the elbow is a hinge joint composed of the distal humerus, which is divided into the capitellum and trochlear articulation; the proximal ulna, which articulates with the trochlea and is composed of a coronoid process and an olecranon process, forming the greater sigmoid notch; and the proximal radius, which articulates with the capitellum as well as with the proximal ulna, which is constrained by the annular ligament. Bony stability of the elbow joint is confined to the coronoid trochlear articulation and the radiocapitellar joint. The olecranon process offers little varus-valgus stability, assuming ligamentous competency is maintained, and then only in complete extension (Fig. 16-1).[19]

Cadaver studies as well as clinical studies have demonstrated that the olecranon can be surgically removed without violating elbow stability up to the insertion of the anterior oblique ligament of the medial collateral ligament complex.[27] The joint capsule with the brachialis anterior and the triceps posterior is normally thin and offers little stability.

Capsular thickness, however, can change markedly in pathologic injury states, producing an elbow flexion contracture.

Ligamentous Structures

The primary ligament support of the elbow is the **medial collateral ligament** complex. The origin of the medial collateral ligament is medial and inferior to the medial epicondyle with a fanned insertion from the coronoid through the olecranon process. The medial collateral ligament is composed of the thickened parallel fibers of the anterior oblique portion of the ligament. They are organized so that some fibers remain taut throughout the entire arch of flexion and extension of the elbow. The fan-shaped posterior oblique is less well developed, taut in flexion, and lax in extension. A small nonfunctional transverse ligament is present on the ulnar attachment

---

Medial collateral ligament components

- Anterior oblique—thick parallel fibers
- Posterior oblique—fan shaped
- Transverse—nonfunctional

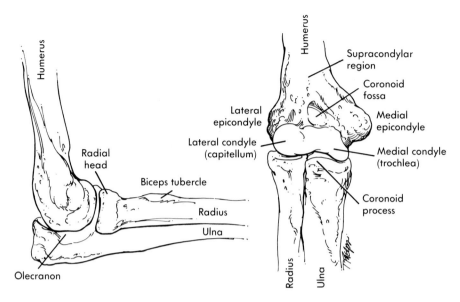

FIG. 16-1. Osseous anatomy of the elbow joint.

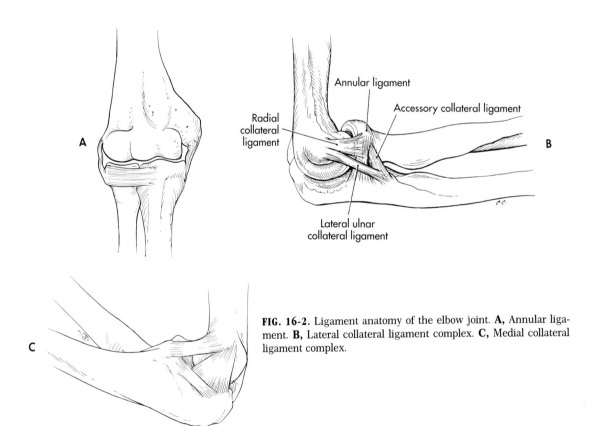

FIG. 16-2. Ligament anatomy of the elbow joint. **A,** Annular ligament. **B,** Lateral collateral ligament complex. **C,** Medial collateral ligament complex.

of the medial collateral ligament. The medial collateral ligament complex is reinforced by the flexor muscle mass origin.

The **lateral collateral ligament** complex of the elbow has four ligamentous components as described by O'Driscoll et al[24]: the radial collateral ligament originates from the lateral epicondyle and inserts into the annular ligament; the annular ligament, arises and inserts on the ulna at the radial notch; the lateral ulnar collateral ligament stabilizes the posterior lateral aspect of the radiocapitellar joint, originates from the epicondyle, and inserts on the tubercle of the crest of the supinator on the ulna; the accessory lateral collateral ligament arises from the annular ligament and inserts on the tubercle of the

supranator; and the entire lateral collateral ligament complex is further reinforced by the anconeus muscle laterally (Fig. 16-2).[20,24]

Lateral collateral ligament complex

- Radial collateral ligament
- Annular ligament
- Lateral ulnar collateral ligament
- Accessory lateral collateral ligament

BIOMECHANICS OF ELBOW STABILITY

Biomechanically, valgus elbow stability primarily depends on the integrity of the medial collateral ligament, of which the primary stabilizing factor is the anterior oblique component.[27] This is present in response to the valgus load placed on the elbow in everyday activities and accentuated in throwing sports. Lateral joint stability has two components: the stability provided by the annular ligament, which maintains the relationship of the radial head to the proximal radioulnar joint (this ligament is critical in forceful flexion-supination activities), and the lateral collateral ligament complex. Varus elbow joint forces are rare, and therefore the lateral collateral ligament is not commonly stressed. The lateral ligament anatomy reflects this. The radiocapitellar joint acts as a secondary constraint to valgus stress.

Restraints to valgus stress

- Medial collateral ligament—anterior oblique component
- Radiocapitellar joint—secondary restraint

Therefore the stability of the elbow joint is contingent on the bony relationship of the radiocapitellar articulation, the trochlear-ulnar joint with its coronoid process, and an intact medial and lateral collateral ligament complex. Alterations in any of these elements may produce pain, weakness, limitation of motion, or instability.

Additional support about the elbow is formed by the muscle envelope, particularly the flexor-pronator mass and extensor tendon origins of the wrist. Various forms of acute overuse muscle strain exist (see Chapter 17). Medial epicondylitis, lateral epicondylitis, triceps tendinitis, and biceps tendinitis may result from an overload or overuse syndrome. Treatment consists of rest, brace or strap support, and antiinflammatory medications followed by strengthening and range of motion programs. Initial ice treatment followed by heat modalities is beneficial. Cortisone injection to a specific site is used sparingly. In the athlete with chronic elbow pain, overuse injuries must be considered both as a primary diagnosis as well as in the differential diagnosis of elbow instability.

SKELETALLY IMMATURE ATHLETES

Children's elbow injuries are usually seen as a result of trauma to the elbow. The result is either fracture or dislocation. The diagnosis and treatment of these injuries are not within the scope of this chapter. It is sufficient to say that closed treatment is usually effective for reduction of the fractures or dislocations, followed by healing and range of motion recovery. Occasionally open reduction internal fixation or percutaneous pins are required in displaced fractures about the elbow.

Little League Elbow

Little league elbow is an all-inclusive term that may encompass a variety of pathologic problems within the elbow.[3,8] Localized elbow pain at the medial epicondyle associated with a diminished ability to throw suggests a medial epicondyle stress lesion. Usually benign and responding to simple rest, it can, with continued valgus stress such as throwing or a fall, produce an epicondylar avulsion fracture.[34]

Medial Epicondyle Fractures

Medial epicondyle fractures in children may signify a greater problem of acute elbow instability. This fracture is usually associated with a fall and is often nondisplaced. If displacement is present, instability can exist. In the younger child the entire medial epicondylar fragment is avulsed and contains the medial collateral ligament. If the valgus gravity stress test is positive, surgical repair is indicated.[34] Failure to obtain accurate replacement may result in marked instability of the elbow. Also the fracture fragment may become entrapped within the joint, preventing reduction. This is seen radiographically as a widened ulnar trochlear joint (Fig. 16-3).

In the older child the epiphysis is in the process of closing. Avulsion fracture fragments may be small and may not necessarily involve the medial collateral ligament. Instability is less likely. Unless instability can be demonstrated with the gravity valgus stress test, these fractures may well be treated conservatively (Fig. 16-4). Acute valgus instability with demonstrated tear of the medial collateral ligament has been successfully treated conservatively. However, if return to competitive level athletics is expected and the involved elbow is the dominant arm, performance may be better ensured with surgical repair. Displaced epicondylar fractures are reattached with either Kirschner wires in the young child or a cancellous screw in the adolescent. The medial collateral ligament is evaluated and repaired as indicated.

Lateral Elbow Pain

Lateral elbow pain in a child or young adolescent suggests lateral epicondylitis; however, this is relatively rare. More common is **osteochondritis dissecans** or osteochondrosis of the radiocapitellar joint.[25] The basic pathologic state is avascular necrosis of either the capitellum or radial head or both. The diagnosis is made by suspicion, the presence of an elbow flexion contracture, and radiographic findings. Treatment consists of rest and withdrawal from throwing activities. Continued throwing activities deform the articular surfaces and can produce

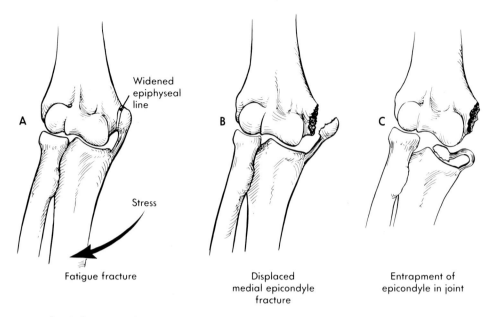

FIG. 16-3. Valgus stress lesions in children. **A,** Stress fracture. **B,** Fracture of epicondyle. **C,** Fracture displaced into joint.

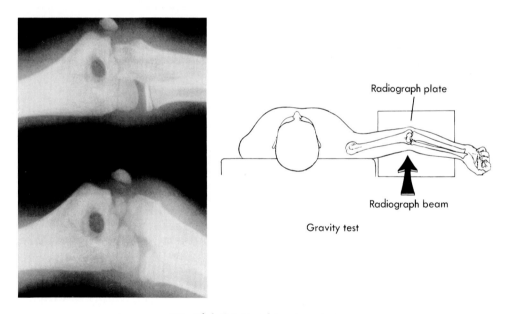

FIG. 16-4. Gravity valgus stress test.

permanent joint irregularities or exfoliate loose bodies (Fig. 16-5).

Anterior or Posterior Pain

Pure anterior or pure posterior pain is rarely seen in the child or adolescent unless fracture dislocation is present.

ADULT INJURIES
Anterior Elbow Pain

As the adolescent matures and sports participation becomes more sophisticated, the injuries tend to be more localized and more severe. Of these, anterior elbow pain associated with hyperextension injuries suggests brachialis muscle or anterior capsular tears with or without joint subluxation. In addition, a capsular flexion contracture may result from bleeding and fibrosis within the

---

Anterior flexion contracture in pitchers

- Repeated anterior capsule injury
- Flexor mass hypertrophy
- Repeated medial collateral ligament injury

capsule. This anterior flexion contracture is often seen in professional baseball pitchers, resulting in part from compensatory hypertrophy of the flexor forearm mass and repeated injury to the anterior capsule and medial ligament structures of the elbow. As medial ligament support is lost, the forearm drifts into valgus and posterior impingement of the olecranon into the olecranon fossa may occur (Fig. 16-6).[15] The result is loose body formation.

Biceps Tendinitis and Rupture

Biceps tendinitis at the elbow level is uncommon. However, with hyperextension or repetitive forceful pronation-supination activities, the musculotendinous junction or tendon insertion on the radial tuberosity may be damaged. Occasionally violent extension or forceful flexion against immovable objects produces a distal biceps tendon avulsion. This is easily identified by the loss of biceps tendon function and a palpable defect at the elbow. The characteristic loss of supination strength is present (Fig. 16-7).

Diagnosis of distal biceps tendon rupture must be differentiated from a **disruption of the annular ligament** with anterior dislocation of the radial head. This also may occur after forceful flexion of the elbow against resis-

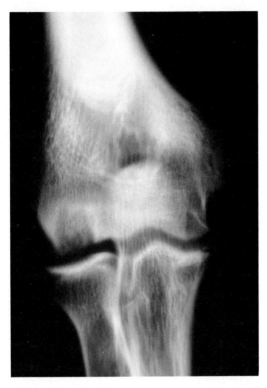

FIG. 16-5. Osteochondritis dissecans of the capitellum.

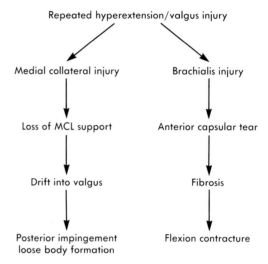

FIG. 16-6. Anterior elbow pain.

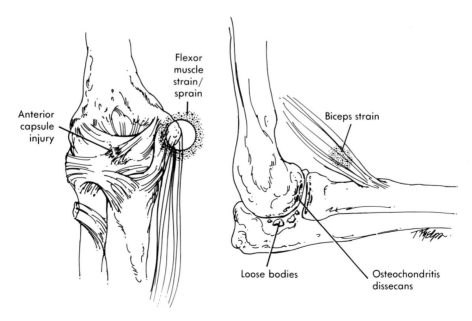

FIG. 16-7. Causes of anterior elbow pain.

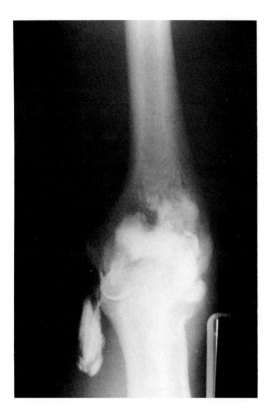

FIG. 16-8. Positive elbow arthrogram with acute medial collateral ligament tear.

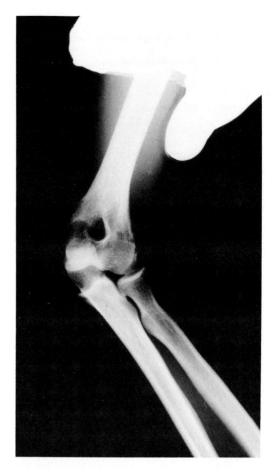

FIG. 16-9. Manual valgus stress radiograph.

tance. The diagnosis of dislocation is easily made radiographically.

Both conditions warrant surgical reconstruction. Anchor suture or pull-out wire reattachment of the avulsed biceps tendon to the radial tuberosity requires the forearm to be in supination and the elbow in 90-degree flexion. Protection for 6 weeks is required. Following this, active flexion, active extension, and protected passive extension for an additional 2 weeks are recommended. A 3- to 6-month period from competitive sports activity is necessary before full activities are instituted.

Annular ligament tears are similarly protected to allow appropriate healing of the repaired or reconstructed annular ligament.

Complications of heterotopic bone formation in radioulnar synostosis with loss of pronation-supination may occur with surgical intervention of these injuries.

Medial Elbow Pain

Acute medial elbow pain may occur from either epicondylitis with bone or muscle lesions. Actual **rupture of the flexor forearm mass** is rare and limited almost entirely to the activity of throwing or elbow dislocation. Its diagnostic signs are ecchymosis and hemorrhage of the medial elbow with a palpable muscle defect. Magnetic resonance imaging (MRI) may be useful in diagnosis.

Acute **rupture of the medial collateral ligament** has been reported in javelin throwers[31]; however, baseball pitchers and other throwing athletes can occasion-

ally sustain this lesion. The clinical diagnosis is made by demonstrating instability of the elbow to valgus stress associated with pain localized to the medial aspect of the elbow. This diagnosis may be confirmed by the use of elbow arthrography showing extravasation of dye along the torn ligament (Fig. 16-8).[11,18] However, stress radiographic examination of the elbow is usually adequate unless the instability to stress is masked by spasm of the intact forearm flexor muscle mass (Fig. 16-9).

Ulnar Neuritis

Repetitive medial elbow joint injury may occur from activities such as unrestrained throwing. This can result in an ulnar traction spur medially and secondary ulnar neuritis. Pain, numbness, tingling along the course of the ulnar nerve distribution, and (in severe cases) intrinsic muscle function loss may be present. Acute ulnar neuritis in the absence of other elbow injury may be managed with rest, antiinflammatory medications, and protection. If the sensory deficits persist and interfere with competitive athletics, the diagnosis should be confirmed by nerve conduction tests and electromyography (EMG). Decompression is indicated by clinical assessment and confirmed by electrodiagnostic studies. Ulnar nerve compression is treated by either simple fascial decompression of the ulnar nerve within the cubital tun-

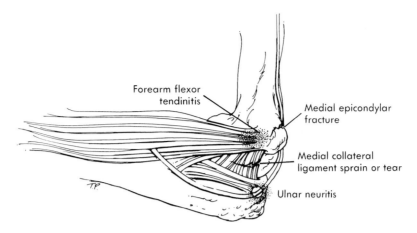

FIG. 16-10. Causes of medial elbow pain.

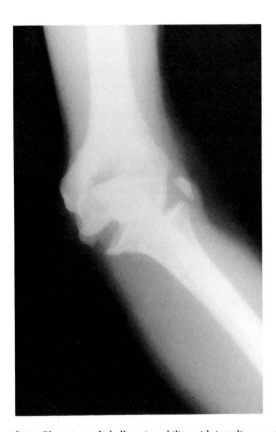

FIG. 16-11. Chronic medial elbow instability with intraligamentous heterotopic calcification.

nel or anterior transposition of the nerve either submuscularly or subcutaneously (Fig. 16-10).[9]

Acute Medial Stress Injuries

Acute medial stress injuries to the elbow may require medial reconstruction of either fractures or the medial collateral ligament.[10] In these instances decompression of the ulnar nerve or anterior transposition is indicated to prevent damage to the nerve from acute bleeding, swelling, chronic scar fibrosis, and cubital tunnel compression.

Heterotopic Bone Islands

Medial or lateral joint line ossicles within the substance of the collateral ligaments are seen in competitive throwing athletes. These ossicles do not represent loose body formation and in general should not be removed. Instead, they are heterotopic bone islands within the substance of the collateral ligaments and represent healed incomplete collateral ligament tears (Fig. 16-11). If removal of these heterotopic bone islands within the medial collateral ligament is contemplated, extreme care should be taken to evaluate the status of the medial collateral ligament and to ensure that incompetency of the collateral ligament does not result following resection. This heterotopic lesion, left unmolested, does not usually restrict motion. We have unfortunately seen those patients who have had this procedure performed with resultant unstable elbows after "a loose body was removed." In fact, the entire medial collateral ligament complex was inadvertently resected (Fig. 16-12).

Heterotopic bone present in the anterior capsule may compromise range of motion. Actually it may form a bony bridge across the anterior capsule with a rigid contracture. The anterior lesion must be clearly distinguished from the medial ossicle. Excision of the anterior bone lesion may be indicated for improved range of motion.

Medial Collateral Ligament Rupture

Acute medial collateral ligament ruptures are seen normally in two instances: dislocations and throwing sports.[23] In both instances the acute tear represents primary avulsion from its origin on the medial epicondyle in about 70% of the cases. In an additional 20% the avulsion is distal at the insertion of the ligament on the ulna. The remaining 10% are midsubstance tears.[27]

Acute medial collateral ligament rupture

- Avulsion from epicondyle—70%
- Avulsion from ulna—20%
- Midsubstance tears—10%

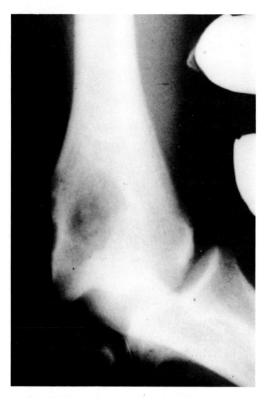

FIG. 16-12. Gross instability of the elbow after heterotopic calcification removal and medial collateral ligament disruption.

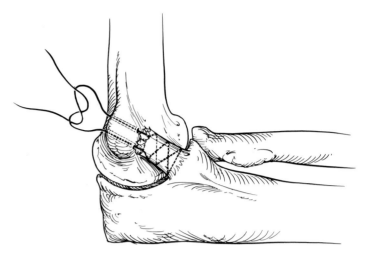

FIG. 16-13. Reattachment of the avulsed medial collateral ligament to the medial epicondyle.

Repair depends on the site and type of tear.[30] A medial epicondyle avulsion tear is repaired by the use of drill holes through the undersurface of the medial epicondyle after periosteal roughening of the medial epicondyle. The ligament is brought snugly to and tied over the epicondyle. Distal lesions are reattached using either drill holes and sutures or staples (Fig. 16-13).

Midsubstance tears are repaired with mattress or figure-eight sutures. In all instances proper tension is restored by placing the elbow at 30 degrees of flexion and suturing the ligament in place. The forearm flexor mass is then reattached over the repaired ligament.

The ulnar nerve, if not symptomatic, is simply decompressed through the flexor carpi ulnaris distally and proximally by resection of the intermuscular septum. If there is clinical evidence of ulnar neuropathy before surgery, then appropriate external neurolysis and anterior transposition are performed. With the anterior submuscular transposition I prefer to position the nerve alongside the median nerve rather than in the subcutaneous or intramuscular position. The flexor mass is not sutured about the nerve.

Medial collateral ligament repair techniques

- Epicondyle avulsion—repair through drill holes
- Midsubstance tear—mattress or figure-eight sutures
- Ulna avulsion—reattach through drill holes or staple
- Always—tension ligament at 30 degrees

The wound is drained and placed in a posterior splint for 7 days. A cast brace protecting varus-valgus stress but allowing flexion with extension block to within 30 degrees is used for 1 month. For 2 additional months the cast brace is used, but the extension block is removed. When full flexion-extension is achieved, strengthening exercises are allowed in the second 3-month period (Fig. 16-14). Resumption of throwing activities may begin at 6 months and be maximized over the course of a year. Return to competitive athletics is delayed for 1 year.[2]

Postoperative regimen

- Posterior splint—7 days
- Cast brace (30 to 120 degrees)—4 weeks
- Cast brace (0 to 120 degrees)—8 weeks
- Begin strengthening after range of motion returns (usually at 12 weeks)
- Light throwing for a short distance
- Moderate to full throwing at regular distance
- Resume throwing at 6 months

Varus Instability

Varus instability is uncommon; however, varus instability in association with anterior radial head dislocation and annular ligament disruption is seen occasionally. The athlete initially complains of a popping sensation on the lateral aspect of the elbow with associated pain. During forceful flexion or supination the radial head dislocates anteriorly. There may also be an associated varus instability that can be demonstrated on varus stress radiographs (Fig. 16-15).

Acutely these injuries may be repaired by reattaching the annular ligament to its origin with sutures to bone or using the pull-out wire technique. In addition, the lateral collateral ligament complex of the elbow must be evaluated and reconstructed, when necessary, to its ep-

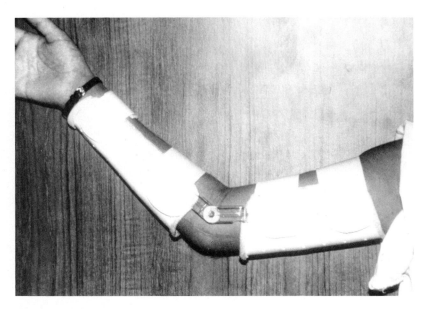

FIG. 16-14. Cast brace on the elbow.

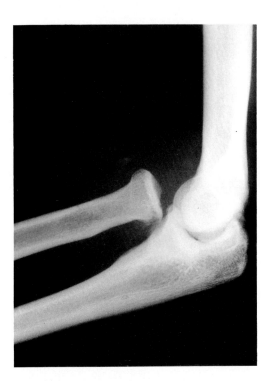

FIG. 16-15. Anterior dislocation of the radial head.

icondylar origin, the proximal ulna, or the annular ligament. Radial head subluxation has been identified in association with incomplete radial head fractures and lateral collateral ligament injury or instability of the elbow. This is discussed later in this chapter.

Lateral and Medial Muscle Injuries

Acute rupture of the lateral extensor or medial flexor muscle origin is associated with severe pain. A popping or snapping about the elbow is described. In the competitive athlete these acute ruptures of the lateral exten-

sor origin or medial flexor origin are best repaired surgically.

Acute rupture of the flexor-pronator mass occurs in the athlete. This is often disguised and treated as medial epicondylitis with or without fracture and medial collateral ligament tear. Complete muscle rupture can occur and may be documented on MRI evaluation. If major muscle tear is present, repair or reattachment of the flexor-pronator muscle mass to the medial epicondyle is performed.

Posterior Interosseous Nerve Compression

Chronic lateral epicondylitis (tennis elbow) is not discussed in this chapter (see Chapter 17). However, compression of the posterior interosseous nerve by the supinator arcade (the arcade of Frosche) must be differentiated from acute and chronic lateral epicondylitis. Acute entrapment or compression of the posterior interosseous nerve is associated with elbow fractures or massive soft-tissue injuries. Swelling may produce nerve compression, which is reflected in an inability to extend the thumb and fingers. Because the posterior interosseous nerve is a motor nerve to the common finger extensor muscles and thumb extensor, a pure motor palsy results. Posterior interosseous nerve palsy in association with elbow fractures treated closed should recover function. However, following open fracture fixation, particularly with proximal radius and radial head fractures, surgical identification of the posterior interosseous nerve is made. It is important to assess the possibility of nerve contusion vs. transsection or rupture. Nerve repair or cable nerve graft is performed if nerve rupture is detected.

Neural entrapment, particularly of the lateral antebrachial cutaneous nerve or the terminal portion of the musculocutaneous nerve, may present as lateral elbow pain and burning and should be differentiated from lat-

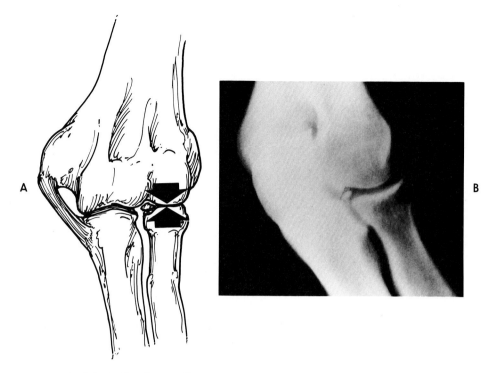

FIG. 16-16. Radial head–capitellum compression loose bodies. **A,** Drawing. **B,** Radiograph.

eral epicondylitis and posterior interosseous nerve entrapment syndrome.

Loose Bodies

Bone changes may result from focal osteochondritis dissecans or diffuse avascular necrosis of the radial head or capitellar joint. When the medial collateral ligament is incompetent, compression of the lateral radiocapitellar joint may occur with loose body formation. These loose bodies in the lateral joint may cause a mechanical block to radial head rotation or a fixed flexion contracture. The loose body can be removed arthroscopically or by an open surgical procedure. Loose body excision rarely resolves the flexion contracture but may provide pain relief and correct joint locking (Fig. 16-16).

Arthroscopy of the elbow has been used for diagnosis of elbow injury, synovectomy, and removal of loose bodies.[12] Currently it has not been expanded past this because of the narrow anatomic confines of the joint. Chondroplasty, olecranon decompression ostectomy, or radial head decompression resection may be performed in selected cases (see Chapter 15).

Attenuated Medial Collateral Ligament

Chronic valgus instability is most commonly seen in the professional throwing athlete, specifically the professional baseball pitcher. Attenuation of the medial collateral ligament occurs because of chronic repetitive valgus load during the throwing act. The elbow carrying angle drifts into an increasing valgus position, which is documented in more than 30% of professional baseball pitchers. As this occurs, the medial tip of the olecranon process may impinge on the wall of the olecranon fossa,

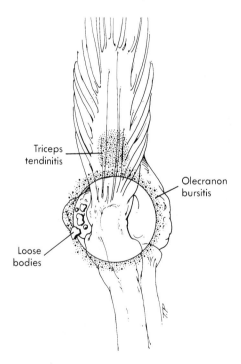

FIG. 16-17. Causes of posterior elbow pain.

causing development of either osteophytes on the medial olecranon tip or loose body formation within the olecranon fossa.[15] Wilson et al[33] has described this as a valgus hyperextension overload in the pitching elbow. Joint debridement and olecranon impingement osteotomy may relieve the symptoms (Fig. 16-17).[33]

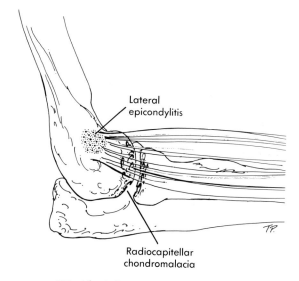

FIG. 16-18. Causes of lateral elbow pain.

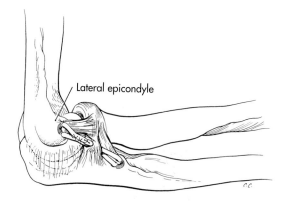

FIG. 16-19. Reconstruction of the lateral ulnar collateral ligament with tendon graft.

Similarly, valgus stress can cause an attenuated medial collateral ligament with resultant lateral radiocapitellar joint compression. Osteophytes and lateral loose bodies occur because the radiocapitellar joint acts as a secondary defense mechanism to valgus stress (Fig. 16-18). Open or arthroscopic joint debridement with loose body excision may be indicated.

Radial head or capitellar resection is done only with caution because once significant bony alterations are performed within the elbow joint, an athlete's professional career may well be terminated. This is particularly true if medial ligament incompetency is missed and subsequent lateral elbow surgery further accentuates elbow instability.

Lateral Collateral Ligament Rupture

Acute lateral collateral ligament rupture occurs with complete dislocation of the elbow. The annular ligament component may remain intact as the dislocation occurs. Radial head fracture with dislocation may also involve the lateral collateral ligament complex. Damage to the lateral collateral ligament complex has been reported with overzealous common extensor origin release for lateral epicondylitis or tennis elbow as well as excessive exposure for radial head fracture resection and repair.

Subsequent instability of the lateral aspect of the elbow may result as either a posterolateral rotatory subluxation or posterolateral instability of the elbow joint. This may be independent from the radial head instability, as seen with an insufficient annular ligament. The **lateral pivot-shift test,** as described by Nestor, O'Driscoll, and Morrey[22] helps identify this point of instability. Acute repair of the lateral ligament complex is performed in a similar fashion to the medial collateral ligament complex.[22] Late reconstruction with the palmaris longus tendon or appropriate fascial graft similarly mimics the medial collateral ligament reconstruction process. Chronic laxity is uncommon, however, because of the less common varus stress patterns about the elbow. If present,

reconstruction using tendon graft is performed in a similar manner to the medial collateral ligament. The lateral ulnar collateral ligament is reconstructed from the lateral epicondyle to the tubercle of the proximal ulna (Fig. 16-19).

Rehabilitation is similar also to the medial collateral ligament program with a wrist brace and a 30-degree extension block for 1 month. The postoperative regimen remains the same for the lateral collateral complex repair or reconstruction.

Posterior Elbow Problems

Posterior elbow pain may be seen with **olecranon bursitis,** which can be inflammatory or infectious. Generally these are managed conservatively with rest, protection, and antiinflammatory medications. If, however, aspiration is performed, it is recommended that the area be prepared surgically and a large bore needle, after lidocaine (Xylocaine) infiltration through the skin, be inserted through subcutaneous tissue into the olecranon bursa. This allows the needle tract to seal, decreases the incidence of infection, and decreases the incidence of fistula formation through the thin skin. Chronic persistent bursitis or infected bursitis is surgically incised and drained or totally excised.

Triceps tendinitis with spur formation on the olecranon tip can be seen acutely as an overuse extension phenomenon. Additionally **valgus extension overload syndrome** produces posterior elbow pain because of olecranon impingement into the olecranon fossa of the distal humerus. Loose body formation may occur, causing pain and locking as well as blocking of motion. Surgical removal is indicated. At the same time, decompression of the posterior olecranon may be performed.

Triceps rupture is uncommon but when seen should be reconstructed, because the professional athlete with such a rupture will lose power extension. Reconstruction may be performed with repair of the triceps or by tendon grafting procedures through the triceps tendon into the olecranon. Rehabilitation is similar to the biceps reattachment with protected active motion, and no resistive motion until satisfactory healing has occurred.

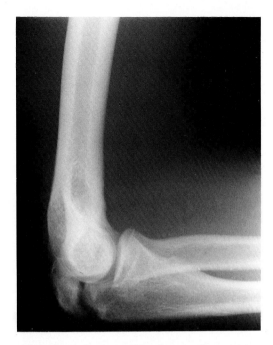

FIG. 16-20. Stress fracture of the olecranon in an adolescent.

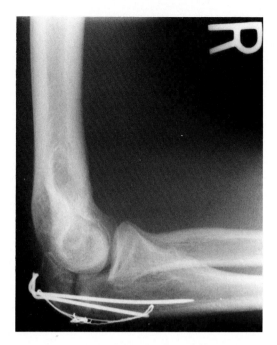

FIG. 16-21. Open reduction with internal fixation of an olecranon fracture with K-wire and tension-band technique.

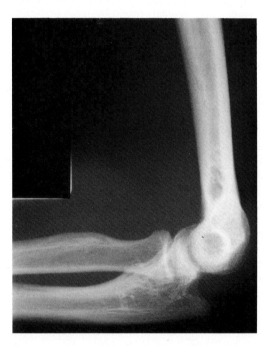

FIG. 16-22. Excision of olecranon with stable elbow because of preservation of the anterior oblique component of the medial collateral ligament.

Olecranon fractures may be seen as stress fractures in the young athlete or as acute fractures in the mature athlete (Fig. 16-20). Olecranon fractures without concomitant injury about the elbow may be treated, if nondisplaced, with extension immobilization until healed. If the fracture is displaced, open reduction or internal fix-

ation (Fig. 16-21) and excision of the olecranon process are options (Fig. 16-22).[1,7]

ACUTE FRACTURES AND DISLOCATIONS

Anteroposterior stability of the elbow joint is the function primarily of an intact coronoid process and integrity of the medial and lateral collateral ligaments. The capsule offers little support against the stresses of acute flexion or extension. In addition, the anterior muscular groups (the brachialis and biceps) do little to maintain anteroposterior stability in the face of forced hyperextension.

Elbow dislocations are generally an injury of hyperextension[32] with a fall on the outstretched or extended arm, although dislocation may occur in flexion. Flexion dislocation is often associated with radial head fractures. The olecranon process is forced into the olecranon fossa and levers the trochlea over the coronoid process. In the course of this traumatic event the medial collateral ligament is usually ruptured and the lateral collateral ligament also disrupted. If the dislocation is simple without associated fractures, reduction may result in a stable elbow if the forearm flexors, extensors, and annular ligament have maintained their continuity. In these cases early motion is resumed and the ultimate prognosis is good.[13,17]

Elbow dislocations that are complex and involve fractures of the bony stabilizing forces about the elbow present a much more difficult problem (Fig. 16-23). Medial collateral ligament rupture, when associated with radial head or capitellar fracture dislocation, creates a significant instability pattern that cannot completely be corrected on either the medial or lateral side of the elbow

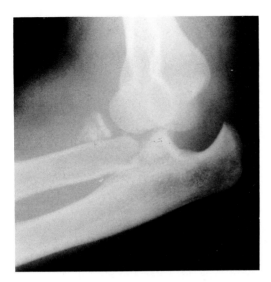

FIG. 16-23. Complex fracture dislocation of the elbow.

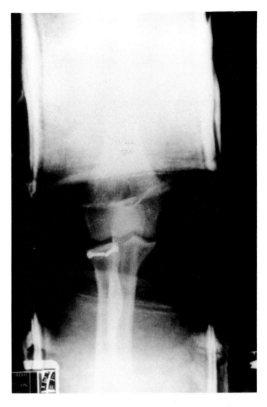

FIG. 16-24. Open reduction with internal fixation of a radial head fracture to preserve lateral elbow stability.

alone for maximum functional return. Attempts to preserve capitellar fracture fragments and radial head fracture fragments with internal fixation are performed (Fig. 16-24). Medial collateral ligament repair is performed. In severe comminuted cases of radial head fractures in which the radial head is removed, a Silastic spacer may be used.[29] Silastic spacer alone does not provide adequate lateral stability against valgus forces if medial collateral ligament support is absent. Silastic spacers also produce additional problems of particulate synovitis and fatigue fractures within the prosthesis. We use the Silastic radial head as a lateral stint to support the medial collateral ligament repair in those cases where there is loss of both stabilizers. The lateral collateral ligament complex is also repaired.

Silastic radial head spacers

- May be used in severe comminuted radial head fractures
- Do not provide adequate lateral stability against valgus stress if used alone and medial collateral ligament support is absent
- May cause silicone synovitis
- May go on to fatigue fractures

Coronoid fractures additionally must be addressed in fracture dislocation injuries with reconstruction of the coronoid if it involves greater than the anterior 20%, which allows for the insertion of the capsule and brachialis. The remainder of the coronoid allows for the insertion of the anterior oblique ligament as a stabilizing factor in the elbow and must be reconstructed for stability (Fig. 16-25).[26]

Reagan and Morrey[26] have classified coronoid fractures into three groups. Groups I and II (less than 10% and less than 50%, respectively) usually do not need open reduction with internal fixation but should suggest

the possibility of elbow dislocation that has been reduced. Group III fractures (greater than 50%) often require open reduction with internal fixation of the coronoid fracture fragment for anteroposterior stability and an early motion program. All types may have had an associated dislocation of the elbow that has been spontaneously reduced.

Acute **radial head fractures** must be managed appropriately with minimal immobilization and early motion for the nondisplaced or Grade I, fracture. A Grade II or III fracture in the competitive athlete presents a more difficult problem. Many advocate open reduction and internal fixation using screw or pin fixation. This is followed by early motion. A Grade IV comminuted fracture-dislocation often ends a career in competitive athletics. Removal of comminuted radial head fractures, stabilization of the elbow joint, and evaluation of the wrist joint

---

Radial head fractures in athletes

- Nondisplaced or Grade I—minimal immobilization and early motion
- Grade II—open reduction and internal fixation and early motion
- Grade III—open reduction and internal fixation and early motion if possible
- Grade IV (comminuted)—radial resection; check distal joint (Essex-Lopresti injury); guarded prognosis for sports

NOTE: Check for medial collateral ligament instability.

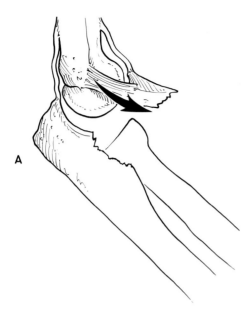

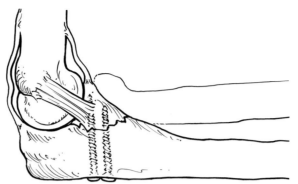

FIG. 16-25. A, Fracture coronoid with dislocation. **B,** Open reduction with internal fixation of a coronoid fracture for stability.

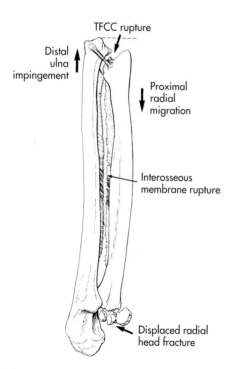

FIG. 16-26. Essex-Lopresti lesion with fractured radial head, interosseous membrane, and triangular fibrocartilage complex rupture resulting in longitudinal axial instability of the forearm.

for distal ulnar dislocation is mandatory in these injuries. Prognosis is guarded, and chronic residual elbow pain as well as restriction of motion persists.

Longitudinal Axial Instability of the Forearm

Displaced or comminuted radial head fractures require evaluation of the forearm interosseous membrane and the distal radial-ulnar joint for stability. If both structures are disrupted, longitudinal axial instability exists with proximal migration of the radial head fracture into the

capitellum and distal ulnar impingement into the carpus. Kirchner pin fixation of the joint and radial head reconstruction or a Silastic spacer is used until interosseous membrane healing occurs. This injury constitutes the Essex-Lopresti lesion.[6] If simple radial head excision is performed, forearm instability and proximal migration of the radius with significant wrist symptoms and impingement result (Fig. 16-26).

VASCULAR INJURIES/COMPARTMENT SYNDROME

Acute vascular insufficiency or rupture of the brachial artery is rare; however, in cases of supracondylar fractures or fracture dislocations of the elbow, consideration of vascular injury must be made (Fig. 16-27).[5,14] Appropriate monitoring of pulses, Doppler evaluation, and indicated arteriography allow early diagnosis and treatment. Nerve entrapment may likewise occur and requires surgical correction.[16] Compartment syndrome is evaluated through clinical examination and pressure monitoring of the compartments.[21] Fasciotomy, to include the lacertus fibrosus at the elbow is indicated in the deteriorating patient with compartment syndrome or when there are appropriate pressure readings using either the wick catheter or the blood pressure gauge monitoring of intracompartmental pressures. At the level of the elbow the brachial artery needs to be visualized and decompressed, as do the median nerve, radial nerve, and on occasion the ulnar nerve.

REHABILITATION

Rehabilitation of the elbow varies according to the injury and the pathologic condition involved. Medial and lateral epicondylitis rehabilitation programs are extensively outlined in Chapter 19. Fracture rehabilitation programs likewise have been outlined. Ligament reconstruction stresses controlled mobilization while protecting against deforming forces.[10] Clinical and biomechan-

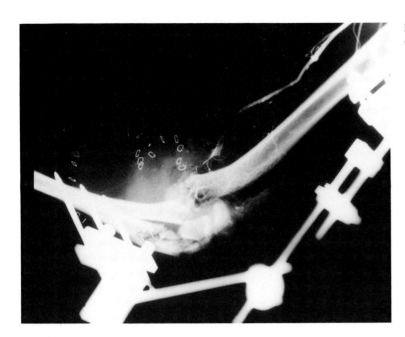

FIG. 16-27. Arteriogram with occlusion of the brachial artery in severe fracture about the elbow.

ical factors as well as physiology of ligament and bone healing must be considered in the rehabilitation process. Maximized healing and motion must be obtained before competitive athletics are resumed.

Rehabilitation issues regarding the elbow must be specific for the injury, age of the patient, type of sports activity involved, and level of competition. Each reconstruction has a specific rehabilitation program and has been outlined under issues of rehabilitation in the individual sections of the chapter.

REFERENCES

1. Adler S, Fay GF, MacAusland WR: Treatment of olecranon fractures, indications for excision of the olecranon fracture, repair of the triceps tendon, *J Trauma* 2:597, 1962.
2. Bennett JB, Green MS, Tullos HS: Surgical management of chronic medial elbow instability, *Clin Orthop* 278:62, 1992.
3. Brodgon BG, Crow NF: Little Leaguer's elbow, *Am J Roentgenol* 8:671, 1960.
4. DeHaven KE, Evarts CM: Throwing injuries of the elbow in athletes, *Orthop Clin North Am* 1:801, 1973.
5. Eliason EL, Brown RB: Posterior dislocation at the elbow with rupture of the radial and ulnar arteries, *Ann Surg* 106:1111, 1937.
6. Essex-Lopresti P: Fractures of the radial head with distal radioulnar dislocation, *J Bone Joint Surg* 33(B):244, 1951.
7. Gartsman GM, Sculco TP, Otis JC: Operative treatment of olecranon fractures: excision or open reduction with internal fixation, *J Bone Joint Surg* 63A(5):718, 1981.
8. Gugenheim et al: Little League survey: the Houston study, *Am J Sports Med* 4:189, 1976.
9. Indelicato P et al: Correctable elbow lesions in professional baseball players, *Am J Sports Med* 7(1):72, 1979.
10. Jobe FW, Stark H, Lombardo SJ: Reconstruction of the ulnar collateral ligament in athletes, *J Bone Joint Surg* 68A(8):1158, 1986.
11. Johanson O: Capsular and ligament injuries of the elbow joint: a clinical and arthrographic study, *Acta Chir Scand* 287(suppl):17, 1962.
12. Johnson LL: *Diagnostic and surgical arthroscopy,* St Louis, 1981, Mosby.
13. Josefsson O, Johnell D, Gentz CF: Long-term sequelae and simple dislocation of the elbow, *J Bone Joint Surg* 66A(6):927, 1984.
14. Kerin R: Elbow dislocation and its association: vascular disruption, *J Bone Joint Surg* 51A(4):756, 1969.
15. King JW, Brelsford HF, Tullos HS: Analysis of the pitching arm of the professional baseball pitcher, *Clin Orthop* 67:116, 1969.
16. Mannenfelt L: Median nerve entrapment after dislocation of the elbow: report of a case, *J Bone Joint Surg* 50B:152, 1968.
17. Mehlhoff T et al: Treatment of simple elbow dislocation in the adult, ASES and AAOS, San Francisco, *J Bone Joint Surg* 70A:244, 1988.
18. Mink JH, Eckardt JJ, Grant TT: Arthrography in recurrent dislocation of the elbow, *Am J Radiol* 136:1242, 1981.
19. Morrey BF: Anatomy of the elbow joint. In Morrey BF (ed): *The elbow and its disorders,* Philadelphia, 1985, WB Saunders.
20. Morrey BF, An KN: Functional anatomy of the ligaments of the elbow, *Clin Orthop* 201:84, 1985.
21. Mubarak SJ et al: Acute compartment syndrome: diagnosis and treatment with the aid of the wick catheter, *J Bone Joint Surg* 60A:1091, 1978.
22. Nestor B, O'Driscoll SW, Morrey BF: Surgical stabilization for lateral rotatory instability of the elbow, *J Bone Joint Surg* 74A:1235, 1992.
23. Norwood LA, Shook JA, Andrews JR: Acute medial elbow ruptures, *Am J Sports Med* 9(1):16, 1981.
24. O'Driscoll SW et al: The anatomy of the lateral ulnar collateral ligament, *Clin Anat* 5:296, 1992.
25. Pappa AM: Elbow problems associated with baseball during childhood and adolescence, *Clin Orthop* 164:30, 1982.
26. Reagan W, Morrey BF: Fractures of the coronoid process and the ulna, *J Bone Joint Surg* 71A:1348, 1989.
27. Schwab GH et al: Biomechanics of elbow instability: the role of the medial collateral ligament, *Clin Orthop* 146:42, 1980.
28. Slocum DB: Classification of elbow injuries from baseball players, *Am J Sports Med* 6:62, 1978.
29. Swanson AB, Jaeger SH, LaRochelle D: Comminuted fracture of the radial head: the role of the silicone-implant replacement arthroplasty, *J Bone Joint Surg* 63A:1039, 1981.
30. Tullos HS et al: Factors influencing elbow instability. In Murray DG (ed): *AAOS instructional course lectures,* vol 8, St Louis, 1982, Mosby.
31. Waris W: Elbow injuries in javelin throwers, *Acta Chir Scand* 93:563, 1946.
32. Wheeler DK, Linscheid RL: Fracture dislocations of the elbow, *Clin Orthop* 50:95, 1967.
33. Wilson FD et al: Valgus extension overload in the pitcher's elbow, *Am J Sports Med* 11:83, 1983.
34. Woods GW: Elbow instability and medial epicondyle fractures, *Am J Sports Med* 5:23, 1977.

CHAPTER 17

Overuse Injuries of the Elbow

Frank A. Cordasco
James C. Parkes, II

Athletic injuries of the elbow are common and often lead to significant disability. These injuries occur in a broad spectrum of activities but are reported to have a particularly high incidence in baseball, racquet sports, football, and track and field events such as javelin throwing.* With proper treatment, technique, and conditioning the athlete can return to his or her former level of participation and perform satisfactorily. Overuse injuries can be divided into four groups: (1) musculotendinous, (2) articular, (3) ligamentous, and (4) neural entrapment lesions.

MUSCULOTENDINOUS INJURIES

There are essentially four areas where musculotendinous overuse injuries can occur. These are defined by their anatomic location—lateral, medial, posterior, and anterior.

Lateral Musculotendinous Injuries

The common extensor muscles centered around the extensor carpi radialis brevis span the wrist and elbow and originate from the lateral epicondyle of the humerus. This musculotendinous unit is particularly susceptible to overuse injuries resulting from participation in racquet sports.† Tennis elbow, originally described as lawn-tennis elbow,[60] has become a popular term for the description of lateral epicondylitis. The characteristic age of onset is between 35 and 50 years, and the overall male/female ratio is usually equal.[72,73] Lateral epicondylitis is directly related to activities that increase the tension and hence the stress of the wrist extensor and supinator muscles. These muscular contractile overloads may occur concentrically or eccentrically. This is clearly an overuse problem characterized by excessive forearm use with respect to intensity and duration.

Although Cyriax[20] correctly concluded that the origin of the extensor carpi radialis brevis was the major site of pathology in tennis elbow, it was nearly 30 years later in 1964 when Goldie[36] detailed pathologic changes in the subtendinous tissue adjacent to the lateral elbow. Subsequently Nirschl and Pettrone[72] described the essential

---

*References 2, 3, 5, 8, 13, 21, 22, 45, 49, 53, 81, 82, 95, 96, 102, and 105.
†References 10-12, 20, 27, 32, 36, 42, 52, 70, and 73.

pathologic condition as angiofibroblastic hyperplasia. Regan et al[84] recently demonstrated a histopathologic picture of hyalin degeneration with neovasculature. Thus the surgical pathologic condition reveals an aborted effort of healing and hyalin degeneration, without evidence of inflammation.

Clinical Picture

The patient generally complains of pain along the lateral aspect of the elbow. Tenderness is localized to the lateral epicondyle and origin of the extensor carpi radialis brevis. Passive volar flexion of the wrist with the elbow extended increases the pain, as does active dorsiflexion of the wrist against resistance. Radiographs of the elbow are generally negative, although in approximately 20% a small calcific deposit may be noted laterally in the region of the epicondyle.

Treatment

Initial treatment is directed at relief of pain and begins with the time-honored modalities of rest and application of cold. Nonsteroidal antiinflammatory agents are started and physical therapy may be considered. If pain relief is not achieved in a short time, a steroid injection is appropriate because the patient may be incapable of progressing in the rehabilitation program. Generally we use 2.5 to 5 ml of 0.5% bupivacaine (Marcaine) without epinephrine combined with 20 to 40 mg of methylprednisolone (Depo-Medrol). This solution is instilled below the extensor carpi radialis brevis just anterior and slightly distal to the lateral epicondyle. Care is taken to avoid superficial placement of the injection because hypopigmentation and subcutaneous atrophy may result. More than two or three steroid injections per year is inappropriate and probably harmful, since cellular death and potential weakening of the surrounding normal tissues have been documented.[97] Once symptoms have begun to resolve, the patient can be started on a more aggressive physical therapy program designed to increase strength and flexibility. Isotonic and isokinetic exercises can be incorporated into a strength and endurance exercise program before return to sport.[73] At this stage an evaluation of the training technique can be helpful. Improper stroke mechanics have been noted commonly. For example, the athlete may begin the backhand stroke by leading with the elbow rather than the body and shoulder. The correct technique with respect to the sport not only enhances performance but is less likely to cause injury.[73] Equipment (particularly in the racquet sports) may play an important role in the pathomechanics of this overuse syndrome. A larger head racquet, medium string

tension (55 to 60 lb), lighter racquet material, and appropriate grip size have been noted to minimize excessive forces.[70,73] In selecting proper handle size, Nirschl[70] has used the distance from the midpalmar crease to the ring finger. Finally, counterforce bracing has been helpful in the conservative management of tennis elbow.[30,44] In our experience this conservative program has been successful in over 90% of patients and similar results have been noted in the literature.[72]

Surgery is considered in those patients who have persistent pain for at least 1 year despite a high-quality conservative program as outlined above. Surgery should not be considered unless a positive injection test (pain relief with a steroid injection) has been demonstrated.

The surgical treatment of lateral epicondylitis has included release of the extensor aponeurosis at the level of the lateral epicondyle,[42,61] release of the extensor aponeurosis as well as the orbicular ligament,[10] lengthening of the extensor carpi radialis brevis tendon in the distal forearm,[32] resection of the radial nerve to the lateral epicondyle,[52] lengthening of the extensor carpi radialis brevis proximally,[92] excision of the pathologic tendinous tissue,[69,72] and percutaneous extensor tenotomy.[7,107] We have found the technique as described by Nirschl and Pettrone[72] to be efficacious (see p. 799). Surgery is performed on an outpatient basis using regional or local anesthesia. The patient is started on early gentle range of motion exercises and progressed through a rehabilitation program similar to the regimen used preoperatively. For recreational racquet sports, gentle ground strokes are begun 6 to 8 weeks from the time of surgery. Counterforce brace protection is used until full strength has returned as documented by isokinetic testing. Full return to sport averages 3 to 5 months postoperatively. This program has yielded 85% good to excellent results with respect to pain relief and function. These results compare favorably with those reported in the literature.[10,11,69,72,107]

Morrey[63] has provided the only description of the causes of failure, the method of assessment, and results of reoperation. He classified the failure of surgical treatment of lateral epicondylitis into two types. The Type 1 failure is one in which the patient describes symptoms identical to those that were noted before the original surgery. Three basic factors can result in a Type 1 failure: improper patient selection, incomplete or improper diagnosis, and an inadequate or incomplete surgical procedure. The latter factor was the most common cause of failure in Morrey's series. Incomplete or improper diagnosis generally results when the differential diagnosis has not been entirely considered. Additional causes of lateral elbow pain include anconeus compartment syndrome,[1] degenerative arthrosis,[27] lateral ligament instability,[74] and posterior interosseous nerve entrapment.* A Type 2 failure is characterized by patient complaints that differ from those voiced before the index procedure. The causes of Type 2 failure consist primarily of surgically introduced, or iatrogenic, injury, which includes synovial

---

Return to tennis after musculotendinous injuries

- Larger head racquet
- Medium string tension
- Lighter racquet material
- Appropriate grip size

---

*References 16, 24, 46, 67, 86, 87, and 103.

fistula, adventitial bursa, and lateral collateral ligament insufficiency. Yerger and Turner[107] noted synovial fistulas as a complication following percutaneous extensor tenotomies. If a surgeon is faced with a failed surgical treatment of refractory lateral epicondylitis, Morrey[63] has described an extremely straightforward algorithm, which should be used in the assessment of these patients.

Medial Musculotendinous Injuries

Medial epicondylitis may occur independently or may on occasion be associated with lateral tennis elbow.[31,99] The flexor-pronator muscle group originates at the medial epicondyle. Nirschl[71] and Olliviere, Nirschl, and Pettrone[77] have described the pathologic condition as being generally located at the interface between the pronator teres and the flexor carpi radialis. The histopathologic evaluation following the surgical treatment of medial epicondylitis has revealed angiofibroblastic hyperplasia and fibrillary degeneration of collagen.[77]

Clinical Picture

The patient typically describes pain on the medial aspect of the elbow, which is exacerbated when throwing a baseball, or serving or hitting a forehand shot in tennis. Tenderness to deep palpation is located at the medial epicondyle and origin of the flexor-pronator mass. The pain can be reproduced with resisted pronation, resisted volar flexion of the wrist, or by passively extending the wrist with the elbow in extension. Associated ulnar neuropathy at the elbow has been reported in 25% to 60% of patients with medial epicondylitis.[31,71,99] Radiographic evaluation generally does not reveal abnormalities, although occasionally, as with the lateral side, calcific deposits or excrescences may be noted in the region of the medial epicondyle.

Treatment

Nonoperative treatment includes rest, application of cold, use of nonsteroidal antiinflammatory agents, the judicious use of a steroid injection, physical therapy, and counterforce bracing.[31,71]

Rarely, if after 1 year of conservative treatment the patient remains symptomatic, outpatient surgery may be considered. Little information is available on the surgical treatment of medial epicondylitis. Two recent reports have documented a high success rate following debridement and resection of the degenerative tendon tissue.[31,77] Gabel and Morrey[31] noted a poor outcome in cases with associated ulnar neuropathy. We have used the approach as described by Nirschl beginning with a 4-cm incision centered over the medial epicondyle (see p. 801).[71,77] For isolated medial epicondylitis an elliptical incision is used to resect the pathologic tissue, which is generally located at the interface between the flexor carpi radialis and pronator teres. An attempt is made to close the resection defect to avoid subsequent weakness.[77,99] Postoperatively early range of motion exercises are started and the patient is progressed much the same as with the lateral epicondylitis group. Full return to sport is noted in most cases 4 to 5 months postoperatively.

Posterior Musculotendinous Injuries

The posterior region is less commonly involved than the lateral and medial areas. The triceps muscle tendon unit is overloaded in sports that involve repetitive forceful extension of the elbow, such as throwing and racquet sports, gymnastics, shot putting, javelin throwing, boxing, and weight lifting.

Clinical Picture

The patient's symptoms are referred to the posterior aspect of the elbow. On examination the patient has tenderness just superior to the attachment of the triceps on the olecranon or actually on the olecranon where the tendon attaches. There may also be some mild swelling over the tender area. If the physician has the patient attempt to forcefully extend the elbow against resistance, the pain increases. Radiographic evaluation of the elbow does not generally reveal any significant findings.

Treatment

Rest and a short course of nonsteroidal, antiinflammatory medication usually decreases the pain in 5 to 7 days. The patient then begins a program of rehabilitation to increase the strength and flexibility of the elbow extensor muscles. Steroid injections in this area are to be avoided because experience has shown that this can lead to triceps tendon rupture.[97] The physician should communicate with the athlete's coach so that proper mechanics training can be instituted. If this program is followed, the results are successful.

Anterior Musculotendinous Injuries

The anterior area is the least commonly involved region, although injury in this area may be seen in athletes who participate in sports that require repetitive flexion with forced extension. This includes bowling, weight lifting, and gymnastics. In these sports the biceps and brachialis muscle tendon units are repeatedly stressed and overloaded. This repetitive microtrauma can lead to clinical problems.

Clinical Picture

The patient complains of pain along the anterior aspect of the elbow. Localized tenderness may be found along the course of the biceps tendon. Resisted supination or flexion of the elbow increases the pain. Radiographic evaluation usually does not reveal pathologic findings. Occasionally an acute distal biceps rupture may be suspected, often following steroid injections into the tendon. Anterior swelling and tenderness are present. A palpable gap can be noted in the usual location of the distal biceps tendon. Weakness of elbow supination and flexion is profound.

Treatment

For patients with symptoms of microtrauma and tendinitis, nonsteroidal antiinflammatory medication, rest, and rehabilitation have generally been effective. Steroid injections are avoided because of the potential of steroids

to contribute to tendon rupture.[97] Repair of acute distal biceps tendon ruptures is reviewed in Chapter 16.

ARTICULAR INJURIES

Chronic repetitive stress syndromes have an impact on the articular surfaces of the elbow and can result in subsequent impaired function.[2,3,8] Articular injuries in the form of chronic stress osteophyte formation[9,37] and loose body formation[6,9,62,104] may occur in the competitive athlete of any age. Gore et al[37] have demonstrated that repetitive elbow stress in sports can result in osseous manifestations, which include bony hypertrophy, loose bodies, osteophytes, traction spur formation, osteochondral defects, epiphyseal and apophyseal hypertrophy, fragmentation, and avulsion. Injury can be seen medially, laterally, posteriorly, or in a combination of all these areas.

Medial Compartment Injuries

In throwing and racquet sports the medial aspect of the joint is subjected to repetitive valgus tension stress.[53,64,104] The medial epicondyle serves as the origin of the flexor-pronator muscle mass as well as the anterior band of the medial collateral ligament.[64,66]

Athletes who repeatedly subject the elbow to valgus stress develop strong tension forces on the medial epicondyle. This occurs predominantly during the late cocking and early acceleration phases of the throw (Fig. 17-1). This area is particularly prone to injury in young athletes before the medial epicondylar apophysis fuses.[105] Several studies have documented the radiographic changes that are often present in this region in a significant number of Little League athletes.*

Clinical Picture

Usually the patient is a young adolescent who has been throwing or playing racquetball or tennis. He or she complains of pain along the medial aspect of the elbow. The discomfort is increased in intensity during athletic participation. Tenderness is present over the medial epicondyle, and an elbow flexion contracture of 5 to 15 degrees may be present.

Radiographs can demonstrate a number of abnormalities, including widening of the apophyseal line, enlargement of the apophysis, and fragmentation of the apophysis.[9,37]

Radiographic findings in adolescent athletes with medial elbow pain

- Widening of the apophyseal line
- Apophyseal enlargement
- Fragmentation of the apophysis

Less commonly, the athlete experiences acute pain and is unable to play. In this situation examination reveals swelling and tenderness of the medial aspect of the elbow. Gentle valgus stress at 20 to 30 degrees of flexion demonstrates instability when compared with the normal elbow. Radiographic examination reveals partial or complete avulsion of the epicondyle.[37,105]

Treatment

In the athlete with a chronic problem where no separation or less than 1 mm of separation is present, initial treatment includes the use of nonsteroidal antiinflammatory medication. This program usually leads to decreased symptoms in 3 to 6 weeks. This should be followed by a rehabilitation program to increase strength and flexibility. Results of this treatment regimen are almost always successful.

In acute cases, where there is greater than 3 mm of separation of the epicondyle, open reduction and internal fixation with unthreaded K-wires, suture, or screw fixation is indicated.[9,105]

Lateral Compartment Injuries

The lateral compartment is subjected to significant compressive stress, particularly in sports such as tennis, baseball, gymnastics, racquetball, and javelin throwing. These activities tend to place a valgus stress on the elbow, causing tension forces medially and compression forces laterally.† Lateral compression forces involve the

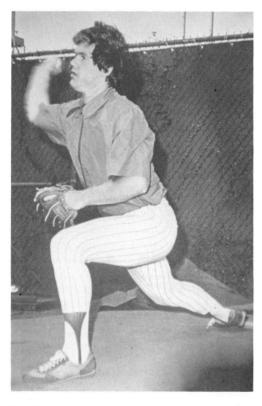

FIG. 17-1. Extreme valgus stress on the elbow as the pitcher is throwing in the acceleration phase. There is medial tension and lateral posterior compression stress. This combination leads to many clinical problems in the elbows of throwing athletes.

---

*References 2, 3, 9, 13, 37, and 95.
†References 2, 3, 8, 9, 37, 53, 81, and 95.

radial head and the capitellum. This repetitive compressive stress across the radiocapitellar joint can lead to degeneration of the articular cartilage of the radial head, capitellum, or both. This may result in loose body formation (Fig. 17-2). In children, the epiphyses are sensitive to compression stress, and osteochondritis can develop (Fig. 17-3).[80,106]

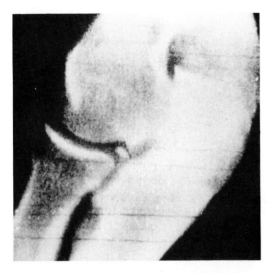

FIG. 17-2. Loose body in the lateral compartment, secondary to compression of the radial head against the capitellum.

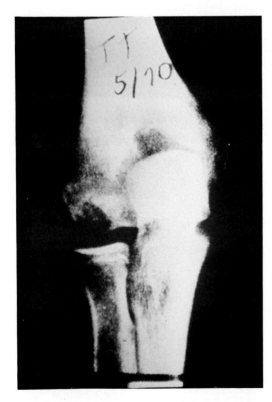

FIG. 17-3. Radiolucent area in the capitellum is secondary to repetitive compression stress of the radial head against the capitellum.

Loose Body Formation

Repetitive valgus stress resulting in compression at the radiocapitellar joint can lead to injury of the articular cartilage surfaces and loose body formation. Loose bodies can arise from the radial head or capitellum.[9,37,104]

Clinical picture. The patient's chief complaint is pain in the elbow, which is associated with catching and clicking. No single traumatic event is usually recalled. However, some patients may experience a locking episode with the elbow sticking at a certain point in flexion. Often, they must shake or toggle it to regain motion from the fixed position.

Examination discloses crepitus during passive range of motion testing. Occasionally a loose body can be palpated laterally between the radial head and capitellum.

Radiographs reveal loose bodies anteriorly in the radiocapitellar joint (Fig. 17-2). However, often when one surgically explores these patients, more fragments are found than are revealed on radiographs because of the large number of pure cartilage (unossified) bodies.

Treatment. Loose bodies can be successfully removed arthroscopically or if necessary via a small lateral arthrotomy. Postoperatively the arm is placed in a soft dressing and motion is instituted at once. After approximately 6 weeks of active range of motion exercises, a strengthening program can be started. First, isometric exercises are performed, followed by isotonic and isokinetic exercises. The patient can begin to compete again 12 to 16 weeks after surgery. Unless the radiocapitellar joint has severe articular cartilage damage, the outlook for return to full activity is quite good.[45,75,105]

Osteochondritis Dissecans of the Radiocapitellar Joint

Compression forces in repetitive microtrauma at the radiocapitellar joint may produce vascular insufficiency, which is presumed to be the etiology for osteochondritis dissecans in the adolescent.[80,106] Osteochondritis generally affects the capitellum, although signs of aseptic necrosis have been found in the radial head.[2,95]

Clinical picture. The typical patient presents in early adolescence with the insidious onset of dominant elbow pain and a flexion contracture of 10 to 15 degrees. Radiographic evaluation often reveals a lucency in the capitellum (Fig. 17-3). Fragmentation and loose body formation may also be present. Occasionally the initial radiograph may be normal and magnetic resonance imaging (MRI) in these cases may define early injury. Late radiographic changes include hypertrophy of the radial epiphysis and flattening of the radial head or capitellum.[9,37]

Treatment. If loose bodies are present, the decision to proceed with surgery is clearly supported.[45,75] Arthroscopic removal of loose bodies is generally the treatment of choice with the occasional need of a limited arthrotomy for large osteochondral loose bodies. In the absence of loose bodies 6 weeks of rest is indicated. If the pain and flexion contracture persist beyond 6 weeks, further diagnostic studies including computed tomography (CT) arthrography or MRI can be helpful to determine if fragmentation or separation has occurred. Ultimately ar-

throscopy provides the definitive diagnosis.[9,75] The treatment plan is formulated based on the disease stage. Once separation of the fragment has occurred, healing is unlikely and excision of the fragment is preferred. When the lesion is large, attempted reattachment via open reduction and internal fixation with multiple K-wires,[45] bone graft pegs,[9] and biodegradable pins may be considered.

Posterior Compartment Injuries

In sports such as tennis, baseball, racquetball, and javelin throwing, posterior compartment injuries are frequently noted. Valgus stress combined with repetitive hyperextension causes impingement of the posteromedial olecranon tip into the olecranon fossa (Fig. 17-4), resulting in osteophyte formation, fragmentation, and the subsequent development of loose bodies.[6,9,37,104] Less commonly this repetitive impingement can lead to a stress fracture of the olecranon.

Loose Body and Osteophyte Development

Osteochondral loose bodies must be differentiated from accessory ossicles, a persistent apophysis, and other pathologic manifestations.[15,40,62]

Clinical picture. The patient complains of pain in the posterior aspect of the elbow. It may be associated with clicking and grating. Occasionally the elbow will lock in a fixed position and the patient will have to shake it to restore motion. On examination, crepitus can be felt over the posterior aspect of the elbow as the elbow is flexed and extended. Active extension is limited, because the osteophytes and loose bodies prevent full extension. Tenderness is apparent posteriorly along the margins of the olecranon, and on occasion loose bodies may be palpable in the same area. Radiographic examination reveals marginal osteophytes and enlargement of the olecranon. In addition, one or more loose bodies can often be seen (Fig. 17-5).

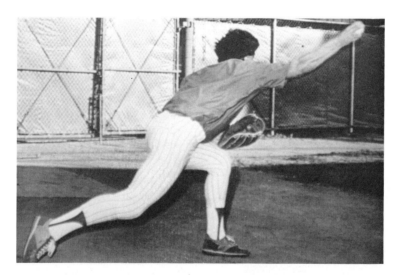

FIG. 17-4. In the follow-through and release phases of throwing, the elbow is forcefully extended, further compressing the olecranon into the olecranon fossa.

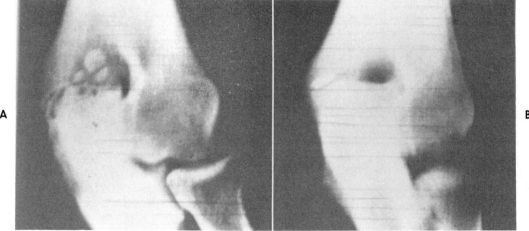

FIG. 17-5. A, Loose bodies in the posterior compartment. **B,** Fracture of a bony prominence on the medial aspect of the olecranon secondary to impaction of this region against the olecranon fossa.

Treatment. If no loose bodies are present, a period of rest plus judicious use of nonsteroidal antiinflammatory medication can usually decrease the symptoms in 7 to 14 days. A complete rehabilitation program is begun when symptoms are improved. Generally, in 4 to 6 weeks, the patient can resume athletic participation. The coaching staff and trainers should stress good mechanics to avoid a recurrence.

When patients have persistent symptoms or in those cases in which loose bodies are present, arthroscopic decompression for posterior impingement is helpful. This procedure includes debridement of olecranon osteophytes as well as removal of loose bodies if present (Fig. 17-6).[75,104] A small lateral arthrotomy may be necessary to complete the procedure. This approach avoids violating the triceps tendon. Range of motion exercises are begun in the early postoperative period. Subsequently, progressive range of motion and strengthening exercises are instituted. Usually in 12 to 16 weeks the patient can resume athletic activity.

Stress Fracture of the Olecranon

A stress fracture of the olecranon is uncommon but can occur in sports such as baseball, tennis, and racquetball where repetitive forceful extension of the olecranon into the olecranon fossa occurs.

Clinical picture. The patient presents with the gradual onset of pain in the posterior aspect of the elbow. The pain steadily increases in severity to the point that performance is affected. At this point the patient usually seeks medical attention.

Tenderness is present over the olecranon, and full extension is difficult to obtain. Forced extension against resistance usually increases the pain.

Findings on plain radiographs are generally negative. A bone scan reveals an increased uptake in the olecranon, and lateral tomograms or MRI may reveal the stress fracture line.

Treatment. Treatment consists of splinting the elbow for 4 to 6 weeks. This is followed by a progressive rehabilitation program to increase range of motion and strengthening exercises. Usually in 4 to 6 months the patient can return to full activity. If there is a nonunion, the area can be bone grafted, but this step is usually not necessary.

LIGAMENTOUS INJURIES

Recurrent elbow instability in the athlete has been essentially limited to medial collateral ligament pathology.[18,48-50,104] Chronic valgus instability due to attenuation of the anterior band of the medial collateral ligament is usually seen in throwers, particularly pitchers, and appears to be due to repetitive microtrauma.[18,50] The pitching motion is a dynamic activity taking less than $\frac{3}{100}$ of a second from late cocking to ball release, generating angular velocities which approach 6000 degrees per second and baseball speeds of greater than 90 miles per hour (Fig. 17-1).[82]

Recently the recognition of the importance of the lateral ulnar collateral ligament and the diagnosis of posterolateral rotatory instability,[65,74] has led to the development of a global spectrum of elbow instability.[76] This classification scheme is divided into three stages, which share an essential lesion involving the lateral ulnar collateral ligament (Fig. 17-7). Stage 1 is posterolateral rotatory instability and consists of a disruption of the lateral ulnar collateral ligament. Stage 2 is characterized by

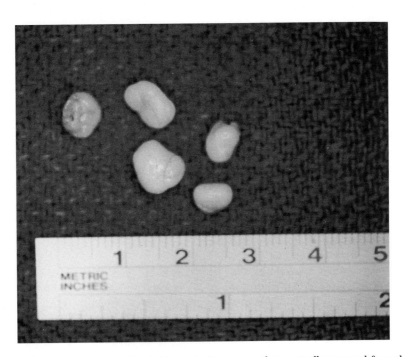

FIG. 17-6. These multiple osteochondral loose bodies were arthroscopically removed from the posterior compartment of the elbow of a 22-year-old pitcher.

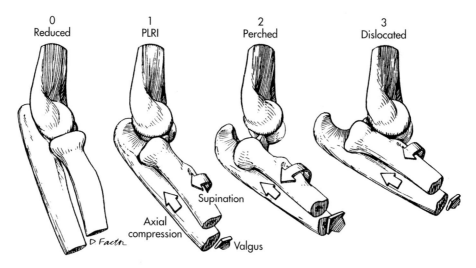

FIG. 17-7. Classification of elbow instability correlating with the pathoanatomic stages of capsuloligamentous disruption. Forces and moments responsible for displacements are illustrated. *PLRI*, Posterolateral rotatory instability. (From O'Driscoll SW et al: *Clin Orthop* 280:195, 1992.)

the additional disruption of the anterior and posterior capsule resulting in a "perched" subluxation. Stage 3 is divided into Stage 3a, in which the anterior band of the medial collateral ligament is intact, and stage 3b, in which the entire medial collateral complex is disrupted. Posterior dislocation occurs in both stages. O'Driscoll and colleagues[74,76] believe that posterolateral rotatory instability may be the most common pattern of elbow dislocation.

In the context of athletic injuries, chronic deficiency of the lateral ulnar collateral ligament appears to occur subsequent to a complete elbow dislocation in most cases, but it may occasionally occur following an elbow subluxation or sprain.[68,74] Unlike throwing injuries in which repetitive valgus stress may result in attenuation of the medial collateral ligament,[18,48-50,53,104] repetitive varus stress rarely occurs at the elbow and thus chronic lateral ulnar collateral ligament injury is as a result particularly uncommon.[68,74,76]

Medial Capsuloligamentous Injuries

The anterior band of the medial (ulnar) collateral ligament has been demonstrated to be the primary structure resisting valgus stress at the elbow.[64,65,88] In the general population acute injury to the medial collateral ligament rarely results in recurrent instability of the elbow.[54,64] Repetitive microtrauma in athletes from the valgus stress that occurs in the late cocking and early acceleration phases of the throwing motion can compromise the integrity of the medial collateral ligament.[18,50,82] The osseous articulation of the elbow contributes little to medial stability with the arm in this position.[43,64-66,88,89]

Clinical Picture

The patient typically has a history of repetitive overhand throwing activities and complains of pain along the

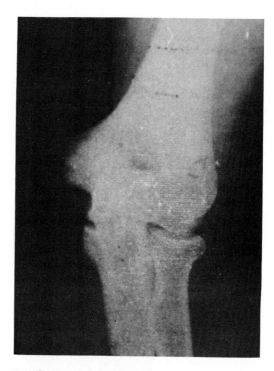

FIG. 17-8. Spurring of the ulnohumeral joint and calcification in the region of the medial collateral ligament. This is secondary to tension stresses placed on this aspect of the elbow.

medial aspect of the elbow, particularly during the late cocking and early acceleration phases of the throwing motion. Occasionally the patient may describe associated paresthesias in the ulnar nerve distribution. On examination tenderness is elicited over the medial collateral ligament commonly at the distal insertion and occasionally in a more diffuse distribution. A positive Tinel's sign at the cubital tunnel may be present, since associated ul-

nar nerve symptoms can occur in 40% of patients.[18,34] Valgus stress is applied to the elbow at 20 to 30 degrees of flexion, and local pain, tenderness, and end-point laxity are assessed. Standard radiographs may identify hypertrophy of the humeral condyle and posteromedial olecranon,[53,104] calcification within the medial collateral ligament, marginal osteophytes of the ulnohumeral (Fig. 17-8) or radiocapitellar joints, or loose bodies in the posterior compartment.

Treatment

Treatment of athletes with chronic medial collateral ligament injury begins with rest and nonsteroidal anti-inflammatory medication. With resolution of symptoms, rehabilitation should be instituted with emphasis on flexibility and strength. Overview of the athlete's mechanics, which may include video assessment, should then be evaluated with the coaching staff and trainers. This treatment regimen has been successful.[5,18] If periods of rest and rehabilitation have failed to result in a resolution of symptoms, the athlete may be a candidate for surgery.

Operative management consists of repair or reconstruction. In the case of an acute rupture, surgical repair can be considered; however, the indications are extremely limited. The avulsed ligament should be without evidence of calcification, and if there is any question as to the quality of the tissue, reconstruction should be performed. The use of an autologous palmaris longus tendon graft has been demonstrated to be biomechanically satisfactory.[83] We have used the technique for reconstruction of the medial collateral ligament as described by Jobe et al.[18,50] One of us (JCP) has been successful in returning professional players to their sports using this technique.

Lateral Capsuloligamentous Injuries

It has been well established that posterior dislocation of the elbow rarely results in recurrent instability.[14,39,78,93,94] The recent description of posterolateral rotatory instability and the recognition of the importance of the lateral ulnar collateral ligament has improved our understanding of the pathomechanics in this area.[65,74] Although chronic lateral collateral ligament instability is extremely uncommon, it can occur subsequent to a complete posterior dislocation and has been observed after a discrete varus injury to the elbow.[68,74,76] Of note, it has also occurred as an iatrogenic complication following release of the common extensor tendon for lateral epicondylitis.[63]

Clinical Picture

O'Driscoll, Bell, and Morrey[74] and Nestor and colleagues[68] have reported their experience with this particular pathologic entity. Their typical patient presented with a spectrum of complaints ranging from recurrent dislocations to subtle mechanical symptoms of locking, catching, snapping, and clicking. They have described the **lateral pivot-shift test,** which is best performed in the supine position. The forearm is supinated and axial compression as well as a valgus moment are applied to

the elbow during flexion (Fig. 17-7). This results in a typical apprehension response and reproduces the patient's symptoms.[74] Radiographic evaluation is generally negative.

Treatment

Once the diagnosis of posterolateral rotatory instability has been made, O'Driscoll, Bell, and Morrey[74] Nestor, O'Driscoll, and Morrey[68] recommend that one seriously consider repair or reconstruction of the lateral collateral ligament. Nonoperative treatment may include physical therapy as well as a hinged brace with an extension block or with the forearm in full pronation. The surgical technique for ligament repair is performed via a Kocher approach and involves the plication of the anterior capsule and posterior capsule as well as an advancement of the lateral collateral ligament complex using a Bunnell suture.[68] The ligament reconstruction is performed via a similar approach using an autologous palmaris longus tendon graft.[68]

NEURAL ENTRAPMENT LESIONS

Neural entrapment lesions associated with athletic activities may be related to a number of etiologic factors.* In some cases the nerve entrapment is but one component in a spectrum of disorders affecting the athlete and one must consider these other problems closely.[26,33,34,49] Whenever nerve compression lesions at the elbow are considered, the differential diagnosis must include the possibility of compression lesions at other levels such as the cervical spine, brachial plexus, and wrist.[33,101]

Ulnar Nerve Entrapment

Ulnar nerve compression may occur as a result of direct trauma, traction, compression, recurrent subluxation or dislocation, and osseous degenerative changes.† In athletes ulnar nerve irritation is likely to develop secondary to mechanical factors that occur during the late cocking and early acceleration phases of the throwing motion.[25,26,33,34,49] In this setting ulnar neuritis appears to be one component of a spectrum of pathology that affects the medial side of the elbow and includes medial instability and medial epicondylitis.

Feindel and Stratford[28] proposed the term **cubital tunnel syndrome** to identify a specific anatomic site for entrapment of the ulnar nerve and to differentiate this entity from tardy ulnar nerve palsy, which was associated with posttraumatic deformities. The ulnar nerve is a terminal division of the medial cord of the brachial plexus and passes from the anterior compartment of the brachium into the posterior compartment through the arcade of Struthers, located 8 cm proximal to the medial epicondyle.[90] The cubital tunnel is a fibroosseous ring, the roof of which is formed by a fascial sheath described by Osborne.[79] It has been shown that the cubital tunnel changes contour and volume during elbow range of motion.[4] The ulnar nerve can therefore be compromised by

---

*References 23, 25, 26, 33-35, 38, 41, 57, 86, 87, and 108.
†References 4, 17, 23, 35, 53, 59, and 98.

any swelling that occurs within the canal or with inflammatory changes that result in thickening of the fascial sheath.[4,33,79]

Clinical Picture

The patient generally describes medial elbow pain associated with numbness and tingling in the ulnar nerve distribution. Paresthesias may be present with radiation from the medial epicondyle distally along the ulnar aspect of the forearm and into the fourth and fifth fingers. These sensory symptoms usually precede the development of motor deficits. Physical examination is significant for tenderness at the cubital tunnel, which may include the medial epicondyle. Tinel's sign is generally present at the cubital tunnel. Although subluxation of the ulnar nerve may occur in as many as 16% of asymptomatic individuals,[17] the presence of ulnar nerve subluxation or dislocation should be assessed in the patient with symptoms, since it may contribute to injury.[33,34] An evaluation for the presence of medial collateral ligament insufficiency and medial epicondylitis should be performed, since there can be significant overlap particularly in the population of throwing athletes.[26,34,49]

Radiographs may demonstrate osseous pathology such as hypertrophy of the humerus and olecranon, osteophytes, calcifications in the region of the medial collateral ligament (Fig. 17-9), and loose bodies. A cubital tunnel view should be included in the radiographic series.[101] Particularly in the athletic population, electrodiagnostic studies are frequently negative.[23,26,33]

The possibility of nerve compression lesions at other levels should always be considered, and the differential diagnosis includes cervical radiculopathy, brachial plexus injury, a Pancoast tumor, compression at Guyon's canal,[33,101] and shoulder subluxation resulting in traction paresthesias.[19]

Treatment

If the patient presents early after onset of symptoms, treatment should include rest, antiinflammatory medications, protective padding, and occasionally the use of extension night splints. This should be followed by a rehabilitation program before return to sport. If the patient remains symptomatic despite a conservative program, surgery is generally recommended. It should be noted that, although physical findings other than local tenderness may be minimal and electrodiagnostic tests are rarely positive, good to excellent results may be obtained by anterior transposition of the nerve in the throwing athlete.[25,26,33,108]

The surgical treatment options include decompression alone[79] and subcutaneous, intramuscular, or submuscular transposition.[47,55,56,108] Medial epicondylectomy has been used as a decompression technique particularly in patients with posttraumatic structural joint changes; however, it is not advisable in athletes due to the vulnerability of the humeral attachment of the medial collateral ligament.[34] We prefer the stabilized subcutaneous transposition, which creates a new medial septum posterior to the transposed nerve.[25,26,33] Careful protection of medial brachial and antebrachial cutaneous nerves

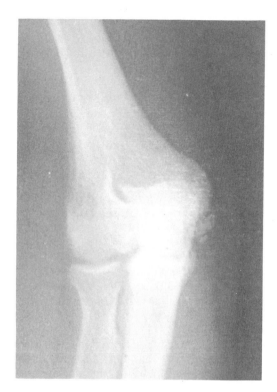

FIG. 17-9. Calcification inferior to the medial epicondyle, which can contribute to the development of ulnar neuropathy. These represent either avulsions from the medial epicondyle or calcifications in the medial collateral ligament or both.

must be maintained throughout the procedure. Potential injury located at any of the classic sites of compression should be addressed to avoid persistent neural compromise. Early range of motion exercises are encouraged. It has been demonstrated that those patients with more severe preoperative findings, which include motor deficits and positive electrodiagnostic studies, have less favorable outcomes.[29] We have found the stabilized subcutaneous transposition (Figs. 17-10 and 17-11) to yield satisfactory results in 85% of patients.

Radial Nerve Entrapment

Entrapment of the radial nerve, specifically the posterior interosseous nerve, occurs within the radial tunnel and has been defined as the basis of two distinct syndromes.[24,33,58,86] Patients with the diagnosis of **radial tunnel syndrome** are said to present with pain and without evidence of motor weakness,[33,57,58,86] whereas patients with **posterior interosseous nerve compression** develop motor weakness in the absence of pain.[33] These compressive neuropathies are extremely uncommon, and therefore controversy has been generated in the literature resulting in some degree of confusion.*

The importance of radial nerve compression within the context of sports medicine arises when considering the differential diagnosis of lateral epicondylitis. The distinction between lateral epicondylitis and radial nerve—spe-

---

*References 33, 57, 58, 85-87, 91, and 100.

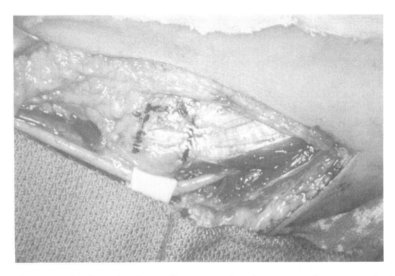

FIG. 17-10. Ulnar nerve has been freed up and is now ready to be transposed anterior to the fascial sling.

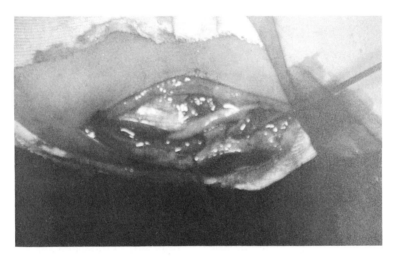

FIG. 17-11. Ulnar nerve is positioned anterior to the fascial sling, which serves as a new medial septum.

cifically posterior interosseous nerve—entrapment has been evaluated during the last 3 decades.* The issue is complicated by the fact that lateral epicondylitis may coexist with posterior interosseous nerve entrapment in approximately 5% of individuals.[103]

The radial nerve enters the anterior compartment of the brachium by piercing the lateral intermuscular septum at the spiral groove level of the humerus. The radial nerve divides into the superficial radial nerve and posterior interosseous nerve at the radiocapitellar joint level.[33,58] Several structures within the radial tunnel may be responsible for compression of the posterior interosseous nerve. These structures include fibrous bands, which are anterior to the radial head, the radial recurrent fan (leash of Henry), the tendinous margin of the extensor carpi radialis brevis muscle, the arcade of

Frohse, and the distal border of the superficial supinator muscle.[33,57,58] The most common site of compression is said to be the arcade of Frohse, which is the strong proximal border of the superficial belly of the supinator muscle.[33,57,58]

Clinical Picture

The patient typically presents with lateral elbow pain, which is localized to the proximal extensor compartment and occasionally radiates distally to the wrist. The pain is exacerbated by activities and often racquet sports are implicated. Nocturnal pain may be present. The physical examination reveals tenderness to deep palpation at the level of the arcade of Frohse just distal to the radial head. Lister, Belsole, and Kleinert[58] described the so-called middle finger test as pathognomonic of radial tunnel syndrome; however, we have noted pain elicited by this maneuver in approximately 30% of patients with lateral epicondylitis. Additional findings include pain upon

---

*References 16, 24, 46, 63, 67, 86, and 103.

resisted supination of the extended forearm and pain with passive pronation of the forearm and full wrist flexion. Tenderness is generally not elicited by palpation of the lateral epicondyle and origin of the extensor carpi radialis brevis as seen in the typical lateral epicondylitis. Radiographs are generally negative and electrodiagnostic studies have been minimally helpful. Morrey[63] has described a reliable triad, which he has found helpful in making the diagnosis of posterior interosseous nerve entrapment. This triad includes precise localization of pain at the arcade of Frohse reproduced by direct palpation, aggravated by resisted supination, and relieved with injection of 2 ml of lidocaine. In evaluating the patient with atypical lateral elbow pain, a local injection of 1 to 2 ml of lidocaine in the region of the lateral epicondyle should be performed and the early response should be noted. If the injection at the epicondyle does not completely relieve the pain and if the physical examination suggests posterior interosseous nerve entrapment, a second injection with lidocaine is performed in the region of the arcade of Frohse. The use of sequential injections in this way can help to distinguish lateral epicondylitis from posterior interosseous nerve entrapment in the unusual patient with an atypical presentation.[33,63]

Treatment

Symptoms are generally relieved by rest, nonsteroidal antiinflammatory agents, and the avoidance of positions of compromise. In some cases splinting may be utilized to enforce rest and additionally provide relief of symptoms. The elbow should be splinted in flexion with the forearm in supination and the wrist in dorsiflexion. In the rare patient who does not respond to conservative measures, operative decompression may be considered. We prefer the extensile anterolateral approach; a posterolateral approach may be used as well, and the transbrachioradialis approach is favored by some.[33] The anterolateral approach is particularly appropriate when the exact area of compression cannot be determined from the preoperative evaluation. In this case all possible compressive structures should be evaluated and released as indicated. Results have been mixed in that satisfactory pain relief has been reported to range from two thirds to nearly all patients in several series.[58,85,86,91]

Pronator Teres Syndrome

Compressive neuropathy of the median nerve proximal to the carpal canal, known as the pronator teres syndrome, may develop as a result of a thickened ligament of Struthers, sharpened lasertus fibrosis, pathology within the pronator tunnel, and a tendinous edge of the flexor digitorum superficialis arch.[38,51] Athletic activities that involve repetitive pronation of the forearm, such as baseball and racquet sports, may initiate irritation of the median nerve at this level, although the pronator teres syndrome is quite rare.

Clinical Picture

The patient may describe an aching discomfort and easy fatigability of the muscles of the forearm as well as numbness in the distribution of the median nerve. These symptoms may be exacerbated by activities that require repetitive pronation, as in the practicing of tennis serves. Nocturnal awakening may be present but is much less common than in carpal tunnel syndrome.[38] Physical examination is significant for tenderness of the proximal part of the pronator teres.

Forceful pronation of the forearm against resistance may generate paresthesias in the distribution of the median nerve. A positive Tinel's sign at the proximal aspect of the pronator teres has been noted in approximately half of the patients.[38,51] Hypertrophy of the proximal forearm muscles, particularly the pronator teres, may be observed. A depression in the contour of the forearm superficial to the lasertus fibrosis may be present as well.[38] As with other nerve compression syndromes, electrodiagnostic studies are generally negative.

Treatment

Rest, modification of activities with particular emphasis on the avoidance of repetitive pronation exercises, and the use of nonsteroidal antiinflammatory medications usually result in a cessation of symptoms. In the unusual patient who does not respond to this management, surgical exploration of the median nerve and a thorough evaluation of all potential sites of compression may be indicated. The results following decompression have been variable.[38,51]

SUMMARY

Athletes commonly develop overuse injuries of the elbow, which can significantly limit their ability to perform. Injuries can be grouped into four general categories, including musculotendinous injuries, articular surface injuries, ligamentous injuries, and neural entrapment lesions. The physician with a good working knowledge of anatomy, pathophysiology, biomechanics, principles of rehabilitation, and treatment options can be successful in returning the injured athlete to his or her former level of participation.

REFERENCES

1. Abrahamsson SO et al: Lateral elbow pain caused by anconeous compartment syndrome: a case report, *Acta Orthop Scand* 58:589, 1987.
2. Adams JE: Injury to the throwing arm: a study of traumatic changes in the elbow joints of boy baseball players, *Calif Med* 102:127, 1965.
3. Adams JE: Bone injury in very young athletes, *Clin Orthop* 58:129, 1968.
4. Apfelberg DB, Larson SJ: Dynamic anatomy of the ulnar nerve at the elbow, *Plast Reconstr Surg* 51:79, 1973.
5. Barnes DA, Tullos HS: An analysis of 100 symptomatic baseball players, *Am J Sports Med* 6:63, 1978.
6. Bassett LW et al: Post-traumatic osteochondral "loose body" of the olecranon fossa, *Radiology* 141:635, 1981.
7. Baumgard SH, Schwartz DR: Percutaneous release of the epicondylar muscles for humeral epicondylitis, *Am J Sports Med* 10:233, 1982.
8. Bennett GE: Shoulder and elbow lesions distinctive of baseball players, *Ann Surg* 126:107, 1947.
9. Bennett JB: Articular injuries in the athlete. In Morrey BF (ed): *The elbow and its disorders,* Philadelphia, 1993, WB Saunders.
10. Bosworth DH: The role of the orbicular ligament in tennis elbow, *J Bone Joint Surg* 37A:527, 1955.

11. Boyd HD, McLeod AC: Tennis elbow, *J Bone Joint Surg* 55A:1183, 1973.
12. Briggs CA, Elliott DG: Lateral epicondylitis: a review of structures associated with tennis elbow, *Anat Clin* 7:149, 1985.
13. Brodgon BG, Crow NF: Little leaguer's elbow, *Am J Roentgenol* 8:671, 1963.
14. Burgess RC, Sprague HH: Post-traumatic posterior radial head subluxation: two case reports, *Clin Orthop* 186:192, 1984.
15. Burman MS: Unusual locking of the elbow joint by the sesamum cubiti and a free joint body, *Am J Radiol* 45:731, 1941.
16. Capener N: The vulnerability of the posterior interosseous nerve of the forearm: a case report and anatomical study, *J Bone Joint Surg* 48B:770, 1966.
17. Childress HM: Recurrent ulnar nerve dislocations at the elbow, *Clin Orthop* 108:168, 1975.
18. Conway JE et al: Medial instability of the elbow in throwing athletes: surgical treatment by ulnar collateral ligament repair or reconstruction, *J Bone Joint Surg* 74A:67, 1992.
19. Cordasco FA et al: Management of multidirectional instability, *Oper Techn Sports Med* 1(4):293, 1993.
20. Cyriax JH: The pathology and treatment of tennis elbow, *J Bone Joint Surg* 18:921, 1936.
21. DeHaven KE, Evarts CM: Throwing injuries of the elbow in athletes, *Orthop Clin North Am* 1:801, 1973.
22. DeHaven KE et al: Symposium: throwing injuries to the adolescent elbow, *Contemp Surg* 9:65, 1976.
23. Del Pizzo W, Jobe FW, Norwood L: Ulnar nerve entrapment syndrome in baseball players, *Am J Sports Med* 5:182, 1977.
24. Dewey P: The posterior interosseous nerve and resistant tennis elbow, *J Bone Joint Surg* 55B:435, 1973.
25. Eaton RG: Anterior subcutaneous transposition. In Gelberman RH (ed): *Operative nerve repair and reconstruction*, Philadelphia, 1991, JB Lippincott.
26. Eaton RG, Crowe JF, Parkes JC III: Anterior transposition of the ulnar nerve using a noncompressing fasciodermal sling, *J Bone Joint Surg* 62A:820, 1980.
27. Emery SE, Gifford JF: One hundred years of tennis elbow, *Contemp Orthop* 12:53, 1986.
28. Feindel W, Stratford J: The role of the cubital tunnel and tardy ulnar palsy, *Can J Surg* 1:287, 1958.
29. Foster RJ, Edshage S: Factors related to the outcome of surgically managed compressive ulnar neuropathy at the elbow level, *J Hand Surg* 6:181, 1981.
30. Froimson AI: Treatment of tennis elbow with forearm support band, *J Bone Joint Surg* 53A:183, 1971.
31. Gabel GT, Morrey BF: Medial epicondylitis: surgical management, influence of ulnar neuropathy, *J Shoulder Elbow Surg* 3(1):511, 1994.
32. Garden RS: Tennis elbow, *J Bone Joint Surg* 43B:100, 1961.
33. Gelberman RH, Eaton RE, Urbaniak JR: Peripheral nerve compression, *J Bone Joint Surg* 75A:1854, 1993.
34. Glousman RE: Ulnar nerve problems in the athlete's elbow, *Clin Sports Med* 9:365, 1990.
35. Godshall RW, Hansen CA: Traumatic ulnar neuropathy in adolescent baseball pitchers, *J Bone Joint Surg* 53A:359, 1971.
36. Goldie I: Epicondylitis lateralis humeri (epicondylalgia or tennis elbow): a pathogenetic study, *Acta Chir Scand Suppl* 339:7, 1964.
37. Gore RM et al: Osseous manifestations of elbow stress associated with sports pitchers, *Am J Roentgenol* 134:971, 1980.
38. Hartz CR et al: The pronator teres syndrome: compressive neuropathy of the median nerve, *J Bone Joint Surg* 63A:885, 1991.
39. Hassmann GC, Brunn F, Neer CS II: Recurrent dislocation of the elbow, *J Bone Joint Surg* 57A:1080, 1975.
40. Henderson MS, Jones HT: Loose bodies in joints and bursae due to synovial osteochondromatosis, *J Bone Joint Surg* 5:400, 1923.
41. Herrick RT, Herrick S: Ruptured triceps in a power lifter presenting as cubital tunnel syndrome: a case report, *Am J Sports Med* 15:514, 1987.
42. Hohmann G: Das Wesen und die Behandlung des Sogenannten tennisellenbogenes, *Munch Med Wehnschr* 80:250, 1933.
43. Hotchkiss RN, Weiland AJ: Valgus stability of the elbow, *J Orthop Res* 5:372, 1987.
44. Ilfeld FW, Field SM: Treatment of tennis elbow: use of a special brace, *JAMA* 195(2):67, 1966.
45. Indelicato PA et al: Correctable elbow lesions in professional baseball players: a review of 25 cases, *Am J Sports Med* 7:72, 1979.
46. Jalovarra P, Lindholm RV: Decompression of the posterior interosseous nerve for tennis elbow, *Arch Orthop Trauma Surg* 108:243, 1989.
47. Janes PC, Mann RJ, Farnworth TK: Submuscular transposition of the ulnar nerve, *Clin Orthop* 238:225, 1989.
48. Jobe FW, Kvitne RS: Elbow instability in the athlete, *Inst Course Lect* 40:17, 1991.
49. Jobe FW, Nuber G: Throwing injuries of the elbow, *Clin Sports Med* 5:621, 1986.
50. Jobe FW, Stark H, Lombardo SF: Reconstruction of the ulnar collateral ligament in athletes, *J Bone Joint Surg* 68:1158, 1986.
51. Johnson RK et al: Median nerve entrapment syndrome in the proximal forearm, *J Hand Surg* 4:48, 1979.
52. Kaplan EB: Treatment of tennis elbow (epicondylitis) by denervation, *J Bone Joint Surg* 41A:147, 1959.
53. King JW, Brelsford HJ, Tullos HS: Analysis of the pitching arm of the professional baseball pitcher, *Clin Orthop* 67:116, 1969.
54. Kuroda S, Sakamaki K: Ulnar collateral ligament tears of the elbow joint, *Clin Orthop* 208:266, 1986.
55. Learmonth JR: A technique for transplanting the ulnar nerve, *Surg Gynecol Obstet* 75:792, 1942.
56. Leffert RD: Anterior submuscular transposition of the ulnar nerve by the Learmonth technique, *J Hand Surg* 7:147, 1982.
57. Lister GD: Radial tunnel syndrome. In Gelberman RH (ed): *Operative nerve repair and reconstruction*, Philadelphia, 1991, JB Lippincott.
58. Lister GD, Belsole RD, Kleinert HE: The radial tunnel syndrome, *J Hand Surg* 4:52, 1979.
59. MacNicol MF: The results of operation for ulnar neuritis, *J Bone Joint Surg* 61B:159, 1979.
60. Major HP: Lawn-tennis elbow, *Br Med J* 2:557, 1883.
61. Michele AA, Krueger FJ: Lateral epicondylitis of the elbow treated by fasciotomy, *Surgery* 39:277, 1956.
62. Milgram JW: The development of loose bodies in human joints, *Clin Orthop* 124:292, 1977.
63. Morrey BF: Reoperation for failed surgical treatment of refractory lateral epicondylitis, *J Shoulder Elbow Surg* 1:47, 1992.
64. Morrey BF, An KN: Articular and ligamentous contributions to the stability of the elbow joint, *Am J Sports Med* 11:315, 1983.
65. Morrey BF, An KN: Functional anatomy of the ligaments of the elbow, *Clin Orthop* 201:84, 1985.
66. Morrey BF, Tanaka S, An KN: Valgus stability of the elbow: definition of primary and secondary constraints, *Clin Orthop* 265:187, 1991.
67. Morrison DL: Tennis elbow and radial tunnel syndrome: differential diagnosis and treatment, *J Aust Orthop Assoc* 80:823, 1981.
68. Nestor B, O'Driscoll SW, Morrey BF: Surgical stabilization for lateral rotatory instability of the elbow, *J Bone Joint Surg* 74A:1235, 1992.
69. Neviaser TJ et al: Lateral epicondylitis: results of out-patient surgery and immediate motion, *Contemp Orthop* 11:43, 1985.
70. Nirschl RP: Tennis elbow, *Orthop Clin North Am* 4:787, 1973.
71. Nirschl RP: Medial tennis elbow, surgical treatment, *Orthop Trans* 7:298, 1983.
72. Nirschl RP, Pettrone F: Tennis elbow: the surgical treatment of lateral epicondylitis, *J Bone Joint Surg* 61A:832, 1979.
73. Nirschl RP, Sobel J: Conservative treatment of tennis elbow, *Phys Sports Med* 9:42, 1981.
74. O'Driscoll SW, Bell DF, Morrey BF: Posterolateral rotatory instability of the elbow, *J Bone Joint Surg* 73A:440, 1991.
75. O'Driscoll SW, Morrey BF: Arthroscopy of the elbow, *J Bone Joint Surg* 74A:84, 1992.
76. O'Driscoll SW et al: Elbow subluxation and dislocation: a spectrum of instability, *Clin Orthop* 280:186, 1992.

77. Olliviere CO, Nirschl RP, Pettrone FA: Surgical treatment for medial tennis elbow tendinosis—a prospective analysis. Paper presented at the American Shoulder and Elbow Surgeons, ninth open meeting, San Francisco, Feb 21, 1993.

78. Osborne G, Cotterill P: Recurrent dislocation of the elbow, *J Bone Joint Surg* 48B:340, 1966.

79. Osborne GV: The surgical treatment of tardy ulnar neuritis, *J Bone Joint Surg* 39B:782, 1957.

80. Panner HJ: A peculiar affection of the capitulum humeri resembling Calvé-Perthes disease of the hip, *Acta Radiol* 10:234, 1928.

81. Pappas AM: Elbow problems associated with baseball during childhood and adolescence, *Clin Orthop* 164:30, 1982.

82. Pappas AM, Zawacki RM, Sullivan TJ: Biomechanics of baseball pitching: a preliminary report, *Am J Sports Med* 13:216, 1985.

83. Regan WD et al: Biomechanical study of ligaments around the elbow joint, *Clin Orthop* 271:170, 1991.

84. Regan WD et al: Microscopic histopathology of chronic refractory lateral epicondylitis, *Am J Sports Med* 20:746, 1992.

85. Ritts GD, Wood MB, Linscheid RL: Radial tunnel syndrome: a ten-year surgical experience, *Clin Orthop* 219:201, 1987.

86. Roles NC, Maudsley RH: Radial tunnel syndrome: resistant tennis elbow as a nerve entrapment, *J Bone Joint Surg* 54B:499, 1972.

87. Rossum JV et al: Tennis elbow: a radial tunnel syndrome? *J Bone Joint Surg* 60B:197, 1978.

88. Schwab GH et al: Biomechanics of elbow instability: the role of the medial collateral ligament, *Clin Orthop* 146:41, 1980.

89. Sojbjerg JO, Oveson J, Nielsen S: Experimental elbow instability after transection of the medial collateral ligament, *Clin Orthop* 218:186, 1987.

90. Spinner M, Kaplan EP: The relationship of the ulnar nerve to the medial intermuscular septum in the arm and its clinical significance, *Hand* 8:239, 1976.

91. Steichen JB, Mulbry LW, Christensen AW: Radial tunnel syndrome: clinical experience and results of treatment, *Orthop Trans* 12:4, 1988.

92. Stovall PB, Beinfield MS: Treatment of resistant lateral epicondylitis of the elbow by lengthening of extensor carpi radialis tendon, *Surg Gynecol Obstet* 149:526, 1979.

93. Symeonides PP et al: Recurrent dislocation of the elbow: report of three cases, *J Bone Joint Surg* 57A:1084, 1975.

94. Trias A, Comeau Y: Recurrent dislocation of the elbow in children, *Clin Orthop* 100:74, 1974.

95. Tullos HS, King JW: Lesions of the pitching arm in adolescents, *JAMA* 220:264, 1972.

96. Tullos HS et al: Unusual lesions of the pitching arm, *Clin Orthop* 88:169, 1972.

97. Unverferth LJ, Olix ML: The effect of local steroid injection on tendon, *Am J Sports Med* 1:31, 1973.

98. Vanderpool DW et al: Peripheral compression lesions of the ulnar nerve, *J Bone Joint Surg* 50B:792, 1968.

99. Vangsness T, Jobe F: The surgical treatment of medial epicondylitis, *Orthop Trans* 12:733, 1988.

100. Verhaar J, Spaans F: Radial tunnel syndrome: an investigation of compression neuropathy as a possible cause, *J Bone Joint Surg* 73A:539, 1991.

101. Wadsworth TG: The external compression syndrome of the ulnar nerve at the cubital tunnel, *Clin Orthop* 124:189, 1977.

102. Waris W: Elbow injuries in javelin throwers, *Acta Chir Scand* 93:563, 1946.

103. Werner CO: Lateral elbow pain and posterior interosseous nerve entrapment, *Acta Orthop Scand Suppl* 174:1, 1979.

104. Wilson FD et al: Valgus extension overload in the pitching elbow, *Am J Sports Med* 11:83, 1983.

105. Woods GW, Tullos HS, King JW: The throwing arm: elbow injuries, *Am J Sports Med (Sports Safety Suppl)* 1:4, 1973.

106. Woodward AH, Bianco AJ: Osteochondritis dissecans of the elbow, *Clin Orthop* 110:35, 1975.

107. Yerger B, Turner T: Percutaneous extensor tenotomy for chronic tennis elbow: an office procedure, *Orthopaedics* 8:1261, 1985.

108. Zemel NP, Jobe FW, Yocum LA: Submuscular transposition/ulnar nerve decompression in athletes. In Gelberman RH (ed): *Operative nerve repair and reconstruction*, Philadelphia, 1991, JB Lippincott.

CHAPTER 18 Degenerative Joint Disease of the Elbow

John J. Brems

History and physical examination

Radiographic evaluation

Management

Summary

The elbow is a complex joint having freedom of motion along both the transverse and longitudinal planes. Despite its mechanical complexity and despite the tremendous biomechanical forces to which it is subjected in throwing sports, it is remarkably resistant to progressive degenerative joint disease. That degenerative arthritis of the elbow is extremely rare is testified to by the fact that less than 5% of the elbow arthroplasties performed at the Mayo clinic were done for primary degenerative arthritis.[6,7] Goodfellow and Bullough[1] described the pattern of aging of the elbow articular cartilage and found consistent age-related findings at the radiocapitellar joint, but they found only limited changes at the articular cartilage of the humeroulnar joint.

Muscle strain, ligament sprains, and generalized overuse syndromes are frequent conditions encountered by the athlete but do not lead to degenerative joint disease. Loose bodies, frequently seen in the elbow, may lead to wear and degenerative changes and should not be ignored. Untreated loose bodies may lead to "three body wear" with severe rapid damage to the articular surfaces.[3]

HISTORY AND PHYSICAL EXAMINATION

The most consistent patient complaint is limitation of elbow motion, manifested primarily as a flexion contracture. This contracture may be either bone in origin, as in olecranon impingement from hypertrophic spurring,

---

Findings in elbow degenerative joint disease

- Flexion contracture
- Loss of terminal flexion
- Forearm atrophy
- Limitation of forearm rotation (variable)
- Crepitus

---

or it may be soft tissue in origin from a tight anterior capsule or a contracted brachialis or biceps muscle.

The athlete may complain of medial joint pain from a chronic inflammation or sprain of the medial ligament complex, consisting of the anterior and posterior oblique ligaments. Stretching of the ligaments may lead to increased compression at the radiocapitellar joint laterally. This may result in a fragmentation of the lateral joint articular surfaces with resultant formation of loose bodies and, later, degenerative disease. The patients may complain of pain posteriorly and along the medial olecranon border. King, Brelsford, and Tullos[2] found a high incidence of degenerative changes in this area in baseball pitchers.

Forearm atrophy may be present on the affected extremity, but generally this is difficult to assess and is of limited value in patient evaluation.

When examining range of motion, in addition to the flexion contracture, there is usually loss of maximal flexion when compared with the uninvolved extremity (Fig. 18-1). In degenerative disease this is most likely secondary to radial head osteophytes that impinge on the anterior distal humerus. A tight posterior capsule or triceps contracture may also limit flexion. Loose bodies and the pain of joint incongruity may limit the observed motion (Fig. 18-2).

Pronation and supination motions may likewise be limited to varying degrees, depending on the location of the degenerative change. It is important for the examiner to initially measure the pronation and supination passively. Active motion causes increased compression of the articular surfaces and may increase pain, resulting in an apparent loss of motion greater in degree than would be seen with passive examination. Similarly, when evaluating the joint for crepitus, the examiner must remember that active motion may increase the crepitus that may otherwise go undetected. Needless to say, a careful neurologic examination is mandatory.

RADIOGRAPHIC EVALUATION

A minimum of anteroposterior (AP) and lateral views are required for evaluating the elbow. The AP view is performed with the elbow in extension and the lateral view with the elbow in 90 degrees of flexion. In degenerative joint disease the examiner looks for joint space narrowing and hypertrophic bone changes (Fig. 18-3). Occa-

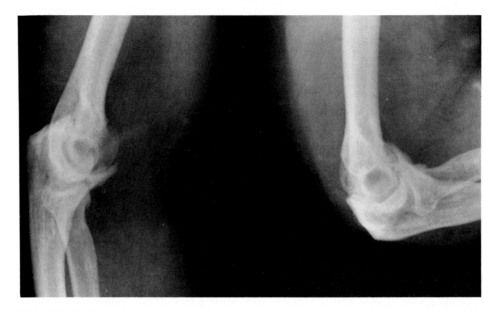

FIG. 18-1. Radiograph taken in the lateral projection shows the maximal extension and flexion obtained in this elbow with severe degenerative arthritis. The common cause of loss of extension is osteophytes on the olecranon process or loose bodies in the olecranon fossa. A tight anterior capsule or brachialis and biceps contractures also limit extension. Flexion is usually limited by osteophytes on the radial head and in the area of the coronoid process. Additionally, soft-tissue contractures involving the triceps or posterior capsule can limit flexion.

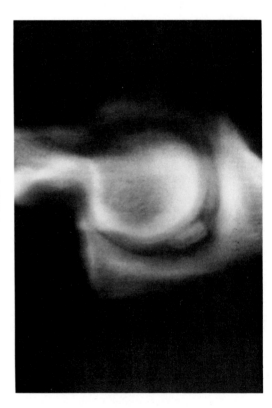

FIG. 18-2. Arthrotomogram of the elbow of an active National Football League lineman. This technique is superior for defining the size and location of loose bodies. Not all loose bodies are calcified and ossified, and this technique of arthrotomography can demonstrate these types of cartilagenous loose bodies.

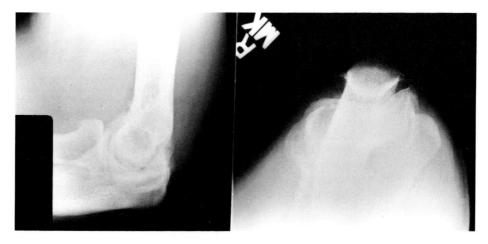

FIG. 18-3. Two views of an active National Football League lineman, showing severe arthritis of the elbow. The most characteristic changes are osteophytes on the radial head and on the coronoid and olecranon processes. The axial view clearly shows the degenerative process involving the olecranon process.

sionally a joint effusion may be seen by the presence of the anterior and posterior fat pad signs.

The most common area for joint space narrowing is at the radiocapitellar joint. Hypertrophic new bone may be seen at the articular margins of the radial head and neck and around the olecranon process, especially on its medial side. Loose bodies may be seen anywhere in the joint but most commonly are found in the olecranon fossa or on the lateral side of the joint. Double contrast arthrotomography is especially helpful in identifying intraarticular loose bodies.

MANAGEMENT

Operative management is only rarely indicated for primary degenerative joint disease about the elbow. For the most severe cases where pain and disability is unresponsive to nonoperative management, either fascial arthroplasty or arthrodesis may be indicated. The gross instability following resection arthroplasty makes this procedure unsatisfactory except in severe sepsis or tuberculosis. Total joint replacement or hemiarthroplasty has only limited use in the surgical management of degenerative disease of the elbow in the active athletic patient. Indications and contraindications are well outlined by Morrey.[4,5] Arthroscopic joint debridement is in its infancy, and adequate data are not available to recommend its widespread use in the arthritic elbow (see Chapter 15).

Nonoperative management of degenerative joint disease of the elbow must initially attempt to control pain. Pain management may consist of the use of oral antiinflammatory agents, together with splinting to decrease tissue edema. In more severe cases intraarticular corticosteroids may be given. Once pain has abated, range of motion exercises and general muscle conditioning begins. Adjustable splints may be fabricated with thermoplastic materials in which range of motion in flexion and extension are controlled (Fig. 18-4). These splints should be worn at night and may be worn during activities to

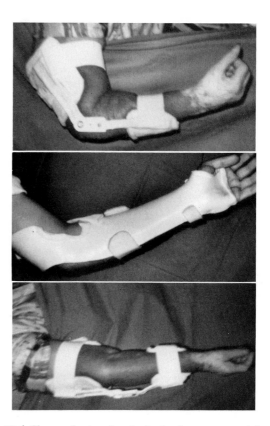

FIG. 18-4. Thermoplastic splints in the fixed position or with hinges provide significant relief of pain in the arthritic elbow. They may be used as resting night splints, or with hinges they may be worn during certain activities to provide increased stability and to limit motion to the more painless arc.

resist extremes of motion that may otherwise cause or aggravate symptoms.

When intraarticular corticosteroids are used, they are most easily instilled via the lateral side in the radiocapitellar joint. Physical therapy modalities include instruc-

tion in active range of motion exercises to the limit of pain and general muscle strengthening using isometric and isotonic techniques.

SUMMARY

Management of degenerative joint disease about the elbow fortunately is not a common problem. Few orthopaedic surgeons are faced with active patients who have advanced arthritis, and the literature offers little guidance in their management. The vast majority appear to respond satisfactorily to nonoperative management, and surgical intervention should remain the management of last resort.

REFERENCES

1. Goodfellow JW, Bullough PG: The pattern of aging of the articular cartilage of the elbow joint, *J Bone Joint Surg* 49B:175, 1967.
2. King JW, Brelsford HJ, Tullos HS: Analysis of the pitching arm of the professional baseball pitcher, *Clin Orthop* 67:116, 1969.
3. Morrey BF: Loose bodies. In Morrey BF (ed): *The elbow and its disorders*, 1985, Philadelphia, WB Saunders.
4. Morrey BF: Reconstructive procedure of the elbow. In Morrey BF (ed): *The elbow and its disorders*, 1985, Philadelphia, WB Saunders.
5. Morrey BF (ed): *The elbow*, New York, 1994, Raven Press.
6. Morrey BF et al: Total elbow arthroplasty: a five-year experience at the Mayo Clinic, *J Bone Joint Surg* 63A:1050, 1981.
7. Ortner DJ: Description and classification of degenerative bone changes in the distal joint surfaces of the humerus, *Am J Phys Anthrop* 28:139, 1968.

CHAPTER 19

Rehabilitation of Elbow Injuries

Fred L. Allman, Jr.
Carolyn A. Carlson

The basic power unit of performance is the muscle-tendon unit; therefore most elbow problems that arise during or as a result of athletic activity are related to muscular activity. The main offender is a dynamic overload to this unit. The resulting injuries may be acute, subacute, or chronic. In addition, injuries may occur over an extended period of time as the result of the late effects of repetitive microtrauma.

Injuries to the elbow and subsequent rehabilitation must include restoration of all the basic qualities of muscle function. Clinically, there are three basic qualities of muscle function.

1. *Strength*—the ability of a muscle to contract
2. *Elasticity*—the ability of a muscle to give up contraction and to yield to passive stretch
3. *Coordination*—the ability of a muscle to cooperate with other muscles in proper timing and with appropriate power and elasticity

It is usually possible to explain a deficiency in muscle action as the consequence of one, two, or all three of these basic qualities of muscle function.

A muscle acts from an elongated position because the elastic force of the muscle augments a contractible force. A muscle contracts best from its full length. Overuse or overloading leads to fatigue, and with fatigue the muscle relaxes more slowly and more incompletely than normal. It then enters a state of myostatic contracture in which injuries are likely to occur. The resulting injury might be a minor strain to the muscle or tendon. If repeated strains occur, actual tears may take place in the muscle. Attempts at repair result in fibrosis, which may in turn result in a permanent loss of elbow extension.

Although rest, ice, and gentle massage are helpful, the main effort in treatment and rehabilitation should be directed to the cause of the condition rather than to the resultant effect. The muscle-tendon unit must be slowly and gradually strengthened to withstand the stress of athletic participation without producing an undue overload. Rehabilitation therefore must consist primarily of restoration or improvement in the quality of the impaired muscle function. If the muscle is weak, it must be strengthened. If the muscle is inelastic, the elasticity must be improved. If the muscle has lost its proper timing and synchronous action, the goal should be to restore proper coordination. The problem may be related to all three qualities—strength, elasticity, and coordination.

For the athlete with an elbow injury, especially in the throwing and racquet sports, rehabilitation must extend beyond the upper extremity, trunk, and lower extremities, and rehabilitation must also be directed to these areas. An alteration of function involving any of these regions will likely lead to further and more prolonged problems. Therefore total body fitness must be one of the goals of rehabilitation.

RATIONALE FOR REHABILITATION FOR SPECIFIC ELBOW CONDITIONS
Tension Overload

Tension overload injuries occur in both throwing and racquet sports, as well as in weight training.

Medial Tension Overload

In baseball the most common injury is a tear or partial avulsion of one of the tendons or muscle insertions, often the result of medial overload produced by the valgus strain on the elbow (see Chapter 16).

In football the windup is less than in baseball, the forward fling is shorter, and the follow-through is in a different arc and not as powerful.

Hammer throwing and shot-putting place tremendous traction stress on the heavy muscles of the elbow and shoulder because of the momentum of the follow-through and the heavier projectile that is being propelled.

The javelin is released with a powerful extension of the elbow and with forcible pronation of the forearm. The pronation is extreme and it is necessary to prevent the whip of the javelin. In the follow-through the thrower may almost completely turn around.

Tension overload is seen frequently early in the season. Tightness develops on the medial aspect of the involved elbow. The medial muscle mass becomes tense and sore, and temporarily there is a loss of extension. If activity is allowed to continue while the athlete is in a state of myostatic contracture, more serious injury is likely to occur because fibrosis results from multiple tearing throughout the muscle with resultant permanent loss of elbow extension.

The aim of rehabilitation in this condition is to slowly and gradually strengthen the muscle-tendon unit to withstand the stress without producing an undue overload.

Lateral Tension Overload

In tennis or other racquet sports, lateral tension overload is likely to occur. This is often referred to as *lateral epicondylitis*. This condition is primarily caused by intrinsic and extrinsic overload at the extensor aponeurosis.

Lateral Compression Injuries

Lateral compression injuries are the result of impaction of the head of the radius against the capitellum in the act of throwing. Roughening and degeneration of the articular cartilage often result from repeated injury.

More than 50 years ago Shands showed that trauma to hyaline cartilage produced a definite hyperplasia. The margins and the tip of the olecranon and the adjacent surfaces of the condyle of the humerus are constantly traumatized by the act of throwing. The result produces a definite osteochondritis with exfoliation of the articular cartilage, which may in turn produce loose bodies, synovial thickening, and semiattached cartilaginous masses that obstruct and limit extension of the elbow.

Minor abnormalities in valgus-varus alignment of the ulna can result in impingement of the tip of the olecranon against the walls of the fossa as full extension is approached.

Rehabilitation for lateral compression injuries is helpful in the early stages of injury but has considerable limitation after osteophytes, loose bodies, and articular cartilage damage have occurred. Therefore the aim should be to detect lateral compression injuries early and to begin rehabilitation before more pronounced changes occur.

Extension Injuries

Extension injuries are relatively common in the throwing sports but especially so in pitchers. Extension injuries are probably secondary to medial tension and lateral compression in that, as noted previously, these two mechanisms cause increased valgus with abnormal wear and tear on the medial side of the olecranon process and articulate cartilage damage on the lateral side because of impaction.

Chronic intermittent overload by the extensor mechanism, however, can in itself result in hypertrophy of the ulna, the humerus, and the triceps muscle. If allowed to continue over a prolonged period of time, hypertrophy of the ulna and distal humerus results in a decrease in the size of the olecranon fossa, thus producing abnormal wear and loose body formation.

REHABILITATION PRINCIPLES

After injury or surgical procedure, initial rehabilitation is directed toward maintaining and regaining a normal range of motion. Gentle, active range of motion includes flexion, extension, pronation, and supination of the forearm. Gentle, slow, passive stretching for both extension and flexion is begun. For the elbow healing from surgery or for those with major soft-tissue or osseous damage such as dislocated elbows, care is taken to avoid early aggressive stretching because of the risk of traumatic myositis ossificans.

Forearm musculature flexibility is improved by passively stretching the extensor musculature (flexion with pronation) and the flexor-pronator group (passive extension with supination).

Initial strengthening is achieved by low-resistance, high-repetition biceps and triceps curls. Pronation and supination are also improved through use of a hammer or similar tool to produce greater torque throughout the range of motion.

Proper technique is emphasized with the patient concentrating on number of repetitions rather than amount of weight lifted.

Finally, grip and shoulder exercises are initiated. For grip, patients may use a tennis ball for frequent isometric exercise. Many other grip devices are adequate as well. The shoulder may be exercised with free weights using a low-weight, high-repetition protocol. Strengthening exercises are conducted in straight anatomic and functional planes. For some individuals, primarily athletes, a well-structured machine program such as Nautilus may be used. Occasionally, in the late postoperative phase of rehabilitation, the elbow may require more aggressive stretching, especially for flexion contracture. Ideally the patient performs this independently, beginning with a good warm-up and then high-repetition exercise, followed by passive stretching with a dumbbell in the affected hand and positioning the elbow to allow for maximal flexor pronator stretch. As is the rule in the ini-

tial postoperative phase, ice is applied immediately after exercise.

Rehabilitation of the elbow focuses on strength and flexibility of the prime movers and stabilizers, as well as on conditioning of the entire upper extremity.

ELBOW REHABILITATION PROGRAMS
The Baltimore Therapeutic Equipment

The Baltimore Therapeutic Equipment (BTE) is a versatile, computerized system that may be used to provide quantitative analysis of the following:
1. Maximal isometric strength
2. Maximal work capacity (strength over time)
3. Maximal vs. submaximal effort

This single compact instrument has a number of attachments and is designed to provide for specific repetitive motions against measurable resistances over a measurable period of time.

A number of different weight-lifting modes may be simulated as well as functional motions that are the key to athletic performance. The machine's capacity is limited only by the imagination of the clinician.

Regarding the elbow, the BTE may be used for the following:
1. Evaluate strength
2. Provide various strength and training modes
3. Simulate athletic activity before return to play

For the competitive athlete the BTE assists the clinician in providing a complete rehabilitation program, and it is an effective adjunct to free weights and machines.

Figs. 19-1 to 19-4 demonstrate the use of the BTE.

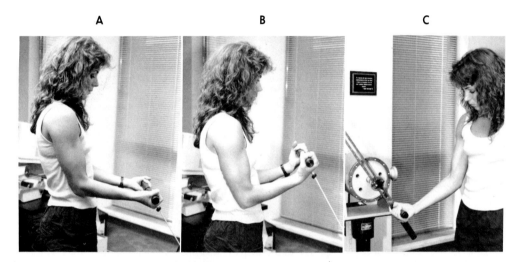

FIG. 19-1. A and **B,** Elbow flexion (pulley method). **C,** BTE evaluation of elbow flexion (bar method).

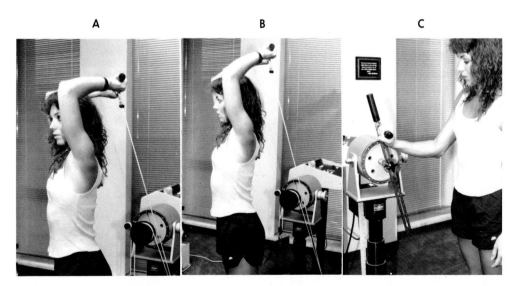

FIG. 19-2. A and **B,** Elbow extension (pulley method). **C,** Elbow extension (bar method) BTE evaluation.

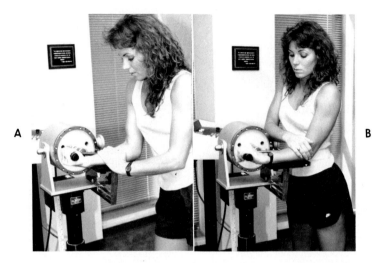

FIG. 19-3. A, Wrist flexion. **B,** BTE evaluation of wrist extension.

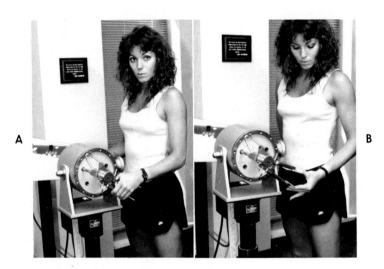

FIG. 19-4. Evaluation of grip **(A)** and pinch grip (BTE) **(B).**

Proprioceptive Neuromuscular Facilitation

Proprioceptive neuromuscular facilitation (PNF) patterns for the upper extremity incorporate elbow, wrist, and hand motion in functional, repetitive, and concentric actions. These patterns allow application of graded resistance by the therapist in functional patterns not applicable by machines. In certain cases of elbow rehabilitation, PNF may be the initial means of beginning a strengthening program as well as providing motion and isometric exercise to other joints in the affected extremity.

Functional Training

Two recent additions to our upper extremity rehabilitation program are the Stairmaster Crossrobics 2650 UE Kayak Conditioning System (Fig. 19-5) and the Stairmaster Gravitron 2000 AT Upper Body Exercise System (Fig. 19-6). These two machines are capable of achiev-

ing a functional training response: (1) precise control of the load (the level of resistance you have to overcome while exercising); (2) a wide range of loads; (3) precise control of velocity (the speed at which you must perform the exercise movement); and (4) a wide range of velocities. This training significantly improves functional capacity by inducing systemic adaptations that increase specific performance-related factors (endurance, speed, strength, and power).

REHABILITATION PROTOCOLS

Specific protocols exist to rehabilitate the competitive athlete, the recreational or weekend athlete, and the active Little League athlete as well.

Program I is designed to rehabilitate the competitive athlete as quickly and effectively as possible through use of the BTE. This requires the patient to be seen in the

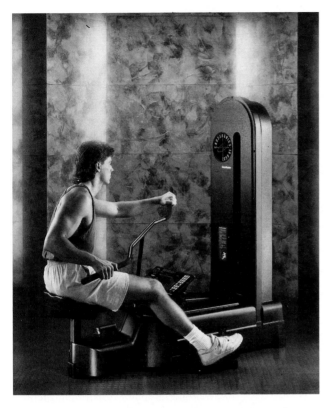

FIG. 19-5. StairMaster Crossrobics 2650 UE Kayak Conditioning System. (Courtesy StairMaster Sports/Medical Products, Inc.)

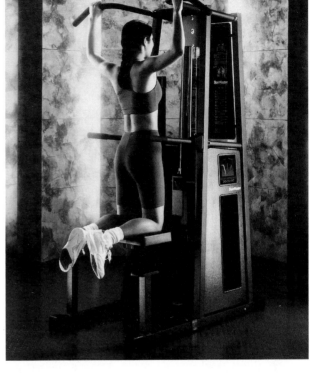

FIG. 19-6. StairMaster Gravitron 2000 AT Upper Body Exercise System. (Courtesy StairMaster Sports/Medical Products, Inc.)

clinic three times per week for intensive work on the BTE, free weights, and machines for total upper body conditioning. Other mechanical devices that can provide a variety of strength-training techniques can also be used.

Program II considers the recreational athlete or amateur who has access to a fitness facility or collegiate training room. In this situation athletes may use free weights at home and the gym, and they may use upper body machines at the fitness facility.

Program III covers a home program for those individuals who do not have easy access to a fitness facility or training room and do not require intensive physical therapy.

Each program achieves the desired result of greater strength, flexibility, and overall performance but is designed to meet the needs of the individual.

Elbow Rehabilitation Program I

I. *Initial evaluation*—includes history and mechanism of injury
  A. BTE strength assessment
    1. Elbow flexion, extension
    2. Wrist flexion, extension
    3. Forearm pronation, supination
    4. Grip
    5. Pinch grip
  B. Grip strength—Jamar hand dynamometer (Fig. 19-7)

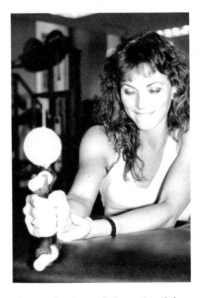

FIG. 19-7. Grip evaluation with Jamar hand dynamometer.

  C. Active range of motion (AROM)
    1. Elbow
    2. Wrist
    3. Fingers
  D. Girth—upper arm and forearm

II. *Exercise program*
A. Specific to elbow and forearm
1. BTE—elbow flexion, extension
2. a. BTE—forearm pronation, supination, flexion, and extension
b. BTE—grip
c. BTE—motion specific to sport (e.g., tennis, baseball, golf)
3. Free weights—low-weight, high-repetition exercise (to alternate with BTE)
a. Elbow flexion, extension—dumbbells 3 sets of 10 repetitions
b. Wrist flexion, extension—light dumbbells, e.g., heavy hands, 3 sets of 10 repetitions
c. Forearm pronation, supination—hammer, tennis racquet, bar weighted at one end 3 sets of 10 repetitions
B. General upper body conditioning
1. Nautilus or exercise machines (e.g., Crossrobics 2650 UE or Gravitron 2000 AT)
a. Shoulder—deltoids, trapezius, shoulder girdle musculature
b. Chest—pectorals, anterior deltoid
c. Arms—forearm curl machine
d. Theraband exercises for shoulder rotator cuff
C. Flexibility
1. Forearm—extensors, flexors
a. Gentle passive stretch
2. Shoulder—anterior, posterior musculature
a. Overhead stretch (for latissimus and extensors)
b. Extension/pectoral stretch for anterior shoulder and chest muscles
c. Horizontal adduction stretch for posterior deltoid and rotator cuff muscles
III. *Modalities*
A. Heat
1. Before beginning exercise
2. Subacute or chronic phase
B. Ice
1. After exercise session for 20 minutes
2. Ice massage—directly to painful area using circular motion for approximately 5 to 10 minutes
3. As needed for pain and swelling control
IV. *Protocol specifics*
A. Frequency—three times per week
B. Location—sports medicine clinic or physical therapy department
C. Duration
1. Approximately 1½ hr visits
2. One month, then reevaluation
D. Reevaluation
1. BTE strength testing
2. Jamar grip testing
3. AROM measurements
E. Conditions necessary for return to play
1. Pain-free
2. Equal strength bilaterally

3. Equal AROM or girth (upper arm and forearm)

Elbow Rehabilitation Program II

I. *Initial evaluation*—includes history and mechanism of injury
A. BTE strength assessment
1. Elbow flexion, extension
2. Wrist flexion, extension
3. Forearm pronation, supination
4. Grip
5. Pinch grip
B. Grip strength—Jamar hand dynamometer
C. AROM measurements
1. Elbow
2. Wrist
3. Fingers
D. Girth—upper arm and forearm
II. *Exercise program*
A. Specific to elbow and forearm
1. Free weights—low weight, high repetition
a. Elbow flexion, extension 3 sets of 10 repetitions
b. Wrist flexion, extension 3 sets of 10 repetitions (beginning with 1 or 2 lb)
c. Forearm pronation, supination 3 sets of 10 repetitions (using a hammer, racquet, or other end-weighted device)
2. Theraband exercises elbow flexion, extension, pronation, supination
B. Upper body conditioning (Figs. 19-8 and 19-9)
1. Nautilus or exercise machines (e.g., Crossrobics 2650 UE or Gravitron 2000 AT)
a. Shoulder—deltoid, trapezius, shoulder girdle musculature, compound shoulder, shoulder shrug, rowing torso combined pullover torso/arm
b. Chest—pectorals, anterior deltoid (combined chest machine)
c. Arms—biceps/triceps machine
2. Theraband—rotator cuff exercise
C. Flexibility—gentle passive stretching
1. Forearm—flexors and extensors
2. Shoulder—anterior and posterior musculature
D. Home program
1. Dumbbells, free weights
2. Theraband
3. Practice sport-specific motions before return to play
III. *Modalities*
A. Heat
1. Before exercise
2. Subacute or chronic phase
B. Ice
1. After exercise for 20 minutes
2. Alternative—ice massage to affected area 5 to 10 minutes
3. As needed for pain control

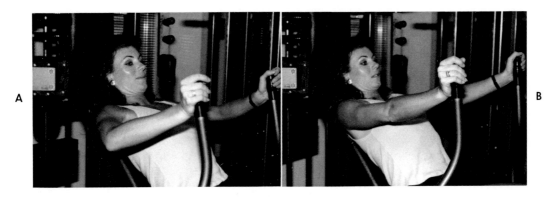

FIG. 19-8. Chest press on Nautilus equipment.

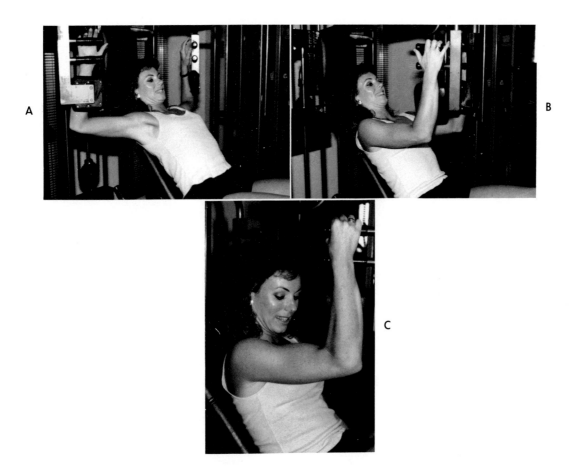

FIG. 19-9. Pectoral flys on Nautilus equipment.

IV. *Protocol specifics*
  A. Frequency
    1. Daily home program every day at first; as weight increases, decrease to program three times per week
    2. Clinic, training room, gym—three times per week
  B. Location
    1. Clinic, training room
    2. Home
  C. Duration
    1. 1-hour gym visits
    2. Approximately 30 minutes home program
  D. Reevaluation
    1. BTE strength test
    2. Grip strength—Jamar hand dynamometer
    3. AROM measurements
  E. Conditions necessary for return to play
    1. Pain-free
    2. Equal strength bilaterally (or within 10%)
    3. Equal AROM and/or girth of upper arm and forearm

Elbow Rehabilitation Program III

I. *Initial evaluation*—includes history and mechanism
  A. BTE strength assessment—as time permits
    1. Elbow, wrist, forearm musculature
    2. Grip
  B. Grip strength—Jamar hand dynamometer
  C. AROM measurements
  D. Girth—upper arm and forearm
II. *Exercise program*
  A. Specific to elbow and forearm
    1. Free weights—low-weight, high-repetition dumbbells, heavy hands
      a. Elbow flexion, extension 3 sets of 10 repetitions (Fig. 19-10)
      b. Wrist flexion, extension 3 sets of 10 repetitions (Fig. 19-11)
      c. Forearm pronation, supination 3 sets of 10 repetitions (Fig. 19-12)
    2. Theraband—isometric resistive exercise
      a. Elbow flexion, extension 3 sets of 10 repetitions

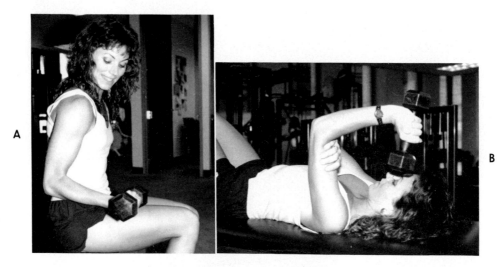

FIG. 19-10. A, Elbow flexion using free weights. **B,** Elbow extension using free weights.

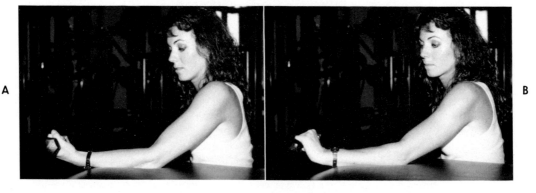

FIG. 19-11. A, Wrist flexion with free weights. **B,** Wrist extension with free weights.

b. Forearm pronation, supination 3 sets of 10 repetitions
B. Upper body conditioning
  1. Free weights
    a. Shoulder
      (1) Super 7 progressive resistive exercises: active resistive straight plan range of motion
      (2) Shrugs
  2. Theraband
    a. Rotator cuffs—internal and external rotation
C. Flexibility—gentle, passive stretching
  1. Forearm—flexors and extensors
  2. Shoulder—anterior, posterior musculature
D. Sports
  1. Practice motion of sport-specific activity
  2. Gradual return to play

III. *Modalities*
  A. Heat—as needed before exercise or sport
  B. Ice
    1. After exercise or sport for 20 minutes
    2. Alternative—ice massage to affected area 5 to 10 minutes
    3. As needed for pain control
IV. *Protocol specifics*
  A. Frequency—daily home program (daily initially; as weights increase, decrease frequency to three times per week)
  B. Location—home
  C. Duration—once per day, approximately 30 to 45 minutes
  D. Reevaluation
    1. BTE strength test (if performed initially)
    2. Grip strength—Jamar hand dynamometer
    3. AROM measurements

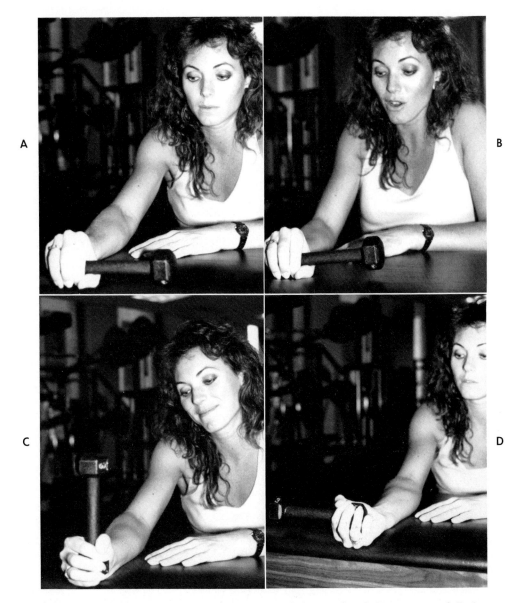

FIG. 19-12. Forearm exercises. **A** and **B,** Pronation with free weights. **C,** Forearm neutral. **D,** Supination with free weights.

E. Conditions necessary for return to play
1. Pain-free
2. Equal strength bilaterally (or within 10%)
3. Equal AROM and/or girth of upper arm and forearm

HOME REHABILITATION PROGRAMS

An important component of any elbow rehabilitation program is the home program. These programs are designed to allow the athlete to gain strength and flexibility with the use of minimal equipment. The home program reinforces the exercise regimen performed at the rehabilitation center and prevents regression of the athlete's progress by avoiding days in inactivity. Home programs are often designed to meet specific rehabilitation needs. Often a general program can be used and portions of it tailored to meet each patient's needs. A more specific program is often used for lateral tennis elbow.

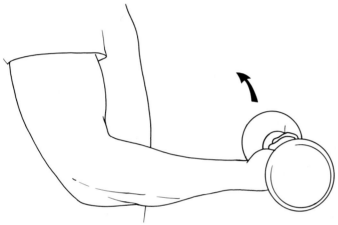

General Home Elbow Program

1. *Elbow flexion (curls)*—Weight in hand; arm at side; slowly bend elbow, bring hand to the palm-up position. Hold 2 to 3 seconds, return to starting position. Three sets of 10 repetitions.

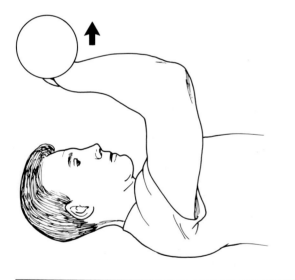

2. *Elbow extension (triceps curls)*—Supine; arm raised toward ceiling; weight in hand; support arm with opposite hand. Slowly allow elbow to bend, then straighten elbow out; return to bent position to start again. Three sets of 10 repetitions (Fig. 19-10, *B*).

3. *Forearm pronation/supination*—Grasp hammer (or similar light resistance); forearm supported; rotate hand to palm down position; return to starting position and rotate to palm-up position. Return to starting position; repeat 3 sets 10 repetitions (Fig. 19-10).

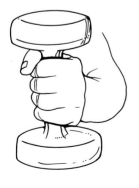 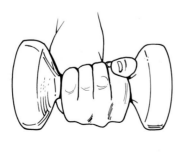 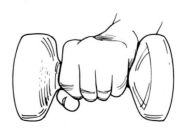

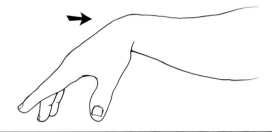

4. *Forearm stretching*—With arm in extended position, palm down, apply pressure to back of hand; feel stretch along top of forearm.

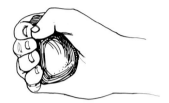

5. *Gripping exercise*—Carry an old tennis ball or other grip device and grip it frequently.

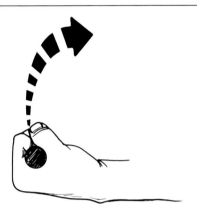

6. *Wrist curls and extensions*—Weight in hand, forearm supported, bend wrist in palm-up position, then palm down. Three sets 10 repetitions.
   Wrist flexion—Place the wrist in a palm-up position, supported at the edge of a table or on your knee, so that only the hand is allowed to move. Grasp the weighted dumbbell (2 lb) or weighted bag. Perform the exercise as follows:
   a. Flex (bend upward) the wrist as far as possible.
   b. Hold 2 to 3 seconds.
   c. Lower fully; repeat up to 15 repetitions.
   d. Increase weight if 15 proper repetitions can be performed with no pain at the site of injury.
      Wrist extension—Performed in similar fashion to flex exercise except palm faces down. Start with 2 lb.

Home Rehabilitation for Tennis Elbow
Hot or Cold

Using either ice or moist heat can provide relief from pain. Both have similar physiologic responses that are desired. Therefore use the modality in small time quantities, *although often.*

Ice is recommended for an acute, inflamed stage. Moist heat may be more comfortable for a chronic, sore period. (You can be in an acute stage even though the injury has been around for a long time.) Perform ice massage (water frozen in a paper cup) right on the area of pain for 5 minutes. Use moist heat (hot towels) as above for 5 minutes.

Stretching

Extend arm, straighten elbow. Let hand fall palm down. Grasp involved hand with noninvolved hand and pull down, bending wrist. You should feel a pull along the top of the forearm and into the area of pain. Hold for a count of 20; repeat five times.

Exercise

With elbow bent and wrist supported do the following:
1. Weight held in hand. Palm down. Raise wrist/hand up slowly and lower slowly.

2. Palm up. Bend wrist up slowly; lower slowly.
3. Thumb up. Bend wrist up.
For all exercises do 20 repetitions three to five times a day. Begin with 1 lb and *increase as tolerated.*
   1. Stretch again.
   2. Ice again.
   3. Also, squeeze tennis ball throughout the day.
   4. Take lessons, if appropriate.
   5. Check handle grip and size and weight of racquet.

PREVENTION OF ELBOW AND SHOULDER PROBLEMS

Over the years we have developed a set of guidelines that we give to our throwing athletes to prevent elbow and shoulder problems. These apply for young athletes, recreational athletes, and professional athletes. These guidelines include the following:
   1. Begin warm-up early enough to avoid being hurried.
   2. Adjust warm-up period to weather conditions.
   3. Gradually work up to maximal efficiency.
   4. Concentrate on complete relaxation following each pitch.
   5. Do not expose pitching arm to draft.
      a. Wear long-sleeved sweat shirt.
      b. Wear jacket when not pitching.

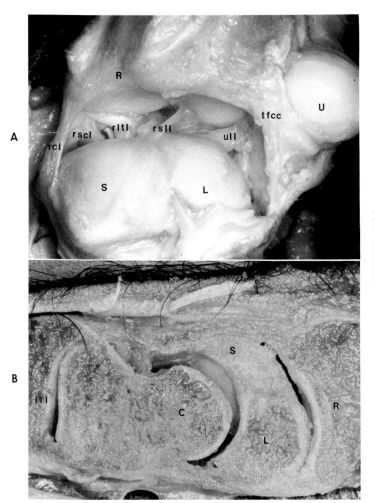

FIG. 21-3. **A,** Dorsal view of palmar radiocarpal ligaments. **B,** Sagittal section through center of capitate to illustrate thickness and attachments of palmar ligaments. *C,* Capitate; *L,* lunate; *R,* radius; *rcl,* radial collateral ligament; *rltl,* radiolunate triquetral ligament; *rscl,* radioscaphocapitate ligament; *rsll,* radioscapholunate ligament; *S,* scaphoid; *tfcc,* triangular fibrocartilage complex; *U,* ulna; *ull,* ulnolunate ligament.

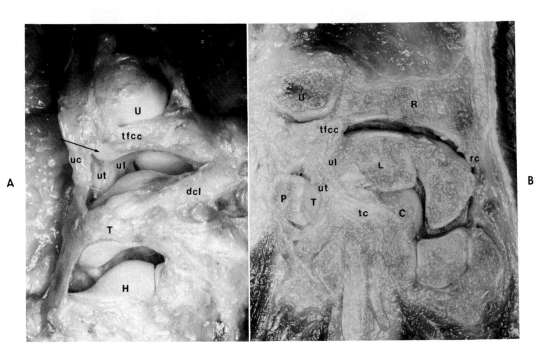

FIG. 21-4. **A,** Dorsal view of ulnar wrist joints and ligaments. **B,** Palmar aspect of ulnocarpal ligaments. *C,* Capitate; *dcl,* dorsal radiocarpal ligaments; *H,* hamate; *L,* lunate; *P,* pisiform; *R,* radius; *rc,* radial collateral ligament; *T,* triquetrum; *tfcc,* triangular fibrocartilage complex; *uc,* ulnar collateral ligament; *ul,* ulnolunate ligament; *ut,* ulnotriquetral ligament, continues as *tc,* triquetral capitate ligament; *arrow,* ulnar styloid.

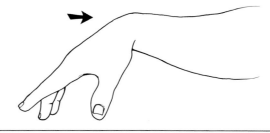

4. *Forearm stretching*—With arm in extended position, palm down, apply pressure to back of hand; feel stretch along top of forearm.

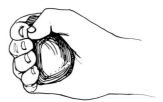

5. *Gripping exercise*—Carry an old tennis ball or other grip device and grip it frequently.

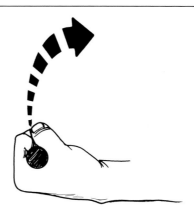

6. *Wrist curls and extensions*—Weight in hand, forearm supported, bend wrist in palm-up position, then palm down. Three sets 10 repetitions.

Wrist flexion—Place the wrist in a palm-up position, supported at the edge of a table or on your knee, so that only the hand is allowed to move. Grasp the weighted dumbbell (2 lb) or weighted bag. Perform the exercise as follows:

a. Flex (bend upward) the wrist as far as possible.
b. Hold 2 to 3 seconds.
c. Lower fully; repeat up to 15 repetitions.
d. Increase weight if 15 proper repetitions can be performed with no pain at the site of injury.

Wrist extension—Performed in similar fashion to flex exercise except palm faces down. Start with 2 lb.

Home Rehabilitation for Tennis Elbow
Hot or Cold

Using either ice or moist heat can provide relief from pain. Both have similar physiologic responses that are desired. Therefore use the modality in small time quantities, *although often.*

Ice is recommended for an acute, inflamed stage. Moist heat may be more comfortable for a chronic, sore period. (You can be in an acute stage even though the injury has been around for a long time.) Perform ice massage (water frozen in a paper cup) right on the area of pain for 5 minutes. Use moist heat (hot towels) as above for 5 minutes.

Stretching

Extend arm, straighten elbow. Let hand fall palm down. Grasp involved hand with noninvolved hand and pull down, bending wrist. You should feel a pull along the top of the forearm and into the area of pain. Hold for a count of 20; repeat five times.

Exercise

With elbow bent and wrist supported do the following:
1. Weight held in hand. Palm down. Raise wrist/hand up slowly and lower slowly.

2. Palm up. Bend wrist up slowly; lower slowly.
3. Thumb up. Bend wrist up.

For all exercises do 20 repetitions three to five times a day. Begin with 1 lb and *increase as tolerated.*
1. Stretch again.
2. Ice again.
3. Also, squeeze tennis ball throughout the day.
4. Take lessons, if appropriate.
5. Check handle grip and size and weight of racquet.

PREVENTION OF ELBOW AND SHOULDER PROBLEMS

Over the years we have developed a set of guidelines that we give to our throwing athletes to prevent elbow and shoulder problems. These apply for young athletes, recreational athletes, and professional athletes. These guidelines include the following:
1. Begin warm-up early enough to avoid being hurried.
2. Adjust warm-up period to weather conditions.
3. Gradually work up to maximal efficiency.
4. Concentrate on complete relaxation following each pitch.
5. Do not expose pitching arm to draft.
   a. Wear long-sleeved sweat shirt.
   b. Wear jacket when not pitching.

6. Do not attempt to pitch in presence of illness, injury, or when under undue mental tension.
7. Report shoulder or elbow pain immediately and discontinue pitching until after complete evaluation. (Under proper circumstances, you may be able to play another position.)
8. Do not practice throwing at home.
9. Do not shag fly balls and throw them in from the outfield if you are not properly warmed up.
10. Do not pitch more often than the league rules permit.
11. Do not pitch in more than one league.
12. After any layoff, regardless of cause or duration, be sure to resume activity gradually and do not attempt to throw hard or in a game until full recovery has been reached.

RETURN-TO-SPORTS CRITERIA

Return-to-sports activity follows a sequence much like the rehabilitation program. Initially the motion necessary for the specific sport is performed without weight, with the athlete monitoring technique in the mirror and paying close attention to detail. In the throwing sports, once pain is gone, throwing is allowed, with a gradual increase in the amount of time spent throwing. Again, technique is of the utmost importance in this phase. If over the course of several sessions pain does not recur, the athlete may begin to increase velocity. Throughout this final phase, as during early rehabilitation, there must be adequate warm-up, exercise (sport), and cool-down phases. The importance of a general conditioning program cannot be overemphasized. As early as possible with a given injury to the elbow, patients are strongly encouraged to maintain or increase their aerobic fitness and strength of the sound extremities. This facilitates a safe and rapid return to athletic competition or recreational activities.

SUMMARY

The elbow allows for fairly simple and direct methods of rehabilitation because four basic motions are present. On a more subtle level is the soft-tissue response to trauma about the elbow. Hence the clinician must pay close attention to any change in level of pain, any reproducible pain, or minimal changes in range of motion. These may be indicators of early myositis ossificans, irritation of the ulnar nerve in the cubital tunnel, or the radial nerve in the arcade of Frohse. Most often, discontinuing the aggravating activity resolves the pain.

CHAPTER 20 Athletic Training and Protective Equipment

Robert C. Reese, Jr.
T. Pepper Burruss
Joseph Patten

A variety of elbow injuries in the athlete can be managed with application of appropriate taping and protective padding. These techniques are an adjunct to the usual modes of treatment of both acute and chronic elbow injuries. These modalities can permit an earlier return to sports if used in a judicious manner and monitored by trained sports medicine personnel.

TAPING TECHNIQUES

Athletic tape can be used at the elbow for hyperextension injuries or as part of treatment for mild valgus injuries. In both instances tape is applied to restrict an undesired motion. For moderate to severe injuries, in which a significant limited range of motion is required, a plastic orthosis with hinges may be more appropriate.

In general, elbow-taping techniques work best after the swelling has resolved. Taping is then used to protect the athlete on return to participation. At all times close supervision of the athlete is maintained because neurovascular problems can potentially arise with elbow injuries and their treatment.

Hyperextension Injuries

The hyperextension taping technique is designed to limit elbow extension after a hyperextension injury. It is a useful technique in mild injuries and provides mild restriction of elbow extension.

Technique

The arm is usually shaved from the shoulder to the wrist. A pad is placed in the crease of the elbow after pe-

troleum jelly has been applied to the undersurface of the pad (Fig. 20-1). This lubricated pad prevents tape burns around the flexion crease of the elbow. Tape adhesive spray is next applied to the surrounding area to provide better adherence of the tape and underwrap material to the skin.

Underwrap material is placed circumferentially around the elbow, beginning distally at the midforearm and continuing proximally to the midarm (Fig. 20-2). Anchor strips are applied with elastic tape on the proximal and distal portions of the underwrap (Fig. 20-3).

The elbow is held at approximately 30 degrees, and crossing strips (x-strips) of standard cloth adhesive tape are applied along the anterior (flexion) portion of the elbow (Fig. 20-4, *A*). These strips, which cross the elbow anteriorly, limit elbow extension by virtue of their application with the elbow held in flexion. These crossing strips, or checkreins, are applied in an alternating fashion until the anterior aspect of the elbow is covered (Fig. 20-4, *B*).

Anchor strips of cloth adhesive tape are now placed on the elbow in a circumferential fashion, at both the midpoint of the arm and midpoint of the forearm, to anchor the checkreins at the proximal and distal limits of the tape job (Fig. 20-5).

A layer of elastic tape is now used to secure and solidify the entire tape application. The elastic tape is applied circumferentially from distal to proximal as one continuous, overlapping strip of tape (Fig. 20-6). A short piece of cloth tape is placed proximally to affix the elastic tape in place at the proximal portion of the tape job.

This completed taping technique permits elbow flexion but limits elbow extension as a result of the cloth adhesive tape applied anteriorly on the elbow with the elbow in a flexed position.

Variations

The checkrein pattern (cloth adhesive butterfly) can be prepared ahead of time to facilitate the application of the tape job in the locker room (Fig. 20-7). This is accomplished by applying the adhesive tape in the crossing pattern onto a smooth, clean surface that allows the tape to be carefully lifted off as a single unit after completion of the taping scheme. The entire checkrein unit

347

FIG. 20-1. Lubricated pad is placed in elbow flexion crease to prevent tape burns.

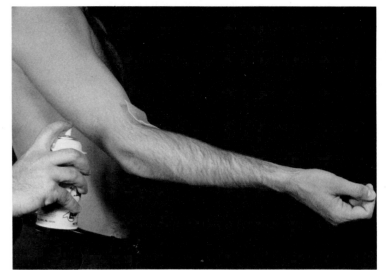

FIG. 20-2. Underwrap applied.

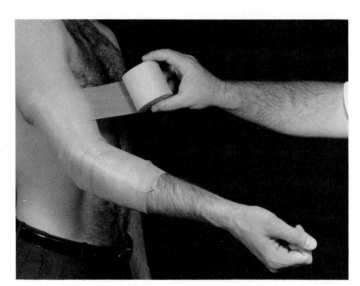

FIG. 20-3. Anchor strips at proximal and distal limits of tape area.

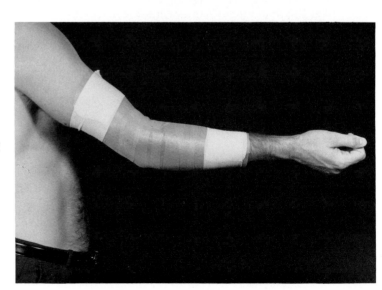

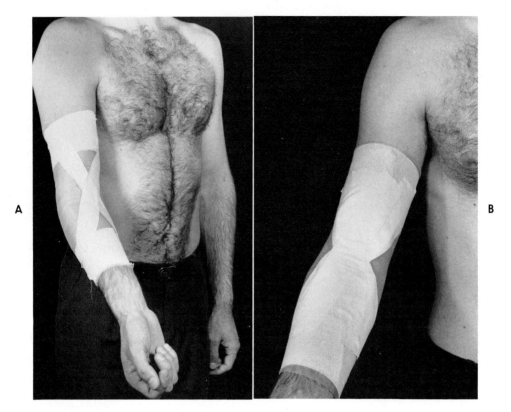

FIG. 20-4. A, Checkreins (x-strips) applied anteriorly to limit extension. **B,** Elbow is covered anteriorly with a series of checkreins.

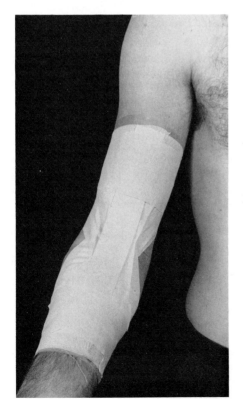

FIG. 20-5. Anchor strips applied at midpoint of arm and forearm to secure checkreins.

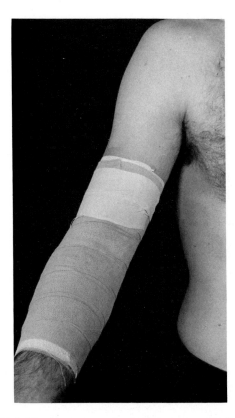

FIG. 20-6. Elastic tape is used to bind entire tape application.

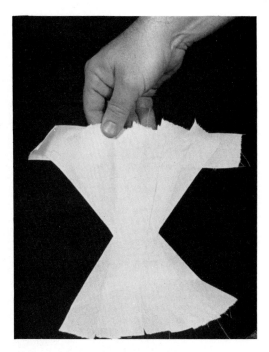

FIG. 20-7. Tape butterfly or x pattern of checkreins can be prepared on a smooth, clean surface to facilitate application.

can then be applied directly to the arm and anchored in place as previously described.

Another technique variation includes the use of a crimped piece of cloth adhesive tape to provide additional bulk and strength to the tape technique. This crimped strip is placed longitudinally along the anterior aspect of the elbow (Fig. 20-8) and is secured with anchor strips at the proximal and distal portions of the tape. A small space can initially be left between the body of the tape job and the crimped piece of tape. This crimped tape is then incorporated into the entire tape job.

The use of moleskin can also improve the ability of the taping technique to restrict extension. Moleskin can be costly, however, and its use is recommended when budget considerations permit. The moleskin is applied as an anterior longitudinal checkrein across the flexion crease (Fig. 20-9). After application of the moleskin, elastic tape is used circumferentially to hold the moleskin in place. The key to this technique is making certain the moleskin is well anchored proximally and distally by cloth adhesive tape.

In addition to a direct longitudinal anterior strut, x-shaped checkreins can also be fabricated out of 1½-inch moleskin. These are applied in a similar fashion as an x-shaped checkrein made from cloth tape but in a smaller number because the moleskin cannot conform as well as the less bulky elastic tape. The moleskin ends should overlap to have the moleskin adhere to the previous strip and provide integrity to the tape technique. As additional layers of moleskin are added, the flexibility of

the elbow is diminished because of the bulk and strength of the moleskin. This provides the greatest limitation of elbow extension possible with taping and provides great stability and integrity of the taping technique. Of course, as with the use of moleskin in any fashion, elastic tape is applied to seal the entire tape job.

Medial and Lateral Elbow Support

Occasionally, elbow taping techniques can enhance treatment of mild valgus elbow injuries. This is appropriate in situations in which minimal laxity is present, swelling is not readily apparent, and protective support without great bulk is desired.

For this technique longitudinal strips (checkreins) are applied along the medial or lateral aspect of the elbow. This is done after the standard preparation and prewrapping of the elbow (Fig. 20-10). If protection against valgus forces is sought, the longitudinal strips are placed medially. If varus protection is the goal, the strips should be applied along the lateral side of the elbow. These strips can provide some support to the elbow when external valgus or varus loads are applied. For situations in which moderate or great forces are anticipated, however, more stability and protection are offered by a hinged orthosis and the orthosis is the better choice.

PROTECTIVE EQUIPMENT
Elbow Pads

Elbow pads are some of the most basic and frequently used protective pads in athletic participation (Fig. 20-11). Essentially, the pads provide cushioning for the portions of the elbow that can be injured by direct contact.

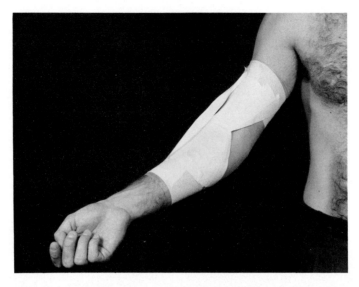

FIG. 20-8. Crimped adhesive tape applied anteriorly for additional strength.

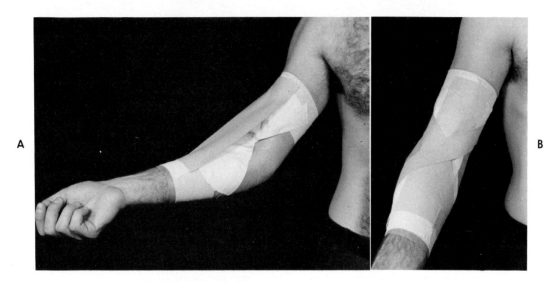

FIG. 20-9. A and **B,** Moleskin applied anteriorly for strength.

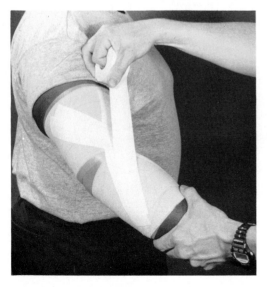

FIG. 20-10. Checkreins applied medially or laterally can provide some support to resist varus or valgus stress.

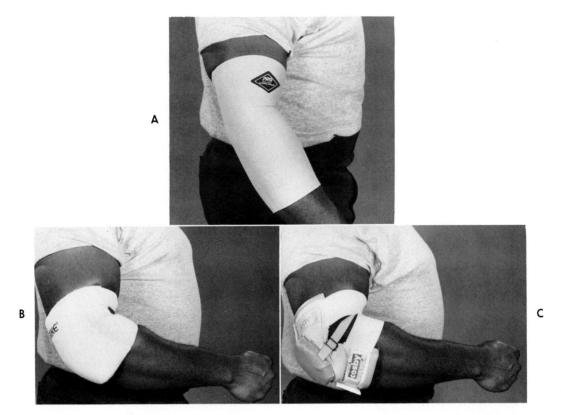

FIG. 20-11. Elbow pads are designed to protect the olecranon bursa and proximal ulna. **A,** Neoprene. **B,** Cloth and foam. **C,** Leather, foam, and cloth.

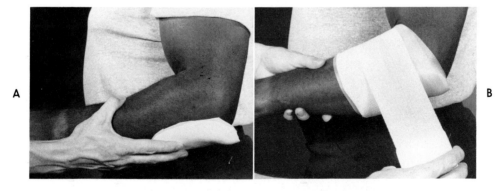

FIG. 20-12. A, Hard plastic shell can be fabricated to protect the proximal ulna. **B,** Care must be taken to allow elbow motion.

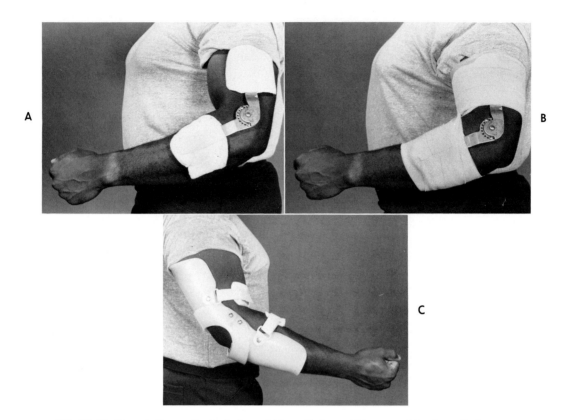

FIG. 20-13. Hinged elbow orthosis. **A,** Lateral hinge. **B,** Lateral hinge taped in place. **C,** Posterior hard shell with elbow hinge.

Most commonly, the olecranon bursa is the site of the contusion and traumatic bursitis, so the bulk of the padding is concentrated posteriorly.

Most elbow pads are a combination of foam rubber and elastic. A variety of foam densities are available, from very light open and closed cell foam rubbers to dense viscoelastic polymers such as Sorbothane. Some pads incorporate donut-shaped foam rings that provide more protection to the region.

Occasionally, a hard shell pad that takes repeated contact over the proximal ulna and olecranon process is needed for an athlete. These can be custom fabricated with thermomoldable plastic, such as Orthoplast, and built with appropriate padding and relief areas (Fig. 20-12). They are fixed in place with circumferential elastic and cloth adhesive tape around the forearm. The shells are not taped proximal to the elbow flexion crease, so as to permit elbow motion.

Great care should be taken in selecting prefabricated elbow pads or in fabricating a hard shell for elbow protection. Ill-fitting pads provide little or no protection if they slip up or down the arm. Pads with too much bulk anteriorly limit elbow flexion and restrict the athlete. The choice of pads should ultimately take into consideration the sport, the athlete's size, and the athlete's needs in terms of protective capability.

Elbow Orthoses

Hinged elbow orthoses can be extremely useful in athletics. Most commonly, these braces are used following a hyperextension sprain or a posterior elbow dislocation. In this setting the orthosis can be used to permit flexion and limit elbow extension, protecting the anterior structures (capsule and tendons) from further injury.

Orthoses can be designed with medial and lateral hinges or with either a single medial or a single lateral hinge (Fig. 20-13). Double-hinged orthoses provide the most rigidity and are often used initially following injury. Often the medial hinge is removed to permit the athlete easier use of the arm, while the lateral hinge is left in place. In any case these metal hinges need to be adequately padded to prevent injury to other athletes.

The hinges often are adjustable, and the range of motion desired can be set by the treating individual. Hinged orthoses can be built as a unit, with permanently attached plastic shells for securing the hinge to the extremity. The hinge itself can be applied with underwrap and athletic tape if less bulk is desired.

PART IV Wrist and Hand

CHAPTER 21

Anatomy of the Forearm, Wrist, and Hand

George P. Bogumill

SKIN AND SUBCUTANEOUS TISSUE
Forearm

The skin of the forearm is thick and hairy on the dorsal radial aspect and fairly thin and hairless on the ulnar flexor aspect. The amount of subcutaneous fat varies greatly among individuals and is held loosely to the deep fascia by the vessels and nerves that penetrate the fascia to extend into the subcutaneous tissue and skin. The subcutaneous fat and overlying skin strip readily from the deep fascial layer. Most of the veins and lymphatics draining the hand travel in this subcutaneous layer, as do the superficial sensory nerves.

Dorsal Hand

The skin of the hand is frequently injured because of its exposed position; it is the most frequently unprotected point of contact of the body with the environment. The skin on the dorsum of the hand is loose and elastic to allow for the increased length needed for simultaneous flexion of wrist and digits. The larger surface area needed during flexion must be considered when placing skin grafts on the dorsum of the hand. The flexible elastic skin over the dorsum of the hand and fingers, particularly over the metacarpophalangeal joints, tears easily because of its thinness and lack of deep attachments. Between the skin and extensor tendons lies the subcutaneous space, a potential space with sparse fatty subcutaneous tissue that readily fills with lymphatic fluid and accounts for the major dorsal swelling following any trauma, infection, or other insult to the hand or fingers. In this subcutaneous space over the dorsum of the hand lie the dorsal venous arches; draining them are the major veins extending proximally into the forearm.

Palmar Hand

On the palm of the hand the skin is thick, hairless, and usually callused to varying degrees. It has numerous nerve endings and sweat glands. It is held in place during grasp by numerous short vertical fibrous septa extending from the palmar aponeurosis into the deeper layers of the skin (Fig. 21-1). The blood supply to palmar skin is conveyed by numerous short vessels that pass through the palmar aponeurosis with the fibrous septa. Skin loss is common after traumatic shearing or surgical elevation of palmar skin flaps for transposition.

The palmar aponeurosis has longitudinal fibers that run from the wrist crease to the skin of the distal palm with extensions to the side of the proximal phalanges. Eight septa pass from the deep surface to anchor the aponeurosis to the anterior interosseous fascia and form canals for lumbrical muscles, digital vessels, and nerves (Fig. 21-7).

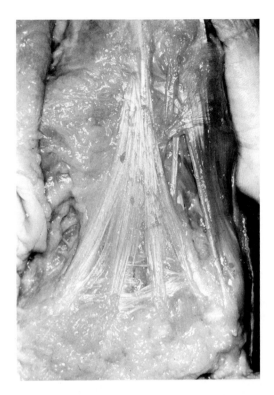

FIG. 21-1. Palmar aponeurosis. Longitudinal fibers begin as a continuation of the palmaris longus and end in the palmar skin over the metacarpophalangeal joint. Transverse fibers are present at the level of the distal palmar crease and the finger webs. The numerous small nubbins remaining on the anterior surface are the cut ends of septa and vessels that anchor and nourish the palmar skin.

Digits

The palmar skin of the digits is also thicker and less distensible than the dorsal skin. It is held in place primarily by the retaining ligaments of the digits (Cleland[4] and Grayson[7]) on the midlateral line of the fingers.[11] The pulp of the finger in the distal segment is held in place by numerous septa and blood vessels connecting the skin to the periosteum of the distal phalanx. This effectively provides padding of the end of the finger without slippage of the skin during grasp. The skin of the fingertip has numerous nerve endings of different types, sensitive to pressure, light touch, and pain.

On the dorsum of the terminal segment of the finger are the nail bed and plate. The nail bed is thin, with its deeper layers continuous with the periosteum of the distal phalanx. The nail bed and matrix are readily torn when the phalanx is fractured, resulting in open contaminated fractures with the proximal portion of the nail displaced over the eponychium.

BONES AND JOINTS
Forearm

The skeleton of the forearm is composed of the radius and the ulna, which are attached firmly to each other in a way that allows smooth rotation of the forearm through an arc of 180 degrees. At the proximal end they are attached by the annular and quadrate ligaments, which hold the radial head against the proximal ulna; the combination articulates with the humerus to form the elbow joint. They also articulate at their distal ends to form the distal radioulnar joint separated from the radiocarpal joint by the triangular fibrocartilage complex (TFCC) (Fig. 21-2, B). A major component holding the two bones together in all positions of elbow flexion and forearm rotation is the interosseous membrane, recently demonstrated to have a thick condensation in its central portion that remains taut in all positions of forearm rotation.

There is intense interest at present in the relative lengths of the radius and the ulna, particularly as related to Kienböck's disease, and many operations have been devised to adjust their length and relationship to the carpus and to each other. Whether these operations will stand the test of time is uncertain.

Wrist

The wrist is the region that connects the distal forearm to the hand. Its boundaries are somewhat imprecise, depending on the purposes of description. It consists of the distal radius and ulna, the proximal ends of the five metacarpals, and the eight intercalated carpal bones, conventionally described in two rows of four bones each (Fig. 21-2, A and B). The eight bones also have been described and evaluated kinematically as being arranged in columns[16]; these are less obvious anatomically.

The carpal bones are bound to each other, and to the radius and metacarpals (Fig. 21-2, B and C), by a complex array of ligaments that are difficult to define (Figs. 21-3 and 21-4). These ligaments show a fair amount of variability from wrist to wrist and are given a variety of names by different authors.[9,14,17] The mobility of the wrist is determined by the shapes of the bones making up this complex, as well as by the attachments and lengths of the various ligaments.[10] This complex osteoligamentous array allows a large range of motion limited at the extremes by a combination of bony shape and ligamentous attachment. With the exception of the pisiform, there are no muscles originating or inserting directly onto the carpal bones. Therefore wrist movements are purely passive, being both permitted and restrained by the complex shape and ligamentous attachments of the various bones; the carpus acts as a freely moving intercalated segment between forearm and hand. The long wrist flexors and extensors cross the carpus to insert into the metacarpal bases. Thus the position of the wrist at any given moment depends on a summation of forces applied by muscle pull, external resistance, the osseous configuration, and ligament attachments.[8,17] The axes of flexion-extension and radial-ulnar deviation pass through the head of the capitate.

Large portions of the surface of the carpal bones are covered with articular cartilage (Fig. 21-5). The ligamentous attachments are the sites for vascular access to nourish the individual carpal bones. When these ligaments are disrupted, the vessels frequently are also disrupted, with variable effects on the individual bones.

The fibrous capsule, lined by synovium, divides the

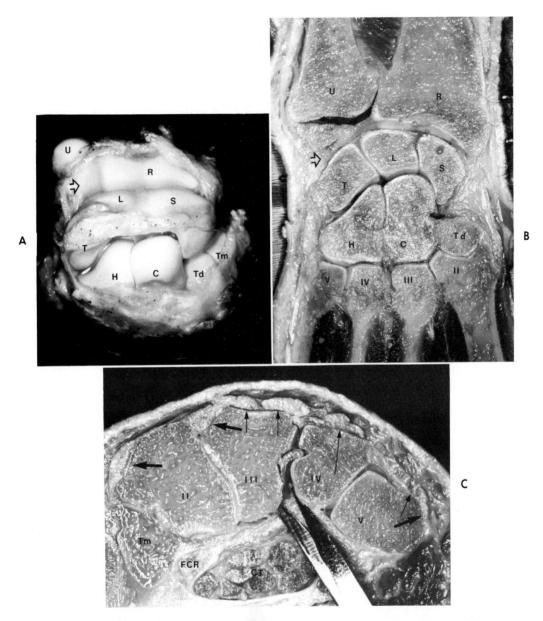

FIG. 21-2. A, Dorsal view of radiocarpal and midcarpal joints. Proximal surfaces of scaphoid, lunate, and triquetrum are joined by intercarpal ligaments that separate radiocarpal and midcarpal joints. **B,** Coronal section through midcarpus. Intercarpal ligaments bind carpals together in proximal and distal rows. Triangular fibrocartilage complex separates distal radioulnar from radiocarpal joint. Note ununited ulnar styloid. **C,** Transverse section through bases of second through fifth metacarpals to illustrate strong interosseous ligaments and proximal palmar arch. *C,* capitate, *CT,* carpal tunnel; *FCR,* flexor carpi radialis; *H,* hamate; *L,* lunate; *R,* radius; *S,* scaphoid; *T,* triquetrum; *Tm,* trapezium; *Td,* trapezoid; *U,* ulna; *heavy arrows,* wrist extensors; *light arrows,* finger extensors; *open arrow,* triangular fibrocartilage complex; *II* to *V,* metacarpals.

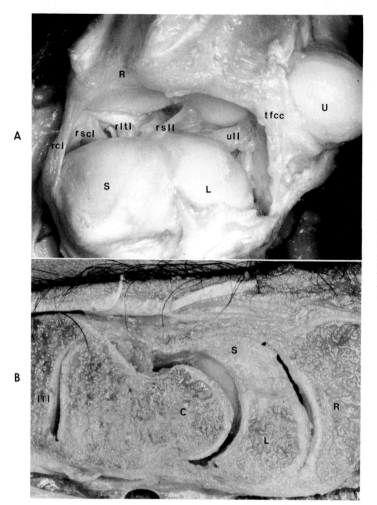

FIG. 21-3. A, Dorsal view of palmar radiocarpal ligaments. **B,** Sagittal section through center of capitate to illustrate thickness and attachments of palmar ligaments. *C,* Capitate; *L,* lunate; *R,* radius; *rcl,* radial collateral ligament; *rltl,* radiolunate triquetral ligament; *rscl,* radioscaphocapitate ligament; *rsll,* radioscapholunate ligament; *S,* scaphoid; *tfcc,* triangular fibrocartilage complex; *U,* ulna; *ull,* ulnolunate ligament.

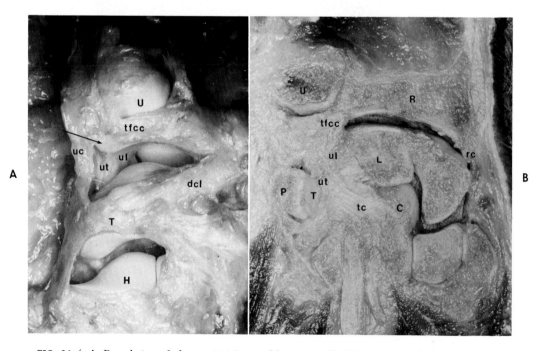

FIG. 21-4. A, Dorsal view of ulnar wrist joints and ligaments. **B,** Palmar aspect of ulnocarpal ligaments. *C,* Capitate; *dcl,* dorsal radiocarpal ligaments; *H,* hamate; *L,* lunate; *P,* pisiform; *R,* radius; *rc,* radial collateral ligament; *T,* triquetrum; *tfcc,* triangular fibrocartilage complex; *uc,* ulnar collateral ligament; *ul,* ulnolunate ligament; *ut,* ulnotriquetral ligament, continues as *tc,* triquetral capitate ligament; *arrow,* ulnar styloid.

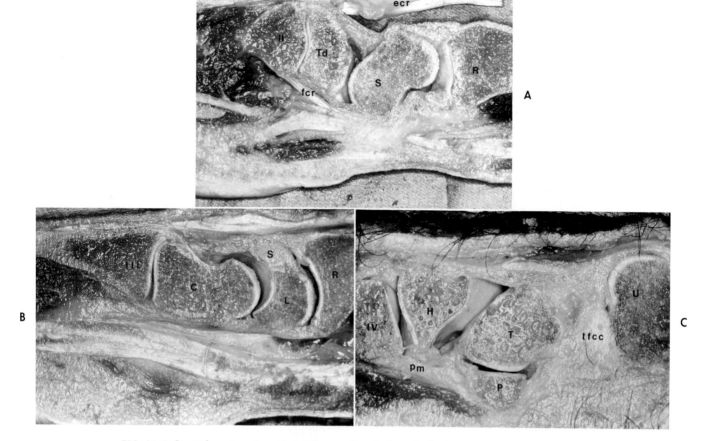

FIG. 21-5. Sagittal sections through radial, central, and ulnar thirds of wrist joint to illustrate carpal relationships and ligaments. **A,** Section through scaphoid. Note insertion of flexor carpi radialis into base of second metacarpal. **B,** Section through capitolunate joint. **C,** Section through triquetrohamate joint. *C,* Capitate; *ecr,* extensor carpi radialis longus and brevis; *fcr,* flexor carpi radialis; *H,* hamate; *L,* lunate; *P,* pisiform; *pm,* pisometacarpal ligament; *R,* radius; *S,* scaphoid; *Td,* trapezoid; *T,* triquetrum; *tfcc,* triangular fibrocartilage complex; *U,* ulna; *II, III,* and *IV,* metacarpals.

complex into a series of joints that are separate from each other in the normal wrist but may communicate as the individual ages (e.g., distal radioulnar joint with the radiocarpal joint).[13]

Hand

The metacarpal region of the hand is somewhat longer than the carpal area and comprises most of the length and breadth of the palm and dorsum of the hand. The first, fourth, and fifth metacarpals are mobile at their basilar attachment, whereas the second and third metacarpals are relatively immobile and constitute the so-called fixed point of the hand. The shape of the metacarpals and their relationships to the carpus provide for a longitudinal arch as well as two transverse arches, one at the base of the metacarpals, which are firmly anchored to each other by short interosseous ligaments and joint capsules (Fig. 21-2, *C*), and one at the metacarpal heads. These arches are primarily adaptive in function and allow the palm of the hand to be placed around objects of

varying sizes and to still maintain contact and grasp. When the fingers are flexed individually, their tips are directed toward the tuberosity of the scaphoid, a useful bit of information that allows determination and control of rotation during fracture treatment. This distal transverse arch is flattened when all fingers are flexed simultaneously.

Digits

Metacarpophalangeal Joints

There are three phalanges in each finger and two in the thumb. The base of the proximal phalanx articulates with the metacarpal head to form the metacarpophalangeal joint. Although the head of the metacarpal is rounded and the base of the phalanx concave, the fit is not congruent but quite loose. The integrity of the joint is maintained by the collateral ligaments, volar plate, and joint capsule; motion is allowed in flexion, extension, abduction, adduction, and, to a limited extent, rotation. The proximal attachment of the collateral ligament to the

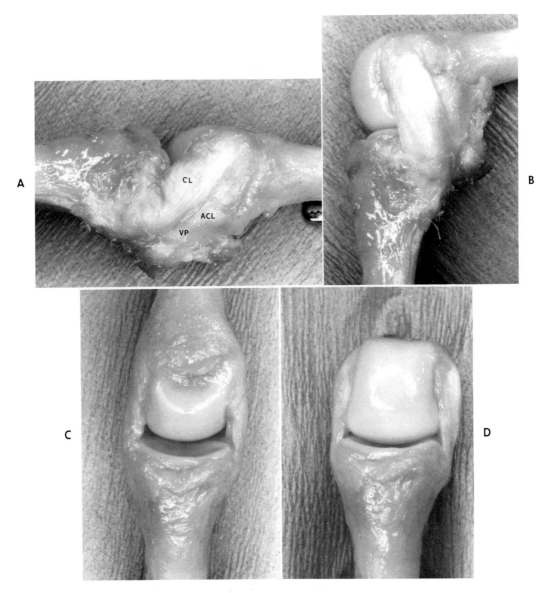

FIG. 21-6. Lateral and dorsal views of collateral ligaments of metacarpophalangeal joint of finger. Cord portion of ligament is lax in extension, allowing separation of joint surfaces (**A** and **C**) but becomes taut as the phalanx glides around the metacarpal head (**B** and **D**). The reverse is true for the accessory collateral ligament. *ACL,* Accessory collateral ligament attached to the volar plate; *CL,* collateral ligament (cord portion); *VP,* volar plate.

head of the metacarpal is dorsal to the axis of flexion and extension (Fig. 21-6). The collateral ligament is relatively lax when the joint is extended, allowing distraction of the joint surfaces. As the phalanx glides toward the palm around the head of the metacarpal during flexion, the slack in the ligament disappears; when the joint is fully flexed, the ligament is at its maximal tension. Thus positioning the fingers in flexion is useful to help reduce and control rotation of metacarpal fractures during healing. Injuries of the hand should be splinted with the metacarpophalangeal joints flexed to prevent shortening of the ligaments during the immobilization period with consequent loss of proximal phalangeal flexion.

The portion of the ligament that tightens with flexion is the cord portion attaching from bone to bone. The accessory collateral ligament, or fan portion, extends from the metacarpal heads to the sides of the volar plate and remains tighter in full extension than it does in full flexion. The volar plates attach firmly to the base of the proximal phalanx and, with the cord and fan portions of the collateral ligaments, form a pocket for articulation with the metacarpal head (Fig. 21-6). Also attaching to the sides of the volar plate, connecting the volar plate of one finger with the next, are the deep transverse metacarpal ligaments (Fig. 21-7, *B* and *C*). Joining this juncture are attachments of the A-1 flexor pulley, as well as the in-

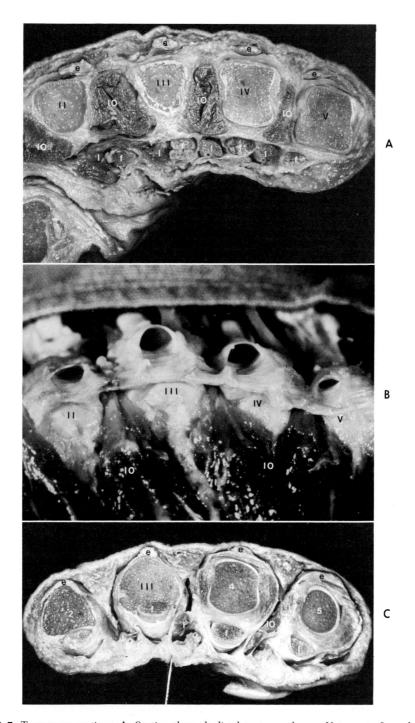

FIG. 21-7. Transverse sections. **A,** Section through distal metacarpal area. Note septa from deep surface of palmar aponeurosis to anterior interosseous membrane, creating compartments for lumbricals and digital nerves and vessels. These septa are commonly involved with Dupuytren's contracture but seldom with trauma. **B,** Dissection to illustrate relationship of volar plate of metacarpophalangeal joints to deep transverse metacarpal ligaments and A-1 pulleys. **C,** Transverse section through metacarpophalangeal joint level. Note extensor hoods, collateral ligaments, volar plate, and flexor pulleys, connected by deep transverse metacarpal ligaments. *e,* Finger extensor tendons; *f,* finger flexor tendons; *IO,* interosseous muscles; *l,* lumbrical muscles; *II* to *V,* metacarpals; *2, 4,* and *5,* proximal phalanges.

sertion of the transverse portion of the extensor hood. Thus at the sides of the volar plate there is an extensive array of fibrous bands, blending and mingling to provide a substantial structure.

Interphalangeal Joints

The proximal and distal interphalangeal joints have a different configuration than the metacarpophalangeal joint. The head of the proximal phalanx is almost circular in the sagittal plane but is broad and straight in the coronal plane. The cord and fan portions of the collateral ligaments remain taut in all positions of the joint and effectively restrict abduction and adduction. In the child they attach to the epiphysis and metaphysis, providing a measure of stability to the growth plate.[2] Extending proximally from the volar plate and the base of the middle phalanx is a band of fibers that attaches to the shaft of the proximal phalanx at the attachment of the A-2 pulley. This band acts as a checkrein to prevent hyperextension of the proximal interphalangeal joint.[3] Hypertrophy of this band is commonly seen after injury to the proximal interphalangeal joint and results in severe flexion contractures. Passing beneath this fibrous band are transversely oriented branches that arise from the digital arteries, extend to the distal end of the proximal phalanx, and enter into the proximal interphalangeal joint.

Thumb Articulations

The thumb skeleton is considerably different from that of the fingers. The bones are shorter, broader, and heavier. They consist of one metacarpal and two phalanges, rather than three (Fig. 21-8). The **trapezial metacarpal joint** at the base of the thumb is reciprocally biconcavoconvex (saddle shaped), which allows for motion in flexion, extension, abduction, adduction, and some rotation because the ligaments and fit of the joint are relatively loose. There is a significant volar-ulnar ligament that holds the base of the metacarpal to the base of the second metacarpal and trapezoid. It is this ligament that holds the smaller fracture fragment of an intraarticular Bennett's fracture in place. The orientation of the thumb is approximately 90 degrees pronated from the orientation of the rest of the digits; this can be increased to nearly 180 degrees so that the pulp of the thumb opposes the pulp of the index and middle fingers. The tip of the thumb can be brought to the tip, or even to the base, of each of the fingers by the ability of the thumb metacarpal to be rotated at its base.

The **thumb metacarpophalangeal joint** is an articulation between the rounded head of the metacarpal and the concave surface of the base of the proximal phalanx. This joint, too, is relatively lax but not as lax as the finger metacarpophalangeal joints. It has heavier radial and ulnar collateral ligaments. The volar plate contains two sesamoids at the insertions of the adductor pollicis, flexor pollicis brevis, and abductor pollicis brevis. Displacement of a sesamoid seen on a radiograph indicates serious disruption of the joint ligaments.

The **interphalangeal joint** of the thumb articulates with the rounded head of the proximal phalanx in such a manner that flexion provides for increasing pronation of the distal phalanx as flexion increases. The movement at this joint is primarily hinge because of the relatively broad shape of the joint surfaces in the coronal plane compared to the circular shape in the sagittal plane. There is often enough laxity of this joint to allow an amount of hyperextension that varies from individual to individual. It usually flexes almost 90 degrees and can hyperextend from 15 to 90 degrees and still be entirely within a normal range. The metacarpophalangeal joint conversely has a variable amount of flexion from individual to individual; some persons have almost none, and others have a range from hyperextension to 90 degrees of flexion.

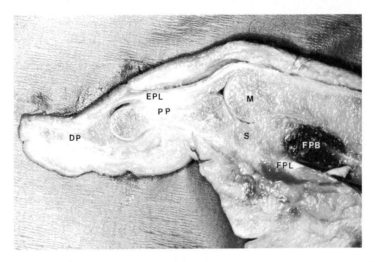

FIG. 21-8. Sagittal section of thumb. Volar plate of metacarpophalangeal joint is thickened by a sesamoid bone at the blended insertions of abductor pollicis brevis with flexor pollicis brevis into the volar plate and proximal phalanx. If the plate is displaced on radiograph, it usually indicates major disruption of the joint. *DP,* Distal phalanx; *EPL,* extensor pollicis longus; *FPB,* flexor pollicis brevis; *FPL,* flexor pollicis longus; *M,* metacarpal; *PP,* proximal phalanx; *S,* sesamoid.

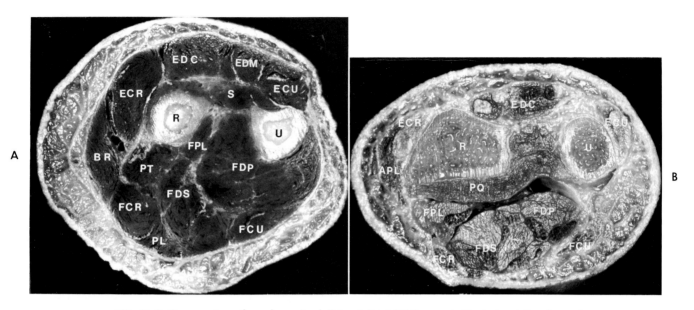

FIG. 21-9. Cross sections through proximal **(A)** and distal **(B)** forearm to illustrate relative size and position of flexor and extensor muscle groups. *APL,* Abductor pollicis longus; *BR,* brachioradialis; *ECR,* extensor carpi radialis brevis and longus; *ECU,* extensor carpi ulnaris; *EDC,* extensor digitorum communis; *EDM,* extensor digiti minimi; *EPL,* extensor pollicis longus; *FCR,* flexor carpi radialis; *FCU,* flexor carpi ulnaris; *FDP,* flexor digitorum profundus; *FDS,* flexor digitorum superficialis; *FPL,* flexor pollicis longus; *PL,* palmaris longus; *PQ,* pronator quadratus; *PT,* pronator teres; *R,* radius; *S,* supinator; *U,* ulna.

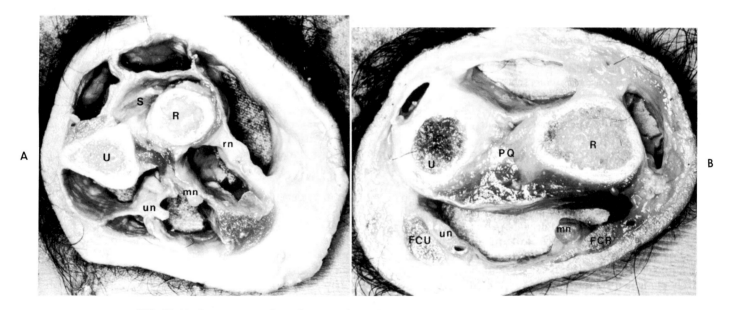

FIG. 21-10. Cross sections through proximal and distal aspects of forearm with most muscle bellies removed, to illustrate the intermuscular septa forming compartments that contain muscles, nerves, and vessels. The septa also serve to increase the surface area for origin of muscle fibers of the flexor and extensor muscle groups. Note vulnerability of nerves to expansion of muscles with increased pressure in compartments. **A,** Proximal forearm. Note median and ulnar nerves. **B,** Distal forearm, with fewer compartments because most muscle bellies have been replaced by tendons. *FCR,* Flexor carpi radialis; *FCU,* flexor carpi ulnaris; *mn,* median nerve; *PQ,* pronator quadratus; *R,* radius; *rn,* radial nerve; *S,* supinator; *U,* ulna; *un,* ulnar nerve.

FLEXOR MUSCLE SYSTEM
Forearm

The flexor-pronator muscle group takes its origin from a common tendon attached to the medial epicondyle of the humerus, as well as from the numerous intermuscular septa between the various muscle groups. The muscle bellies are proximally located in the forearm with the tendons beginning in the substance of the muscle. In the distal third of the forearm much of the muscle tissue has been replaced by tendon (Fig. 21-9). This configuration is felt to account partly for the difference in success rates of replantations through the proximal vs. distal forearm. The muscles are conventionally described in several layers, with the pronator teres, flexor carpi radialis, palmaris longus, and flexor carpi ulnaris being in the superficial layer; the flexor digitorum superficialis comprises an intermediate but still fairly superficial layer. The flexor pollicis longus, flexor digitorum profundus, and pronator quadratus remain deeply placed in the forearm, since they originate from the radius and ulna, respectively. Because of the inelastic nature of the fibrous septa between the muscle groups, any swelling of injured muscle will quickly result in worsening ischemia, most pronounced in the deepest muscles, that is, flexor pollicis longus and flexor digitorum profundus (Fig. 21-10).

Flexor muscle layers

Superficial
- Pronator teres
- Flexor carpi radialis
- Palmaris longus
- Flexor carpi ulnaris

Intermediate
- Flexor digitorum superficialis

Deep
- Flexor pollicis longus
- Flexor digitorum profundus
- Pronator quadratus

The **pronator teres,** the most proximal of this entire group of muscles, crosses obliquely from the medial epicondyle of the humerus to the middle of the shaft of the radius, where it ends in a fairly short broad tendon and inserts onto the radial aspect of the middle of the shaft, just distal to the insertion of the supinator. When using this muscle for transfer, the short tendon can be effectively elongated by raising some of the adjacent periosteum in continuity with the tendon; the muscle can thus reach the back of the forearm in the commonly used transfer to the extensor carpi radialis brevis for wrist extension in radial nerve palsies. It is innervated by the median nerve, which passes between the humeral and ulnar heads of this muscle to enter the proximal forearm.

The **flexor carpi radialis** ends near the middle of the forearm in a tendon that travels with the radial artery to the level of the wrist. Here it passes in a separate synovial-lined tunnel across the carpus, lying in a groove in the trapezium and inserting into the second metacarpal base with a frequent slip to the third.

By leaving the distal insertion intact, the tendon can be detached from the muscle in the forearm and pulled distally, where it is balled up and used to fill the space left by removing the arthritic trapezium. By attaching the tendon to the first metacarpal, a new volar-ulnar ligament for the thumb is constructed, providing for stability between the first and second metacarpals.[3a]

The **palmaris longus** is present in approximately 85% of forearms. It ends as a long, flat, slender tendon that is inserted into superficial layers of the flexor retinaculum at the wrist. Its fibers continue into the palmar aponeurosis; it is innervated by the median nerve.

The **flexor carpi ulnaris** originates with the common flexor tendon from the medial humeral epicondyle, as well as an extensive origin from the ulnar shaft and medial intermuscular septum. The muscle fibers extend almost to the wrist (Figs. 21-9, *B,* and 21-10, *B*), a feature that makes it easy to distinguish the tendon from ulnar nerve when both are lacerated in the distal forearm. The flexor carpi ulnaris tendon inserts into the pisiform and from there, via the pisohamate and pisometacarpal ligaments, into the hamate and fifth metacarpal, respectively. The ulnar nerve enters the proximal forearm between the humeral and ulnar heads of origin of this muscle; at this point it is subject to compression by a transversely placed band of fibers connecting the two heads and attaching to the medial humeral epicondyle and olecranon. This band of fibers is lax in extension of the elbow joint, but as the joint flexes the olecranon process moves away from the medial epicondyle and this fibrous band then becomes taut over the nerve (Fig. 21-11).

The pisohamate ligament forms the floor of Guyon's canal, and the roof is formed by a prolongation of fibers from the transverse retinacular ligament. Guyon's canal transmits the ulnar artery, vein, and nerve from forearm to palm.

The **flexor digitorum superficialis, flexor pollicis longus,** and **flexor digitorum profundus** give rise to tendons in the middle of the forearm, which then traverse the carpal tunnel.

Carpal Tunnel

The carpal tunnel is formed on three sides by carpal bones forming a **C** on transverse section. The **C** is converted into a **D** by the flexor retinaculum, which closes the volar aspect (Fig. 21-12). The retinacular ligament is approximately 2.5 cm (1 inch) long from proximal to distal; it attaches to the triquetrum and hook of the hamate on the ulnar side and to the tuberosities of scaphoid and trapezium on the radial side. The carpus and flexor retinaculum thus form a rigid-walled tunnel lined by synovium, through which pass the nine tendons of the flexor digitorum superficialis, flexor digitorum profundus, and flexor pollicis longus muscles and the median nerve.

Palm and Digits

As the tendons of the finger and thumb flexors cross the palm, they lie on the anterior surface of the anterior

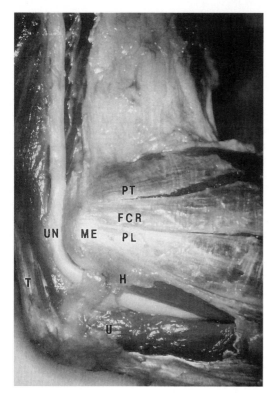

FIG. 21-11. Ulnar nerve crossing elbow to enter forearm between two heads of origin of flexor carpi ulnaris muscle. Note the transverse fascial band between the two heads of the flexor carpi ulnaris, which can become tight enough in elbow flexion to cause compression of the ulnar nerve. *FCR*, Flexor carpi radialis; *H*, humeral head of origin of flexor carpi ulnaris; *ME*, medial epicondyle of humerus; *PL*, palmaris longus; *PT*, pronator teres; *T*, triceps; *U*, ulnar head or origin of flexor carpi ulnaris; *UN*, ulnar nerve.

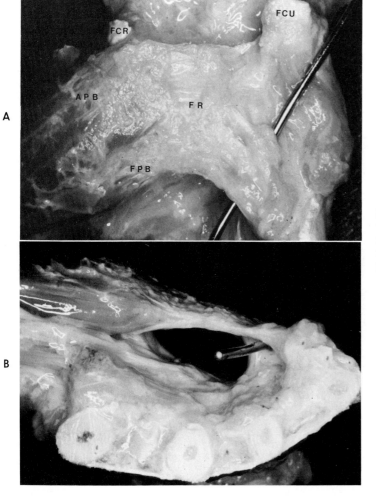

FIG. 21-12. Anterior (**A**) and transverse (**B**) views of carpal tunnel. Probe lies in unnamed tunnel for deep branch of ulnar artery and nerve. *APB*, Abductor pollicis brevis; *FCR*, flexor carpi radialis; *FCU*, flexor carpi ulnaris; *FPB*, flexor pollicis brevis; *FR*, flexor retinaculum.

interosseous membrane, a sheet of fascia that separates them from the interosseous muscles (Fig. 21-7, *A*). The long thumb flexor and the flexors to the little finger reside in a continuous digital tenosynovial sheath beginning proximal to the wrist and ending at the base of the terminal phalanx of the digit. The index, middle, and ring fingers have similar tenosynovial sheaths in the fingers, but the sheaths do not extend proximal to the level of the distal palm, forming a cul-de-sac just proximal to the A-1 pulley by reflecting from the pulley onto the tendon.

Each finger has a series of pulleys recently redescribed by Doyle and Blythe[5] and others and designated annulus 1 through 5 and cruciate 1 through 3. Pulleys A-1 to A-3 are located at the level of the metacarpophalangeal joint volar plate (A-1), proximal phalanx (A-2), and volar plate of the proximal interphalangeal joint (A-3). The A-3 pulley is somewhat inconstant and seldom substantial.

Pulley sites in digits

- A-1: metacarpophalangeal joint
- A-2: proximal phalanx
- A-3: proximal interphalangeal joint
- A-4: middle phalanx
- A-5: distal interphalangeal joint

The A-4 pulley is attached to the middle phalanx, and the A-5 pulley, when present, is at the level of the volar plate of the distal interphalangeal joint. The pulleys are lined on their inner surface by the parietal layer of synovium, which reflects onto the tendon at the profundus insertion and just proximal to the A-1 pulley as a visceral layer of synovium. The space between is filled with synovial fluid to lubricate and nourish the tendons. A mesotenon conveys blood vessels to the tendons; it is discontinuous in the fingers and represented by the vincula longus and brevis of each tendon (Fig. 21-13). Vessels enter the tendons on their dorsal surface and remain in the dorsal half as they extend up and down the length of the tendon.[1,12] In the thumb there are two pulleys: a transverse one at the level of the metacarpophalangeal joint and an oblique one across the volar aspect of the proximal phalanx (Fig. 21-14, *B*).

Pulley sites in thumb

- Transverse: metacarpophalangeal joint
- Oblique: proximal phalanx

As the finger flexor tendons approach the A-1 pulley, the superficialis tendon is anterior to the profundus, but it divides to pass around either side of the profundus to become dorsal. At the distal end of the proximal phalanx, the fibers of each half of the superficialis rejoin and decussate with each other behind the profundus tendon in such a manner that the profundus cannot be compressed and hindered in its gliding by longitudinal pull on the superficialis. Each half of the superficialis tendon spirals around the profundus tendon, decussates dorsal to it at the proximal interphalangeal joint level, and inserts into the middle of the shaft of the middle phalanx, not to its

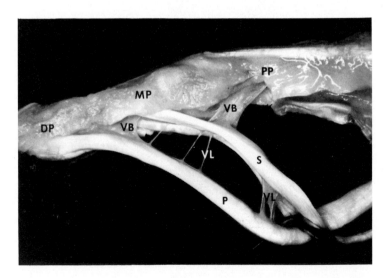

FIG. 21-13. Flexor tendon mechanism in the finger. The flexor digitorum superficialis tendon splits in distal palm to permit passage of flexor digitorum profundus; the two halves rejoin and decussate dorsal to the profundus at proximal interphalangeal joint level. The vincular vessels enter the tendons dorsally. *DP,* Distal phalanx; *MP,* middle phalanx; *P,* flexor digitorum profundus; *PP,* proximal phalanx; *S,* flexor digitorum superficialis; *VB,* vinculum breve; *VL,* vinculum longum. (From Pettrone, F (ed): *Symposium of upper extremity injuries in athletes,* St Louis, 1986, Mosby.)

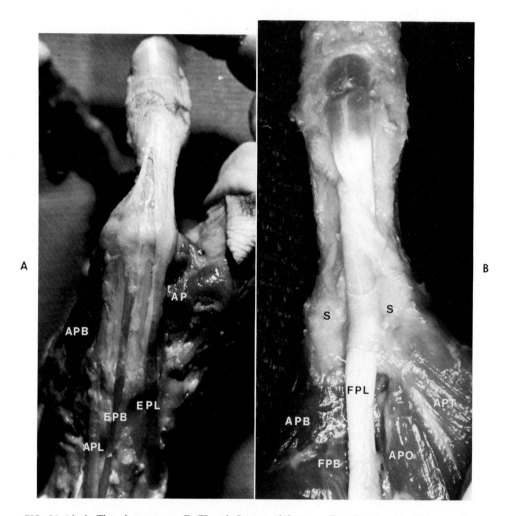

FIG. 21-14. A, Thumb extensors. **B,** Thumb flexors. Abductor pollicis brevis and adductor pollicis are primary flexors of metacarpophalangeal joint but send extensions into the extensor pollicis longus to form a hood over the proximal phalanx and assist extension of the interphalangeal joint. Note oblique flexor pulley over proximal phalanx, which must be avoided when doing trigger thumb release. Sesamoid bones are present in volar plate at conjoined sites of insertions of abductor and adductor with flexor pollicis brevis. *AP,* Adductor pollicis; *APO,* adductor pollicis, oblique head; *APT,* adductor pollicis, transverse head; *APB,* abductor pollicis brevis; *APL,* abductor pollicis longus; *EPB,* extensor pollicis brevis; *EPL,* extensor pollicis longus; *FPB,* flexor pollicis brevis; *FPL,* flexor pollicis longus; *S,* sesamoid bones in volar plate.

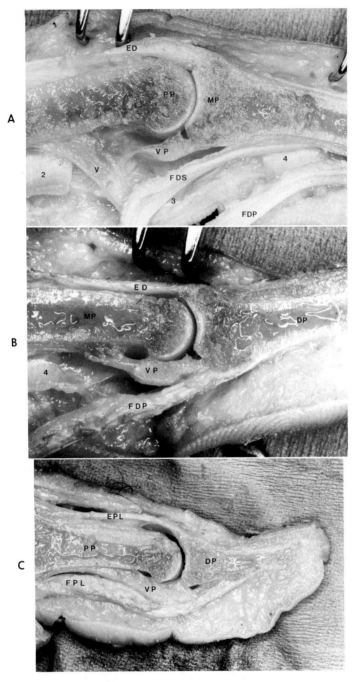

FIG. 21-15. A, Sagittal section through proximal interphalangeal joint of middle finger. Central slip of extensor blends with dorsal capsule and inserts into dorsal lip of middle phalanx. Flexor digitorum superficialis inserts into midshaft of middle phalanx. **B,** Sagittal section through distal interphalangeal joint of middle finger. Extensor and flexor insert into base of distal phalanx. **C,** Sagittal section through interphalangeal joint of thumb. Extensor pollicis longus inserts into dorsal base of distal phalanx, but flexor pollicis longus inserts well distal on shaft of distal phalanx. Note that volar plate contains a sesamoid bone. *2, 3,* and *4,* Annular flexor pulleys; *DP,* distal phalanx; *ED,* extensor digitorum; *EPL,* extensor pollicis longus; *FDP,* flexor digitorum profundus; *FDS,* flexor digitorum superficialis; *FPL,* flexor pollicis longus; *MP,* middle phalanx; *PP,* proximal phalanx; *V,* vinculum; *VP,* volar plate.

base (Fig. 21-15, *A*). Thus fractures of the base of the middle phalanx are not displaced by muscle pull. The profundus passes through this decussation to reach its attachment to the volar base of the distal phalanx (Fig. 21-15, *B*); fractures of the volar lip of the distal phalanx often are displaced by muscle pull. The decussation is a very important part of the gliding mechanism for the flexor digitorum profundus and should not be removed or damaged during tendon repair. The long thumb flexor passes through transverse and diagonal pulleys[6] and inserts closer to the terminal end of the distal phalanx than do the finger flexors (Fig. 21-15, *C*).

EXTENSOR MUSCLE SYSTEM
Forearm

The extensor-supinator muscles, like the flexors, take their origin as a partially differentiated muscle mass from the distal humerus. The brachioradialis and radial wrist extensors originate as muscular fibers without intervening tendon from the lateral aspect of the distal third of the humerus and lateral epicondyle. The brachioradialis

is primarily an elbow flexor and has no direct function on the wrist or hand, although it may assist pronation or supination to the middle position of forearm rotation. The extensor carpi radialis longus and brevis muscles insert by large tendons into the dorsal radial aspects of the bases of the second and third metacarpals, respectively (Fig. 21-2, *C*). They are active wrist extensors and radial deviators of the hand and contribute significantly to power grip. Wrist and finger motions are synergistic; to obtain maximal wrist extension, one must flex the fingers. Active wrist extension and stabilization during power grip allow greater force to be applied by the finger flexors. When the wrist extensors are paralyzed, grip is markedly weakened. The brachioradialis and extensor carpi radialis longus and brevis are innervated by the radial nerve proximal to the elbow joint.

The remainder of the extensor muscles originate in the proximal forearm from a conjoined tendon attaching to the lateral epicondyle and from the radius, ulna, and interosseous membrane. There is also an extensive origin from septa between the individual muscle groups (Fig. 21-10). Tendons originate from this muscle mass in the

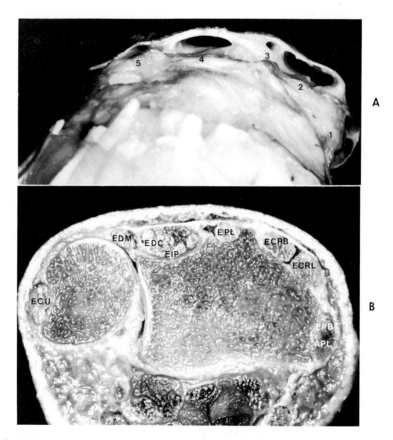

FIG. 21-16. A, Extensor retinaculum to illustrate septa and compartments after tendons have been removed. Note first compartment has a septum dividing it in half. **B,** Cross section through distal radioulnar joint to illustrate extensor compartments with tendons in situ. Compartments 1 through 5 are attached to the distal radius; compartment 6 with the extensor carpi ulnaris is attached to the ulna, and thus extensor carpi ulnaris functions as a wrist adductor when forearm is pronated. *APL*, Abductor pollicis longus; *ECRB*, extensor carpi radialis brevis; *ECRL*, extensor carpi radialis longus; *ECU*, extensor carpi ulnaris; *EDC*, extensor digitorum communis; *EDM*, extensor digiti minimi; *EIP*, extensor indicis proprius; *EPB*, extensor pollicis brevis; *EPL*, extensor pollicis longus.

middle of the forearm and extend distally toward their insertions. As the tendons cross the wrist, they pass through compartments in the extensor retinaculum complex, which binds them to the dorsal radius and ulna (Fig. 21-16) and provides for function without bowstringing. At the wrist level the tendons are enclosed in synovial sheaths that extend a short distance proximal and distal to the retinaculum. Over the metacarpals a loose paratenon forms a mesotenon to convey blood supply to the tendons.

Extensor Retinaculum

The extensor retinaculum complex is a thickening of distal forearm fascia by transversely placed fibers that are attached to the radial aspect of the distal radius; they cross the distal radius and carpus dorsally to blend with the ulnar collateral ligament and the fascia of the hypothenar eminence. From the deep surface of the retinaculum pass a number of short strong fibrous bands (Fig. 21-16), attaching the retinaculum firmly to the distal radius and making a series of synovial-lined compartments or tunnels through which pass the extensor tendons.

The first compartment is the most radial, and through it pass the abductor pollicis longus and extensor pollicis brevis tendons. These may be as few as two or as many as six or seven because the abductor pollicus longus may have multiple tendon slips. The compartment may be a single large compartment or, more commonly, incompletely septate. The combination of multiple tendons and partial septations may be the cause of de Quervain's stenosing tenosynovitis.

Through the second compartment pass the two radial wrist extensors, and through the third compartment passes the extensor pollicis longus. The second and third compartments are separated by Lister's tubercle to which the extensor retinaculum is firmly attached, and just distal to which the second and third compartments become one.

Extensor compartments

1: Abductor pollicis longus
   Extensor pollicis brevis
2: Extensor carpi radialis longus
   Extensor carpi radialis brevis
3: Extensor pollicis longus
4: Extensor digitorum communis
   Extensor indicis proprius
5: Extensor digiti minimi
6: Extensor carpi ulnaris

Through the fourth compartment pass the tendons of the extensor digitorum communis superficially and the deeper extensor indicis proprius, which frequently has muscle fibers present almost to the level of the compartment.

The fifth compartment is attached to the distal radius or to the dorsal ligament of the distal radioulnar joint and transmits the double tendons of the extensor digiti minimi.

The sixth compartment is attached solely to the distal ulna, where it covers a deep groove containing the extensor carpi ulnaris (Fig. 21-16, *B*). When the forearm is in supination, the tendon is on the dorsal aspect of the forearm. With pronation, as the radius rotates around the distal ulna carrying its attached hand, the extensor carpi ulnaris remains in place since the ulna does not rotate. Thus the tendon remains on the ulnar aspect of the wrist and is no longer a wrist extensor but functions as an adductor to stabilize the wrist when opening the thumb for grasp. The extensor carpi ulnaris inserts into the dorsal aspect of the fifth metacarpal base.

Dorsal Hand

As the extensors to the fingers traverse the dorsal aspect of the metacarpal area, they are bound together by a sheet of intertendinous fascia and also by tendon bundles (juncturae tendinum) that pass from one tendon to an adjacent one (Fig. 21-17, *A*). This combination creates an extensor plane that is bounded on superficial and deep surfaces by potential spaces that contain veins, lymphatics, and superficial nerves (Fig. 21-17, *B* and *C*) and can be easily distended by fluid. The space superficial to the tendons can be obliterated without significant alteration of function, because even though the skin becomes adherent to the tendons, they can glide and carry the adherent skin along. However, if the subaponeurotic space deep to the tendons is obliterated by infection or scar tissue, the tendons become adherent to the immobile bones or the fascia covering the interosseous muscles, and the tendons are no longer able to glide. This is frequently seen following burns or other trauma to the extensor tendons, resulting in an extension contracture of the metacarpophalangeal joints.

Extensor Hood Mechanism

When the extensor tendons reach the distal end of the metacarpal, they enter into the complex array of the extensor hood.[15] Sagittal fibers extend from the sides of each extensor tendon to pass toward the palm alongside the capsule of the joint and the collateral ligament and insert into the sides of the volar plate of the metacarpophalangeal joint (Fig. 21-18, *A* and *C*). Traction on these fibers produces extension of the proximal phalanx of the finger. Distal to the sagittal fibers are transverse and oblique fibers that originate from the interosseous and lumbrical muscles and blend into the sides of the extensor tendon over the proximal phalanx (Fig. 21-18, *A*, *B*, and *D*). These facilitate flexion of the metacarpophalangeal joint by forming a hood over the top of the proximal phalanx. As the extensor tendon complex approaches the proximal interphalangeal joint, the central group of fibers divides into three distinct portions, with the central slip continuing across the proximal interphalangeal joint and inserting into the dorsal base of the middle phalanx. The other two slips diverge to the radial and ulnar aspects of the joint, respectively, where they join fibers from the interosseous and lumbrical muscles to form the lateral bands. Oblique fibers from interosseous and lumbrical muscles also separate and blend with the three portions of the central slip to compose a strong insertion

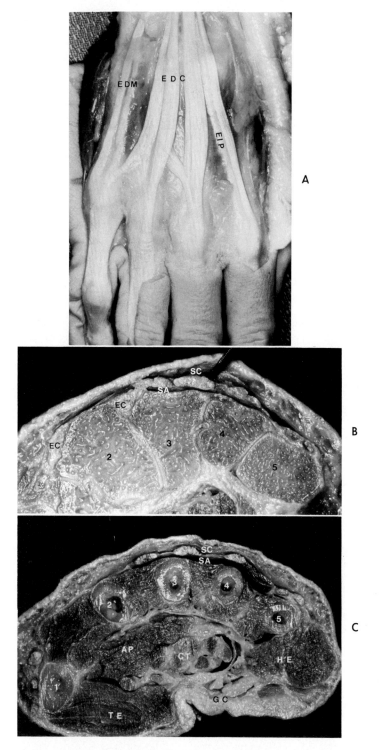

FIG. 21-17. A, Extensor tendon plane across dorsum of hand. Juncturae tendinum and fascia bind tendons into unit. Note that double tendon of extensor digit minimi coming through separate (fifth) compartment of extensor retinaculum is augmented distally by junctura from ring finger extensor. **B,** Cross section through bases of metacarpals to illustrate extensor tendon plane and subcutaneous (with probe) and subaponeurotic spaces. **C,** Cross section through midpalm. Note extensor plane and spaces allowing free gliding. *AP,* Adductor pollicis; *CT,* carpal tunnel; *EC,* extensor carpi radialis longus and brevis; *EDC,* extensor digitorum communis; *EDM,* extensor digiti minimi; *EIP,* extensor indicis proprius; *GC,* Guyon's canal; *HE,* hypothenar eminence; *SA,* subaponeurotic space; *SC,* subcutaneous space; *TE,* thenar eminence; *1* to *5,* metacarpals.

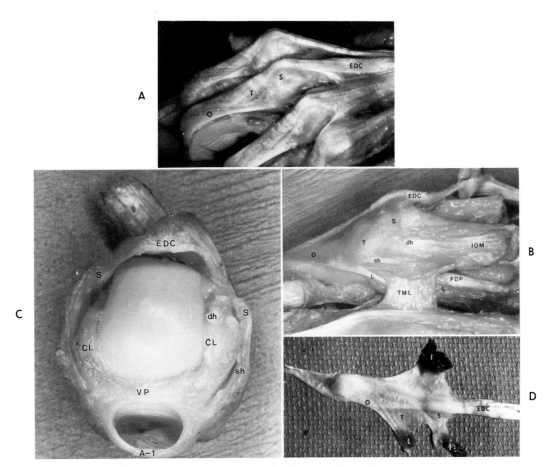

FIG. 21-18. Extensor hood mechanism of the fingers. **A,** Long extensor tendon blends with fibers from interossei and lumbricals to provide flexion and extension at metacarpophalangeal joint, as well as extension at interphalangeal joints. **B,** Radial view of metacarpophalangeal joint of long finger demonstrating deep and superficial portions of second dorsal interosseous muscle relationship to extensor hood. Deep portion inserts into proximal phalanx, and superficial portion blends into extensor hood and lateral band and lumbrical. **C,** End-on view of long finger metacarpal head illustrating relationship of extensor hood, collateral ligaments, volar plate, and A-1 pulley. **D,** Dorsal view of an extensor hood illustrates blending of tendon fibers from extrinsic and intrinsic extensors. *A-1,* First annular pulley; *CL,* collateral ligament; *dh,* deep head, second dorsal interosseous muscle; *EDC,* extensor digitorum communis; *FDP,* flexor digitorum profundus; *IOM,* second dorsal interosseous muscle; *L,* lumbrical; *O,* oblique fibers from intrinsic muscle that extend interphalangeal joints; *S,* sagittal fibers from long extensor that extend proximal phalanx; *sh,* superficial head, second dorsal interosseous muscle; *T,* transverse fibers from intrinsic muscle that flex proximal phalanx; *TML,* transverse metacarpal ligament; *VP,* volar plate. (**A** and **D** from Pettrone F (ed): *Symposium of upper extremity injuries in athletes,* St Louis, 1986, Mosby.)

into the proximal phalanx and continue as the lateral bands to attach into the dorsal lip of the proximal portion of the distal phalanx. These intersecting fibers do not contain elastic fibers, but by their basket-weave effect they allow for some give and take with movement of the different joints. At the proximal interphalangeal joint level the lateral bands lie dorsal to the flexion-extension axis and thus extend the proximal interphalangeal joint. The lateral bands slide toward the palm during flexion to permit simultaneous flexion of proximal and distal interphalangeal joints (Fig. 21-19). When the central slip is ruptured, the lateral bands slide anterior to the flexion-extension axis and are held there by fibers of the trans-

verse retinacular ligament. They can no longer extend the proximal interphalangeal joint; when extension is attempted, the proximal interphalangeal joint flexes more and the distal interphalangeal joint receives all the extensor power producing the boutonnière deformity. With time, adhesions develop and the deformity is no longer passively correctable.

The interosseous muscles are short and bulky with limited excursion but excellent power. They are the primary flexors of the metacarpophalangeal joints and make up approximately 50% of the strength of power grip. On the radial side of the index and middle fingers, most of the first and second dorsal interosseous muscles insert

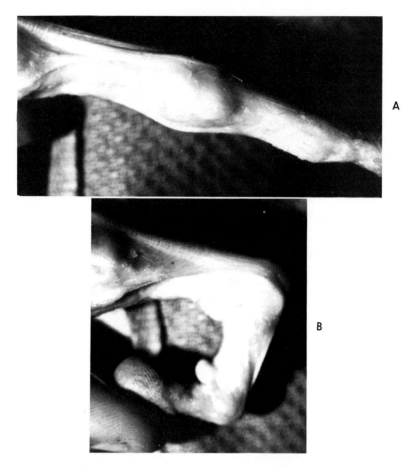

FIG. 21-19. Side view of extensor hood position over proximal interphalangeal joint. **A,** Extension. **B,** Flexion. Lateral bands normally slip volar during flexion; they may be retained there by the transverse retinacular ligament if central slip is ruptured.

directly into the proximal phalanx (Fig. 21-18, *B*) and thus function as powerful abductors to resist thumb forces during pinch.

This intricate arrangement of the extensor hood permits the beautiful and complex interplay between extrinsic flexors and extensors and the interosseous and lumbrical muscles to provide the almost infinite variability in positioning the digital joints and segments for function. With the metacarpophalangeal joint flexed, the long extensor becomes the primary extensor of the proximal interphalangeal and distal interphalangeal joints, augmented by tenodesis effect and wrist position. If the metacarpophalangeal joint is extended or hyperextended, the long extensor of the finger no longer has enough excursion remaining to extend the interphalangeal joints. Conversely, if the interosseous muscles have used up their excursion by flexing the metacarpophalangeal joints fully, they no longer have enough remaining excursion to extend the interphalangeal joints fully. Thus there is a balance between the interosseous muscles and the long extensors of each digit that interact to provide the delicate balance available to have any degree of flexion or extension available to any joint of the finger, regardless of the position of more proximal and distal joints. This is the basis for the intrinsic plus or intrinsic minus configurations and contractures that develop when one set of muscles is paralyzed by radial or ulnar palsies.

The three thumb extensors are the abductor pollicis longus, which attaches into the base of the first metacarpal; the extensor pollicis brevis, which blends with the dorsal capsule over the metacarpophalangeal joint and inserts into the base of the proximal phalanx with a frequent contribution continuing to the distal phalanx; and the extensor pollicis longus, which passes the metacarpophalangeal joint on its ulnar aspect and inserts into the base of the distal phalanx (Figs. 21-14, *A,* and 21-15, *B*). The extensor pollicis longus is augmented over the proximal phalanx by contributions from the abductor pollicis brevis and adductor pollicis to form an extensor hood over the dorsum of the joint, which functions much as the extensor hood of the fingers. The adductor pollicis and abductor pollicis brevis are flexors of the metacarpophalangeal joint of the thumb and extensors of the interphalangeal joint. This function is often seen in opposition of the thumb and in pinch.

NERVES

Superficial Nerves

The forearm and hand are supplied by a number of cutaneous nerves, some of which are continuations of those supplying sensation in the arm and around the elbow while others limit their cutaneous distribution to the hand. The **musculocutaneous nerve** emerges at the lateral border of the biceps tendon and continues into the forearm as the lateral antebrachial cutaneous nerve. It divides into dorsal and volar branches that supply sensation to the radial aspect of the forearm from elbow to wrist, where they blend with the cutaneous supply of the superficial radial nerve. Injuries of either nerve can cause similar symptoms of pain and paresthesias over the base of the thumb.

The **medial antebrachial cutaneous nerve** is a branch from the medial cord of the brachial plexus. It supplies the skin of the medial aspect of the forearm over the flexor muscle mass from elbow to wrist. It is important to realize that it is the medial antebrachial cutaneous nerve that supplies this area of the forearm because so often inexperienced persons assume that this area of the forearm is supplied by the ulnar nerve. Occasionally, one end of the ulnar nerve is sutured to an end of the antebrachial cutaneous nerve, not realizing that there should be two nerves repaired following a laceration above the elbow that results in anesthesia of the ulnar aspect of both the forearm and hand.

The **superficial radial nerve** passes down the forearm deep to the brachioradialis muscle and emerges near the wrist on the dorsal aspect of the tendon of that muscle (Fig. 21-20). It winds around the distal radial aspect of the wrist to supply the base of the thenar eminence on the palmar side, as well as the dorsal aspect of the thumb web and a variable area on the dorsum of the index, middle, and occasionally ring finger metacarpals and proximal phalanges. These branches cross the wrist superficially in the area of the anatomic snuffbox and are frequently injured during operations for de Quervain's stenosing tenosynovitis. They are easily visible, and one is usually palpable as it crosses the extensor pollicis longus tendon at the level of the snuffbox. The superficial radial nerve supplies most of the dorsum of the thumb to the eponychial level. On the fingers, the nerve extends approximately to the level of the proximal interphalangeal joint, dorsally. The distal two segments of the fingers are supplied with sensation by dorsal branches of the volar digital nerves, and thus a volar digital block would provide adequate anesthesia to operate on the nail bed or the distal interphalangeal joint.

The remainder of the dorsum of the hand has cutaneous innervation from the **dorsal branch of the ulnar nerve,** which originates several inches proximal to the wrist flexion crease in the volar forearm. The dorsal branch travels with the main ulnar nerve to the level of the ulnar styloid where it crosses the ulnar collateral ligament and extensor carpi ulnaris tendon to attain the back of the hand (Fig. 21-21). Here it supplies the dorsum of the proximal segments of the ring and little fingers with a frequent contribution to the middle finger. It also supplies a variable amount of the skin over the ulnar metacarpals.

The **palmar cutaneous branch of the median nerve** arises from the median nerve several centimeters above the proximal wrist flexion crease (Fig. 21-22) and passes distally to provide cutaneous sensation to a variable sized area of the thenar eminence. Damage to this branch often creates a neuroma that can produce painful paresthesias and hypersensitivity.

Deep Nerves

All three deep nerves in the hand and forearm enter the forearm between two heads of one of the forearm muscles and supply both motor and sensory innervation.

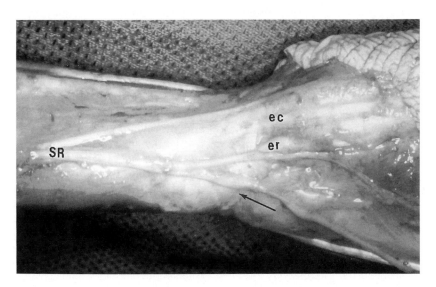

FIG. 21-20. Superficial radial nerve. Nerve penetrates deep fascia dorsal to the tendon of brachioradialis and divides into branches to thumb and dorsal hand. *ec,* Extensor digitorum communis; *er,* extensor carpi radialis longus; *SR,* superficial radial nerve. Arrow indicates tip of radial styloid.

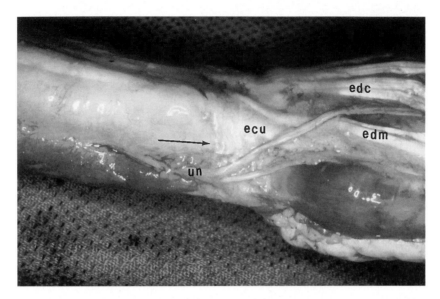

FIG. 21-21. Dorsal sensory branch of ulnar nerve. The branch originates several inches proximal to the wrist joint, stays volar to distal ulna, and reaches the dorsum of the hand by crossing the ulnar collateral ligament distal to the ulnar styloid. *ecu,* Extensor carpi ulnaris; *edc,* extensor digitorum communis; *edm,* extensor digiti minimi; *un,* ulnar nerve. Arrow indicates tip of ulnar styloid.

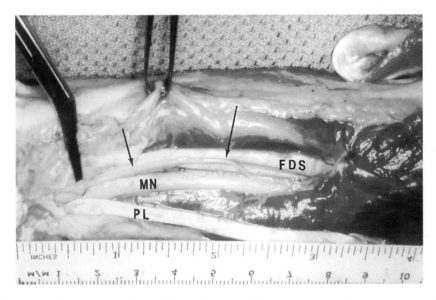

FIG. 21-22. Palmar cutaneous branch of median nerve. Originates from median nerve 2½ inches proximal to wrist flexion crease and penetrates the deep fascia of distal forearm to supply sensation to the base of the thenar eminence. *FDS,* Flexor digitorum superficialis; *MN,* median nerve; *PL,* palmaris longus.

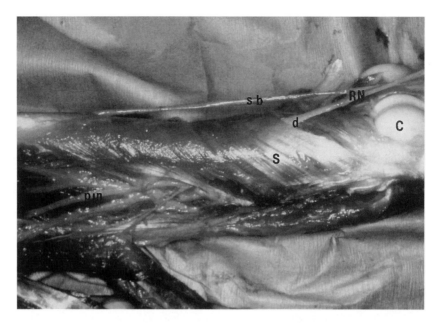

FIG. 21-23. Radial nerve enters forearm with the motor branch passing between humeral and ulnar heads of supinator. *C,* Capitellum; *d,* deep (motor) branch of radial nerve; *pin,* posterior interosseous nerve; *RN,* radial nerve; *S,* supinator muscle; *sb,* superficial (sensory) branch of radial nerve.

Radial Nerve

The radial nerve enters between the deep and superficial layers of the supinator muscle to reach the back of the forearm (Fig. 21-23). As it exits the supinator it divides into a number of short nerves that pass directly posterior to enter the deep surface of the extensors of the fingers and the extensor carpi ulnaris. The remainder of this nerve continues as the posterior interosseous nerve, which travels on the posterior aspect of the interosseous membrane with the posterior interosseous artery to the level of the wrist, ending in the capsule of the wrist joint or in an extensor digitorum brevis manus if one is present. The posterior interosseous nerve provides motor innervation to the abductor pollicis brevis, extensor pollicis longus, extensor pollicis brevis, and extensor indicis proprius.

Ulnar Nerve

The ulnar nerve enters the forearm between the humeral and ulnar heads of the flexor carpi ulnaris (Fig. 21-11). At this point it is subject to compression by a transverse band between these two heads. It continues distally between the flexor carpi ulnaris and the flexor digitorum profundus muscle bellies, supplying both muscles with several branches, one in the proximal forearm and one more distally. It supplies the muscle bellies of the flexor digitorum profundus to ring and little fingers, occasionally to the middle finger, but seldom to the index finger. As the ulnar nerve approaches the wrist, it lies deep to the tendon of the flexor carpi ulnaris adjacent to the ulnar artery and vein. With these vessels it enters Guyon's canal, where it divides into three major branches (Fig. 21-24), one of which is sensory in the form of common and proper digital nerves to the two

sides of the little finger and the ulnar side of the ring finger (Fig. 21-25). It frequently blends with a branch of the median nerve to supply the radial side of the ring finger. A second branch supplies the muscles of the hypothenar eminence, and a third branch winds around the hook of the hamate through a special unnamed canal in the flexor retinaculum (see Fig. 21-12) and winds its way across the bases of the proximal metacarpals in company with the deep arterial arch. As it crosses the palm from ulnar to radial, it sends branches to the palmar and dorsal interosseous muscles of each space, to the lumbrical muscles of the same fingers supplied by the ulnar nerve in the forearm (i.e., to the ring and little fingers and possibly the middle finger). It passes between the two heads of the adductor pollicis to end in the first dorsal interosseous muscle.

Median Nerve

The median nerve passes beneath the lacertus fibrosus before it enters the forearm between the humeral and ulnar heads of the pronator teres (Fig. 21-26), where it is subject to compression. It then passes beneath the proximal origin of the flexor digitorum superficialis as it originates from radius and ulna and a loop of intervening fascia; this could also be a site of nerve compression. The anterior interosseous branch arises from the medial aspect of the median nerve near the hiatus in the pronator teres and joins the anterior interosseous artery, to pass distally between the radius and ulna to its termination in the pronator quadratus and wrist joint capsule. Along the way it sends muscle branches to the flexor pollicis longus and digitorum profundus to the index finger. The remainder of the median nerve passes distally in the forearm attached to the underside of the flexor digitorum

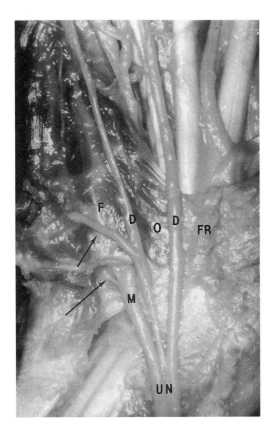

FIG. 21-24. Ulnar nerve crossing wrist at Guyon's canal. Just proximal to the wrist the nerve divides into three portions: (1) sensory to the small and ulnar half of ring finger; (2) motor branches to the muscles of the hypothenar eminence; and (3) deep motor branch to the interossei and varying muscles of the thenar eminence. *D*, Digital sensory nerves to ring and small fingers; *F*, flexor digiti minimi; *FR*, flexor retinaculum; *M*, deep motor branch passing around hook of hamate to enter depths of the proximal palm; *O*, opponens digiti minimi; *UN*, ulnar nerve. Arrows indicate motor branches to hypothenar muscles.

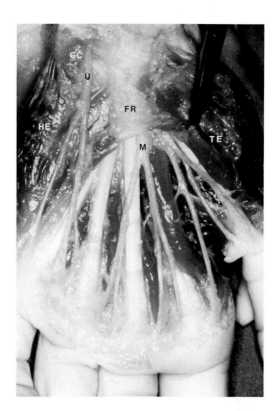

FIG. 21-25. Dissection of median and ulnar nerves in palm. Vessels have been removed. Note motor branches to first and second lumbricals from common digital nerves to index and middle fingers. Median nerve emerges from distal end of flexor retinaculum (carpal tunnel). Ulnar nerve is more superficial in Guyon's canal (opened). *FR*, Flexor retinaculum; *GC*, Guyon's canal; *HE*, hypothenar eminence; *M*, median nerve; *TE*, thenar eminence; *U*, ulnar nerve.

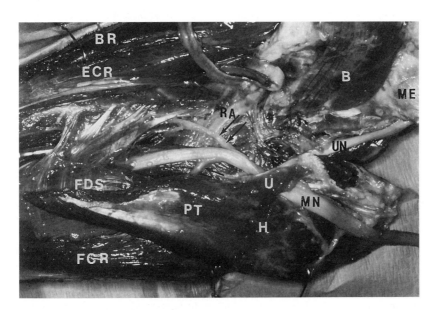

FIG. 21-26. Median nerve crossing elbow to enter forearm between two heads of origin of pronator teres. Flexor-pronator muscle group origin detached and reflected from medial humeral epicondyle. *B*, Brachialis muscle; *BR*, brachioradialis; *ECR*, extensor carpi radialis longus and brevis; *FCR*, flexor carpi radialis; *FDS*, leash of origin of flexor digitorum superficialis; *H*, humeral head of pronator teres; *MN*, median nerve; *PT*, pronator teres; *RA*, radial artery; *U*, ulnar head of pronator teres; *UN*, ulnar nerve; *single arrow*, motor branch of median nerve to flexor-pronator group; *double arrow*, anterior interosseous nerve.

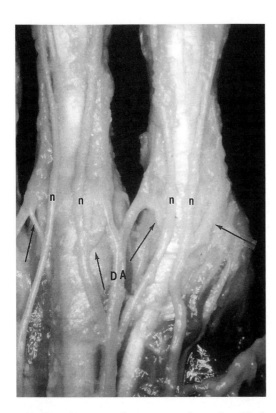

FIG. 21-27. Digital nerves and arteries to index and middle fingers. Note that common digital artery branches more distal than the nerve in the palm. *DA,* Common digital artery; *n,* proper digital nerves. Arrows indicate dorsal branches of each volar digital nerve, which supply sensation to the dorsum of the finger at and distal to the proximal interphalangeal joint.

superficialis. One must be aware of this fact when the muscle is injured or tendons are being taken for transfer, because the nerve mingles with the tendons in the distal part of the forearm and could be injured (Fig. 21-22). The nerve then passes beneath the flexor retinaculum at the wrist, where it is frequently subject to compression, causing carpal tunnel syndrome. As it exits the carpal tunnel, a branch arises laterally and winds around or through the distal portion of the flexor retinaculum to enter the thenar muscles and supply the abductor pollicis brevis, opponens pollicis, and in most cases, one or both heads of the flexor pollicis brevis. The median nerve then terminates by forming a number of branches that become the common and proper digital nerves to the thumb, index, and middle fingers and one branch to the ring finger (Fig. 21-25). The branch to the radial aspect of the thumb passes directly across the metacarpophalangeal flexion crease in the volar midline of the thumb and can be easily injured in approaches for trigger thumb release. The more ulnar branch lies on the base of the thumb metacarpal. This is the nerve that may be traumatized in bowlers and undergo interstitial fibrosis similar to Morton's neuroma in the foot.

The common digital nerves provide motor branches to index and middle finger lumbrical muscles (Fig. 21-25) before they divide in each web space to form proper dig-

ital nerves to each side of each finger. This division is proximal to the division of the common metacarpal arteries, which makes digital transpositions easier (Fig. 21-27).

The proper digital nerves travel beside the flexor tendon sheaths to the same digit. At the level of the metacarpophalangeal joint, each volar digital nerve sends a branch obliquely across the sides of the proximal phalanx to reach the dorsal aspect of the terminal two segments of the digit (Fig. 21-27). Thus the dorsal innervation to middle and distal phalanges of each finger is supplied by the proper digital nerve. This is not true for the thumb, where most of the supply of the dorsal aspect comes from the superficial radial nerve.

The common digital nerves travel with the digital arteries along the side of the finger, just below the midlateral line, where they are held in place by Cleland's and Grayson's ligaments. A midaxial incision would thus place the neurovascular bundle in the volar skin flap. This is a safe incision to use to approach the side of the finger or the flexor sheath except at the proximal portion of the proximal phalanx, where the dorsal branch is heading dorsally across the side of the digit.

VESSELS
Arteries

The **brachial artery** is a direct continuation of the axillary. It enters the forearm by passing beneath the lacertus fibrosus, where it may be compressed with injuries to the distal humerus or elbow. It divides into radial and ulnar arteries after giving off recurrent branches that join in the anastomosis about the elbow.

The **radial artery** crosses superficial to the pronator teres and progresses distally down the forearm on the volar aspect of the distal radius, providing a nutrient artery to the radius and a number of muscle branches. A dorsal branch passes toward the ulna at the level of the carpus and gives off several dorsal metacarpal arteries. As the radial artery turns dorsally to cross the anatomic snuffbox it divides into superficial and deep branches. The superficial branch crosses the thenar eminence to join the terminal end of the superficial branch of the ulnar artery in forming the superficial arterial arch in the palm. The deep branch continues through the anatomic snuffbox deep to the thumb extensors, where it is very vulnerable to injury in approaches to the scaphoid or in procedures on the basal thumb joint. It passes between the two heads of the first dorsal interosseous muscle at the proximal ends of the first and second metacarpals to enter the deep surface of the palm, where it gives proper digital branches to the thumb and the radial aspect of the index finger. It continues between the two heads of the adductor pollicis, travels across the bases of the metacarpals, sending branches into the carpal tunnel to supply the synovium and carpal bones, and joins the deep branch of the ulnar artery to make up the deep arterial arch (Fig. 21-28). Extending distally from this arch are metacarpal branches that communicate at the web space with digital arteries from the superficial arch. This frequently is the route of arterial supply to the fingers

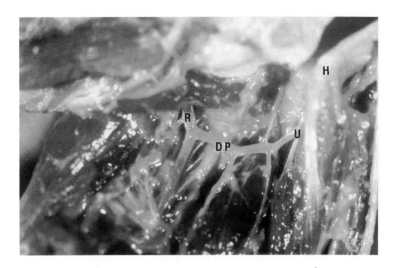

FIG. 21-28. Deep palmar arterial arch. Metacarpal arteries pass distally on the interossei and communicate with common digital branches from the superficial arch in the web spaces. Branches also pass proximally into the carpal tunnel to supply the synovium and wrist joint capsule. *DP,* Deep palmar arterial arch; *H,* hook of the hamate bone; *R,* Deep branch of radial artery entering palm between two heads of adductor pollicis; *U,* deep branch of ulnar artery passing around the hook of the hamate bone.

when the ulnar artery is occluded, which often occurs in the *hypothenar hammer* syndrome.

The **common interosseous artery** originates from the ulnar artery soon after it arises as one of the terminal divisions of the brachial artery and travels to the upper end of the interosseous membrane. Here it divides into anterior and posterior interosseous arteries that pass distally on either surface of the interosseous membrane to the level of the wrist joint, where they may again communicate with each other and with other vessels in an anastomosis around the carpus.

The **ulnar artery,** after providing the common interosseous artery, progresses distally between the flexor carpi ulnaris and flexor digitorum profundus muscles in company with the ulnar nerve. At the level of the wrist joint it enters Guyon's canal, where it divides into superficial and deep branches. The superficial branch passes radially beneath the palmar aponeurosis just at the distal end of the carpal tunnel, where it ends by joining the superficial branch of the radial artery near the thenar eminence. Frequently this communication is absent and the ulnar artery takes an oblique course across the palm, ending in the common digital artery to the web space between the index and middle fingers. The superficial branch is subcutaneous for a short distance between its exit from Guyon's canal and the edge of the palmar aponeurosis. At this site it is subject to trauma in using the heel of the hand to strike objects. From the superficial arch arise several common digital arteries that then divide into proper digital arteries to supply each side of the fingers. The tip of the index finger may be supplied solely by a branch from the radial artery or entirely by a branch from the ulnar artery. In this situation, occlusion of the radial or ulnar artery might result in ischemic necrosis of a portion of the tip of the finger. The deep branch of

the ulnar artery, given off in Guyon's canal, travels with the deep branch of the ulnar nerve through a canal in the origin of the hypothenar muscles from the hook of the hamate (Fig. 21-12). It passes across the bases of the metacarpals to join the deep branch of the radial artery to form the deep arch that lies approximately 1 cm proximal to the superficial arch.

Veins

Veins are numerous in the fingers and thumb where they run longitudinally in the subcutaneous fatty tissue. When they approach the web spaces they pass dorsally onto the back of the hand and empty into a dorsal venous arch over the distal portions of the metacarpals. From the radial and ulnar ends of this arch larger collecting veins arise and traverse the radial and ulnar aspects of the forearm to the cubital area, where the more ulnar vein passes deep to join the brachial vein. The more radial vein crosses the cubital fossa as the antecubital vein and continues proximally as the cephalic vein. There is usually a large connection between these two at the level of the proximal forearm.

Lymphatics

Lymphatics tend to follow the veins and drain dorsally onto the back of the hand. There is an extensive network in the subcutaneous space on the back of the hand and forearm. Any insult to the fingers will quickly be reflected in edema of the back of the hand; this has to be carefully evaluated to avoid confusion with an abscess following a purulent tenosynovitis of a finger. There are no lymph nodes in the hand or forearm. There is a first node evident in the epitrochlear region above the medial epicondyle of the humerus, and then the major drainage is into the axillary nodes.

REFERENCES

1. Amadio PS, Jaeger SH, Hunter JM: Nutritional aspects of tendon healing. In Hunter JM et al (eds): *Rehabilitation of the hand*, ed 2, St Louis, 1984, Mosby.
2. Bogumill GP: A morphologic study of the relationship of collateral ligaments to the growth plate in the digits, *J Hand Surg* 8:74, 1983.
3. Bowers WH et al: The proximal interphalangeal joint volar plate. I. An anatomical and biomechanical study, *J Hand Surg* 5:79, 1980.
3a. Burton RI, Pellegrini VD, Jr: Surgical management of basal joint arthritis of the thumb. Part II. Ligament reconstruction with tendon interposition arthroplasty, *J Hand Surg* 11A:324, 1986.
4. Cleland FRS: On the cutaneous ligaments of the phalanges, *J Anat Physiol* 12:526, 1878.
5. Doyle JR, Blythe W: The finger flexor tendon sheath and pulleys: anatomy and reconstruction. In *AAOS symposium on tendon surgery in the hand*, St Louis, 1975, Mosby.
6. Doyle JR, Blythe WF: Anatomy of the flexor tendon sheath and pulleys of the thumb, *J Hand Surg* 2:149, 1977.
7. Grayson J: The cutaneous ligaments of the digits, *J Anat* 75:164, 1940.
8. Mayfield JK: Wrist ligamentous anatomy and pathogenesis of carpal instability, *Orthop Clin North Am* 15:209, 1984.
9. Mayfield JK, Johnson RP, Kilcoyne RF: The ligaments of the human wrist and their functional significance, *Anat Rec* 186:417, 1976.
10. Mayfield JK, Johnson RP, Kilcoyne RF: Carpal dislocation: pathomechanics and progressive perilunar instability, *J Hand Surg* 5:226, 1980.
11. Milford L: *Retaining ligaments of the digits of the hand*, Philadelphia, 1968, WB Saunders.
12. Ochiai N et al: Vascular anatomy of flexor tendons. I. Vincular system and blood supply of the profundus tendon in the digital sheath, *J Hand Surg* 4:321, 1979.
13. Palmer AK: The distal radioulnar joint: anatomy, biomechanics and triangular fibrocartilage complex abnormalities, *Hand Clin* 3(1):31, 1987.
14. Palmer AK, Werner FW: The triangular fibrocartilage complex of the wrist: anatomy and function, *J Hand Surg* 6:153, 1981.
15. Smith RJ: Intrinsic muscles of the fingers: function, dysfunction, and surgical reconstruction. In AAOS: *Instructional course lectures*, vol 24, St Louis, 1975, Mosby.
16. Taleisnik J: The ligaments of the wrist, *J Hand Surg* 1:110, 1976.
17. Taleisnik J: Wrist: anatomy, function and injury. In AAOS: *Instructional course lectures*, vol 27, St Louis, 1978, Mosby.

ADDITIONAL READINGS

Bogumill GP: Functional anatomy of the forearm and hand. In Petrone FA (ed): *AAOS symposium on upper extremity injuries in athletes*, St Louis, 1986, Mosby.

Bogumill GP: Anatomy of the wrist. In Lichtman DL (ed): *The wrist and its disorders*, Philadelphia, 1988, WB Saunders.

Kanavel AB: *Infections of the hand: a guide to the surgical treatment of acute and chronic suppurative processes in the fingers, hand and forearm*, ed 7, Philadelphia, 1939, Lea & Febiger.

Laudsmeer JMF: *Atlas of anatomy of the hand*, Edinburgh, 1976, Churchill Livingstone.

Spinner M (ed): *Kaplan's functional and surgical anatomy of the hand*, ed 3, Philadelphia, 1984, JB Lippincott.

Taleisnick J: *The wrist*, New York, 1985, Churchill Livingstone.

Tubiana R (ed): *The hand*, vol I, Philadelphia, 1981, WB Saunders.

CHAPTER 22

Diagnostic and Surgical Arthroscopy of the Wrist

Terry L. Whipple

LOADING PATTERNS OF THE WRIST IN SPORTS

The wrist is a complex joint capable of motion in three planes. It provides the foundation for force transfer from the hand and postures the hand for fine motor activity and power grip.

In sports the wrist may sustain injury through any of four principal mechanisms: traction, weight bearing, twisting, and impact.[4]

Traction

Throwing and swinging motions apply a traction force to the wrist. In all throwing activities the wrist moves from a position of extension and radial deviation toward flexion and ulnar deviation—a motion also common to racquet sports, golf, and batting. The weight of a ball, club, or the hand itself applies traction to the wrist throughout the motion of throwing or swinging. Most of this traction is applied through the abductor pollicis longus, extensor pollicis brevis, and the radial wrist extensors, while a counterforce is applied through the flexor carpi ulnaris. If a supinating motion is involved, as in throwing a curve ball or undercutting a tennis forehand, the extensor carpi ulnaris stretches through its retinaculum over the distal ulna. Overuse syndromes therefore usually relate to these specific muscle tendon units or to the ligaments that support the pisiform.[3,17,32,38,39] Excessive throwing or swinging of racquets, bats, or clubs may cause extensor carpi ulnaris tendinitis, de Quervain's stenosing tenosynovitis, or occasionally sprains of the pisotriquetral ligament or stress fractures of the pisiform. Intraarticular injuries of the wrist are not commonly associated with throwing or swinging motions.[1,2,9,27,31]

Weight Bearing

In sports such as gymnastics, weight lifting, shotputting, and distance cycling the wrist bears heavy compression loads. Torque may also be applied during compression. In gymnastics, support of the gymnast's entire body weight through the wrist is required for floor exercises, parallel bars, vaulting, and aerial rings. In body building or competitive weight lifting, compressive loads through the wrist may greatly exceed body weight. These loads are usually transferred with the forearm pronated and the wrist in extension and radial deviation. Most of the stress is applied to the palmar structures, which include the flexor carpi ulnaris–pisiform–triquetrum complex, the volar ulnocarpal ligaments, the volar radiocarpal ligaments, and the thicker palmar aspect of the scapholunate ligament. Hyperextension of the wrist dorsiflexes the lunate but forces it in a palmar direction. Dislocation of the lunate may occur in weight-bearing activity as a result of rupture of the volar radiocarpal ligaments and the intrinsic ligaments of the proximal carpal row. The volar radiocarpal ligaments are well developed as an evolutionary reflection of our quadruped ancestors.

Articular lesions may develop on the head of the capitate or the volar lip of the radius (Fig. 22-1), and the volar ulnocarpal ligament is sometimes avulsed from the ulna or the central disk of the triangular fibrocartilage complex (TFCC). Alternatively, tears through the central disk may occur parallel to its volar margin (Fig. 22-2 and Plate 11).*

---

*References 5, 6, 8, 11, 15, and 18.

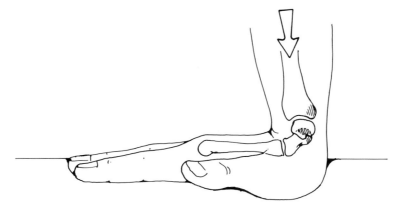

FIG. 22-1. Axial loading of the wrist in dorsiflexion. Axial loading can produce articular lesions on the volar lip of the radius or the dorsal aspect of the head of the capitate (*shaded areas*).

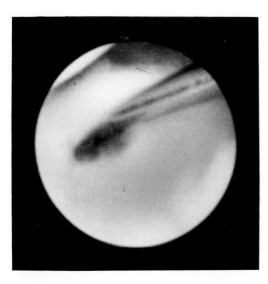

FIG. 22-2. Right wrist. Arthroscopic view of a linear tear in the volar aspect of the TFC articular disk. The tear runs parallel to the volar radioulnar ligament.

Twisting

Most pronation and supination motions are functions of the elbow and forearm. The wrist translates this motion through the distal radioulnar joint, resulting in tension on the volar and dorsal radioulnar ligaments, which attach to the base of the ulnar styloid. These structures are at risk to excessive passive pronation or supination (Fig. 22-3).[22,23,26]

Twisting injuries are not uncommon in wrestling and gymnastics. Again, parallel bars, floor exercises, and aerial rings pose the greatest threat in gymnastics. Forceful pronation and supination are motions that are uncommon in other sports. Twisting injuries to the wrist are more often associated with industrial accidents involving rotating machinery or hand tools. If the force is dissipated distally, the volar ligaments between the triquetrum and hamate may tear, resulting in midcarpal instability. Disruption of the saddle joint between the hamate and triquetrum causes a form of midcarpal instability wherein the hamate drops palmward in supination and the proximal pole of the hamate crosses the articular surface of the lunate in extreme ulnar deviation.[7,15,23] This injury can be devastating.

Impact

The most unpredictable form of impact loading results from falls that can occur in any athletic activity. Falls on the outstretched hand usually load the palmar aspect of the wrist. A shearing force progresses from the ulnar to the radial side of the wrist as body weight is applied (Fig. 22-4). Virtually any structure of the wrist can be injured in a fall, but the most common injuries are fractures of the distal radius with or without disruption of the distal radioulnar joint, fractures of the ulnar styloid, fractures of the waist of the scaphoid, tears of the lunotriquetral or scapholunate ligaments, tears of the triangular fibrocartilage, and tears of the volar radiocarpal ligaments.* If the neck of the capitate articulates with the dorsal edge of the lunate in hyperextension of the wrist, excessive force may produce a transverse fracture of the capitate, although this is infrequent.

Falls on the flexed wrist put stress on the dorsal side. Common injuries include avulsion of the dorsal capsule from the lunate or the distal radius, tears of the scapholunate ligament, fractures of the scaphoid, and flexion fractures of the distal radius (Fig. 22-5).[12,21,24]

Seemingly minor dorsal or volar capsule sprains may result in eventual ganglion formation through a process of mucoid degeneration.

More controlled impact loading to the wrist occurs with any sport in which the hands are used for offensive or defensive purposes. Examples include combat sports such as boxing and martial arts. In these sports the wrist is usually loaded in either of two ways. In boxing, axial loads through the metacarpals are transferred to the carpus through the capitate, lunate, and proximal pole of the scaphoid. If excessive, such forces may result in chondromalacic changes on the articular cartilage of the

---

*References 5, 6, 13, 15, 18, and 24.

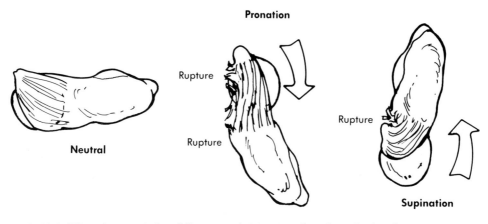

FIG. 22-3. When the wrist is forcefully pronated, injuries to the volar radioulnar ligament may occur. "Ulna dorsal" instability of the distal radioulnar joint may also be present. Hypersupination injuries may rupture the dorsal radioulnar ligament, which is rolled at the base of the ulnar styloid.

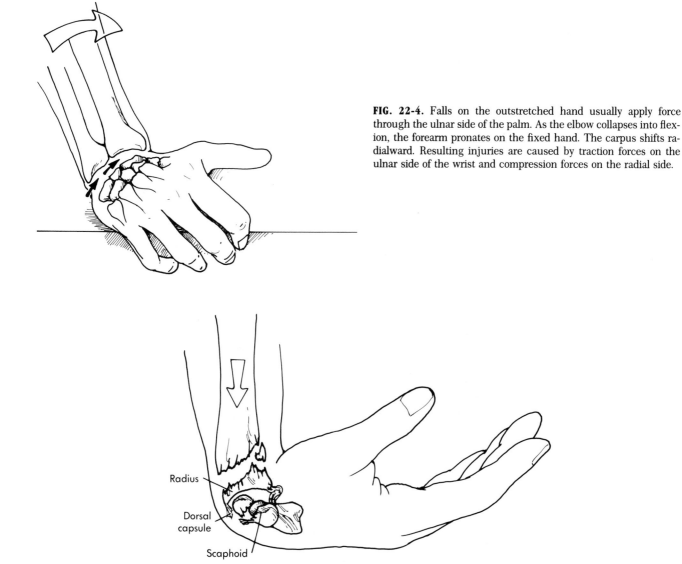

FIG. 22-4. Falls on the outstretched hand usually apply force through the ulnar side of the palm. As the elbow collapses into flexion, the forearm pronates on the fixed hand. The carpus shifts radialward. Resulting injuries are caused by traction forces on the ulnar side of the wrist and compression forces on the radial side.

FIG. 22-5. Falls on the wrist in flexion produce dorsal soft-tissue injuries or fractures of the distal radius, frequently with a volar butterfly fragment.

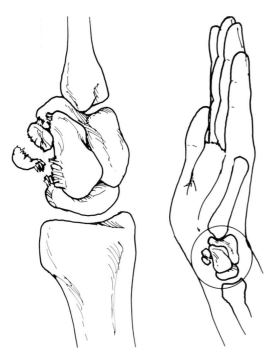

FIG. 22-6. Impact load applied to the palmar ulnar aspect of the wrist may fracture the pisiform or tear the pisotriquetral or the piso-hamate ligaments.

head of the capitate or on the convex surfaces of the lunate and scaphoid. The loading pattern is controlled by stabilization of the carpus with the extensor and flexor tendons. Forces applied with the wrist malpositioned or unstabilized stretch the intercarpal ligaments, especially the dorsal aspect of the scapholunate ligament. Fractures of the proximal pole of the scaphoid may occur, or small bone fragments may be avulsed at the insertion of the scapholunate ligament.

Impact loading also occurs on the ulnar side of the wrist in combat sports. Most offensive actions load the palmar aspect of the ulnar side of the wrist along the base of the fifth metacarpal or in the region of the pisiform. Defensive maneuvers more often load the dorsal ulnar aspect of the wrist when absorbing or deflecting the blows of an opponent.

Palmar ulnar impact injuries may fracture the pisiform or tear its ligamentous attachment to the triquetrum or hamate (Fig. 22-6). The saddle joint of the triquetrum and hamate is also at risk, and fractures of the fifth metacarpal are common. Impact injuries applied directly to the base of the palm may fracture the hook of the hamate.[19]

Defensive injuries to the dorsal ulnar aspect of the wrist usually involve the extensor carpi ulnaris retinaculum, the ulnar styloid, and the lunotriquetral ligament. Less commonly the dorsal ligamentous aspect of the TFCC may be torn or avulsed from the central articular disk.

Athletic injuries to the ulnar side of the wrist usually involve soft tissues. Injuries on the radial side are more likely to involve bone and articular cartilage.[6,8,23]

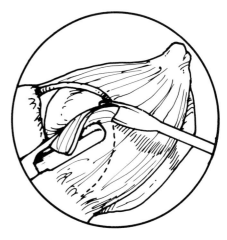

FIG. 22-7. Representation of arthroscopic excision of the radial central aspect of the TFC articular disk with a miniature banana blade arthroscopy knife and grasping forceps.

ARTHROSCOPY AND ITS ROLE IN WRIST DISORDERS

The value of wrist arthroscopy in sports injuries lies in its potential for achieving the most satisfactory long-term treatment results with decreased treatment morbidity when the alternative would be either a prolonged non-operative treatment with less precise anatomic repair of injured tissues or an extensive surgical exposure. Arthroscopy also has an advantage in the professional or high-performance amateur athlete in achieving a more rapid return to competition because it facilitates obtaining an earlier definitive diagnosis. When appropriate, arthroscopy also allows minimally invasive surgical treatment.

Wrist arthroscopy is a recently developed modality. Although attempted sporadically since 1975 in the United States and Japan, it was not until 1985 that the technique was refined sufficiently, that diagnostic arthroscopic examination became a practical consideration, and that surgical procedures under arthroscopic control were attempted with predictable, favorable expectations.[25,36,37]

Equipment

Because the interosseous spaces between the radius and proximal carpal row and between the proximal and distal carpal rows are limited, an arthroscope with an outermost diameter of 3 mm or less is necessary for a comprehensive arthroscopic examination. In small athletes, especially petite females, smaller scopes with an outside sheath diameter of 2.5 mm or less are advantageous in the radiocarpal and midcarpal spaces because they enable examination of the joint thoroughly without traumatizing the articular surfaces. The smaller scopes are essential for inspection of the scaphoid-trapezium-trapezoid (STT) joint and the distal radioulnar joint.

With larger scopes in the 5-mm diameter range, a larger portal can be made to place the tip of the scope just inside the joint and view from side to side. This af-

fords a larger field of view but limited access to the volar structures and midcarpal articular surfaces. Larger scopes may be useful for an occasional wrist examination when the cost of smaller instruments is not warranted but is no substitute for the smaller scopes if wrist arthroscopy is to be practiced regularly.

Because the smaller diameter arthroscopes contain more fragile optics that can easily break, shorter arthroscope lengths are recommended to reduce the bending forces applied. High-sensitivity, lightweight microchip video cameras are essential to provide a magnified image. The lighter weight microchip cameras place less force on the small-diameter arthroscopes than do heavier tube cameras, and the more sensitive microchip designs perform best with smaller diameter scopes carrying fewer fiberoptic light bundles.

Wrist arthroscopy equipment

- Small-diameter arthroscope (3 mm or less)
- High-sensitivity microchip video camera
- Small grasping devices, scissors
- Miniature sharp knives
- Miniature motorized equipment
- Cordless wire driver
- Disposable pinch pump inflow system

Small grasping devices, cutting forceps, and miniature sharp knives are available to facilitate surgical procedures in the wrist. These tools make it possible to retrieve loose bodies or debride small fragments of tissue from the joint and can be used to excise portions of the triangular fibrocartilage articular disk (Fig. 22-7). Miniaturized tips that fit powered arthroscopic instrumentation are also available and are indispensible for ensuring a clear visual field and efficient removal of any thin or filmy tissue (Fig. 22-8).

A small, preferably cordless wire driver can be used to

stabilize carpal bones or fracture fragments under arthroscopic control.

A disposable inflow system has been developed with a specially designed pinch chamber in the sterile field that introduces 2 to 3 mm of irrigant under pressure when needed (Fig. 22-9). This helps keep the joint distended and obviates the need for cumbersome syringes and stop-

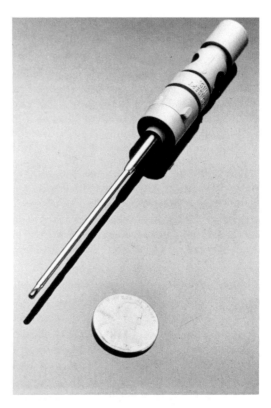

FIG. 22-8. This 2-mm shaver tip is helpful for the removal of small cartilage fibers and filmy synovial tissue from the joint. (Linvatec, Inc, Largo, Fla.)

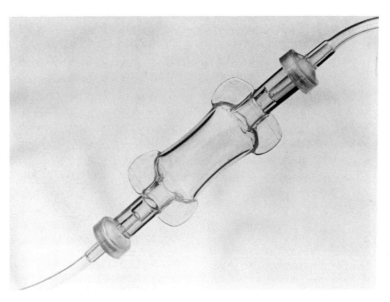

FIG. 22-9. This 2-mm pinch chamber near the end of the inflow tubing allows rapid introduction of additional irrigating solution when needed. (Linvatec, Inc, Largo, Fla.)

cocks. Expensive mechanized pumps have not been found necessary in this small joint.

Wrist arthroscopy is a technically demanding procedure. Appropriate instrumentation definitely makes the procedure easier and enhances the surgeon's successful performance.

Operating Room Environment

The surgical team should be coordinated and well rehearsed when undertaking arthroscopy of the wrist. The patient is positioned supine with the shoulder abducted 60 to 90 degrees and supported on a hand table or an arm board (Fig. 22-10). The elbow is flexed 90 degrees with the forearm vertical. Sterile finger traps are applied to the index and long fingers for most procedures, but if a pathologic condition is suspected on the ulnar side of the joint, the finger traps should be applied to the ring and little fingers to achieve greater distraction on the ulnar side. Sufficient traction is applied to the finger traps to lift the patient's elbow just off the arm board. This usually requires 7 to 10 pounds of distraction, depending on the patient's size. Distraction equal to the weight of the upper extremity, however, is usually sufficient to distract the radiocarpal and midcarpal spaces for good arthro-

scopic visualization. In patients who have inflammatory arthritis, all four digits may be placed in finger traps to distribute the traction forces and consideration should be given to using less weight.

Video equipment is positioned on the opposite side of the patient. The surgeon sits adjacent to the patient's head, facing the dorsum of the hand. The assistant sits opposite the surgeon at the patient's axilla, facing the palm. This allows the assistant easy access to instruments placed at the end of the hand table, as well as a good view of the video monitor, and the ability to steady the arthroscope and camera for the surgeon when necessary (Fig. 22-11).

Wrist Techniques

Arthroscopic portals for the wrist are most easily identified by the extensor compartments between which they lie.[37] There are five primary portals for the radiocarpal space (Fig. 22-12). The first portal is between the first and second extensor compartments (1-2), just adjacent to the point of intersection of the extensor pollicis longus with the extensor carpi radialis longus. The most important portal for general radiocarpal examination lies between the third and fourth extensor compartments (3-

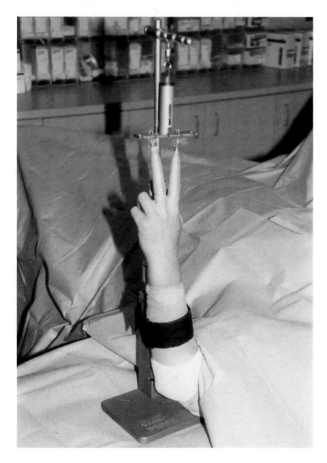

FIG. 22-10. Patient positioned for wrist arthroscopy with traction applied to the index and long fingers through sterile Traction Tower. Electronic and video equipment are arranged on the non-operative side of the patient. (Linvatec, Inc, Largo, Fla.)

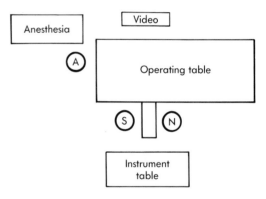

FIG. 22-11. Diagrammatic representation of convenient operating room arrangement. *A,* Anesthesiologist; *S,* surgeon; *N,* nurse assistant.

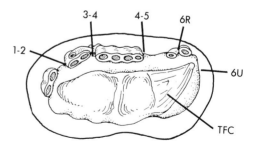

FIG. 22-12. Representation of the arthroscopy portals for the radiocarpal space for the left wrist. Portals are identified between the first and second extensor compartments (*1-2*), the third and fourth extensor compartments (*3-4*), the fourth and fifth extensor compartments (*4-5*), and just to the radial (*6R*) and ulnar (*6U*) sides of the extensor carpi ulnaris.

4). From here most of the articular surfaces of the radiocarpal space and the entire triangular fibrocartilage can be visualized. Between the fourth and fifth extensor compartments (4-5) accessory instruments are introduced to facilitate examination or arthroscopic surgical procedures. Just to the radial side of the extensor carpi ulnaris (6R) or to its ulnar side (6U), an atraumatic plastic inflow cannula is placed. These two ulnar portals are also useful for the arthroscope or for cutting instruments when excising torn flaps of tissue from the triangular fibrocartilage.

There are three useful portals for the midcarpal space. The first lies about 1 cm distal to the 3-4 portal in line with the radial margin of the third ray. This is identified as the midcarpal radial portal. The STT joint can be seen from this portal, as can the articulations between the scaphoid and lunate and also between the lunate and triquetrum. A more ulnar portal between the extensor digitorum communis tendon to the little finger and the extensor digiti quinti is used for accessory or operating instruments. This portal is identified as the midcarpal ulnar portal. Finally, a useful portal occasionally used for accessory instruments in the STT joint interval lies in line with the second metacarpal, just distal to the extensor pollicis longus tendon. This portal is identified as the STT portal. Instruments should enter between the trapezoid and the distal pole of the scaphoid. The radial artery is protected by the intervening extensor carpi radialis longus tendon.

Arthroscopy portals

Radiocarpal space
- Between first and second dorsal compartments (1-2)
- Between third and fourth dorsal compartments (3-4)
- Between fourth and fifth dorsal compartments (4-5)
- Radial aspect of extensor carpi ulnaris (6R)
- Ulnar aspect of extensor carpi ulnaris (6U)

Midcarpal space
- Midcarpal radial
- Midcarpal ulnar
- Scaphoid-trapezium-trapezoid

The distal radioulnar joint can occasionally be entered with a small arthroscope through a portal at the metaphyseal flare of the distal ulna. With the forearm supinated, the dorsal capsule of the distal radioulnar joint is lax and most easily entered, but care must be taken not to injure the extensor tendon to the little finger. It is sometimes possible to advance the arthroscope from this position into the space between the head of the ulna and the proximal surface of the triangular fibrocartilage articular disk to retrieve loose bodies and to inspect or transfix fractures of the ulnar styloid.

The arthroscopic sheath and trocar should always be introduced with a twisting motion to separate the joint capsule fibers in an atraumatic manner. Other instruments should be inserted in a similar fashion. Preferred instruments have tapered or gently pointed tips. Care must be taken to avoid inadvertent introduction of any air bubbles into the joint because they impair visualization.[25,37]

DIAGNOSTIC ARTHROSCOPY

Arthroscopic examination of the wrist is most useful for soft-tissue injuries that cannot be precisely diagnosed through conventional imaging techniques. As more experience is gained, it has become apparent that even definitive diagnoses based on arthrography can be further qualified by arthroscopic examination. Arthroscopic examination also facilitates treatment planning. Leakage of radiographic contrast medium through the triangular fibrocartilage confirms communication between two normally separated spaces but provides no useful information with respect to the mechanical significance or the chronicity of the defect. Tears in the scapholunate or lunotriquetral ligaments may or may not be repairable, but this determination cannot be made on the basis of arthrography alone. Arthroscopic examination is helpful, therefore, if plain radiographs are normal following an acute injury, yet there is reasonable clinical suspicion of an intraarticular soft-tissue injury. Extraarticular tendons, nerves, and vessels cannot be evaluated arthroscopically, of course. Arthrography, isotope scanning, or magnetic resonance imaging (MRI) may be helpful preoperatively in certain circumstances.[5,6,10]

In the radiocarpal space articular surfaces, volar wrist ligaments, and the dorsal wrist capsule can be inspected thoroughly for signs of trauma. The wrist should be flexed and extended while the surgeon watches the motion relationships between the scaphoid and lunate. The scapholunate ligament must be probed thoroughly from the 4-5 portal.

Articular surfaces, the scapholunate, and the lunotriquetral ligaments should be probed thoroughly from the 4-5 portal in search of softening or rupture (Fig. 22-13). Most tears of the scapholunate ligament originate dorsally where the ligament is thinner and may progress to varying degrees toward the volar aspect.*

The triangular fibrocartilage is visualized well from the 3-4 portal or the 6R portal, but the latter vantage is most useful. A probe may be introduced through the 4-5, 6R, or 6U portal. It is often necessary to switch the portals for the arthroscope and probe to facilitate a thorough evaluation of the TFCC. Tears in the central articular disk may be found adjacent to the TFCC's attachment to the sigmoid notch (Type 1-D) in the central portion of the articular disk as in cases of ulnocarpal impingement (Type 1-A), or parallel to the dorsal or volar capsule attachments to the articular disk (Type 1-B).[5,20,22,28]

In an acute injury, inspection of the volar radiocarpal ligaments may disclose hemorrhage or ligament laxity even in wrist extension (Fig. 22-14). Moving the wrist through flexion and extension during the course of arthroscopic examination, as well as extensive probing of the ligaments, helps define the magnitude of these injuries.[6,28]

---

*References 6, 8, 10, 15, 18, 22, and 35.

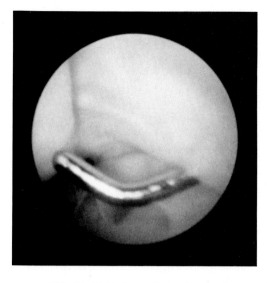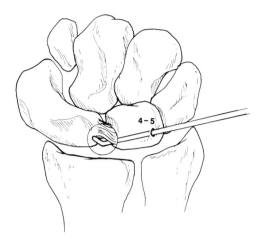

FIG. 22-13. Probe exploring the scapholunate ligament of a right wrist through the 4-5 portal.

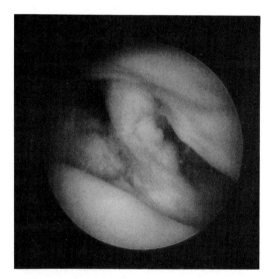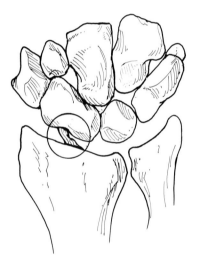

FIG. 22-14. Through the 3-4 portal acute hemorrhage is seen adjacent to a lax volar radiocarpal ligament.

In the midcarpal space the articular surfaces of the scaphoid and capitate can be examined well. In the STT joint articular changes may be found on the distal pole of the scaphoid, at times severe enough to expose subchondral bone.[10]

Structures visualized by wrist arthroscopy

- Articular surfaces
- Volar wrist ligaments
- Dorsal wrist capsule
- Scapholunate ligament
- Lunotriquetral ligament
- Triangular fibrocartilage
- Intercarpal relationships
- Distal radioulnar joint

On the ulnar side of the midcarpal space the tip of the hamate should be inspected thoroughly. It is normally smooth and glistening, and the interval between the hamate and triquetrum permits only a glimpse of the volar ulnocarpal ligaments at best. If this space is widened, if the volar ligaments can be visualized well, and especially if there are erosive changes present on the proximal pole of the hamate, a midcarpal instability is almost certainly present. This injury is characterized by stretch or rupture of the volar ulnocarpal ligament complex extending between the triquetrum and the hamate. In ulnar deviation, at the completion of a golf swing, for example, the tip of the hamate trips across the ulnar edge of the lunate with a discernible "clunk." Midcarpal instability is usually associated with rupture of the lunotriquetral ligament as well.[7,10,14,15]

Finally, from the midcarpal space the orientation of the

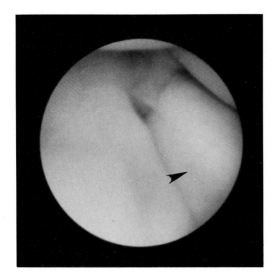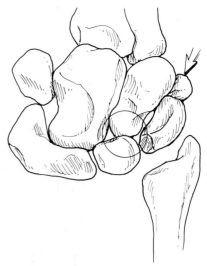

FIG. 22-15. In the midcarpal space of a right wrist, instability between the lunate and triquetrum is evidenced by excessive motion of the triquetrum when external pressure is applied. The lunate articular facet of the triquetrum is seen *(arrow)*.

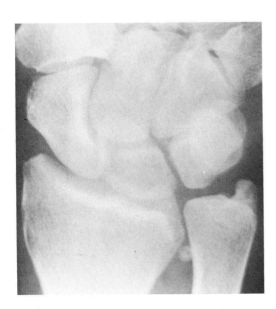

FIG. 22-16. Loose bodies seen in the distal radioulnar joint of the right wrist.

lunate to the scaphoid and the triquetrum should be examined. Each of these carpal bones may be palpated dorsally to test for abnormal anterior-to-posterior translation motion. When all intercarpal ligaments are intact, slight flexion and extension are possible between the scaphoid and lunate and between the lunate and triquetrum. However, this motion is constrained; so the distal articular surface of the proximal row is never grossly irregular. Normally there should be no exposure of the articular surfaces between the lunate and the triquetrum, nor between the scaphoid and the lunate (Fig. 22-15).[6,8,15]

The distal radioulnar joint should be examined if there is suspicion of a pathologic condition. This is a difficult joint to examine arthroscopically. With some experience the degree of distal radioulnar dissociation can be appreciated from translational movements between the bones in extremes of pronation and supination. Loose bodies are occasionally found in this joint as well (Fig. 22-16).[10,15,23]

The volar ulnocarpal ligaments originate from the fovea of the head of the ulna and extend distally blending with the volar edge of the triangular fibrocartilage to form a complex. Avulsion of the ulnocarpal ligaments can sometimes be seen proximal to the triangular fibrocartilage at the base of the ulnar styloid. This injury usually occurs in association with extremes of forceful extension and radial deviation.

ARTHROSCOPIC SURGERY

Arthroscopic surgery is not a new surgical procedure. It is a minimally invasive technique for accomplishing traditional, tested surgical procedures for a variety of wrist disorders, many of which are commonly encountered in athletes. With the reduced morbidity of minimally invasive arthroscopic technique, the indications for surgical treatment of certain disorders might be influenced by the possibility of shortened recuperation periods. Many disorders of the wrist are amenable only to open repair; Type III tears of the TFCC and instability of the distal radioulnar joint are such examples. However, with developing skills and instrumentation, some wrist disorders have become treatable with minimally invasive techniques under arthroscopic control.[33,34]

Articular Cartilage

There is no definitive means of repairing or reversing injuries to hyaline cartilage. The potential for autogenous repair appears to be dependent on the health and responsiveness of remaining chondrocytes and the degree of severity of the injury. Arthroscopic shaving of Outerbridge Grade II and Grade III articular lesions in the knee has

proven to have no reparative benefit for the articular surface. This procedure is believed to be beneficial to the joint, however, by decreasing the inflammatory reaction that is caused by shedded fragments of hyaline cartilage. The procedure has equal therapeutic potential for Grade II and Grade III articular lesions of the wrist, which are common following repeated impact loading or compression loading of this joint. Surface debridement can be accomplished easily with miniaturized shaver tips for motorized instrumentation with virtually no recuperation required. At the same time, hypertrophic or inflamed synovial membranes can be removed.

Full-thickness articular lesions exposing subchondral bone have no potential for spontaneous recovery. It has been demonstrated in other joints, however, that exposure of intraosseous circulation to the surface of the defect produces granulation tissue formation on the exposed subchondral bone. If protected, this granulation

tissue can mature into reasonably firm fibrocartilage and provide some reduction in friction during motion of opposing joint surfaces. This procedure, known as **abrasion arthroplasty,** is a more logical procedure in non–weight-bearing joints of the upper extremity. Short-term benefits of abrading full-thickness defects on articular surfaces of the radius, distal pole of the scaphoid, and proximal tip of the hamate include symptomatic relief. However, a return to sports that involve weight bearing or impact loading on these surfaces should not be recommended.

Small powered burs or curettes are used for removal of superficial subchondral surfaces. Vascular elements are abundant in the distal radius but are apparently sparse in the subchondral bone of the carpals. Drilling exposed carpal surfaces with 0.045-inch K-wires is recommended to access intraosseous vascularity and to minimize removal of normal bone contours (Fig. 22-17).

Intercarpal Ligaments

Many procedures have been devised for chronic severe rotatory subluxation of the scaphoid.[16] Invariably this condition results from a neglected tear of the scapholunate ligament. The radioscaphoidcapitate ligament over which the scaphoid flexes may also be torn or stretched. Rarely do acute injuries result in complete disruption of the scapholunate articulation. Adequate intervention in the acute stage of scapholunate disruption may prevent the eventual consequences of more severe instability. Widening of the scapholunate interval on anterior posterior (AP) radiographs or angulation of more than 15 degrees between the capitate and lunate axes on lateral radiographs is evidence of major scapholunate instability. These changes are rarely seen following acute injury, however, and may reflect chronicity of the scapholunate instability.

Localized tenderness dorsally over the scapholunate junction following an acute injury should raise suspicion of scapholunate ligament disruption. If acute tenderness

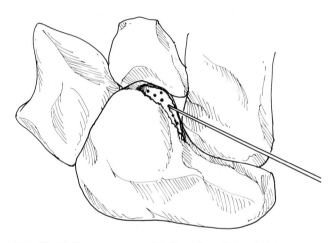

FIG. 22-17. Representation of drilling the subchondral bone with a smooth K-wire in a full-thickness articular defect on the distal pole of scaphoid.

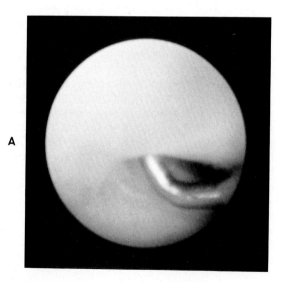
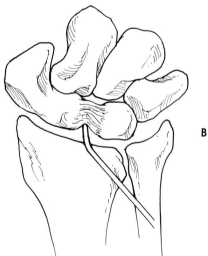

FIG. 22-18. Probe demonstrating a stretch injury to the scapholunate ligament of a right wrist. **A,** Arthroscopic view. **B,** Artist's perspective.

proven to have no reparative benefit for the articular surface. This procedure is believed to be beneficial to the joint, however, by decreasing the inflammatory reaction that is caused by shedded fragments of hyaline cartilage. The procedure has equal therapeutic potential for Grade II and Grade III articular lesions of the wrist, which are common following repeated impact loading or compression loading of this joint. Surface debridement can be accomplished easily with miniaturized shaver tips for motorized instrumentation with virtually no recuperation required. At the same time, hypertrophic or inflamed synovial membranes can be removed.

Full-thickness articular lesions exposing subchondral bone have no potential for spontaneous recovery. It has been demonstrated in other joints, however, that exposure of intraosseous circulation to the surface of the defect produces granulation tissue formation on the exposed subchondral bone. If protected, this granulation

tissue can mature into reasonably firm fibrocartilage and provide some reduction in friction during motion of opposing joint surfaces. This procedure, known as **abrasion arthroplasty,** is a more logical procedure in non–weight-bearing joints of the upper extremity. Short-term benefits of abrading full-thickness defects on articular surfaces of the radius, distal pole of the scaphoid, and proximal tip of the hamate include symptomatic relief. However, a return to sports that involve weight bearing or impact loading on these surfaces should not be recommended.

Small powered burs or curettes are used for removal of superficial subchondral surfaces. Vascular elements are abundant in the distal radius but are apparently sparse in the subchondral bone of the carpals. Drilling exposed carpal surfaces with 0.045-inch K-wires is recommended to access intraosseous vascularity and to minimize removal of normal bone contours (Fig. 22-17).

Intercarpal Ligaments

Many procedures have been devised for chronic severe rotatory subluxation of the scaphoid.[16] Invariably this condition results from a neglected tear of the scapholunate ligament. The radioscaphoidcapitate ligament over which the scaphoid flexes may also be torn or stretched. Rarely do acute injuries result in complete disruption of the scapholunate articulation. Adequate intervention in the acute stage of scapholunate disruption may prevent the eventual consequences of more severe instability. Widening of the scapholunate interval on anterior posterior (AP) radiographs or angulation of more than 15 degrees between the capitate and lunate axes on lateral radiographs is evidence of major scapholunate instability. These changes are rarely seen following acute injury, however, and may reflect chronicity of the scapholunate instability.

Localized tenderness dorsally over the scapholunate junction following an acute injury should raise suspicion of scapholunate ligament disruption. If acute tenderness

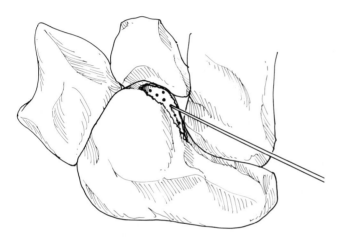

FIG. 22-17. Representation of drilling the subchondral bone with a smooth K-wire in a full-thickness articular defect on the distal pole of scaphoid.

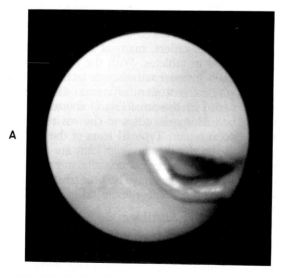
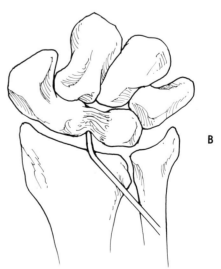

FIG. 22-18. Probe demonstrating a stretch injury to the scapholunate ligament of a right wrist. **A,** Arthroscopic view. **B,** Artist's perspective.

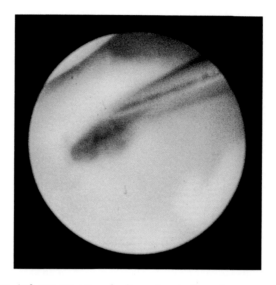

PLATE 11. Right wrist. Arthroscopic view of a linear tear in the volar aspect of the TFC articular disk. The tear runs parallel to the volar radioulnar ligament (Palmer Type I-D).

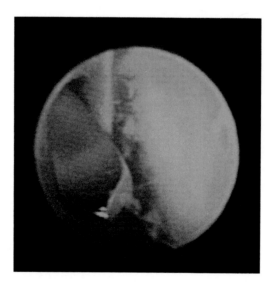

PLATE 12. Arthroscopic view of 0.045-inch smooth K-wire entering the radial wrist capsule adjacent to the proximal pole of the scaphoid.

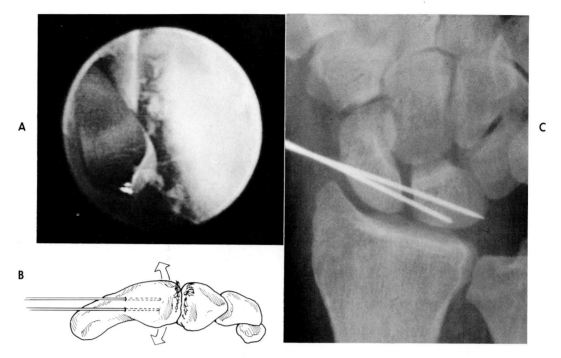

FIG. 22-19. Technique for arthroscopic reduction and internal fixation of an acute scapholunate dissociation injury of the right wrist. **A,** Arthroscopic view of 0.045-inch smooth K-wire entering the radial wrist capsule adjacent to the proximal pole of the scaphoid. **B,** Representation of two K-wires drilled into the proximal pole scaphoid to aid with manipulation and reduction before fixation of the scapholunate interval. **C,** Postoperative radiograph with the scapholunate joint reduced and two K-wires properly positioned to stabilize the joint.

persists after 3 to 4 weeks of immobilization, an arthrogram is indicated. If contrast material flows from the radiocarpal to the midcarpal space through the scapholunate interval, a tear in the scapholunate ligament is confirmed. A negative arthrogram, however, is of little clinical significance. The scapholunate membrane can be stretched enough to cause instability of this joint without complete ligament disruption, just as similar stretch injuries occur in the knee, ankle, and shoulder. If the injury is reduced and immobilized early, healing of the scapholunate ligament is possible. Injury to the scapholunate ligament is confirmed by examination and probing through the 3-4 and 4-5 radiocarpal portals (Fig. 22-18).

To reduce and stabilize the scapholunate interval, two 0.045-inch K-wires are placed transcutaneously into the proximal pole of the scaphoid from the radial side aiming toward the lunate (Fig. 22-19 and Plate 12). The arthroscope is then placed in the midcarpal radial portal to observe the volar articular margins of the scaphoid and lunate in the midcarpal space. The wrist is extended and deviated to the ulnar side to stand the scaphoid vertically. This reduces the scapholunate joint in most cases. Minor adjustment can be accomplished by manipulating one or both of the K-wires or by applying pressure to the scaphoid tubercle. When the articular margins of the scaphoid and lunate are perfectly matched, the K-wires are advanced across the joint into the lunate. Four or five pins should be placed across the scapholunate interval.

Arthroscopic inspection of the midcarpal space and the radiocarpal space will confirm that other articular surfaces have not been violated. An intraoperative radiograph is used to ensure that the pins have been satisfactorily placed. The pins are cut short and the wrist is protected with a cast for 8 weeks.

Although this treatment approach to scapholunate dissociation has not been evaluated by follow-up arthroscopic examination or arthrograms in large numbers of cases, anecdotal relooks have demonstrated that fibrosis between the scaphoid and lunate along the pin tracks provides sufficient stabilization of this interval. Watson[33] has described this concept as a beneficial fibrous union.*

Similar principles are applied for arthroscopic reduction and pin fixation of acute tears of the lunotriquetral ligament and the hamate-triquetral ligament. In these cases K-wires are introduced on the ulnar side of the wrist into the triquetrum and are advanced into the lunate or the hamate as necessary. At least three pins are recommended to avoid rotation of the carpals around the pin axes and to evoke a sufficient fibrous response.[6-8,10,15,21]

Volar and Dorsal Ligament Injuries

As previously discussed, hyperextension or hyperflexion injuries to the wrist may tear or avulse the palmar or dorsal radiocarpal ligaments, respectively. In my experi-

---

*References 6-8, 10, 15, 21, 25, and 33-35.

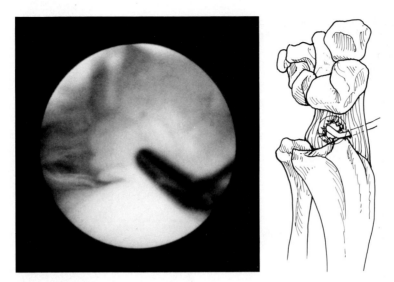

FIG. 22-20. Viewed from the 1-2 portal. Disrupted fibers in the dorsal capsule of a right wrist are probed through the 3-4 portal. Acute injuries demonstrate edema and hypertrophic synovium as well as disrupted fibers.

ence palmar ligaments are more likely to stretch or rupture because dorsal capsular ligaments are more commonly avulsed from their attachment to the radius. Examination of these ligaments is best accomplished through the 1-2 radiocarpal portal with the assistance of a 4-5 placed hook probe.[6,25,36]

Volar radiocarpal ligament injuries are treated by manipulating the wrist under arthroscopic examination to find the position of greatest ligament laxity—usually flexion and slight radial deviation. The wrist is then immobilized in this position for 4 to 6 weeks. A protective, removable gauntlet is recommended thereafter for 3 months, and the wrist should be taped for any athletic endeavor for 6 to 12 months, depending on the severity of the ligament injury. Although experience is insufficient at this time to predict with certainty, neglect of these volar radiocarpal ligament injuries may reasonably be expected to cause dorsal intercalated segmental instability posturing of the lunate.[2,6,14]

Dorsal capsular injuries are treated somewhat differently because they usually entail avulsion from the radius or the lunate. With the wrist in dorsiflexion it is usually possible to visualize the site of avulsion. The dorsal capsule gains attachment to the radius and the carpals immediately adjacent to the articular surface. If there is any undermining of capsule adjacent to the articular margin, ligament avulsion should be suspected. Localized hemorrhage is evident in more acute injuries (Fig. 22-20).

In subacute injuries, with the arthroscope in the 1-2 portal and an accessory bur or curette in the 4-5 or 6R portal, the exposed bone can be abraded to produce bleeding. The wrist should then be positioned in extension with a well-molded cast to relax the dorsal capsule in contact with the freshly abraded bone. Immobilization is recommended for 6 weeks, followed by a protective gauntlet and spica splinting for athletic activities.[18,28] In

chronic dorsal capsule avulsion cases, open reattachment using a suture anchor is the preferred treatment.

Triangular Fibrocartilage Complex

Injuries to the TFCC resulting from impact loading or excessive torque are treated in ways analogous to meniscus tears in the knee. The TFCC provides an opposing articular surface for the ulnar half of the lunate and the triquetrum. By virtue of the insertion of dorsal and volar ulnocarpal ligaments onto the triangular fibrocartilage, this structure also participates in ulnocarpal stability, although the precise mechanism is not well understood. The TFCC has also been credited with contribution to the stability of the distal radioulnar joint, although selective cutting studies have challenged this concept.

Palmer[20] has developed a useful classification of TFCC tears and defects. Central perforations of the triangular fibrocartilage that do not disrupt the peripheral ligamentous attachments or the insertion of the TFCC onto the radius (Types 1-A and 2-A) are of little mechanical consequence. The edges of these injuries can be trimmed smoother if necessary, but little definitive treatment is required.

By contrast, Types 1-B, 1-C, and 1-D injuries to the central disk of the triangular fibrocartilage should be treated more aggressively. Angular Type 1-D tears that create flaps of articular disk may interfere mechanically with wrist flexion and extension or with ulnar deviation. With the arthroscope placed in the 6R portal or the 3-4 portal, unstable flaps of tissue can be excised from the triangular fibrocartilage using miniaturized arthroscopic knives, basket forceps, punches, or certain motorized shaver tips. All unstable tissue should be removed from tears of the central articular disk of the triangular fibrocartilage. This may in many cases convert Type 1-D tears to stable central perforations of the articular disk (Figs. 22-21 and 22-22).

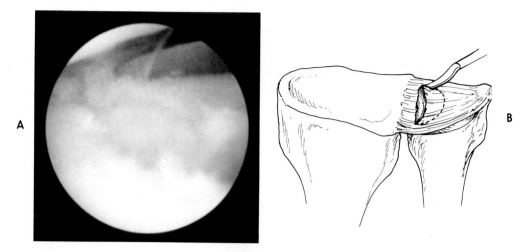

FIG. 22-21. A, Arthroscopic view of miniature banana blade knife excising the unstable portion of a Type 1-A tear in the TFC articular disk, right wrist. **B,** Representation of a Type 1-D tear and the intended line of tissue resection.

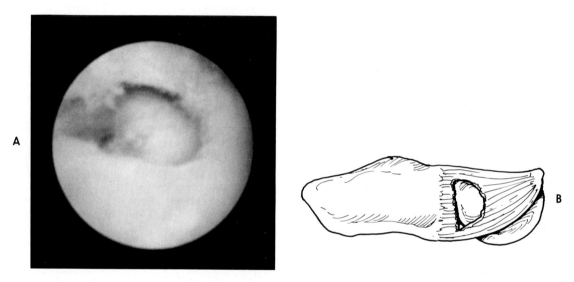

FIG. 22-22. Resected central portion of TFC articular disk. Ulnar head is visible through the defect. **A,** Arthroscopic view. **B,** Artist's perspective.

The wrist may be splinted postoperatively for comfort for a few days, but there is otherwise no contraindication to early return of functioning and competition with protective taping.

Type 1-B tears greater than 3 or 4 mm in length should be treated with suture repair (Fig. 22-23). Arthroscopic repair is possible using a specially designed suture passer and retriever and provides stable reconstitution of the TFCC with excellent results (Fig. 22-24). Precise approaches to the torn complex can be achieved by marking the tear under arthroscopic control with a hypodermic needle. A longitudinal miniature arthrotomy can then be made to directly access the tear by following the path of the needle.[5,15,23,29]

Intraarticular Fractures

There is no substitute for anatomic reduction of articular surfaces in the treatment of intraarticular fractures. To preserve joint mechanics and low friction contact and to decrease formation of adhesions, all fracture fragments containing articular cartilage should be precisely positioned as if assembling a three-dimensional jigsaw puzzle. Arthroscopy has provided a great advantage in the treatment of such fractures of the distal radius. Athletes are susceptible to distal radial fractures from falls on the upper extremity in almost every sport. High-speed or collision sports impart even greater energy with increased risk of fracture comminution. Many fracture fragments have inadequate capsule or ligament attach-

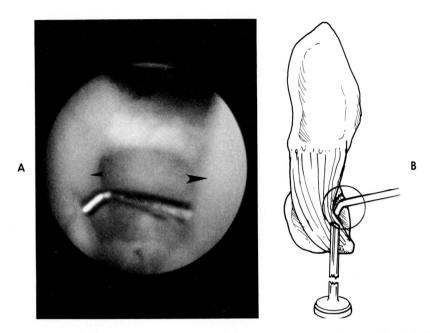

FIG. 22-23. View from the 6R portal of a Palmer Type I-B separation of the articular disk *(large arrow).* **A,** Arthroscopic view. **B,** Artist's perspective.

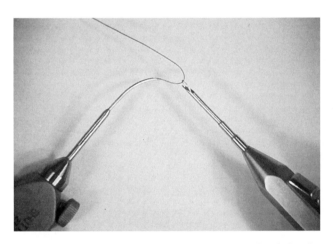

FIG. 22-24. Instruments for suture repair of peripheral detachments of the TFCC. (Linvatec, Inc, Largo, Fla.)

ment to allow manipulative reduction with closed techniques. This problem is typified by the so-called die-punch fracture in which the dorsal portion of the lunate facet of the radius is depressed proximally and impacted.

These fractures are amenable to treatment under arthroscopic control by precise reduction and K-wire fixation of the fracture fragments. This is a tedious procedure, however, and should not be undertaken casually.

Guided by good-quality preoperative radiographs and CT scans of the articular surface if necessary, the distal radius is visualized arthroscopically through the 3-4 or 1-2 portal. Large-volume irrigation is required to evacuate the hemarthrosis. The forearm should be wrapped snugly with a sterile compressive bandage to minimize fluid extravasation into the muscular compartments through fracture planes. This is a precautionary mea-

sure, although the risk is not as great as it might seem. It is important that the irrigation fluid should never be introduced with an inflow rate that is greater than the outflow system can accommodate. This provides adequate lavage of the joint space without forced extravasation into the soft tissues.

Lactated Ringer's solution is recommended not only because it is the most physiologically compatible solution for articular cartilage, but also because it is readily absorbed from soft-tissue compartments if extravasated. By clisis, lactated Ringer's solution is absorbed within minutes. Compartment compression syndromes resulting from closed fractures are usually caused by intramuscular bleeding, producing increased pressure for sustained periods. Arterial perfusion must be compromised for 3 to 4 hours before ischemic changes become irreversible. It is unlikely such compartmental pressure could be maintained by the extravasation of lactated Ringer's solution through articular fracture planes, although awareness of this potential risk should not be underemphasized.

Through accessory portals, small forceps or brushes can be used to remove the fibrin clot that may obscure fracture surfaces. When all fracture lines are well visualized, reduction of the fracture is centered around the largest articular fragment. Smaller fragments are repositioned as much as possible with the assistance of traction and periarticular pressure. Small, smooth K-wires are drilled into fragments that contain minimal soft-tissue attachment and cannot be otherwise manipulated. These K-wires are then used to maneuver the fragments into position to reassemble the articular surface. When fragments are impacted, it may be necessary to free them from one another with a small blunt dissector placed in the fracture planes as a lever (Fig. 22-25). As each fragment is reduced, a K-wire is advanced into the major adjacent fragments to stabilize the fragments. These wires

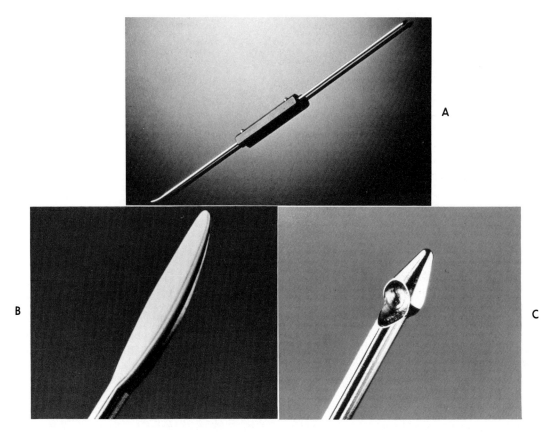

FIG. 22-25. A, Double-ended tool for small-joint arthroscopy. **B,** Curved, flat dissector on one end. **C,** Curette with tapered point on opposite end. (Linvatec, Inc, Largo, Fla.)

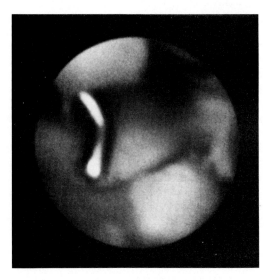

FIG. 22-26. Arthroscopic view of a reduced articular fracture of the distal radius. Intraarticular probe is used to assist with reduction of fragments.

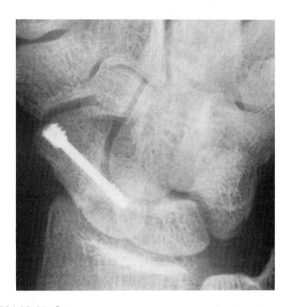

FIG. 22-27. Intraosseous compression screw placed arthroscopically in a nondisplaced fracture of the waist of the scaphoid in a football player, right wrist.

are discreetly placed between tendons so as not to impair finger movement (Fig. 22-26).

When the entire articular surface has been reassembled, an intraoperative radiograph is taken to confirm fracture reduction, joint surface contour, and pin placement. There need be no concern for voids beneath articular surfaces because they fill in during fracture healing with cancellous bone, making grafting unnecessary.

A cast is applied for 2 to 4 weeks, which is then converted to a splint that can be removed for early controlled motion exercises. This regimen facilitates remodeling of the articular surface, mobilizes adjacent joints early, decreases the possibility of intraarticular adhesions, and preserves tendon function. Long-term results from accurate reconstruction of the articular surface following such fractures justify the surgical efforts required.

Nondisplaced fractures of the waist of the scaphoid have been treated successfully with arthroscopic placement of intraosseous screws (Fig. 22-27). The advantage of screw fixation is the early return of the athlete to competition while the fracture is healing without the need for rigid wrist immobilization. Undoubtedly, these fractures would heal otherwise in the vast majority of cases but may require 10 to 20 weeks of cast immobilization. Many contact sports leagues will not permit a player to wear hard casts, however, and the practicality of repeatedly applying latex casts is questionable. Intraosseous screws provide compressed immobilization of fractures of the scaphoid, and permit the athlete to return to competition with simple tape splinting.

The cannulated Herbert-Whipple screw (Zimmer, Inc., Warsaw, Ind.) is ideal for this treatment. The compression jig is easier to use under arthroscopic control, and preliminary K-wire fixation allows the physician to confirm the intended placement of the screw with intraoperative radiographs before drilling the bone.

This treatment modality is recommended for those athletes who are not permitted to wear casts and who desire to return to competition at the earliest possible time. There appears to be little risk and definite advantage to early surgical intervention and internal fixation in properly selected cases of minimally displaced and nondisplaced scaphoid fractures.

Loose Bodies

Osseous loose bodies resulting from acute or repetitive wrist trauma can usually be diagnosed by conventional radiographs. Unossified cartilaginous loose bodies are radiolucent and may present with symptoms of intermittent interference with wrist motion. At arthroscopy, mechanically significant loose bodies can be located and removed with a cupped forceps (Fig. 22-28). Care should be taken to explore by palpation and probing all visible recesses within the joint such as the prestyloid recess and the space of Poirier.

Removal of loose bodies that interfere with the wrist function brings immediate symptomatic relief. Recuperation entails only healing of the skin punctures, which occurs readily within 3 to 7 days. Acute osteocartilaginous fracture fragments too small to be replaced can be removed under arthroscopic control, but the site of origin should be freshened with a curette or bur and the

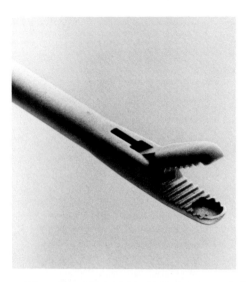

FIG. 22-28. These 2.2-mm cupped grasping forceps are helpful for removing osteocartilaginous loose bodies from the wrist. (Linvatec, Inc, Largo, Fla.)

wrist should be protected for 6 to 8 weeks to allow satisfactory fibrosis of the fracture site. Fracture fragments that are of ample size should be anatomically replaced, which usually requires an arthrotomy. Long-term functional results depend on the preservation of normal joint contours.[30]

SUMMARY

The indication for wrist arthroscopy in athletes is primarily for soft-tissue intraarticular injuries but also includes intraarticular fractures and cases where conventional imaging techniques have failed to delineate the etiology of wrist pain. Surgical intervention with minimally invasive techniques is advantageous in cases of acute intercarpal ligament injury, especially lesions of the scapholunate joint and the lunotriquetral joint. Midcarpal instability and disruption of the triquetral hamate joint occur less frequently but may be problematic for the athlete. Arthroscopic reduction and internal fixation of mild to moderate carpal instability can produce arthrofibrosis sufficient to stabilize these small joints. Arthroscopic reduction and internal fixation of intraarticular fractures is of great advantage in the anatomic restoration of joint surfaces with minimally invasive techniques. This treatment approach facilitates early mobilization of the joints in many cases.

It must be emphasized that arthroscopic surgery of the wrist is not a new procedure but only an advantageous, minimally invasive technique for applying well-established surgical principles of treatment to wrist injuries in appropriately selected cases.

REFERENCES
1. Allum R: Skateboard injuries: a new epidemic, *Injury* 10:152, 1978.
2. Bergfeld JA, Weiker GC, Andrish JT: Soft playing splint for protection of significant hand and wrist injuries in sports, *Am J Sports Med* 10:293, 1982.

3. Burkhart S, Woods M: Post-traumatic recurrent subluxation of the extensor carpi ulnaris tendon, *J Hand Surg* 7A:1, 1982.
4. Burton RL: Overview for athletic upper extremity injuries. In AAOS: *Instructional course lectures,* vol 34, St Louis, 1985, Mosby.
5. Coleman HM: Injuries of the articular disc of the wrist, *J Bone Joint Surg* 42B:522, 1960.
6. Culver JE: Instabilities of the wrist, *Clin Sports Med* 5:725, 1986.
7. Dobyns JH, Sim FH, Linscheid RL: Sports stress syndromes of the hand and wrist, *Am J Sports Med* 6:236, 1978.
8. Dobyns JH et al: Traumatic instability of the wrist. In AAOS: *Instructional course lectures,* vol 24, St Louis, 1975, Mosby.
9. Golfer's wrist, *Br Med J,* December 24-31, p 1622, 1977 (editorial).
10. Green DP: The sore wrist without a fracture. In AAOS: *Instructional course lectures,* St Louis, 1977, Mosby.
11. Gumbs V, Segal D: Bilateral distal radius and ulnar fractures in adolescent weight lifters, *Am J Sports Med* 10:375, 1982.
12. Heiple KG, Freehafer AA, Van't Hof A: Isolated traumatic dislocation of the distal end of the ulna or distal radioulnar joint, *J Bone Joint Surg* 44A:1387, 1962.
13. Lichtman DM, Noble WH, Alexander CE: Dynamic triquetrolunate instability: case report, *J Hand Surg* 9A:185, 1984.
14. Lichtman DM et al: Ulnar midcarpal instability—clinical and laboratory analysis, *J Hand Surg* 6A:515, 1981.
15. Linscheid RL, Dobyns JH: Athletic injuries of the wrist, *Clin Orthop* 196:141, 1985.
16. Linscheid RL, et al: Traumatic instability of the wrist: diagnosis, classification, and pathomechanics, *J Bone Joint Surg* 54A:1612, 1972.
17. Lipscomb A: Baseball pitching injuries in growing athletes, *J Sports Med* 3:25, 1975.
18. Mayfield JK: Mechanism of carpal injuries, *Clin Orthop* 149:45, 1980.
19. McCue F, Baugher H: Hand and wrist injuries in the athlete, *Am J Sports Med* 7:275, 1979.
20. Palmer AK: Triangular fibrocartilage complex lesions: a classification, *J Hand Surg* 14(4):594, 1989.
21. Palmer AK, Dobyns JH, Linscheid RL: Management of post-traumatic instability of the wrist secondary to ligament rupture, *J Hand Surg* 3:507, 1978.
22. Posner M: Injuries to the hand and wrist in athletes, *Orthop Clin North Am* 8:593, 1977.
23. Rainey R, Peautsch M: Traumatic volar dislocation of the distal radioulnar joint, *Orthopedics* 8:898, 1985.
24. Rose-Innes AP: Anterior dislocation of the ulna in the inferior radioulnar joint: case reports, with a discussion of the anatomy of rotation of the forearm, *J Bone Joint Surg* 42B:515, 1960.
25. Roth JH, Poehling GG, Whipple TL: Arthroscopic surgery of the wrist. In Bassett FH III (ed): *Instructional course lectures,* vol 37, Park Ridge, Ill, 1988, American Academy of Orthopaedic Surgeons.
26. Snook GA et al: Subluxation of the distal radio-ulna joint by hyperpronation, *J Bone Joint Surg* 51A:1315, 1969.
27. Stark HH et al: Fracture of the hook of the hamate in athletes, *J Bone Joint Surg* 59A:575, 1977.
28. Taleisnik J: The ligaments of the wrist, *J Hand Surg* 1A:110, 1976.
29. Tehranzadeh J: Ganglion cysts and tear of the triangular fibrocartilage of both wrists in a cheerleader, *Am J Sports Med* 11:357, 1983.
30. Tehranzadeh J, Labosky D: Detection of loose osteochondral fragments by double contrast wrist arthrography, *Am J Sports Med* 12:77, 1984.
31. Torisu T: Fracture of the hook of the hamate by golf swing, *Clin Orthop* 83:91, 1972.
32. Traumatic tenosynovitis of the wrist, *Br Med J,* March 9, p 528, 1977 (editorial).
33. Watson HK: Limited wrist arthrodesis, *Clin Orthop* 149:126, 1980.
34. Watson HK, Hempton RF: Limited wrist arthrodesis: the triscaphoid joint. I, *J Hand Surg* 5A:320, 1980.
35. Weeks P, Young V: A case of painful clicking wrist: a case report, *J Hand Surg* 4A:522, 1979.
36. Whipple TL: Arthroscopic surgery of the wrist. In Chapman MW (ed): *Operative orthopaedics,* Philadelphia, 1988, JB Lippincott.
37. Whipple TL, Marotta JJ, Powell JH III: Techniques of wrist arthroscopy, *Arthroscopy* 2:244, 1986.
38. Wood MB, Dobyns JH: Sports-related extraarticular wrist syndromes, *Clin Orthop* 202:93, 1986.
39. Wood MB, Linscheid RL: Abductor pollicis longus bursitis, *Clin Orthop* 93:293, 1973.

SUGGESTED READINGS
Bell R, Hawkins R: Stress fracture of the distal ulna, *Clin Orthop* 209:169, 1986.
Burton RI, Eaton RG: Common hand injuries in the athlete, *Orthop Clin North Am* 4:809, 1973.
Carr D, Johnson R: Upper extremity injuries in skiing, *Am J Sports Med* 9:378, 1981.
Dauphine RT, Linscheid RL: Unrecognized sprain patterns of the wrist, *J Bone Joint Surg* 57A:727, 1975 (abstract).
Dobyns JH, Linscheid RL: Fractures and dislocations of the wrist. In Rockwood CA Jr, Green DP (eds): *Fractures,* ed 2, Philadelphia, 1975, JB Lippincott.
Ellsasser J, Stein A: Management of hand injuries in a professional football team, *Am J Sports Med* 7:178, 1979.
Flatt AE: Athletic injuries of the hand, *J La State Med Soc* 119:425, 1967.
Howard NJ: Peritendinitis crepitans: a muscle-effort syndrome, *J Bone Joint Surg* 19:447, 1937.
Kalenak A et al: Athletic injuries of the hand, *Am Fam Physician* 14:136, 1976.
Mayfield JR, Johnson RP, Kilcoyne RF: The ligaments of the human wrist and their functional significance, *Anat Rec* 186:417, 1976.
Mino DE, Palmer AK, Levinsohn EM: The role of radiography and computerized tomography in the diagnosis of subluxation and dislocation of the distal radioulnar joint, *J Hand Surg* 8:23, 1983.
Mosher JF: Current concepts in the diagnosis and treatment of hand and wrist injuries in sports, *Med Sci Sports Exerc* 17:48, 1985.
Percy EC: *Injuries to the elbow, wrist, and hand: symposium on athletic injuries,* September, 1967, p 744.
Rayan G: Recurrent dislocation of the extensor carpi ulnaris in athletes, *Am J Sports Med* 11:183, 1983.
Reagan DS, Linscheid RL, Dobyns JH: Lunotriquetral sprains, *J Hand Surg* 9A:502, 1984.
Rettig A: Stress fracture of the ulna in an adolescent tournament tennis player, *Am J Sports Med* 11:103, 1983.
Roser L, Clawson D: Football injuries in the very young athlete, *Clin Orthop* 69:219, 1970.
Sprague B, Justis E: Nonunion of the carpal navicular, *Arch Surg* 108:692, 1974.
Strauss R, Lanese R: Injuries among wrestlers in school and college tournaments, *JAMA* 248:2016, 1982.
Wilson D: The perilous skateboard, *Br Med J,* November 19, 1977, p 1349 (letter).
Youm Y et al: Kinematics of the wrist: I. An experimental study of radial-ulnar deviation and flexion-extension, *J Bone Joint Surg* 60A:423, 1978.

CHAPTER 23 Fractures of the Wrist

Charles P. Melone, Jr.

An increasing fund of knowledge regarding wrist anatomy, kinematics, and pathomechanics has led to important concepts that have considerably enhanced management of the athlete's fractured wrist. Prominent among these is that normal wrist function depends largely on preservation of specific shapes and relationships of multiple bony links (Fig. 23-1). The cuplike and colinear arrangement of the radius, lunate, and capitate (the primary central links) coupled with the skiff-shaped and oblique orientation of the scaphoid (the principal radial link) permits a wide but well-constrained range of flexion and extension distributed over multiple joints. Similarly, integrity of the pyramidal triquetrum (the key ulnar link) and its helicoid articulation with the hamate are essential for intercarpal rotation as well as the synchronous translation that normally occurs between the carpal rows during radial and ulnar deviation. Furthermore, because of their multiple articulations, the bony links are largely covered with hyaline cartilage; hence this vital surface area must remain undisturbed for normal kinematics. Clearly, any fracture that disrupts the relatively complex and unique chondroosseous structure of the wrist poses a serious threat to unimpaired mobility and stability. When fracture occurs, the cardinal rule is prompt restoration of normal configurations and anatomic relationships of the critical bony links.

Bony links of the wrist		
Central link	**Radial link**	**Ulnar link**
Radius	Scaphoid	Triquetrum
Lunate		Hamate
Capitate		

Recognition that precise restoration of skeletal integrity is an absolute prerequisite for maximal recovery after wrist fracture has proved especially beneficial to the injured athlete. In the past, a tendency existed to consider most wrist fractures as trivial incidents with minimal morbidity. Often, a potentially disabling fracture was spuriously dismissed as an innocous bone bruise or chip—often without the benefit of radiography. Like the terminology, treatment was imprecise and recovery predictably compromised. That highly coordinated, powerful flick of the wrist characteristic of the skilled athlete rapidly deteriorated to a painfully weak clunk with the inability to throw, hit, or shoot with strength and dexterity. For some, the long-term consequences proved even more devastating because the more serious fractures resulted in the inevitable sequence of painful wrist instability followed by disabling arthritis. More recently, because of a heightened awareness of the functional significance of the intact wrist and of the serious complications associated with neglected fractures of the carpus and distal radius, such instances of unsatisfactory management have precipitously declined. A casual attitude toward wrist fractures among athletes has been supplanted by an intense concern for precision in diagnosis and treatment. No longer is a rapid return to competition the primary goal of either the sports physician or the injured athlete.

This chapter first discusses established as well as evolving concepts of optimal management and then describes techniques that have continually facilitated treatment of specific fractures incurred by athletes. The objective is to provide rational guidelines for treatment of those fractures prevalent among this highly skilled, select group.

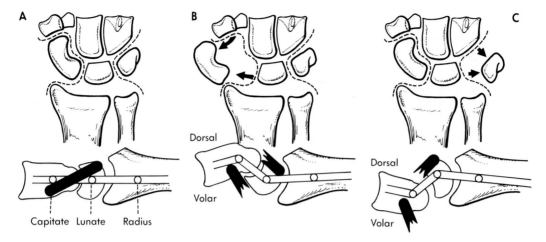

FIG. 23-1. A, Normal wrist function depends largely on preservation of specific shapes and relationships of critical bony links. Integrity of all skeletal components maintains the colinear relationship of the central links as viewed in the sagittal plane. **B,** With destabilization of the scaphoid by fracture, the link system collapses into a predictable dorsal intercalated segment instability (DISI) deformity with excessive dorsal tilting of the lunate. **C,** With destabilization of the triquetrum, the system tends to collapse into a volar intercalated segment instability (VISI) deformity. When wrist fracture occurs, the cardinal rule is to restore anatomic configurations of the disrupted bony links. (Modified from Nathan R, Lester B, Melone CP Jr: *Orthop Rev* 16:80, 1987.)

PRINCIPLES OF MANAGEMENT

Clearly, the acute injury affords the opportune time for restitution of the fractured wrist. In contrast to the unpredictable and often disappointing results of delayed treatment, the prospects for maximal recovery are greatly improved by prompt, skillful management. In the vast majority of cases the prevailing causes of fracture complications—delayed diagnosis, unrecognized fracture displacement, faulty immobilization, errors in operative technique, a premature return to competition—can be avoided by observing basic principles of optimal management.

Diagnostic Considerations

An accurate diagnosis begins with a detailed account of the injury as described by the athlete. The mere mention of certain sports activities should immediately arouse suspicion of specific fractures. For example, football is notorious for the occurrence of scaphoid fractures, skating for distal radius fractures, and stick-handling sports such as baseball, golf, tennis, and hockey for hamate hook (hamulus) fractures. The sport per se is often the first clue to the diagnosis.

Awareness of consistent patterns of injury also facilitates the diagnosis (Fig. 23-2). The usual mechanism is a forcible fall on the outstretched hand that induces a multidimensional force comprising hyperextension, axial compression, ulnar deviation, and intercarpal or radiocarpal supination. In many cases the force impacts on a selective site, causing an isolated fracture of either the carpus or distal radius. Occasionally a similar force results in a simultaneous fracture of the tubercle and the waist of the scaphoid or of the scaphoid and the distal radius. In other cases a greater magnitude of force dis-

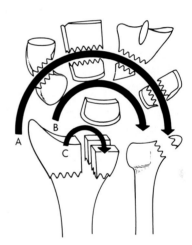

FIG. 23-2. A multidimensional force comprising hyperextension, ulnar deviation, and intercarpal or radiocarpal rotation causes consistent patterns of wrist fracture. *A,* The greater arc injury results in the transscaphoid, transcapitate fracture-dislocation. *B,* The lesser arc injury, traversing the perilunar zone, leads to perilunate or lunate dislocation often associated with fracture of the triquetrum. *C,* Violent compression force transmitted by the carpus disrupts the distal radius articular surface, resulting in predictable types of fracture.

rupts wider but predictable zones of wrist anatomy.[48,60,102] The greater arc injury, initially traversing the scaphoid, results in transscaphoid or transscaphoid-transcapitate perilunate fracture-dislocation; the lesser arc pattern disrupts the major ligamentous support of the wrist, causing perilunate or lunate dislocation, often in association with avulsion fracture of the radial styloid, triquetrum, or ulnar styloid. Thus when a violent fall re-

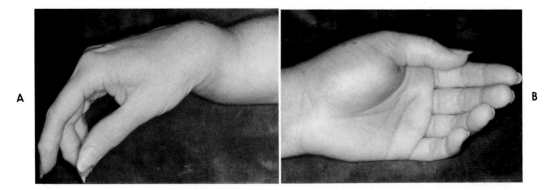

FIG. 23-3. A, Displaced fractures of the distal radius as well as those associated with perilunate injuries often result in readily apparent, characteristic deformity. **B,** Most carpal fractures, however, are associated with minimal disfigurement; nonetheless, careful examination of the carpal surface anatomy invariably pinpoints the site of the pathologic condition. In this case, swelling, bruising, and bony tenderness localized to the thenar eminence are highly suggestive of trapezium fracture.

sults in a painfully swollen wrist, the physician must suspect not only an isolated scaphoid or distal radius fracture, but also a more extensive injury that may require treatment of multiple skeletal and soft-tissue components. Similarly, the physician must recognize that a seemingly insignificant triquetrum fracture may be the only obvious evidence of a serious perilunate disruption that requires surgery for restoration of carpal stability.

Another common mechanism of injury is a direct blow to the palm.[13,61,72,94] A frequent result of this pattern is the hamate hook fracture incurred when the handle of a baseball bat, golf club, tennis racket, or hockey stick forcibly strikes the hypothenar eminence. Less frequently the trapezial ridge fracture results from a similar force transmitted to the base of the thumb. Because both fractures are elusive to routine radiography, they are apt to be overlooked at the time of injury. This problem is considerably lessened with recognition of the common mode of injury, as well as the need for special radiographic views to demonstrate the fracture.

The clinical findings of swelling, tenderness, and limited mobility make the diagnosis increasingly apparent. Perilunate fracture-dislocations and distal radius fractures are characterized by an unmistakable deformity with a pronounced loss of wrist motion (Fig. 23-3). In contrast, most carpal fractures are associated with less obvious, often minimal disfigurement and derangement; localized swelling and bruising with discrete bony tenderness are their distinctive features. Like the classic example of anatomic snuff-box swelling and tenderness as presumptive evidence of a scaphoid waist fracture, hypothenar or ulnar wrist swelling and point tenderness indicate hamate hook or pisiform fractures. Similar findings localized to the thenar eminence suggest a trapezial ridge or scaphoid tubercle fracture. A meticulous examination of the carpal surface anatomy invariably pinpoints the site of the pathologic condition.

Clear visualization of the fracture with appropriate radiographs of good quality confirms the diagnosis. Unlike those of the radius or ulna, acute fractures of the carpus are not readily demonstrated with routine wrist radiography. Special projections are thus an essential part of

the standard evaluation (Fig. 23-4). In addition to posteroanterior (PA), oblique, and lateral views, radiographs for a suspected scaphoid fracture should include radial and ulnar deviation studies and a clenched fist anteroposterior (AP) projection. Forceful ulnar deviation augmented by the clenched fist exerts distraction forces on the scaphoid fragments to illustrate better the fracture, whereas radial deviation, like the oblique view, enhances

---

Special radiographic techniques

Suspected scaphoid fracture
- Radial deviation, anteroposterior (AP) view
- Ulnar deviation, AP view
- Clenched fist, AP view

Suspected hamate hook fracture
- Carpal tunnel view
- Oblique in radial deviation
- Lateral with thumb abducted

Suspected trapezial ridge fracture
- Carpal tunnel view

Suspected pisiform fracture
- Oblique in semisupination
- Ulnar deviation, AP view

---

visualization of fragment displacement. Fracture displacement resulting in carpal instability is best detected on the lateral view that displays abnormal tilting of the lunate with loss of colinear relationships. With minor, albeit significant, scaphoid displacement, this finding is subtle; however, with the transscaphoid perilunate fracture-dislocation, normal relationships are grossly disturbed and the lateral projection graphically depicts the tilted lunate as a spilled teacup (Fig. 23-4, *C* and *D*).

The hamate hook fracture is confirmed by one of several techniques requiring careful positioning of the wrist: a carpal tunnel profile, an oblique view taken with the wrist radially deviated and semisupinated, or a lateral view projected through the first web space with the

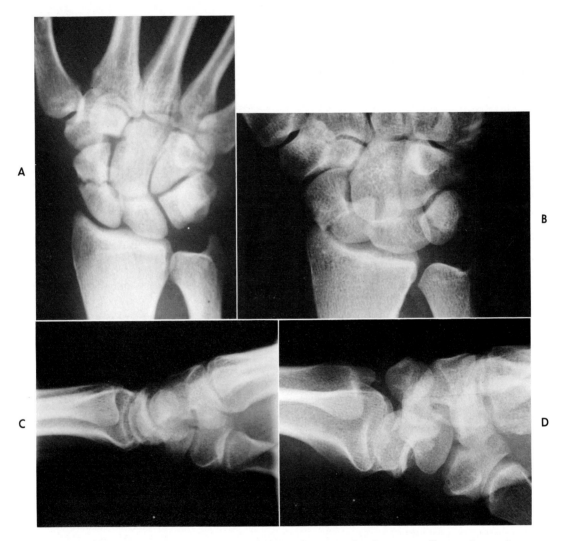

FIG. 23-4. Scaphoid radiography. **A,** Ulnar deviation, by virtue of its distraction effect on the scaphoid, enhances visualization of the fracture. **B,** Radial deviation view clearly demonstrates fracture
instability with displacement of the fragments. Carpal instability resulting from scaphoid displacement is best illustrated on the lateral projection that displays abnormal tilting of the lunate. **C,** Mild
dorsal tilting of the lunate is subtle evidence of fracture instability with displacement. **D,** In contrast, excessive volar tilting of the lunate with its empty articular concavity facing anteriorly (the
spilled teacup sign) is a constant feature of the unstable transscaphoid perilunate fracture-dislocation.
The distal scaphoid fragment displaces dorsally with the capitate, but the proximal pole remains attached to the volarly situated lunate. In all cases of scaphoid fracture displacement, prompt open
reduction with internal fixation is necessary to restore osseous integrity and carpal stability.

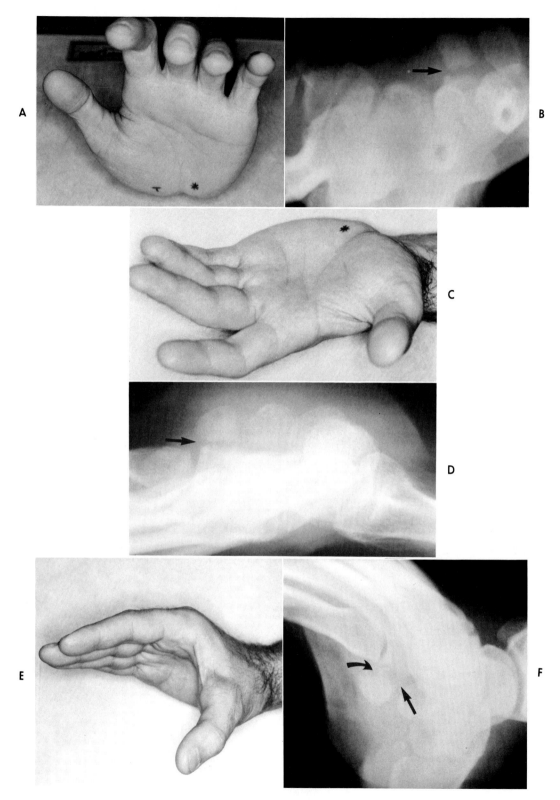

FIG. 23-5. Special radiographic projections are necessary to detect the hamate hook fracture *(arrows)*. **A** and **B,** Carpal tunnel profile taken with the wrist hyperextended. **C** and **D,** Oblique view obtained with the wrist radially deviated and semisupinated. **E** and **F,** Lateral view projected through the first web space with the thumb widely abducted.

thumb abducted (Fig. 23-5). These views occasionally reveal the somewhat confusing presence of a bipartite hamulus, a malformation resulting from separate ossification centers that fail to unite (Fig. 23-6). This incidental finding is distinguished by a discrete, smooth ossicle, usually present bilaterally near the apex of the hook and should not be mistaken for the fracture that invariably occurs near the base of the hook. The same techniques clearly visualize a suspected pisiform fracture; the carpal tunnel projection is the essential view for diagnosis of the trapezial ridge fracture (Fig. 23-7).

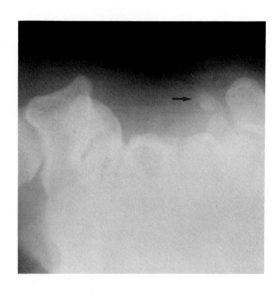

FIG. 23-6. Congenital bipartite hamulus is characterized by a smooth, oval ossicle (*arrow*) located near the apex of the hook and should not be mistaken for a fracture, which invariably occurs at the base of the hook.

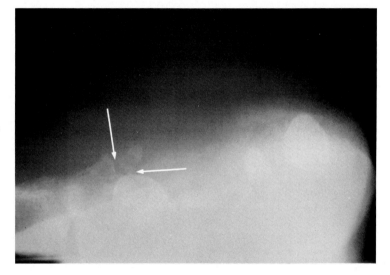

FIG. 23-7. Carpal tunnel profile is the key view for detecting the elusive trapezial ridge fracture (*arrows*).

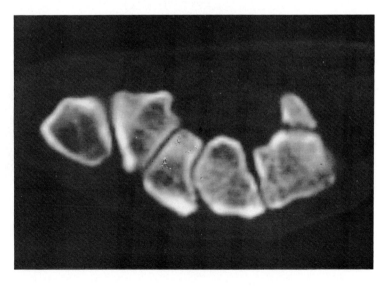

FIG. 23-8. In cases with inconclusive plain radiography, computed tomography is a highly accurate method of demonstrating the hamate hook fracture, which in this case is distracted.

Careful application of these standard radiographic techniques provides sufficient information for optimal management of the vast majority of fractures. Nonetheless, uncertain situations are occasionally encountered; for example, when an acutely fractured hamulus is suspected, painful swelling with limited wrist mobility may preclude the positioning essential to attain unobstructed visualization with special projections. In such instances computed tomography (CT) has proved a highly accurate method of diagnosis (Fig. 23-8).[25,92,94] Tomography has also served as a precise means of assessing both scaphoid fracture displacement and union in cases with inconclusive plain radiographs.[19,20,86] More recently noninvasive magnetic resonance imaging (MRI) has been employed with increasing frequency to assess fracture vascularity when bone grafting for long-standing nonunions with ischemic fragments is contemplated.[75,101] With the potential capacity for preoperatively differentiating viable from necrotic fracture fragments, MRI is apt to prove a valuable prognosticator for successful reconstructive surgery. In contrast to the efficacy of selective radiography, tomography, and occasionally MRI, invasive diagnostic studies are seldom warranted for evaluation of the acutely fractured wrist. It is emphasized that ancillary special studies provide valuable information in specific situations, but they are costly, and indiscriminate usage should never supplant a precise conventional work-up. With awareness of characteristic mechanisms of injury, physical findings, and radiographic features, the overlooked occult wrist fracture of the athlete is an infrequent occurrence.

Fracture Displacement

The importance of early recognition and correction of fracture displacement cannot be overstated. Displacement, the hallmark of the unstable fracture, retards healing and is the major factor predisposing to the serious complications of nonunion, malunion, wrist instability, and degenerative arthritis. Fracture stability must be promptly secured by anatomic reduction coupled with either external or internal fixation. For the more severe wrist fractures open treatment is mandatory for restoration of osseous integrity and wrist stability. Also, the fundamental principle that displaced articular fractures require open reduction and internal fixation for preservation of joint congruity applies to a considerable number of scaphoid, capitate, trapezium, and distal radius fractures.

Uncomplicated healing of either acute or chronic scaphoid fractures relies on exact apposition of fracture fragments. Fragment offset, gapping, mobility, and angulation are radiographic signs of instability that, if uncorrected, severely compromise the healing process. Even minimal angulation, usually dorsally directed and traditionally termed the *humpback* deformity, is apt to result in malunion with serious wrist dysfunction,[3,20,28,32,43] whereas only 1 mm of fragment offset indicates an unstable injury prone to nonunion. Cooney, Dobyns, and Linscheid[18] reported that six (46%) of 13 acute fractures with 1 mm or more displacement failed to unite when treated by closed reduction and cast im-

mobilization. Furthermore, even those which healed led to suboptimal recovery as a result of symptomatic malunion. Weber,[108] also employing closed treatment, found a 55% failure rate for 11 acute fractures with greater than 1 mm offset. Eddeland et al[24] experienced an even greater failure rate (92%) for 25 similarly displaced fractures treated with cast immobilization only. Moreover, Cooney, Dobyns, and Linscheid,[19] in their extensive review of 90 scaphoid nonunions treated with bone grafting, cited residual fragment displacement as the primary cause of failure. The implication of these experiences is clear: precise open reduction with internal fixation is the best means of ensuring uncomplicated scaphoid healing for both the acutely displaced fracture and the chronically displaced nonunion.

For the scaphoid, as well as the capitate, the degree of fracture displacement is proportional to concurrent ligamentous disruption. The widely displaced scaphoid fracture is a key component of the transscaphoid perilunate fracture-dislocation, whereas the markedly rotated capitate neck fracture invariably is associated with the transscaphoid-transcapitate perilunate fracture-dislocation, termed the *scaphocapitate syndrome*. Both types of injury cause a massive derangement of wrist anatomy that must be rectified for preservation of carpal stability. In contrast to increasing dissatisfaction with the results of closed reduction for these transcarpal injuries, evidence is accumulating that a superior recovery can be effected by early open treatment.* Direct visualization facilitates reduction of the displaced fractures and permits meticulous repair of the disrupted ligaments.

The hamate hook fracture is subject to a multitude of deleterious forces that favor displacement and bias healing. This bony projection provides an insertion for the pisohamate ligament, an origin for the opponens digiti quinti as well as the flexor digiti quinti, and an ulnar purchase for the transverse carpal ligament (Fig. 23-9). Because of these strong soft-tissue attachments exerting continuous distraction forces, displacement of the hamate hook is a frequent occurrence. A similar but less common problem occurs with the trapezial ridge fracture because of the distraction force transmitted by the radial attachment of the transverse carpal ligament. In such cases with fracture displacement, union is essentially precluded and prompt excision of the displaced fragment is the most reliable means of affording a rapid, uncomplicated recovery.†

Displacement of the distal radius fracture often is associated with extensive comminution and a major disruption of articular contours. Radiocarpal joint fragmentation and collapse, radial shortening with concomitant loss of distal radioulnar joint congruity, and abnormal radial tilting with radiocarpal and midcarpal malalignment are the hallmarks of the highly unstable injury. Undoubtedly, persistent distortion of these critical articulations is apt to result in a poor outcome following displaced distal radius fractures. Numerous investigators have reported that radiocarpal articular incongruity of

---

*References 31, 44, 46, 71, 76, and 102.
†References 9, 13, 61, 72, 92, and 94.

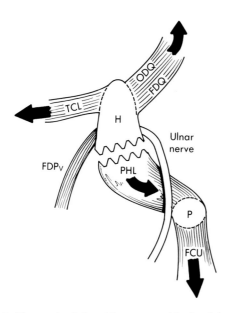

FIG. 23-9. Hamate hook is subject to a multitude of detrimental forces favoring fracture displacement and prejudicing healing. The flexor carpi ulnaris via the pisohamate ligament, the opponens digiti quinti, the flexor digiti quinti, and the transverse carpal ligament exert continuous distraction forces that essentially preclude union of unstable fractures. Because of proximity to the deep motor branch of the ulnar nerve and the deep flexors to the ring and small fingers, the chronic nonunion is prone to cause both compression neuropathy and attritional tendon rupture.

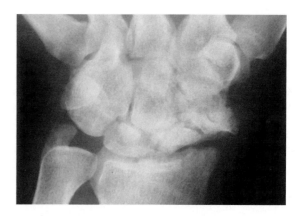

FIG. 23-10. Chronically displaced scaphoid nonunion resulting in the predictable sequence of carpal instability, collapse deformity, and degenerative joint disease.

only 2 mm is prone to serious, and relatively rapid, joint deterioration,* whereas others have cautioned that radial shortening of a seemingly minor extent is apt to cause both distal radioulnar joint instability and ulnocarpal dysfunction.[4,50,56,73] Furthermore, excessive tilting of the distal radius articular surface, either dorsally or less frequently volarly, adversely alters radiocarpal, distal radioulnar, and ulnocarpal joint function, often with considerable impairment.[50,91,98] Although an unsatisfactory reduction occasionally results in satisfactory function, malunion must be recognized as the common factor predisposing to an unfavorable recovery. Clearly, complications are lessened by restoration of articular congruity, radial length, and radial tilt. For most unstable distal radius fractures of the athlete, continuous skeletal traction, also termed *ligamentotaxis*, employing an external fixation device and often supplemented with percutaneous internal fixation Kirschner wires, is necessary to maintain an accurate reduction. For some, open treatment is essential for reduction and fixation of the displaced articular surfaces, as well as repair of concurrent injury to vital periarticular structures.

In many cases persistent fracture displacement profoundly compromises wrist stability. Chronic instability of the key bony links leads to predictable collapse deformities of the wrist, which have been categorized on the basis of lunate displacement (Fig. 23-1).[57] With destabilization of the scaphoid, capitate, or distal radius, the dis-

sociated lunate usually shifts dorsally and the wrist is distorted in a characteristic posture, termed *dorsal intercalated segment instability* (DISI) deformity. With destabilization of the triquetrum the lunate assumes an excessive volar tilt and the system collapses into a *volar flexion intercalated segment* (VISI) deformity. With either deformity kinematics are seriously altered and dysfunction is considerable. This inevitable sequela of uncorrected fracture displacement, namely instability with disabling deformity and ultimately degenerative joint disease (Fig. 23-10), can be prevented by precision management of the acutely injured wrist.

Chronic fracture displacement also poses a serious risk to the integrity of the vital soft tissues transversing the wrist. Owing to alterations in critical anatomic relationships, distal radius malunion and hamate hook nonunion may result in median and ulnar neuropathy.[17,66,94] Similarly, chronically malpositioned or ununited bone fragments are apt to cause attritional ruptures of the flexor or extensor tendons.[9,13,66] Continuous fraying with ultimate rupture of the small finger flexors is a significant complication of chronically ununited hamate hook fractures; ruptures of the deep flexors to the thumb and index finger are associated with malunited distal radius fractures; and rupture of the extensor pollicis longus is liable to result from any malunion or nonunion, which causes a synovitis over the dorsoradial aspect of the wrist. For these ruptures, seldom is a totally satisfactory solution available. The frayed, retracted tendon ends generally preclude direct repair, and restoration of tendon integrity usually requires either intercalated grafts or local transfers, procedures limited in their capacity to restore normal function. The delayed occurrence of predictable soft-tissue injuries must be recognized as an additional consequence of suboptimal primary care.

Fracture Vascularity

The blood supply of the carpus has been extensively studied by numerous investigators employing varying techniques.* Although controversy still exists over cer-

---

*References 5, 30, 51, 68, 70, and 109.

*References 10, 27, 38, 39, 53, 74, 97, and 103.

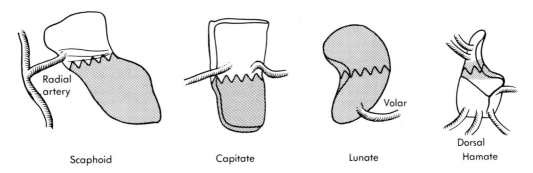

Radial artery

Scaphoid

Capitate

Lunate

Volar

Dorsal

Hamate

FIG. 23-11. Fracture vascularity. Because of deficient circulation, the proximal two thirds of the scaphoid, the proximal capitate, the lunate, and the base of the hamate hook *(shaded areas)* are vulnerable to ischemia and avascular necrosis after fracture. Vascular insufficiency is the basis for the prolonged healing time so frequently associated with carpal fractures.

tain patterns of flow, a consensus prevails that the vascular anatomy of the carpus is a major prognostic factor of fracture healing. Because of relatively insufficient circulation, the proximal two thirds of the scaphoid, the proximal capitate, the entire lunate (in a significant percentage of persons), and the base of the hamate hook are vulnerable to ischemia and avascular necrosis after fracture (Fig. 23-11). Vascular deficiency is, in fact, the basis for the characteristically prolonged healing time of carpal fractures.

Areas vulnerable to avascular necrosis

- Proximal two thirds of the scaphoid
- Proximal capitate
- Lunate
- Base of hamate hook

Because fracture of the vulnerable portion of the scaphoid is the most frequent carpal injury, vascular compromise undoubtedly is a common occurrence and a major consideration in decisions for rational fracture management. Basic to this concept is the need to differentiate fracture ischemia as evidenced by increased radiodensity of the affected area from true avascular necrosis characterized by bone resorption, subchondral fragmentation, and cartilage destruction.* Ischemia, apt to occur with virtually all fractures of the proximal scaphoid as well as those of the capitate, is a transient phenomenon that should not be considered an insuperable obstacle to healing or an irreversible process of carpal destruction. With prompt and continuous treatment, union can be expected in the vast majority of cases and will be followed by revascularization (Figs. 23-20, *H* and *I,* and 23-28, *B*). Fracture healing with vascular ingrowth and new bone formation provides the basis for reconstitution of the devitalized area. Following union, the opaque area of ischemia gradually regains its normal density over a variable period of several or more months. In contrast

avascular necrosis, prone to occur with chronic non-unions exceeding 12 months' duration, is an irreversible precursor of degenerative joint disease.

This critical distinction in fracture vascularity, however, remains a major source of difficulty because current methods of assessment have yet to prove consistently accurate. Concurring with others that radiodensity is not a valid measure of the extent of vascular insufficiency, Green[43] advocated direct visualization of punctate bleeding in cancellous bone found at operation as the best determinant of true avascular necrosis. In his experience with 45 scaphoid nonunions treated by Russe bone grafting, union was consistently achieved when bleeding was clearly visible in the proximal pole. Conversely, with a paucity of punctate bleeding, successful union considerably decreased, and in all cases with a total absence of visible bleeding, nonunion was the rule. He, as did Russe,[84] concluded that if the proximal pole appears nonviable, bone grafting for scaphoid nonunion is prone to failure and an alternative treatment should be considered. Nonetheless, Green acknowledged the limitations of intraoperative scrutiny of pinpoint bleeding as the sole criterion of avascular necrosis and the need for a more objective and consistently reproducible method of vascular analysis.

Toward this end, evidence is accumulating that MRI ultimately may be a superior technique of differentiating ischemia from necrosis. Its noninvasive methodology and its capacity for preoperative rather than intraoperative evaluation are distinct advantages.[75,101] With rapidly increasing accuracy in sensitivity and specificity, MRI has the potential to assess with precision the vascularity of the ununited scaphoid and ascertain its capacity for healing. Further data correlating preoperative imaging with both operative observations and histologic evaluation of biopsy specimens are necessary to determine the efficacy of this promising tool in the management of avascular necrosis.

In my experience structural integrity of the fracture fragments as determined preoperatively by careful scrutiny of quality radiographs and operatively by direct inspection has proved a consistently useful guide to successful surgery for the ununited scaphoid with vascular

---

*References 14, 43, 46, 65, 76, 93, and 111.

increasing number of physicians have permitted an early return to sports activities after certain undisplaced fractures. If the fracture has been judged stable and the acute symptoms of injury have resolved, the athlete resumes competition in a carefully molded silicone wrist cast. Repeated cast changes are necessary to maintain effective immobilization, and careful radiographic surveillance is essential to ensure preservation of fracture stability and uncomplicated healing. With skillful and judicious employment of these techniques, uncompromised healing has been reported for various wrist fractures, including those of the scaphoid.[8,63,82] It needs to be emphasized, however, that for the majority of athletes, unrestrained activity before fracture union constitutes an unacceptable risk of serious complications that should be avoided. Furthermore, even the foremost advocates of early competition with protective casts would agree that, as a general rule, unstable wrist fractures requiring internal fixation should not be prematurely subjected to excessive forces. Despite protection afforded by rubber, fiberglass, or plaster casts, hardware breakage or fracture displacement is apt to occur.

SPECIFIC INJURIES
Scaphoid Fractures

Experience bears out that, with precise management of the most frequently injured and troublesome carpal bone, namely the scaphoid, uncomplicated healing can be achieved in greater than 90% of cases.* Undisplaced fractures usually respond to early continuous immobilization. As long as the fracture is stable, the casting is initiated within 3 to 4 weeks of injury, and the immobilization is effective, union can be expected in the majority of cases.[40,52] It needs to be emphasized, however, that because the slightest displacement essentially precludes uncomplicated healing, the physician must carefully assess the radiographs before concluding that the fracture is undisplaced and suitable for continuous casting. Also, because seemingly stable fractures, especially those of the proximal pole, may subsequently displace after the onset of casting, continual radiographic surveillance is essential during the relatively lengthy period of immobilization. The athlete must be advised that a term of relative inactivity approaching 6 months may prove necessary for optimal recovery and that total compliance is critical to success. The physician should be optimistic that constant surveillance and reassurance are generally rewarded by a favorable outcome.

The criteria for continuous casting are stringent, and adherence to the requisites for success is always difficult and at times impossible, especially in young athletes with a uniformly poor tolerance for long-term casting. Moreover, the need for prolonged immobilization with an uncertain prognosis for union as well as the not infrequent occurrence of delayed displacement are habitual problems of small proximal fractures, recurrent problems that have generated considerable enthusiasm for early surgical intervention. For these troublesome proximal third or proximal fourth fractures in athletes, evidence is accumulating that early open reduction with internal fixation rather than primary casting is the best means of lessening the frequent complications of delayed union, nonunion, and irreparable avascular necrosis with their limited options for salvage.* Personal experience corroborates the favorable reports of others[22,47] that Herbert screw fixation with or without bone grafting is a superior method of treatment for these often termed *insoluble* injuries (Fig. 23-17). It is acknowledged that primary surgery for undisplaced fractures is a highly controversial topic that requires further analysis before definitive recommendations. Nonetheless, early operative treatment has proved an increasingly viable option in the management of carefully selected, complex fractures incurred by the athlete.

The concept of an early return to competition with protective casting for unhealed, undisplaced fractures is attractive to those physicians and athletes experiencing the frustrations so frequently associated with the prolonged treatment of scaphoid injuries. Although the dual objective of active participation and concurrent fracture union has been accomplished in some instances,[82] the ununited scaphoid, regardless of protection, is always vulnerable to the hazardous and unpredictable forces of competitive sports. For the majority of athletes the substantial risk of nonunion with its serious consequences clearly eclipses the transient benefits of a speedy return to sports. As policy consistent with sound judgment, the return to competition employing custom-fit devices for protection of the unhealed scaphoid should be reserved for highly select cases of stable fractures in athletes competing with either minimal risk of further damage or under exigent circumstances. Active participation of a professional athlete with an undisplaced distal third fracture might be permissible, whereas that of a high school football player with a potentially unstable proximal pole fracture is ill advised.

Position for scaphoid fracture immobilization

- Slight wrist volar flexion and radial deviation
- Cast incorporates humeral epicondyles
- Thumb incorporated (to interphalangeal joint)

A clear consensus exists that displaced fractures require open reduction and internal fixation in an anatomic position. For the acute injury uncomplicated by carpal instability, a volar approach (Fig. 23-18) between the flexor carpi radialis and the radial artery affords excellent exposure for reduction and stabilization as well as repair of concomitant scapholunate ligament injury that is apt to occur with the more proximal fractures. Because of longstanding favorable experience, many surgeons still prefer conventional Kirschner wire internal fixation. However, because of its capacity to induce an acceler-

---

*References 12, 19, 22, 24, 29, 32, 46, 48, 65, 84, and 93.

*References 2, 14, 32, 33, 43, 47, 84, 93, and 111.

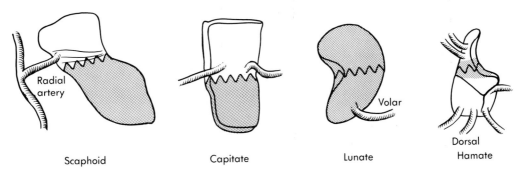

Radial artery

Scaphoid   Capitate   Lunate   Volar   Dorsal Hamate

FIG. 23-11. Fracture vascularity. Because of deficient circulation, the proximal two thirds of the scaphoid, the proximal capitate, the lunate, and the base of the hamate hook (*shaded areas*) are vulnerable to ischemia and avascular necrosis after fracture. Vascular insufficiency is the basis for the prolonged healing time so frequently associated with carpal fractures.

tain patterns of flow, a consensus prevails that the vascular anatomy of the carpus is a major prognostic factor of fracture healing. Because of relatively insufficient circulation, the proximal two thirds of the scaphoid, the proximal capitate, the entire lunate (in a significant percentage of persons), and the base of the hamate hook are vulnerable to ischemia and avascular necrosis after fracture (Fig. 23-11). Vascular deficiency is, in fact, the basis for the characteristically prolonged healing time of carpal fractures.

Areas vulnerable to avascular necrosis

- Proximal two thirds of the scaphoid
- Proximal capitate
- Lunate
- Base of hamate hook

Because fracture of the vulnerable portion of the scaphoid is the most frequent carpal injury, vascular compromise undoubtedly is a common occurrence and a major consideration in decisions for rational fracture management. Basic to this concept is the need to differentiate fracture ischemia as evidenced by increased radiodensity of the affected area from true avascular necrosis characterized by bone resorption, subchondral fragmentation, and cartilage destruction.* Ischemia, apt to occur with virtually all fractures of the proximal scaphoid as well as those of the capitate, is a transient phenomenon that should not be considered an insuperable obstacle to healing or an irreversible process of carpal destruction. With prompt and continuous treatment, union can be expected in the vast majority of cases and will be followed by revascularization (Figs. 23-20, *H* and *I*, and 23-28, *B*). Fracture healing with vascular ingrowth and new bone formation provides the basis for reconstitution of the devitalized area. Following union, the opaque area of ischemia gradually regains its normal density over a variable period of several or more months. In contrast

avascular necrosis, prone to occur with chronic nonunions exceeding 12 months' duration, is an irreversible precursor of degenerative joint disease.

This critical distinction in fracture vascularity, however, remains a major source of difficulty because current methods of assessment have yet to prove consistently accurate. Concurring with others that radiodensity is not a valid measure of the extent of vascular insufficiency, Green[43] advocated direct visualization of punctate bleeding in cancellous bone found at operation as the best determinant of true avascular necrosis. In his experience with 45 scaphoid nonunions treated by Russe bone grafting, union was consistently achieved when bleeding was clearly visible in the proximal pole. Conversely, with a paucity of punctate bleeding, successful union considerably decreased, and in all cases with a total absence of visible bleeding, nonunion was the rule. He, as did Russe,[84] concluded that if the proximal pole appears nonviable, bone grafting for scaphoid nonunion is prone to failure and an alternative treatment should be considered. Nonetheless, Green acknowledged the limitations of intraoperative scrutiny of pinpoint bleeding as the sole criterion of avascular necrosis and the need for a more objective and consistently reproducible method of vascular analysis.

Toward this end, evidence is accumulating that MRI ultimately may be a superior technique of differentiating ischemia from necrosis. Its noninvasive methodology and its capacity for preoperative rather than intraoperative evaluation are distinct advantages.[75,101] With rapidly increasing accuracy in sensitivity and specificity, MRI has the potential to assess with precision the vascularity of the ununited scaphoid and ascertain its capacity for healing. Further data correlating preoperative imaging with both operative observations and histologic evaluation of biopsy specimens are necessary to determine the efficacy of this promising tool in the management of avascular necrosis.

In my experience structural integrity of the fracture fragments as determined preoperatively by careful scrutiny of quality radiographs and operatively by direct inspection has proved a consistently useful guide to successful surgery for the ununited scaphoid with vascular

---

*References 14, 43, 46, 65, 76, 93, and 111.

compromise. Despite obvious radiodensity and a characteristic paucity of punctate bleeding, especially in small proximal fragments, union has been achieved in the vast majority of cases provided the fracture fragments demonstrate normal contours and healthy articular surfaces. For acute fractures and for those nonunions treated within 12 months of injury, uncomplicated healing with revascularization uniformly has occurred.

The major blood supply of the scaphoid arises from the radial artery and enters principally the waist or dorsoradial ridge of the bone. Although the distal scaphoid has an independent circulation, the proximal two thirds of the bone relies on an intraosseous retrograde blood flow and is therefore prone to ischemia with all fractures at or proximal to the waist. Because about 80% of scaphoid fractures occur in this vulnerable area, prolonged healing should be anticipated in most cases. Also, because of the retrograde perfusion, the more proximal the fracture, the greater is the interference with circulation and the time of healing. Union of optimally managed waist fractures averages about 3 months, whereas fractures of the proximal one third or one fourth rarely unite in less than 4 months. In contrast, fractures of the tubercle are generally united within 6 weeks and those of the distal one third within 8 weeks.

The proximal capitate also depends on an intraosseous retrograde blood supply.[103] Like the proximal scaphoid, the head and neck of the capitate are subjected to a major vascular disruption when fractured; hence healing is similarly prolonged, often requiring several months of continuous immobilization. It is estimated that between 8% and 26% of lunates receive their nutrition from one artery, usually entering the volar surface of the bone.[39,53] This paucity of circulation in a substantial number of persons places the fractured lunate at a high risk for pronounced ischemia with an excessive healing time.

Panagis et al[74] have defined the base of the hamate hook, the usual site of fracture, as another potentially high-risk zone of ischemia following trauma. The major portion of the hook and the body derive their blood supply from separate sources that demonstrate few, if any, intraosseous connections. The base of the hook has no independent nutrient vessels and thus is an area of limited vascularity with a diminished capacity for healing.

Failla[27] studied the location, number, and size of vascular foramina in 52 hamate specimens and corroborated a dual but tenuous blood supply for the majority of hamate hooks. In 71% of the specimens he noted nutrient pathways at both the volar tip and the dorsal body. However, in all specimens foramina were absent at the base of the hook, and in 29% foramina were absent in the entire hook. This study, further demonstrating a paucity of circulation, substantiates the vulnerability of the fractured hamulus to avascular necrosis and delayed healing. Clearly the limited vascularity of this critical site of injury unfavorably affects the prospects for union, and at best a lengthy healing process should be anticipated for undisplaced hook fractures treated by immobilization and for those displaced injuries considered amenable to open reduction and internal fixation.

Fracture vascularity is also an important factor in the formulation of plans for surgery. Mainly because of concern about jeopardizing circulation, opinions vary regarding the best approach to the scaphoid. Some surgeons favor a dorsal exposure, whereas others advocate a volar approach for open reduction and internal fixation as well as bone grafting.* Ample evidence now exists that neither approach adversely affects the blood supply provided the critical vascular leash arising from the radial aspect of the bone and attaching to the waist is not disturbed. A direct radial approach through the anatomic snuff-box, however, should be avoided because it not only causes a serious threat to the critical blood supply, but also precludes extensile exposure. The capitate, like the scaphoid, can be safely exposed from either its dorsal or volar surface as long as the crucial and clearly visible vascular network at the distal end of the bone is not sacrificed. Although the dorsal approach to the lunate is preferred because it affords superior exposure and avoids both the key palmar artery and the critical radiocarpal ligaments, experience bears out that the volar approach can be reliably employed when necessary. For example, for the most frequently encountered volarly displaced fractures and dislocations of the lunate, often accompanied by acute median neuropathy, the volar approach is essential not only for precise carpal reduction and capsular repair, but also for nerve decompression (Fig. 23-26). Uncomplicated exposure, of course, is contingent on atraumatic technique that minimizes soft-tissue dissection, thereby avoiding additional and potentially irreversible vascular compromise. In cases of displaced lunate fractures and fracture-dislocations necessitating a volar approach, ischemia has proved transient with a gradual resolution of radiographic density consistently demonstrated following successful soft-tissue and skeletal healing.

Fracture Immobilization

Providing prompt, effective immobilization and avoiding premature discontinuance of immobilization are absolute prerequisites for successful fracture union. Although some debate persists as to what constitutes optimal casting techniques, clearly the mechanism of injury, the type of fracture, and the potential deforming forces must be carefully considered in developing logical guidelines for effective immobilization.

With scaphoid fractures, excessive thumb motion, wrist hyperextension, and ulnar deviation induce forces predisposing to displacement that must be eliminated. This is accomplished by employing a thumb spica cast maintaining the mildly flexed wrist in radial deviation. In addition to impacting the fracture fragments and reducing stress on damaged volar soft tissues, this position of wrist immobilization induces flexion of the lunate, thereby counteracting its tendency for instability with dorsal tilting so frequently associated with scaphoid fractures. The length of the cast is determined by the level and plane of fracture.[40,52,65,105] Most fractures at or prox-

---

*References 19, 20, 28, 44, 46, 65, 71, 84, and 106.

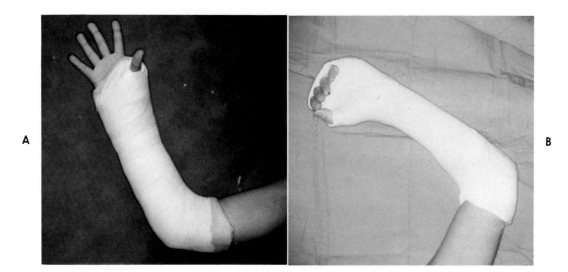

FIG. 23-12. A, Effective immobilization for fractures of the proximal two thirds of the scaphoid maintains the wrist in mild palmar flexion and radial deviation, incorporates the humeral epicondyles to block forearm rotation, and includes the thumb to its interphalangeal joint. **B,** Incorporating the finger metacarpophalangeal joints reduces the enormous compression forces generated by grasping—forces that are especially detrimental to healing of the fractured lunate.

imal to the wrist are oblique to the longitudinal axis of the wrist, an arrangement rendering them particularly susceptible to shearing forces created by forearm rotation and transmitted to the scaphoid by the obliquely oriented radiocarpal ligaments. The deleterious effect of pronation and supination is minimized by extending the cast above the elbow to incorporate the humeral epicondyles (Fig. 23-12, *A*). Thus effective immobilization for fractures of the proximal two thirds of the scaphoid must include the following features: (1) incorporation of the humeral epicondyles to block forearm rotation, (2) incorporation of the thumb to its interphalangeal joint, and (3) maintenance of the wrist in slight palmar flexion and radial deviation.

Substantiating this concept, Gellman et al,[40] in a prospective study comparing casting methods for undisplaced fractures of the proximal two thirds of the scaphoid, clearly demonstrated the efficacy of long arm casting. For 21 fractures treated initially and solely with a short-arm thumb spica cast healing time was relatively prolonged (average 12.7 weeks), delayed union exceeding 4 months occurred in six cases, and nonunion occurred in two. In contrast, for 24 similar fractures treated initially with an above-elbow thumb spica for 6 weeks followed by a short-arm thumb spica until healing was complete, the time to healing was accelerated (average 9.5 weeks) and the incidence of nonunion was eliminated. Moreover, no morbidity resulted from immobilization of the elbow. Such data should serve to reassure the discouraged athlete treated by immobilization that the long arm cast is only a temporary restraint and the most effective means of expediting recovery.

Fractures of the distal third of the scaphoid, as well as those of the tubercle, have a much more adequate blood supply and are subject to far less stress. For these injuries that require less protection, a short-arm thumb spica provides sufficient immobilization.

The lunate fracture, even if undisplaced, should always be considered a precursor of avascular necrosis, fragmentation, and Kienböck's disease. Immobilization must afford maximal protection of this potentially fragile bone. In addition to the same criteria for fractures of the proximal scaphoid, casting of the lunate should include the flexed metacarpophalangeal joints of the fingers (Fig. 23-12, *B*). Incorporation of the most proximal finger joints substantially reduces the enormous compressive forces generated by grasping. These forces, unconstrained and continually absorbed by an ischemic lunate, constitute a major threat to further devitalization with fragmentation.

With hamate hook fractures the deforming forces created by the multiple soft-tissue attachments (Fig. 23-9) need to be neutralized. Comprehensive immobilization is provided by casting the wrist in slight flexion and the metacarpophalangeal joints of the ring and small fingers in acute flexion. The cast also includes the base of the thumb, thereby preventing the distraction force evoked by the thenar musculature and transmitted to the hook via the transverse carpal ligament (Fig. 23-13).

Displaced extraarticular fractures of the distal radius successfully manipulated by closed techniques rely heavily on precise casting for postreduction stability. A well-molded cast is essential to prevent the frequent problem of redisplacement. The cast holds the wrist in mild flexion and incorporates the base of the thumb as well as the humeral epicondyles to militate against detrimental forces occurring at the fracture site. Stability is augmented by selective positioning of the forearm: pronation is employed for Colles' fractures and supination for Smith's fractures. In contrast, extreme positioning of

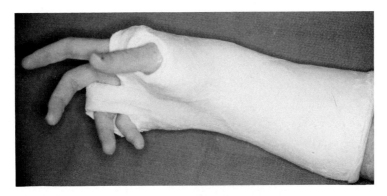

FIG. 23-13. Effective casting for undisplaced hamate hook fractures must neutralize the deforming forces of multiple soft-tissue attachments. The wrist is maintained in mild flexion and the metacarpophalangeal joints of the ring and small fingers in acute flexion. The base of the thumb is also immobilized to prevent distraction forces transmitted via the transverse carpal ligament.

the wrist must be avoided as a potential source of major complications; for example, forced palmar flexion (the Cotton-Loder position) is notorious for causing median nerve compression and disastrous joint contractures of the wrist and digits.

As a basic rule, immobilization must be continued until thorough healing is demonstrated on the radiographs. The essential criterion for union is bony trabeculation across the fracture site with obliteration of the fracture line as illustrated on all radiographic views (Figs. 23-18, *F*, 23-20, *I*, and 23-21, *I*). For distal radius or ulna fractures the healing process is clearly visible; carpal fractures, in contrast, have no appreciable periosteal component to healing, so conspicuous callus formation is seldom present. If the quality of union cannot be ascertained with plain radiographs, an accurate assessment requires tomograms. In fact, because of frequent misinterpretations of plain radiography, it is increasingly advocated that for the most troublesome scaphoid fracture tomography should be considered the definitive method of determining the quality of union. Sole reliance on routine radiographs, with their limited capacity for visualizing intraosseous trabeculation, is liable to an erroneous judgment of fracture union with a premature, hazardous resumption of sports activities.

Because healing is slow in wrist fractures, the time of immobilization often entails a minimum of 8 weeks. The considerable frustration evoked by this lengthy period must be alleviated by repeated reinforcement to the athlete that compliance with appropriate casting is an investment consistently rewarded by a favorable outcome.

Fracture Stabilization
Internal Fixation

For acutely or chronically unstable carpal fractures, Kirschner wires have been the most frequently employed method of internal fixation. Their usage has been consistently accomplished with minimal surgical exposure, few technical difficulties, and a high level of success.[18,19,28,65,93] Their disadvantages, however, are readily apparent: the inability to generate a strong compressive force and the need for an extended period of cast protection often as long as 4 or 5 months, to ensure healing. Despite the relative ease of application and the reliability in maintaining a stable reduction, the use of Kirschner wire fixation has a limited potential to diminish the characteristically protracted treatment regimen for wrist fractures.

In contrast, small compression screws designed specifically for the carpus have the potential for affording rigid fixation and substantially lessening immobilization time and fracture morbidity. Although initial attempts at rigid scaphoid fixation with convential lag screws often were disappointing,[37,59,64] in 1984 Herbert and Fisher[47] reported a highly favorable outcome for 158 scaphoid fractures transfixed with a dual-threaded, headless compression screw. Lacking a protuberant head, the Herbert screw is completely embedded within the scaphoid, thereby eliminating interference with adjacent skeletal and soft tissues. Although its estimated compressive force is less than other carpal screws,[77,90] the distinct advantages of this screw are its intraosseous configuration, its small size (4 mm), and its superior compatability with the unique contours of the scaphoid. The Herbert screw can be inserted either dorsally by a free-hand technique for small proximal pole fractures and fracture-dislocations, or, for the majority of fractures, volarly, employing a guiding jig that rigidly maintains an anatomic reduction while simultaneously facilitating an accurate sequence of drilling, tapping, and screw placement (Fig. 23-14). With either approach Botte et al[10] have demonstrated that meticulous screw placement is unlikely to compromise the precarious vascularity of the scaphoid provided the critical vessels at the radial aspect of the waist are undisturbed. However, the physician should be cautioned that both approaches require a high level of expertise and that technical errors have, in fact, proved the major cause of failure.[2,33,47] Nonetheless, precisely inserted, the Herbert screw has demonstrated with increasing reproducibility the capacity to achieve rigid fixation, to accelerate union, and to enhance recovery.[12,20,22,46] As an increasing fund of experience has

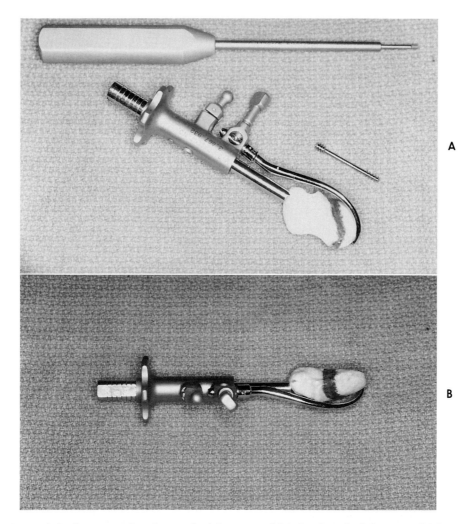

FIG. 23-14. As demonstrated on this scaphoid fracture model (tubercle to the left, proximal pole to the right), the dual threaded Herbert screw is designed for insertion through a guiding jig that maintains anatomic reduction while facilitating drilling, tapping, and screw placement. The jig is attached, **(A),** in the longitudinal axis of the scaphoid and, **(B),** perpendicular to the fracture plane, thereby ensuring accurate intraosseous placement with maximum compression.

corroborated the efficacy of the Herbert screw, for many surgeons, including myself, it currently is the preferred method of scaphoid fixation. Moreover, the scope of its usage has expanded with similar success to other wrist fractures, including those of the capitate, trapezium, hamate body, triquetrum, and radial styloid. Undoubtedly, additional refinements in design, such as cannulated screws with absent or minimally protrusive heads, coupled with less complex techniques of application[32,77,90] will further increase the use of rigid fixation for displaced fractures of the wrist incurred by the athlete.

For unstable distal radius fractures the classic axiom is that reduction is readily achieved but difficult to maintain without supplementary internal or external fixation. When internal fixation is necessary, the Kirschner wire remains the standard method of stabilization. Principally employed for unstable extraarticular fractures, percutaneous Kirschner wire internal fixation is achieved either radially,[15,95] ulnarly[23,79] or more recently intrafocally via

multiple planes in the radius (Kapandji technique).[41,49] Regardless of the technique, with skilled application the wires not only afford secure stabilization but also can be used to facilitate reduction during their placement. Kirschner wires also have been used either alone or in conjunction with external fixators to stabilize articular injuries with moderate displacement. For the more complex irreducible distal radius fractures usually demonstrating dorsal displacement and requiring open reduction, fine wires are the optimal means of securing the comminuted, small-sized articular and metaphyseal fragments. In contrast, the less frequently encountered irreducible distal radius fracture with volar displacement is the optimal situation for fixation with small T or buttress plates (Fig. 23-15).

External Fixation

For highly unstable distal radius fractures usually demonstrating considerable articular disruption, una-

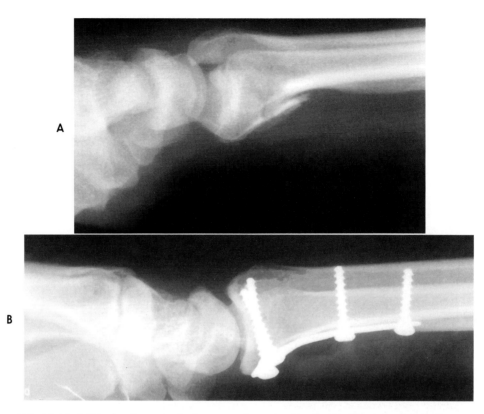

FIG. 23-15. A, Distal radius articular fracture with irreducible volar displacement is optimally suited to open reduction and fixation with a small plate and screws. B, Anatomic reduction and secure plate fixation resulted in uncomplicated union with preservation of articular congruity.

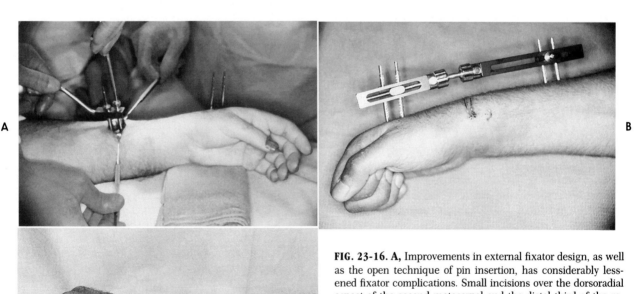

FIG. 23-16. A, Improvements in external fixator design, as well as the open technique of pin insertion, has considerably lessened fixator complications. Small incisions over the dorsoradial aspect of the second metacarpal and the distal third of the radius permit pin insertion under direct visualization that facilitates precise bony purchase and avoids critical soft tissues. B, Sturdy external fixator frame attached to meticulously placed pins maintains an anatomic reduction, which in this case, was augmented by percutaneous Kirschner wire internal fixation. C, Eight weeks after application, when fracture union has occurred, the frame has been detached and the pins, free of complications, are ready for removal.

nimity exists that the external fixator employing continuous distraction (ligamentotaxis) has supplanted other techniques as the preferred method of stabilization. Simplified fixator configurations with less bulk yet enhanced mechanical efficacy have significantly increased use by providing a greater facility for achieving and maintaining complex fracture reduction.[16,36] This increasingly versatile device also permits unobstructed access to wounds as well as secondary adjustments in fracture alignment during the healing process. Furthermore, a sturdy construct serves as a superior method of immobilization until union is complete. With usage of low-profile but strong frames attached to 3- to 4-mm threaded pins securely inserted in bone coupled with improved surgical techniques, the previously high rate of fixator complications has precipitously declined.[16,78,88,109] The formerly frequent occurrence of pin-related problems has been markedly reduced by employment of the limited open technique of pin insertion (Fig. 23-16).[88] Pin placement through small incisions allowing direct visualization avoids critical soft tissues and ensures precise central bony purchase.

Although pins and plaster have proved an effective method of ligamentotaxis,[42,66,78,87] their use is limited by a suboptimal mechanical design, a lack of versatility in fracture management, and a compromised capacity for access to wounds. Nonetheless, owing to the relatively simple methodology, the comparatively low cost, and the satisfactory level of patient acceptance, pins and plaster in select cases remain a useful alternative method of external fixation (Fig. 23-35).

Combined Methods of Fracture Stabilization

For unstable fractures associated with serious wrist instability, combined external fixation and internal fixation have been successfully employed with increasing frequency. The external fixator maintains wrist alignment and provides provisional stabilization while concurrently specific fractures are anatomically reduced by either closed or open techniques and firmly secured by internal fixation.

Fernandez and Ghillani[31] have expanded the scope of external fixation as a method of facilitating exposure, reduction, and repair of complex carpal fracture-dislocations. Combined with Kirschner wire or screw fixation of the carpus, bone grafting, and soft-tissue repairs, the external fixator provides additional stability and free access to wounds. In those injuries characterized by severe soft-tissue disruption, complex revascularization and resurfacing procedures are simplified by preliminary stabilization achieved with the fixator.

In an effort to ensure maintenance of anatomic relationships, Seitz et al[89] have applied combined techniques of stabilization to highly unstable distal radius articular fractures. After a successful reduction is secured by the external fixator, fracture stability is augmented by transcutaneous Kirschner wire internal fixation of the major articular fragments. Transfixion of the radial styloid provides a lateral buttress, whereas transfixion of the lunate facet provides an articular buttress. Employed in a series of 51 unstable injuries, this combined method has considerably lessened the frequent complication of secondary fracture displacement with articular collapse.

Similarly, Raskin and Melone[78] have managed unstable articular fractures of the radius with external fixation and adjunctive percutaneous Kirschner wire internal fixation (Fig. 23-34). After an accurate closed reduction, the external fixator maintains radial length, whereas the Kirschner wires, used not only to stabilize, but also to manipulate key articular fragments, secure articular congruity and radial tilt. Moreover, in those articular injuries irreducible by closed reduction, a combination of open reduction, internal fixation (usually with Kirschner wires), bone grafting, and external fixation are employed to achieve and maintain articular congruity (Fig. 23-36).

For the injured athlete, continuing advances in techniques of fracture stabilization have substantially contributed to a marked improvement in both the speed and quality of recovery as well as a considerable decrease in fracture morbidity.

Return to Competition

Strict guidelines for returning to unrestricted activities are difficult to establish for the athlete who is always vulnerable to injury. A rational decision requires careful consideration of many factors: the type of fracture, the thoroughness of healing, the extent of rehabilitation, and the patient's age, sport, special skills, and level of competition. For fear of reinjury with growth disturbance, an adolescent football player with a distal radius epiphyseal fracture should not resume contact until healing and remodeling of the growth plate are completed and normal function is demonstrated—a period as long as 4 months. In contrast, a professional baseball player might return to the active roster 4 weeks after excision of hamate hook fracture with minimal risk of further damage.

Certain exceptions notwithstanding, the basic requisites for returning to competition are complete healing of the fracture as well as any concomitant soft-tissue injuries and thorough rehabilitation with restoration of a painless, functional arc of wrist motion and near-normal strength. Only with maximal recovery can the risk of reinjury with further impairment be minimized. Also, because of its constant exposure to violent forces, the rehabilitated wrist, whenever possible, should be protected from further trauma. Gloves and rubber casts are usually permissible at all levels of competition, whereas plastic splints and even fiberglass or plaster casts are often allowed in the professional ranks. Custom-fit devices that enhance security against injury yet permit the desired degree of wrist mobility are now available and have become standard equipment for many sports.[6,8,62] With continual improvement in materials and designs, protective gloves and splints will undoubtedly decrease the incidence of wrist fracture and refracture among athletes. For example, a glove with precise contouring and padding of the palm is likely to minimize hamate hook or trapezial ridge fractures; it also lessens the possibility of reinjury at sites previously requiring surgery.

Attempting to lessen the prolonged morbidity so frequently associated with the athlete's fractured wrist, an

increasing number of physicians have permitted an early return to sports activities after certain undisplaced fractures. If the fracture has been judged stable and the acute symptoms of injury have resolved, the athlete resumes competition in a carefully molded silicone wrist cast. Repeated cast changes are necessary to maintain effective immobilization, and careful radiographic surveillance is essential to ensure preservation of fracture stability and uncomplicated healing. With skillful and judicious employment of these techniques, uncompromised healing has been reported for various wrist fractures, including those of the scaphoid.[8,63,82] It needs to be emphasized, however, that for the majority of athletes, unrestrained activity before fracture union constitutes an unacceptable risk of serious complications that should be avoided. Furthermore, even the foremost advocates of early competition with protective casts would agree that, as a general rule, unstable wrist fractures requiring internal fixation should not be prematurely subjected to excessive forces. Despite protection afforded by rubber, fiberglass, or plaster casts, hardware breakage or fracture displacement is apt to occur.

SPECIFIC INJURIES
Scaphoid Fractures

Experience bears out that, with precise management of the most frequently injured and troublesome carpal bone, namely the scaphoid, uncomplicated healing can be achieved in greater than 90% of cases.* Undisplaced fractures usually respond to early continuous immobilization. As long as the fracture is stable, the casting is initiated within 3 to 4 weeks of injury, and the immobilization is effective, union can be expected in the majority of cases.[40,52] It needs to be emphasized, however, that because the slightest displacement essentially precludes uncomplicated healing, the physician must carefully assess the radiographs before concluding that the fracture is undisplaced and suitable for continuous casting. Also, because seemingly stable fractures, especially those of the proximal pole, may subsequently displace after the onset of casting, continual radiographic surveillance is essential during the relatively lengthy period of immobilization. The athlete must be advised that a term of relative inactivity approaching 6 months may prove necessary for optimal recovery and that total compliance is critical to success. The physician should be optimistic that constant surveillance and reassurance are generally rewarded by a favorable outcome.

The criteria for continuous casting are stringent, and adherence to the requisites for success is always difficult and at times impossible, especially in young athletes with a uniformly poor tolerance for long-term casting. Moreover, the need for prolonged immobilization with an uncertain prognosis for union as well as the not infrequent occurrence of delayed displacement are habitual problems of small proximal fractures, recurrent problems that have generated considerable enthusiasm for early surgical intervention. For these troublesome proximal third or proximal fourth fractures in athletes, evidence is accumulating that early open reduction with internal fixation rather than primary casting is the best means of lessening the frequent complications of delayed union, nonunion, and irreparable avascular necrosis with their limited options for salvage.* Personal experience corroborates the favorable reports of others[22,47] that Herbert screw fixation with or without bone grafting is a superior method of treatment for these often termed *insoluble* injuries (Fig. 23-17). It is acknowledged that primary surgery for undisplaced fractures is a highly controversial topic that requires further analysis before definitive recommendations. Nonetheless, early operative treatment has proved an increasingly viable option in the management of carefully selected, complex fractures incurred by the athlete.

The concept of an early return to competition with protective casting for unhealed, undisplaced fractures is attractive to those physicians and athletes experiencing the frustrations so frequently associated with the prolonged treatment of scaphoid injuries. Although the dual objective of active participation and concurrent fracture union has been accomplished in some instances,[82] the ununited scaphoid, regardless of protection, is always vulnerable to the hazardous and unpredictable forces of competitive sports. For the majority of athletes the substantial risk of nonunion with its serious consequences clearly eclipses the transient benefits of a speedy return to sports. As policy consistent with sound judgment, the return to competition employing custom-fit devices for protection of the unhealed scaphoid should be reserved for highly select cases of stable fractures in athletes competing with either minimal risk of further damage or under exigent circumstances. Active participation of a professional athlete with an undisplaced distal third fracture might be permissible, whereas that of a high school football player with a potentially unstable proximal pole fracture is ill advised.

Position for scaphoid fracture immobilization

- Slight wrist volar flexion and radial deviation
- Cast incorporates humeral epicondyles
- Thumb incorporated (to interphalangeal joint)

A clear consensus exists that displaced fractures require open reduction and internal fixation in an anatomic position. For the acute injury uncomplicated by carpal instability, a volar approach (Fig. 23-18) between the flexor carpi radialis and the radial artery affords excellent exposure for reduction and stabilization as well as repair of concomitant scapholunate ligament injury that is apt to occur with the more proximal fractures. Because of longstanding favorable experience, many surgeons still prefer conventional Kirschner wire internal fixation. However, because of its capacity to induce an acceler-

---

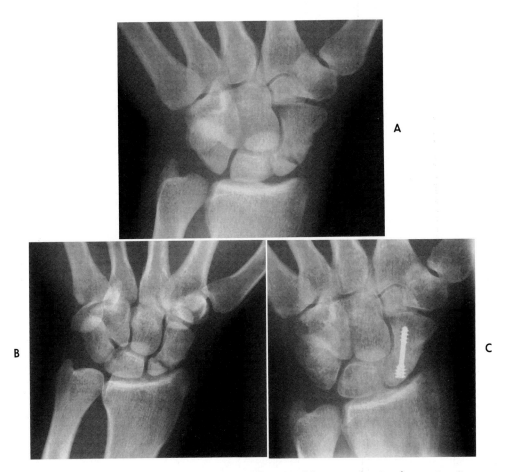

FIG. 23-17. A, Acute scaphoid fracture with a small proximal fragment often is refractory to primary casting and is notorious for complications. **B,** Four weeks after cast immobilization the radiographs demonstrate displacement indicating fracture instability that precludes successful casting. **C,** Stability was promptly restored by open reduction with compression screw fixation, and union occurred 10 weeks later. In carefully selected cases primary open reduction with internal fixation is the preferred method of treatment for this highly complex fracture.

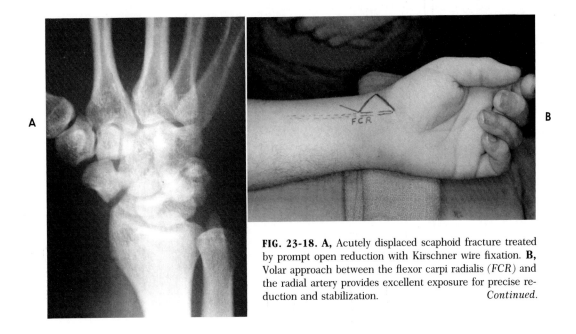

FIG. 23-18. A, Acutely displaced scaphoid fracture treated by prompt open reduction with Kirschner wire fixation. **B,** Volar approach between the flexor carpi radialis *(FCR)* and the radial artery provides excellent exposure for precise reduction and stabilization.   *Continued.*

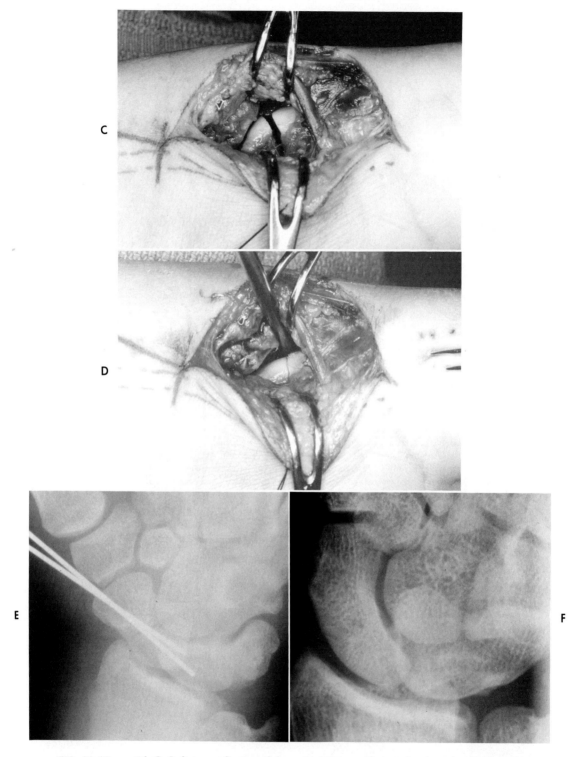

FIG. 23-18, cont'd. C, Judicious reflection of the wrist joint capsule permits clear visualization of widely displaced fracture fragments, which are, **D,** anatomically reduced. **E,** Securely fixed with fine wires. **F,** Twelve weeks after surgery radiographic union is demonstrated.

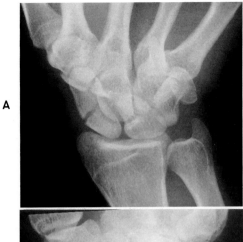

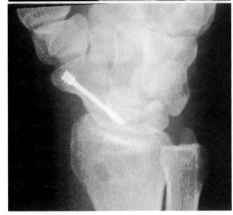

FIG. 23-19. A, Acutely displaced scaphoid fracture treated by open reduction with Herbert screw fixation. **B,** Intraosseous screw affords superior compression and immediately obliterates the fracture site. Although technically more demanding than K-wire fixation, compression screw fixation accelerates union and reduces scaphoid fracture morbidity.

ated union time with a comparable rate of success,[12,22,29,32,47] compression screw fixation, especially with Herbert's design, is rapidly supplanting the Kirschner wire as the primary choice of scaphoid stabilization (Fig. 23-19). Increasing usage has been paralleled by increasing technical expertise and a considerable reduction in fracture morbidity. Nonetheless, even when the fractured scaphoid is secured by rigid fixation, caution is strongly advised against subjecting the injured wrist to the deleterious forces created by unrestricted early motion and premature sports competition. In some instances after screw fixation of both acute and chronic scaphoid fractures, minimal immobilization of 2 to 3 weeks followed by an early return to regular activities within 4 to 7 weeks has been permitted, apparently with no adverse sequelae.[29,47] However, because the athlete is exceptionally liable to reinjury with refracture, a more rational 3- to 4-month period of healing and rehabilitation commensurate with a relatively safe return to sports generally is recommended.

Personal experience with 40 acutely displaced fractures sustained by highly competitive athletes affirms the efficacy of prompt open reduction and secure internal fixation. For the initial 21 fractures, fixation was accomplished with Kirschner wires, whereas subsequently the Herbert screw was used exclusively. In all cases, including eight small proximal pole fractures, uncomplicated radiographic union has occurred, rapid and thorough rehabilitation has been the rule, and return to competition

has ranged between 9 and 16 weeks postoperatively. As expected, the use of screw fixation enhanced union, diminished immobilization time, and expedited the recovery process.

For displaced fractures associated with carpal dislocation (transscaphoid perilunate fracture-dislocation) combined volar and dorsal exposures provide optimal access to the extensive osseous and soft-tissue damage (Fig. 23-20). Through the dorsal approach an anatomic reduction of the scaphoid as well as the disrupted carpal articulations is achieved, and stability is maintained by Kirschner wires alone or in conjunction with screw fixation of the scaphoid. For highly complex fracture-dislocations with excessive soft-tissue injury, an external fixator affords additional stability while concurrently facilitating reduction and maintaining alignment.[31] The volar approach permits repair of the critical soft-tissue injury that invariably involves the major substance of the key radiocarpal ligaments. In my experience this combined surgical approach has consistently resulted in scaphoid union with preservation of carpal stability and a favorable functional recovery. Despite the enormous magnitude of this injury with the inevitable loss of some wrist mobility, most persons are able to resume their former level of activity after completing a comprehensive therapy program. However, the interval between injury and return to activity often exceeds 9 months, and in no case should this seriously injured wrist be prematurely subjected to excessive force.

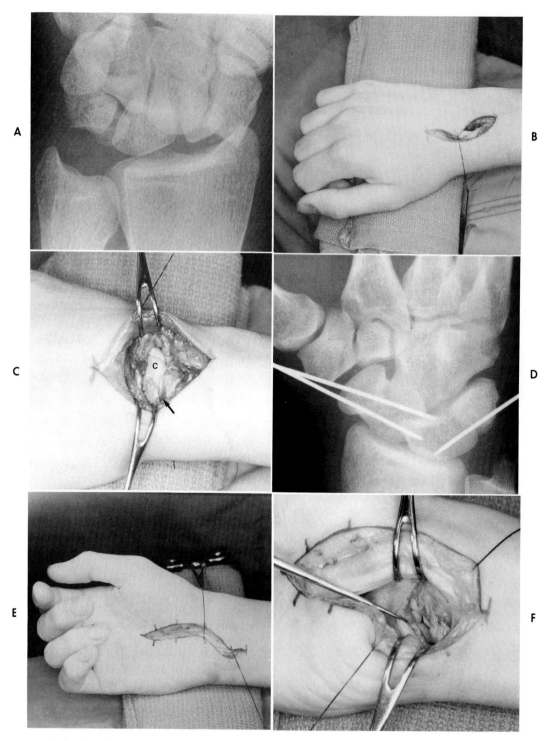

FIG. 23-20. A, Marked scaphoid displacement associated with the transscaphoid perilunate fracture-dislocation. As a preliminary step that considerably facilitates patient comfort and alleviates pressure on contused nerves, the midcarpal dislocation is reduced by closed manipulation. Fracture displacement as well as residual carpal dissociation is then corrected by combined dorsal and volar operative approaches. **B,** The dorsal approach. **C,** The displaced scaphoid (*arrow*) and the residual carpal subluxation (*C*) are clearly identified. **D,** Reduction and stabilization with Kirschner wires. **E,** Volar exposure permits thorough decompression of contused nerves. **F,** Volar exposure also provides access to the critical soft-tissue injury that invariably involves the major substances of the perilunar ligaments (at the tip of the probe).

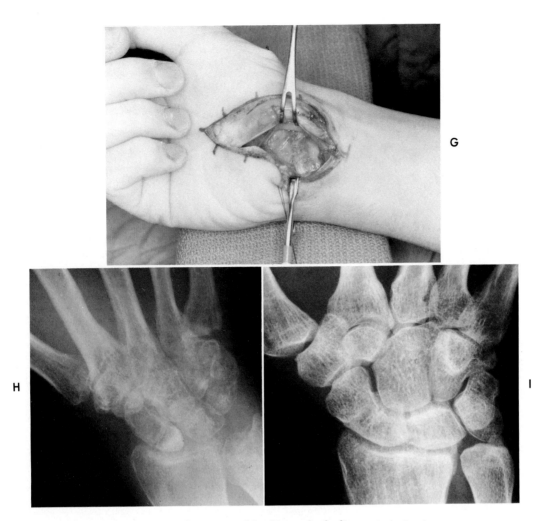

FIG. 23-20, cont'd. **G,** Meticulous repair of the disrupted volar ligamentous structure ensures maximal restitution of midcarpal and lunotriquetral stability. **H,** Eight weeks after surgery the scaphoid proximal pole demonstrates increased radiodensity indicative of ischemia; however, **I,** continuous immobilization results in fracture union with revascularization and preservation of carpal relationships.

Bone grafting as an osteogenic stimulus is indicated for the acutely comminuted fracture, the displaced fracture initially treated 6 or more weeks after injury, and for the chronic nonunion of 4 or more months' duration. Once nonunion, even if relatively asymptomatic, is detected, operative treatment should be recommended as the only reliable means of obtaining healing and preventing the inevitable sequence of carpal instability, progressive deformity, and ultimately disabling osteoarthritis.[58,83] Neither small proximal fragments nor ischemic fragments contraindicate the procedure, which in most cases can be electively planned to cause the least interference with the athlete's career.

Indications for bone grafting

- Chronic nonunion greater than 4 months
- Displaced fractures receiving initial treatment 6 or more weeks after injury
- Acute, displaced comminuted fracture

The operation is performed through a volar zigzag incision that provides excellent access to both the scaphoid nonunion and the distal radius as the bone graft donor site (Fig. 23-21). Fibrous tissue is excised and sclerotic bone debrided at the juncture of the ununited fragments. Both fragments are then excavated, creating a healthy host bed for insertion of the bone graft. The critical and most difficult step of the operation is an anatomic reduction of the fragments; this is essential to achieve uncomplicated endosteal healing as well as to prevent the occurrence of malunion, which must be recognized as an additional and major cause of suboptimal recovery.* Accordingly, for chronically displaced nonunions characterized by the scaphoid humpback deformity with concomitant carpal collapse, a volar opening wedge or interpositional graft is required to elongate the scaphoid and correct the carpal deformity. In such cases the goal is twofold: anatomic restitution of the scaphoid

---

*References 3, 20, 28, 32, 43, and 47.

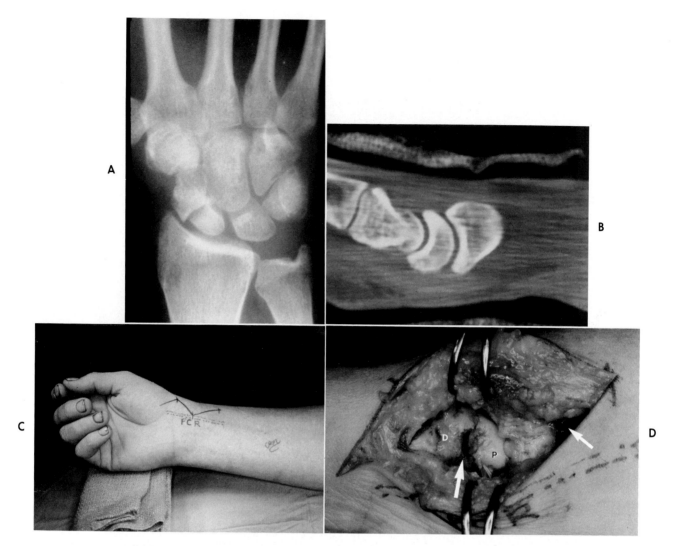

FIG. 23-21. A, Sixteen-month-old scaphoid nonunion. **B,** Same patient with concomitant carpal instability (dorsal intercalated segmental disability [DISI]) treated by bone grafting and adjunctive postoperative pulsing electromagnetic fields. **C,** Volar zigzag incision provides excellent access to both the nonunion and the distal radius as a bone graft donor site. **D,** A wide gap *(left arrow)* filled with fibrous tissue and synovial fluid separates the proximal *(P)* and distal *(D)* fragments. The arrow to the right identifies the distal radius donor site.

and restoration of carpal alignment. A successful outcome depends not only on scaphoid union, but also on preservation of carpal stability. Success is also contingent on a passively correctable deformity, as determined by preoperative radiography and meticulous operative techniques. Stable fixation is accomplished with either Kirschner wires[28,65,93] or small screws* that minimize motion between the graft and its bed, thereby promoting rapid revascularization and union. Postoperatively, cast immobilization must be continued until radiographic union is clearly evident.

In a personal series employing bone grafting and Kirschner wire fixation for 70 consecutive nonunions with a 12-month average interval between fracture and sur-

gery, union occurred in 65 (93%) of the cases. Healing averaged 5 months and consistently was followed by a return to sports 3 to 4 months thereafter. In an effort to accelerate the recovery process, noninvasive electrical stimulation employing pulsing electromagnetic fields (PEMFs) subsequently was added to the postoperative regimen. An analysis of 18 such cases indicated that adjunctive electricity by virtue of its synergism with bone grafting significantly reduced the time to union. Patients receiving PEMF healed more rapidly regardless of fracture location or the presence of ischemic fracture fragments.

This experience combining PEMF stimulation with bone grafting suggests that the use of electricity can safely expedite the athlete's recovery. It also substantiates the opinion of others[1,35] that PEMF stimulation is a

---

*References 12, 20, 22, 29, 47, and 106.

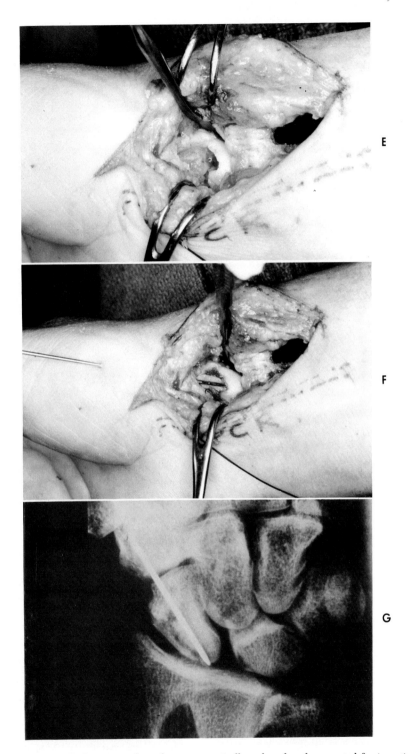

E

F

G

FIG. 23-21, cont'd. E, Fragments have been anatomically reduced and excavated for insertion of the bone graft. **F,** Cancellous bone is packed around a corticocancellous volar wedge graft that elongates the scaphoid and restores carpal alignment. Fixation is achieved with a Kirschner wire. **G,** Radiography after surgery demonstrates an anatomic reduction and obliteration of the fracture with the graft. *Continued.*

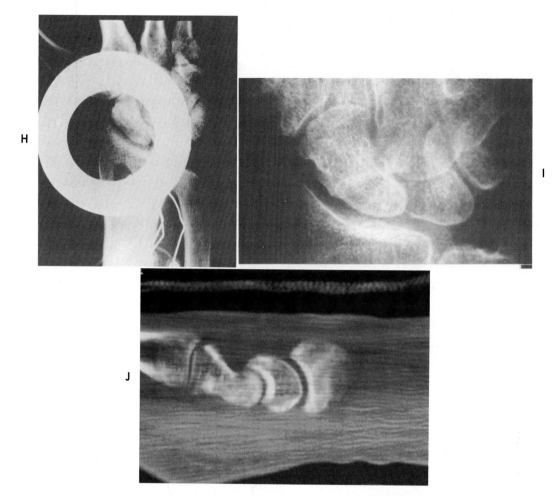

FIG. 23-21, cont'd. H, Five weeks postoperatively the wire has been removed and coils for electric stimulation have been applied to the cast. **I,** Seventeen weeks after surgery radiography demonstrates incorporation of the graft and union as well as, **J,** correction of the DISI carpal deformity. Successful bone grafting requires restoration of both scaphoid integrity and carpal alignment.

useful adjuvant in the treatment of scaphoid nonunion. Nonetheless, because carefully controlled clinical studies are not yet available for critical assessment, the true efficacy of electrical stimulation remains uncertain.

More recently, in a further attempt to diminish the morbidity of scaphoid nonunion, Herbert screw fixation in conjunction with bone grafting has been employed for an additional 30 cases. Significantly, uncomplicated union, confirmed by tomography, has occurred in 28 (93%) of the cases, all of which united within a comparatively rapid period of 12 weeks (Fig. 23-22). Furthermore, successful healing has not been prejudiced by increased radiographic density, small proximal fragments, or the paucity of intraosseous bleeding. This prospective series yields more data supporting the contention that improved techniques of internal fixation can accelerate union and enhance recovery for the athlete with a chronically ununited scaphoid fracture.

Based on the collective experience of the numerous authorities referenced in this chapter, the criteria for op-

timal management of scaphoid nonunion among athletes can be summarized as follows:

1. Existent fracture viability as determined not solely by the presence of intraosseous bleeding but also by the presence of fracture fragment integrity, as evidenced by preservation of normal osseous contours with healthy articular surfaces
2. An anatomic reduction supported by precisely sculptured bone grafting that restores scaphoid as well as adjacent carpal alignment
3. A biocompatible method of internal fixation generating a compressive force with the capacity for maintaining exact apposition of fracture and graft while concurrently promoting rapid revascularization with accelerated union
4. Continuous postoperative immobilization until union is unequivocally verified by precise radiographic techniques
5. Intensive, thorough rehabilitation before resumption of competition

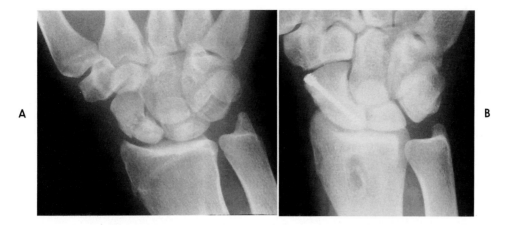

FIG. 23-22. A, Seventeen-month-old scaphoid nonunion treated by volar wedge bone grafting in conjunction with compression screw fixation. **B,** Twelve weeks after surgery, correction of displacement and solid union are demonstrated. Improved methods of bone grafting and screw fixation have enhanced the healing process for both acute and chronic scaphoid fractures.

When confronted with an ununited scaphoid, the physician should make every attempt to preserve osseous integrity of this vital carpal link. For the injured athlete with viable fracture fragments devoid of resorption or articular damage, procedures such as styloidectomy, carpectomy, implant arthroplasty, allograft replacement, and intercarpal arthrodesis should be avoided. These are salvage operations reserved for select cases of irreparable scaphoid injury complicated by painful osteoarthritis.

Hamate Hook (Hamulus) Fractures

Any athlete who vigorously swings a sports device is liable to sustain the impact of the handle against the hypothenar eminence, thereby fracturing the vulnerable hook. Although direct compression of the prominent hamulus is the principal cause of fracture, a concurrent, powerful contraction of the attached hypothenar intrinsic muscles and a violent shearing force generated by the adjacent flexor tendons probably contribute to the mechanism of injury.[107] Because the wrist nearest the handle is susceptible, the nondominant side is typically affected among baseball players and golfers, whereas the dominant side is affected in racquet sports and polo athletes.

The hamate hook fracture truly is a sport-specific problem that undoubtedly can be lessened by preventive measures: coaching to enhance an athlete's stick- or racquet-handling ability, devising more secure grips on sports equipment, and fabricating precisely contoured protective gloves. Nonetheless, the hamulus fracture remains a frequent occurrence that requires prompt treatment to avert the disabling complications of painful nonunion, neuropathy, and flexor tendon injury.

Although some authorities recommend excision of the hamulus for all hamate hook fractures,[94] personal experience as well as that of others[9,110] confirms that healing of undisplaced fractures can occur with continuous casting, and thus immobilization is a viable treatment option for stable injuries. As anticipated, the healing pro-

cess is prolonged and averages between 8 and 12 weeks. Even minimal distraction impedes this process, and, like that of the scaphoid, the hook fracture treated with casting requires continuous radiographic, or preferably tomographic, surveillance to ensure exact apposition of the fracture fragments. As depicted in Fig. 23-8, CT provides unparalleled visualization of the hamulus fracture site and is a superior method of assessing the healing process.[25,92,94]

Whalen, Bishop, and Linscheid[110] reported union in six consecutive cases of acute hamulus fracture treated by continuous immobilization. The mean healing time was 8 weeks with a range from 6 to 19 weeks. They emphasized the formidable challenge of nonoperative treatment and that success demands strict adherence to the following guidelines: first, the fracture must be truly undisplaced as determined by tomography; second, the diagnosis must be early, preferably within the first week of injury; and third, effective casting must be promptly instituted and continued until union is clearly documented. Accordingly, the patient must be willing to comply with a treatment regimen that usually restricts strenuous activities for a minimum of 4 months. For the highly competitive athlete these criteria are often difficult to fulfill because the diagnosis is frequently delayed and the fracture is usually displaced. The relatively prolonged disability imposed by continuous casting is an additional factor limiting its usage among athletes.

With fracture displacement, union by immobilization is precluded and early surgery is essential to minimize morbidity. In an effort to restore normal anatomy, open reduction and internal fixation with or without bone grafting[9,11,107] have been employed, with variable success, for the displaced fracture. Insufficient experience, however, precludes definitive conclusions regarding the use of this method. Nonetheless, the physician should recognize that, even with the most precise techniques of open reduction, internal fixation, and bone grafting the prognosis for osseous healing is decidedly guarded ow-

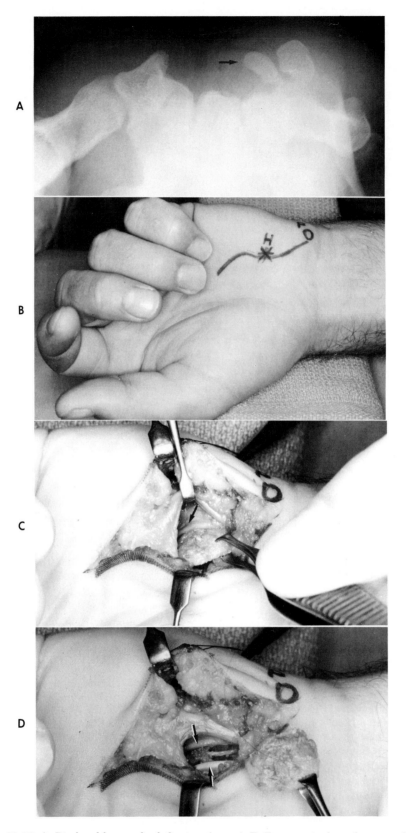

FIG. 23-23. A, Displaced hamate hook fracture *(arrow)*. **B,** Exposure is through a curved palmar incision extending from the hamate *(H)* to the pisiform *(PO)*. **C,** Highly vulnerable motor branch of the ulnar nerve *(arrow)* must be clearly visualized and protected throughout the procedure. **D,** Un-united hook fragment is excised subperiosteally without disturbing the adjacent nerve *(upper arrow)* or flexor tendons to the small finger *(lower arrow)*.

ing to the small size and ischemia of the fracture fragments. Delayed union and nonunion should be considered substantial risks apt to compromise recovery.[9,11]

Clearly, for the hamulus fracture demonstrating acute displacement or nonunion, prompt excision of the hook offers the optimal means of achieving a rapid uncomplicated recovery.* For the athlete treated by hook excision, uniformly good results with short-term immobilization and rapid rehabilitation have been the rule. The operation proceeds as follows: The displaced fragment is exposed through a curved incision extending from the pisiform to the proximal palm along the radial border of the hypothenar eminence (Fig. 23-23). The adjacent soft tissues are carefully preserved as the hook is subperiosteally excised. Throughout the operation the highly vulnerable deep motor branch of the ulnar nerve should be clearly visualized and protected. The raw fracture surface is covered with adjacent periosteal tissues as well as the redundant pisohamate ligament, and soft-tissue connections are restored by suturing the ulnar edge of

---

*References 9, 11, 13, 25, 92, and 94.

the transverse carpal ligament to the fascial origin of the hypothenar muscles. The adjuvant repairs not only reconstitute important soft-tissue attachments, but also lessen postoperative wound sensitivity. Excision of the hook should not be likened to a simple bony debridement. Skillful management of the critical soft tissues in the area of excision is equally important to successful surgery.

After hook excision sports participation with the athlete's preinjury level of skill depends largely on the resolution of hypothenar pain and tenderness, symptoms that tend to persist for several months. The use of custom-fit gloves considerably lessens this problem and facilitates an early return to competition.

Triquetrum Fractures

Triquetrum fractures constitute the second or third most common group of carpal fractures.[11,55] The dorsal marginal fracture resulting from either soft-tissue avulsion or bony impingement is most prevalent among athletes (Fig. 23-24, *A* and *B*) and, despite its frequent failure to unite, seldom requires more than 4 weeks of splint

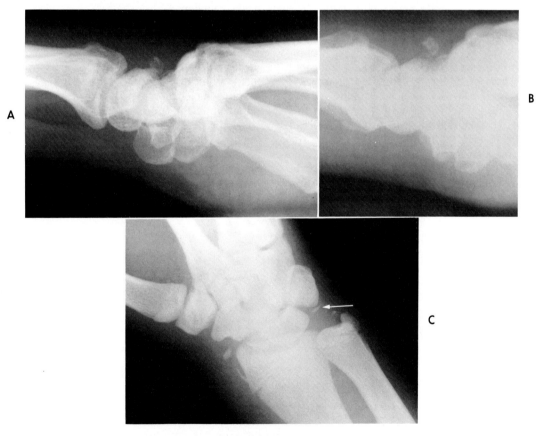

FIG. 23-24. Fractures of the triquetrum. **A,** This dorsal marginal fracture was clinically healed after 4 weeks of splinting. The concept of custom-fit protective casting with an early return to sports often is applicable to this injury, which rapidly becomes asymptomatic and causes no significant alteration of wrist function. **B,** Similar fracture resulting in nonunion. The ununited fragment usually is asymptomatic and has no adverse effect on wrist function. For the occasional painful nonunion, excision of the fragment is the remedy, and several weeks later, competition with protection is permissible as tolerated. **C,** In contrast to the relatively innocuous dorsal fracture, the radiovolar marginal fracture (*arrow*) is a frequent component of serious perilunate fracture-dislocations that require surgery for restoration of carpal stability.

immobilization. At this point the wrist usually is asymptomatic and this relatively innocuous injury can be safely managed by protective splinting or casting, thereby permitting many athletes to resume their sport with minimal risk of further damage. For the occasional case of symptomatic nonunion, excision of the painful ossicle is the remedy.

In contrast to injuries of the dorsal surface, fractures of the radiovolar margin as well as those through the body of the triquetrum usually are associated with perilunate dislocation or fracture-dislocation (Fig. 23-24, C).[32,60] These serious disruptions of carpal anatomy generally require open treatment for reduction of fractures and repair of critical soft tissues. An essential part of the operation is stabilization of the triquetrum by open reduction and internal fixation, or more frequently excision of the small radiovolar fragments and direct repair of the disrupted lunotriquetral capsuloligamentous structure (Fig. 23-20, F and G). Following these serious injuries the athlete's name should remain on the disabled roster for a minimum of 4 months.

Other Carpal Fractures
Lunate Fractures

Sheltered by the enclosure of the radial fossa, the lunate is perhaps the carpal bone least vulnerable to fracture. Stewart and Cross,[96] in their extensive review of lunate injuries, most of which were dislocations, indicated that the acute fracture is rare. Teisen and Hjarbaek[99] evaluated more than 3000 carpal fractures managed over 31 years and documented only 17 acute lunate fractures (0.5% of total). In their series, fracture occurred most frequently through the volar pole, a site apt to disrupt the key volar nutrient artery. Nonetheless, radiographic follow-up, ranging from 4 to 31 years, was available for 11 patients, and failed to demonstrate evidence of resultant avascular necrosis. These investigators concluded that Kienböck's disease was unlikely to result from the isolated acute lunate fracture. Conversely, Beckenbaugh and associates[7] retrospectively identified fracture in 31 of 38 lunates with established Kienböck's osteonecrosis and postulated a causal relationship between the lunate fracture that fails to unite and irreversible avascular necrosis. Although this hypothesis is controversial and the acute fracture is infrequently encountered among athletes, the sports physician must recognize the potential danger of isolated trauma to the lunate, especially in that highly susceptible group with vascular insufficiency and ulnar minus variance.

Lunate fractures must be promptly diagnosed, securely immobilized, and protected from further injury until union is certain (Fig. 23-25). Displaced fractures require early, precise open reduction and internal fixation for restoration of radiocarpal and midcarpal articular congruity as well as for rapid restitution of lunate vascularity (Fig. 23-26). Also, because Kienböck's disease is apt to result from repeated trauma, the athlete with a healed fracture requires protective splinting or casting during subsequent sports participation and constant clinical surveillance.

Trapezium Fractures

Two basic types of trapezium injury are being diagnosed with increasing frequency.[11,21,34,61,72] The vertical body fracture is nearly the mirror image of the Bennett fracture-dislocation (Fig. 23-27, A and B). Instead of the ulnar lip of the thumb metacarpal fracturing, the radial aspect of the trapezium body is split and displaced proximally with the attached metacarpal, disrupting and dislocating the thumb carpometacarpal joint. Through an anterior approach with reflection of the thenar musculature the fracture is reduced and the capsular tissues are

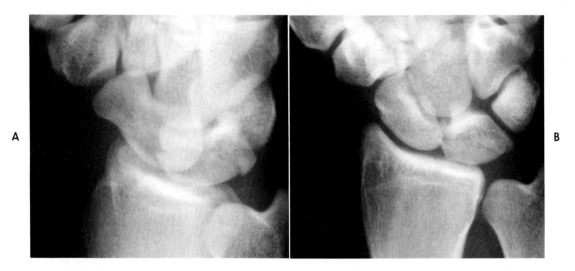

FIG. 23-25. Undisplaced fracture of the lunate in a young athlete with ulnar minus variance. This injury should always be considered a precursor to ischemia, fragmentation, and Kienböck's disease and requires anatomic alignment with prompt immobilization that must be continued until union is certain. In this case, follow-up radiographs demonstrated thorough healing with no evidence of progressive devitalization or fragmentation.

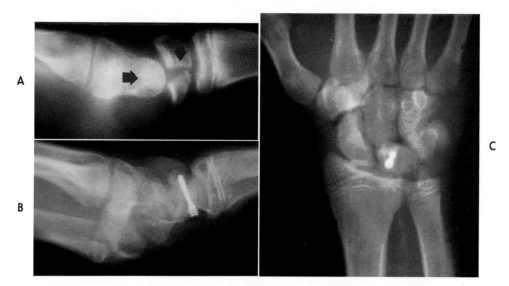

FIG. 23-26. A, Displaced, transverse fracture of the lunate associated with acute median neuropathy. Treatment comprised open reduction, screw fixation, and nerve decompression via a volar approach. **B** and **C,** Postoperatively, lunate anatomy is restored as is adjacent articular congruity. Neither the fracture nor the surgical approach compromised vascularity, and posttraumatic avascular necrosis did not occur.

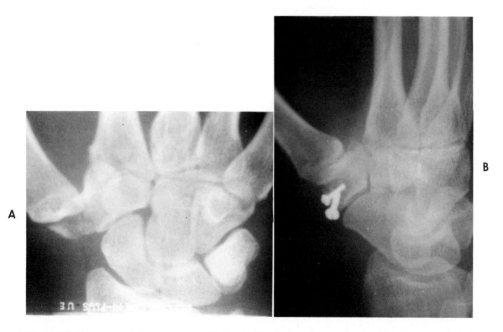

FIG. 23-27. Fractures of the trapezium. **A,** Vertical body fracture resulting in disruption with dislocation of the thumb carpometacarpal joint requires open treatment for both fracture reduction and capsular repair. **B,** Internal fixation with 2-mm lag screws restores fracture stability and joint congruity.   *Continued.*

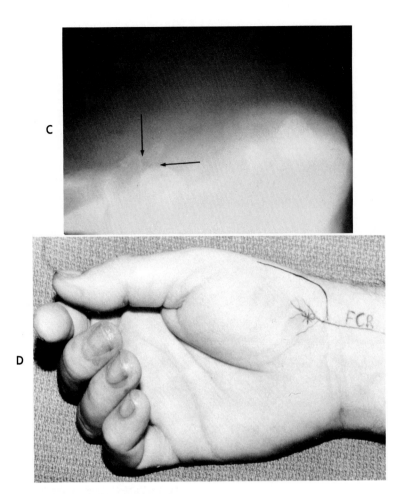

FIG. 23-27, cont'd. **C,** Distracted anterior ridge fracture *(arrows)* is optimally managed by early excision. **D,** Anterior approach bordering the thenar eminence.

repaired, thereby restoring articular congruity and stability. Internal fixation is achieved with either Kirschner wires or small screws.

The anterior ridge fracture is analogous to the hamate hook fracture because minimal distraction precludes healing with cast immobilization, and chronically unhealed fractures are apt to result in neuropathy—in this instance involving the median nerve within the adjacent

---

**Potential complications of trapezial
anterior ridge fracture**

- Nonunion
- Median neuropathy
- Flexor carpi radialis attrition

---

carpal tunnel. Fraying with inflammation or ultimate rupture of the flexor carpi radialis may prove an additional problem. An uncomplicated recovery is facilitated by early excision of the displaced ridge fragment, also employing anterior exposure (Fig. 23-27, *C* to *F*). In

chronic cases with neuropathy or tendinitis the adjacent median nerve and flexor carpi radialis can be decompressed simultaneously. Not infrequently, a considerable degree of wound sensitivity persists for several months after operation and is apt to compromise function. Impairment can be minimized by the use of protective gloves.

Capitate Fractures

Similar to the scaphoid proximal pole fracture, the capitate fracture should be considered inherently unstable because seldom does uncomplicated union occur only with cast immobilization, even if promptly instituted.[103] Delayed union, nonunion, and avascular necrosis characterize a challenging healing process that can be favorably influenced by early surgical intervention. For acute fractures demonstrating any evidence of instability, secure internal fixation with either wires or screws should be strongly considered, and for subacute or chronic injuries supplementary bone grafting is recommended.

Fractures of the head or neck occur most frequently as a key component of the transscaphoid-transcapitate-perilunate fracture-dislocation (scaphocapitate syndrome) or as relatively isolated events. In either instance

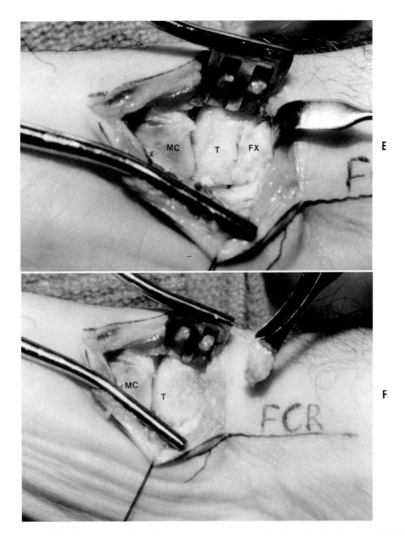

FIG. 23-27, cont'd. E, Reflection of the thenar musculature clearly identifies the fracture. *MC,* Metacarpal of the thumb, *T,* trapezium; *FX,* trapezial ridge fracture. **F,** Ununited fragment (held with the forceps) is excised, and the raw surface of the trapezium is smoothed to minimize postoperative tenderness.

even minor displacement indicates instability that must be corrected by prompt open reduction with internal fixation.[44,76,81,102,103] The scaphocapitate syndrome is characterized by variable displacement of the scaphoid and marked rotation of the capitate head so that its articular surface usually faces the body of the capitate rather than the lunate (Fig. 23-28, *A*). The resultant squared-off appearance of the proximal capitate is a constant radiographic feature of this serious injury that always requires open treatment for restoration of osseous integrity and carpal stability. Through a dorsal approach the proximal capitate is first derotated and stabilized with Kirschner wires or small screws, thereby facilitating anatomic alignment and internal fixation of the scaphoid.[102] Although both bones are substantially devitalized and transient ischemia is frequently demonstrated on the radiographs, an accurate reduction consistently leads to successful union and a favorable outcome. However, a prolonged period in excess of 6 months is required for thorough healing and rehabilitation.

Potential complications of capitate fractures

- Nonunion
- Avascular necrosis
- Carpal collapse
- Traumatic arthritis

Isolated fractures of the capitate are being diagnosed with increasing frequency owing to a heightened awareness of their occurrence coupled with meticulous scrutiny of injury films. The usual site of fracture is the juncture of the body and the neck, and comminution is a relatively common feature (Fig. 23-29). For undisplaced fractures a trial of closed treatment is permissible, but only 1 mm of fragment displacement or distraction is evidence of instability that is optimally managed by prompt surgery. Fractures that are undisplaced but undetected for several weeks as well as those that are grossly dis-

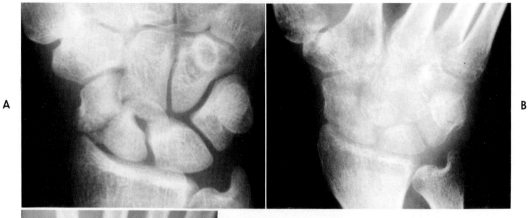

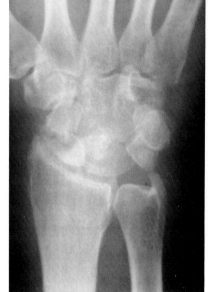

FIG. 23-28. Scaphocapitate syndrome. **A,** Typically the scaphoid fracture is displaced and the capitate head is rotated 180 degrees. The squared-off appearance of the proximal capitate is characteristic of this injury that always requires prompt open reduction and internal fixation for restoration of the severely disrupted carpal anatomy. **B,** Despite transient ischemia of the proximal capitate and scaphoid, both bones united favorably. **C,** In contrast, this untreated scaphocapitate injury resulted in persistent fracture displacement with avascular necrosis and the inevitable sequence of nonunion, carpal collapse, and arthritis.

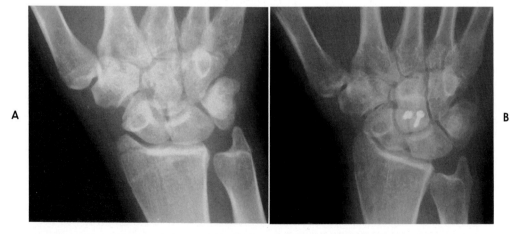

FIG. 23-29. A, Four-week-old capitate fracture through the waist and head demonstrating considerable displacement and comminution. **B,** Open reduction, screw fixation, and supplementary bone grafting restored skeletal integrity as well as articular congruity and resulted in uncomplicated union.

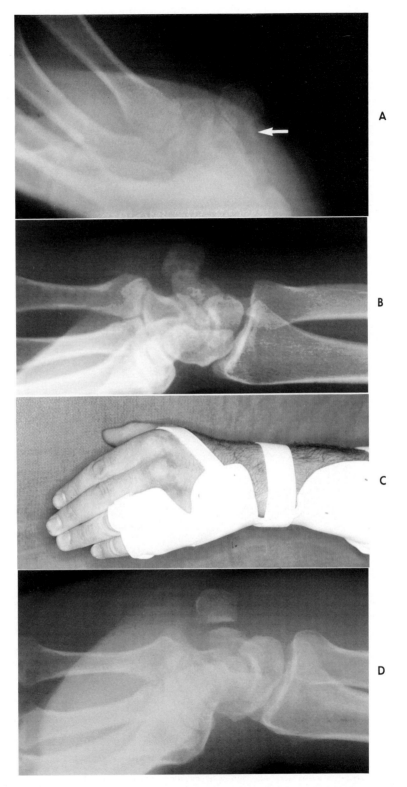

FIG. 23-30. Pisiform fractures. **A,** Minimally displaced avulsion fracture *(arrow).* **B,** Undisplaced body fracture. **C,** These fractures were successfully treated with a contoured splint immobilizing the wrist in mild flexion and the metacarpophalangeal joints of the ring and small fingers in acute flexion. Four weeks after injury a custom-fit rubber cast safely permitted an early return to competition. **D,** Radiograph 6 weeks after injury demonstrates thorough healing of the pisiform body fracture.

placed also require operative treatment to ensure uncomplicated union.

Pisiform Fractures

The pisiform is clearly profiled by the oblique radiograph with the wrist in approximately 30 degrees of supination or the clenched fist AP view with the wrist in ulnar deviation. If undisplaced, pisiform fractures are successfully treated by 3 to 6 weeks of immobilization similar to that used for undisplaced hamate hook fractures (Fig. 23-30). Comminuted fractures or fracture-dislocations causing disruption of the pisotriquetral joint are prone to inadequate healing with persistent pain and are optimally managed by early pisiformectomy (Fig. 23-31).[11,104] Through a small curved incision at the base of the hypothenar eminence the ulnar nerve and artery are carefully protected and the pisiform is subperiosteally excised from the substance of the flexor carpi ulnaris. Redundant soft tissues are secured to the margins of the triquetrum, thereby resurfacing exposed cartilage and preserving ligamentous attachments. The tendon is repaired, and the wound is protected for several weeks postoperatively.

The pisiform fracture, like the dorsal marginal fracture of the triquetrum, causes only a minor interruption of the athlete's career. Following short-term casting of either the undisplaced fracture or the comminuted fracture requiring excision, the injury can be safely managed by protective devices that alleviate residual wound tenderness and permit an early resumption of activity.

Trapezoid Fractures

Trapezoid fractures, like those of the capitate or hamate body, are usually associated with violent injuries that include a major disruption of the adjacent carpometacarpal joint. Operative treatment is indicated for restoration of articular congruity as well as reduction of displaced carpal fragments. The rarely encountered isolated

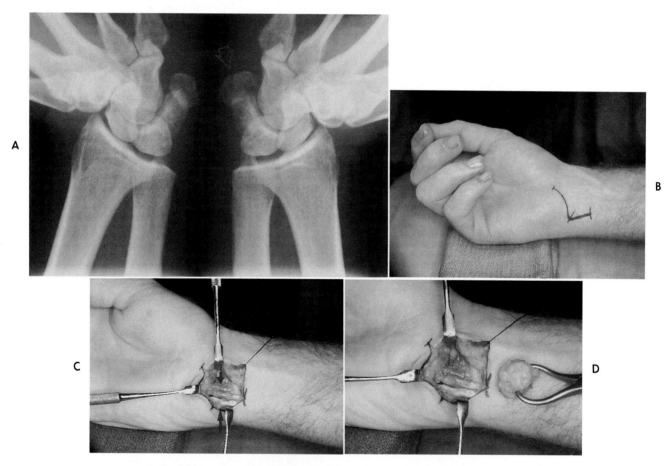

FIG. 23-31. A, For the comminuted pisiform fracture *(arrow)* clearly illustrated on this ulnar deviation, anteroposterior view, early excision is necessary to prevent disability resulting from suboptimal healing with irreversible disruption of the piso-triquetral joint. **B,** Operation is performed through a small incision at the base of the hypothenar eminence with minimal disturbance to the soft-tissue pad. **C,** Exposure of the ulnar neurovascular bundle *(top arrow)* and the flexor carpi ulnaris tendon *(bottom arrow)*, which has been split longitudinally for enucleation of the fractured pisiform. **D,** Excision of the pisiform (held with the forceps) demonstrates a multifragmented, irreversibly damaged articular surface. Side-to-side repair of the flexor carpi ulnaris restores tendon integrity.

fracture of the trapezoid requires only a short term of immobilization because osseous circulation is excellent, as is the prospect for prompt union.

Distal Radius Fractures

Optimal management of distal radius fractures requires differentiation of the relatively low-energy metaphyseal injuries, traditionally termed *Colles' fracture* and *Smith's fracture,* from the more violent injuries that disrupt the distal radius articular surfaces. The articular fractures are prevalent among physically active persons whose wrists are subjected to severe compression forces prone to occur during sports-related activities. The magnitude of force not only disrupts both the radiocarpal and distal radioulnar joint, but also is apt to result in serious concomitant periarticular soft-tissue and skeletal injury. Prominent among these additional injuries are contusions of the median and ulnar nerves, fractures of the scaphoid and distal ulna, and rupture of the scapholunate interosseous ligament.

Optimal management also requires careful assessment of other important fracture characteristics: displacement, stability, and reducibility. Marked displacement with extensive metaphyseal comminution renders the fracture highly unstable and refractory to successful articular restoration by closed reduction alone. Excessive offset, gapping, impaction, and tilting of key articular components are signs of an injury apt to prove irreducible by all methods of closed management. For the unstable articular fracture a method of accurate skeletal fixation is essential for securing fracture reduction and ensuring uncomplicated healing. For those cases with irreducible articular fragments open treatment is the only means of restoring the disrupted articular surfaces as well as repairing the critical periarticular damage.*

Articular Fractures

Axial compression is the key component in the mechanism of the distal radius articular injury (Fig. 23-2, C). The carpus, principally the lunate, forcibly impacts the radial articular fossae, causing predictable patterns of

---

Components of distal radius articular injury

- Radial shaft
- Radial styloid
- Dorsal medial fragment
- Palmar medial fragment

---

fragmentation and displacement.[66] Despite variable comminution, articular fractures comprise four basic components: the radial shaft or metaphyseal fragment, the radial styloid, a dorsal medial fragment, and a palmar medial fragment. To underscore their pivotal position as the cornerstone of both the radiocarpal and radioulnar joints, the medial fragments along with their strong ligamen-

tous attachments to the carpus and the ulnar styloid have been termed the *medial complex.* Displacement of this complex always causes a serious biarticular disruption of the distal radius and is the basis for a classification of articular fractures (Fig. 23-32). Previously, four prevalent fracture patterns of varying severity have been defined[66]; more recently, two additional fracture types have been categorized (Fig. 23-33).[68]

The Type II articular fracture with dorsal displacement, traditionally termed the **die-punch injury,** occurs most frequently and generally has proved amenable to successful reduction by closed techniques and stabilization by external fixation. However, the formulation of more stringent but widely accepted criteria for successful articular restoration has led to recognition that a substantial number of these injuries, termed *Type IIB irreducible fractures,* cannot be satisfactorily managed by closed techniques. Compared with the reducible Type II fracture, the irreducible articular pattern demonstrates greater comminution and displacement of the medial fragments, usually in a dorsal direction, persistent articular step-off or gapping greater than 2 mm, irreversible articular tilting in excess of 20 degrees, and uncorrectable radial shortening exceeding 5 mm. In a continuing assessment of distal radius articular fractures, this increasingly recognized pattern of articular disruption has accounted for 15% of the injuries and, significantly, greater than 70% of those requiring open treatment for preservation of articular congruity.[68]

Another more severe pattern of articular fragmentation, but one that is seldom encountered among athletes, has also been noted to occur with increasing frequency. This serious lesion, termed the *Type V explosion injury,* results from a violent force comprising both axial compression and direct crush that causes profound articular and metaphyseal comminution as well as major soft-tissue trauma that is apt to disrupt skin, nerves, and vascular structures.

Classification of distal radius articular fractures

Type I
- Minimally displaced
- Stable

Type IIA
- Displaced medial complex
- Substantial comminution
- Unstable, reducible

Type IIB
- Greater displacement
- Greater comminution
- Unstable, irreducible

Type III
- Displaced medial complex
- Displaced metaphyseal fragment
- Unstable, irreducible

Type IV
- Wide separation of medial fragments
- Extensive periarticular damage
- Unstable, irreducible

Type V
- Extensive articular, metaphyseal comminution
- Extensive soft-tissue damage
- Unstable, irreducible

---

*References 5, 17, 30, 45, 51, 54, 66, 67, 70, and 109.

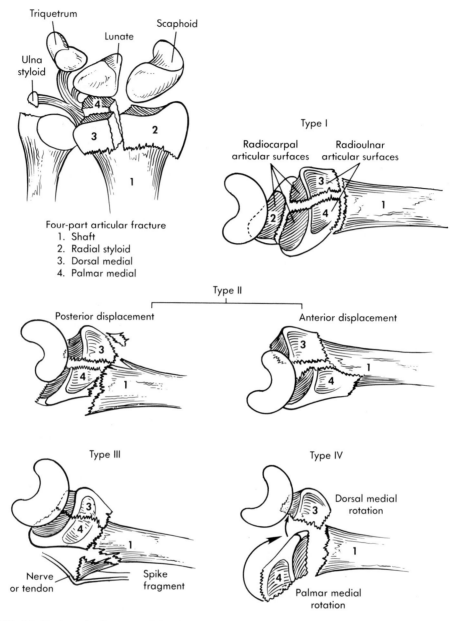

FIG. 23-32. Articular fractures of the distal radius consist of four basic components: (*1*) the radial shaft, (*2*) the radial styloid, (*3*) a dorsal medial fragment, and (*4*) a palmar medial fragment. The key medial fragments and their strong ligamentous attachments to the carpals and ulnar styloid have been termed the *medial complex.* Displacement of this complex is the basis for classification of articular fractures into specific types. The unstable Type II fracture is most frequently encountered among athletes. (From Melone CP Jr: Unstable fractures of the distal radius. In Lichtman DM [ed]: *The wrist and its disorders,* Philadelphia, 1987, WB Saunders.)

Identifying specific fracture components with characteristic patterns of displacement serves as a highly useful guide to management as well as an accurate gauge for prognosis. In all cases, preservation of joint congruity by promptly detecting and correcting predictable articular fragment displacement is the principal prerequisite for a successful outcome.

Author's classification and preferred treatment. For the majority of unstable articular fractures optimal management comprises closed reduction and stabilization with an external fixation device, often in conjunction with percutaneous Kirschner wire internal fixation. It is emphasized that successful usage of the external fixator relies heavily on skillful pin insertion. A precise, limited open technique avoids a multitude of pin problems apt to compromise recovery.

For the irreducible fractures requiring open reduction, internal fixation usually is achieved with fine Kirschner

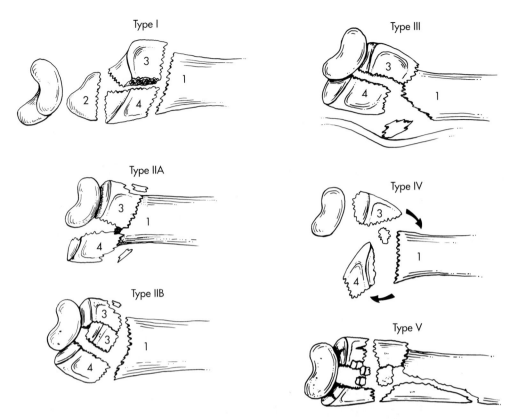

FIG. 23-33. In a continuing assessment of distal radius articular fractures, two additional fracture patterns have been noted with increasing frequency: the Type IIB irreducible die-punch fracture and the Type V explosion fracture. Compared with the Type IIA injury, the Type IIB fracture is characterized by greater comminution and displacement of the medial fragments with articular disruption that is refractory to closed methods of reduction. The Type V fracture results from a severe force comprising both compression and crush that cause extensive comminution, often extending from the articular surface to the diaphysis. (From Melone CP Jr et al: *Orthop Clin North Am* 24:239, 1993.)

wires or occasionally with small plates. Also, for these more serious and highly unstable articular fractures, external fixation and bone grafting often are employed as key constituents of optimal treatment. The external fixator affords additional stability, whereas adjunctive bone grafting provides an articular buttress, restores metaphyseal integrity, and enhances fracture healing.

Type I fractures are minimally displaced, are stable, and are effectively treated by a relatively short period of continuous cast or splint immobilization (usually 4 weeks) followed by a program of progressive remobilization and strengthening supplemented with protective splinting until rehabilitation is complete.

The Type IIA fracture is most frequently encountered among athletes. This fracture is displaced, comminuted, and characteristically unstable. The fracture is also prone to median or ulnar nerve contusion, which is apt to occur in nearly 20% of the cases. Displacement of the articular fragments is either dorsal (the die-punch pattern),[66,68,87] or less frequently volar (a fracture pattern analogous to the Smith Type II or volar Barton's fracture-dislocation).[26,100] It is important to recognize that, regardless of the direction of displacement, the key medial

fragments are not widely separated and are conducive to reduction by traction and manipulation with stabilization by external pins incorporated in either a plaster cast or preferably an external fixation frame.* Successful traction with external pin fixation is contingent on the strength of the ligamentous component of the medial complex, which usually remains intact despite extensive osseous fragmentation.[23] Maintaining these soft tissues under constant tension affords stability to the attached articular fragments.

For Type IIA fractures in athletes the combined technique of an external fixator with supplementary percutaneous Kirschner wire internal fixation has consistently proved a superior method of treatment (Fig. 23-34). In the vast majority of cases accurate restitution of disrupted articular surfaces has been followed by uncomplicated fracture healing, a highly favorable recovery of wrist function, and invariably complete resolution of concomitant neuropathy over a period ranging from several weeks to several months. Owing to the excellent healing capacity of the distal radius as well as an unparal-

---

*References 16, 42, 51, 66, 78, 87, 89, and 109.

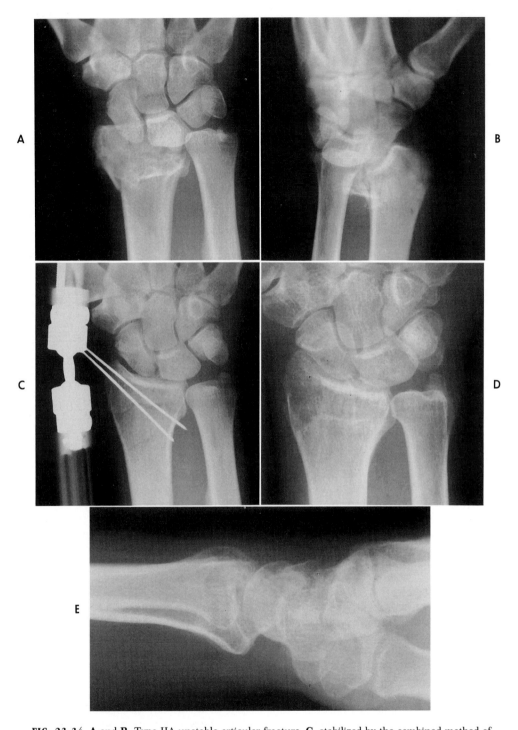

FIG. 23-34. **A** and **B,** Type IIA unstable articular fracture, **C,** stabilized by the combined method of external fixation and adjunctive internal fixation with K-wires. After successful closed reduction, the external fixator maintains radial length whereas the percutaneous K-wires secure articular congruity and radial tilt. **D** and **E,** Postoperatively an accurate restoration of the disrupted articular surfaces is demonstrated.

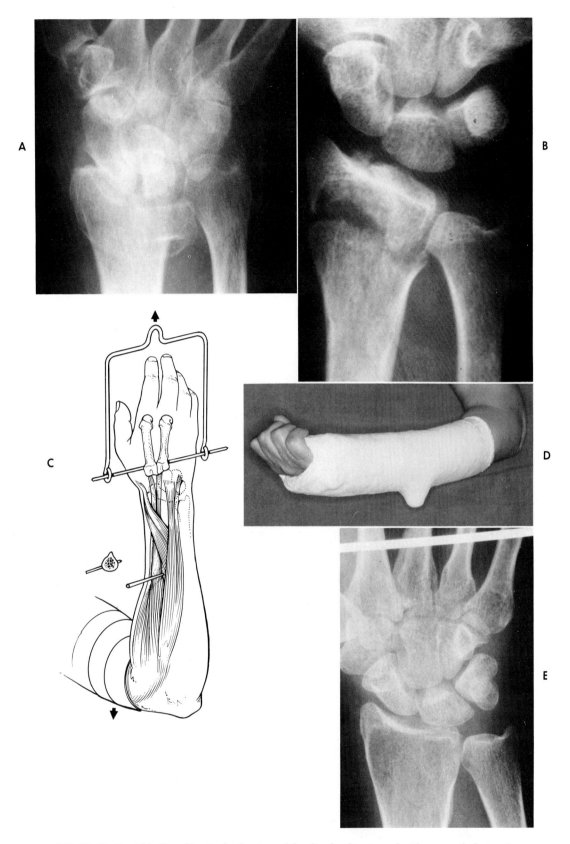

FIG. 23-35. Unstable Type II articular fracture of the distal radius treated with pins and plaster. **A,** Preoperative radiographs demonstrating severe disruption with collapse of the distal radius articular surfaces. **B,** Reduction is achieved and maintained by continuous skeletal traction. **C,** External transfixion pins are passed through the metacarpals and the radius. The radial pin must achieve bicortical purchase but avoid the critical soft tissues of the forearm. **D,** After accurate reduction, the pins are incorporated in a short arm cast that permits immediate active motion of the thumb, fingers, and elbow. **E,** Uncomplicated union with preservation of the articular surfaces is demonstrated 8 weeks after surgery.

leled rehabilitative process, many athletes have returned to competition as early as 3 months after surgery. For less comminuted Type IIA fractures and for unusual situations when an external fixator is neither applicable nor available, pins and plaster are a reliable secondary treatment alternative (Fig. 23-35).

In contrast to the Type IIA injury, restoration of articular congruity in the irreducible Type IIB fracture with dorsal displacement can be accomplished only by open treatment—usually comprising a limited dorsal exposure for articular reduction—and internal fixation with Kirschner wires, supplementary external fixation, and adjunctive iliac bone grafting (Fig. 23-36). The irreducible Type IIB fracture with volar displacement is the articular fracture most suitable for stabilization by plate and screw fixation (Fig. 23-15). In such cases plate fixation is accomplished through a carpal tunnel incision

extended across the ulnar aspect of the wrist, an approach similarly used for Type III and Type IV fractures. In cases with excessive comminution, when plating is impossible, Kirschner wires provide a satisfactory alternative method of fixation.[41]

Type III and Type IV injuries demonstrate more profound fracture instability that is apt to result from sports trauma. The Type III fracture is characterized by displacement of the medial complex as a unit, as well as displacement of an additional spike fragment from the comminuted radial metaphysis. Typically this bony spike projects anteriorly, contusing the median nerve and adjacent tendons. Although the medial fragments can be successfully managed by external fixation, the spike fragment is irreducible by closed methods and necessitates open reduction with internal fixation.

The Type IV fracture constitutes a severe disruption

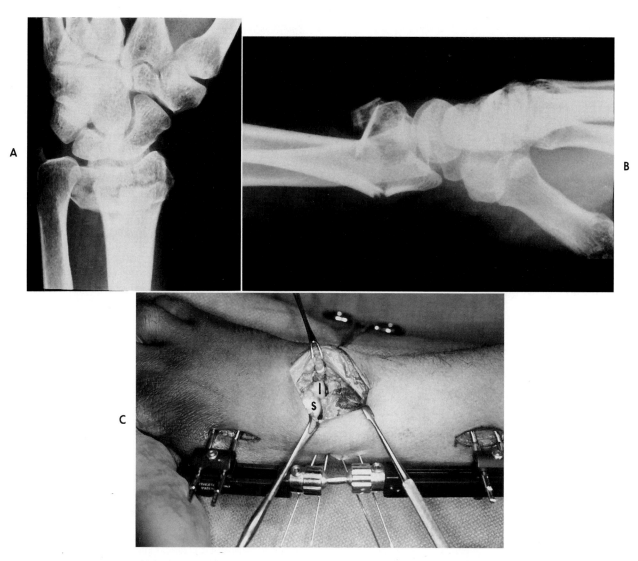

FIG. 23-36. A and **B,** Irreducible Type IIB die-punch fracture with severe radiocarpal and distal radioulnar joint disruption. **C,** Treatment comprised a small dorsal exposure for open reduction of the articular surfaces, K-wire internal fixation, supplementary external fixation, and adjunctive subchondral bone grafting. (S, Scaphoid, L, lunate).

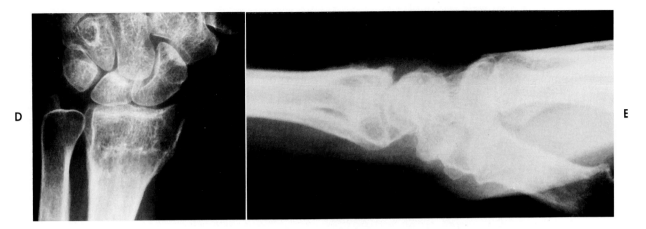

FIG. 23-36, cont'd. D and **E,** Postoperatively the radiographs demonstrate incorporation of the graft with restoration of biarticular congruity.

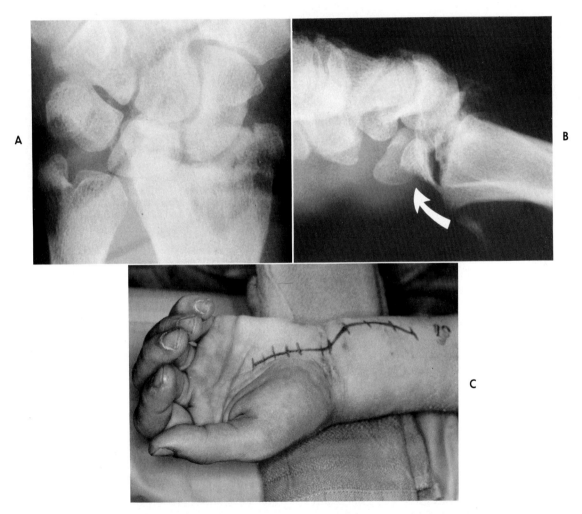

FIG. 23-37. Type IV distal radius articular fracture. **A,** Radiograph demonstrating severe biarticular disruption. **B,** Radiograph showing the palmar medial fragment *(arrow)* rotated 180 degrees. **C,** Open reduction is required for accurate restoration of the articular surfaces and is best achieved through an anterior approach that affords direct access to the displaced fragments, as well as any damaged soft tissues. *Continued.*

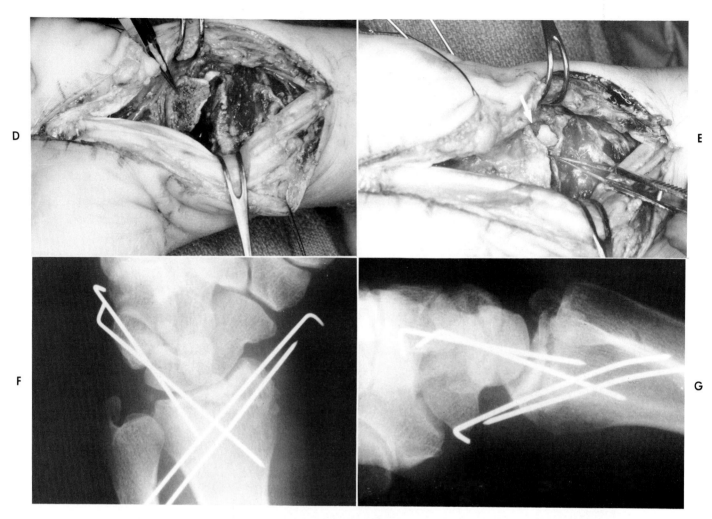

FIG. 23-37, cont'd. D, Widely displaced palmar medial fragment (at the tip of the forceps) is to be, **E,** derotated, reduced, and stabilized with wires to adjacent fragments for restitution of radiocarpal and radioulnar *(arrow)* congruity. **F** and **G,** Following secure stabilization with multiple wires, postoperative radiographs demonstrate an accurate restoration of the distal radius articulations. (From Isani A, Melone CP Jr: *Hand Clin* 4:349, 1988.)

of the distal radius articulations and is always associated with extensive periarticular damage. Characteristically the medial fragments are widely separated or rotated and cannot be accurately realigned by closed manipulation or traction. Open treatment is necessary for restoration of the articular surfaces and repair of concomitant soft-tissue or skeletal injuries (Fig. 23-37).

Inasmuch as the major fracture displacement of both Type III and Type IV injuries usually is volar and the soft-tissue injury occurs within the flexor compartment of the wrist, the volar approach extending from the carpal tunnel to the ulnar aspect of the wrist is the preferential means of surgical exposure. In cases with widely displaced radial styloid fragments, irreducible dorsal medial fragments, displaced scaphoid fractures, carpal dissociation, or extensor tendon injuries, extensile exposure requires a second incision over the dorsum of the wrist. Although the small, comminuted fracture fragments

generally are not suitable for techniques of rigid fixation, secure stabilization can be achieved with multiple Kirschner wires. In those instances with severe comminution, supplementary external fixation and primary bone grafting augment fracture stability and enhance security against collapse of the articular surfaces. Experience bears out that, even for these more serious articular fractures, precise reduction and stabilization of every fracture component in conjunction with meticulous repair of all concomitant injuries are consistently rewarded by a favorable recovery.[67]

For the Type V explosion injury, preparatory stabilization with an external fixator often supplemented with percutaneous Kirschner wires provides a sturdy framework for critical revascularization or resurfacing procedures and serves to maintain skeletal alignment before definitive articular reconstruction.

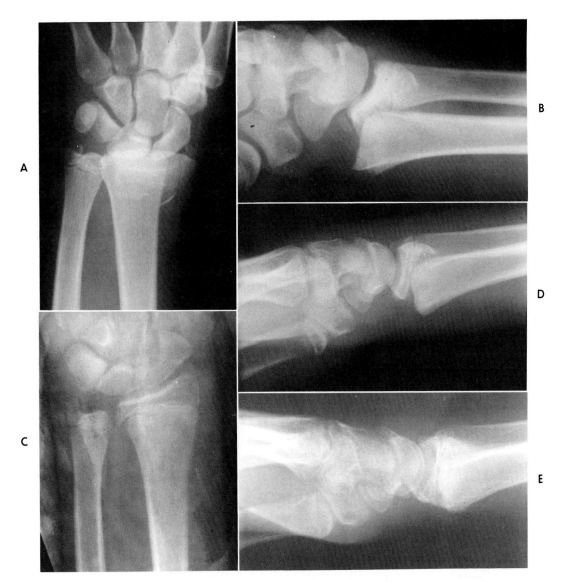

FIG. 23-38. A and **B,** Type II epiphyseal fracture of a 16-year-old football running back. **C,** Closed reduction successfully restores radial length and the normal epiphyseal configuration as viewed on the posteroanterior radiograph. **D,** Despite persistent sagittal displacement, this is a satisfactory reduction that does not require additional and potentially harmful manipulation. **E,** Over several months the remodeling process results in uncomplicated union with restitution of normal radial contours. (From Melone CP Jr, Grad JB: Fractures of the distal ends of the radius and ulna. In Pettrone FA, (ed): *American Academy of Orthopaedic Surgeons symposium on upper extremity injuries in athletes,* St Louis, 1986, Mosby.)

Criteria for accurate articular reduction

Dorsally displaced fractures
- <2 mm articular offset or gapping
- <10 degrees dorsal tilting
- <5 mm radial shortening

Volarly displaced fractures
- <2 mm articular offset
- 0 to 14 degrees volar tilt
- Restoration of colinear carpus
- <5 mm radial shortening

Extraarticular Fractures

Metaphyseal fractures. In contrast to articular fractures, extraarticular injuries principally result from tension forces and tend to be stable after closed reduction and cast immobilization. Facilitated by a regional anesthetic, manipulation of Colles-type fractures is accomplished by axial traction followed by palmar flexion, ulnar deviation, and pronation of the wrist. Smith-type fractures are reduced by traction and supination. Clearly, a stable reduction hinges on the restoration of an intact cortical buttress, either posterior or anterior. If both radial cortices are extensively comminuted, the injury is inherently un-

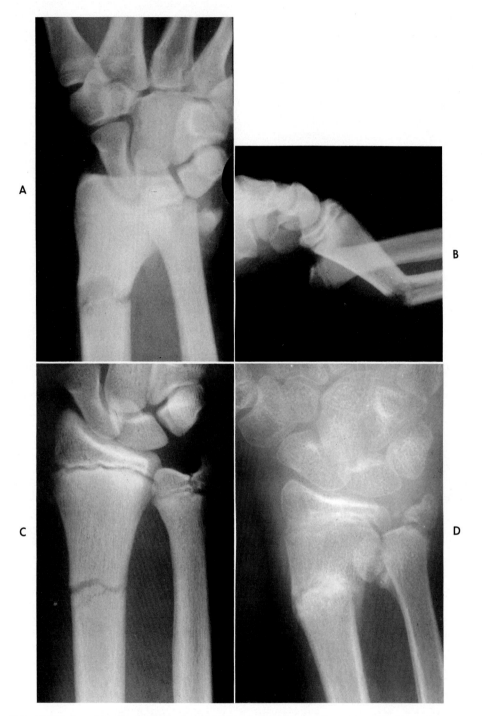

FIG. 23-39. A and **B,** Markedly displaced Galeazzi-equivalent fracture with a Type III epiphyseal injury of the distal ulna incurred by an adolescent hockey player. **C,** Closed reduction results in an anatomic reduction. Radiographic surveillance, however, is mandatory to ensure stability because even minimal epiphyseal displacement requires prompt open reduction with internal fixation. **D,** Untreated Galeazzi-equivalent fracture with a Type IV distal ulna epiphyseal injury resulting in malunion and ultimately growth disturbance with deformity. For this injury, optimal treatment comprises prompt open reduction with internal fixation of the disrupted epiphysis. (From Melone CP Jr, Grad JB: Fractures of the distal ends of the radius and ulna. In Pettrone FA (ed): *American Academy of Orthopaedic Surgeons symposium on upper extremity injuries in athletes,* St Louis, 1986, Mosby.)

stable, and without supplementary fixation loss of reduction is inevitable. In such cases techniques of external fixation and internal fixation, identical to those used for unstable articular fractures, are needed to maintain an accurate reduction.

Epiphyseal fractures. Prevalent among adolescent athletes are injuries of the distal radial epiphysis. An excessive tension force applied to the extended wrist characteristically causes a Type II epiphyseal fracture, or separation. The plane of disruption traverses the growth plate through the zone of cell hypertrophy, and an intact epiphysis along with an attached small metaphyseal fragment (the Thurston-Holland sign) separates from the radial shaft (Fig. 23-38).[85] Because the critical germinal layer of the physis is essentially undisturbed, the prognosis for normal growth after a prompt, accurate reduction is excellent.

Successful reduction can be consistently achieved by gentle closed manipulation and cast immobilization employing techniques similar to those used for adult extraarticular injuries. The fundamental criteria for successful reduction are restoration of normal radial length and preservation of normal configurations of the distal radial epiphysis and radioulnar joint as viewed on the PA radiographs. In the assessment of normal radial length and contour, inspection of comparable radiographs of the uninjured wrist is essential to avoid misinterpretation caused by variations in anatomy or differences in radiographic techniques. In cases with fulfillment of these criteria, the reduction, regardless of persistent sagittal displacement as viewed on the lateral radiographs, should be recognized as satisfactory. One must remember that epiphyseal injuries can occur only in an immature skeleton that always has the potential for considerable remodeling after fracture. As long as radial length is accurately restored, type II fractures demonstrating as much as 50% displacement on the lateral radiograph will consistently remodel to a normal-appearing epiphysis (Fig. 23-38, *D* and *E*). Cast immobilization usually can be discontinued after 4 weeks, but the vulnerable young athlete should not compete in contact sports until fracture remodeling and rehabilitation are complete, about 3 or 4 months.

Distal Ulna Fractures

Fractures of the ulnar styloid, head, or epiphysis seldom occur as isolated events. In the majority of cases they constitute a component of injury that includes a major fracture of the adjacent radius. As a general rule, successful treatment of the fractured radius results in accurate reduction and uncomplicated healing of the ulnar component with a favorable recovery of radioulnar and ulnocarpal joint function. A frequent example of this distinctive fracture pattern is the avulsion fracture of the ulnar styloid that occurs with nearly 90% of unstable distal radius fractures. In such cases the tip of the styloid is avulsed as the distal radius is displaced. Inasmuch as the major attachment of the triangular fibrocartilage complex at the base of the styloid remains intact, neither the styloid fragment nor its frequent failure to unite

appreciably affects recovery, provided the more serious radius fracture is accurately reduced and stabilized.

Less frequently, avulsion of the entire styloid with the attached triangular fibrocartilage occurs, usually in conjunction with either distal third (Galeazzi) or proximal (Essex-Lopresti) fractures of the radius. In cases with clinical and radiographic evidence of distal ulna instability, optimal management must include anatomic reduction and internal fixation of the displaced styloid for restoration of triangular fibrocartilage integrity and radioulnar stability. Secure fixation of the styloid fragment is achieved with Kirschner, tension band, or cerclage wires. For the chronically unstable injury with an ununited, deformed ulnar styloid, excision of the bony fragment and direct suture of the triangular fibrocartilage through drill holes into the distal ulna remnant are the best means of restoring radioulnar stability.

Epiphyseal injuries of the distal ulna, unlike those of the distal radius, are prone to result in Type III or IV fractures (Fig. 23-39). These serious growth plate disruptions invariably occur in association with displaced distal third fractures of the radius; hence the injuries have been termed Galeazzi-equivalent lesions.[69,80] The radial component of the lesion is clearly visualized on routine radiographic projections and usually can be managed by closed manipulation. In contrast, the magnitude of injury to the ulnar component is less apparent but may preclude closed methods of treatment. If careful scrutiny of postreduction radiographs reveals residual epiphyseal displacement, prompt and precise open reduction and internal fixation with fine Kirschner wires are essential to prevent a disabling deformity of the ulna.

SUMMARY

Certain exceptions notwithstanding, the primary prerequisites for optimal management of the athlete's fractured wrist are prompt diagnosis, anatomic and stable reduction, effective immobilization until healing is thorough, and comprehensive rehabilitation of the injured parts. Fulfillment of these fundamental criteria consistently leads to a highly favorable outcome with minimal risk of reinjury. In contrast, a compromise of these principles, especially for the sake of a speedy return to sports, invariably results in suboptimal recovery and, not infrequently, a permanent loss of skills.

The exceptions to the cardinal rule that successful treatment of wrist fractures requires precise restoration of anatomic relationships are specific: displaced hamate hook fractures, displaced trapezial ridge fractures, and comminuted pisiform fractures. In such instances, successful union essentially is precluded, and early excision

---

Fractures treated by early excision

- Displaced hook of hamate
- Displaced trapezial ridge
- Comminuted pisiform

of the displaced fragments is the logical means of facilitating an uncomplicated recovery.

For the more complex fractures requiring stabilization, continual refinements in methods of fixation are considerably diminishing fracture morbidity. The availability of small screws that provide rigid fixation of the carpus is, with increasing consistency, promoting accelerated union and rapid rehabilitation. Well-conceived combinations of low-profile, mechanically efficient external fixators and precisely employed Kirschner wires achieve highly secure fracture stability for the distal radius that similarly enhances recovery with a minimum of complications. Improvements in both design and application of internal and external fixation techniques undoubtedly constitute a major advance in the management of wrist fractures among athletes.

For some athletes the return to competition can be safely expedited by the use of custom-fit protective gloves, splints, or casts. For most, however, the treatment regimen usually entails a minimum of 3 or 4 months. Although the healing and rehabilitation process is often lengthy and may seem costly, particularly in terms of time lost from competition, seldom do athletes regret the investment once they return to their highly skillful activities unencumbered by wrist impairment. Never does the sports medicine physician regret compliance with the principles of optimal care.

REFERENCES

1. Adams BD, Frykman GK, Taleisnik J: Treatment of scaphoid nonunion with casting and pulsed electromagnetic field: a study continuation, *J Hand Surg* 17A:910, 1992.
2. Adams BD et al: Technical factors related to Herbert screw fixation, *J Hand Surg* 13A:893, 1988.
3. Amadio PC et al: Scaphoid malunion, *J Hand Surg* 14A:679, 1989.
4. Aro HT, Koivunen T: Minor axial shortening of the radius affects outcome of Colles' fracture treatment, *J Hand Surg* 16A:392, 1991.
5. Axelrod TS, McMurtry RY: Open reduction and internal fixation of comminuted, intraarticular fractures of the distal radius, *J Hand Surg* 15A:1, 1990.
6. Bassett FH III, Malone T, Gilchrist RA: A protective splint of silicone rubber, *Am J Sports Med* 7:358, 1979.
7. Beckenbaugh RD et al: The natural history of Kienböck's disease and consideration of lunate fractures, *Clin Orthop* 149:98, 1980.
8. Bergfeld JA et al: Soft playing splint for protection of significant hand and wrist injuries in sports, *Am J Sports Med* 10:293, 1982.
9. Bishop AT, Beckenbaugh RD: Fracture of the hamate hook, *J Hand Surg* 13A:135, 1988.
10. Botte MJ et al: Internal vascularity of the scaphoid in cadavers after insertion of the Herbert screw, *J Hand Surg* 13A:216, 1988.
11. Bryan RS, Dobyns JH: Fractures of the carpal bones other than lunate and navicular, *Clin Orthop* 149:107, 1980.
12. Bunker TD, McNamee PD, Scott TD: The Herbert screw for scaphoid fractures: a multicentre study, *J Bone Joint Surg* 69B:631, 1987.
13. Carter PR, Eaton RG, Littler JW: Ununited fractures of the hook of hamate, *J Bone Joint Surg* 59A:583, 1977.
14. Carter PR et al: The scaphoid allograft: a new operation for treatment of the very proximal scaphoid nonunion or for the necrotic, fragmented scaphoid proximal pole, *J Hand Surg* 14A:1, 1989.
15. Clancey G: Percutaneous Kirschner wire fixation of Colles' fractures, *J Bone Joint Surg* 66A:1008, 1984.
16. Cooney WP III: External fixation of distal radius fractures, *Clin Orthop* 180:44, 1983.
17. Cooney WP, Dobyns JH, Linscheid RL: Complications of Colles' fractures, *J Bone Joint Surg* 62A:613, 1980.
18. Cooney WP, Dobyns JH, Linscheid RL: Fractures of the scaphoid: a rational approach to management, *Clin Orthop* 149:90, 1980.
19. Cooney WP, Dobyns JH, Linscheid RL: Non-union of the scaphoid: analysis of the results from bone grafting, *J Hand Surg* 5:343, 1980.
20. Cooney WP et al: Scaphoid nonunion: role of anterior interpositional bone grafts, *J Hand Surg* 13A:635, 1988.
21. Cordrey LJ, Ferrer-Torells M: Management of fractures of the greater multangular, *J Bone Joint Surg* 42A:1111, 1960.
22. DeMaagd RL, Engber WD: Retrograde Herbert screw fixation for treatment of proximal pole scaphoid nonunions, *J Hand Surg* 14A:996, 1989.
23. DePalma AF: Comminuted fractures of the distal end of the radius treated by ulnar pinning, *J Bone Joint Surg* 34A:651, 1952.
24. Eddeland A et al: Fractures of the scaphoid, *Scand J Plast Reconstr Surg* 9:234, 1975.
25. Egawa M, Asai T: Fractures of the hook of the hamate: report of six cases and suitability of computerized tomography, *J Hand Surg* 8:393, 1983.
26. Ellis J: Smith and Barton's fractures: a method of treatment, *J Bone Joint Surg* 47B:724, 1965.
27. Failla JM: Hook of hamate vascularity: vulnerability to osteonecrosis and nonunion, *J Hand Surg* 18A:1075, 1993.
28. Fernandez DL: A technique for anterior wedge-shaped grafts for scaphoid nonunions with carpal instability, *J Hand Surg* 9A:733, 1984.
29. Fernandez DL: Anterior bone grafting and conventional lag screw fixation to treat scaphoid nonunions, *J Hand Surg* 15A:140, 1990.
30. Fernandez DL, Geissler WB: Treatment of displaced articular fractures of the radius, *J Hand Surg* 16A:375, 1991.
31. Fernandez DL, Ghillani R: External fixation of complex carpal dislocations: a preliminary report, *J Hand Surg* 12A:335, 1987.
32. Fisk GR: The wrist, *J Bone Joint Surg* 68B:396, 1984.
33. Ford DJ et al: The Herbert screw for fractures of the scaphoid, *J Bone Joint Surg* 69B:124, 1987.
34. Freeland AE, Finley MD: Displaced vertical fracture of the trapezium treated with a small cancellous lag screw, *J Hand Surg* 9A:843, 1984.
35. Frykman GK et al: Treatment of nonunited scaphoid fractures by pulsed electromagnetic field and cast, *J Hand Surg* 11A:344, 1986.
36. Frykman GK et al: Comparison of eleven external fixators for treatment of unstable wrist fractures, *J Hand Surg* 14A:247, 1989.
37. Gasser H: Delayed union and pseudarthrosis of the carpal navicular: treatment by compression-screw osteosynthesis: a preliminary report on twenty fractures, *J Bone Joint Surg* 47A:249, 1965.
38. Gelberman RH, Menon J: The vascularity of the scaphoid bone, *J Hand Surg* 5:508, 1980.
39. Gelberman RH et al: The vascularity of the lunate bone and Kienböck's disease, *J Hand Surg* 5:272, 1980.
40. Gellman H et al: Comparison of short and long thumb-spica casts for nondisplaced fractures of the carpal scaphoid, *J Bone Joint Surg* 71A:354, 1989.
41. Greatting M, Bishop A: In intrafocal (Kapandji) pinning of unstable fractures of the distal radius, *Orthop Clin North Am* 24:301, 1993.
42. Green DP: Pins and plaster treatment of comminuted fractures of the distal end of the radius, *J Bone Joint Surg* 57A:304, 1975.
43. Green DP: The effect of avascular necrosis on Russe bone grafting for scaphoid nonunion, *J Hand Surg* 10A:597, 1985.
44. Green DP, O'Brien ET: Open reduction of carpal dislocations: indications and operative techniques, *J Hand Surg* 3:250, 1978.

45. Hastings H III, Leibovic SJ: Indications and techniques of open reduction–internal fixation of distal radius fractures, *Orthop Clin North Am* 24:309, 1993.

46. Herbert TJ: Use of Herbert bone screw in surgery of the wrist, *Clin Orthop* 202:79, 1986.

47. Herbert TJ, Fisher WE: Management of the fractured scaphoid using a new bone screw, *J Bone Joint Surg* 66B:114, 1984.

48. Johnson RP: The acutely injured wrist and its residuals, *Clin Orthop* 149:33, 1980.

49. Kapandji A: Bone fixation by double percutaneous pinning: Functional treatment of non-articular fractures of the lower end of the radius, *Ann Chir Main* 30:903, 1976.

50. Kazuki K, Kusunoki M, Shimazu A: Pressure distribution in the radiocarpal joint measured with a densitometer designed for pressure-sensitive film, *J Hand Surg* 16A:401, 1991.

51. Knirk JL, Jupiter JB: Intra-articular fractures of the distal end of the radius in young adults, *J Bone Joint Surg* 68A:647, 1986.

52. Langhoff O, Andersen JL: Consequences of late immobilization of scaphoid fractures, *J Hand Surg* 13B:77, 1988.

53. Lee MLH: Intraosseous arterial pattern of the carpal lunate bone and its relationship to avascular necrosis, *Acta Orthop Scand* 33:43, 1963.

54. Leung KS et al: Ligamentotaxis and bone grafting for comminuted fractures of the distal radius, *J Bone Joint Surg* 71B:838, 1989.

55. Levy M et al: Chip fractures of the os triquetrum, *J Bone Joint Surg* 61B:355, 1979.

56. Lidström A: Fractures of the distal end of the radius: a clinical and statistical study of end results, *Acta Orthop Scand (Suppl)* 41:1, 1959.

57. Linscheid RL et al: Traumatic instability of the wrist: diagnosis, classification and pathomechanics, *J Bone Joint Surg* 54A:1612, 1972.

58. Mack GR et al: The natural history of scaphoid non-union, *J Bone Joint Surg* 66A:504, 1984.

59. Maudsley RH, Chen SC: Screw fixation in the management of the fractured carpal scaphoid, *J Bone Joint Surg* 54B:432, 1972.

60. Mayfield JK, Johnson RP, Kilcoyne RF: Carpal dislocations: pathomechanics and progressive periulnar instability, *J Hand Surg* 5:226, 1980.

61. McClain EJ, Boyes JH: Missed fractures of the greater multangular, *J Bone Joint Surg* 48A:1525, 1966.

62. McCue FC, Miller GA: Soft-tissue injuries to the hand. In Pettrone FA (ed): *Symposium on upper extremity injuries in athletes,* St Louis, 1986, Mosby.

63. McCue FC et al: Hand and wrist injuries in the athlete, *Am J Sports Med* 7:275, 1979.

64. McLaughlin HL, Parkes JC: Fracture of the carpal navicular (scaphoid) bone: gradations in therapy based upon pathology, *J Trauma* 9:311, 1969.

65. Melone CP Jr: Scaphoid fractures: concepts of management, *Clin Plast Surg* 8:83, 1981.

66. Melone CP Jr: Articular fractures of the distal radius, *Orthop Clin North Am* 15:217, 1984.

67. Melone CP Jr: Open treatment for displaced articular fractures of the distal radius, *Clin Orthop* 202:103, 1986.

68. Melone CP Jr: Distal radius fractures: patterns of articular fragmentation, *Orthop Clin North Am* 24:239, 1993.

69. Mikić ZK: Galeazzi fracture-dislocations, *J Bone Joint Surg* 57A:1071, 1975.

70. Missakian ML et al: Open reduction and internal fixation for distal radius fractures, *J Hand Surg* 17A:745, 1992.

71. Moneim MS, Hofammann KE III, Omer GE: Transscaphoid perilunate fracture-dislocation: result of open reduction and pin fixation, *Clin Orthop* 190:227, 1984.

72. Palmer AK: Trapezial ridge fractures, *J Hand Surg* 6:561, 1981.

73. Palmer AK, Werner FW: The triangular fibrocartilage complex of the wrist: anatomy and function, *J Hand Surg* 6:153, 1981.

74. Panagis JS et al: The arterial anatomy of human carpus. II. The intraosseous vascularity, *J Hand Surg* 8:375, 1983.

75. Perlik PC, Guilford WB: Magnetic resonance imaging to assess vascularity of scaphoid nonunions, *J Hand Surg* 16A:479, 1991.

76. Rand JA, Linscheid RL, Dobyns JH: Capitate fractures: a long-term follow-up, *Clin Orthop* 165:209, 1982.

77. Rankin G et al: A biomechanical evaluation of a cannulated compressive screw for use in fractures of the scaphoid, *J Hand Surg* 16A:1002, 1991.

78. Raskin KB, Melone CP Jr: Unstable articular fractures of the distal radius: comparative techniques of ligamentotaxis, *Orthop Clin North Am* 24:275, 1993.

79. Rayhack J: The history and evolution of percutaneous pinning of displaced distal radius fractures, *Orthop Clin North Am* 24:287, 1993.

80. Reckling FW: Unstable fracture-dislocation of the forearm (Monteggia and Galeazzi lesions), *J Bone Joint Surg* 64A:857, 1982.

81. Richards R, Paitich CB, Bell RS: Internal fixation of a capitate fracture with Herbert screws, *J Hand Surg* 15A:885, 1990.

82. Riester JN et al: A review of scaphoid fracture healing in competitive athletes, *Am J Sports Med* 13:159, 1985.

83. Ruby LK, Stinson J, Belsky MR: The natural history of scaphoid non-union: a review of fifty-five cases, *J Bone Joint Surg* 67A:428, 1985.

84. Russe O: Fracture of the carpal navicular: diagnosis, nonoperative treatment, and operative treatment, *J Bone Joint Surg* 42A:759, 1960.

85. Salter RB, Harris WR: Injuries involving the epiphyseal plate, *J Bone Joint Surg* 45A:587, 1963.

86. Sanders WE: Evaluation of the humpback scaphoid by computed tomography in the longitudinal axial plane of the scaphoid, *J Hand Surg* 13A:182, 1988.

87. Scheck M: Long-term follow-up of treatment of comminuted fractures of the distal end of the radius by transfixation with Kirchner wires and cast, *J Bone Joint Surg* 44A:337, 1962.

88. Seitz WH, Froimson AI, Leb RB: Reduction of treatment-related complications in the external fixation of complex distal radius fractures, *Orthop Rev* 20:169, 1991.

89. Seitz WH et al: Augmented external fixation of unstable distal radius fractures, *J Hand Surg* 16A:1010, 1991.

90. Shaw JA: A biomechanical comparison of scaphoid screws, *J Hand Surg* 12A:347, 1987.

91. Short WH et al: A biomechanical study of distal radial fractures, *J Hand Surg* 12A:529, 1987.

92. Smith P III et al: Excision of the hook of the hamate: a retrospective survey and review of the literature, *J Hand Surg* 13A:612, 1988.

93. Stark HH et al: Treatment of ununited fractures of the scaphoid by iliac bone grafts and Kirschner-wire fixation, *J Bone Joint Surg* 70A:982, 1988.

94. Stark HH et al: Fracture of the hook of the hamate, *J Bone Joint Surg* 71A:1202, 1989.

95. Stein A, Katz S: Stabilization of comminuted fractures of the distal inch of the radius: percutaneous pinning, *Clin Orthop* 108:174, 1975.

96. Stewart MJ, Cross H: The management of injuries of the carpal lunate with a review of sixty cases, *J Bone Joint Surg* 50A:1489, 1968.

97. Taleisnik J, Kelly PJ: The extraosseous and intraosseous blood supply of the scaphoid bone, *J Bone Joint Surg* 48A:1125, 1966.

98. Taleisnik J, Watson HK: Midcarpal instability caused by malunited fractures of the distal radius, *J Hand Surg* 9A:350, 1984.

99. Teisen H, Hjarbaek J: Classification of fresh fractures of the lunate, *J Hand Surg* 13B:458, 1988.

100. Thomas FB: Reduction of Smith's fracture, *J Bone Joint Surg* 39B:463, 1957.

101. Trumble TE: Avascular necrosis after scaphoid fracture: a correlation of magnetic resonance imaging and histology, *J Hand Surg* 15A:557, 1990.

102. Vance RM, Gelberman RH, Evans EF: Scaphocapitate fractures: patterns of dislocations, mechanisms of injury and preliminary results of treatment, *J Bone Joint Surg* 62A:271, 1980.

103. VanderGrend R et al: Intraosseous blood supply of the capitate and its correlation with aseptic necrosis, *J Hand Surg* 9A:677, 1984.

104. Vasilas A, Grieco RV, Bartone NF: Roentgen aspects of injuries to the pisiform bone and pisotriquetral joint, *J Bone Joint Surg* 42A:1317, 1960.

105. Verdan C, Narakas A: Fractures and pseudarthrosis of the scaphoid, *Surg Clin North Am* 48A:1083, 1968.

106. Warren-Smith CD, Barton NJ: Non-union of the scaphoid: Russe graft vs Herbert screw, *J Hand Surg* 13B:83, 1988.

107. Watson HK, Rogers WD: Nonunion of the hook of the hamate: an argument for bone grafting the nonunion, *J Hand Surg* 14A:486, 1989.

108. Weber ER: Biomechanical implications of scaphoid waist fractures, *Clin Orthop* 149:83, 1980.

109. Weber SC, Szabo RM: Severely comminuted distal radial fracture as an unsolved problem: complications associated with external fixation and pins and plaster techniques, *J Hand Surg* 11A:157, 1986.

110. Whalen JL, Bishop AT, Linscheid RL: Nonoperative treatment of acute hamate hook fractures, *J Hand Surg* 17A:507, 1992.

111. Zemel NP et al: Treatment of selected patients with an ununited fracture of the proximal part of the scaphoid by excision of the fragment and insertion of a carved silicone-rubber spacer, *J Bone Joint Surg* 66A:510, 1984.

CHAPTER 24 Ligamentous Injuries of the Wrist in Athletes

John F. Jennings
Clayton A. Peimer

The functional role of the hand and wrist in sports makes them particularly vulnerable to injuries sustained as a result of direct trauma or constant repetitive activity. Diagnosis and treatment are especially difficult because of the complexity of the multiple integrated articulations of the radius, ulna, and carpal bones.[32] Success demands specific diagnosis-related treatment to achieve maximum function, avoid unnecessary delays, and prevent further injury.[56]

The historically common diagnosis of a wrist ligament "sprain" after an injury is often spurious. Such a diagnosis can actually be dangerous because it ignores possible structural derangement and, as a consequence, chronic instability may develop secondary to an undiagnosed ligament injury.[58] Every effort should be made to diagnose the wrist injury accurately so that proper treatment can be instituted to preserve the athlete's skills at an optimal level.[26,110] The surgeon who would treat such problems needs a thorough understanding of wrist anatomy and biomechanics as well as diagnostic and treatment modalities.

This chapter describes the anatomy of the wrist with respect to the bony structures and ligaments, as well as their kinematics. The mechanisms and patterns of car-

pal instabilities are detailed, and the diagnostic and treatment protocols for specific injuries are presented.

ANATOMY
Osseous Anatomy

There are two rows of carpal bones. Beginning radially, the proximal row consists of the scaphoid, lunate, triquetrum, and pisiform bones, although the last is really a sesamoid of insertion for flexor carpi ulnaris. The distal row includes trapezium, trapezoid, capitate, and hamate bones. Structurally, the wrist positions the hand and transmits forces between the hand and forearm.[26] Wrist function requires a coordinated interaction of bones independently and as groups, depending on their osseous anatomy and soft-tissue attachments.

All the muscles that initiate wrist motion insert at a site distal to the wrist, making the carpus an intercalated segment, as described by Landsmeer.[67] In fact, because the distal carpal row moves in syndesmotic union with the hand, it is really just the proximal row that is an intercalated segment.[134]

Scaphoid

The scaphoid, the only bone that traverses the midcarpus, acts as a link between the proximal and distal carpal rows. Gilford, Bolton, and Lambrinudi[43] in 1943 and later Linscheid et al[74] noted that the two carpal rows should be unstable in compression either by extrinsic forces or by (intrinsic) muscle loads, unless they are secured by a mechanical stop, a function supplied by the bridging effect of the scaphoid.[60,61,75,114]

Lunate

The lunate bone is wedge shaped in sagittal section. The volar (palmar) pole is longer and wider than the dorsal pole.[60,61] This configuration makes the lunate tend toward dorsiflexion (i.e., the distal surface points dorsally). The lunate articulates proximally with the radius and distally with the capitate, serving to transmit forces between them.

Triquetrum and Hamate

The triquetrum articulates with the lunate radially and the hamate distally. The surface facing the hamate has an inferior, shallow, paddle-shaped facet. The hamate has a helicoidal medial articular facet.[120] In ulnar deviation, therefore, the triquetrum descends beneath the hamate as if going down a spiral staircase and moves distally toward the fifth metacarpal, allowing the ulna to move closer to the hand. In radial deviation the reverse occurs; the triquetrum ascends this inclined plane and moves proximally into the space between the ulna and the fifth metacarpal.

Trapezium, Trapezoid, and Capitate

These three bones are syndesmotic. They, as well as the hamate, support the metacarpals at the mobile (first, fourth, and fifth) and immobile (second and third) carpometacarpal joints, and they transmit forces to the forearm via the bones of the proximal carpal row.

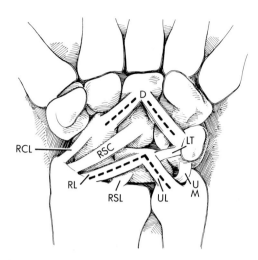

FIG. 24-1. Volar wrist ligaments. *RCL,* Radial collateral ligament; *RSC,* radioscaphocapitate ligament; *RL,* radiolunate ligament; *RSL,* radioscapholunate ligament; *LT,* lunotriquetral ligament; *UL,* ulnolunate ligament; *UM,* ulnocarpal meniscus homologue; *D,* deltoid or V ligament.

Ligamentous Anatomy

The volar ligaments of the wrist are the major stabilizers. Taleisnik[118] has divided them into two major groups: extrinsic ligaments, which connect the carpus and radius or metacarpals, and the intrinsic ligaments, which originate and insert entirely on the carpal bones (Fig. 24-1).

Volar wrist ligaments

Extrinsic ligaments
- Carpus to radius
- Carpus to metacarpals

Intrinsic ligaments
- Intercarpal

Volar Radiocarpal Ligaments

There are two layers of volar radiocarpal ligaments, one superficial and one deep.[79,118] The superficial fibers assume an inverted V-shape with apex at the capitate, and from radial to ulnar these fibers consist of the radioscaphocapitate, radiolunate, and radioscapholunate ligaments. Recent evidence confirms that the radioscapholunate ligament may actually be the neurovascular supply to the scapholunate interosseous ligament and not as important a palmar stabilizer as previously thought.[12] The radial collateral ligament is the most lateral of the volar radiocarpal ligaments, and because it is actually more volar than lateral, it probably does not truly function as a collateral ligament. In lower primates the ulna styloid articulates with the triquetrum. In humans a cartilaginous structure, the **ulnocarpal meniscus homolog,** is interposed between the ulna and triquetrum; there is no direct ligamentous connection between the ulna and the carpus.[70,118] This cartilage meniscus is sep-

arate from the **triangular fibrocartilaginous complex** (TFCC), although both attach to the dorsoulnar corner of the radius. The TFCC is connected to the carpus by the ulnolunate ligament, which secures the dorsoulnar radius to the volar carpus. The volar and radial corner of the radius is connected to the carpus by the deep (volar) radiocarpal ligaments. Therefore the carpus can be seen as suspended from the radius; the head of the ulna is not really part of the wrist joint itself.[43,99,118,128] The ulnar collateral ligament represents a thickening of joint capsule on the ulnar side rather than a true ligament.[60]

Volar radiocarpal ligaments

- Radioscaphocapitate
- Radiolunate
- Radioscapholunate
- Radial collateral

Intrinsic Ligaments

The intrinsic ligaments of the wrist originate and insert on the carpal bones. These volar ligaments, which are thicker and stronger than the dorsal ligaments, are further divided into short, intermediate, and long ligaments.

The **short intrinsic ligaments,**[118] which include the trapeziotrapezoidal, the trapeziocapitate, and the capitohamate, bind together the four bones of the distal row into a single, functional whole.

Intrinsic wrist ligaments

Short
- Trapeziotrapezoidal
- Trapeziocapitate
- Capitohamate

Intermediate
- Scaphotrapezium
- Scapholunate
- Lunotriquetral

Long
- Deltoid

The **intermediate intrinsic ligaments**[57,118] connect the trapezium to the scaphoid and then to the bones of the proximal carpal row. These include the scaphotrapezium, the scapholunate, and the lunotriquetral ligaments. The triquetrum is more firmly attached to the lunate than the scaphoid, thereby causing the lunate to dorsiflex when it descends the hamate spiral and volar flex as it ascends.

Of the two **long intrinsic ligaments**[79,118,120] the volar (which is more important) has been referred to as the "deltoid," "radiate," "arcuate," and "V" ligament. The volar ligament stabilizes the capitate and may fan out proximally (from the capitate) to the scaphoid, lunate, and triquetrum. Often the central point of this deltoid fan ligament is absent, and there are attachments only to the scaphoid and triquetrum, forming an inverted V with the distal lunate in the middle of the opening.

Dorsal Radiocarpal Ligament

The dorsal radiocarpal ligament, or radiolunate triquetrum ligament, originates on the dorsal rim of the radius and inserts on the scaphoid, lunate, and triquetrum.[120] Further support is provided by the extensor tendon compartments.

Dorsal Intercarpal Ligament

The dorsal intercarpal ligament originates from the triquetrum and inserts dorsally into the scaphoid and trapezium.[120]

Summary

In summary the major ligaments of the wrist are volar and intracapsular and cannot be readily visualized by the surgeon.[48,70,79] These volar ligaments are arranged in a double V, with the capitate at the apex of the broad V and the lunate at the apex of the smaller V. Between these there may be an area of potential weakness, the **space of Poirier,** which is not present in persons with deltoid or radiate ligaments connecting the capitate to the lunate. Navarro[91,92] and Taleisnik[120] believed that this lunocapitate ligament "defect" might explain carpal subluxation. In individuals with systemic articular laxity or hypermobility syndromes, patterns of carpal instability can be produced as a consequence of volar or dorsal stress in the normal wrist.[62,116,120]

KINEMATICS

The kinematics of the normal wrist have been studied and reported by many investigators.* The wrist is functionally more complex than might be inferred by the fact that it is characterized by two (transverse) rows of carpal bones. There are different perspectives on functional anatomy, and the clinician needs to understand them. The traditional concept was simply that the carpus was made up of two rows of carpal bones traversed by the scaphoid. Gilford, Bolton, and Lambrinudi[43] noted that this "link joint" would be unstable in compression were it not for the scaphoid's bridging across the midcarpus.

In 1935 Navarro[91,92] proposed his theory of the columnar carpus, noting that the wrist is not made of transverse articulations but of three separate longitudinal columns (Fig. 24-2, *A*). He postulated that there is a **central flexion-extension column** composed of the lunate, capitate, and hamate; a **lateral mobile column** constituted by the scaphoid, trapezoid, and trapezium; and a **medial rotatory column** made up of the triquetrum (and pisiform). Navarro[92] stressed the fundamental role of the medial column in hand rotation. Taleisnik[118] modified this theory by suggesting that the central column should be expanded to include the lunate *and* all the bones of the distal carpal row (since they are intimately connected by the short intrinsic ligaments and move as one unit) (Fig. 24-2, *B*). He eliminated the pisi-

---

*References 6, 19, 29, 33, 75, 81, 111, 128, 129, 136, and 138.

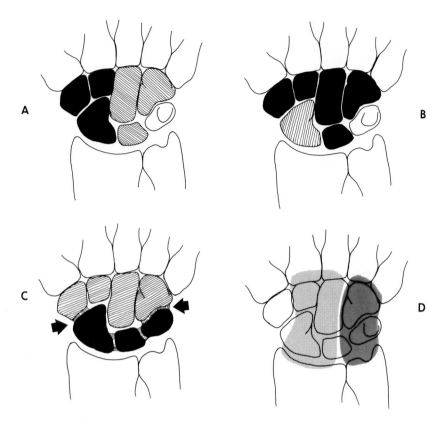

FIG. 24-2. Schematic concepts of carpal bone kinematic relationships. **A,** Navarro columnar wrist theory.[91] **B,** Taleisnik's columnar wrist model.[118] **C,** Lichtman et al. oval ring concept of carpal links.[71] **D,** Weber's longitudinal columnar theory of carpal mechanics.[134,135]

form from the medial column because it does not participate in integrating carpal motion. The central column is thought to be the main link of flexion and extension; the mobile scaphoid is still believed to stabilize the midcarpus when dorsiflexed and to allow mobility with volar flexion; triquetral motion on the hamate functions as the pivot around which carpal rotation occurs.

In 1980 Lichtman et al[71] studied several cases of ulnar midcarpal instability. They proposed an oval ring theory, conceptualizing the carpus as a dynamic ring (Fig. 24-2, C). They thought the lunate should not be considered part of the rigid central column because there is considerable mobility between the capitate and the lunate in all wrist motions. With motion and load bearing[126] the distal row moves as one unit. In ulnar deviation the helicoidal geometry of the triquetrohamate joint causes dorsiflexion of the entire proximal carpal row. In radial deviation the entire row volar flexes in response to forces initiated at the scaphotrapezial joint.[2] Therefore their physiologic model would be a ring with two mobile links—the scaphotrapezial joint and the rotatory triquetrohamate joint—and any break in this ring (across bone *or* ligament) would result in destabilization and abnormal motion (carpal instability).[2,18,71]

Weber[134] introduced the longitudinal columns theory in 1984, combining bone and ligament supports into two columns (Fig. 24-2, *D*). The **force-bearing column** consists of the distal radius, the proximal two thirds of the scaphoid, the lunate, the trapezoid, and the bases of

the second and third metacarpals. The **control column** consists of the distal ulna, TFCC, triquetrum, hamate, and bases of the fourth and fifth metacarpals. He points out that the forces generated by the hand are ultimately directed radially via bony and ligamentous anatomy, first toward the scaphoid and lunate and then to the distal radius. (Forces applied from an ulnar position are also directed in this fashion as the compliant TFCC yields, allowing the radius to accept the load.)[134,135] The medial control column depends on the triquetrohamate articulation, with movement at the helicoidal hamate surface causing dorsiflexion or volar flexion of the remainder of the proximal carpal row, which is accommodated at the scaphotrapeziotrapezoidal (STT) joint.

In summary, the radiocarpal and midcarpal joints both contribute to total flexion-extension and radioulnar deviation.* Flexion-extension motions require that the lunate and capitate move together (i.e., in the same direction). For radial and ulnar deviation the kinematics become much more complex. In radial deviation, as the distal row approaches the radial styloid, the scaphoid volar flexes (becomes more vertical) to prevent impingement against the radial styloid, allowing for increased motion. The attached lunate also volar flexes, and as the triquetrum ascends the spiral hamate groove it further adds to lunate flexion. In ulnar deviation the triquetrum descends on the hamate and into dorsiflexion; the lunate (attached)

and scaphoid also dorsiflex. Stability is maintained throughout because of the precise articular configurations and the intrinsic and extrinsic ligamentous support systems.[115]

MECHANISM AND PATTERNS OF CARPAL INSTABILITIES

Watson and Black[131] noted that, if the carpal bones were unencumbered by ligamentous constraints, they would *not* assume the normal wrist position. Because of its larger volar pole, if alone, the lunate would tend to remain dorsiflexed, but the unlinked scaphoid would tend to remain volar flexed (vertical). Bony anatomy is constrained in such a way that the ligaments maintain predetermined interactive vectors. In a large sense instability problems arise because of the difference between constrained normal and bony neutral anatomy. A specific injury results from several nonindependent factors. These include the characteristics of the injuring force, its magnitude, rate of loading, and direction; the position of the hand at impact, including all secondary angulatory and rotatory changes produced by temporal progression of the injury; and the relative strengths of the carpal bones and ligaments.[120] In general, the most frequent carpal injuries and dislocations are caused by an axial load directed proximally onto the palm (as in a fall),

---

Factors in carpal injuries

- Magnitude of injury force
- Rate of load application
- Force direction
- Position of hand
- Angulatory and rotatory changes as injury develops
- Bone strength
- Ligament strength

---

which produces combined hyperextension, ulnar deviation, and intercarpal supination and results in destruction of the radial bones and/or ligaments.[26,77,78,80] Instabilities in the ulnar carpus are likely to be caused by destructive forces applied to the ulnar side of the wrist, and these are believed to be associated with palmar flexion and intercarpal pronation.[131,134]

Carpal injuries represent a spectrum of bony and ligamentous damage, and the terminology describing them depends on whether there are fractures associated with ligament disruption(s). If there is a major carpal dislocation without fracture, it is typically either a dislocation of the carpus around the lunate, with the lunate remaining in alignment (dorsal or volar *peri*lunate dislocation) or a dislocation of the lunate that is palmar (rarely dorsal) to the radius. When there is a fracture associated with the dislocation, descriptive (diagnostic) terminology includes the name of the bone *fractured* (e.g., *transscaphoid* perilunate, *transscaphoid transcapitate* perilunate). Although perilunate and lunate injuries were historically considered separate entities, they are actually part of a continuum; the final radiographic picture depends on the aggregate of all forces (Fig. 24-3). The anatomic and biomechanical data show that there is progressive perilunar instability generally seen as four stages, each associated with further ligamentous injury as the carpus is progressively torn from the lunate.[77,78,80]

The instability patterns may be separated functionally into static and dynamic deformities.[49,119,120] Static or dissociative instabilities are apparent radiographically. Misplaced and widened intercarpal spaces are possibly as easy to find as a missing tooth—if only one takes the time to look. The dynamic or nondissociative instabilities may not be readily seen and will only be reproduced with the wrist in motion (patients may often assume such positions at will).[119] Routine radiographs from such patients will be normal, and at the least, static views in maximal deviation or cineradiographs (i.e., videofluoros-

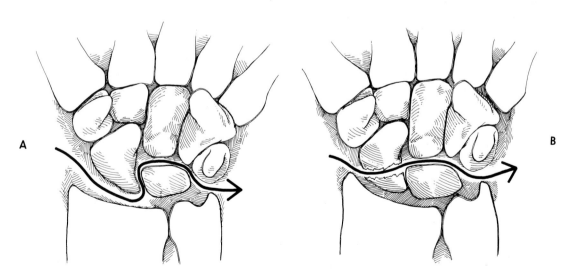

FIG. 24-3. Destructive forces are spent through the ligamentous and bony anatomy depending on exact position of hand at impact, rate of loading, and secondary peritraumatic events. **A,** Pure ligamentous perilunate disruption. **B,** Transosseous (transscaphoid, in this case) perilunate osteoligamentous disruption.

copy) are needed to reveal this group of (possibly incomplete) carpal instabilities.[6,54,119]

We find that Taleisnik's classifications based on columnar carpus theory are useful for grouping different injuries. We generally follow his terminology in discussing the diagnosis and management of pathologic conditions of the wrist ligament.

DIAGNOSIS

Evaluation of the injured wrist, especially in those without evidence of fracture on x-ray examination, presents a challenge to the treating physician. Whether acute trauma or chronic pain is the presenting complaint, it is essential to employ a logical, sequential approach to establish a correct diagnosis and to make specific treatment recommendations.

History and Physical Examination

The single most useful means of achieving the correct diagnosis is by taking a careful history. One needs to ascertain both the mechanism and hand/wrist position at injury[8] (e.g., "Was the hand extended or flexed?") and the current functional and symptomatic complaints (e.g., "What motion reproduces the pain?" or "Does pain occur during downswing or follow-through?"). In athletes these injuries are often witnessed by professional personnel (e.g., trainers, team physicians) or can be evaluated before the onset of inflammation and associated muscle spasm allowing insight into a diagnosis that is not readily available at a later time.[66]

Next, inspection of the injured wrist may reveal areas of swelling, synovitis, hematoma, or ecchymosis that can give important clues to the underlying pathologic condition. Careful, sometimes tedious, palpation of topographic anatomy is essential. Particular attention must be directed to sites of pain, clicks, and snaps, especially in those patients with chronic problems. A logical and thorough (circumferential) pattern is most important, and the use of a pencil eraser may help localize complaints precisely to individual bony interspaces.[8,121]

The final step in the physical examination is an attempt to stress each symptomatic joint to reproduce the patient's symptoms, comparing positive findings to the unaffected, opposite side. Asking the patient to perform whatever motion produces the symptoms while listening *and* gently palpating for abnormal crepitance or bony motion may also be helpful. One may inject an isolated carpal joint with lidocaine (Xylocaine) in a further effort to localize complaints and confirm with the athlete the site of chronic discomfort, noting changes in symptoms or static grip strength after injection (grip strength is an important measure of pain and dysfunction). The history and physical examination serve to localize injuries. A variety of diagnostic imaging modalities may then be employed to verify or achieve a diagnosis.

Radiographic Assessment
Routine Wrist Survey

Initially, four standard views of the wrist should be taken, including posteroanterior (PA), lateral, radial oblique, and scaphoid axial projections.[30,32] On a normal

PA view all articular surfaces should be parallel and all joint spaces symmetric, measuring about 1 to 2 mm. Three smooth arcs can be drawn along the carpal articular surfaces: one along the proximal aspect of the scaphoid, lunate and triquetrum; another along the distal concavity of these bones; and a third along the proximal margins of the capitate and hamate. A break in an arc or significant isolated joint space widening indicates potential ligamentous disruption.[16] The wrist must also be held in neutral position to evaluate ulnar variance,[96,97] since correlation exists between ulnar variance and a variety of specific wrist injuries, which are detailed below.

Standard wrist views for assessment of ligament injury

- Posteroanterior
- Lateral
- Radial oblique
- Scaphoid axial

The true lateral, with the wrist in neutral (no flexion-extension and no radial or ulnar deviation), is essential in determining axial alignment. The longitudinal axis of the radius, lunate, and capitate is normally colinear. Loss of this alignment is consistent with possible ligamentous disruption. Three angles are commonly measured to assist in diagnosis.[45,83] The **scapholunate angle** is formed by the longitudinal axes of the scaphoid and lunate, and in normal wrists it can range from 30 to 60 degrees. Angles over 70 degrees are consistent with scapholunate dissociation, and angles of less than 30 degrees often represent ulnar instabilities (Fig. 24-4).[26,74] The **capitolunate angle,** formed by the longitudinal axes of the capitate and lunate, is normally colinear. An angle of more than about 15 degrees (dorsal or volar) indicates instability (Fig. 24-5). The **radiolunate angle** is

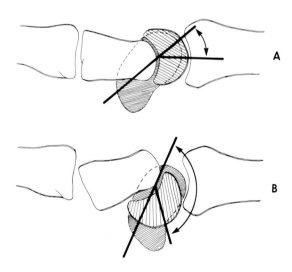

FIG. 24-4. Scapholunate angle measurement is made on the lateral radiograph. **A,** Normal scapholunate angle is 30 to 60 degrees. **B,** Pathologic scapholunate angle where scaphoid is vertical and lunate in subluxation palmward measures over 70 degrees.

formed by the longitudinal axes of the radius and lunate (also colinear) and measures the amount of dorsiflexion or palmar flexion of the proximal carpal row on the radius. (Fig. 24-6).[74]

Wrist instability has been further classified and clarified by Linscheid et al,[74] who divided instabilities into dorsal and volar intercalary segment instability patterns,

based on the capitolunate angle as seen on true lateral radiographs.

Five patterns of carpal instability can be determined from these radiographs (Table 24-1).[16] **Dorsal intercalated segmental instability (DISI)** occurs when the intercalated segment, the lunate, is dorsiflexed and the scaphoid is volar flexed (Fig. 24-7). The scapholunate angle is greater than 70 degrees, and the capitate translocates dorsal to the midaxis of the radius (Fig. 24-4).

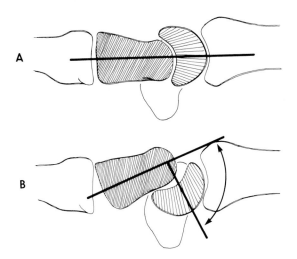

FIG. 24-5. Capitolunate angle is best measured on lateral radiographs. **A,** Normal capitolunate angle is 0 to 15 degrees and in this view with the wrist neutral, the capitate, lunate, and radius are colinear (0 degrees). **B,** Pathologic capitolunate angle of more than +15 degrees (as in this view of a dorsal intercalated segmental instability deformity) or greater than −15 degrees with the lunate volar flexed (in volar intercalated segmental instability deformity, not shown).

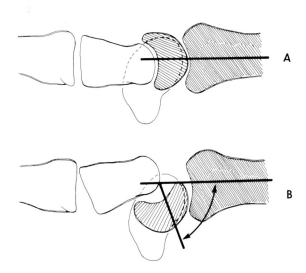

FIG. 24-6. Radiolunate angle is measured on true lateral radiographs. **A,** Normal radiolunate angle with the wrist neutral and the bones colinear. **B,** In dorsal intercalated segmental instability deformity the lunate is in subluxation palmward and dorsiflexed; the angle is greater than 30 degrees.

TABLE 24-1 Carpal instability patterns

	Normal	Dorsiflexion Instability	Palmar Flexion Instability	Ulnar Translocation	Dorsal Subluxation	Palmar Subluxation
Scapholunate angle	30-60 degrees	60-80 degrees = borderline >80 degrees = abnormal	<30 degrees	Normal	Normal	Normal
Capitolunate angle	0-30 degrees	Normal	>30 degrees	Normal	Normal	Normal
Comments		Lunate tipped dorsally; scaphoid tipped toward palm	Lunate and scaphoid tipped toward palm	>50% lunate medial to radius on posteroanterior view with hand in neutral	Shift of carpals dorsal to midplane of radius on lateral view	Shift of carpals anterior to midplane of radius on lateral view

From Gilula LA, Weeks PM: Post-traumatic ligamentous instabilities of the wrist, *Radiology* 129:641, 1978; adaptation courtesy of Weissman BN, Sledge CB: The wrist. In Weissman BN, Sledge CB: *Orthopedic radiology*, Philadelphia, 1986, WB Saunders.

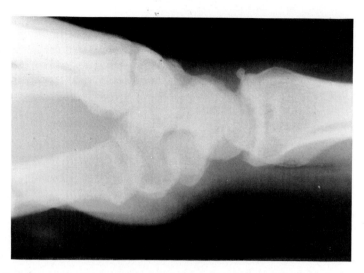

FIG. 24-7. Dorsal intercalated segmental instability deformity seen on this lateral radiograph includes dorsal subluxation of the capitate, lunate dorsiflexion with palmar subluxation, and a vertical scaphoid (the scaphoid is, technically speaking, volar flexed); the scapholunate, capitolunate, and radiolunate angles are all abnormal.

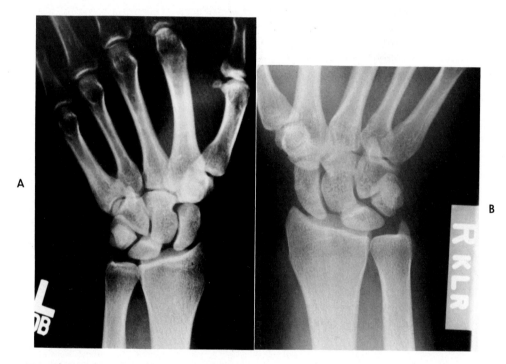

FIG. 24-8. A, PA radiograph of the left wrist in a 27-year-old soccer player who fell and landed on his left palm and complained of pain; note abnormal widening of the scapholunate interval. **B,** Comparison views of the right wrist were obtained demonstrating the same scapholunate separation of over 3 mm in this uninjured wrist ("David Letterman sign"). He recovered with only splint support.

The opposite condition is **volar intercalated segmental instability (VISI).** Both lunate and scaphoid are volar flexed. The scapholunate angle is less than 30 degrees. The capitate moves volar while its distal portion tilts dorsally, resulting in a capitolunate angle greater than 15 degrees. **Dorsal and palmar subluxation** is also determined on the lateral views when the midaxis of the lunate and carpus is dorsal or palmar to the mid-axis of the radius. On the PA film **ulnar translocation** can be determined if greater than 50% of the lunate is medial to the radius with the wrist in neutral position, leaving a widened space between the radial styloid and scaphoid.

It is important to look for soft-tissue swelling on such films.[27,28,55] Fracture of the volar lip or styloid of the radius disrupts continuity of the important volar ligaments

and should make the physician wary of potential associated instability.[48] There is a strong association of ulnar minus variance (ulna shorter than radius) and potential ligament injury. In all cases the radiographs should reveal symmetric and uniform interspaces, unbroken contours, and bony architecture.* We do not routinely order a full bilateral instability series, but we do correlate any positive findings with those of the opposite wrist, if needed (Fig. 24-8).

Supplementary Static Views

Specialized views should be obtained if a suspicious area is not sufficiently detailed with the routine survey or if obviously symptomatic joints appear benign. These additional static views may include a carpal tunnel projection to delineate the hamulus, oblique views between neutral and full pronation to visualize the ulnar side of the carpus, and a 30-degree semisupinated view to show the palmar aspect of the triquetral surface, pisiform, and pisotriquetral joints.

Supplementary static projections

- Carpal tunnel view
- Oblique views
- 30-degree semisupinated view

Abnormal instability patterns noted on plain radiographs are referred to as dissociative or static instabilities. If the routine x-ray scans are normal and abnormal carpal alignment is demonstrated only with positional change or wrist motion, it is referred to as a nondissociative or dynamic instability.

Videofluoroscopy

With standard views read as normal, in the face of significant symptoms, or if there is sufficient suspicion, we proceed with motion views. Perhaps better than the standard instability series[44,46] is videofluoroscopy.[82] With the wrist in motion abnormal gaps between parallel articular surfaces can be identified and recorded. The wrist can be moved from radial to ulnar deviation, with or without clenched fist views or compression, and spot films can be obtained. The wrist can be optimally positioned during these maneuvers, and it has been noted that gaps in the joints may actually be more apparent between the extremes of radial and ulnar deviation seen on standard instability series. Studying the films in slow motion may also yield subtle signs of irregularity in the normally smooth motion of various carpal joints.[26]

Ligament instability series

- Posteroanterior (neutral, radial deviation, ulnar deviation)
- Lateral (neutral, radial deviation, ulnar deviation)
- Bilateral anteroposterior clenched fist

---

*References 30, 45, 54, 74, 137, and 138.

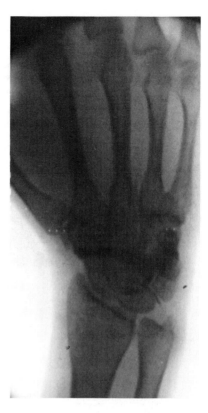

FIG. 24-9. Digital subtraction arthrogram following midcarpal injection in this 19-year-old cheerleader with chronic ulnar wrist pain following a fall from a pyramid reveals abnormal dye leakage via a lunotriquetral ligament tear. Subsequent radiocarpal and radioulnar injections were normal.

Arthrography

Arthrography with or without digital subtraction is a useful technique for delineating both acute and chronic ligamentous injuries.[69,89] There is a strong correlation between ulnar side wrist pain and perforations; no such correlation exists for radial wrist pain.[76] Normally there is no communication between the midcarpal, radiocarpal, and radioulnar joint spaces. Injection of dye individually into each of these compartments can be followed (fluoroscopically), with and without wrist motion, to evaluate the presence of abnormal communications within the carpal ligaments and TFCC.[69] Digital subtraction is used to eliminate both bone and previously injected dye densities to produce a more thorough examination (Fig. 24-9).[76] Recently, because a high prevalence of bilateral abnormalities has been noted on arthrogram, some have suggested routine comparative views of the opposite wrist, particularly for those with minimal symptoms[20] and unexpected sites of leaks.

Magnetic Resonance Imaging

Magnetic resonance imaging (MRI) is beginning to show great promise in the evaluation of wrist pain. With the development of new surface coils and computer software technology, it may surpass all other noninvasive methods.[31] High-resolution MRI is now comparable to arthrography in evaluating TFCC and scapholunate lig-

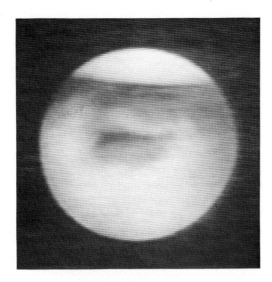

FIG. 24-10. Arthroscopic view of partial midbody triangular fibrocartilaginous complex tear in a symptomatic 19-year-old basketball player following a twisting injury while slam dunking (the lunate is seen at the top). This lesion was successfully treated by arthroscopic debridement.

ament injuries[139]; lunotriquetral injuries, however, are frequently missed.[76]

Tomograms, Bone Scans, and Computed Tomography Scans

Tomograms and bone scans are not particularly helpful in diagnosing ligamentous injury, although they may be beneficial in defining or excluding osseous injuries (such as hamulus fracture) not revealed on plain radiographs. However, because many ligamentous injuries occur in association with fractures, these techniques are useful in visualizing an occult fracture in suspected association with ligamentous instability. The computed tomography (CT) scan is the standard for evaluating distal radioulnar joint alignment and congruity.[11,87]

Arthroscopy

The role of arthroscopy continues to evolve in the diagnosis and treatment of athletic wrist injuries.[66] The technique is detailed in Chapter 22. We have used the arthroscope to evaluate and treat both chronic and acute ligamentous disruptions. Visually the physician can verify anatomic defects and determine correct alignment with percutaneous pinning techniques. It is an excellent tool for evaluating and treating many TFCC lesions (Fig. 24-10), and for identifying concomitant degenerative and partial injuries in those with associated ligamentous disruption.

MECHANISM, DIAGNOSIS, AND TREATMENT OF SPECIFIC INJURIES

This section defines and describes specific pathologic problems with respect to their anatomy and kinematics, diagnosis and imaging, and recommended treatment. Acute injuries of the wrist should be reduced and stabi-

lized. Our own experience, as well as many reports in the literature, does not support open repairs rather than accurate percutaneous pinnings of purely intraarticular ligament tears in all cases.

Scapholunate Dissociation Instability

The most frequently identified carpal instability is scapholunate dissociation. Scapholunate ligamentous injuries may be as common as scaphoid fractures. The most significant problem with these injuries is a delay in making the diagnosis.[26,56,58,119] Treatment often does not begin until several months after injury, when full-blown static instability has developed. In the meantime, potential degenerative changes or ligament scarring may have already occurred, and the possibility of restoring normal wrist function has dramatically diminished.[26,49,56,58] We cannot overemphasize the importance of *suspecting* scapholunate dissociation, making the diagnosis promptly, and thereby greatly improving the ultimate outcome of these injuries.

Kinematics

The scaphoid (mobile column) palmar flexes (becomes vertical) to permit normal radial deviation. The scaphoid is linked to the lunate by the scapholunate interosseous and radioscapholunate ligaments, and the lunate also is brought into palmar flexion as the capitate moves relatively palmar (muscle load-induced compression further assists to tilt the lunate).[111] As long as the triquetrolunate ligament is intact, the triquetrum moves from its low (dorsiflexed) position on the hamate upward into palmar flexion. There is disagreement as to whether these forces initiate mechanically at the STT or at the triquetrohamate joint. A break in the scaphoid-to-lunate link still allows the scaphoid-to-palmar flex in response to loads, gravity, and radial deviation, but the lunate (which has the natural tendency to dorsiflex because of its bony geometry) would not be moved. The result is a palmar flexed (vertical) scaphoid and a dorsiflexed lunate and triquetrum. (The capitate rides high on the lunate, dorsal to the axial plane of the radius.) The lunate is now an intercalated segment that is dorsiflexed. The scaphoid is vertical and usually described on the lateral radiograph as a part of the DISI or as rotatory scaphoid subluxation.

Mechanism

The proposed mechanism of injury is usually a fall on or blow to the outstretched hand with impact at the thenar eminence resulting in hyperextension, ulnar deviation, and intercarpal supination. Progressive loading by this mechanism was reproduced by Mayfield, Johnson, and Kilcoyne[80] creating a reproducible pattern of ligament failure.

The first ligament to go is the radial collateral ligament, progressing to the radiocapitate, and then the scapholunate interosseous ligament, creating Stage I, or scapholunate, instability. With a continuation of the force vector, the tear extends between the capitate and lunate (Stage II), and then around the lunate to rupture the lunotriquetral ligament creating lunotriquetral instability (Stage III). Finally, disruption of the dorsal radio-

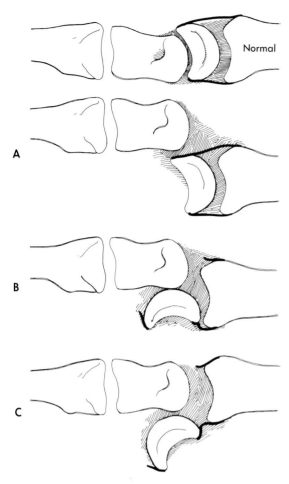

FIG. 24-11. Kinematic stages of progressive disruption (pure ligament and osteoligamentous) in perilunate and lunate disruption. **A,** Perilunate. **B,** Transition from perilunate to lunate dislocation. **C,** True lunate dislocation.

carpal ligament occurs, resulting in volar lunate dislocation. The end result of this progressive perilunar dislocation leaves the lunate suspended only on its volar radial and ulnar ligamentous attachments. With further carpal motion the lunate is forced out through the space of Poirier and winds up with its concave surface facing proximally (Fig. 24-11).

This mechanism does not account for all injuries but is probably the most common. Because of the differing maximal elongation lengths of the extrinsic and intrinsic ligaments, a variety of injury patterns can result. The more stout scapholunate interosseous ligament may rupture, whereas the more plastic extrinsic ligaments stretch,[103] offering some residual stabilizers to prevent static instability patterns on early radiographs. In time, with further attenuation, this partial dynamic instability may become static and lead to arthrosis as a result of altered kinematics. Therefore it is imperative that any athlete with radial wrist pain after trauma be carefully evaluated for both scaphoid fracture and possible ligamentous injury.

A widening of the scapholunate space and rotatory subluxation does not develop unless the scapholunate in-

terosseous ligament and either the restraining scaphotrapezial or palmar radiocarpal ligaments are divided,[14,15] which explains the normal findings on x-ray scans of athletes with significant pain (and the need for a high index of suspicion).

If rotatory scaphoid subluxation is not diagnosed, the capitate descends proximally between the scaphoid and lunate. As the normal force-bearing column of Weber[134] is disrupted, the articular contact characteristics of the radiocarpal joints change. The radioscaphoid articulation moves dorsal and radial and becomes more elliptical[15]; the lunate maintains a more spherical contact, but in its dorsiflexed posture only the narrowest dorsal portion intervenes between the capitate and radius. Greater transmission of compressive and shear forces begins at the radioscaphoid articulation. The end result is the eventual development of radioscaphoid and later capitolunate arthritis, the **scapholunate advanced collapse (SLAC) deformity** appreciated on late x-ray studies.[130] The more spherical radiolunate articulation may be more tolerant of abnormal joint motion,[15] with the radiolunate joint commonly spared from the arthrosis.

Although some with low-demand hands may not develop significant symptoms,[36] the associated pain, weakness, and loss of motion would devastate an athlete. Because of the natural history of this problem, we treat the earliest stages of scapholunate ligament injuries to prevent the more advanced static and collapse deformities from developing.

Diagnosis

In the acute stage, after obtaining a thorough history, one should be aware of the diagnosis in any athlete complaining of dorsoradial wrist pain, with swelling and tenderness in the region of the anatomic snuffbox.

Chronic problems are generally associated with (milder) intermittent symptoms related to certain activities, especially those requiring rotation or deviation of the wrist. Palmer, Dobyns, and Linscheid[96] noted that 100% of their patients who had diagnosed ligamentous disruption experienced wrist pain, 91% had decreased grip strength, 71% demonstrated decreased motion, and one third experienced clicking of the wrist. The clicking has been described as a catch-up clunk—as the wrist moves from radial to ulnar deviation, the lunate and triquetrum move synchronously, but the scaphoid is left behind in palmar flexion.[33,55,131] As the radial side of the carpus elongates further, the scaphoid suddenly jumps into place, catching up with the lunate. Many patients with ligamentous instability have been found to have a diffuse ligamentous laxity of many joints, including those of the opposite extremity.[120]

Dynamic instabilities can be suspected in those with pain in the anatomic snuffbox and normal x-ray scans. Dynamic instabilities can often be diagnosed using **Watson's scaphoid test:** the examiner places four fingers of one hand on the distal radius and the thumb on the scaphoid tuberosity while the wrist is postured in ulnar deviation (elongating the scaphoid). Pressure is directed dorsally with the thumb at the volar scaphoid, while the wrist is radially deviated. Pressure on the scaphoid, which prevents it from becoming vertical, drives the

proximal pole dorsally if the ligaments are not intact. Pain is the hallmark of a positive test, although sometimes the dorsal movement of the scaphoid can actually be seen to move dorsally.[131]

The scaphoid shift test, a modification of Watson's test, relies on a relaxed wrist in neutral position to slight radial deviation (10 degrees), with direct posterior force applied to the scaphoid tubercle. Findings can be correlated with the opposite wrist.[68]

Radiographic Assessment

There are several radiographic methods for diagnosing scapholunate dissociation. However, we recommend the instability series as especially helpful.[44-46] If fluoroscopy is available, then examination under fluoroscopy with motion and compression should be performed, as previously described.

Suggestive findings on PA projections include a scapholunate space greater than 2 mm (in any event, not greater than other intercarpal spaces). Marked gaps are obvious and are remembered when termed a "David Letterman" sign (or "Terry-Thomas"[41] or "Leon Spinks" sign[55]) (Fig. 24-8). The scaphoid may appear foreshortened and have a superimposed cortical ring because of the end-on projection of its now vertical proximal pole. Blatt[14] suggests measuring the ring to proximal distance with both wrists in neutral. The distance from the proximal portion of the ring to the proximal pole of the scaph-

---

Radiographic signs of scapholunate dissociation

- Scapholunate interval >2 to 3 mm
- Foreshortened scaphoid
- Cortical "ring" sign
- Scapholunate angle >70 degrees

---

oid is reduced by at least 4 mm, or is no greater than 7 mm, or both, when compared with the opposite (normal) wrist.

On lateral films (Figs. 24-4 to 24-7), the capitate, third metacarpal, and radius are normally colinear, with the scaphoid at 30 to 60 degrees. From this perspective, with the lunate in dorsiflexion (DISI), the scaphoid is in a vertical position (>65 to 70 degrees).[74] Motion studies reveal the abnormal catch-up clunk, and the lunate remains dorsiflexed throughout motion, since the palmar flexing influence of the scaphoid has been lost. Arthrograms offer some information for cases that are otherwise difficult to diagnose.[98] We use diagnostic arthroscopy on those patients with suspected injuries but equivocal radiographic findings.

Treatment

Acute injuries. In those patients complaining of a painful wrist in the region of the scapholunate joint, who have negative x-ray studies and a suspicious history, we advocate 2 to 3 weeks of cast immobilization with x-ray studies at 10 days to rule out occult scaphoid fracture,

or bone scan after 48 to 72 hours after fracture when an early diagnosis is required.

Controversy exists regarding proper management of acute scapholunate dissociation. Many authors feel strongly that only open treatment is proper.[54,55] Others, including us, believe that closed reduction (sometimes with arthroscopic verification) and Kirschner wire (K-wire) fixation are effective, if properly performed and if followed by maintenance with gauntlet cast support for 8 weeks.[49,105] Those who advocate open treatment argue the merits of a dorsal approach alone vs. combined dorsal and volar approaches. The two-incision approach allows the surgeon to both evaluate the reduction dorsally and repair the volar ligament through a separate volar incision.[55] The paradox[80] is that, although wrist dorsiflexion is the position of bony reduction, this configuration further produces separation and displacement of the palmar ligaments. The problem is overcome by reducing the scaphoid in wrist dorsiflexion, pinning it to the capitate and/or lunate, but then immobilizing the wrist in mild palmar flexion to facilitate apposition of the torn ligaments.[55,120] Hand therapy is begun 8 weeks after repair/reduction, but impact loading is restricted for another 8 weeks.

After reduction of perilunate or lunate dislocations, rotatory scaphoid subluxation frequently becomes apparent in follow-up radiographs. We prefer to pin most cases acutely to avoid this complication. If diagnosed late, open reduction may often be required. In the presence of transosseous perilunate dislocations, the dynamic tendency to instability resulting from the ligamentous disruption is a likely cause of scaphoid nonunion.[90]

Chronic injuries. Treatment of chronic scapholunate dissociations can be difficult. Operations to stabilize the carpal architecture have been described.* Initial attempts at using tendon grafts for reconstruction of the scapholunate ligament were unreliable.[47,96,117,120] Recent reports indicate that a more comprehensive four-bone ligament reconstruction (radius, lunate, capitate, and scaphoid) may hold more promise,[4] as have reports of osteoligamentous stabilization procedures for those with a subacute (no degenerative changes) DISI deformity.[25,73] Blatt[13] proposed reconstruction (especially for nondissociative instabilities) using a dorsal wrist capsular flap sutured to the distal pole of the scaphoid. The purpose of this procedure is to achieve more motion than can be expected from limited intercarpal arthrodeses. He performs this operation when a relatively unblemished scaphoid can be reduced easily to anatomic position at surgery. A thumb spica is used for immobilization for 2 months, and then hand therapy is initiated. No forceful stress is permitted for 4 to 6 months postoperatively. He reports neither radioscaphoid nor STT degenerative changes with an average 7½-year follow-up. Reasonable wrist range of motion and grip strength are also achieved. We currently recommend this technique in those patients without static deformities, but further follow-up is necessary to determine its long-term efficacy and its role in those with static deformities.[14a]

---

*References 7, 13, 39, 63, 65, 96, and 130.

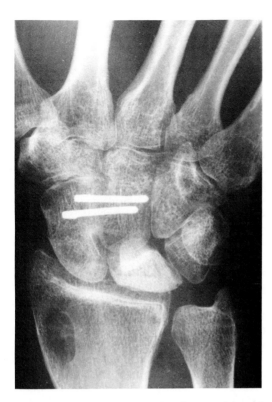

FIG. 24-12. Posteroanterior radiographs of successful scaphocapitate arthrodesis in a 22-year-old squash player with Stage II Kienböck's disease.

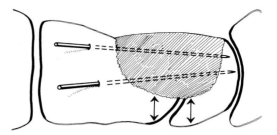

FIG. 24-13. Diagramatic representation of generic intercarpal arthrodesis, preserving original (reduced) intercarpal spaces by retaining the palmar third of cortex and cartilage, but tightly packing the curetted interspace generously with autogenous bone graft.

Many authors now prefer limited intercarpal fusions to treat chronic scapholunate dissociation (Fig. 24-12).[59,101,104,123,133] In reconstructing the force-bearing column, Weber[135] believed it would make sense to link the scaphoid to the lunate to transfer force from the capitate to the radius. However, a successful scapholunate arthrodesis is most difficult to achieve[52,123] because of the small contact surface area and the considerable forces applied to the segments. In 1967 Peterson and Lipscomb[101] proposed STT fusion. Later popularized by Watson et al,[133] this procedure is used to reconstruct the scaphoid as a midcarpal strut, to restore carpal height, and to retain triquetral lunate motion (thus keeping more carpal motion).[55,63,65] The key is accurate reduction of the scaphoid to the level of the dorsiflexed lunate and restoration of the scapholunate unit to its normal position before pinning the scaphoid to the capitate. Recent reports indicate a roughly 20% incidence of progressive carpal arthrosis with STT fusion despite attention to detail in achieving reduction.[40,64] Because the entire distal carpal row is a single bony unit and the objective is to transmit forces from capitate through scaphoid and lunate to the radius, it makes equal mechanical sense to fuse the scaphoid to the capitate.[34,35,84] We prefer a scaphocapitate fusion, because it is easier to perform than other intercarpal fusions. The joint is also in the operative area where most of the surgical dissection takes place.[104] Experimentally, incorporation of the lunate in the fusion may diminish the load borne by the scaphoid

fossa.[127] Recent clinical studies indicate that good early results can be achieved with scaphocapitolunate (SCL) fusion in spite of a theoretical decrease in range of motion.[109] For all limited arthrodeses it is essential to preserve original intercarpal spaces by retaining the palmar third of cortex and cartilage but by tightly packing each curetted interspace with a generous bone graft (Fig. 24-13). We initially stabilize these bones with K-wires and power bone staples (3M Company, Minneapolis) and remove the wires at about 6 weeks. The use of titanium staples allows us to mobilize these wrists sooner, even as bone bridging is progressing, because of the stability added by the internal fixation (Figs. 24-12 and 24-14, *B*).

Medial Carpal Instabilities

Medial instabilities involve the ligaments attached to the medial or rotatory column in Taleisnik's kinematic model, including lunotriquetral and triquetrohamate or midcarpal instability. Although the lateral (radial) carpus is bridged by the scaphoid (control rod of Gilford), the ulnar carpus lacks such a bony bridge and relies on the volar arcuate **V** ligament for stabilization.[71,118] In normal ulnar deviation the triquetrum descends distally under the palmar surface of the hamate and moves into a dorsiflexed posture. Because the lunate-triquetrum unit is functionally inseparable, similar to an ulnar version of the bridging scaphoid,[5] the palmar movement and dorsiflexion of the triquetrum are transmitted to the attached lunate, resulting in smooth, synchronous dorsiflexion of the entire proximal carpal row. Sectioning the lunotriquetral ligament would exclude the dorsiflexing influence of triquetrum on the lunate. The resulting volar flexed lunate and scaphoid seen with a dorsiflexed triquetrum is the typical VISI pattern deformity seen only on lateral radiographs. This deformity may be dynamic, visualized only in such cases with axial compression, or as a static deformity in those with severe or chronic injuries.[120] Viegas et al[127] have correlated static and dynamic deformities seen radiographically with sectioning of the lunotriquetral interosseous ligament and surrounding palmar lunotriquetral and dorsal radiocarpal ligaments. In the presence of midcarpal instabilities, it is the loss of influence of the bony geometry of the triquetrohamate joint on the lunate that allows VISI deformity to develop.[2]

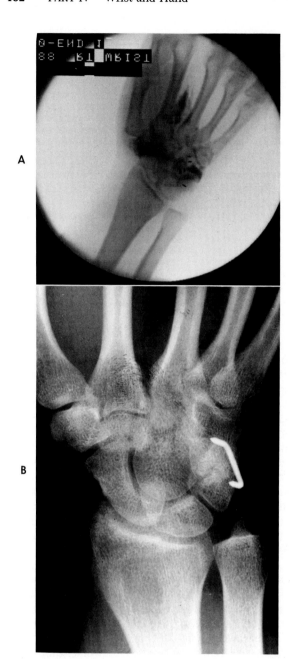

FIG. 24-14. A, Abnormal digital subtraction arthrogram following midcarpal injection demonstrating dye leakage across the hamotriquetral joint. **B,** This young female gymnast was successfully treated by triquetrohamate intercarpal arthrodesis.

Triquetrohamate (Midcarpal) Instabilities
Mechanism

Lichtman's oval ring concept of carpal kinematics dictates that a break in the ring at the triquetrohamate joint would result in instability of the midcarpus.[17] Laxity of either arm of the arcuate ligament due to trauma, attenuation, or generalized ligamentous laxity is usually the cause of midcarpal laxity. Many patients recall no specific injury, and ligamentous laxity of the opposite wrist is often found.* A classification system for midcarpal in-

*References 2, 3, 18, 59, 71, 116, and 131.

stability has been described based on cause (intrinsic or extrinsic) and direction of subluxation. In essence there are two types[72]:

1. **Palmar midcarpal instability** (most common) results from laxity of the ulnar arm of the arcuate ligament and the dorsal radiolunotriquetral ligament, which decreases the influence of the spiral triquetrohamate joint on the proximal row due to poor bone contact. At neutral position of the wrist the proximal row follows gravity and the scaphoid and remains volar flexed, causing palmar displacement of the distal row. The proximal row then remains in volar flexion until the last few degrees of ulnar deviation, when increased contact of the triquetrohamate joint forces the entire proximal row to snap into dorsiflexion,[3] a phenomenon which is accompanied by an audible clunk.

2. **Dorsal midcarpal instability** results from laxity of the radial arm of the arcuate and radioscaphocapitate ligaments.[72] The capitate is in dorsal subluxation on the lunate with the wrist at neutral, and the proximal row maintains a DISI posture throughout radial and ulnar deviation. In radial deviation the dislocation may be reduced by palmar directed force on the metacarpals.[3]

Diagnosis

The presenting complaint is often a painful clunk that occurs during activities involving pronation of the forearm and ulnar deviation of the wrist.[2,18] A volar sag may be visible at the midcarpal joint and tenderness found over the triquetrohamate joint. Many patients can actively reproduce the painful clunk as they move from neutral to extreme ulnar deviation. In those who cannot, where the diagnosis is suspected, a clinical test has been described by Lichtman et al.[72] To examine the right wrist, the examiner's left hand holds the patient's forearm in a pronated position. With the wrist in neutral deviation, the examiner's right hand grasps the patient's hand and, with the thumb, exerts palmarly directed pressure on the dorsal wrist, at the level of the distal capitate. The wrist is then simultaneously axially loaded and ulnarly deviated. The test is positive when a painful clunk occurs with ulnar deviation that reproduces the patient's symptoms.

Lunotriquetral rupture, TFCC tears, ulnar abutment syndrome, and subluxation of the distal radioulnar joint potentially may also produce painful clicks on the ulnar aspect of the wrist.[18] After completion of the history and physical examination, radiographic studies are warranted.

Causes of clicks in the ulnar area

- Triquetrohamate instability
- Lunotriquetral rupture
- Triangular fibrocartilaginous complex tears
- Ulnar abutment syndrome
- Distal radioulnar joint subluxation

Radiographic Assessment

Because medial carpal instabilities are frequently dynamic, standard (static) PA, lateral, radial, and ulnar deviation views are often within normal limits. The most helpful diagnostic tool in evaluating midcarpal instabilities is the cineradiograph (videofluoroscopy).[2,18] Typically, in these cases, as the patient moves from the volar flexed physiologic VISI of radial deviation toward the ulna, there is a sudden snap of the proximal carpal row into DISI nearing the limits of ulnar deviation. The failure of a smooth transition from physiologic VISI to physiologic DISI is typical of midcarpal instability. Tears may also be demonstrated by arthrogram (Fig. 24-14, A).

Treatment

Patients with chronic, mild triquetrohamate instabilities may have an associated synovitis that does not require surgery. For athletes seen early after injury, anti-inflammatory medications and local injections of steroids are justified only if frank dissociation cannot be definitely diagnosed.[2,71,120] The defined acute tear may be treated by percutaneous pinning and gauntlet cast or by a long arm cast (forearm in supination and wrist in neutral) for 6 to 8 weeks; we prefer pins in most instances.

Authors have various opinions regarding surgery for chronic pathologic conditions. Taleisnik[120] recommends capsulodesis (tenodesis) for patients who will not place excessive loads upon the wrist or for those whose grip strength is less than 40 kg and who will not have frequent, high loads applied, criteria that are rarely met in the injured athlete. Lichtman attempted several types of soft-tissue reconstructions but found these unsuccessful.[2,18,72] Volar capsular reefing procedures directed at the attenuated arcuate and associated volar[122] and dorsal ligaments[125] were also found unreliable. If the wrist is symptomatic, supportive treatment fails in a participating athlete (except, perhaps, chess players), and soft-tissue procedures should *not* be considered reliable. Midcarpal arthrodesis, either triquetrohamate or triquetrohamate-capitate-lunate, is the best stabilization method. Long-term follow-up studies are not yet available to evaluate secondary deformities, and one can predict diminished wrist mobility after intercarpal fusion.[35,84]

During an operation for arthrodesis the triquetrohamate joint, or triquetro-hamate capitate-lunate joint, is approached from the dorsum. The dorsal half to two thirds is decorticated, and the bones are reduced and pinned. With direct vision the physician must verify that the midcarpal subluxation has been eliminated as the wrist goes through a full passive range of motion. Autogenous radius metaphyseal bone graft is harvested (through a separate incision) and densely packed to obliterate the interspace. The basic principle of limited arthrodesis is always the same: restore but do not change the normal spacial relationships between carpal bones with fusion (Fig. 24-13).[132]

Lunotriquetral Instabilities

The triquetrum is securely tethered to the lunate by the lunotriquetral ligament. This functional unit has been considered a mirror image of the scaphoid when congenital coalitions occur. Although there is considerable motion between the mobile scaphoid and lunate, the lunate and triquetrum are functionally inseparable.[5] Triquetral descent under the hamate during ulnar deviation causes volar displacement and dorsiflexion of the triquetrum. By virtue of the strong ligamentous attachments of the proximal row, there is a synchronous dorsiflexion of the remainder of the proximal portion of the oval ring (the physiologic DISI). Attenuation or rupture of the lunotriquetral ligament eliminates the controlling influence of the triquetrum, and the naturally volar flexing scaphoid, with its intact scapholunate ligament, brings the lunate into a volar flexed attitude, thereby creating the typical VISI deformity. On the lateral radiograph of such cases the volar flexed lunate and scaphoid are seen concurrently with a dorsiflexed triquetrum in *both* radial and ulnar deviation.

Mechanism

The exact mechanism of injury is uncertain. Lunotriquetral dissociation may represent a *forme fruste* of Stage III perilunar instability, in which the scapholunate or transscaphoid component has healed.[3] Isolated lunotriquetral injury may result from hyperpronation of the hand on the forearm.[55,80,120] Weber[134,135] believed that such injuries are caused by impact on the dorsum of a palmar flexed hand and that, characteristically, the palmar fibers (radiolunotriquetral ligament) are spared. He presumed that these palmar fibers become the rotational axis as a VISI deformity develops. If the lunate is free to flex in a palmar direction at the same time as the scaphoid, the triquetrum dorsiflexes as it is forced by the capitate to move ulnarly and down the hamate; under such circumstances a static VISI deformity may develop.

Diagnosis

Diagnosis can be difficult soon after injury, before a VISI pattern develops radiographically. The athlete may recount a history that includes falling on an outstretched hand in radial deviation. Or he or she may tell of being struck on the back of the hand and seeking treatment for pain along the ulnar side of the wrist. Tenderness may be elicited at the lunotriquetral joint, frequently with associated weakness, but there may not be a click produced by passively loading the wrist and moving from ulnar to radial deviation.[2,108,134,135]

The **ulnar snuff-box test** can help distinguish between lunotriquetral and isolated TFCC injuries. Lateral pressure is applied in the sulcus distal to the ulnar head that is formed by the extensor carpi ulnaris and flexor carpi ulnaris tendons; if it reproduces the patient's pain, a problem of the lunotriquetral joint should be suspected.[5] The **lunotriquetral ballotement test**[108] requires stabilization of the lunate with the examiner's thumb and index finger and shucking the pisiform and triquetrum palmarward and dorsally with the other hand to determine the presence of laxity, pain, and crepitance. Like diagnoses of midcarpal instabilities, differential diagnoses include TFCC tears, triquetrohamate tears, subluxation or dislocation of the radioulnar joint, subluxation of extensor carpi ulnaris tendon, and ulnocarpal abutment.

Radiographic Assessment

Isolated lunotriquetral ligament injury will not cause a static VISI deformity. Concommitant sectioning of the dorsal radiotriquetral and scaphotriquetral ligaments consistently produces the static VISI deformity seen on plain radiographs.[53] Standard films are typically normal; however, an associated VISI deformity on the lateral view must be identified where both the scaphoid and lunate are volar flexed, but the triquetrum is dorsiflexed and distal on the hamate. The PA view shows a break in continuity in the carpal arcs at the triquetrolunate joint.[108,120] Disruption of the normal radiographic sinusoidal curve from the lunotriquetral to the capitatohamate joints should also arouse suspicion.[5] Since lunotriquetral tears may be part of an **ulnar impaction syndrome (UIS)**, ulnar variance should be evaluated on plain radiographs.[96] UIS is usually associated with neutral or positive ulnar variance. Bone scans can be confirmatory if increased uptake is noted over the distal ulna and proximal lunate.[102] We find that the most useful test is an arthrogram, which usually demonstrates the ligament tear (leak) and associated pathologic condition.

Arthroscopy is now playing a larger role in evaluating chronic lunotriquetral injuries. It permits reliable evaluation of the lunotriquetral ligament in addition to direct inspection of the TFCC and all articular surfaces.[66] Synovitis, chondromalacia, and other evidence of ulnocarpal impaction can be readily evaluated. In confusing cases arthroscopy shortens the diagnostic workup and permits simultaneous debridement, resulting in a more rapid return to the playing field.

Treatment

Athletes who have acute partial tears, including significant injuries that do not yet show static VISI deformity on radiograph, should be immobilized for 6 to 8 weeks with a long arm cast positioning the wrist in ulnar deviation and dorsiflexion. The plaster should be molded to apply palmar pressure on the pisiform.[108,111]

In the presence of static VISI deformity the scaphoid and lunate must be immobilized in a dorsiflexed position to match the triquetrum and consequently to reverse the clinical deformity. Acute complete disruptions should be fixed internally. Although open ligament repair is sometimes advocated,[2,108] we believe that percutaneous pinning under fluoroscopic control is sufficient if maintained for 8 weeks. For chronic cases, we agree with Lichtman, who recommends lunotriquetral arthrodesis for static deformities or nondissociative instabilities unresponsive to conservative care. Although excellent results have been obtained with ligament reconstruction,[37] in our hands lunotriquetral arthrodesis preserves the intercarpal relationships and has proven most reliable.

Proximal Carpal Instabilities (Ulnar Translocation)

Ulnar translocation has been found after trauma.[74,77,120] Rayhack et al[107] described several cases in detail, in which three of eight patients were injured during athletics.

Diagnosis

Hyperextension associated with substantial torque, possibly pronation of the forearm on a fixed hand, is postulated as a mechanism for ulnar translation.[107] Cadaver dissections by Rayhack et al[107] revealed that the carpus could not be translocated toward the ulna until all insertions of the palmar radiocarpal ligaments are disrupted. At examination, acute injuries are associated with massive swelling and striking loss of strength. The carpus may be obviously unstable because of radioulnar pressure directed to the second metacarpal or triquetrum; redisplacement occurs with release of pressure (Fig. 24-15).

Radiographic Assessment

The diagnosis of ulnar translocation cannot be determined by clinical means alone; specific radiographic findings include ulnar displacement of the carpus on the radius with less than half of the lunate within the lunate fossa. The distance between the radial styloid and scaphoid is increased, and the lunate blocks ulnar deviation. Most important, McMurtry,[81] Rayhack et al,[107] and Chamay[21] described the measurement of the carpal ulnar distance or the carpal translation index. If an erroneous diagnosis of scapholunate dissociation is made, an associated increase in the scapholunate interval influences the treatment and outcome.

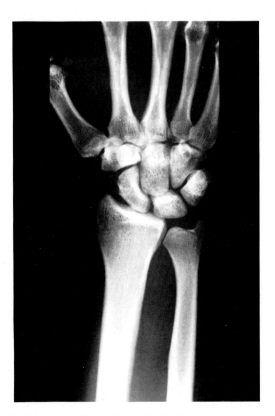

FIG. 24-15. Acute radiocarpal shift (with ulnar translation) in a 19-year-old woman who fell while competitively skateboarding. Note the increased radioscaphoid space. She was treated by open reduction, pinning of the scaphoid and lunate to the radius, plus repair of the dorsal and volar ligaments and capsule.

Treatment

Initially the injury should be reduced and the reduction should be held in a cast or splint until plans for surgery have been made. Closed reduction alone is inadequate. Primary ligament repair and internal stabilization are highly recommended. For chronic cases, radiolunate arthrodesis is performed because ligamentous stabilizations have proved futile.[55,96,120]

Dorsal and Palmar Subluxations

There are few reports of palmar translocation in the literature, and none pertain to athletic activities.[10] Dorsal translocation is frequently secondary to malunited fractures of the distal radius or rheumatoid arthritis. Treatment should be directed at correcting the malangulation of the articular surface of the radius by osteotomy if the articular surface is intact. If the articular surface is noncongruent or degenerated, limited fusion of the involved joint(s) is best.

Diagnosis

Lateral radiographs demonstrate that the lunate and capitate are dorsal or volar to the articular surface of the radius, differing from perilunate dislocations, which are characterized by an intact radiolunate relationship except that the capitate is dorsal.

Treatment

When isolated and not associated with radial fractures, this injury needs open reduction, pinning, and ligament repair or reconstruction. Late cases will undoubtedly require radius–proximal row arthrodesis to achieve adequate stabilization.

Ligamentous Disruptions of the Distal Radioulnar Joint

Although ligamentous disruptions of the distal radioulnar joint have been recognized for nearly two centuries, only in the past decade have we gained a detailed understanding of the anatomy and biomechanics of this joint. The additional information should lead to improved treatment of athletes who sustain injuries to it. Besides the causative athletic endeavor, it is important to consider the patient's vocational and avocational goals as future treatment may depend on them.

Mechanism

The TFCC, which is the major stabilizer of the distal radioulnar joint, is composed of the triangular fibrocartilage, ulnar meniscus homolog, ulnar collateral ligament, dorsal and volar radioulnar ligaments, the ulnolunate and ulnotriquetral ligaments, and the extensor carpi ulnaris tendon sheath.[99,100] Because many of these individual structures are poorly defined in the clinical setting, they have been grouped into one complex, which arises from the ulnar aspect of the lunate fossa[17,100] and suspends the carpus from the distal radius. The complex inserts into the base of the ulnar styloid, and the volar aspect of the TFCC is very strongly attached to the lunotriquetral interosseous ligament and triquetrum. The TFCC is thick along its dorsal and volar edges, but thin in the cen-

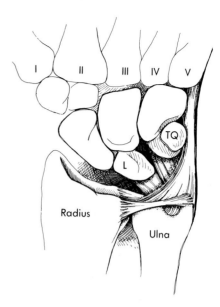

FIG. 24-16. Triangular fibrocartilage complex comprises the triangular fibrocartilage, ulnar meniscus homologue, ulnar collateral ligament, dorsal and volar radioulnar ligaments, ulnolunate and ulnotriquetral ligaments, and extensor carpi ulnaris; it is a major stabilizer of the distal radioulnar joint.

ter in the region of the lunate/TFCC articulation (Fig. 24-16).[100] The peripheral dorsal, volar, and ulnar portions of the TFCC are vascular and have the potential to heal. The central 80% and radial attachment are avascular.[9,22]

Triangular fibrocartilage complex

- Triangular fibrocartilage
- Ulnar meniscus homolog
- Ulnar collateral ligament
- Dorsal and volar radioulnar ligaments
- Ulnolunate ligament
- Ulnotriquetral ligament
- Extensor carpi ulnaris tendon sheath

The forearm can rotate approximately 150 degrees at the distal radioulnar joint. The radius (and hand) rotates about the ulnar head, which is not immobile during this rotation, as was once believed. Ray, Johnson, and Jameson[106] demonstrated that the distal ulna abducts 8 to 9 degrees with pronation and adducts with supination. The ulnar head moves dorsally in pronation and volarward in supination.[124] In addition, Palmer and Werner[99] and Friedman et al[42] have demonstrated that the ulnar head moves slightly distally (positive variance) with pronation and with grip. It moves proximally with supination and grip release. Pronation therefore causes the ulna to abduct and to move dorsally and distally, and supination causes the distal ulna to adduct and move volarward and proximally in relation to the radius. Stability throughout a range of motion and axial loading is dependent on both

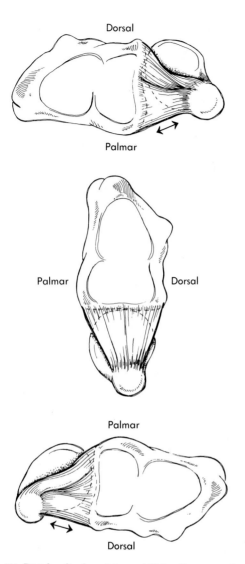

Dorsal

Palmar

Palmar   Dorsal

Palmar

Dorsal

FIG. 24-17. Distal radioulnar joint stabilizing ligaments (triangular fibrocartilage complex). Some fibers are taut in all forearm positions, such that injury of the volar fibers allows dorsal displacement while the ulna is in pronation and the reverse in supination.

TFCC integrity and bony congruence. The volar aspect of the TFCC is taut in pronation and relaxed in supination; the reverse is true for its dorsal aspect, which is taut in supination and relaxed in pronation, thereby resisting subluxation (with the ulnocarpal ligaments) throughout forearm rotation (Fig. 24-17).

Distal radioulnar joint mechanics

Pronation
- Distal ulna abducts
- Ulnar head moves dorsally
- Ulnar head advances distally

Supination
- Distal ulna adducts
- Ulnar head moves volarward
- Ulnar head advances proximally

The TFCC, the pronator quadratus, and the interosseous membrane are also important in cushioning and transmitting ulnar axial loads. Disruption of a portion of the TFCC may allow instability, and excision of the entire TFCC causes nonphysiologic increases in loading of the radius. Palmer and Werner [98] demonstrated that ulnar variance (the relative length of the ulna compared to that of the radius) also has dramatic effects on the amount of load borne by the ulna. Shortening the length of the ulna by 2.5 mm decreases the force borne by the distal ulna from 20% to 4% of the total force of the forearm. Increasing the length of the ulna by 2.5 mm increases the force borne by the ulna to 42% of the total. Such changes in transmission of load are significant in the development of early arthrosis at contact points.

Diagnosis

A history of wrist extension and forearm hyperpronation is commonly described by those who can recall the events leading to the injury. Typical examples of the incidents affecting athletes involve falling on the outstretched hand or "straight arming" an opponent in football or rugby.[50] In the presence of an acute injury, instability of the ulnar head, swelling, crepitance, or pain with volar-directed compression of the ulna can be observed. If there is no acute injury, it is necessary to localize the site of the pathologic abnormality by palpating the area. The differential diagnosis includes radioulnar or radiocarpal arthritis, extensor carpi ulnaris subluxation, ulnocarpal impingement, or impaction, and medial and midcarpal instabilities. The athlete should describe when his or her pain occurs, and the physician should then attempt to reproduce the circumstances with manipulation. In the presence of instability, most often dorsal subluxation of the ulna (whatever the anatomic basis), a painful clunk often accompanies the passive maneuver. There are now a variety of imaging techniques that can assist in achieving an accurate diagnosis.

Radiographic Assessment

The lack of truly standardized PA and lateral views for evaluation of the distal radioulnar joint has contributed to the difficulty in evaluating films identifying dorsal or volar subluxation if the diagnosis is not clinically obvious. Bowers[17] recommends that the PA film be taken with the shoulder abducted to 90 degrees, elbow flexed 90 degrees, and the hand flat on each set. Both radial and ulnar styloids should be at the extreme medial and lateral edges on the radiograph. The lateral is taken with the shoulder at zero degrees abduction, with the elbow flexed to 90 degrees, and with the x-ray tube at a right angle to the wrist. Besides looking for evidence of fracture or subluxation, **ulnar variance** should be assessed because it may influence diagnosis and care. The hand should remain relaxed because a clenched fist can potentially alter the measured ulnar variance.[113] *Positive variance* is more often associated with TFCC injury and impaction, and *negative variance* is associated with Kienböck's disease and posttraumatic carpal instability. Trispiral tomograms can be helpful in identifying small fractures not seen in plain films.

We find that the CT scan is the most reliable method

for assessing distal radioulnar joint congruence. Mino, Palmer and Levinsohn[87,88] compared radiographs to CT scans for evaluating the distal radioulnar joint. The CT scan obviates the problem of achieving neutral wrist rotation on a plain film. The wrist of an acutely injured athlete can thereby be evaluated while still splinted, without regard to wrist position. MRI is now thought to be extremely helpful in evaluating the TFCC but less reliable in identifying associated lunotriquetral injuries.[11,31]

Arthrography

Arthrography is an excellent method for identifying defects (tears) in the TFCC. Many patients have degenerative tears in the TFCC that were not caused by acute trauma. Degenerative defects and secondary ulnolunate abutment develop into synovitis secondary to cartilaginous erosion.[85,99] Wrist pain may be secondary to impaction (abutment), which is the real problem that needs to be addressed (not the tear, which may well be asymptomatic). At the time of an acute injury the TFCC may be avulsed from the ulna, and contrast will leak into the subcutaneous tissues around the ulna or from the triquetral recess proximally across the TFCC into the distal radioulnar joint.[50,95] Central TFCC tears also are usually easy to demonstrate. Avulsion at the radial margin of the TFCC is clearly appreciated following both radiocarpal and distal radioulnar injections.

Arthroscopy

Because tears visualized on arthrography may be traumatic or degenerative and because their identification does not necessarily pinpoint the cause of wrist pain in the athlete, arthroscopy has an important place in evaluating the injured wrist, including the distal radioulnar joint and TFCC. Palmer[94] has classified various TFCC defects based on their cause (traumatic or degenerative) and their location (central, radial, peripheral). The probable cause can usually be determined by arthroscopic assessment, and associated synovitis or chondromalacia may affirm the diagnosis of ulnocarpal impaction. With the ability to debride avascular flaps and to repair peripheral defects, the arthroscope can be an indispensable adjunct for diagnosis and treatment of TFCC lesions.[93]

Treatment

The TFCC has three important functions: it is a major stabilizer of the distal radioulnar joint; it serves as a cushion or load bearer for transfer of ulnar axial loads; and it is a major stabilizer of the ulnar carpus and hand on the forearm. Posttraumatic clinical assessment should address which functions have been altered, and treatment should proceed accordingly.

If an athlete has sustained an acute injury and seeks treatment with a fresh history and physical examination suggestive of subluxation or dislocation of the distal ulna, primary treatment should focus on achieving and maintaining reduction. Such injuries usually result from avulsion of the TFCC from the ulnar styloid base or from the distal radius, and therefore the forearm should be immobilized. If dorsal ulnar subluxation has occurred, the forearm is placed in full supination with the elbow at 90 degrees. For a volarward dislocated ulna the wrist is im-

mobilized in pronation and the elbow at 90 degrees. Joint congruity in the cast must be checked with CT scan. If closed reduction is not successful, operative intervention is warranted. If the ulnar styloid is fractured *and* if it is a large enough fragment, it may be approximated with tension band wires or compression screw; the TFCC itself can be reapproximated with sutures or intraosseous wires.[17,51] The lunotriquetral ligament in all these cases should be evaluated to exclude associated injury.[99]

Acute perforations of the central portion of the TFCC are believed to be rare.[50,85,95] Those that are seen usually have neutral or positive ulnar variance.[86,95] Most become asymptomatic with conservative care. However, some patients complain of persistent wrist pain and clicking. If the clinical diagnosis is ulnar impaction syndrome and x-ray scans demonstrate positive ulnar variance, an ulnar shortening osteotomy can be recommended without any further diagnostic workup. With negative or neutral ulnar variance, arthrography and/or arthroscopy are performed to evaluate degenerative changes in the TFCC, the ulnar head, and lunate to determine whether impaction exists and if ulnar osteotomy is needed.[23] Consideration should also be given to wafer resection of the distal ulna to achieve decompression and to allow for TFCC debridement.[38] If no impaction exists, then debridement of the flap should be all that is necessary. If the physician is not skilled with the wrist arthroscope, open debridement may be performed, although recovery is prolonged.

Treatment of the older athlete who has chronic wrist pain secondary to (an old) TFCC tear, is initially conservative, consisting of splint support, nonsteroidal antiinflammatory drugs (NSAIDs), and local injection. If these measures are not successful, the same workup is recommended, and treatment options are the same. Some authors advise complete excision of the disk,[24] but based on the functions of the TFCC, we believe that total excision should be avoided if at all possible. Recent studies indicate that significant kinematic and structural changes occur when more than two thirds of the articular disk is removed.[1] We therefore recommend limited central excision of the TFCC in traumatic and degenerative lesions.[1]

Bowers[17] has described many of the soft-tissue approaches used in reconstruction of the chronically unstable distal radioulnar joint, using portions of flexor carpi ulnaris, extensor carpi ulnaris, and extensor retinaculum, but we have not been consistently pleased with long-term results of such procedures for younger athletes. Accurate initial assessment prevents such difficult and unsatisfactory choices in the vigorous athlete. For athletes with chronic injuries and degenerative changes of the articular surfaces, we prefer a partial or complete (Darrach) ulnar head resection, although in certain cases some authors advise ulnar shortening and lunotriquetral fusion.[95]

SUMMARY

Although they involve a wide spectrum of anatomy and pathologic conditions, acute carpal ligament injuries can be accurately diagnosed and effectively treated. Restora-

tion of optimal function requires a careful and detailed examination in conjunction with proper imaging studies to establish the site and degree of damage. Healthy athletes deserve our best efforts. With early treatment and supervised rehabilitation, most are able to resume their previous activities.

ACKNOWLEDGMENT

The authors thank Fran Sherwin, M.A., for her editorial assistance.

REFERENCES

1. Adams BD: Partial excision of the triangular fibrocartilage complex articular disk: a biomechanical study, *J Hand Surg* 18A:334, 1993.
2. Alexander CE, Lichtman DM: Ulnar carpal instabilities, *Orthop Clin North Am* 15:307, 1984.
3. Alexander CE, Lichtman DM: Triquetrolunate and midcarpal instability. In Lichtman DM (ed): *The wrist and its disorders,* Philadelphia, 1988, WB Saunders.
4. Almquist EE et al: Four bone ligament reconstruction for treatment of chronic complete scapholunate separation, *J Hand Surg* 16A:322, 1991.
5. Ambrose L, Posner MA: Lunotriquetral and midcarpal joint instability, *Hand Clin* 8(4):653, 1992.
6. Arkless R: Cineradiography of normal and abnormal wrists, *Am J Roentgenol* 96:837, 1966.
7. Armstrong GWD: Rotational subluxation of the scaphoid, *Can J Surg* 11:306, 1968.
8. Beckenbaugh RD: Accurate evaluation and management of the painful wrist following injury, *Orthop Clin North Am* 15:289, 1984.
9. Bednar MS, Arnoczky SP, Weiland AJ: The microvasculature of the triangular fibrocartilage complex: its clinical significance, *J Hand Surg* 16A:1101, 1991.
10. Bellinghausen HW et al: Posttraumatic palmar carpal subluxation, *J Bone Joint Surg* 65A:998, 1983.
11. Beltran J, Shankman S, Schoenberg NY: Ligamentous injuries to the wrist: imaging technique, *Hand Clin* 8(4):611, 1992.
12. Berger RA, Kauer JMG, Landsmeer JMF: Radioscapholunate ligament: a gross anatomic and histologic study of fetal and adult wrists, *J Hand Surg* 16A:350, 1991.
13. Blatt G: Capsulodesis in reconstructive hand surgery—dorsal capsulodesis for the unstable scaphoid and volar capsulodesis following excision of the distal ulna, *Hand Clin* 3:81, 1987.
14. Blatt G: Scapholunate instability. In Lichtman DM (ed): *The wrist and its disorders,* Philadelphia, 1988, WB Saunders.
14a. Blatt G, Nathan R: *Dorsal capsulodesis for rotary subluxation of the scaphoid—a review of the long-term results,* Paper presented at the American Society for Surgery of the Hand 47th Annual Meeting, Phoenix, Nov 1992.
15. Blevens AD et al: Radiocarpal articular contact characteristics with scaphoid instability, *J Hand Surg* 14A:781, 1989.
16. Bond JR, Berquist TH: Radiologic evaluation of hand and wrist motion, *Hand Clin* 7:1, 1991.
17. Bowers WH: The distal radioulnar joint. In Green DP (ed): *Operative hand surgery,* ed 2, New York, 1988, Churchill Livingstone.
18. Brown DE, Lichtman DM: Midcarpal instability, *Hand Clin* 3:135, 1987.
19. Brumfield RH, Champoux JA: A biomechanical study of normal functional wrist motion, *Clin Orthop* 187:23, 1984.
20. Cantor RM, Stern PM, Wyrich JD: *Selective bilateral wrist arthrography,* Paper presented at the American Society for Surgery of the Hand 47th Annual Meeting, Phoenix, Nov 1992.
21. Chamay A, Pellasanta D, Vilaseca A: Radiolunate arthrodesis: factors of stability for the rheumatoid wrist, *Ann Chir Main* 3:5, 1983.
22. Chidgey LK et al: Histologic anatomy of the triangular fibrocartilage, *J Hand Surg* 16A:1084, 1991.

23. Chun S, Palmer AK: The ulnar impaction syndrome: follow-up of ulnar shortening osteotomy, *J Hand Surg* 18A:46, 1993.
24. Coleman HM: Injuries of the articular disc at the wrist, *J Bone Joint Surg* 42:522, 1960.
25. Conyers DJ: Scapholunate interosseous reconstruction and imbrication of palmar ligaments, *J Hand Surg* 15A:690, 1990.
26. Culver JE: Instabilities of the wrist, *Clin Sports Med* 5:725, 1986.
27. Curtis DJ: Injuries of the wrist: an approach to diagnosis, *Radiol Clin North Am* 19:625, 1981.
28. Curtis DJ et al: Importance of soft tissue evaluation in hand and wrist trauma: statistical evaluation, *Am J Radiol* 142:781, 1984.
29. Cyriax EF: On the rotatory movements of the wrists, *J Anat* 60:199, 1926.
30. Czitrom AA, Dobyns JH, Linscheid RL: Ulnar variance in carpal instability, *J Hand Surg* 12A:205, 1987.
31. Dalinka MK et al: Magnetic resonance imaging of the wrist, *Hand Clin* 7(1):87, 1991.
32. Dobyns JH, Linscheid RL: Editorial comment: carpal bone injuries, *Clin Orthop* 149:2, 1980.
33. Dobyns JH et al: Traumatic instability of the wrist. In AAOS: *Instructional course lectures,* vol 24, St Louis, 1975, Mosby.
34. Reference deleted in proofs.
35. Douglas DP, Peimer CA, Koniuch MP: Wrist motion after simulated limited intercarpal arthrodesis—an experimental study, *J Bone Joint Surg* 69A:1413, 1987.
36. Fassler PR, Stern PJ, Kiefhaber TR: Asymptomatic SLAC wrist: does it exist? *J Hand Surg* 18A:682, 1993.
37. Favero KJ, Bishop AT, Linscheid RL: *Lunotriquetral ligament disruption: a comparative study of treatment methods,* Paper presented at The American Society for Surgery of the Hand 46th Annual Meeting, Orlando, 1991.
38. Feldon P, Terrono AL, Belsky MR: Wafer distal ulna resection for posttraumatic disorders of the distal radioulnar joint, *J Hand Surg* 17A:731, 1992.
39. Fisk GR: An overview of injuries of the wrist, *Clin Orthop* 149:137, 1980.
40. Fortin PT, Louis DS: Long term follow-up of scaphoid-trapezium-trapezoid arthrodesis, *J Hand Surg* 18A:675, 1993.
41. Frankel VH: The Terry-Thomas sign, *Clin Orthop* 129:121, 1977.
42. Friedman SL et al: The change in ulnar variance with grip, *J Hand Surg* 18A:713, 1993.
43. Gilford WW, Bolton RH, Lambrinudi C: The mechanism of the wrist joint with special reference to fractures of the scaphoid, *Guy's Hosp Rep* 92:529, 1943.
44. Gilula LA: Carpal injuries: analytic approach and case exercises, *Am J Radiol* 133:503, 1979.
45. Gilula LA, Weeks PN: Post-traumatic ligamentous instability of the wrist, *Radiology* 129:641, 1978.
46. Gilula LA et al: Roentgenographic diagnosis of the painful wrist, *Clin Orthop* 187:52, 1984.
47. Glickel SZ, Millender L: Results of ligamentous reconstructions for chronic carpal instability, *Orthop Trans* 6:167, 1982.
48. Green DP: Carpal dislocations and instabilities. In Green DP (ed): *Operative hand surgery,* ed 2, New York, 1988, Churchill Livingstone.
49. Green DP, O'Brien ET: Classification and management of carpal dislocations, *Clin Orthop* 149:55, 1980.
50. Hamlin C: Traumatic disruption of the distal radioulnar joint, *Am J Sports Med* 5:93, 1977.
51. Hermansdorfer JD, Kleinman WB: Management of chronic peripheral tears of the triangular fibrocartilage complex, *J Hand Surg* 16A:340, 1991.
52. Homs S, Ruby LK: Attempted scapholunate arthrodesis for chronic scapholunate dissociation, *J Hand Surg* 16A:334, 1991.
53. Horii E et al: A kinematic study of lunotriquetral dissociations, *J Hand Surg* 16A:355, 1991.
54. Howard FN, Fahey T, Wojcik E: Rotatory subluxation of the navicular, *Clin Orthop* 104:134, 1974.
55. Howard FN et al: Symposium: carpal instability, *Contemp Orthop* 4:107, 1982.

56. Isani A, Melone CP: Ligamentous injuries of the hand in athletes, *Clin Sports Med* 5:757, 1986.
57. Johnston HM: Varying positions of the carpal bones in the different movements at the wrist. I. Extension, ulnar and radial flexion, *J Anat* 41:109, 1907.
58. Jones WA: Beware the sprained wrist—the incidence and diagnosis of scapholunate instability, *J Bone Joint Surg* 70B:293, 1988.
59. Kauer JMG: The interdependence of carpal articulation chains, *Acta Anat* 88:481, 1974.
60. Kauer JMG: Functional anatomy of the wrist, *Clin Orthop* 149:9, 1980.
61. Kauer JMG: The mechanism of the carpal joint, *Clin Orthop* 202:16, 1986.
62. Kirk JA, Ansell BN, Bywaters EGL: The hypermobility syndrome, *Ann Rheum Dis* 26:419, 1967.
63. Kleinman WB: Management of chronic rotatory subluxation of the scaphoid by scaphotrapeziotrapezoid arthrodesis—rationale for the technique, postoperative changes in biomechanics, and results, *Hand Clin* 3:113, 1987.
64. Kleinman WB, Carroll C: Scaphotrapeziotrapezoid arthrodesis for treatment of static and dynamic scapholunate instability: a ten-year perspective on pitfalls and complications, *J Hand Surg* 15A:408, 1990.
65. Kleinman WB, Steichen JB, Strickland JW: Management of chronic rotatory subluxation of the scaphoid by scaphotrapeziotrapezoid arthrodesis, *J Hand Surg* 7:125, 1982.
66. Koman LA, Mooney JF, Poehling GG: Fracture and ligamentous injuries of the wrist, *Hand Clin* 6:3, 1990.
67. Landsmeer JMF: Studies in the anatomy of articulation, *Acta Morphol Neerl Scand* 3:287, 1961.
68. Lane LB: The scaphoid shift test, *J Hand Surg* 18A:366, 1993.
69. Levinsohn EM et al: Wrist arthrography: value of the three-compartment injection technique, *Skeletal Radial* 16:539, 1987.
70. Lewis OJ, Hamshere RJ, Bucknill TN: The anatomy of the wrist joint, *J Anat* 106:589, 1970.
71. Lichtman DM et al: Ulnar midcarpal instability—clinical and laboratory analysis, *J Hand Surg* 6:515, 1981.
72. Lichtman DM et al: Palmar midcarpal instability: results of surgical reconstruction, *J Hand Surg* 18A:307, 1993.
73. Linscheid RL, Dobyns JH: Treatment of scapholunate dissociation, rotatory subluxation of the scaphoid, *Hand Clin* 8(4):645, 1992.
74. Linscheid RL et al: Traumatic instability of the wrist diagnosis, classification and pathomechanics, *J Bone Joint Surg* 54A:1612, 1972.
75. MacConaill MA: The mechanical anatomy of the carpus and its bearings on some surgical problems, *J Anat* 75:166, 1941.
76. Manaster BJ, Mann RJ, Rubenstein S: Wrist pain: correlation of clinical and plain film findings with arthrographic results, *J Hand Surg* 14A:466, 1989.
77. Mayfield JK: Patterns of injury to carpal ligaments: a spectrum, *Clin Orthop* 187:36, 1984.
78. Mayfield JK: Wrist ligamentous anatomy and pathogenesis of carpal instability, *Orthop Clin North Am* 15:209, 1984.
79. Mayfield JK, Johnson RP, Kilcoyne RF: The ligaments of the human wrist and their functional significance, *Anat Rec* 186:417, 1976.
80. Mayfield JK, Johnson RP, Kilcoyne RF: Carpal dislocations: pathomechanics and progressive perilunar instability, *J Hand Surg* 5:226, 1980.
81. McMurtry R et al: Kinematics of the wrist: an experimental study of radial/ulnar deviation and flexion-extension, *J Bone Joint Surg* 60A:423, 1978.
82. Metz VM, Gilula LA: Is this scapholunate joint and its ligament abnormal? *J Hand Surg* 18A:746, 1993.
83. Metz VM et al: Variability in measurements of carpal bone angles on lateral wrist radiograph, *J Hand Surg* 16A:893, 1991.
84. Meyerdierks EM, Mosher JF, Werner FW: Limited wrist arthrodesis: a laboratory study, *J Hand Surg* 12A:526, 1987.
85. Mikic ZDJ: Age changes in the triangular fibrocartilage complex of the wrist joint, *J Anat* 126:367, 1978.
86. Milch H: Cuff resection of the ulna for malunited Colles' fracture, *J Bone Joint Surg* 23:311, 1941.
87. Mino DE, Palmer AK, Levinsohn EN: The role of radiography and computerized tomography in the diagnosis of subluxation and dislocation of the distal radioulnar joint, *J Hand Surg* 8:23, 1983.
88. Mino DE, Palmer AK, Levinsohn, EN: Radiography and computerized tomography in the diagnosis of incongruity of the distal radio-ulnar joint, *J Bone Joint Surg* 67A:247, 1985.
89. Moneim MS, Omer GE: Wrist arthrography with acute carpal injuries, *Orthopaedics* 6:299, 1983.
90. Monsivais JJ, Nitz PA, Scully TJ: The role of carpal instability in scaphoid non-union: casual or causal? *J Hand Surg* 11B:201, 1986.
91. Navarro A: *Anales del Instituto de Clinica Quirurgica y Cirugia Experimental,* Imprenta Artistica de Dornaleche, 1935, Montevideo.
92. Navarro A: *Anatomia y fisiologia del carpo,* An Inst Clin Quir Cir Exp, 1935, Montevideo.
93. Osterman AL, Terrill RG: Arthroscopic treatment of triangular fibrocartilage complex lesions, *Hand Clin* 7(2):277, 1991.
94. Palmer AK: Triangular fibrocartilage complex lesions: a classification, *J Hand Surg* 14A:594, 1989.
95. Palmer AK: The distal radioulnar joint: anatomy, biomechanics, and triangular fibrocartilage complex abnormalities, *Hand Clin* 3:31, 1987.
96. Palmer AK, Dobyns JH, Linscheid RL: Management of posttraumatic instability of the wrist secondary to ligament rupture, *J Hand Surg* 3:507, 1978.
97. Palmer AK, Glisson RR, Werner FW: Ulnar variance determination, *J Hand Surg* 7:376, 1982.
98. Palmer AK, Levinsohn EN, Kuzma GR: Arthrography of the wrist, *J Hand Surg* 8:15, 1983.
99. Palmer AK, Werner FW: The triangular fibrocartilage complex of the wrist—anatomy and function, *J Hand Surg* 6:153, 1981.
100. Palmer AK, Werner FW: Biomechanics of the distal radioulnar joint, *Clin Orthop* 187:26, 1984.
101. Peterson HA, Lipscomb PR: Intercarpal arthrodesis, *Arch Surg* 94:127, 1967.
102. Pin PG et al: Management of chronic lunotriquetral ligament tears, *J Hand Surg* 14A:77, 1989.
103. Pin PG et al: Coincident rupture of the scapholunate and lunotriquetral ligaments without perilunate dislocation: pathomechanics and management, *J Hand Surg* 15A:110, 1990.
104. Pisano SM et al: Scaphocapitate intercarpal arthrodesis, *J Hand Surg* 16A:328, 1991.
105. Rask MR: Carponavicular subluxation: report of a case treated with percutaneous pins, *Orthopedics* 2:134, 1979.
106. Ray RD, Johnson RJ, Jameson RN: Rotation of the forearm: an experimental study of pronation and supination, *J Bone Joint Surg* 33A:993, 1951.
107. Rayhack JN et al: Post-traumatic ulnar translation of the carpus, *J Hand Surg* 12A:180, 1987.
108. Reagan DS, Linscheid RL, Dobyns JH: Lunotriquetral sprains, *J Hand Surg* 9A:502, 1984.
109. Rotman MB et al: Scaphocapitolunate arthrodesis, *J Hand Surg* 18A:26, 1993.
110. Ruby LK: Common hand injuries in the athlete, *Clin Sports Med* 2:609, 1983.
111. Ruby LK et al: Relative motion of selected carpal bones: a kinematic analysis of normal wrist, *J Hand Surg* 13A:1, 1988.
112. Sarrafian SK, Melamed JL, Goshgarian GN: Study of wrist motion in flexion and extension, *Clin Orthop* 126:153, 1977.
113. Schuind FA et al: Changes in wrist and forearm configuration with grasp and isometric contraction of elbow flexors, *J Hand Surg* 17A:698, 1982.
114. Sebald JR, Dobyns JH, Linscheid RL: The natural history of collapsed deformities of the wrist, *Clin Orthop* 104:140, 1974.
115. Stuchin SA: Wrist anatomy, *Hand Clin* 8(4):603, 1992.
116. Sutro CJ: Hypermobility of bones due to "over-lengthened" capsular and ligamentous tissues, *Surgery* 21:67, 1947.
117. Taleisnik J: Wrist: anatomy, function and injury. In AAOS: *Instructional course lectures,* St Louis, 1975, Mosby.
118. Taleisnik J: The ligaments of the wrist, *J Hand Surg* 1:110, 1976.
119. Taleisnik J: Post-traumatic carpal instability, *Clin Orthop* 149:73, 1980.

120. Taleisnik J: *The wrist,* New York, 1985, Churchill Livingstone.
121. Taleisnik J: Pain on the ulnar side of the wrist, *Hand Clin* 3:51, 1987.
122. Trumble T et al: Kinematics of the ulnar carpus related to the volar intercalated segment instability pattern, *J Hand Surg* 15A:384, 1990.
123. Uematsu A: Intercarpal fusion for treatment of carpal instability: a preliminary report, *Clin Orthop* 144:159, 1979.
124. Vesely DG: The distal radio-ulnar joint, *Clin Orthop* 51:75, 1967.
125. Viegas SF, Pogue DJ, Hokanson JA: Ulnar sided perilunate instability: an anatomic and biomechanic study, *J Hand Surg* 15A:268, 1990.
126. Viegas SF et al: The effects of various load paths and different loads on the load transfer characteristics of the wrist, *J Hand Surg* 14A:458, 1989.
127. Viegas SF et al: Evaluation of the biomechanical efficacy of limited intercarpal fusions for the treatment of scapholunate dissociation, *J Hand Surg* 15A:120, 1990.
128. Volz RG, Leib N, Benjamin J: Biomechanics of the wrist, *Clin Orthop* 149:112, 1980.
129. VonBonin G: A note on the kinematics of the wrist joint, *J Anat* 63:259, 1919.
130. Watson HK, Ballet FL: The SLAC wrist: scapholunate advanced collapse pattern of degenerative arthritis, *J Hand Surg* 9A:358, 1984.
131. Watson HK, Black DN: Instabilities of the wrist, *Hand Clin* 3:103, 1987.
132. Watson HK, Goodman ML, Johnson TR: Limited wrist arthrodesis. II. Intercarpal and radiocarpal combinations, *J Hand Surg* 6:223, 1981.
133. Watson HK, Hempton RF: Limited wrist arthrodeses. I. The triscaphoid joint, *J Hand Surg* 5:320, 1980.
134. Weber ER: Concepts governing the rotational shift of the intercalated segment of the carpus, *Orthop Clin North Am* 15:193, 1984.
135. Weber ER: Wrist mechanics and its association with ligamentous instabilities. In Lichtman DM (ed): *The wrist and its disorders,* Philadelphia, 1988, WB Saunders.
136. Wright RD: A detailed study of the movement of the wrist joint, *J Anat* 70:137, 1935.
137. Youm Y, Flatt AE: Kinematics of the wrist, *Clin Orthop* 149:21, 1980.
138. Youm Y et al: Kinematics of the wrist. I. An experimental study of radial-ulnar deviation and flexion-extension, *J Bone Joint Surg* 60A:423, 1978.
139. Zlatkin MB et al: Chronic wrist pain: evaluation with high resolution MR imaging, *Radiology* 173:723, 1989.

CHAPTER 25 Wrist Pain

Adolph J. Yates, Jr.
E.F. Shaw Wilgis

The injured wrist of the athlete deserves careful evaluation. Many vague wrist "sprains" improve with conservative therapy and no more specific diagnosis. Wrist sprain, however, should be a diagnosis of exclusion and one that is used less often as sophistication with wrist evaluation improves. The missed scaphoid fracture or undiagnosed ligamentous instability can lead to prolonged impairment and the need for more complicated treatment. The identification of a specific pattern of injury can lead to better-directed care and, when appro-priate, more focused surgical intervention. The results should be an earlier and a safer return to the patient's avocation and avoidance of permanent disability.

Not making a diagnosis carries some significance. In one study[54] 40% of young women with vague wrist pain, followed for a median of 13 years, continued to have pain without any evidence of psychiatric or emotional distur-bance. Such a lingering morbidity in a young population calls for a sharpening of the skills of all clinicians asked to care for the injured wrist. Successful treatment re-quires a correct diagnosis; being knowledgeable of the scope of injury affecting the wrist and the variety of tools needed to define that injury makes achieving the right diagnosis more likely.

The complexity of the wrist makes it uniquely vulner-able to many modes of injury. Anatomically the wrist in-cludes the region between the metacarpals and the dis-tal radius and ulna. Its functions are to position the hand in space and to transmit forces to and from the hand and forearm[16]; few sports do not make demands on these functions. The wrist is required to provide multiaxial mo-tion while bearing forces across its many joints. At the same time it acts as the narrow conduit for the nerves, vessels, and tendons of the most important human or-gan of function—the hand.

HISTORY

A careful history is the beginning of any evaluation of a wrist injury. Often the examiners must rely on the his-tory to pinpoint the site, type, and degree of pain and any motions that exacerbate the discomfort. Previous injury to the wrist should be elicited; injuries whose scale is out of proportion to the mechanism of injury may be the re-sult of an old underlying instability. An example is car-pometacarpal dislocation from light contact in a patient with a previous injury to the same joint from a higher energy accident. What causes or exacerbates the pain of the acute injury can help establish its dynamic compo-nents.

A chronic presentation needs careful questioning about any intervening therapy, its success, and any wax-ing and waning of the pain. The exact mechanism of in-jury may not be available. A history of the patient's sports involvement, including athletic participation in other seasons, as well as work activity is necessary. Most ar-ticular injuries result from excessive loading of the wrist, such as a fall while in dorsiflexion, ulnar deviation, and

carpal supination. Thus it is important to ascertain a traumatic event, however trivial it may seem. The wrist may also absorb injury by excessive use of muscle, be it a single overuse trauma or repetitive activity. Certain sports are associated with specific injuries, such as handlebar palsy,[21,56] catcher's hand,[7,36] and bowler's thumb.[20] The patient's position in team sports should be determined. Riester and associates' study of football players[52] showed a 1 in 100 incidence per season of scaphoid fractures; interestingly, they also showed an 8:3 ratio of defensive to offensive players.

PHYSICAL EXAMINATION

Guided by a careful history, the physician begins examination of the wrist with inspection. The contralateral wrist should be inspected for comparison and should be included throughout the examination as a reference for the involved wrist. Areas of swelling and deformity should be observed, as well as small puncture wounds, lacerations, and old scars. The examiner should record active and passive flexion, extension, pronation, supination, and radioulnar deviation and compare these motions to the contralateral wrist. A careful neurovascular examination is also essential, using two-point discrimination; observation of changes in color, temperature, perspiration, and pulse; and Allen's test. The paths and sensory distributions of the sensory branch of the radial nerve, the dorsal branch of the ulnar nerve, and the palmar cutaneous branch of the median nerve should be checked for neuromata or dysesthesias to light touch.

The history should guide the palpation of the injured wrist. It is important to localize the anatomic point of maximal tenderness. This site can guide the examiner toward anatomic derangements. Each of the carpal bones, the distal radius and the ulna, and the base of the metacarpals should be palpated both volarly and dorsally, as should the anatomic snuffbox, lunate, hamate, triquetrum, distal ulna, distal radioulnar joint, distal pole of the scaphoid, and pisiform. Palpation of the carpal tunnel with its median nerve and flexor tendons should be coupled with palpation of the ulnar nerve and artery in Guyon's canal. The remaining flexor and extensor tendons should also be palpated in their various routes for tenderness, crepitus, or subluxation.

Passive and active range of motion should be observed, as well as the limitations imposed by pain. Palpation over the radioulnar, radiocarpal, ulnocarpal, intracarpal, and carpometacarpal joints during motion can reveal clicks and hesitations. A click alone does not mean a pathologic condition; however, a painful click may have clinical significance, often reflecting carpal instabilities. A painful click as the wrist is forced into palmar flexion and radial deviation is associated with the proximal pole of the scaphoid moving into subluxation dorsally over the rim of the radius, a sign of scapholunate dissociation. The clicks associated with ulnar instability usually occur with ulnar deviation and rotation.

Special tests can be useful in wrist examination. **Finkelstein's test** is used to evaluate the first dorsal compartment (containing the abductor pollicis longus and extensor pollicis brevis) for tendinitis. The examiner holds the thumb flexed and abducted and then deviates the wrist ulnarward, stretching those tendons. A positive test elicits pain over the first dorsal compartment.

Wrist examination: special tests

- Finkelstein's test
- Phalen's test
- Watson's test (scaphoid shift)
- Injection tests
- Scaphoid compression test
- Grip strength

Phalen's test consists of permitting the wrist to drop into a palmar flexed position for 60 seconds to duplicate the symptoms of carpal tunnel syndrome when Tinel's sign is inconclusive. **Watson's test,** or the scaphoid shift,[62] has been described by several authors[5,24] and involves using the fingers to apply pressure over the distal dorsal radius while using the thumb to apply pressure over the palmar distal pole of the scaphoid. The wrist is then put through radial deviation. A painful click in the area of the scaphoid denotes a positive test; the click is secondary to dorsal subluxation of the scaphoid and is considered a sign of scapholunate instability. Watson[61] has shown, however, that 20% of 1000 randomly selected normal subjects had a positive scaphoid shift, and of these, only half were symptomatic.

Suspected scaphoid fractures are traditionally examined by palpation of the anatomic snuffbox. The **scaphoid compression test** is done by compressing the first ray longitudinally. It has been shown to have both good sensitivity and specificity; an added advantage is that it can be performed with a cast in place, and a negative test correlates to a healed fracture.[11]

Another important diagnostic tool is the injection of a local anesthetic at the point of greatest tenderness. Generally, 1% to 2% lidocaine injected into the point of tenderness can help localize the anatomic derangement and dictate therapeutic options. The examiner should assess the range of motion and grip strength before and after injection. Steroid injections, when appropriate, can accompany such injections.[24]

A final special test is the use of **grip strength testing,** especially in chronic wrist pain. As a screening test it has been reported to show a correlation between a decrease in grip strength and either a positive bone scan or confirmed injury.[18]

RADIOGRAPHY

Radiographs are the next step in evaluating the wrist. The importance of routine posteroanterior (PA) and lateral radiographs in the neutral position cannot be overemphasized. Various diagnostic algorithms have been proposed for acute[32,34] and chronic[12,34] wrist pain. They all emphasize the importance of the history, physical examination, and basic radiographs with special views as

the routine start of the wrist evaluation; more expensive imaging studies are reserved for when the diagnosis is not evident from routine films.

With **PA radiographs** the scaphoid and the distance between the carpal bones can be assessed. A gap of 3 mm or more between the scaphoid and lunate is abnormal and indicates a tear of the scapholunate interosseous ligament. A supinated, clenched-fist anteroposterior (AP) radiograph accentuates this gap. A foreshortening of the scaphoid and the ring sign, which is the distal tubercle seen head-on, both suggest palmar flexion of the scaphoid. A widened space between the lunate and triquetrum may denote a tear of the lunatotriquetral ligament.

Radiographic normal limits

- Scapholunate gap (posteroanterior): <3 mm
- Scapholunate angle (lateral): 30 to 70 degrees

On the **lateral radiograph** an angle between the long axis of the scaphoid and the lunate greater than 70 degrees is abnormal and consistent with scapholunate dissociation. An angle of 30 degrees or less is also abnormal and could signify ulnocarpal instability. Lateral radiographs in full flexion and extension complement PA radiographs in radial and ulnar deviation when the examiner is assessing carpal instability.[24] Comparison radiographs of the contralateral wrist are valuable.

Special plain radiographs can further elucidate pathologic conditions. A **carpal tunnel view,** which is a radiograph with the wrist in full extension, fingers extended, and the beam in front of the third metacarpal, helps the examiner visualize fractures of the hook of the hamate. The pisotriquetral area can be better seen with lateral radiographs of the hand and forearm in 10 to 15 degrees of supination.[24] **Couno and Watson's special view**[17,24] offers better visualization of the carpometacarpal joints; this is a lateral view taken with 30 degrees of supination and 20 to 30 degrees of ulnar deviation. The scaphotrapeziotrapezoid (STT) joint is better seen with the supinated oblique.[34]

Additionally, **fluoroscopy** and **cineradiography** allow the physician to view the wrist while it is in motion and are the best techniques for demonstrating dynamic instability patterns. Coupling fluoroscopy with **arthrography** is also useful. Videotape fluoroscopy can be particularly helpful with obscure pain.[27] It is most commonly done by injecting contrast into the radiocarpal joint at the radial stylus; potential injury is represented by a communication through the scapholunate or lunotriquetral ligaments, or through the triangular fibrocartilage complex (TFCC). Because of unidirectional defects, injections into the midcarpal and distal radioulnar joints have also been recommended.[65,68] Digital subtraction arthrography is not useful if there is motion[65] but potentially increases the yield of the procedure; one study showed a high correlation of ulnar-sided perforations

with ulnar-sided pain, and less so with radial lesions and radial-sided pain.[37] The same study showed a lower than expected incidence of scapholunate perforation (26%) in the presence of scapholunate dissociation.[37] **Double contrast arthrography** has been described as useful in diagnosing loose foreign bodies.[60]

With vague wrist complaints, **bone scans** are a useful screening device. A positive scan can localize lesions and dictate further diagnostic workup, whereas a negative scan confirms the absence of articular pathologic conditions. Cases of fractures or intrinsic ligament ruptures have an abnormal scan 95% of the time, as opposed to wrists without definable injury having a normal scan rate of 96%.[49] Bone scans are less useful for partial ligament injuries and synovitis.[49] Sports enthusiasts pose at least one special scintigraphic challenge; a false positive scan of an asymptomatic wrist has been reported in an athlete that returned to fencing between injection and imaging.[29]

Trispiral tomography has replaced laminar tomography for more careful evaluation of possible fractures or cases of avascular necrosis.[51] Acute and chronic fractures of the scaphoid and the hamate and the early sclerotic or cystic changes of avascular necrosis of the scaphoid, lunate, and hamate are often seen on such tomographic views when not visualized on plain radiographs. It is important that the clinician specify that both AP and lateral views are needed. An alternative approach is the use of computed tomography (CT); this depends on the availability and the quality of the scanner and its resolution. It offers much of the same information as above and is probably the best way to evaluate the distal radioulnar joint.[46]

Magnetic resonance imaging (MRI) of the wrist is still evolving but has the advantage of soft-tissue definition and no radiation exposure. It has been shown effective in evaluating ganglion cysts, fractures of the hamate, nonunions of the scaphoid, the compression of the median nerve in carpal tunnel syndrome,[64] and carpal avascular necrosis.[15] When used to evaluate the TFCC, it has reported values of accuracy ranging from 89% to 95% when compared with arthrography and 90% to 95% when compared with arthroscopy/arthrotomy.[23,55,69] Although constantly improving, MRI in vitro is inferior to three-compartment digital subtraction arthrography for the interosseous ligaments and the TFCC.[25] **Cine MRI** as a research tool has been used by Mandelbaum[38] to find subtle dynamic instabilities in the distal radioulnar joint in gymnasts.

The various modalities of radiography available require the clinician to consider time and cost and to use the history and physical examination to selectively guide decisions. Incidental and misleading findings are possible in any study, especially arthrography and bone scans, and must be coupled with a leading diagnosis and not obtained in shotgun fashion.

ARTHROSCOPY

Diagnostic and therapeutic arthroscopy can be used in the patient with acute or chronic wrist pain. Effective in-

strumentation would include a 2.7-mm scope, a mini shaver, and a probe. In the acute situation, if conventional examination and radiographic technique fail to reveal the pathologic condition, an arthroscope can be inserted in the radiocarpal region between the digital extensor tendons and wrist extensor tendons in the fluid-filled and distracted wrist joint in an appropriately anesthetized patient. Appropriate visualization of the articular surface of the radius and ulna and triangular fibrocartilage complex can be made. The scaphoid and interligamentous structures between the scaphoid and lunate and triquetrum can be inspected and probed through a probe inserted on the ulnar aspect of the wrist. The arthroscope can then be introduced deeply, and the volar ligaments can be inspected. Small ligamentous tears can be shaved, and synovium can be removed with a mini shaver.

The midcarpal joint can also be inspected arthroscopically and the ligaments probed for diagnostic purposes.

For chronic pain diagnostic arthroscopic surgery can be combined with therapeutic arthroscopic surgery if necessary. Therapeutic surgery for the most part consists of synovectomy and a shaving of ligamentous tears. This has been a valuable addition for the patient with unexplained or undiagnosed wrist pain and, in many cases, can help evaluate the situation before planning definitive treatment. For example, if a patient is considering a procedure within the wrist joint, such as an intercarpal arthrodesis, the articular surfaces should be inspected and a prediction made as to whether the treatment would be appropriate on a long-term basis. We have found this to be particularly useful in evaluating the treatment of scaphoid nonunion and concomitant radioscaphoid arthritis. Visualization of the radioarticular surface will direct our treatment depending on the presence or absence of articular damage.

Wrist arthroscopy has the potential to become the gold standard for evaluation of chronic wrist pain. Dynamic maneuvers during arthroscopy have been shown to be more sensitive than radiographs in discovering scapholunate dissociation and may show "preradiographic" lesions.[19] Pathologic findings believed to be potentially diagnostic were found in around 95% of two series of chronic wrist injuries[30,44]; in posttraumatic cases, however, it has been reported that arthroscopy revealed injury that was a plausible source of symptoms only 70% of the time.[1]

DIFFERENTIAL DIAGNOSIS OF WRIST PAIN

The following is not an exhaustive listing of pathologic conditions of the wrist. It reviews the more common problems of the wrist likely to occur from trauma or overuse, especially in a sports setting. To simplify the array of conditions, the derangements are catalogued into two broad groups. Articular injuries include all bony and ligamentous conditions isolated to the carpus, whereas extraarticular injuries pertain to lesions of the tendons, nerves, and vessels that cross the carpus.

Fractures
Scaphoid

The most common of the carpal bones to be fractured is the scaphoid, accounting for approximately 70% of carpal fractures.[3] It occurs in a 1:10 ratio to fractures of the distal radius but occurs more frequently in the younger sports-related population.[14] Waist fractures of the scaphoid have been shown to be caused by pressure to the radial aspect of the palm with the wrist in dorsiflexion.[63] The scaphoid bridges the two carpal rows, making it more prone to injury with falls onto the outstretched distal palm.[63] Diagnosis of this fracture begins with heightened suspicion. Any pain in the radiocarpal area should be suspected of being a scaphoid fracture. A partial differential diagnosis includes fractures of the trapezium or radial styloid, de Quervain's disease, and osteoarthritis of the first carpometacarpal joint.[11] Palpable tenderness of the scaphoid, either on the volar side or in the anatomic snuffbox, necessitates 2 weeks' immobilization, even with normal radiographs. At both the initial presentation and the 2-week follow-up, the scaphoid series as described previously is the first line of x-ray evaluation. If a fracture is not seen on plain radiographs at that time and if the patient continues to have tenderness, tomograms or bone scan can be obtained to confirm the diagnosis. MRI can also be helpful in establishing the diagnosis of scaphoid fracture and has the added advantage of reverting to normal with bony union.[28]

The reason for such concern with this fracture is its predilection to go on to delayed union or nonunion and, more important, to the high incidence of avascular necrosis (AVN) associated with scaphoid fractures. The scaphoid has a single interosseous artery, and 70% of the blood supply to the proximal pole depends on one dorsal branch of the radial artery.[22] As a result, 30% of middle-third fractures and close to 100% of proximal fractures go on to AVN.[22,67]

Scaphoid fractures can be classified by the timing of their presentation, their anatomic location, their configuration, and the amount of initial displacement. The fracture that is seen 2 hours after injury differs from the one that is seen 2 weeks after injury and differs even more from the one that is seen 2 months after injury. Anatom-

---

Distribution of scaphoid fractures

- Middle third: 70%
- Proximal third: 20%
- Distal third: 10%

---

ically, 70% of scaphoid fractures occur through the middle third; 20% proximally; and 10% through the distal third.[53] Some authors have classified the fracture by its configuration, either being a horizontal oblique, transverse, or vertical oblique fracture; the clinical significance is that the last of these three is considered unstable.[53] Another commonly used criterion for stability is the degree of initial displacement.

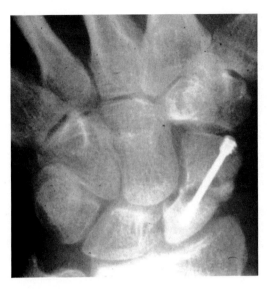

FIG. 25-1. Scaphoid fracture internally fixed with a Herbert screw.

The significance of the various classifications is both prognostic and therapeutic. Prognostically, a delayed presentation, a proximal-third fracture, or one that is displaced has a higher likelihood of going on to nonunion or AVN. These types of fractures may warrant more prolonged immobilization, long arm casting, and possibly more aggressive early surgical intervention (Fig. 25-1).

**Prognostic factors for nonunion
or avascular necrosis**

- Delayed presentation
- Proximal-third fracture
- Displacement

The nondisplaced, stable fracture can be initially treated with a short arm–thumb spica cast in slight palmar flexion and slight radial deviation.[14,67] The cast should be changed every 3 to 4 weeks to ensure a good fit, and radiographs should be taken frequently to guarantee adequate position. Average duration of immobilization is about 3 months.[14,67] The displaced fracture first needs reduction through longitudinal traction and is then casted in a long arm spica cast.[14] If the reduction is adequate, the same stipulations apply as above, and the long arm cast can be converted to a short arm cast at about the sixth or eighth week. Inability to reduce the fracture is an indication for surgery. Once the fracture is thought to be healed, the patient can resume activity wearing a rigid splint for at least the first 2 months.[67] Riester and associates,[52] Cabrera and McCue,[7] and Bergfield and associates[2] have all reported successful treatment of football players with acute scaphoid fractures in soft but rigid Silastic or silicone casts that allowed them to continue their sports participation. The decision to al-

low contact sports during the period of initial immobilization should be individualized not only to the fracture pattern, but more importantly, to the needs and level of competition of the athlete, with his or her full participation in the decision and understanding of the risks involved.

Triquetrum

The triquetrum is the second most fractured carpus.[3] Chip or avulsion fractures are the most common. Body fractures are unusual in the athlete.[67] The dorsal chip fracture is most common and is thought to be secondary to hyperflexion, ulnar deviation, and impingement on the ulnar styloid.[6,33] Splinting for 4 to 6 weeks is usually sufficient and allows the patient to return to sports.[6,33] Occasional nonunions of the chip fracture types require excision when symptomatic.[6]

Hamate

The hamate is a less frequently fractured carpal bone. The hook of the hamate, however, is particularly prone to injury in club and racquet sports such as golf, baseball, and tennis. The classic and often seen example of method of injury is the dubbed golf swing; the force of the swing is blocked by the ground, transmitted up the shaft of the club, and levered against the hypothenar area of the top of the hand, causing a hook of the hamate fracture.[6,67] A history of such an injury or pain in the hypothenar area should lead to special views such as the carpal tunnel view. An oblique view with the wrist in supination can show a lateral profile of the fracture. Both CT and MRI have been used to show this fracture as well (Fig. 25-2).[64] Plaster immobilization of these fractures has been reported to result in only a 46% rate of healing[8]; this leads many authors to suggest the option of early excision of the hook fragment, which can lead to a much earlier return to activity.[6,8,9,57,67]

Hook of hamate evaluation

- Carpal tunnel view
- Oblique view with wrist in supination
- Computed tomography
- Magnetic resonance imaging

Lunate

Fractures of the other carpal bones are less common, but certain aspects should be considered. Compression fractures of the lunate from repetitive trauma that interrupts the blood supply have been suggested as the cause of Kienböck's disease, or avascular necrosis of the lunate. The minor repetitive trauma of sports can also cause this disease with little to differentiate those patients from occupational cases than a younger age and less ulnar variance.[43]

The diagnosis is indicated by well-localized pain over the lunate and a secondary decrease in the range of motion in the involved wrist. Early radiographs may appear

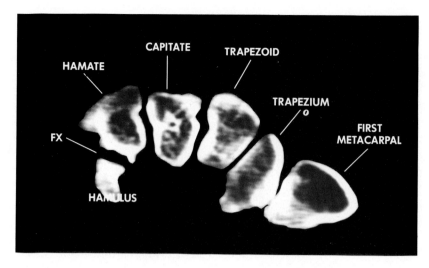

FIG. 25-2. Computed tomography scan depicting fracture of the hook of the hamate.

normal, despite definitive symptoms; tomograms and bone scans are the next step and often uncover early changes despite normal plain radiographs. Treatment of Kienböck's disease is beyond the scope of this chapter. However, patients with suspected and unconfirmed Kienböck's disease can be treated with a short arm cast for several weeks. The definitive surgical therapy of this entity is controversial. In Nakamura's et al series,[43] seven out of 10 athletes returned to sports after a variety of treatments including conservative management, shortening of the radius, lateral closing osteotomy of the radius, and proximal row carpectomy.

Pisiform

Fractures of the pisiform are usually secondary to direct trauma.[6,67] These are usually best treated with a short arm cast for 3 to 6 weeks.[6,67] Occasionally posttraumatic arthrosis may necessitate excision, with postoperative recovery lasting about 8 weeks.[67]

Trapezium

The trapezium is usually injured by a blow to the adducted thumb or a fall on the hyperextended wrist in radial deviation.[6,67] Nondisplaced avulsion or vertical fractures can be treated conservatively with casting; displaced vertical fractures, however, are best treated by internal fixation either by percutaneous pinning or by open reduction, the choice depending on the size and reducibility of the fracture.[6,67]

Capitate

Capitate fractures can occur as an isolated entity; they may, however, be a sign of scaphocapitate fracture as the result of continuing deforming hyperextension after the more typical fracture of the scaphoid and subsequent impingement of the radius.[58] For isolated capitate fractures conservative therapy consisting of splinting or casting will suffice.[6] If reduction is not possible, open reduction and internal fixation are necessary.[67] The capitate is an-

other of the carpal bones at risk for AVN after fracture. Both AVN and posttraumatic arthrosis may require midcarpal arthrodesis.[6]

Trapezoid

The trapezoid is the least frequently fractured carpus. It responds well to casting for 3 to 6 weeks. Again, late posttraumatic arthrosis may indicate fusion.[6]

Ligament Injuries and Instability

The intercalated wrist is without intrinsic musculature. Its dynamic and static stability depends on intracapsular ligaments, interosseous ligaments, and the inherent stability of the different joint configurations. The major volar intracapsular ligaments are the radiocapitate, the radiotriquetral, and the radioscaphoid; the important dorsal intracapsular ligament is the dorsal radiocarpal ligament.[16,39] The interosseous ligaments run circumferentially around each carpal row, primarily giving rotational stability from one carpal bone to another.[16]

Wrist instability from injury to these ligaments is an intricate topic. The instability may be seen on examination as tenderness in a certain area alone or as a painful click such as in Watson's test, described previously. If static instability exists, then plain radiographs will reveal gaps in the carpal rows, particularly the scapholunate area or the triquetrolunate area on AP or oblique views. On normal lateral views the lunate lies within a 0- to 15-degree arc of longitudinal alignment between the radius and the capitate. A collapse that results in dorsiflexion of the lunate is referred to as a **dorsal intercalated segmental instability (DISI).** When the instability results in palmar flexion of the lunate, it is referred to as a **volar intercalated segmental instability (VISI).** Such angulations reflect disruption of the interosseous ligaments on either side of the lunate responsible for rotational control. In a DISI configuration the failed ligament is the scapholunate ligament, which allows volar tilt of the scaphoid and dorsal angulation of the lunate. The oppo-

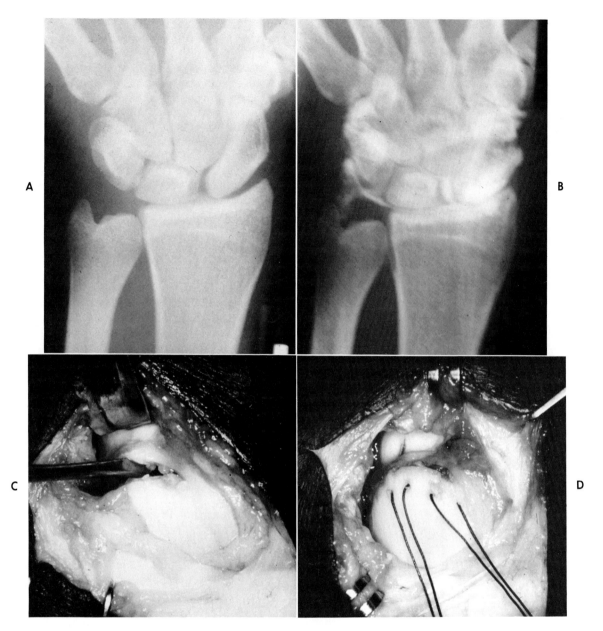

FIG. 25-3. A, Scapholunate ligament rupture. **B,** Arthrogram showing dye in the scapholunate space.
C, The ligament rupture at surgery. **D,** Operative repair of the scapholunate ligament.

site is true of the lunotriquetral ligament, or sometimes the triquetrohamate ligament, the failures of which can cause the VISI configuration. These are gross simplifications of what can be more complicated injuries involving many other structures or fractures. These injuries can be arranged into (1) radial instabilities, which center around injuries to and around the scaphoid; and (2) ulnar instabilities, which involve the lunotriquetral or midcarpal joints.[16]

Differentiating lunotriquetral instability from ulnar impaction syndrome (UIS) is not always simple. Some ways to differentiate the two are that ulnar variance tends to be neutral or positive in UIS; lunotriquetral injuries usually have an identifiable wrist injury in the history; in UIS arthrographic evidence of TFCC injury generally precedes lunotriquetral perforations; and bone scans in UIS show increased uptake of the distal ulna and the lunate.[50] Ulnolunate ligament disruption is another source of reported ulna-sided pain.[41]

Bridging radial and ulnar instability is a sequence of injuries known as progressive perilunar instability.[16,39,40] This sequence is a result of progressive hyperextension, ulnar deviation, and supination, causing circumferential injury to the ligaments surrounding the lunate, starting with the scapholunate ligament, which is stage 1.[16,39,40] The next ligament to be injured is the capitolunate or stage 2, followed by the triquetrolunate. Stage 3 permits dorsal perilunate dislocation. Stage 4 is disruption of the dorsal radiocarpal ligament; this allows volar dislocation of the lunate itself.[16,39,40]

If plain or motion radiographs fail to show the instability, options still include cineradiography and fluoroscopy. If strong clinical suspicion exists for wrist instability, then arthrography can be useful in showing disruptions of the proximal row interosseous ligaments. Once the particular instability has been demonstrated, care must be taken to rule out any associated nondisplaced fractures.

The care of the acutely unstable wrist is controversial, with recommendations ranging from simple immobilization to percutaneous fixation, to open reduction and ligament repair (Fig. 25-3). A conservative approach would be to reduce and hold the wrist immobilized in a cast for 6 to 12 weeks, relying on frequent radiographs to ensure continued reduction; pin fixation would be reserved for failure to hold position.[16] Green[24] believed that neither is stable enough for successful treatment of the acute scapholunate dissociation, and he recommended immediate surgical repair of the ligament.

DISI deformity in association with a displaced scaphoid nonunion has been reported to be a consequence of the bony deformity and not an injury of the scapholunate ligament.[42] Cases exist, however, of confirmed scapholunate ligament injury found at surgery concomitant with scaphoid fractures; such an injury pattern should be considered if there is persistent DISI deformity even with correction of scaphoid fracture with nonunion angulation.[4]

If such an injury is seen later or if it becomes a chronic instability, splinting with the soft cast as described by Bergfield and associates[2] and other authors can provide symptomatic relief. For chronic instability, nonsteroidal antiinflammatory drugs (NSAIDs) and steroid injections may provide significant relief. Surgery is indicated for those patients for whom conservative treatment fails. The various ligament repairs and arthrodeses are beyond the scope of this discussion.

Radioulnar Joint and the Triangular Fibrocartilage Complex

Injuries to the radioulnar joint are easily confused with radiocarpal and carpocarpal complaints. Rotation that causes pain in this area, especially forced resisted pronation that recreates the patient's complaint, suggests injury to the radioulnar joint.[24,46] It needs to be distinguished from ulnocarpal impingement in ulnar-positive wrists, as well as ulnocarpal pathologic conditions. In addition to actual fractures through this area and radioulnar dissociations, the triangular fibrocartilage complex can be torn, causing pain. The triangular fibrocartilage complex is the complicated harness that radiates from the lunate fossa of the radius to the ulna and up to the edges of the ulnar wrist and fifth metacarpal[46]; it acts as a sling, "supporting the distal ulnar carpus and radius from the distal ulna."[46,48]

Diagnostic studies that can aid in evaluating the distal radioulnar joint include CT scans to evaluate possible dissociation, bone scans to help validate clinical suspicions of arthrosis in this area, and arthrograms to help diagnose tears in the triangular fibrocartilage complex. Extrusion of contrast into the radioulnar area is a fre-

quent incidental finding and should not be considered pathognomonic unless coupled with a strong clinical suspicion based on history and examination.[24]

Radioulnar dissociation, ulnocarpal arthrosis, ulnar impingement, and questions of ulnar-positive or -minus wrists can be addressed as chronic problems; they are best treated symptomatically and with splints before entertaining the option of surgery such as arthroplasty or Darrach or Lauenstein procedures. Of more immediate importance is the athlete with a suspected acute triangular fibrocartilage complex tear. Green[24] believed that this is unlikely to have predictably good results if treated operatively at a later time; thus he recommended immediate long-arm casting for 4 to 6 weeks, regardless of the time of athletic season.

Arthroscopic evidence of a TFCC injury in the patient with ulna-sided pain does not automatically explain the symptoms. Taleisnik[59] has argued that arthroscopic debridement of the TFCC should not become a "therapeutic wastebasket"; in making this request he points out other potential sites for pain such as pisotriquetral arthritis, extensor carpi ulnaris injury, ulnocarpal impingement, occult ganglions, and chondromalacia of the head of the ulna. Palmer[47] has proposed a classification system for injury to the TFCC based on the two broad categories of traumatic and degenerative. The classification leads to his treatment recommendations for TFCC injuries that do not respond to conservative measures: never excise the TFCC entirely; limit debridement of horizontal tears; approximate avulsions or midsubstance injuries either through positioning or open repair followed by immobilization; and treat degenerative lesions by ulnar shortening.

Carpometacarpal Injuries

The ulnar four carpometacarpal joints are not commonly involved in sports-related injuries. Their sturdy ligaments and capsules are more likely to be injured in more violent events such as motor vehicle accidents and industrial injuries.[26] Dislocations of these joints are reducible but frequently require open pinning to guarantee stability.[26] Chronic sprains of the same joints can be pinpointed with lidocaine injections.[24,26] The lateral carpometacarpal view is described above and may be helpful in identifying small fractures, arthritis, and subluxation.[17] Although splints may help symptomatically, the procedure of choice is arthrodesis.[26]

Tendinous Injuries

Repetitive motion of the wrist in throwing, lifting, and contact sports can result in various forms of tendinitis, tenosynovitis, and tendon subluxation. Clinically, there is tenderness localized to the involved tendon. Pain is accentuated by passive stretch of the involved tendon. Radiographs are usually normal except for occasional calcifications around the involved tendon sheath.

Dorsal Tendinitis

Dorsal tendinitis is usually secondary to overuse, not infrequently from the backhand of racquet sports. It is manifested by swelling, erythema, and pain with resisted

motion over the tendons involved.[7,66] The second dorsal compartment, containing the radial wrist extensors, and the sixth compartment, containing the extensor carpi ulnaris, are the most common sites of such inflammation after the first compartment (de Quervain's disease).[7,66] Treatment consists of splinting, NSAIDs, activity modification, and eventually strengthening of the involved muscles and is usually effective. Special care should be taken with tendinitis of the third compartment, especially with a history of previous injury; the inflammation may be secondary to posttraumatic deformity of Lister's tubercle following fracture and requires surgery to avoid rupture of the extensor pollicis longus.[66]

de Quervain's Disease

de Quervain's disease represents tenosynovitis of the first dorsal compartment. The first dorsal compartment contains the abductor pollicis longus and extensor pollicis brevis. These tendons are particularly prone to tendinitis from repetitive hand and wrist motions; bowling is a common example. On physical examination there is tenderness and swelling at the radial styloid. There may be a thickened, inflamed cyst over the first dorsal compartment as well. A positive Finkelstein's test is highly suggestive for this condition. If de Quervain's disease is treated early, the treatment is the same as for other dorsal compartments, consisting of rest, splinting, and oral NSAIDs. Steroid injections, if coupled with rest, can also be effective. If conservative therapy fails or if the condition is allowed to progress to a chronic state, surgical decompression becomes necessary. During surgery a search for anatomic abnormalities is important; failure to recognize a separate canal for the extensor pollicis brevis or multiple slips of the abductor pollicis longus may yield an unsatisfactory result.

Recurrent Subluxation of the Extensor Carpi Ulnaris Tendon

Subluxations of the extensor carpi ulnaris rarely are seen as an acute injury.[7] They represent tears of the retinacular restraints of the sixth dorsal compartment, allowing the extensor carpi ulnaris to repeatedly escape its groove and producing snapping symptoms.[24,66] Such a snapping sensation can be felt by palpation over the sixth compartment when the wrist is supinated while in ulnar deviation. Various authors recommend surgical reconstruction of the tendon's restraints if conservative therapy fails.[24,66] Chronic ulna-sided pain from a partial rupture of the extensor carpi ulnaris tendon has been reported; removal of an ulnar ridge, debridement, and tendon sheath reconstruction led to a successful outcome.[13]

Intersection Syndrome

Intersection syndrome is described by Wood and Dobyns[66] and is suggested by pain, crepitus, and a squeaky sensation in the area of the radial dorsal forearm where the abductor pollicis longus and the extensor pollicis brevis cross over the radial wrist extensors. It is common among weight lifters and various types of rowers.[66] The treatment is the same as with other tendinitis problems (i.e., rest, NSAIDs, splinting, and, when needed, steroid

injection) and is usually effective.[66] It is mentioned here to be distinguished from the tendinitis of the more proximal dorsal compartments.

Flexor Tendinitis

The flexor carpi ulnaris is the most common of the flexor tendons to be afflicted with tendinitis.[66] The treatment for this tendon as well as other flexor tendons is similar to that of the extensor tendons, namely, rest, splinting, and NSAIDs.

The flexors of the digits, because of their location within the carpal tunnel, can both mimic and cause carpal tunnel syndrome. Conservative treatment can be successful, but the workup should also consider median nerve compression. If there is no relief of symptoms, both carpal tunnel release and synovectomy of the flexors may be necessary.[7,66] Symptomatic restrictive thumb-index flexor tenosynovitis presents with or without carpal tunnel syndrome and is diagnosed by index finger flexion with thumb flexion across the palm; all have hypertrophic synovium connecting the flexor pollicis longus and the index profundus tendons, and half have tendinous connections.[35] In the Mayo Clinic series[35] describing the above incidence of anomalies, 13 of the 17 patients were helped with surgery and none had long-term relief with steroid injection.

Nerve Compression
Carpal Tunnel Syndrome

Any sports activity requiring repeated hand and wrist motion can cause carpal tunnel syndrome and compression of the median nerve. Symptoms usually consist of pain in the wrist area radiating to three and a half radial digits; there may also be complaints of paresthesias in the same area, often with nocturnal intensification. On examination, positive Tinel's sign over the carpal tunnel, positive Phalen's test, decreased sensation over the median nerve distribution, and signs of thenar motor weakness are all diagnostic. Conservative therapy, consisting of splinting and NSAIDs, can be curative. However, if there is no improvement or if there is any question as to the diagnosis, electromyography and nerve conduction studies can be useful. Persistent symptoms despite treatment and signs of motor weakness are indications to proceed with operative decompression.

Guyon's Canal Syndrome

The ulnar nerve corollary to the carpal tunnel is Guyon's canal. This is another site of potential nerve compression, although less commonly seen. It is a problem seen with cyclists because of the compression of their grips, thus the name "handlebar palsy."[21,56] Although the ulnar nerve does not have to share this small space with the many flexor tendons that sometimes compress the carpal tunnel, it does course through this area with the ulnar artery, and pathologic conditions of the ulnar artery can either mimic or cause ulnar nerve compression. Ganglions can cause compression of the ulnar nerve as well.[31]

Positive Tinel's sign (paresthesias of one and a half ulnar digits) with or without signs of motor branch involve-

TABLE 25-1 Wrist injuries and initial treatment in the athlete

Injury	Treatment
Fractures	
Scaphoid, nondisplaced	Short arm–thumb spica cast; possible surgery
Scaphoid, displaced	Long arm–thumb spica cast; possible surgery with Herbert screw
Triquetrum (chip)	Splint for 4-6 weeks
Hamate (body)	Splint for 4-6 weeks; open reduction internal fixation (ORIF) if displaced
Hamate (hook)	Consider early excision if symptomatic
Lunate	Short arm cast
Trapezium, nondisplaced	Cast for 6 weeks
Trapezium, displaced	Pin, possible ORIF
Capitate	Splint or cast for 6 weeks
Trapezoid	Cast for 3-6 weeks
Ligamentous Injuries	
Acute DISI, VISI, perilunate injuries	Controversial; options include (1) reduction with cast, (2) pin, (3) ligament repair
Chronic DISI, VISI, perilunate injuries	NSAIDs, splint, injection; consider limited fusion
Acute triangular fibrocartilage complex	Long arm cast for 4-6 weeks
Chronic triangular fibrocartilage complex	Splint, NSAIDs, possible flap debridement
Carpometacarpal Dislocation	
Acute injury	Pin, possible ORIF
Tendinous Injuries	
Dorsal and volar tendonitis, de Quervain's disease	NSAIDs, splint, rest
Nerve Injuries	
Carpal tunnel, Guyon's canal	NSAIDs, splint, rest
Ulnar Artery Thrombosis	Excision of segment
Ganglion	Splint, NSAID

ment is diagnostic. Treatment should initially be conservative, including modification of activity, splinting, and the use of NSAIDs. Again, electromyograms and nerve conduction studies may be useful, especially when there is a possibility of more proximal involvement. Failure to respond to conservative treatment is an indication for surgical decompression.[7,66]

Other Causes of Wrist Pain

Vascular Injuries

Repetitive trauma to the ulnar artery along its course through Guyon's canal to its digital branches can cause both thrombosis and aneurysm; this has been called "catcher's hand,"[7,36] but it is also seen in cyclists[45] and handball players.[7] A careful vascular examination, with the use of Doppler ultrasound, can usually make the diagnosis without arteriography.[7] This condition can be asymptomatic but most often occurs with paresthesias in the ulnar nerve distribution. Vasospastic or vasoocclusive symptoms that afflict the digits may also exist. Treatment is surgical, usually with resection of the involved segment.[7,66] Reanastomosis is made if there is no tension,[7] but this and grafting remain controversial.[66] Both the radial artery and persistent median artery can be seen with traumatic thrombosis or aneurysm, the latter causing median nerve neuritis; these are rare injuries.[66]

Ganglions

Ganglions can occur from either intraarticular or extraarticular origins. Diagnosis is usually from palpation,

but pain without mass may be the presenting complaint of an occult dorsal ganglion; articular injection with lidocaine can help make this diagnosis but not definitively.[24] There has been a recent report of the use of MRI to locate ganglions, and this may be of use in such a situation.[64] Extraarticular ganglions most frequently arise from the flexor carpi radialis tendon sheath, the digital extensors, and the roof of the first dorsal compartment.[66] Treatment involves rest and splinting, but again, if there is no improvement, surgical excision may be necessary.

Growth Plate Injuries

Growth plate abnormalities of the distal radius and ulna in adolescent male gymnasts have been reported; the etiology proposed was Salter type stress fractures of the growth plate, with resolution after rest.[10] These may be related to the positive ulna variance reported by Mandelbaum[38] in collegiate gymnasts.

SUMMARY

The preceding discussion of wrist injuries is not unique to athletes. On the contrary, nonathletic injuries to the wrist in each of the above categories far outnumber sports-related ones. There is no dramatic and uniquely sports-related injury in the wrist, such as the anterior cruciate ligament of the knee or the recurrent dislocation of the shoulder. There is, however, a shift in the spectrum of injury because of the younger age of the population involved; the athlete will fracture the scaph-

oid or injure one of its tendons in a fall rather than suffer a Colles' fracture; he or she is more prone to tendinitis from overuse than from underlying arthritis. Expectations are different as well; the athlete's demands for full and immediate functional recovery of the injured part are greater than the industrial-related accident or the same injury in the elderly.

The vast majority of the injuries described can be treated conservatively, and even contact sports can be resumed wearing the soft casts described.[2,7,52] Certain exceptions must be kept in mind. Green[24] believed that injuries to the distal radioulnar joint, in particular a tear in the triangular fibrocartilage complex, should be placed in a long-arm cast immediately; he also stated that disruption of the scapholunate ligament deserves immediate surgical repair. More than one author agrees that hook of the hamate fractures can cause prolonged disability unless they are simply excised on presentation, thus allowing full recovery in as soon as 6 weeks.[6,10,57,67] The return to full contact with a soft cast for a football player with a scaphoid fracture is proposed by some.[2,7,52] Table 25-1 outlines various injuries of the wrist, conservative vs. more immediate surgical therapy, and recommendations as far as return to activity.

The most important point in taking care of the athlete with a wrist injury is recognition of those injuries that carry possible long-term disability without dramatic initial deformity. Wrist "sprains" do exist but should remain a diagnosis of exclusion.

REFERENCES

1. Adolfsson L: Arthroscopy for the diagnosis of post-traumatic wrist pain, *J Hand Surg* 17B:46, 1992.
2. Bergfield JA et al: Soft playing splint for protection of significant hand and wrist injuries in sports, *Am J Sports Med* 10:293, 1982.
3. Borgeskov S et al: Fracture of the carpal bones, *Acta Orthop Scand* 37:276, 1966.
4. Braithwaite IJ, Jones WA: Scapho-lunate dissociation occurring with scaphoid fracture, *J Hand Surg* 17B:286, 1992.
5. Brown DE, Lichtman DM: The evaluation of chronic wrist pain, *Orthop Clin North Am* 15:185, 1984.
6. Bryan RS, Dobyns JH: Fractures of the carpal bones other than lunate or navicular, *Clin Orthop* 149:107, 1980.
7. Cabrera JM, McCue FC III: Nonosseous athletic injuries of the elbow, forearm and hand, *Clin Sports Med* 6:681, 1986.
8. Carroll RE, Lakin JF: Fracture of the hook of the hamate: acute treatment, *J Trauma* 34:803, 1993.
9. Carter PD, Eaton RO, Littler JW: Ununited fracture of the hook of the hamate, *J Bone Joint Surg* 59A:583, 1977.
10. Carter SR et al: Stress changes of the wrist in adolescent gymnasts, *Br J Radiol* 61:109, 1988.
11. Chen SC: The scaphoid compression test, *J Hand Surg* 14B:323, 1985.
12. Chidgey LK: Chronic wrist pain, *Orthop Clin North Am* 23:49, 1992.
13. Chun S, Palmer AK: Chronic ulnar wrist pain secondary to partial rupture of the extensor carpi ulnaris tendon, *J Hand Surg* 12A:1032, 1987.
14. Cooney WP, Dobyns JH, Linscheid RL: Fractures of the scaphoid: a rational approach to management, *Clin Orthop* 149:90, 1980.
15. Cristiani G: Evaluation of ischemic necrosis of carpal bones by magnetic resonance imaging, *J Hand Surg* 15B:249, 1990.
16. Culver JE: Instabilities of the wrist, *Clin Sports Med* 5:725, 1986.
17. Cuono CB, Watson HK: The carpal boss: surgical treatment and etiologic considerations, *Plast Reconstr Surg* 63:88, 1979.
18. Czitrom AA, Lister GD: Measurement of grip strength in the diagnosis of wrist pain, *J Hand Surg* 13A:16, 1988.
19. Dautel G, Goudot B, Merle M: Arthroscopic diagnosis of scapho-lunate instability in the absence of x-ray abnormalities, *J Hand Surg* 18B:213, 1993.
20. Dobyns JH et al: Bowler's thumb: diagnosis and treatment. A review of seventeen cases, *J Bone Joint Surg* 54A:751, 1972.
21. Finelli PF: Handlebar palsy, *N Engl J Med* 292:702, 1975 (letter).
22. Gelberman RH et al: The arterial anatomy of the human carpus. I. The extraosseous vascularity, *J Hand Surg* 8:367, 1983.
23. Golimbu CN: Tears of the triangular fibrocartilage of the wrist: MR imaging, *Radiology* 173:731, 1989.
24. Green DP: The sore wrist without a fracture. In Stauffer ES (ed): *AAOS instructional course lectures,* vol 34, St Louis, 1985, Mosby.
25. Gundry CR et al: Is MR better than arthrography for evaluating the ligaments of the wrist? in vitro study, *Am J Radiol* 154:337, 1990.
26. Gunther SF: The carpometacarpal joints, *Orthop Clin North Am* 15:259, 1984.
27. Hankin FM et al: Dynamic radiographic evaluation of obscure wrist pain in the teenage patient, *J Hand Surg* 11A:805, 1986.
28. Imeda T et al: Magnetic resonance imaging in scaphoid fractures, *J Hand Surg* 17B:20, 1992.
29. Jackson ML, Goldfarb R, Ongseng F: The offensive wrist, *Clin Nucl Med* 11(2):130, 1986.
30. Kelly EP, Stanley JK: Arthroscopy of the wrist, *J Hand Surg* 15B:236, 1990.
31. Kuschner SH, Gelberman RH, Jennings C: Ulnar nerve compression at the wrist, *J Hand Surg* 13A:577, 1988.
32. Larsen CF et al: An algorithm for acute wrist trauma: a systematic approach to diagnosis, *J Hand Surg* 18B:207, 1993.
33. Levy M et al: Chip fractures of the os triquetrum, *J Bone Joint Surg* 61B:355, 1979.
34. Linn MR, Mann FA, Gilula LA: Imaging the symptomatic wrist, *Orthop Clin North Am* 21:515, 1990.
35. Lombardi RM, Wood MB, Linscheid RL: Symptomatic restrictive thumb-index flexor tenosynovitis: incidence of musculotendinous anomalies and results of treatment, *J Hand Surg* 13A:337, 1988.
36. Lowrey CW, Chadwick RO, Waltman EN: Digital vessel trauma from repetitive impact in baseball catchers, *J Hand Surg* 1:236, 1976.
37. Manaster BJ, Mann RJ, Rubenstein S: Wrist pain: correlation of clinical and plain film findings with arthrographic results, *J Hand Surg* 14A:466, 1989.
38. Mandelbaum BR: Wrist pain syndrome in the gymnast: pathogenic, diagnostic, and therapeutic considerations, *Am J Sports Med* 17:305, 1989.
39. Mayfield JK: Wrist ligamentous anatomy and pathogenesis of carpal instability, *Orthop Clin North Am* 15:209, 1984.
40. Mayfield JK, Johnson RP, Kilcoyne R: Carpal dislocation: pathomechanics and progressive perilunar instability, *J Hand Surg* 5:226, 1980.
41. Mooney JF, Poehling GG: Disruption of the ulnolunate ligament as a cause of chronic ulnar wrist pain, *J Hand Surg* 16A:347, 1991.
42. Nakamura R et al: Scaphoid nonunion with DISI deformity, *J Hand Surg* 16B:156, 1991.
43. Nakamura R et al: Sports-related Kienböck's disease, *Am J Sports Med* 19:88, 1991.
44. North ER, Meyer S: Wrist injuries: correlation of clinical and arthroscopic findings, *J Hand Surg* 15A:915, 1990.
45. Nullander LH, Nalebuff EA, Kodson E: Aneurysms and thrombosis of the ulnar artery in the hand, *Arch Surg* 105:686, 1972.
46. Palmer AK: The distal radioulnar joint, *Orthop Clin North Am* 15:321, 1984.
47. Palmer AK: Triangular fibrocartilage complex lesions: a classification, *J Hand Surg* 14A:594, 1989.
48. Palmer AK, Werner FW: The triangular fibrocartilage complex of the wrist: anatomy and function, *J Hand Surg* 6:153, 1981.
49. Pin GP et al: Role of radionuclide imaging in the evaluation of wrist pain, *J Hand Surg* 13A:810, 1988.

50. Pin PG et al: Management of chronic lunotriquetral ligament tears, *J Hand Surg* 14A:77, 1989.
51. Posner MA, Greenspan A: Trispiral tomography for the evaluation of wrist problems, *J Hand Surg* 13A:175, 1988.
52. Riester JN et al: A review of scaphoid fracture healing in competitive athletes, *Am J Sports Med* 13:159, 1985.
53. Russe O: Fracture of the carpal navicular, *J Bone Joint Surg* 47A:759, 1980.
54. Ryley JP, Langstaff RJ, Barton NJ: The natural history of undiagnosed wrist pain in young women, *J Hand Surg* 17B:51, 1992.
55. Schweitzer ME et al: Chronic wrist pain: spin-echo and short tau inversion recovery MR imaging and conventional and MR arthrography, *Radiology* 182:205, 1992.
56. Smail DF: Handlebar palsy, *N Engl J Med* 292:322, 1975 (letter).
57. Stark HH et al: Fracture of the hook of the hamate in athletes, *J Bone Joint Surg* 59A:575, 1977.
58. Stein F, Siegel MW: Naviculocapitate fracture and syndrome: a case report and new thoughts on the mechanism of injury, *J Bone Joint Surg* 51A:391, 1968.
59. Taleisnik J: Clinical and technological evaluation of ulnar wrist pain, *J Hand Surg* 13A:801, 1988 (editorial).
60. Tehranzadeh J, Labosky DA: Detection of intraarticular loose osteochondral fragments by double contrast wrist arthrography: a case report of a basketball injury, *Am J Sports Med* 12:177, 1984.
61. Watson H et al: Rotary subluxation of the scaphoid: a spectrum of instability, *J Hand Surg* 18B:62, 1993.
62. Watson HK, Ashmead D IV, Makhlouf MV: Examination of the scaphoid, *J Hand Surg* 13A:657, 1988.
63. Weber ER, Chao EY: An experimental approach to the mechanism of scaphoid wrist fractures, *J Hand Surg* 3:142, 1978.
64. Weis KL, Beltran J, Lubbers LM: High-field MR surface coil imaging of the hand and wrist. II. Pathologic correlations and clinical relevance, *Radiology* 160:147, 1986.
65. Wilson AJ, Mann FA, Gilula LA: Imaging the hand and wrist, *J Hand Surg* 15B:153, 1990.
66. Wood MB, Dobyns JH: Sports related extraarticular wrist syndromes, *Clin Orthop* 202:93, 1986.
67. Zemel NP, Stark HH: Fractures and dislocations of the carpal bones, *Clin Sports Med* 5:705, 1986.
68. Zinberg EM et al: The triple-injection wrist arthrogram, *J Hand Surg* 13A:803, 1988.
69. Zlatkin MB et al: Chronic wrist pain: evaluation with high-resolution MR imaging, *Radiology* 173:723, 1989.

CHAPTER 26 Hand Injuries

Martin A. Posner

The hand, by virtue of its many functional capabilities and vulnerable anatomic position, is susceptible to a wide variety of sports-related injuries. The incidence of these injuries is difficult to determine because there are few available data. Even in segments of the population where

483

statistics have been compiled, the accuracy is questionable. In organized college sports, for example, statistics have been collected for injuries considered to be significant, that is, preventing the athlete from participating in a sport for at least 1 week.[95] However, many athletes with a variety of serious injuries to the hand continue to play with a cast or brace. Technically these athletes are not considered disabled, so the available data underestimate the true incidence of injuries. However, the data are helpful in indicating those college sports in which the hand is particularly at risk; they include football, gymnastics, wrestling, and basketball.

Sports with higher risk of hand injury

- Football
- Gymnastics
- Wrestling
- Basketball

Regardless of the patient's age or level of proficiency—occasional recreational athlete, serious amateur competitor, or paid professional—all hand injuries require a careful medical evaluation, including appropriate radiographs. Without early and accurate assessment, healing is delayed. A relatively simple problem that could be successfully treated with a splint or cast may progress to a chronic condition requiring complicated surgery. More important, the surgery necessitated by this delay may fail to restore normal mobility or strength, which may prevent the athlete from ever being able to resume full sport participation.

A wide variety of injuries can affect the hand in athletics. Even common abrasions or contusions should not be quickly dismissed as trivial because local swelling, ecchymoses, and tenderness may indicate a more serious injury to underlying structures. This chapter discusses injuries involving muscle-tendon units, ligaments, and bones at specific anatomic regions in the fingers and thumb.

Fingers

CARPOMETACARPAL JOINT AREA

Anatomy

The carpometacarpal joints of the fingers comprise the articulations between the trapezoid, capitate, and hamate, and the bases of the second through fifth metacarpals. Though the trapezium articulates with the radial aspect of the second metacarpal, it is primarily involved with stability and mobility of the first metacarpal and is discussed in the section on the thumb.

The anatomic configuration of the ligaments and the articular surfaces of the finger metacarpals and their contiguous carpal bones form two functional units, one being stable and the other mobile. The carpometacarpal joints of the index and middle fingers are stable, and their metacarpals comprise the longitudinal arch of the hand. The carpometacarpal joints of the ring and little fingers are mobile, with the fifth metacarpal having greater mobility than the fourth. The differences in mobility are due to the unique configuration of the articular surfaces of the joints. The articular surface of the base of the fourth metacarpal is divided into a radial and ulnar portion by a proximal ridge. The ulnar portion articulates with the hamate at a facet that has a quadrangular or semilunar outline and is flat in the transverse axis.[50] The ulnar portion of the hamate is shallow and articulates with the base of the fifth metacarpal, which is convex in the dorsovolar axis and concave in the radioulnar axis. The corresponding surfaces of the hamate and fifth metacarpal resemble the saddle configuration of the basal joint of the thumb. This accounts for the greater mobility of the fifth metacarpal, particularly with respect to flexion and extension.[154]

The functional aspects of the stable and mobile components of the carpometacarpal joints are easily appreciated when the position of the metacarpal heads is observed during finger motion. In complete extension the metacarpal heads of the second and third metacarpals remain stable. However, there is progressive flexion of the heads of the fourth and fifth, resulting in a curved arch. The heads of all of the finger metacarpals make up the distal transverse arch. The curvature of this arch is similar to that of the proximal transverse arch, which is composed of the distal row of carpal bones and is completely rigid.

Muscle-Tendon Injuries

Strains are injuries to muscle-tendon units. Strains can be divided into acute and chronic types, depending on the nature of the forces and the duration of their application. When the cause of injury is a single forceful contraction of the muscle against resistance (overexertion) or when the muscle is suddenly stretched beyond its normal extensile range (overstretching), the result is an acute strain. A chronic strain is caused by excessive use beyond the muscles' fatigue quotient.

Acute strains are classified as first, second, or third degree, depending on the magnitude of the injury to the muscle-tendon unit. Rarely is the tendon itself damaged, provided it is healthy. More commonly damage is to the muscle belly, the musculotendinous junction, or the site of the tendon's insertion into bone.[126] In a first-degree, or mild, strain there is local muscle or tendon irritation, but no loss of strength or mobility. Treatment is primarily symptomatic and consists of rest and avoidance of active motion. A second-degree, or moderate, strain occurs when there is actual damage to a portion of the muscle-tendon unit that compromises its strength. There may be a partial tear of the muscle itself or a partial avulsion of the tendon at its bone insertion. Protection is important in this type of injury to prevent further damage. A third-degree strain is the most severe and is characterized by a complete rupture of a portion of the muscle-tendon unit.

Chronic strains are caused by overuse, which usually occurs over a prolonged period. However, such strains may also occur following a single, prolonged ac-

tivity. Though by definition a chronic strain is not caused by an acute injury, it may be initiated by one that is not adequately treated. The symptoms of a chronic strain are varied and depend on the area of the muscle-tendon unit that is affected. If the muscle itself is fatigued, a myositis develops, which leads to secondary spasm. Similar irritation can occur to the musculotendinous junction, anywhere along the course of the tendon, or at the site of the tendon's insertion into bone. If the tendon is irritated in its course through a sheath where it is surrounded by tenosynovium, tenosynovitis develops. Initially, there may be local tenderness and swelling over the sheath. In more severe cases a fluid exudate develops that can cause adhesions between the tendon and its sheath and interfere with the normal gliding motion of the tendon. Crepitation, sometimes referred to as *snowball crepitation*, can often be palpated with active tendon motion in such cases.[141] If untreated, tenosynovitis can progress until the tendon becomes entrapped within its sheath, which affects mobility of the joint.

In the wrist it is important to differentiate tenosynovitis from an underlying problem involving the wrist liga-ments or carpal bones. This is relatively simple when dealing with tenosynovitis of the abductor pollicis longus and extensor pollicis brevis tendons in the first dorsal tendon compartment (de Quervain's tenosynovitis). The problem becomes more difficult when tenosynovitis involves one of the wrist extensors, particularly the extensor carpi ulnaris. Local pain and tenderness may not be due to inflammation of the tendon, but rather a problem involving the triangular fibrocartilage complex. Injection of the tendon sheath with lidocaine helps differentiate between the two conditions.

Accurate and early diagnosis of tenosynovitis of the digital extensors is important. This is particularly true when the extensor pollicis longus is affected, because this tendon tends to rupture. This complication is rarely seen with a tenosynovitis of any other extensor tendon. An exception might be tenosynovitis of the extensor digiti quinti proprius, which is more likely to occur in a chronic arthritic disorder such as rheumatoid arthritis than after an injury.[170] The extensor pollicis longus is vulnerable because it is a relatively thin tendon that passes through a narrow curved tunnel around Lister's

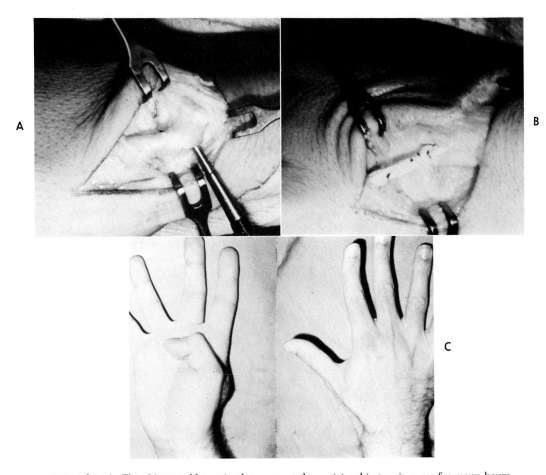

FIG. 26-1. A, This 30-year-old tennis player reported practicing his tennis serve for many hours. Within several days he developed swelling over the dorsal aspect of his wrist and then noted inability to extend the interphalangeal joint of his thumb. At surgery the ruptured extensor pollicis longus tendon ends were joined by an area of scarred tenosynovium. **B** and **C,** Tendon transfer using the extensor indicis proprius to the distal stump of the ruptured tendon was carried out. This restored excellent thumb mobility.

tubercle. If the swelling that occurs with tenosynovitis persists, it can damage the blood supply to the tendon and lead to rupture. Usually this problem occurs after a Colles fracture, more commonly when the fracture is minimally displaced or even nondisplaced than when there is severe displacement of the fragments.[59] The explanation for this seeming paradox is that in a nondisplaced fracture of the distal end of the radius the tendon sheath remains intact and the swelling that occurs with any fracture compromises circulation to the tendon. Conversely, with a severely comminuted and displaced fracture the sheath is more likely to be torn. This allows greater freedom of the tendon, and it is therefore less likely to be affected by local swelling. Although an extensor pollicis longus tenosynovitis leading to rupture usually results from chronic overuse, which has been referred to as *drummer boy's palsy*, it can also follow sustained activity over a relatively brief period. It has also been observed in a tennis player who, while practicing his serve for many hours, repetitively snapped his wrist into flexion (Fig. 26-1). Although the interval between activity and tendon rupture was hours in this particular individual, the interval is more likely to be days or weeks. Prompt recognition of tenosynovitis of this tendon is therefore important to prevent rupture.

Regardless of the tendon involved or the area of the muscle-tendon unit that is irritated, treatment for a chronic strain is basically rest. The use of a wrist splint as well as nonsteroidal antiinflammatory medication is also helpful. Injection of a steroid into the involved tendon sheath may also be effective. Soluble steroids such as dexamethasone are preferable to insoluble steroids, which tend to leave a deposit. Repeated injections should be avoided. It is questionable whether this treatment should be used for tenosynovitis of the extensor pollicis longus because the steroid itself may contribute to tendon rupture. If conservative measures fail and the tenosynovitis persists, surgery is necessary to release the tendon sheath and excise any hypertrophic tenosynovium. For de Quervain's tenosynovitis the sheath is excised, leaving a narrow strip volarly to serve as a shelf to prevent later subluxation of the abductor pollicis longus. Frequently the extensor pollicis brevis lies within its own sheath, separated from the abductor pollicis longus by a distinct fibrous septum. Failure to recognize this situation can occur, since the abductor pollicis longus usually comprises multiple slips, and the most dorsal one can be confused with the extensor pollicis brevis, which generally is a thin tendon. It is critical to release not only the sheath over the extensor pollicis brevis, but also any septum between it and the abductor pollicis longus. Although excising the sheath over the first tendon compartment is an effective procedure, excising the sheaths over the other tendon compartments would be ill advised because of the likelihood of causing tendon subluxation. For the extensor carpi ulnaris in the sixth compartment, this would tend to occur with forearm rotation. When tenosynovectomies are necessary for the tendons in the second through sixth compartments, the sheaths should be closed, but in a fashion that does not restrict tendon gliding.

Inflammation of the flexor tendons is also common,

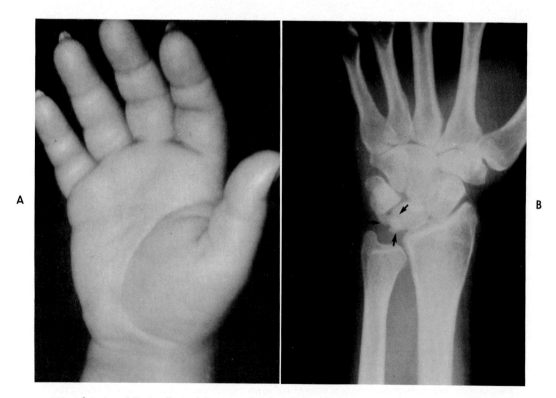

FIG. 26-2. A and **B,** Swelling of the entire hand with marked tenderness and erythema in the area of the pisiform. Radiographs show a large calcific deposit *(arrows)*.

and the clinical presentation depends on the area that is involved. Flexor tenosynovitis within the carpal tunnel would not only cause pain and limited mobility of the fingers, but would also likely result in compression of the median nerve. This problem has been observed in athletes whose sport requires repetitive pulling (e.g., rowing) or pressure applied to the palms for prolonged periods (e.g., cycling). The most effective treatment is cessation of the activity and rest. The flexor tenosynovitis usually subsides fairly rapidly, which also relieves the symptoms of the median nerve compression. In athletes whose carpal tunnel is developmentally shallow or whose problem is chronic, improvement following conservative treatment may be limited. If symptoms persist or weakness develops in the intrinsic muscles, surgical decompression and neurolysis of the nerve are required.

With overuse of the wrist flexors, it is usually the flexor carpi ulnaris that is strained. Inflammation of this tendon causes symptoms and physical findings that can be dramatic, particularly when there is a calcific deposit. Clinically there is redness, increased warmth, and swelling that may extend into the hand and proximally into the forearm. Local tenderness is usually intense and the diagnosis is often confused with cellulitis or lymphangitis (Fig. 26-2). However, there is never any local lymph-

adenopathy or other general signs of infection, such as a fever with a calcific tendinitis. The diagnosis is established by a radiograph that shows a calcific deposit, usually near the insertion of the tendon into the pisiform.[33,129] The most effective radiographic projection is an oblique view of the wrist that permits the pisiform bone to be seen in profile. There is no correlation between the intensity of the patient's symptoms and clinical signs, and the size of the calcium deposit. The cause of the calcification remains unclear. Some believe that there is an area of necrotic tissue in the tendon caused by some minor trauma, and that into this area of decreased vascularity calcium salts are precipitated. Treatment consists of needling the deposit with a short 25-gauge needle and injecting a local anesthetic mixed with a soluble steroid such as dexamethosone. Care must be taken to avoid traumatizing the ulnar artery or nerve during this injection. It is questionable whether the steroid increases the efficacy of needling the deposit, though it may aid in reducing the local inflammation. Clinical improvement is usually rapid, with pain, tenderness, and erythema subsiding within 24 to 48 hours. Repeat radiographs 1 week later usually show a significant, if not complete, resorption of the deposit. Surgical excision of the calcium deposit is rarely necessary.

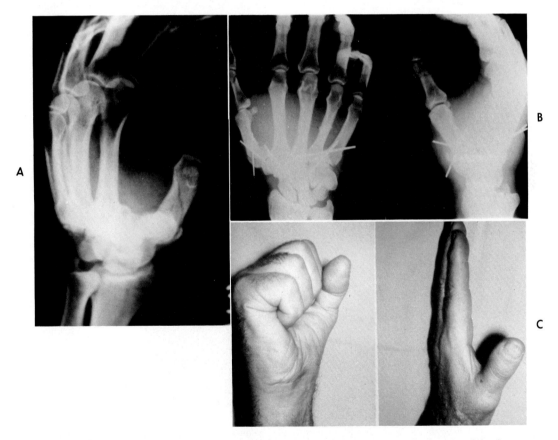

FIG. 26-3. A, Acute dislocation to the carpometacarpal joints of all fingers and a fracture of the first metacarpal. **B,** Following closed reductions the carpometacarpal joints were stabilized using Kirschner wires, which were inserted percutaneously. Open reduction and internal fixation were necessary for the fractured first metacarpal. **C,** Active range of motion exercises were started soon after surgery, and the patient regained complete digital mobility.

Ligament Injuries
Acute Injuries

Ligament injuries at the carpometacarpal joints are usually associated with subluxations or dislocations. Avulsion fractures of the bases of the metacarpals or adjacent carpal bones frequently accompany these injuries. There is usually marked swelling over the dorsal aspect of the hand; however, there may be no obvious deformity, and the severity of the injury may initially go unrecognized. Routine anteroposterior (AP) and lateral radiographs may fail to demonstrate the pathologic condition. Oblique radiographs in different projections are often required to profile the injured joint(s) adequately. The vast preponderance of these dislocations are dorsal and, if recognized early, can be easily reduced by manipulation. However, the propensity for redislocation is high, particularly for the second and third metacarpals, because of contraction of the extensor carpi radialis longus and brevis tendons.[164] The fourth and fifth metacarpals tend to be more stable after reduction, although they may also redislocate, particularly the fifth due to the pull of the extensor carpi ulnaris. Plaster immobilization is inadequate as the sole method of treatment after reduction, and percutaneous Kirschner wire fixation of the injured joint(s) is recommended (Fig. 26-3). Care must be taken in the placement of the wires to avoid injuring the extensor tendons to the fingers, the sensory branches of the radial nerve, or the dorsal sensory branch of the ulnar nerve. The wires need not transfix the radiocarpal joint and, if possible, they should also avoid transfixing of the midcarpal joint. The wrist is splinted, but the splint is removed several times each day for active range of motion exercises. Unrestricted movements for the digits are encouraged immediately after reduction and fixation. The wires are left in place for a minimum of 8 weeks. Close follow-up is required for months after removal of the wires, because later subluxations can occur.

Subluxation or dislocation of the carpometacarpal joint of the little finger may be accompanied by a comminuted fracture at the base of the metacarpal. If there is displacement of the metacarpal, it is usually more ulnar than dorsal, because of the direction of pull of the extensor carpi ulnaris. Operative reduction and internal fixation of these fractures are required to restore articular congruity and reduce the risk of later arthritis.[15]

Chronic Injuries

Injuries to the carpometacarpal joints that are not adequately treated at the time of the acute trauma frequently lead to chronic instability and arthritis, which is likely to seriously compromise hand function. There are pain and deformity at the involved joint(s), which weakens grip strength (Fig. 26-4). With involvement of the index and middle metacarpals, arthrodesis restores stability to joints that normally are functionally stable (Fig. 26-5). When secondary arthritic changes develop at the carpometacarpal joint of the little finger, a resectional arthroplasty has been recommended to maintain mobil-

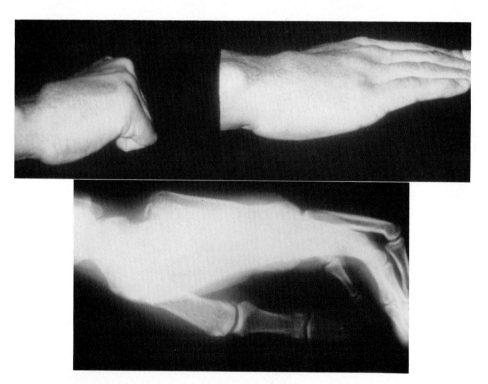

FIG. 26-4. Chronic dorsal dislocations (more than 1 year) involving the carpometacarpal joints of the ring and little fingers in a 19-year-old college wrestler who never had any treatment at the time of his injury. He was disturbed by the obvious deformity and also complained of pain and weakness of grasp, which prevented him from continuing with his sport. Both joints were reduced and arthrodesis was performed with the fifth in slightly more flexion than the fourth. Grip strength was restored and he resumed wrestling.

ity.[130] However, an arthrodesis eliminates pain more predictably and does not cause any significant functional impairment if the joint is fused in about 30 degrees of flexion. Fusing the joint in this position maintains the normal curvature of the distal transverse metacarpal arch with the clenched fist. Though the patient is unable to completely flatten the palm with finger extension, this rarely causes any functional impairment (Fig. 26-6).

METACARPAL AREA
Anatomy

The second, third, fourth, and fifth metacarpals function as stabilizers between the carpus and fingers. They form a functional unit that is separate from the role of

the first metacarpal. The longitudinal axis for all the finger metacarpals is slightly bowed with a dorsal convexity, but each bone has distinct characteristics in shape and size. Though the head of the third metacarpal is frequently the most prominent with the clenched fist, it is not necessarily the longest metacarpal. The second metacarpal is usually as long as, if not longer than, the third.[154] The apparent greater length of the third metacarpal is because its articulation with the carpus is at a more distal level than the other metacarpals. The fourth metacarpal is shorter than the third, and the fifth is the shortest. Each metacarpal is stabilized proximally by the carpometacarpal ligaments, distally by the deep transverse metacarpal ligaments, and centrally by the interossei muscles. A fracture to a single metacarpal is there-

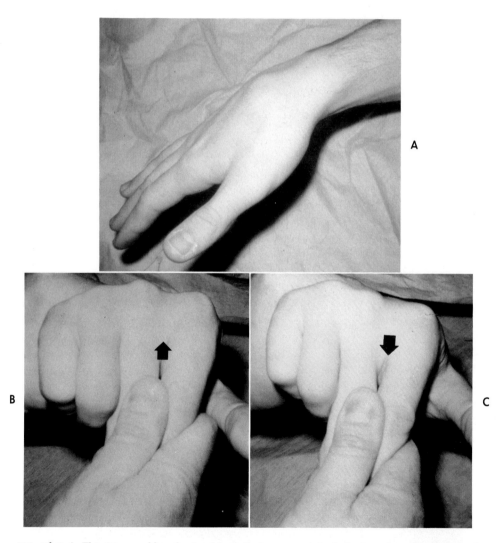

FIG. 26-5. A, This 24-year-old professional football player complained of pain at the carpometacarpal joints of his index and middle fingers. He recalled an injury to the area 1 year earlier that was never treated. Both joints were tender, and the bases of the second and third metacarpals were in dorsal subluxation. **B** and **C,** Instability at the involved carpometacarpal joints was readily apparent by moving the fingers up and down with their metacarpophalangeal joints flexed. The normal curvature of the transverse metacarpal was distorted.

Continued.

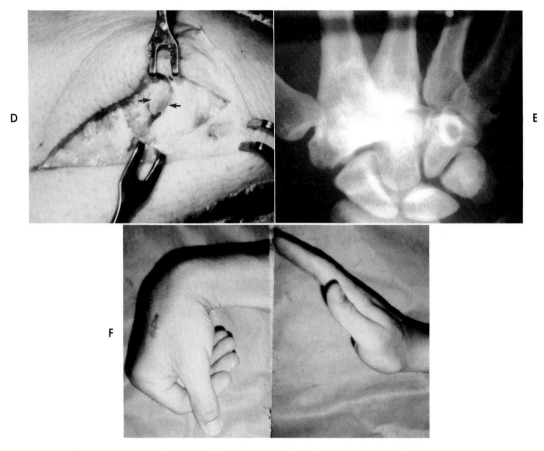

FIG. 26-5, cont'd. D, At surgery, there were arthritic changes with erosive changes in the cartilaginous surfaces of the joints. E and F, Arthrodesis was carried out on both joints, eliminating the previous pain. Postoperative wrist motions were only slightly impaired.

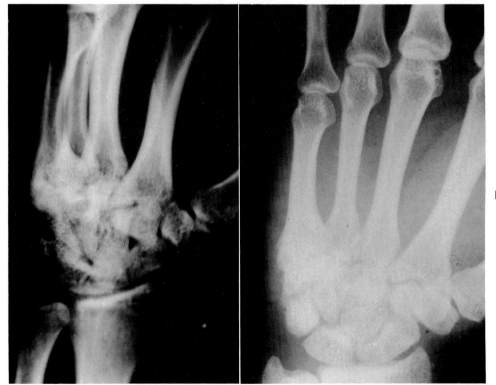

FIG. 26-6. A, Traumatic arthritis of the carpometacarpal joints of the ring and little fingers after untreated intraarticular fractures of the bases of the fourth and fifth metacarpals. Mobility at both joints was limited and painful. B, Arthrodesis of both joints was carried out, eliminating both pain and the deformity.

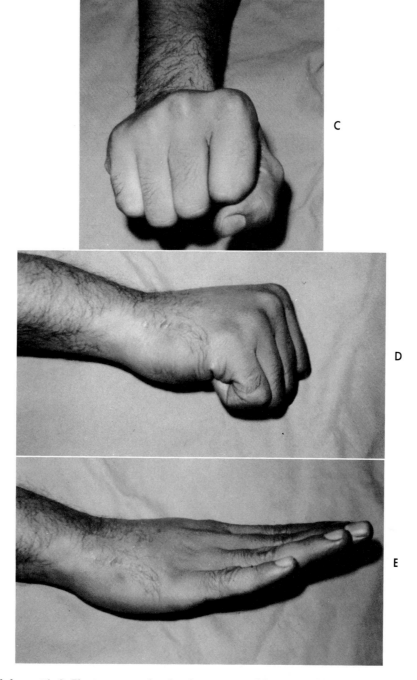

FIG. 26-6, cont'd. C, The joints were fused in flexion to avoid flattening of the transverse metacarpal arch when the patient clenched a fist. **D,** The patient regained full mobility. **E,** In extension he could not completely flatten his palm, which did not cause any functional impairment.

fore inherently stable, particularly when one of the central metacarpals (third or fourth) is injured because it receives additional support from its adjacent border metacarpal (second or fifth). The interossei muscles provide a muscular environment for the bones, which accommodates posttraumatic edema to a greater degree than in the finger itself. They also serve to protect the gliding of the flexor and, more notable, the extensor tendons. This is because viscoelastic tissue resistance usually does not develop to the degree that would result in tendon adherence. Fractures of the metacarpals are therefore considered to be more benign than phalangeal fractures.[185] Nevertheless, trauma to this area of the hand is serious and requires careful attention.

Muscle-Tendon Injuries

Extrinsics

Acute injuries. Injuries to the muscle-tendon units affect either the tendons of the extrinsic forearm muscles or the intrinsic muscles, which are located entirely in the hand. Acute extrinsic strains usually involve the flexor tendons and follow sudden overstretching. The tendon most commonly fails at its bony insertion, but ruptures in the palm do occur. Though tendons that rupture within their substance can rarely be successfully repaired, an exception is sometimes seen with rupture of a flexor profundus in the area of origin of its lumbrical muscle. The frayed tendon ends can sometimes be excised without sacrificing too much tendon length and the repair site covered using the lumbrical.

Chronic injuries. Chronic extrinsic strains are caused by overuse and are commonly manifested by tenosynovitis at the wrist level, which is discussed in the previous section.

Intrinsics

Acute injuries. Strains of the intrinsic muscles in the palm usually result from overuse. These injuries predominate over similar strains to the extrinsics. Strains of the intrinsics are common in sports that require repetitive gripping, such as tennis, golf, and rowing.[56] Initially the athlete with intrinsic muscle fatigue complains of aching, tiredness, or cramping in the hand. Recovery is usually prompt with rest and cessation of the activity, and there are usually no residual sequelae. Continued overuse, however, may lead to more severe and persistent symptoms and in some cases can actually result in fibrosis and contracture of the injured muscle(s). Acute intrinsic muscle injuries can also result from closed direct trauma, particularly to the most vulnerable dorsal aspect of the hand. There may be swelling and even hemorrhage within the muscles. Early recognition is important. As soon as the acute swelling subsides, exercises are started to reduce the risk of later contractures. The objective of the exercises is to stretch the intrinsic muscle. This can be accomplished by two methods: either by holding the metacarpophalangeal joint(s) in maximum extension and having the patient actively and passively flex the interphalangeal joints; or by holding the interphalangeal joints in flexion, usually with an elastic strap, and having the patient actively and passively extend the metacarpophalangeal joint(s). The assistance of a hand therapist is important in fabricating the necessary exercise devices and in monitoring the patient's compliance with the program.

Chronic injuries. If unrecognized, intrinsic muscle injuries can progress to fibrosis, resulting in contractures. The classic deformities of an intrinsic plus hand with flexion contractures of all metacarpophalangeal joints and extension contractures of all interphalangeal joints are more commonly encountered after severe crush or burn injuries than after athletic injuries. The intrinsic contractures seen in the athlete are rarely as severe. The findings are more apt to be subtle, sometimes with no obvious deformity to the finger(s). The patient may even be able to move the finger(s) completely but complains of stiffness or tightness with flexion. The intrinsic contractures in these cases may involve just a few muscles, sometimes those within a single intermetacarpal area. Such contractures frequently result from a fracture of a single metacarpal, but they can also occur in the absence of fracture. The realization that isolated intrinsic contractures occur and may exist even in the presence of complete digital mobility is important to make the diagnosis.

The contractures are demonstrated by a careful physical examination. Testing for intrinsic contractures is strictly a passive test that requires the examiner to maximally extend and even hyperextend the metacarpophalangeal joint to put the intrinsic muscle under maximal stretch. The proximal interphalangeal joint is then passively flexed. The test can determine if the intrinsic tightness is on both sides of a finger or just on one side. This is determined by not simply hyperextending the metacarpophalangeal joint, but also deviating it radially and ulnarly before flexing the proximal interphalangeal joint. This is useful when evaluating a localized injury that damages the intrinsic muscles in a single intermetacarpal area. For example, an injury to the area between the third and fourth metacarpals can damage the third dorsal and second volar interossei muscles, and contractures of these muscles would affect function of the middle and ring fingers. The excursion of the intrinsic on either side of each finger is compared. For the middle finger, the metacarpophalangeal joint is hyperextended and then deviated radially before the proximal interphalangeal joint is passively flexed. If the third dorsal interosseous was contracted, flexion of the joint would be limited because the muscle is under maximum stretch. Conversely, when the hyperextended metacarpophalangeal joint is deviated ulnarly, the third dorsal interosseous is relaxed and its contracture would not be obvious. Since the second dorsal interosseous is undamaged, passive flexion of the proximal interphalangeal joint would not be affected. The same procedure is carried out for the ring finger, differentiating the contracture of the second volar interosseous on the radial side of its metacarpal from the unaffected fourth dorsal interosseous on the ulnar side. It is important that passive flexion of the proximal interphalangeal joints is also tested with the metacarpophalangeal joints in flexion. If the problem is limited to the intrinsic, passive flexion of the proximal interphalangeal joints would not be affected. If it is, there must be other problems affecting the extrinsic tendon or joint capsule.

Isolated contractures of the first dorsal interosseous on the radial side of the index or of the intrinsics in the hypothenar area on the ulnar side of the fifth metacarpal are less common. Because these muscles are bounded by a metacarpal on only one side, they are not as confined as the intrinsics in the intermetacarpal areas. They are therefore not as susceptible to the effects of swelling and hemorrhage.

Fractures

A variety of forces can produce a fracture of a metacarpal shaft, including indirect compression, torsion, or a direct blow that damages the overlying soft tissues.

Careful clinical examination is the essential first step in treatment and should always precede radiographs. Rotation, angulation, and shortening at the fracture site can often be diagnosed by simply observing the resting position of the injured finger as well as its relationship to the adjacent fingers at rest and during gentle active motions. This is particularly true when there is malrotation, which may not be evident on routine radiographs. It has been estimated that for each degree of malrotation at the fracture site as much as 5 degrees of malrotation will occur at the fingertip.[142] Thus a fracture that is rotated only 5 degrees can result in 1.5 cm of digital overlap, an obviously unacceptable condition that requires correction.[58]

The vast majority of metacarpal fractures can be successfully managed by closed measures. Though circular plaster casts are frequently applied in hospital emergency departments for these fractures, they are unnecessary and often troublesome to deal with in follow-up visits. Effective immobilization for the acute fracture is more easily provided by applying a padded aluminum splint on the volar aspect of the injured digit and then incorporating it into a plaster splint with the wrist held in slight dorsiflexion. The splint is applied with the patient's forearm in supination and the wrist resting on a gauze roll to achieve the desired position of slight wrist dorsiflexion. The aluminum splint is bent to conform to the position of the wrist and finger, with the metacarpal joint in acute flexion to minimize the risk of a later extension contracture. The splint is sandwiched between a sufficient number of plaster splints, which stabilizes both the splint and the wrist joint. The aluminum splint is always molded to the finger and never the reverse. The normal capsular laxity of a metacarpophalangeal joint in extension may permit a malrotated or angulated fracture to appear to be reduced if the finger is manipulated to a splint that has been molded to conform to the normal positions of the adjacent uninjured fingers. The improvement in alignment or rotation of the injured finger would be illusory because when the splint is removed, the deformity would persist. With stable fractures active range of motion exercises can be started within 7 to 10 days. The splint is removed several times each day for these exercises and then reapplied and worn at all other times. With less stable fractures the total period of immobilization may have to be longer before active exercises are begun but should never exceed 3 weeks. If immobilization for longer than 3 weeks is necessary, the fracture should have been treated with some type of internal fixation.

With each follow-up visit the clinical appearance of the finger out of the splint is checked and new radiographs obtained to determine if there has been any displacement at the fracture site. Splint immobilization is continued, allowing for periodic daily exercises, until there is radiographic evidence of complete healing. The initial aluminum and plaster splint can be changed after a week or two when swelling has subsided to a splint fabricated by a hand therapist out of thermoplastic materials. Plastic splints are lighter in weight and easier for the patient to remove for the exercise program. Immobilization of uninjured fingers during the healing process should be avoided.

Oblique/Spiral Fractures

Metacarpal fractures are classified as oblique/spiral, transverse, or comminuted. Oblique/spiral fractures are the most common type. These fractures result from a rotational force on the bone and have a tendency to displace, resulting in overriding of the fragments and shortening. The displacement may not be present at the time of acute injury, but occur a week or two later. Therefore these fractures require attentive follow-up care. When there is displacement, various techniques have been recommended for internal fixation. Kirschner wires probably are the most popular, and two or more parallel wires drilled across the fracture site usually provide fixation (Fig. 26-7). Percutaneous insertion of the wires at either the fracture site or through the head of the bone and down its medullary cavity has been suggested.[16,34,113,157] The technique is safer for oblique fractures of the second and fifth metacarpals than for similar fractures of the third and fourth metacarpals, in which there is greater danger of impaling an extensor tendon(s) with the wire. Drilling the wire down the medullary cavity of the bone can cause scarring of the joint capsule and extensor tendon hood and, unless other wires are inserted across the fracture, may not control rotation.[150,151] If longitudinal wires are used, they should be inserted at the sides of the metacarpal head in the area of origin of the collateral ligaments, thus avoiding damage to its articular surface.[139] The most effective method of wire placement, which I prefer, is surgery. The risk of an open procedure is far outweighed by clearly visualizing the fracture, obtaining an anatomic reduction, and precisely inserting the wires. Two or more small screws can be substituted for the wires, and they are, in fact, preferable because they provide more rigid fixation. It is important that the length of the fracture is at least twice the width of the bone (Fig. 26-8).[58] Short oblique fractures can also be treated with a screw inserted in a lag mode, but it must be supplemented with a neutralization plate applied to the dorsal surface of the bone.

Transverse Fractures

Transverse fractures differ from oblique or spiral fractures in several ways. They tend toward greater overriding, which accentuates the deformity; however, once reduced, they are more stable because the fracture ends are compressed together. Another difference may be the rate of healing, which is slower for a transverse midshaft fracture, because the fracture surfaces are small and in the cortical diaphyseal portion of the bone (Fig. 26-9). These fractures may result in angulation, which is usually dorsal. Though this angulation rarely interferes with gliding of the extensor tendons, it can cause an imbalance at the metacarpophalangeal joint, producing a claw-type deformity with finger extension. In addition, the head of the fractured metacarpal becomes more prominent in the palm and may interfere with grasp. Opinions vary as to the degree of angulation that is acceptable for each metacarpal. Up to 10 degrees of angulation for the second and third metacarpals is tolerated by most au-

Text continued on p. 499.

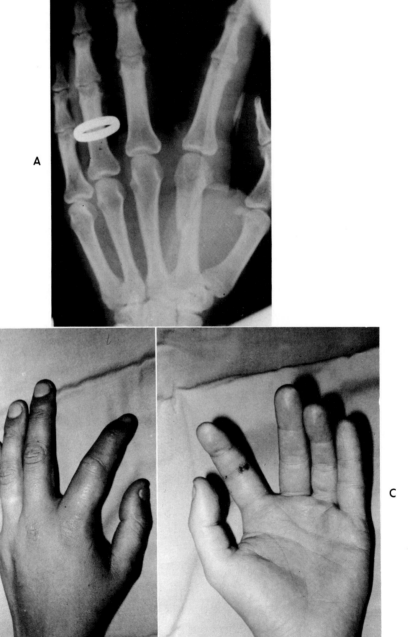

FIG. 26-7. A to **C,** Oblique fracture of the second metacarpal causing an obvious rotational deformity of the finger.

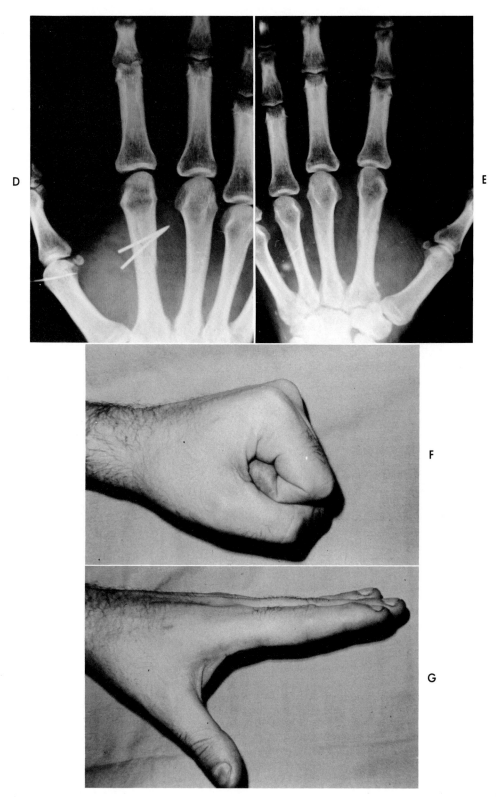

FIG. 26-7, cont'd. D and **E,** Rigid internal fixation was obtained using multiple Kirschner wires, which resulted in healing within 8 weeks. **F** and **G,** The patient started active range of motion exercises within 10 days of surgery and regained complete digital mobility.

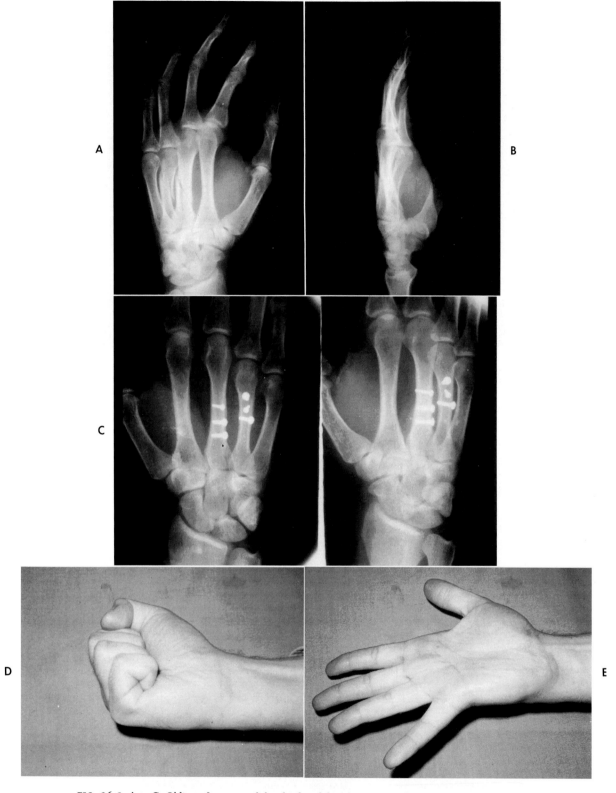

FIG. 26-8. A to **C,** Oblique fractures of the third and fourth metacarpals were fixed using 1.5- and 2-mm cortical screws. The fractures were sufficiently oblique to permit three screws in each bone. The screws were inserted in a lag fashion to obtain maximum compression of the fractures. **D** and **E,** Since rigid fixation of each bone was obtained, active range of motion exercises were begun a week after surgery and the patient regained complete mobility. A protective splint was worn until there was radiographic evidence of bone healing.

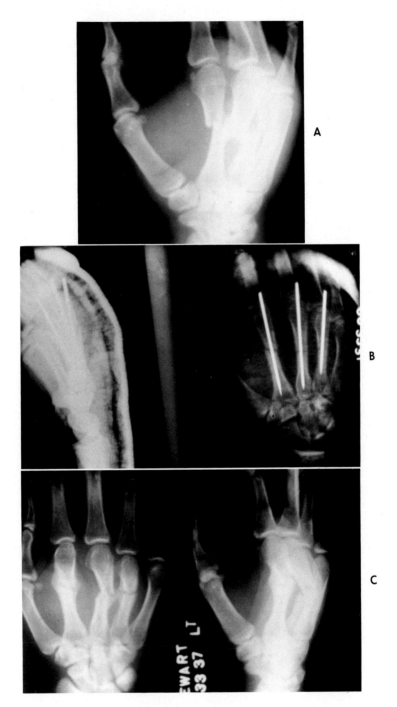

FIG. 26-9. A and **B,** Transverse fractures of the second, third, and fourth metacarpals were stabilized using intramedullary wires inserted through the metacarpal heads. Though the fractures were successfully stabilized using this technique, inserting wires through joints will result in capsular scarring and lead to joint stiffness. It is a method of treatment that should be avoided. The surgeon who treated this patient was apparently aware of this risk, and removed the wires after only 6 weeks. **C,** The fractures had not sufficiently healed and therefore collapsed. Transverse fractures in the diaphyseal portion of a metacarpal take longer to heal than similar fractures in the metaphyseal area of the bone. Stabilizing these fractures with small plates and screws would have been the preferred method of treatment.

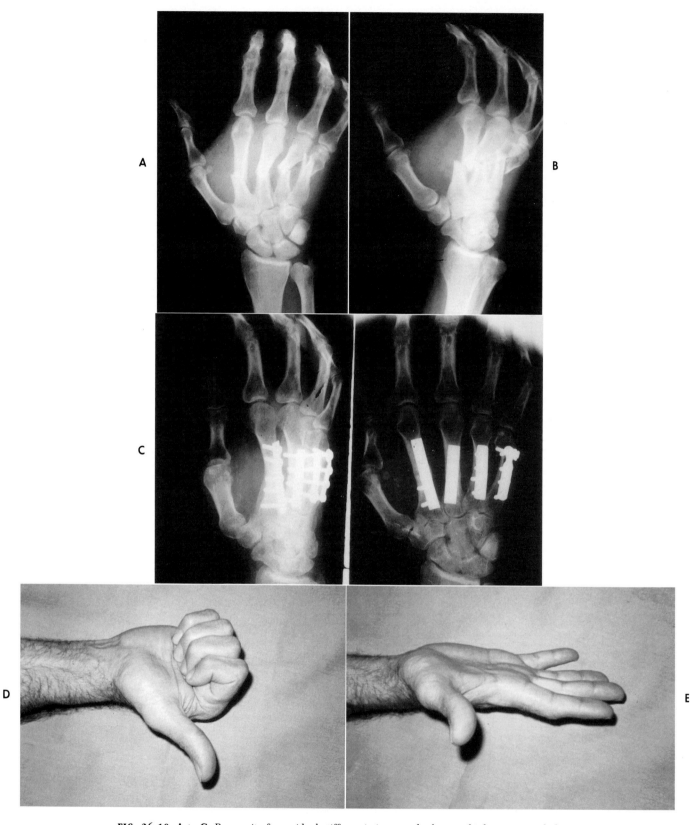

FIG. 26-10. A to **C,** Propensity for residual stiffness is increased when multiple metacarpals have been fractured. It is particularly important in these injuries to provide rigid fixation, which permits early active range of motion exercises. The use of dorsal plates and screws is an effective method of fixation for transverse fractures, as in this patient who fractured his second through fifth metacarpals. A T-plate was used for the fracture of the fifth metacarpal because it was through the neck portion of the bone. **D** and **E,** Postoperative mobility was only minimally repaired.

thors, whereas acceptable angulation for the mobile fourth and fifth metacarpals ranges from 20 degrees for the fourth to 35 degrees for the fifth.[55,171] Shortening is generally not a significant problem for a single shaft fracture because of the tethering effect of the deep transverse metacarpal ligaments, which are attached to the adjacent intact metacarpals. Some authors claim that shortening never poses a functional problem,[12,28] whereas others recommend that it be corrected.[74] Though the published figures for what is considered acceptable angulation and shortening provide convenient reference points, they should not be applied to every case. Each patient's fracture must be treated with a complete understanding of the demands placed on the athlete's hand in the particular sport. For the amateur or professional boxer, any angulation of a fractured metacarpal, whether it be the stable second or mobile fifth, requires correction. The tremendous compressive forces applied to the hand in boxing will likely refracture any metacarpal if it is allowed to heal in angulation. Shortening of a metacarpal would be equally damaging, particularly if it involves either the second or third. The knuckle of the adjacent uninjured metacarpal would become more prominent, exposing its extensor tendon and joint capsule to risk of injury. Metacarpal shortening would also be detrimental to individuals in whom precision and coordinated finger movements are important. Pianists, the ultimate athletes with respect to dexterity and endurance in hand function, fall into this category.

Most transverse fractures can be successfully managed by closed manipulation. If closed reduction cannot be achieved, surgery is necessary. As with oblique frac-

tures, various methods for internal fixation are available, including Kirschner wires, cerclage wiring, a plate, or a combination of methods.[68,80,116,187,188] A plate applied to the dorsal surface of the bone provides excellent rigidity and is particularly useful where there are multiple fractures (Fig. 26-10).[139]

Comminuted Fractures

In severely comminuted fractures the problems of fixation are increased. Frequently there is shortening of the metacarpal, which must be restored to its normal length. This is accomplished by applying longitudinal traction to the finger and then stabilizing the distal fracture fragment into the adjacent intact metacarpals using Kirschner wires that are drilled at a right angle to the bone. It is important that a minimum of two wires be inserted. If only a single wire is inserted, flexion will occur at the fracture site rather than at the metacarpophalangeal joint as the distal fracture fragment rotates around the wire. Usually a dynamic flexion splint is applied within a week to facilitate flexion exercises. If there is a large gap at the fracture site, a bone graft may be required as soon as swelling subsides and active finger motions are restored (Fig. 26-11).

METACARPOPHALANGEAL JOINT AREA
Anatomy

The metacarpophalangeal joints of the fingers are the most proximal joints in a series of four separate triarticular chains that face the palm and thumb to achieve prehension. Though the joints within each triarticular chain

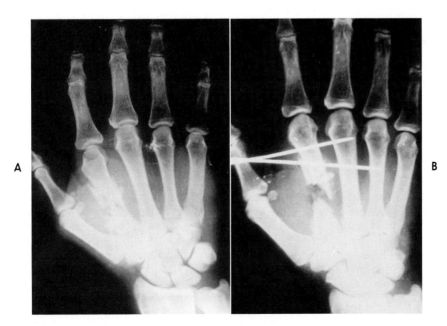

FIG. 26-11. A and **B,** This comminuted fracture of the second metacarpal resulted in shortening of the bone. Metacarpal length was restored by longitudinal traction on the finger and then stabilizing the distal fracture fragment into the adjacent metacarpals using two Kirschner wires. By using two wires rotation of the metacarpal was prevented and allowed more effective flexion at the metacarpophalangeal joint.

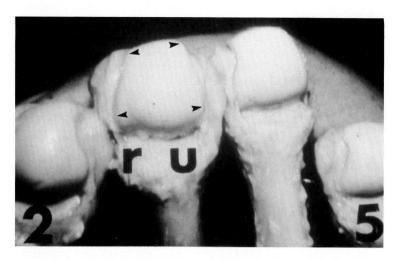

FIG. 26-12. Frontal view of the metacarpophalangeal joints of the fingers. The metacarpal heads are trapezoidal in configuration. They are narrower dorsally than volarly, and the collateral ligaments are shown to be taut in full flexion.

have structural differences, they function as a unit to facilitate flexion and prevent hyperextension.[45] The metacarpophalangeal joint is formed by an asymmetric spherodial head of the metacarpal, which articulates against the broad, concave base of the proximal phalanx. It is a multiaxial condyloid joint that permits flexion, extension, abduction, adduction, and, to a slight degree, circumduction. The asymmetry of the head is apparent when it is viewed in different projections: it is flattened transversely and wider volarly than dorsally. In the frontal plane the head curves smoothly on its radial side but stops abruptly on its ulnar side (Fig. 26-12). This asymmetry is most obvious in the second and third metacarpals and is responsible for the tendency of the proximal phalanges of these two fingers to drift ulnarly with flexion.[45] Flexion-extension movements of the metacarpophalangeal joints do not occur about a single axis, but rather about a series of axes, which lie on an arc that moves in a palmar direction with increasing joint flexion.

The supporting structures for each joint consist of a capsule dorsally, a glenoid fibrocartilage plate volarly, and a combination of ligaments, sagittal bands, and intrinsic tendons laterally. The dorsal capsule is thin and is reinforced by fibers from the overlying extensor tendon(s). These fibers permit gliding of the extensor apparatus and stabilize the tendon in a midline position over the joint.[154] The capsule is lax to facilitate a wide range of flexion, and it forms a large bursa that extends proximally for a distance of 15 to 20 mm along the dorsal aspect of the metacarpal. At the joint line the synovial membrane of the capsule folds inward to form a meniscal cushion. Its function is unknown. It may prevent the dorsal capsule from being trapped between the joint surfaces during extension, or it may improve joint congruity in an area where the surface of the phalangeal head is small.[45]

The volar aspect of the capsule consists of a thick fibrocartilaginous structure, the volar plate. Its distal portion is thick, rigid, and cartilaginous and moves volar to the head with flexion and extension. It is firmly anchored into the volar surface of the proximal phalanx. Proximally, the plate is thin, flexible, and membranous. With joint flexion, it folds like the bellows of an accordion between the metacarpal head and the cartilage portion of the plate. The anterior part of the plate forms the posterior wall of the fibrous tendon sheath at the level of the A-1 pulley. The volar plates are interconnected by the deep transverse metacarpal ligaments.

Laterally the ligament support for the metacarpophalangeal joint is composed of two parts, the collateral ligaments and the accessory collateral ligaments (Fig. 26-13). The collateral ligaments arise from eccentrically located tuberosities on the sides of the metacarpal head and insert on lateral tuberosities on the proximal phalanx, near its volar surface. Asymmetry exists in these ligaments. The radial fibers are thicker and stronger and run in a more oblique direction than the ulnar fibers. These differences produce passive axial rotation of the finger, which goes from supination in the extended position to pronation as it is flexed. This also contributes to the tendency for the finger to deviate in an ulnar direction.[105] Both collateral ligaments are dorsal to the flexion-extension axis for these joints. Because this axis moves volarly with joint flexion, the collateral ligaments are lax in extension and become increasingly taut as the proximal phalanx flexes. They must also diverge to accommodate the wider width of the metacarpal head on its volar side, which is another reason they become taut with joint flexion. Therefore lateral movement is greatest in extension and becomes increasingly limited with progressive flexion. The collateral ligaments also stabilize the joint in its flexion-extension arc. Without these ligaments the tremendous flexion force on the proximal phalanx sup-

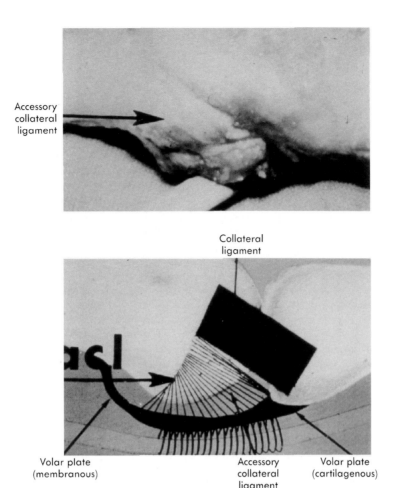

FIG. 26-13. Anatomic and diagramatic views of the lateral aspect of a metacarpophalangeal joint.

plied by the extrinsic flexor tendons and intrinsic muscles (interossei and lumbricals) would result in volar subluxation of the joint.[54,171]

The accessory collateral ligaments originate on the sides of the metacarpal head volar to the origins of the collateral ligaments. They insert on the borders of the glenoid fibrocartilage plate. The accessory collateral ligaments are volar to the flexion-extension axis of the joint. They are lax in flexion and taut in extension, the reverse for the collateral ligaments. The accessory collateral ligaments, by their suspensory action on the volar plate, stabilize the flexor tendons with joint flexion. Additional lateral stability for the metacarpophalangeal joints is provided by the intrinsic muscles and sagittal fibers of the dorsal tendon mechanism.

Tendon Injuries

Subluxation of the extensor tendon from its midline position over the dorsal aspect of a metacarpophalangeal joint usually results from forceful deviation of the finger in an ulnar direction. The middle finger is most frequently affected because of the unique anatomic relationship of its extensor tendon to the dorsal hood. There

is not the intimate connection between tendon and the transverse fibers of the hood that exists for other fingers; rather, the extensor tendon in the middle finger lies on top of the hood, to which it is only loosely connected. Consequently, there is a defect in continuity between the radial intrinsic muscle and the extensor tendon, which leaves the tendon vulnerable to displacement. The force required to cause this displacement is greatest in full extension and full flexion and decreases during the first 60 degrees of flexion.[99]

An extensor tendon subluxation can also occur from a direct blow to the knuckle, such as striking a hard object with the clenched fist. Involvement of the middle finger and displacement of the tendon in an ulnar direction is also seen with this type of injury, but not with the same frequency as with sudden forceful deviation of the finger. Regardless of the mechanism of injury, the diagnosis requires a careful examination because swelling over the injured joint may obscure the position of the tendon and its displacement may go unrecognized. The examiner should follow the direction of the tendon from its more proximal portion over the metacarpal, where it can be more easily palpated. When there is swelling and

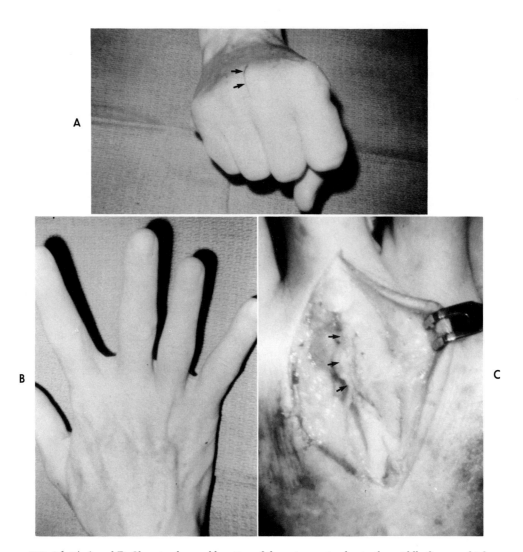

FIG. 26-14. A and **B,** Chronic ulnar subluxation of the extensor tendon to the middle finger, which is obvious with the joint in full flexion. Even in extension there was slight ulnar deviation of the finger, because the extensor tendon was not in its normal midline position. **C,** The hood was explored through a curved incision and the sagittal fibers (*arrows*) repaired, restoring the tendon to its normal midline position. *Continued.*

the tendon cannot be palpated, subluxation should be suspected. Once the diagnosis is established, there are two treatment options. If the tendon is relocated with extension of the metacarpophalangeal joint, a volar splint is used for 3 to 4 weeks. The metacarpophalangeal joints of the fingers are immobilized in full extension, but the interphalangeal joints should not be immobilized. If necessary, a soft, wide catheter is placed to the displaced side of the tendon to help maintain it in its correct position. The other treatment option is surgery, which is indicated for severe subluxation of the tendon, particularly when it remains subluxed with finger extension. Repair of the torn sagittal fibers will effectively restore the tendon to its normal position.[78,99]

In chronic cases direct repair of the torn fibers may also be possible after excision of the scar tissue at the site of hood disruption (Fig. 26-14). If necessary, a relaxing incision is made in the sagittal fibers on the ulnar side of the tendon to relocate it into its proper position. If the radial portion of the hood is so deficient or scarred as to preclude repair, some form of tether must be used to centralize the tendon. Various techniques have been proposed including rerouting a juncturae tendinum or splitting the extensor tendon and rerouting that tendon slip around the radial collateral ligament or lumbrical muscle.[32,118,188,192] Regardless of which procedure is carried out, care must be taken to ensure that the repair is secure enough to resist recurrence of the subluxation when the finger is passively flexed at surgery.[42]

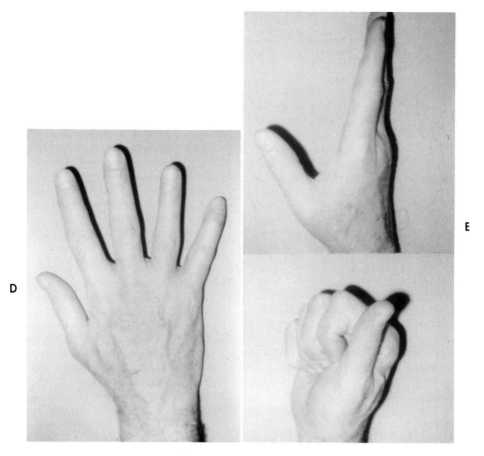

FIG. 26-14, cont'd. D and **E,** Postoperatively the tendon was restored to its normal position over the joint, and the previous ulnar deviation of the finger in extension was eliminated.

Ligament Injuries

In general, ligaments in the mobile joints of the hand have two important functions: to permit normal joint motion and to provide stability against abnormal motions. When the force toward an abnormal motion exceeds the power of the ligament to prevent it, a sprain occurs. Sprains therefore result from overstress, as opposed to contusions, which result from a direct blow to a ligament. When stress is applied to a ligament, it initially tenses to withstand the force. However, at some point the ligament fails, resulting in damage to its fibers. The extent of damage depends on the force and duration of its application.

There are three categories of sprains. First-degree sprain is the mildest. Only a few fibers of the ligament are damaged, and its strength is not compromised. It is therefore unnecessary to protect the ligament and treatment is entirely symptomatic. The patient is usually able to resume full activities within 1 to 2 weeks. In second-degree, or moderate, sprain a greater portion of the ligament is torn and some functional loss usually results. The joint is stable with active motion, but some laxity can be demonstrated with stress testing. Because part of the ligament remains intact, treatment is directed toward protection. If the joint is immobilized, the damaged por-

tion of the ligament should be expected to heal, because the torn fibers are in close proximity to each other. Despite adequate protection, some second-degree sprains do not heal and, though there may be no appreciable joint instability, the patient may continue to complain of pain and tenderness. Surgery is sometimes necessary for these cases. The third-degree, or severe, sprain occurs when the ligament is completely torn, either within its substance or at one end of its bony attachments. When it is damaged at either attachment, it sometimes avulses with a bone fragment. This has been referred to as a sprain-fracture.[141] Though a fracture fragment is present, the injury is primarily to the ligament, and it is to the ligament that treatment must be directed. With third-degree sprains the stabilizing function of the ligament is lost and the joint is unstable. When subluxations or dislocations with clinical or radiographic evidence of joint incongruity are evident, the sprain must be third degree. Frequently the initial subluxation or dislocation spontaneously reduces, leaving a joint that is stable with active motion and has no incongruity. Stress testing in these cases demonstrates gross instability.

Though the treatment for third-degree sprains depends on the specific ligament disrupted, several general

principles should be followed. The primary objective is to restore stability. Therefore it is advisable to immobilize the joint for several weeks. This is followed by active range of motion exercises and protection for 2 to 3 months. Avoidance of immobilization to reduce the likelihood of later joint stiffness may succeed, but at the risk of continued instability. If stiffness develops after treatment, it is preferable to instability and usually easier to treat.[18]

Surgery is required for third-degree sprains in the following situations. The first is failure to restore normal articular congruity after reduction of a subluxation or dislocation. This is evident on AP and lateral radiographs. A second indication is unstressed instability. If the joint fails to remain in alignment with active motion, then there are interposed tissues within the joint or the disruption of capsular structures is of such magnitude that it requires surgical exploration and repair. A third indication for surgery is an articular fracture fragment that remains widely displaced. In all likelihood the avulsed ligament is attached to this fragment, and its displaced position usually precludes the possibility of healing with stability. Even when the fracture fragment has not widely displaced, surgery may still be indicated when the fragment is large and its displacement has resulted in significant articular incongruity.

Volar Plate

Ligament injuries to the metacarpophalangeal joints are uncommon, but when they occur they usually follow sudden hyperextension, which results in a dorsal dislocation. The index finger is involved most commonly,[6,134] followed by the little finger. The volar plate ruptures at its membranous connection to the metacarpal and shifts dorsally with the proximal phalanx, to which it remains attached. The plate becomes entrapped behind the dorsal aspect of the metacarpal head. The metacarpal is further trapped by taut structures on both radial and ulnar sides of its neck. In dislocation of the index finger the lumbrical muscle is radial and the flexor tendons are ulnar; in dislocation of the little finger both the lumbrical muscle and flexor tendons are to the radial side and the conjoined tendon of the hypothenar intrinsic muscles to the ulnar side.[5,95] Rarely the torn volar plate, while still attached to the dislocated phalanx, is not displaced behind the metacarpal head but remains volar to it. A closed reduction is readily achievable in these situations. First the wrist is flexed to relax the flexor tendons. Then pressure is applied to the dorsal aspect of the base of the proximal phalanx in a distal and volar direction, sliding the joint into flexion. Care must be taken not to apply traction on the joint or to hyperextend the digit initially, because this maneuver might shift the plate dorsally. The plate could then pass over the metacarpal head, converting an incomplete subluxation into a complete and irreducible dislocation.[43]

The complete dislocation, often termed complex because of the number of anatomic structures that block its reduction, was first described by Farebeuf in 1876 and introduced into the English literature by Barbard in 1901. It was not until 1957 that Kaplan[95] published his classic article describing its clinical and anatomic features. The finger is flexed at its interphalangeal joints and slightly hyperextended at its metacarpophalangeal joint (Fig. 26-15). The finger is also deviated toward the adjacent fingers and the palmar skin is characteristically dimpled or puckered at the proximal palmar crease. Dorsally a defect can be palpated proximal to the phalanx. In an incomplete subluxation there is no lateral deviation of the finger because the proximal phalanx, which may be hyperextended up to 90 degrees, lies directly dorsal to the metacarpal head.[72] Radiographs show widening of the joint space on the AP view and an obvious dislocation on the lateral view. Because the sesamoid bones of the fingers are embedded within the volar plate, their presence within the joint on the lateral radiographic view is pathognomonic of a complex dislocation.[138,184]

The classical surgical approach is carried out via a midaxial incision along the side of the joint (radial for the index finger and ulnar for the little finger), which is then curved into the palmar crease. Meticulous care must be taken with the skin incision because of the risk of severing the neurovascular bundle, which is tented over the metacarpal head. The radial neurovascular bundle is vulnerable for the index finger dislocation, and the ulnar neurovascular bundle is vulnerable for the little finger dislocation. The structure that is most responsible for preventing relocation is the volar plate, which is interposed between the base of the phalanx and the metacarpal head. The plate must be removed from this position before reduction can be achieved. The first step is to relieve the tension of the flexor tendons, and this is accomplished by releasing the A-1 pulley of the tendon sheath. With the tendons retracted, an attempt is made to extricate the plate with the aid of a probe. This is possible if, at the time of the dislocation, the plate tears not only from its proximal attachment but also from its lateral connection to the adjacent deep transverse metacarpal ligament. Frequently the lateral attachment does not tear completely, and the portion that remains intact must be released by an incision along the lateral edge of the plate. The plate can then be restored to its normal position. It is unnecessary to reattach the plate to the periosteum at the neck of the metacarpal. Because of the complexity of the volar approach and the danger of injury to the neurovascular bundles, a dorsal surgical approach, which was the approach originally recommended by Farebeuf, is the preferred procedure.[14] A longitudinal incision is made in the joint capsule and the displaced volar plate is immediately apparent. Restoring the plate back to its original position is easily accomplished using a probe or small elevator. Active exercises must begin on the first postoperative day because of the inverse relationship between the time of postoperative immobilization and the ultimate range of motion of the joint.[125] A dorsal block splint is used to protect against hyperextension for the first 2 weeks. If there is still any concern about redislocation, a dynamic flexion splint is used for an additional week or two. The elastic on the splint should be a sufficient tension to prevent hyperextension, but not full extension, during exercises.

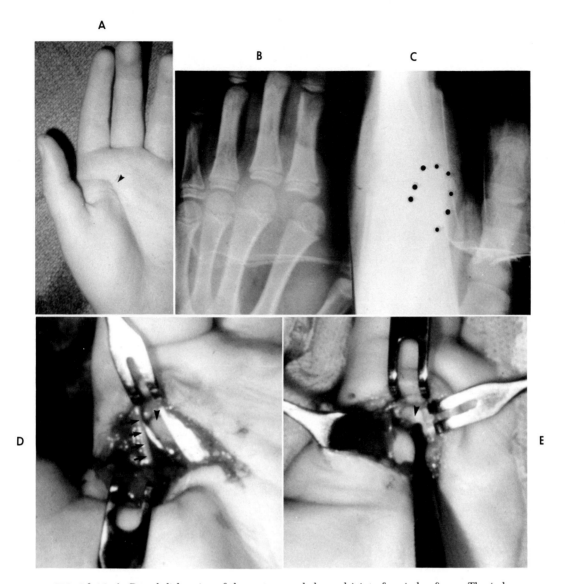

FIG. 26-15. A, Dorsal dislocation of the metacarpophalangeal joint of an index finger. The index finger was adducted against the adjacent middle finger and the palmar skin was puckered *(arrow)* in the palmar crease. **B** and **C,** Lateral radiographs show the proximal phalanx to be dorsal to the metacarpal head. In the oblique view there is abnormal widening of the joint space. **D,** At surgery care must be taken when making skin incisions because the radial neurovascular bundle *(small arrows)* is tented over the head of the metacarpal *(large arrow)* and can easily be inadvertently cut. **E,** The volar plate *(arrow)* is displaced posterior to the head of the metacarpal and is the major structure that prevents reduction.

Collateral Ligaments

Collateral ligament sprains of the metacarpophalangeal joints are rare for several reasons. The joints are protected by their recessed position in the palm and support is provided by adjacent fingers. In addition, the anatomic configuration of the ligaments permits the fingers to deviate in extension. The mechanism of injury is forced lateral deviation, almost always in an ulnar direction and usually with the joint in some flexion. The degree of joint flexion at the moment of injury is a determining factor in the severity of the sprain. In full extension normal ligament laxity will more likely dissipate a laterally or ulnarly directed force than if that same force is applied to the joint in full flexion when the ligament is taut.

The diagnosis of these sprains is frequently delayed. The patient, though experiencing pain, often does not appreciate the seriousness of the injury if joint motions are not impaired. After weeks and sometimes months of discomfort, the patient finally seeks medical attention. By that time there is little if any swelling, and the joint appears deceptively benign. However, careful examination

Text continued on p. 510.

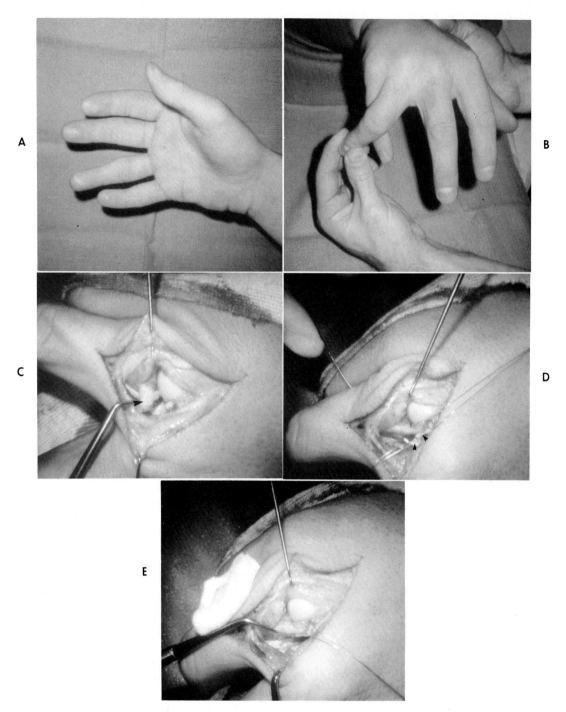

FIG. 26-16. A and **B,** This 28-year-old professional basketball player ruptured the radial collateral ligament of the metacarpophalangeal joint of his right ring finger. At rest the finger deviated toward the little finger. Stress testing with the joint flexed showed marked instability. **C** to **E,** At surgery the volar two thirds of the ligament *(large arrow)* ruptured proximally and was reattached to the metacarpal. The dorsal one third of the ligament *(small arrow)* was reattached using a pull-out wire suture into a slot made in the proximal phalanx. Padding was placed beneath the button to avoid skin ulcer. **F** and **G,** The dorsal capsule *(arrow)* was then sutured to the repaired ligament. This was followed by closure of the dorsal hood. **H** to **L,** The patient regained complete mobility and stability of his finger. He was allowed to play basketball within 1 month of his surgery wearing a small splint that blocked full extension as well as lateral deviation of the finger.

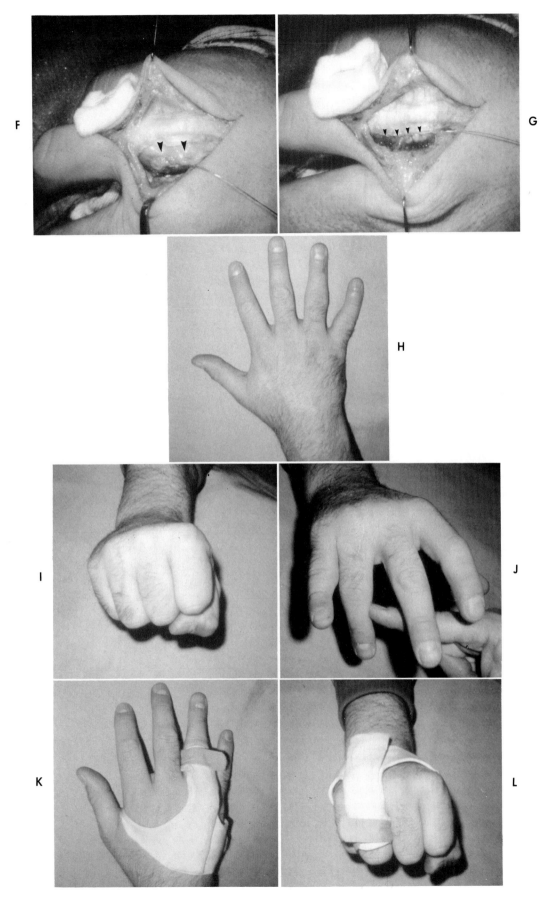

FIG. 26-16, cont'd. For legend see opposite page.

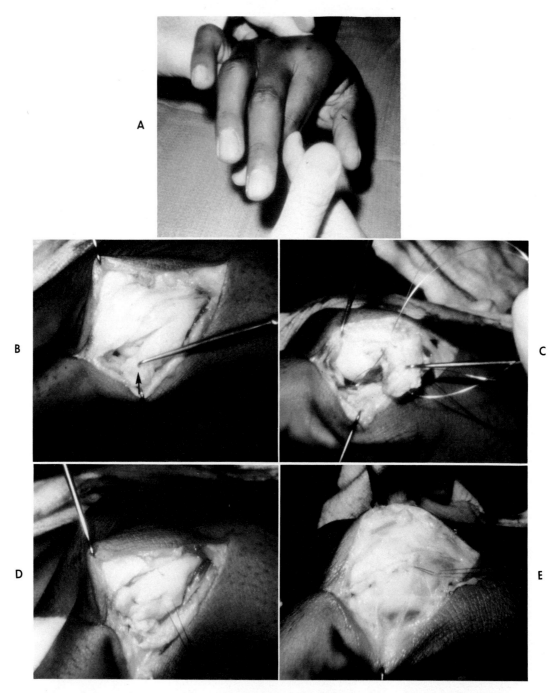

FIG. 26-17. A, Chronic instability of the metacarpophalangeal joint of the index finger in a 28-year-old professional football player. **B** to **D,** The ligament *(arrow)* had ruptured from the proximal phalanx and was reinserted into the bone using a pull-out wire suture. **E,** The dorsal hood was then repaired.

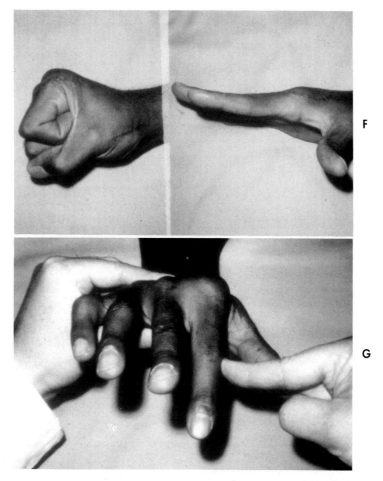

FIG. 26-17, cont'd. F and **G,** Because this patient was a pass receiver, care was taken to avoid producing a flexion contracture, since extension of the joint was more important than flexion. He regained excellent mobility as well as stability of the finger.

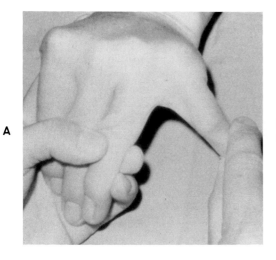

FIG. 26-18. A, Chronic instability of the metacarpophalangeal joint of the little finger caused by a rupture of the radial collateral ligament.

Continued.

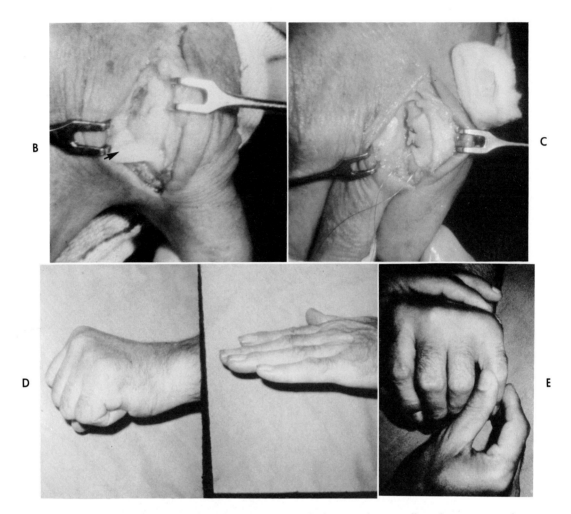

FIG. 26-18, cont'd. B and **C,** At surgery the ligament had ruptured proximally and was reinserted into the metacarpal using a pull-out wire suture. The dorsal capsule *(large arrow)* was then repaired and the dorsal hood closed *(small arrows).* **D** and **E,** Postoperatively the patient regained complete mobility and stability.

shows tenderness over the injured ligament and, more important, instability with stress testing. The evaluation is carried out by passive motion of the joint radially and ulnarly, in full extension as well as full flexion. Normally there is considerable laxity in full extension, but little in full flexion. Gross instability in the flexed position demonstrates a third-degree sprain. In some third-degree sprains the diagnosis is obvious by simple observation of the deviated position of the finger (Fig. 26-16). Arthrography is also a useful diagnostic technique.[86]

Ligament injuries of these joints have received scant attention in the literature and, though they have been reported to occur most frequently in the ring and little fingers, they may occur in any finger.[44,86] Surgery is usually necessary when there is gross instability. If possible, the torn collateral ligament is reinserted into the bone from which it avulsed, which occurs with equal frequency at the phalanx or metacarpal (Figs. 26-17 and 26-18). In some situations, particularly chronic cases, it may be necessary to reconstruct a new ligament using a

tendon graft (e.g., palmaris longus). Care must be taken to reestablish the normal configuration of the ligament. Reconstruction so that the ligament is taut in full extension should be avoided because it is likely to result in an extension contracture of the joint. Though this might not pose a problem to the athlete whose fingers are often in an extended position (e.g., the basketball player or football pass receiver), it would be disabling to the athlete whose sport requires using a clenched fist (e.g., the boxer). It is preferable to reconstruct the ligament in such a way that it is taut with the joint in about 60 degrees of flexion. Following the period of postoperative immobilization and therapy, a protective splint, similar to what is used after a second-degree sprain, is often used to protect the joint from reinjury for several additional months (Fig. 26-19).

Dorsal Capsule

Direct trauma to the dorsal aspect of a knuckle is common and usually causes a contusion, which heals within

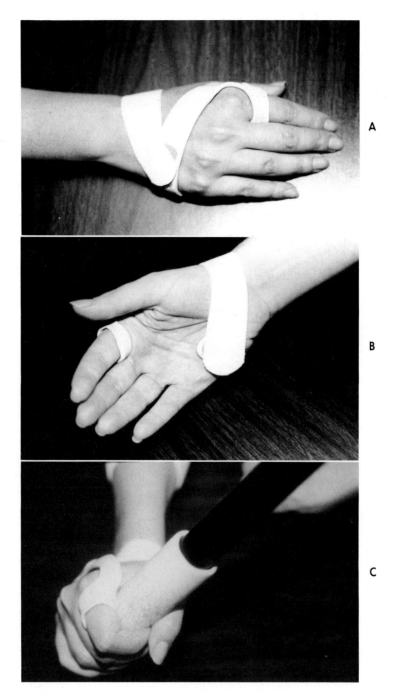

FIG. 26-19. **A,** Second-degree injury to the radial collateral ligament of the metacarpophalangeal joint of the finger treated with a protective splint. **B** and **C,** The splint prevents ulnar deviation of the index finger and can be worn under a mitten, permitting the patient to resume skiing.

a week or two. With greater trauma there is a tear in the dorsal hood involving either the radial or ulnar sagittal fibers. If the radial sagittal fibers are torn, the extensor tendon is displaced in an ulnar direction. This would resemble the tendon subluxation that occurs with forced ulnar deviation of a finger, as previously discussed. An even more severe blow to the knuckle or repetitive blows occurring during one episode or over a long period can damage the underlying dorsal joint capsule and actually cause it to rupture. These injuries can occur in any sport in which the knuckles are subjected to local direct trauma, such as amateur and professional boxing and karate.[153]

It is important to differentiate a capsular tear from the less severe injury to the sagittal fibers of the dorsal hood. Though an injury to the dorsal hood may respond to non-

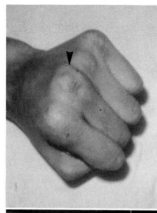

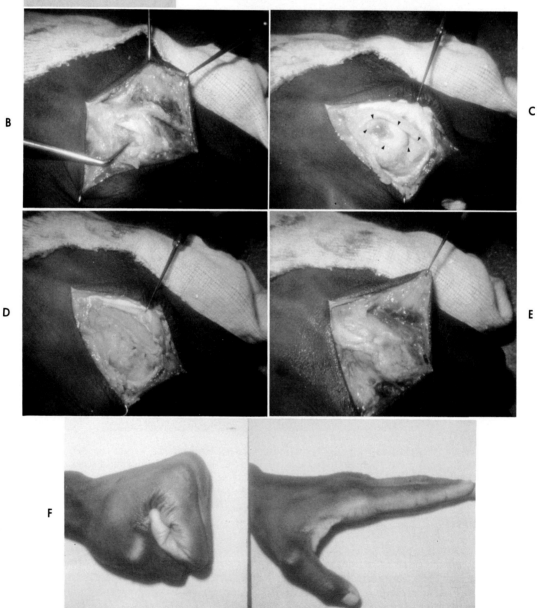

FIG. 26-20. A, This 21-year-old Olympic gold medal winner in boxing complained of chronic pain over the metacarpophalangeal joint of his middle finger. The extensor tendon *(arrow)* was displaced ulnarly, and there was a palpable defect directly over the head of the underlying metacarpal. **B,** At surgery a curved incision was made over the joint, and when skin flaps were mobilized the metacarpal head was clearly visible *(probe).* **C,** The tear in the hood was incised further proximally and distally to visualize the joint capsule, which was torn *(small arrows)* over a distance of more than 2 cm. **D,** The capsule, which was adherent to the underlying dorsal hood, was mobilized and then repaired with fine 4-0 nylon sutures. **E,** The dorsal hood was then repaired. **F,** The patient regained full digital flexion and continued with his successful professional career, becoming world champion.

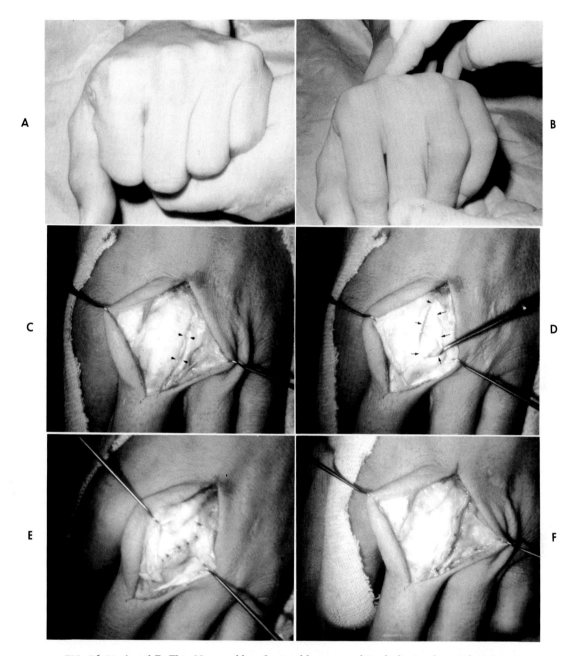

FIG. 26-21. A and **B,** This 22-year-old professional boxer complained of pain of more than 1 year's duration over the metacarpophalangeal joint of his middle finger. Following each bout he reported pain and swelling that took weeks to subside. Though the extensor was in its normal midline position at rest, it was easily shifted rapidly, and a defect was palpable in the underlying capsule. **C,** At surgery an incision *(arrows)* was made to the radial side of the extensor tendon through a scarred, but intact, dorsal hood. **D,** With the hood retracted, there was a large defect *(arrows)* in the capsule. **E** and **F,** The capsule was repaired and the dorsal hood closed.

operative treatment, particularly if there is only slight displacement of the tendon, a dorsal capsular tear usually requires surgery (Fig. 26-20). The position of the extensor tendon may aid in the differential diagnosis. In some situations when the capsule is torn on its ulnar aspect, the tendon is deviated radially. This would be exceedingly rare if the injury was confined to the hood. The most important clinical finding is a palpable defect over

the joint, which represents the site of the tear. This is a consistent finding even when the tear is in the midline and there is no tendon subluxation. In these situations the tendon can be shifted to one side, usually the radial, to allow palpation of the defect (Fig. 26-21). At surgery there is scarring either over the tendon itself, or more commonly in the radial or ulnar sagittal fibers. An incision is made in the scarred area of the hood, which is

then retracted to permit inspection of the underlying capsule, which is always torn in a longitudinal direction. Though the torn edges of the capsule may be retracted and adherent to the hood, they can be mobilized by sharp dissection and brought together for repair. Contractures of the torn capsule have not been observed, probably because the tears are never transverse. Any ragged edges of the capsule are sharply excised; however, before this is done care must be taken to ensure that the edges of the capsule can be brought together for repair without limiting passive flexion of the joint. Following capsular repair with fine nonabsorbable sutures, the incision in the sagittal fibers is closed, and if necessary the extensor tendon is relocated into its normal midline position. Postoperatively the joint is immobilized in flexion. This position is particularly important for boxers. Though a residual flexion contracture would not pose any functional impairment in making a fist, a mild extension contracture might end the athlete's career. Active exercises are started 3 weeks after surgery, and punching is avoided for at least 6 months. In athletes for whom clenching a fist is not as important, the joint is immobilized in less flexion postoperatively.

Fractures

Fractures of the distal portion of a metacarpal are more likely to involve the neck of the bone than its intraarticular head. A fracture of the metacarpal neck usually results from a direct blow with the clenched fist. Typically the fracture is angled dorsally because of the direction of the impact and the deforming force of the interossei muscles. The angulation can result in several problems: the head, which is tilted volarly, can cause a painful prominence in the palm that interferes with grasp; there may be a tendon imbalance similar to but less severe than that which occurs with angulated fractures in the midshaft of the bone; and finally extension at the metacarpophalangeal joint is restricted equivalent to the degree of volar tilt of the head.[185] The latter problem is usually of little functional significance, because the normal hyperextension of the metacarpophalangeal joints that exists in many patients negates any loss of extension. As with the indications for treatment of angulated shaft fractures, various figures have been proposed as being acceptable depending on the particular metacarpal that is fractured. Greater angulation can generally be tolerated for the fourth and especially the fifth metacarpal because of the mobility of their carpometacarpal joints, which diminishes the effect of the palmar protrusion of the heads of the bones during grasp. The acceptable degree of angulation depends not simply on a numeric value but on the specific functional requirements of each patient.

**Problems stemming from residual angulation
of metacarpal neck fractures**

- Metacarpal head in palm; painful and interferes with grip
- Tendon imbalance
- Loss of metacarpophalangeal extension

Though slight angulation in a fourth or fifth metacarpal neck fracture may not be annoying to a basketball or football player, it may compromise the effectiveness of a baseball pitcher and have dire consequences for a boxer.

Frequently, metacarpal neck fractures can be treated by closed reduction. The metacarpophalangeal joint of the injured finger is flexed completely, which relaxes the deforming force of the intrinsic muscles. More important, this maneuver tightens the collateral ligaments, which stabilize the fractured metacarpal head, and upward pressure on the proximal phalanx levers the head back into alignment. First recommended by Jahss,[87] this is an effective technique for reducing a fracture; however, it should never be used as a method for immobilization because it will result in proximal interphalangeal joint stiffness or even pressure necrosis over the extensor mechanism at that joint. If closed reduction is not successful or if the reduction is unstable, surgery is necessary. Kirschner wire fixation of the fracture is an effective method, either alone or in combination with a dorsal tension band wire.

Though intraarticular fractures are less common than metacarpal neck fractures, they are potentially more serious and often lead to joint stiffness. These fractures are classified depending on anatomic involvement and include small osteochondral fragments, intraarticular fractures that are oblique (sagittal), vertical (coronal), or horizontal (transverse), comminuted fractures, and those associated with ligament avulsions.[124] Avulsion fractures may be small, and special radiographic views may aid in their visualization, including the Brewerton view.[106] This view, which was originally designed to demonstrate early erosive changes in the metacarpal heads in patients with rheumatoid arthritis, is taken with the dorsal aspects of the fingers on the radiographic cassette, the metacarpophalangeal joints flexed 65 degrees, and the roentgen beam angled from a position 15 degrees to the ulnar side of the hand.[24] Treatment for intraarticular fractures frequently requires surgery to restore articular congruity. The use of Kirschner wires is an effective method of fixation. Postoperatively the joint is immobilized in flexion, and active range of motion exercises are started within a week or two to minimize joint stiffness. In severely comminuted fractures of the metacarpal head, skeletal traction through the proximal phalanx may be required to maintain the length of the bone.

Intraarticular fracture patterns

- Osteochondral fragments
- Oblique (sagittal)
- Vertical (coronal)
- Horizontal (transverse)
- Associated with ligament avulsions

PROXIMAL PHALANGEAL AREA
Anatomy

In contradistinction to the metacarpal area of the palm, the phalangeal areas in the fingers are not protected by

overlying muscles and are in closer contact with the tendons. At the proximal phalangeal level the bone is virtually encircled by tendons, with the flexor tendons on their volar aspect and the extensor tendon mechanism laterally and dorsally. A cross-section through this level demonstrates the intimate association between bone and surrounding tendons and the limited area through which the tendons glide. Any disturbance in these gliding pathways causes tendon adherence and subsequent loss of mobility. The area is therefore vulnerable to the pernicious effects of edema.

Tendon Injuries

Aside from lacerations, tendon problems in this area are usually caused by closed trauma. The normally restricted area in which the tendons glide can easily become more limited by adhesions, which may develop with or without a concomitant fracture. The problems are magnified with a fracture because of the likelihood for greater scarring and the fact that even slight bony displacement may further interfere with the gliding pathways of the tendons. Adhesions may involve the extrinsic or intrinsic components of the dorsal tendon mechanism, or they may affect the flexor tendons on the volar aspect of the digit.

Scarring of an extrinsic extensor tendon is most likely to occur as the tendon passes under the retinaculum at the wrist level or over the dorsal aspect of the hand, where it may become adherent to a metacarpal. At these locations the limited excursion of the tendon prevents simultaneous flexion of the metacarpophalangeal and proximal interphalangeal joints of a finger. This dorsal tenodesis prevents flexion of the proximal interphalangeal joint when the metacarpophalangeal joint is actively or passively flexed. When the proximal interphalangeal joint flexes, the reverse situation occurs at the metacarpophalangeal joint and it goes into extension or even hyperextension. Clinically the patient is able to actively flex the proximal interphalangeal joint if the metacarpophalangeal joint is extended and vice versa. Simultaneous flexion of both joints is impossible. When the extrinsic extensor becomes adherent over the proximal phalanx, the tenodesis affects flexion at only one joint, the proximal interphalangeal joint. Scarring of the dorsal tendon mechanism may also involve and be limited to its intrinsic components, the lateral bands. Clinically the test for intrinsic tightness will be positive. As discussed in the section on intrinsic contractures at the metacarpal level, testing for tight intrinsics is a passive examination, and it is important that the patient not try to assist the examiner by actively flexing the finger. Active flexion of the finger may mask a mild degree of intrinsic tightness, and the problem may go unrecognized. On the volar surface of the proximal phalanx adhesions are more likely to involve the flexor superficialis tendon, where the broad area of the Camper chiasma is in closer contact with the bone than is the flexor profundus tendon. Clinically, extension of the proximal interphalangeal joint is limited because of the tethering effect of the adhesions between tendon and bone. If the profundus tendon is spared, motions at the distal interphalangeal joint are not affected.

Treatment for adhesions of the flexor and extensor tendons should be preventive by encouraging early range of motion exercises after any injury. The use of dynamic splints is often effective. For chronic cases in which adhesions are permanent and refractory to therapy, surgical tenolysis is required. With respect to the dorsal tendon mechanism, adhesions involving the extrinsic tendon component are released and the patient is started on an early program of active and passive exercises. With involvement of one or both lateral bands of the intrinsic component of this mechanism, the band(s) together with its oblique fibers are excised, but the transverse fibers are preserved. When surgery is required for adhesions involving the flexor system, tenolysis of the flexor superficialis tendon may not be adequate, because the tendon may be too badly damaged to permit its salvage. Excision of the tendon is often warranted in such cases. As with extensor tendon releases, early active range of motion exercises are started immediately after surgery. Flexion exercises against resistance or the use of a forceful dynamic extension splint should be avoided for several weeks if the vinculum longus to the profundus had to be sacrificed during tenolysis or if excision of the flexor superficialis was necessary. Circulation to the profundus would be compromised in such cases and there would be a danger of it rupturing.

Fractures

Treatment of fractures of the proximal phalanx is difficult because of the necessity of restoring alignment and maintaining stability of the bone to facilitate early exercises (Fig. 26-22). Various classifications can be used for these fractures, including the anatomic region of the bone that is damaged and whether the fracture is intraarticular.[88] This discussion groups fractures according to location: base, shaft, and neck and head regions.

Base Fractures

Fractures of the base are frequently angulated volarly because of the pull of the intrinsic muscles. The degree of angulation is difficult to visualize by lateral radiograph because the proximal phalanges of the uninjured fingers are superimposed on the film. An oblique radiograph is helpful, but it may fail to show the true severity of the angulation. Unfortunately many of these fractures heal in malunited positions, which seriously compromises prehension.[36] Active extension at the proximal interphalangeal joint is diminished because the dorsal tendon mechanism is relaxed, and active flexion may also be affected by the increase in excursion that is required of the flexor tendons as they pass around the volar convexity at the fracture site. Flexion may also become limited at the metacarpophalangeal joint as contractures develop in the collateral ligaments.

Volar angulation of the fracture is often noticed by a depression on the dorsal aspect of the bone, which can be palpated as the examiner's finger moves across the metacarpophalangeal joint and along the dorsal aspect of the phalanx. Reduction of the fracture is achieved by acutely flexing the metacarpophalangeal joint, which relaxes the intrinsics and stabilizes the proximal fragment

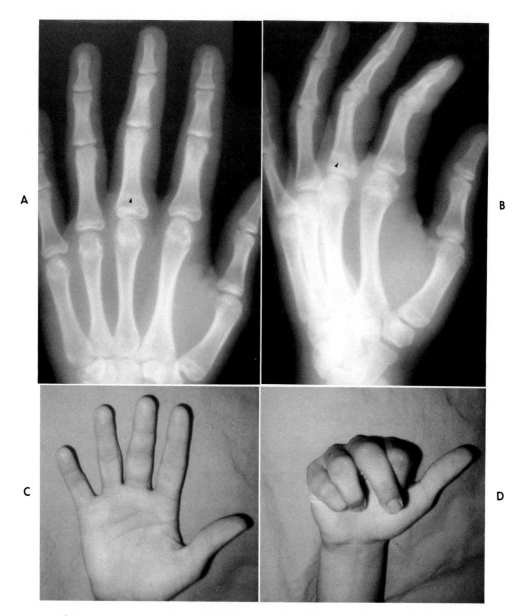

FIG. 26-22. A and **B,** Careful clinical examination of an injured digit is the essential first step in the treatment of any fracture. The oblique fracture at the base of the proximal phalanx of the middle finger *(arrows)* appears nondisplaced in these AP and oblique radiographs. **C** and **D,** Clinical examination showed an obvious rotational deformity of the digit, which was corrected by nonoperative measures.

by tightening the collateral ligaments. The proximal interphalangeal joint is then placed in complete extension to relax the central extensor tendon, thereby further neutralizing any muscle imbalance.[185] The distal fracture fragment is then flexed, correcting the angulation. The digit is immobilized, maintaining the metacarpophalangeal joint in acute flexion and the proximal interphalangeal joint in slight flexion, not exceeding 30 degrees. This immobilization is the safe position because it reduces the likelihood of contractures at both joint levels. This position should be differentiated from the position of function, in which the metacarpophalangeal joints are

in only slight flexion and the interphalangeal joints in greater flexion. The position of function would be appropriate for fusions of these joints, but not suitable for preventing contractures. If the fracture cannot be reduced and stabilized in almost an anatomic position, internal fixation is necessary. Though percutaneous wires inserted across the flexed metacarpophalangeal joint and down the medullary cavity of the phalanx has been recommended,[9] the technique will likely cause scarring in the dorsal tendon mechanism. Inserting the wires to either side of the central tendon and only into the proximal phalanx is less likely to cause these problems. If per-

7

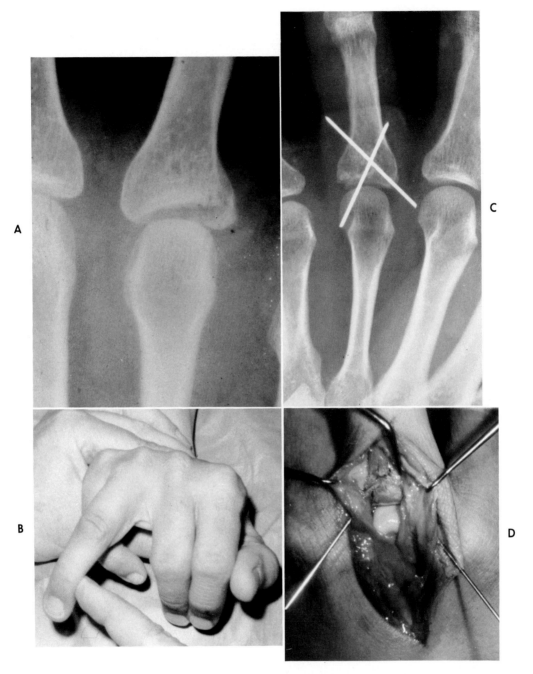

FIG. 26-23. A and **B,** This intraarticular fracture of the base of the proximal phalanx resembled a collateral ligament injury with apparent instability of the metacarpophalangeal joint. **C** and **D,** Open reduction and internal fixation of the fracture were necessary. The Kirschner wires were inserted into the sides of the phalanx, avoiding any further damage to the joint.

cutaneous wires do not achieve the desired result, the fracture should be opened and wires inserted under direct vision.

Salter-Harris Type II epiphyseal fractures are common injuries in children and usually involve the little finger. If there is lateral deviation at the fracture, reduction is accomplished in the same manner as in adults. A pencil is placed in the web space, which provides leverage for manipulation of the fracture. Rarely is any in-

ternal fixation required. If it is, a single, thin, nonthreaded Kirschner wire is drilled percutaneously across the epiphyseal plate. Removing the wire within 3 weeks is unlikely to cause any growth damage.

With respect to **intraarticular fractures at the base of the phalanx,** the same method of reduction applies as for nonarticular fractures. However, the likelihood for surgery to restore articular congruity is greater, particularly if the fragment is sizable and associated with joint

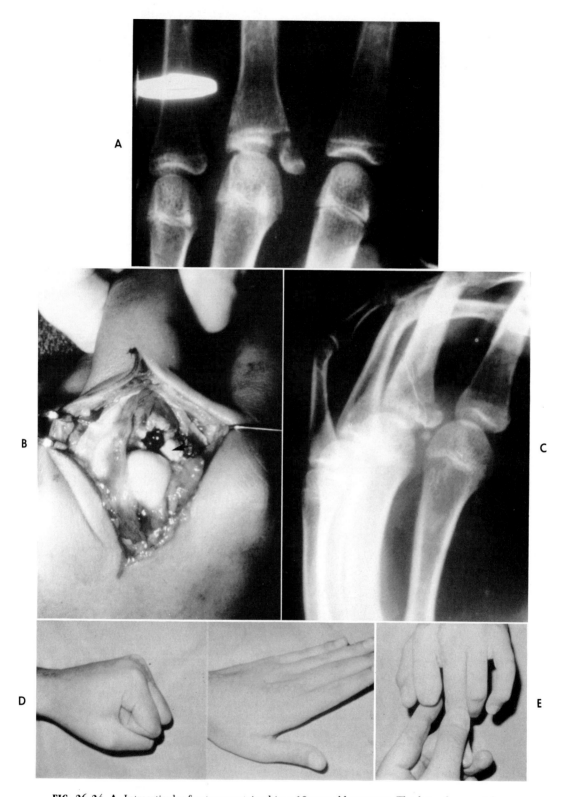

FIG. 26-24. A, Intraarticular fracture sustained in a 16-year-old gymnast. The bone fragment from the epiphysis was displaced and rotated. **B** and **C,** At surgery the collateral ligament, as anticipated, was attached to the bone fragment (*arrow*), which was reattached into the phalanx with a wire suture. **D** and **E,** The gymnast regained complete mobility and stability of the finger.

instability (Fig. 26-23).[139] Intraarticular fractures are also seen in children (Salter-Harris Type III) and occur more commonly than those at the base of the middle phalanx as a result of differences in the insertions of the collateral ligaments at these two joint levels. The collateral ligaments for the proximal phalanx insert exclusively into the epiphysis, whereas the insertion of the ligaments at the middle phalanx extend further distally (Fig. 26-24).[13] If surgery is required, it is best carried out through a curved incision to one side of the metacarpophalangeal joint. The transverse and sagittal fibers are incised and the extensor tendon retracted. The underlying capsule is then opened to allow visualization of the fracture site. The bone fragment with its attached collateral ligament is then stabilized using a Kirschner wire, wire suture, or small screw. A straight dorsal incision, which splits the extensor tendon, should be reserved for operative reduction of displaced T-shaped fractures that cannot be adequately visualized by either a radial or ulnar approach.[55,156] This tendon-splitting incision, though it provides excellent visualization of the entire dorsal and lateral aspects of the phalanx, tends to cause greater scarring and adherence of the extensor mechanism, thereby limiting restoration of mobility. Meticulous closure of the periosteum and tendon as separate layers will reduce but not eliminate the risk of later adhesions.

Shaft Fractures

Shaft fractures may be transverse, oblique, spiral, or comminuted.[7] The spiral type may actually be intraarticular, extending into the proximal interphalangeal joint. If unrecognized and allowed to heal in this position, the fracture spike can block joint flexion. As with any fracture, a complete radiographic examination in-

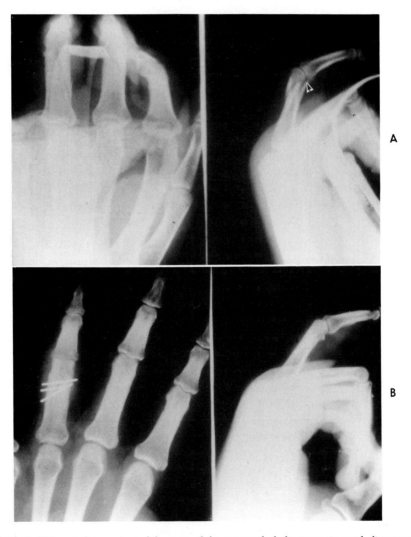

FIG. 26-25. A, This spiral comminuted fracture of the proximal phalanx was in good alignment in the posteroanterior radiograph. However, the lateral radiograph showed displacement with a spike of the proximal fragment (*arrow*) abutting against the base of the middle phalanx. **B,** An anatomic reduction was obtained after surgery, and rigid internal fixation with Kirschner wires permitted early active range of motion exercises. Cortical screws could not be used because the fracture was comminuted.

cluding a direct lateral view is mandatory. Proper radiographs at the time of the injury demonstrate any problem and often make later, more difficult reconstructive surgery unnecessary (Fig. 26-25).

Most shaft fractures are nondisplaced and can be managed by splint immobilization. Early active range of motion exercises within 3 weeks are important if function is to be restored.[27,181] As fracture healing progresses, the digit is protected until there is complete union. This can be achieved by strapping the injured finger to an adjacent finger (buddy taping). Although this is a satisfactory method of protection, it is not a successful method for stabilizing a fracture immediately after the acute injury. Return to full activity should not be permitted until there is radiographic evidence of complete healing.

If the fracture cannot be reduced, internal fixation is required. Percutaneous wires enjoy considerable popularity, and various clamps that stabilize the fractures as well as facilitate introduction of the wires have been devised.[11,69,139] However, these methods often fail to achieve a complete reduction, and wire placement may interfere with joint motions (Fig. 26-26).[8] If a fracture is in an unsatisfactory position and reduction and internal fixation are required, the reduction should be anatomic and the fixation precise. This is best achieved by surgery in which an incision is made in the midaxial line on either the radial or ulnar side of the bone. The side of the finger on which the midaxial incision is made matters little for a transverse fracture, and only surgical convenience need be considered. For an oblique fracture, however, it is important to make the incision on the side to which the distal fragment has displaced. In this manner

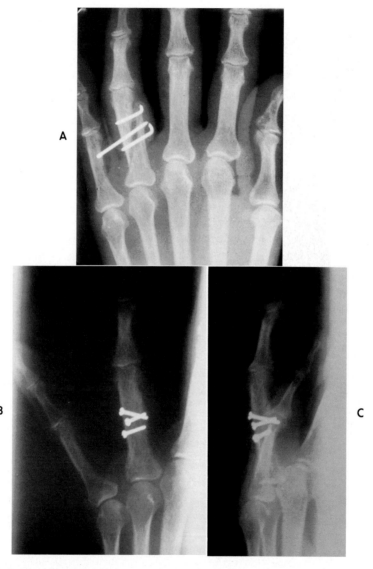

FIG. 26-26. A, This oblique fracture of the proximal phalanx was treated at another hospital with percutaneous pins. When seen 2 weeks later the fracture was obviously in an unsatisfactory position. **B** and **C,** Open reduction and internal fixation using cortical screws were immediately carried out, which would have been the preferred treatment initially.

the unstable distal fragment can be accurately reduced and fixed to the stable proximal fragment. Failure to make the incision of the proper side of the finger seriously interferes with visualizing the fracture site and makes it virtually impossible to achieve a rigid and anatomic reduction unless a second midaxial incision is made on the opposite side of the finger. The extensor tendon mechanism is retracted dorsally, and the bone is subperiosteally exposed. If the proximal portion of the bone must be exposed and the lateral band cannot be adequately retracted dorsally, an incision is made through the oblique and transverse fibers, and the lateral band is retracted in the volar direction. After the fracture is stabilized, the lateral band can be resutured using fine (5-0 or 6-0) monofilament nylon.

Various techniques for fixation can be used depending on the nature of the fracture, as well as the experience of the surgeon. For oblique and spiral fractures, Kirschner wires are effective. If possible, the wires are inserted in a frontal plane between the flexor and extensor tendons so that the pins do not interfere with the gliding of the tendons. Because fractures may take many weeks and sometimes months to unite, there is no urgency to remove the wires. As a general principle, wires that are left in place for an indefinite period are cut off beneath the skin. Wires that will be removed at a specific time (usually within a few weeks) can be left protruding through the skin. Included in the latter category are wires that transfix joints. Oblique and spiral fractures can also be rigidly fixed using small cortical screws, and generally they are preferable to Kirschner wires provided that the fracture is not comminuted and the length of the fracture is at least twice the width of the bone.[80,127,128]

With transverse fractures a variety of methods have also been employed, including crossed Kirschner wires, interosseous wiring combined with a single wire, or tension band fixation on the dorsal or tension side of the bone. The use of a plate and screws, though technically feasible, is rarely necessary. The relative bulk of these devices applied to a small bone with limited soft tissue coverage tends to interfere with tendon gliding.

Neck and Head Fractures

Fractures of the distal end of the phalanx involve either the intraarticular neck portion of the bone or the intraarticular condyles. **Phalangeal neck fractures** are more common in children than adults. Displacement of the phalangeal head can be severe, often exceeding 90 degrees. In the AP radiographs the rotated head presents an ovoid appearance similar to a metacarpal head epiphysis.[40] Because there is no epiphysis at this end of the phalanx, this radiographic sign should alert the examiner to a serious problem. The lateral radiograph clearly demonstrates that the phalangeal head is not only displaced dorsally, but also rotated so that its articular surface faces dorsally and its fractured side volarly. An attempt should be made to manipulate the displaced head back into position by applying firm digital pressure to the dorsal aspect of the acutely flexed joint.[139] Surgery for this fracture is difficult because of the small size of the

phalangeal head fragment and the limited area available for stabilization. The fracture is exposed through a midaxial incision, and, if possible, crossed Kirschner wires are drilled across the fracture site. The first wire is drilled from the head into the proximal shaft. In young children the phalangeal head is very small and there may be room for only a single wire. If the thinnest caliber Kirschner wire is still too wide, a straight needle can be substituted. The problem of fixation is not as difficult in adults, in whom the larger bone fragment permits other techniques to be used, including intraosseous wiring.[114] Although it has been reported that there is no appreciable remodeling of these fractures and any residual angulation is unacceptable,[8,112] this is not the situation in children. As long as there is no rotation of the head, remodeling does occur with bone growth since the angulation is in the axis of joint motions. Naturally, the younger the child at the time of injury, the greater the likelihood for remodeling.

Condylar fractures are either unicondylar or bicondylar. Unicondylar fractures are common in athletic injuries, and unfortunately delayed treatment is common because good joint mobility often remains.[174] Lateral inclination of the finger soon becomes obvious as the joint tilts toward the side of the displaced condyle. Open reduction and internal fixation of the displaced condyle are necessary using either Kirschner wires or a lag screw (Fig. 26-27).[38] The fracture is exposed either by a midaxial incision and dorsal retraction of the lateral band, or by a curved incision and entering into the joint between the central slip and the lateral band. Care is taken not to disturb the insertion of the central slip or damage the collateral ligament, which provides the blood supply to the condylar fragment.[127,128] Bicondylar fractures present even a greater surgical challenge. The two condyles are first stabilized to each other, then fixed to the shaft of the bone. The surgical approach is, by necessity, an extensive one, and some permanent loss of mobility should be anticipated with these fractures.

PROXIMAL INTERPHALANGEAL JOINT AREA
Anatomy

In no other area of the hand is the anatomy as complex and interrelated as at the proximal interphalangeal joint. Though each anatomic structure in this area is important to the function of the others, the extensor tendon system and the joint capsule deserve special attention because of the frequency of injuries to both and the deleterious effect these injuries have on function.

The extensor system is actually a fascial-tendon expansion with both extrinsic and intrinsic components. At the proximal interphalangeal joint the entire expansion lies dorsal to the axis of the joint with its central tendon (extrinsic component) inserting at the base of the middle phalanx and its two lateral tendons, the lateral bands (intrinsic components), continuing distally and joining to form a single tendon. The insertion of this terminal extensor tendon into the base of the distal phalanx is more secure than is the insertion of the central tendon into the middle phalanx. All the tendons that make up

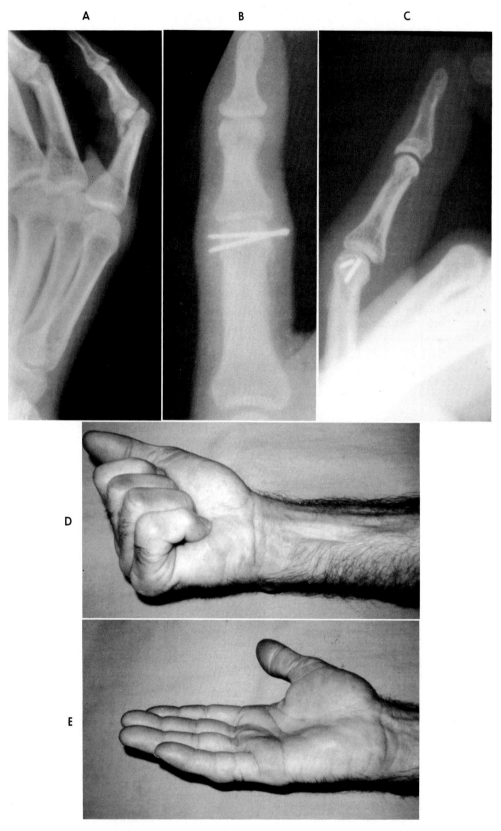

FIG. 26-27. A, Intercondylar fracture of the proximal phalanx, which was untreated for 2 weeks. **B** and **C,** Open reduction and internal fixation were required. During the operation the collateral ligament to the fracture fragment was not disturbed. **D** and **E,** Postoperative mobility.

the extensor mechanism and their fascial connections have fixed and critical lengths, and only a few millimeters of displacement, shortening, or lengthening often result in a diminution of their power and deformity of a finger.[26] Because the three joints within each finger are an intercalated linkage system, a deformity at the proximal interphalangeal joint usually produces deformities at the metacarpophalangeal and distal interphalangeal joints. The limited tolerance for change in the length of any part of the extensor mechanism is not shared by the flexor system, where there is an independent flexor (flexor digitorum superficialis and profundus) for each interphalangeal joint.

The proximal interphalangeal joint itself is a hinge or ginglymus joint, permitting a wide range of motion in a flexion-extension arc ranging from 100 to 110 degrees. The articular surfaces consist of the head of the proximal phalanx, which has two condyles of almost perfect curvature separated by a shallow intercondylar grove.[45] The articular surface of the middle phalanx is broad, and its anatomic features are the reciprocal of the proximal phalanx, consisting of two depressions separated by a median ridge. The joint surface of the proximal and middle phalanges form a tongue-and-groove configuration that facilitates movement in the sagittal plane but resists lateral or rotational motions. In the transverse plane the joint surfaces are about equal, but in the sagittal plane the base of the middle phalanx covers only half of the head of the proximal phalanx.[45] Thus in extension a considerable portion of the condyles of the proximal phalanx protrudes volarly and can easily be palpated.

Laterally the interphalangeal joint is supported by two layers of soft tissue. The more superficial layer is thin and consists of the transverse and oblique fibers of the retinacular ligaments of Landsmeer and the intermediate bundle of the Cleland ligament.[37] The deeper layer, which is much thicker, consists of collateral ligaments that are quadrangular and arise from small fossae on the sides of the head of the proximal phalanx and insert into the volar one third of the middle phalanx and into the distal margins of the volar plate. The collateral ligaments are 2 to 3 mm thick, and their widths at origin and insertion are almost half their length.[46] Some of the ligaments fibers run in a more oblique direction and insert into the sides of the volar plate, forming the accessory collateral ligaments. Unlike the ligaments at the metacarpophalangeal joint level, whose tension depends on the position of the joint, the ligament tension at the proximal interphalangeal joints varies little from extension to flexion.

The volar plate, or glenoid fibrocartilage, forms the floor of the joint. Though similar to the plate at the metacarpophalangeal joint, the volar plate at the proximal interphalangeal joint has several distinct differences. The distal attachment of its thick cartilaginous portion is only at its lateral margins, where it becomes confluent with the insertion of the collateral and accessory collateral ligaments. These attachments into the lateral volar tubercles of the middle phalanx at the critical corners provide the main resistance against hyperextension of the joint.[17,21] The central portion of the distal end of the

plate, making up more than three fourths of its width, has no firm insertion into the phalanx, which in this area consists of the volar tubercle of the median ridge. The plate attachment in this area is to the periosteum on the metaphyseal portion of the bone, which gives the plate a meniscoid character. This configuration facilitates movement of the plate away from the base of the middle phalanx during flexion.[21,61] Proximally the plate thins in its central portion, which allows passage for important capsular vessels.[67] The lateral portions are much thicker. They attach to ridges on the phalanx just proximal to the condyles, inside the walls of the distal portion of the second annular (A-2) pulley, and confluent with the origin of the proximal portion of the first cruciate (C-1) pulley.[21] These proximal attachments, referred to as the lower fibers of the capsule[103] or the check-rein ligaments,[46] produce a swallow-tail configuration at the proximal portion of the plate.[21] Dorsally the joint capsule is intimately connected with the extensor apparatus, and it is difficult to separate the two. The central tendon not only functions as an active extensor of the joint but also serves as a dorsal ligament.[45]

Tendon Injuries
Acute Boutonnière Deformity

Tendon injuries at the proximal interphalangeal joint are usually closed and almost always involve the central slip of the extensor tendon mechanism. Aside from injuries to the terminal extensor tendon at the distal interphalangeal joint, which is discussed in a subsequent section, injuries to the central tendon are the most common closed tendon injuries in athletes.[27,121] They result from direct trauma to the tendon or from sudden forced flexion of the joint. Often the athlete neglects to seek immediate medical attention or, if attention is sought, an accurate diagnosis may not be made. Initially there may be only a paucity of objective clinical findings. The joint may be only slightly swollen and there may be little or no loss of active extension. A boutonnière deformity may not be present. However, after a week or two, as the lateral bands slip volarly, the characteristic deformity becomes obvious.

An index of suspicion and a careful physical examination are necessary if an accurate diagnosis is to be made at the time of the injury and prompt, effective treatment is to be instituted. Localization of the area of maximum tenderness is important; it will be over the insertion of the central tendon into the base of the middle phalanx. Though any loss of joint extension is significant, it is not by itself pathognomonic of tendon injury. A more important clue to the injury may be obtained by observing active and passive flexion at the distal interphalangeal joint after first stabilizing the proximal interphalangeal joint in extension. With disruption of the central tendon, even slight volar slippage of the lateral bands significantly compromise active and passive flexion at the distal joint.[22] Radiographs are usually negative except in those rare cases in which the tendon avulses from the dorsal base of the phalanx with a fragment that can be clearly visualized on a lateral radiograph. If the radiographs are negative, treatment is to splint the proximal interphalan-

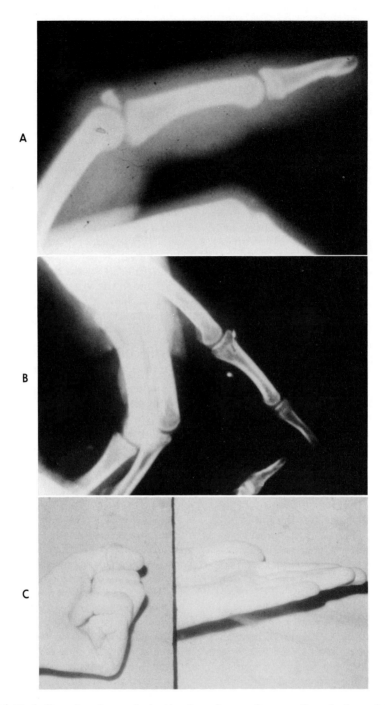

FIG. 26-28. A, Central tendon avulsed with a large fracture fragment from the base of the middle phalanx, resulting in an acute boutonnière deformity. **B,** The fragment was reattached with the cerclage wire. **C,** Postoperative mobility.

geal joint in full extension, leaving the distal interphalangeal joint free. Active and passive flexion exercises for the distal interphalangeal joint are encouraged to prevent contracture of the retinacular ligaments.[151] Continuous splinting for the proximal interphalangeal joint is maintained for 4 to 5 weeks, followed by periodic splinting for an additional 2 weeks. During this time active range of motion exercises are encouraged for the other two joints

in the finger. Only in those rare cases of avulsion fracture is surgery required for the acute injury. If the fragment is large enough, a transverse drill hole is made in it as well as in the phalanx, and the fracture is then reattached using a 30- to 32-gauge wire (Fig. 26-28). If the fragment is small, the wire suture is passed through the central tendon rather than the fragment and then anchored to the phalanx. The wire suture must be passed

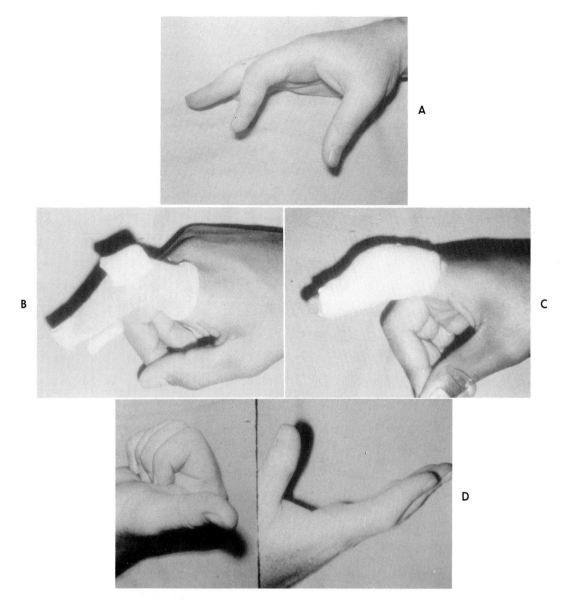

FIG. 26-29. A, Closed injury to the extensor tendon at the proximal interphalangeal joint that occurred 6 weeks earlier. **B** and **C,** Serial plaster casts were applied each week to correct the secondary joint contracture. The casts were applied with padding limited only to the pressure areas over the dorsal aspect of the proximal interphalangeal joint and the volar aspect of the distal interphalangeal joint. **D,** After four serial casts the patient regained complete flexion at both interphalangeal joints with only a slight impairment in extension at the proximal interphalangeal joint.

deep to the lateral bands before it is threaded through the phalanx to avoid limiting the excursion of the lateral bands.

Subacute Boutonnière Deformity

If the injury is untreated for several weeks, contractures develop at both interphalangeal joints. In this subacute stage it may be possible to improve passive extension of the proximal interphalangeal joint by the use of serial casts, which are changed weekly, or by dynamic splints. After joint extension is achieved, the digit is splinted for several weeks with the proximal interphalan-

geal joint in extension but the distal joint free. Active range of motion exercises are then encouraged for all joints. These patients usually regain satisfactory function of the injured finger without surgery, though mobility is rarely completely restored (Fig. 26-29).

Chronic Boutonnière Deformity

When the condition is chronic, the flexion contracture at the proximal interphalangeal joint and extension contracture at the distal interphalangeal joint have become rigid. The chronic boutonnière deformity is among the most difficult and challenging problems to treat. The

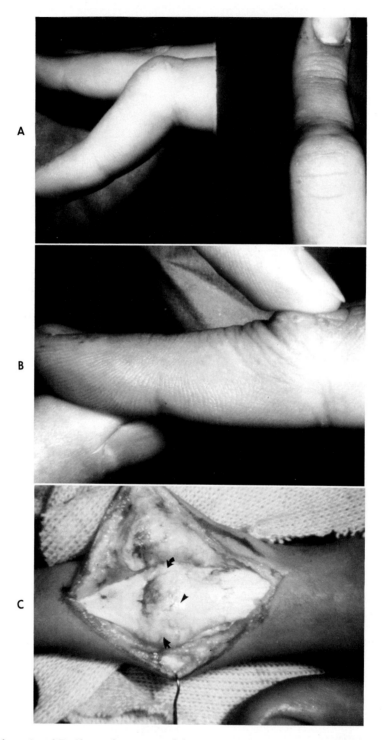

FIG. 26-30. A and **B,** Chronic boutonnière deformity in a young patient with full passive extension of the proximal interphalangeal joint, an ideal situation for reconstructive surgery. **C,** The central tendon was scarred and retracted *(small arrow)* and both lateral bands *(curved arrows)* were subluxed volar to the axis of motion at the joint.
Continued.

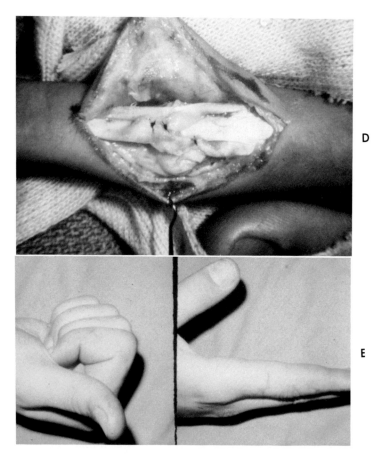

FIG. 26-30, cont'd. D, The lateral bands were replaced dorsally and the central tendon advanced. Sutures were placed in the extensor mechanism distal to the joint level to avoid producing a later extension contracture. **E,** Postoperative mobility.

original injury confined to the central extensor tendon has progressed to volar displacement and fixation of the lateral bands, fibrosis with shortening of the transverse and oblique retinacular ligaments, and contractures of the collateral ligaments at both interphalangeal joints. Essentially there are two problems: an incompetent extensor tendon mechanism and a flexion contracture at the proximal interphalangeal joint. Though it is technically feasible to treat both problems with a single operation, namely a capsulectomy at the proximal interphalangeal joint to restore full passive extension and a reconstruction of the tendon mechanism, the result would be poor. Postoperative care following a capsulectomy, which involves early active and passive exercises, is radically different from that following tendon reconstruction, which requires that the digit be immobilized for several weeks. Capsulectomy and tendon reconstruction carried out together would in all likelihood convert the stiff flexed finger into a stiff extended one.

The primary objective with a chronic boutonnière deformity is to improve passive joint mobility by nonoperative measures. If this can be achieved, then the only problem remaining is the damaged extensor tendon, which then can be improved by surgery. Serial casts followed by dynamic splints are used to treat the joint con-

tractures. Passive extension at the proximal interphalangeal joint must be restored before surgery for the tendon problem can be considered.

A variety of surgical techniques are available to reconstruct the tendon, and all have the same goals—to advance the scarred and retracted central extensor tendon to the level of its normal insertion at the base of the middle phalanx and to relocate the displaced lateral bands to their normal position dorsal to the axis of motion at the proximal interphalangeal joint (Fig. 26-30). The extension or hyperextension at the distal interphalangeal joint can be managed either by passive flexion of the joint and fixation in a more functional flexed position with a Kirschner wire for several weeks or, if the joint cannot be manipulated, by division of the terminal extensor tendon. A mild flexion contracture at the distal joint is much more functional than a hyperextension contracture.

If the joint contractures do not respond to conservative measures and remain rigid, a two-stage procedure is required. Capsulectomy is the first procedure, and after satisfactory passive mobility is restored, the dorsal tendon mechanism is reconstructed. This two-stage procedure is rarely indicated because of the prolonged period of rehabilitation required, usually a minimum of 6

months. Before this extensive reconstructive program is considered, the boutonnière deformity should be causing a significant disability. Equally important is that the patient must have a complete understanding of the complexity of the problem, the limited objectives of the surgical procedures, and the necessity for complete cooperation in the postoperative therapy. In some cases for which two-stage procedure is planned, the function of the extensor mechanism improves sufficiently after capsulectomy, and a second operation is unnecessary.

Pseudoboutonnière Deformity

Pseudoboutonnière deformity is often confused with boutonnière deformity. The two deformities bear a superficial resemblance in that the proximal interphalangeal joint is in a flexed position in both. The difference can be distinguished by observing the distal interphalangeal joint: there is an extension or hyperextension contracture in the boutonnière deformity, but normal mobility in the pseudoboutonnière deformity.[161] The two deformities also differ in their mechanism of injury and the time it takes for joint contractures to appear. Boutonnière deformity results from damage to the central extensor tendon, and joint contractures develop soon after the injury. In contrast, pseudoboutonnière deformity follows a hyperextension injury, which tears the volar capsule of the proximal interphalangeal joint. The flexion contracture develops as a later complication.[119,121,123] Rarely a severe and chronic pseudoboutonnière deformity can develop into a boutonnière deformity as the central slip elongates over the flexed proximal interphalangeal joint, which permits the lateral bands to slip volarly. Secondary contractures of the retinacular ligaments then develop, limiting flexion at the distal interphalangeal joint, and the transformation is completed.

Initial treatment for pseudoboutonnière deformity involves active and passive exercises and the use of dynamic extension splints to restore extension at the proximal interphalangeal joint. If the proximal interphalangeal joint contracture is rigid and disabling, surgical release followed by early exercises is necessary. Because there is no damage to the dorsal tendon mechanism in these cases, the prognosis for regaining mobility is better than after surgery for a boutonnière deformity.

Ligament Injuries

Injuries to the ligaments at the proximal interphalangeal joint are among the most common affecting the hand. Their incidence is impossible to establish because medical attention is rarely sought for most of them. Many dislocations spontaneously reduce or are reportedly snapped back into place by the injured athlete. Medical attention is usually sought only because the finger remains painful, swollen, and stiff weeks after the injury. These athletes frequently describe their injury as a *jammed finger*, which may represent a spectrum of diagnoses ranging from a mild first-degree sprain to a third-degree sprain resulting in instability, subluxation, dislocation, or even a fracture-dislocation of the joint. Obviously, a delay of weeks in treating an unstable joint or

a fracture-dislocation results in a serious and permanent impairment. Fortunately, most chronic *jammed fingers* represent first- or second-degree sprains, and no appreciable harm is caused by the delay in treatment. The athlete is often concerned by the persistent joint swelling, and he must be informed that it may take up to 18 months for the swelling to reach a point of maximum improvement. With severe injuries some permanent enlargement of the joint should be anticipated.

Volar Plate

Acute injuries. Injuries to the volar plate occur most commonly in sports activities, in either the recreational amateur athlete or professional.[67] The volar plate is the primary static restraint limiting joint extension. Experimental studies in fresh anatomic specimens show that when stress is applied slowly to the joint, there is a gradual attenuation of the proximal attachments.[17,18] If this stress is continued, the middle phalanx dislocates dorsally, taking with it the volar plate, which can then be entrapped over the head of the proximal phalanx and block reduction. Because a slow hyperextension force is an unusual mechanism of injury, proximal disruption and entrapment of the plate within the joint represent a clinical rarity. When these unusual dislocations do occur, a lateral radiograph view shows persistent incongruity of the joint following attempted reduction (Fig. 26-31).[73,101]

With rapid loading of the joint, which is the usual method of injury, the plate fails at its distal insertion. Two types of distal ruptures are encountered, and each may occur with or without avulsion of a bone flake from the metaphyseal area of the middle phalanx.[17,18] In the Type I rupture the damage is confined to the thin center portion of the plate, and its important corner attachments remain intact. Though these injuries may be initially painful and cause swelling and stiffness, there is no instability with stress testing. Overtreatment must be avoided. If immobilization is used, it should be for a brief period, not exceeding 1 week. Buddy taping for an additional 1 or 2 weeks is all that is required for these injuries. If the hyperextension force on the joint continues, the distal lateral attachments at the plate rupture and the lateral capsule tears between the accessory collateral and collateral ligaments, producing the Type II injury. The middle phalanx can then shift dorsally, hinging on the origins of the collateral ligaments. If the split in the lateral capsule is incomplete, the joint will be hyperextended, sometimes as much as 70 to 80 degrees. However, the articular surfaces remain in contact as the middle phalanx articulates with the dorsal aspect of the head of the proximal phalanx.[43] When the lateral capsular tear is more severe, the middle phalanx actually dislocates dorsally, producing a bayonet alignment with the proximal phalanx. A closed reduction can usually be achieved by simply pushing the displaced middle phalanx over the head of the proximal phalanx. Traction should be avoided, because it could cause entrapment of soft tissues within the joint and prevent reduction.[18] There is rarely any lateral instability after reduction, because the

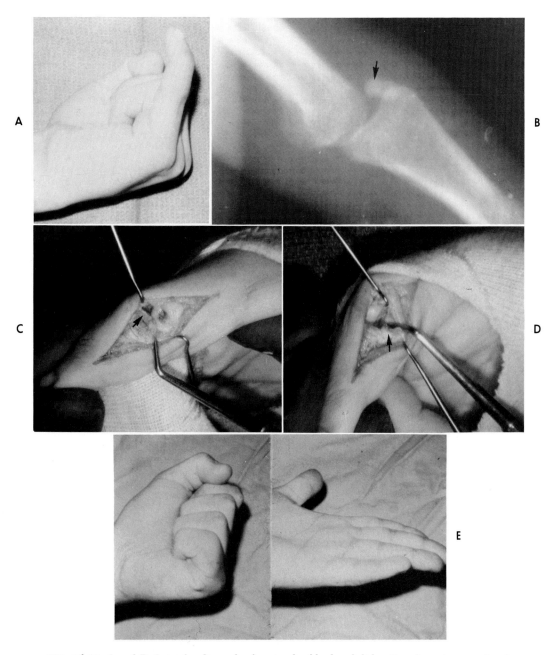

FIG. 26-31. A and **B,** Lateral radiograph of an irreducible dorsal dislocation shows incongruity of the joint. The small bone fragment was attached to the volar plate, which had detached proximally and was dorsal to the head of the proximal phalanx. **C** and **D,** At surgery the plate, which was interposed between the joint, prevented reduction. As soon as it was mobilized *(arrow)*, the subluxation was reduced. **E,** Postoperative mobility.

collateral ligaments remain intact.[17,18,21,46,94] Treatment involves the use of a dorsal block splint. This prevents the joint from extending the last 20 to 30 degrees but permits active and even passive flexion exercises. The presence of an avulsion fracture in Type II injury may even be considered fortunate because the patient will usually receive medical treatment. Problems occur with Type II injuries with no chip fracture because volar instability of the joint often goes unrecognized. Without

appropriate dorsal block splinting, subluxation of the joint may continue and progress to chronic volar instability.

Occasionally a compressive force on the joint or an axial force on the partially flexed finger may cause the volar base of the middle phalanx to shear dorsally against the condyles of the proximal phalanx. This results in a fracture-dislocation, which is often the most complex and difficult to treat intraarticular fracture encountered

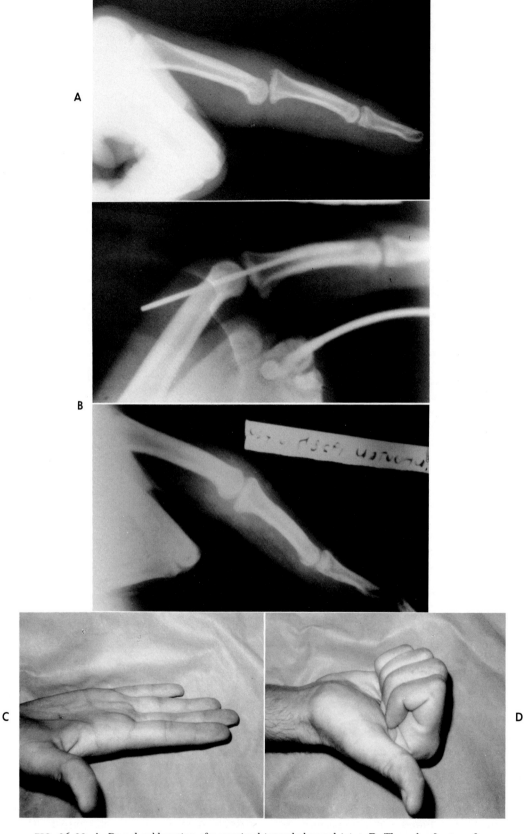

FIG. 26-32. A, Dorsal subluxation of a proximal interphalangeal joint. **B,** The volar fracture fragment was small, and the joint was easily reduced by manipulation and percutaneously wired for 3 to 4 weeks. **C** and **D,** The joint remained stable. The patient regained complete digital mobility.

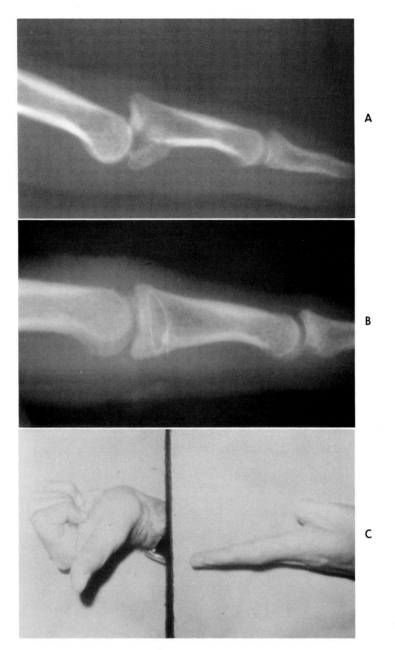

FIG. 26-33. A, Intraarticular fracture of the base of the middle phalanx resulted from a shear force. **B,** Articular congruity was restored by an open reduction and cerclage wire fixation of the fracture fragment. **C,** Postoperative mobility.

in hand trauma.[85] Except for some swelling, the finger may look normal after the injury. Unfortunately the athlete frequently neglects to seek immediate medical attention, which complicates treatment and compromises the ultimate return of joint mobility.

The extent of articular disruption at the base of the middle phalanx determines stability following reduction. Instability is not a problem with small avulsion fractures because the volar plate and only a small portion of the collateral ligaments have disrupted. However, instability should be anticipated with larger fragments that make up a third or more of the articular surface. This is be-

cause most if not all of the collateral ligament insertions into the middle phalanx have been detached. The restraining forces on the middle phalanx are lost, and dorsal bone subluxation occurs. Surgery is necessary, and if possible the volar fragment is reattached using a Kirschner wire or interosseous wire suture (Figs. 26-32 and 26-33).

Frequently the volar fragment is severely comminuted, precluding any reattachment. In these situations the fragments can be excised and the volar plate advanced into the defect of the base of the middle phalanx (Fig. 26-34).[46] A Bruner-type zigzag incision is made on

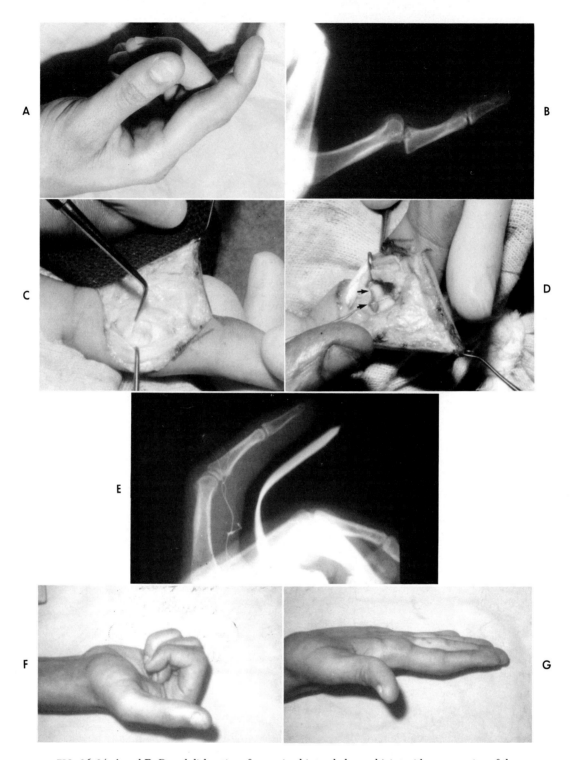

FIG. 26-34. A and **B,** Dorsal dislocation of a proximal interphalangeal joint with compression of the volar one third of the base of the middle phalanx. **C,** Through a volar approach, the joint was explored. With the tendons retracted, the plate was visualized. It had avulsed distally with several small bone fragments and retracted *(probe).* **D** and **E,** The volar plate was reattached into the middle phalanx using a pull-out wire suture, and the digit was immobilized for 3 to 4 weeks before active range of motion exercises were started. **F** and **G,** Postoperative motions of the digit were satisfactory.

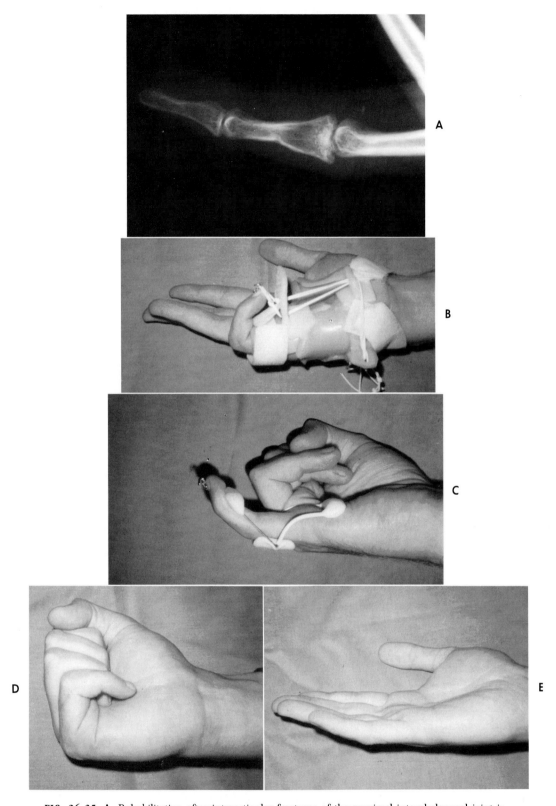

FIG. 26-35. A, Rehabilitation after intraarticular fractures of the proximal interphalangeal joint is lengthy requiring the cooperation of the patient to exercise effectively. **B** and **C,** Frequently dynamic flexor and extensor splints are used to facilitate the exercise program after fracture healing. This dynamic flexion splint has a flexion block at the metacarpophalangeal joint to permit the flexor tendons to exert their full force on the proximal interphalangeal joint. **D** and **E,** Rarely is complete mobility restored to the injured joint, but it is usually in a functional range.

the volar aspect of the digit with the apex of the incision at the midaxial point on either the radial or ulnar side of the proximal interphalangeal flexion crease. A triangular skin flap is elevated, and both neurovascular bundles are identified and protected. The tendon sheath between the A-2 and A-4 pulleys is then excised to permit retraction of the flexor tendons and inspection of the joint. The volar plate can be retracted proximally and the middle phalanx extended to allow visualization of the defect in its articular surface. Division of any remaining portions of the collateral ligaments facilitates the exposure. Small fragments are debrided from the joint as well as from the distal portion of the plate. The joint is then reduced and stabilized in slight flexion (about 30 degrees) using a thin, nonthreaded Kirschner wire. The volar plate is then inserted into the defect in the base of the middle phalanx using a pull-out wire suture. Proper placement of this suture is critical to the procedure. It should first be threaded into the plate with its two ends emerging from the distal corners and then passed into corresponding drill holes that have been made in the lateral margins of the articular defect in the middle phalanx. The wires exit on the dorsal aspect of the bone, and traction on them pulls the plate snugly into the defect. Postoperatively the finger is immobilized for 3 weeks. The wire is then removed and active range of motion exercises begun. Passive flexion also should be encouraged, but passive extension should be avoided for several more weeks. If at that time there is an extension deficit greater than 35 degrees, a dynamic extension splint can be used. Though mobility is rarely restored completely, this difficult operation restores volar stability as well as a satisfactory range of motion (Fig. 26-35).

An alternative procedure is to use a skeletal traction device. Its application is based on the fact that a single axis of rotation of flexion/extension is located between the dorsal and palmar bundles of the collateral ligaments at their origin, on the sides of the head of the proximal phalanx. The device maintains reduction, provides distraction, which permits reduction of the fracture fragments by ligamentoaxis, protects the joint surface from compressive loading, and, most important, allows for immediate active and passive exercises. The procedure is simpler than an operative repair.[79]

Chronic injuries. Chronic injuries to the volar plate involve either an unrecognized fracture-dislocation or volar instability. Treatment for a chronic fracture-dislocation depends on the condition of the joint surfaces. If secondary degenerative arthritic changes have not yet developed, the contracted capsule is released and the volar plate advanced, as for the acute injury. In selected cases an osteotomy of the malunited fracture at the base of the middle phalanx can be considered to salvage some joint function. Once arthritic changes develop, surgical options are either implant arthroplasty or arthrodesis, with arthrodesis being the preferred treatment for the active athlete.

Chronic volar instability is an unusual and interesting condition. There is considerable conjecture why instability develops rather than the more commonly encountered flexion contracture. One theory is that the sparse vascularity at the distal insertion of the plate results in insufficient bleeding to cause scarring after rupture, which would permit adherence of the plate to the bone from which it avulsed.[140] This would explain the tendency for poorer healing when the plate avulses without a fragment from the metaphyseal area of the middle phalanx. The absence of a bone fragment indicates that there was no fracture bleeding, and without bleeding there is less likelihood for scarring.[18] In addition, if the joint is not immobilized after the acute injury or if there are multiple hyperextension injuries, any small clots that form may be washed away by the flow of the synovial fluid between the joint and flexor tendon sheath. The ruptured plate fails to heal and rounds off, similar to what occurs to the ends of flexor tendons severed within their sheaths.[17,83]

With chronic volar instability, the middle phalanx hyperextends, and its articular surfaces frequently get caught in a position on the dorsal aspect of the head of the proximal phalanx. Slight passive flexion is required to unlock the joint before it can be actively flexed. The objective of treatment is to restore a volar restraint to complete joint extension. Various surgical procedures have been described: reattaching the avulsed plate into the middle phalanx,[80,144] shifting a portion of the proximal part of the collateral ligament volarly on the head of the proximal phalanx,[102] and reconstructing a plate substitute using either a free tendon graft[2] or the flexor superficialis tendon in the finger.[97,107,183]

I prefer to use the flexor superficialis tendon because of its strength (Fig. 26-36). A midaxial incision is made along the side of the finger that is most convenient for the surgeon: radial side for the index and middle fingers and ulnar side for the ring and little fingers. The tendon sheath between the A-2 and A-4 pulleys is excised and the flexor tendons retracted, with care taken to avoid damage to their vincula. The ruptured plate is clearly visible with its smooth distal edge. The joint is then fixed in a slightly flexed position of 20 to 30 degrees with a thin, nonthreaded Kirschner wire. A transverse trough is made with a power bur across the diaphyseal portion of the proximal phalanx, and the dorsal surface of the flexor profundus tendon is scraped with a scalpel blade to encourage adhesions between it and the bone. Two drill holes are made in the lateral margins of the trough, and the entire flexor superficialis tendon is then sutured into the trough with a pull-out wire suture. The suture in the tendon should be placed in such a way that it will pull the tendon snugly into the trough. There is no danger of pulling the tendon too tightly, because the degree of joint flexion has already been fixed by the transarticular Kirschner wire. The ends of the wire suture are then tied over padding on the dorsal surface of the phalanx to avoid pressure sores on the skin. The edge of the superficialis tendon is sutured to the edge of the volar plate, thereby adding further reinforcement. After 3 weeks the wire is removed and active exercises including passive flexion are begun. The objective is a joint that has full flexion but is prevented from extending completely by the tenodesis effect of the flexor superficialis tendon.

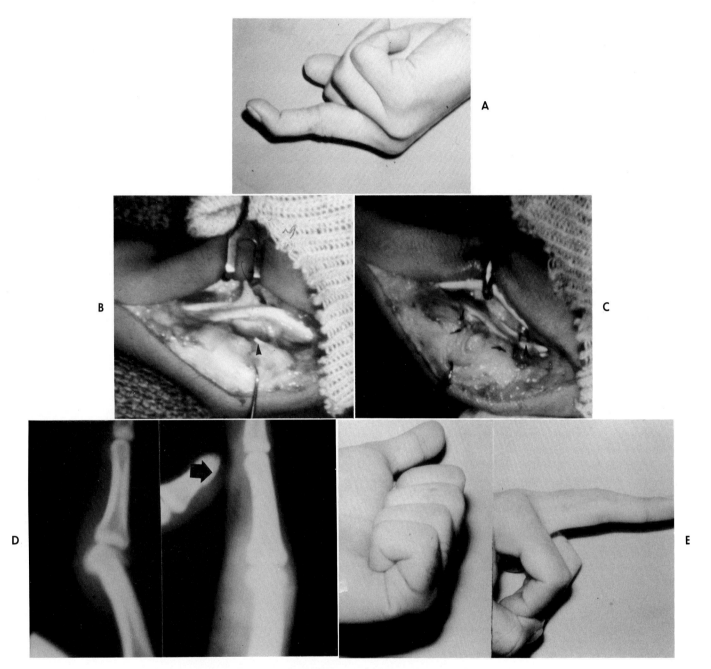

FIG. 26-36. A, Chronic volar instability of the proximal interphalangeal joint in a baseball player. The middle phalanx would frequently get caught in the hyperextended position and the patient would have to passively unlock it to permit flexion. **B,** At surgery the volar plate was seen to be torn distally. **C,** The flexor superficialis tendon *(arrow)* was attached into a trough made in the proximal phalanx with the proximal interphalangeal joint in 20 to 30 degrees of flexion. The edge of the tendon was also sutured to the edge of the volar plate. **D,** Comparison of preoperative and postoperative lateral radiographs. Preoperatively the joint was unstable with active extension. Postoperatively hyperextension was eliminated even to passive forces. (Arrow indicates direction of force of examining finger.) **E,** The patient regained complete mobility. The 20-degree deficit to full extension was insignificant.

Collateral Ligaments

Acute injuries. Lateral dislocation of a proximal interphalangeal joint results after a rupture of one collateral ligament, usually the radial, and most if not all of the insertion of the volar plate.[121,158] The joint hinges laterally on the intact collateral ligament. Usually the dislocation can be easily reduced, and the torn ligament resumes its normal position. Though only one of the collateral ligaments remains intact, the joint is relatively stable because of the congruity of the tongue-and-groove configuration of its articular surfaces and the compressive effect provided by the intact flexor and extensor tendon systems. After reduction the joint should be immobilized for 2 to 3 weeks in slight flexion. Additional protection

can be achieved by buddy taping to the finger on the side of the ligament rupture for several additional weeks. In those dislocations which are reduced spontaneously, the joint appears deceptively normal. However, stress testing readily demonstrates instability and the need for immobilization. Surgery is indicated in those rare acute cases in which reduction cannot be achieved or if the joint redislocates with active motion.

Chronic injuries. Chronic lateral instability is rare. It is usually seen in athletes who report multiple dislocations or whose previous injuries never received adequate treatment. Clinically there is slight enlargement of the joint on the side of the damaged ligament, which is most frequently the radial collateral ligament. Stress testing

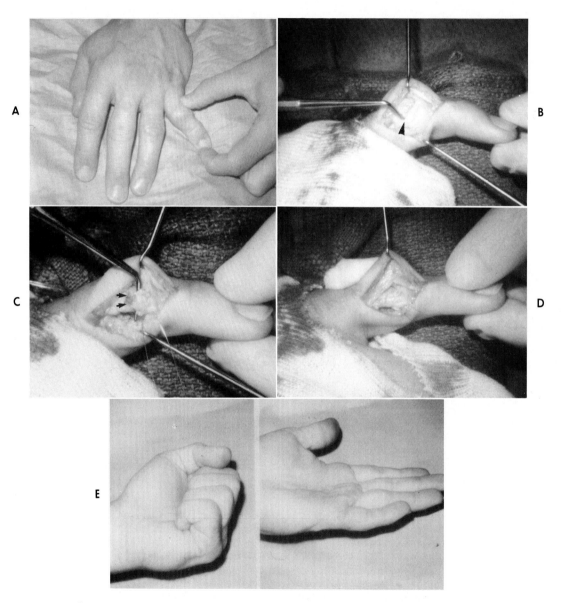

FIG. 26-37. A, Chronic lateral instability of the proximal interphalangeal joint of the little finger in an athlete who reported multiple ulnar dislocations, none of which received any treatment. **B,** Collateral ligament was scarred and attenuated proximally *(probe)*. **C** and **D,** Trough was made in the side of the head of the phalanx *(small arrow)*, and the normal portion of the ligament was reinserted into the bone. **E,** Postoperatively, stability and mobility were restored.

readily demonstrates the degree of instability, and if it is greater than 20 degrees it usually indicates a complete disruption of the collateral ligament.[100] In mild cases buddy taping to the adjacent digit during sports activities may suffice. In more severe cases requiring surgery the procedure depends on the operative findings. If possible, the avulsed collateral ligament is reinserted into the phalanx. This may be feasible even in chronic cases because the ligament rarely ruptures in its midsubstance (Fig. 26-37). Usually the most volar and proximal fibers of the ligament tear first, followed by the dorsal fibers, because the joint is laterally angulated. If there is no rec-

ognizable ligament tissue, a new ligament must be reconstructed using either a portion of the volar plate[53] or the flexor superficialis tendon (Figs. 26-38 and 26-39).[107]

Volar Dislocations

Volar dislocation is far less common than either dorsal or lateral dislocation. This is fortunate because volar dislocation tends to cause residual joint stiffness. The injury results from sudden forceful flexion of the middle phalanx or from violent torsional injury to the joint. When the force is primarily flexion, the head of the prox-

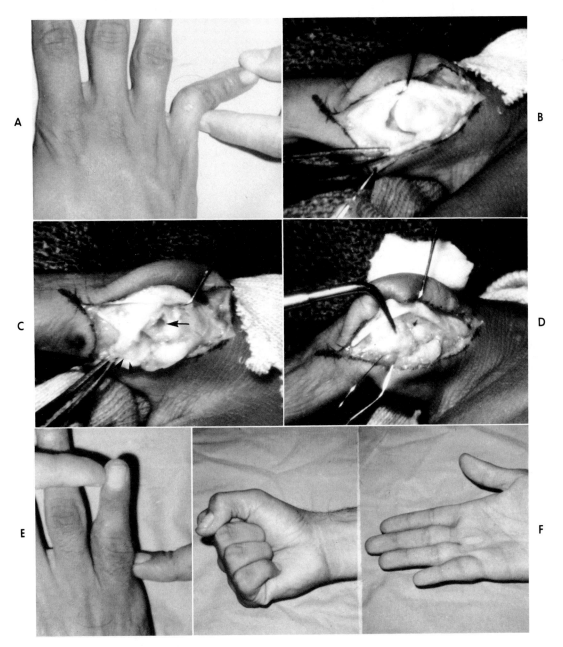

FIG. 26-38. A, Chronic lateral instability. **B,** At surgery there was no recognizable ligamentous tissue. **C,** Portion of the volar plate (*arrow*) was mobilized, and a trough (*arrow*) was made in the side of the head of the phalanx. **D,** The volar plate (under the probe) was attached into the side of the bone using a pull-out wire suture. **E and F,** Postoperatively mobility and stability were restored.

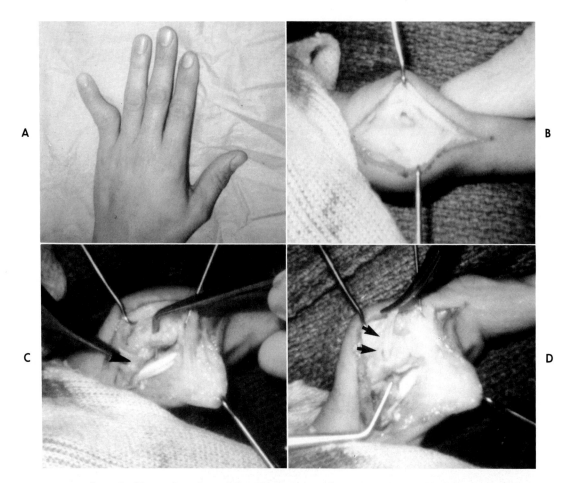

FIG. 26-39. A, Chronic lateral instability. **B,** At surgery there was scarring of both the collateral ligament and volar plate, and neither structure was suitable to reconstruct the ligament. **C,** Hole *(probe)* was drilled in the head of the phalanx, and one slip of the flexor superficialis tendon was detached proximally *(arrow).* **D,** The tendon was passed through the head of the phalanx and sutured into the side of the middle phalanx.

imal phalanx ruptures through the extensor tendon mechanism, tearing the central slip. Reduction can usually be achieved by closed measures and must be confirmed by radiographs, particularly a lateral view showing congruity of the joint surfaces. Though some authors recommend surgery to repair the central slip,[127,172] the preferred treatment is the same as for the closed acute boutonnière deformity.

When the mechanism of injury is primarily a torsional force, it results in disruption of one collateral ligament and partial avulsion of the volar plate. As the middle phalanx rotates volarly, the condyle of the proximal phalanx causes a longitudinal tear in the extensor mechanism, usually between the central slip and the ipsilateral lateral band. The lateral band slips volar to the condyle and entraps it, resulting in an irreducible dislocation (Fig. 26-40). In some situations the tear is between the central slip and the contralateral lateral band, and both the central slip and ipsilateral lateral band become entrapped (Fig. 26-41).[90,133,136,155] The radiographs in these cases

do not show a complete dislocation, as in those injuries where the central slip is torn. However, a lateral radiograph shows incongruity of the joint, and the proximal and middle phalanges project differently. One of the phalanges appears in a lateral projection, whereas the other appears slightly oblique because of the rotational deformity of the joint. Closed reduction should be attempted with the metacarpophalangeal and proximal interphalangeal joints in flexion to relax the displaced lateral band. The joint is then rotated and extended, which may allow the lateral band to slip back into its normal position.[43] Usually this maneuver is unsuccessful and surgery is necessary. A curved incision is made over the dorsal aspect of the joint with the apex of the incision at the midaxial line on the side where the ligament disrupted. The displaced and entrapped portion of the extensor mechanism, the lateral band, and possible the central slip are liberated. This can usually be accomplished by use of a blunt instrument such as a dental probe. If the collateral ligament is found to have avulsed cleanly from the

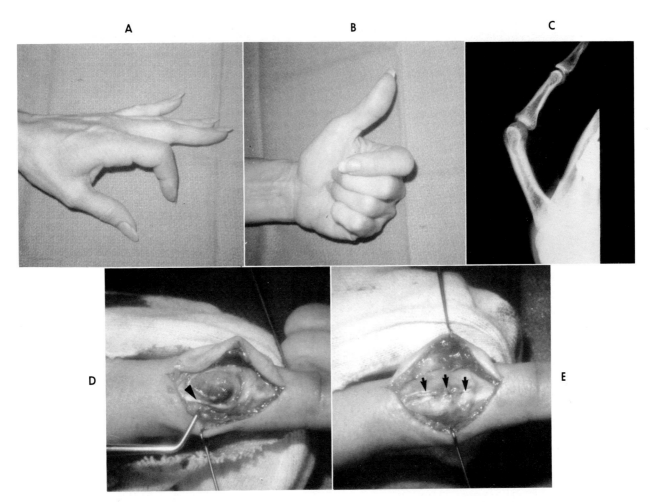

FIG. 26-40. **A** and **B,** This irreducible volar dislocation followed a twisting injury to the index finger. The finger was obviously malrotated. **C,** Lateral radiograph of the finger showed incongruity of the proximal interphalangeal joint. The proximal phalanx appeared rotated compared to the middle and distal phalanges indicative of interposed tissue. **D,** At surgery the radial collateral ligament was torn, and the radial lateral band *(arrow)* was dislocated volar to the radial condyle of the head of the phalanx. **E,** Following reduction the rent in the dorsal hood *(arrows)* was repaired.

bone, it can be resutured. However, this is rarely the situation, and the ligament usually appears frayed. Attempting to reapproximate it with multiple sutures is likely to result in increased scarring and therefore should be avoided. The longitudinal tear in the dorsal tendon mechanism should be sutured with fine 5-0 nonabsorbable nylon sutures. Because the extensor mechanism is intact, active range of motion exercises can be started within 1 week. Paradoxically, the prognosis is far better after an irreducible dislocation that requires surgery than after a reducible dislocation, since in the former the extensor mechanism is displaced but not disrupted. Therefore repair of the central tendon is unnecessary and immobilization of the joint is for a brief period.

Dorsal Capsule

Though chronic volar instability can result from injuries to the volar plate and chronic lateral instability can result from injuries to the collateral ligaments, chronic dorsal instability never occurs. Although there is a joint capsule dorsally, it is thin and ineffective as a dorsal stabilizer. The central extensor tendon, by virtue of its strength and wide insertion, functions both as the important active extensor of the joint and its dorsal ligament. If the central tendon is damaged as the result of a traumatic avulsion or laceration or if it becomes attenuated, its function as both an active extensor and a dorsal stabilizer is lost, and a boutonnière deformity develops. Dorsal instability is therefore not clinically possible.

MIDDLE PHALANX AREA
Anatomy

The middle phalanx has several distinct anatomic differences from the proximal phalanx. Besides being shorter, its volar surface is not as concave as the proxi-

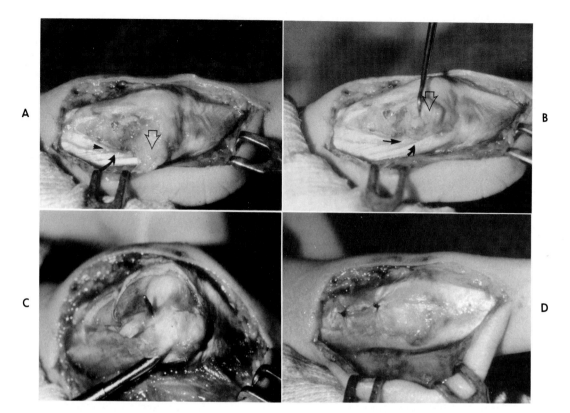

FIG. 26-41. A and **B,** Irreducible volar dislocation with both the central slip *(small arrow)* and radial lateral band *(large arrow)* dislocated beneath the condyle at the phalanx. The collateral ligament *(open arrow)* was torn from its insertion into the middle phalanx. **C,** The central tendon (under the probe) remained intact. **D,** After reduction the tear between the lateral band that was not displaced and the central tendon was a sutured with fine, nonabsorbable sutures.

mal phalanx, and its dorsal surface is flatter. The lateral crest in the shaft portion of the bone, where the slips of the flexor digitorum superficialis insert, are also thicker, rougher, and wider.[154] The base of the bone is much wider than its shaft, and on its dorsal aspect is a ridge that separates the base from its articular surface. In the middle of the ridge is a prominent tubercle for attachment of the central extensor tendon. The ridge extends volarly to each side, where it ends with tubercles onto which the collateral ligaments insert. The head of the bone is similar to the configuration of the head of the proximal phalanx.

Tendon Injuries

Acute injuries to the extensor tendon mechanism in this area are rare, except for lacerations. Secondary adhesions after blunt trauma or fractures are more common. A similar paucity of closed injuries is encountered in the flexor tendons, though rare avulsions of the flexor superficialis tendon have been reported after hyperextension injuries.[23,65]

Fractures

Fractures of the middle phalanx tend to be more transverse than at the proximal phalanx.[25,139] Most fractures occur distal to the insertion of the flexor superficialis tendon, which results in flexion of the proximal fragment and extension of the distal fragment. If the fragment occurs proximal to the insertion of the superficialis but distal to the insertion of the central extensor slip, the reverse deformity occurs with extension of the proximal fragment and flexion of the distal fragment. With fractures in the middle of the bone, the angulation may be in either direction, and this may be more a result of the direction of the trauma than of the pull of the flexor superficialis tendon.[23,65] Closed reduction for these angulated fractures can usually be accomplished. If the fracture is stable, the digit is immobilized with the metacarpophalangeal joint in acute flexion and the proximal interphalangeal joint in slight flexion. Because the fractures are in the cortical diaphyseal portion of the bone, healing is slow. Though active range of motion exercises are started within 2 to 3 weeks, the digit must be protected until there is radiographic evidence of complete healing, which may take 10 to 12 weeks or even longer. For those unstable fractures internal fixation, usually with Kirschner wires, is required.

DISTAL INTERPHALANGEAL JOINT AREA
Anatomy

A distal interphalangeal joint is a hinge, or ginglymus, joint whose articular and capsular components are similar to those of a proximal interphalangeal joint, but with

certain distinct variations. The head of the middle phalanx is bicondylar and fits snugly into the concave surface of the base of the distal phalanx. The condyles of the middle phalanx in the middle finger are symmetric, and the longitudinal axes for both middle and distal phalanges are in a straight line. In the index, ring, and little fingers, however, the condyles of the middle phalanges are more asymmetric in their widths, anteroposterior dimensions, and projections. The difference in condylar projections accounts for the ulnar deviation of the index finger toward the middle finger and the radial deviation of the ring and little fingers toward the middle finger seen in many individuals. Differences also exist in the extension-flexion arcs between the interphalangeal joints. Passive hyperextension exists in the distal interphalangeal joint, but not at a proximal interphalangeal joint, and this is reflected in the distance that the cartilage over the head of the middle phalanx extends proximally. A reciprocal situation exists with flexion, which is less at a distal interphalangeal joint. This is consistent with the more limited cartilage over the volar aspect of the head of a middle phalanx as compared to the head of a proximal phalanx.[154] With respect to the capsular structures, the check-rein configuration of the ligaments that tether the volar plate at a proximal interphalangeal joint is not present distally, and this permits passive joint hyperextension. The location of the insertion of the flexor profundus and superficialis tendons may explain the differences in flexion between the interphalangeal joints. The insertion of the flexor superficialis tendon is several millimeters distal to the base of the middle phalanx. When the tendon contracts, the insertion moves away from the proximal interphalangeal joint, increasing its mechanical advantage. The flexor profundus insertion, however, because of its closer proximity to the joint, does not have this advantage.[46] Dorsally the synovium and joint capsule are in intimate contact with and virtually inseparable from the terminal extensor tendon. The insertion of the tendon is not limited to the dorsal tubercle at the base of the distal phalanx as it is with the insertion of the central tendon into the base of the middle phalanx. Rather, its insertion is over a wide area extending to the nail matrix. The skin around the distal interphalangeal joint is firmly fixed by the Cleland ligaments.

Tendon Injuries
Extensor Tendons

Acute injuries. Injuries to the terminal extensor tendon are common in athletes, particularly those who catch or hit a ball (e.g., baseball, football, basketball, and volleyball). The usual history is a ball striking the extended finger, forcing the distal interphalangeal joint into acute flexion. The vast majority of these injuries are closed and result in acute stretching or rupture of the terminal extensor tendon or its avulsion from the base of the distal phalanx, often with a small bone fragment. The patient complains of pain, swelling, and tenderness over the dorsal aspect of the joint and notices its flexed position. The deformity is frequently referred to as a mallet or baseball finger, but both terms are misnomers. The finger does not actually resemble a mallet, and numerous activities

besides baseball can be responsible for the problem. A more accurate and descriptive term is *drop finger*.[1] The distal joint is flexed because of the relatively unopposed action of the flexor profundus tendon. The damaged terminal extensor tendon slides proximally, increasing the extension forces at the proximal interphalangeal joint. In loose-jointed patients a secondary hyperextension deformity may develop at this joint, and with the flexed position at the distal joint the finger assumes a swan-neck appearance.

Treatment for the acute injury is splinting of the distal joint in extension or slight hyperextension not exceeding 10 to 15 degrees for 6 weeks. Application of the splint to the dorsal aspect of the joint is usually more comfortable and functional than a splint on the volar aspect because it allows for tactile sensibility at the pulp.[120] Commercial splints are also available, but they tend to cover the volar aspect of the digit tip and may pose more of a functional impairment than a dorsally applied splint. It is important that the joint not be splinted in severe hyperextension, which causes the dorsal skin to blanch because of the risk of causing an ulcer in that area. This is more likely to occur immediately after the injury, when there may be considerable swelling. It is important that the joint be maintained in extension at all times. The patient should be seen periodically to check for any skin irritation. When the splint is changed, the joint is maintained in extension. The cooperative and reliable patient can be instructed in the technique of changing the splint without allowing the distal joint to inadvertently flex. The proximal interphalangeal joint is not immobilized and should be exercised to prevent stiffness. After 6 weeks the splint is removed several times each day for active range of motion exercises and the splint can be discontinued after another 2 weeks. Occasionally it may be an unrealistic burden for a patient to maintain an extension splint for the many weeks necessary for effective treatment. In these situations a Kirschner wire can be drilled across the joint to maintain it in full extension, and the patient can resume most activities.[71]

Surgery is reserved for injuries in which there is an open laceration[51,175] or a fracture with volar subluxation in the distal phalanx.[39,191] Subluxations with fractures are likely to occur when the dorsal fragment is large. In these situations the loss involves not only the dorsal support of the extensor tendon, but also the lateral support provided by both collateral ligaments, which remain attached to the dorsal fragment. Surgery is not indicated solely on the basis of the size of the dorsal fragment or the distance of its displacement. In the absence of any subluxation, it should be avoided because of its propensity to cause scarring of the matrix with nail deformity and joint stiffness. Even displaced avulsion fractures heal with satisfactory remodeling of the articular surface (Fig. 26-42). A dorsal beak may persist in these cases but is rarely symptomatic. With subluxations of the distal phalanx, however, there is no alternative but to reduce the joint and transfix it with a Kirschner wire. If the avulsed fragment is large, it can also be stabilized with a separate wire.

A drop finger can also be caused by a forced hyperex-

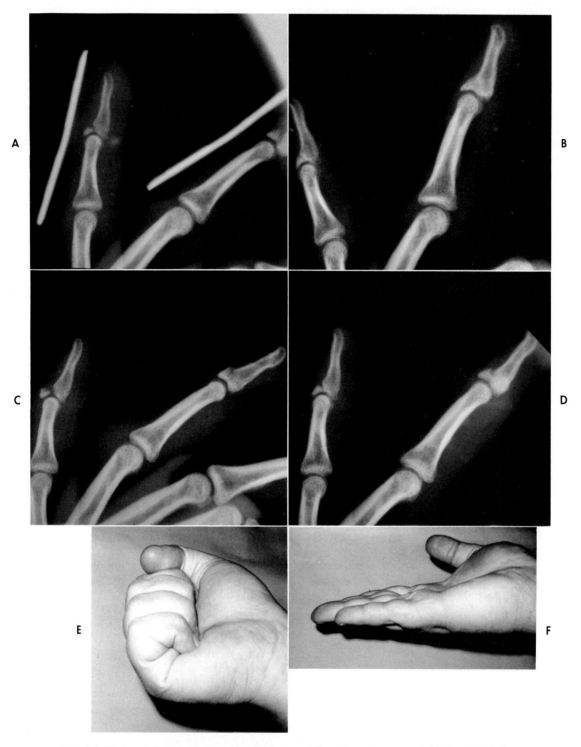

FIG. 26-42. A and **B,** "Drop" ring and little fingers with avulsion fractures of the distal phalanges were treated by dorsal extension splints. Surgery was unnecessary since neither injured phalanx was in volar subluxation. **C,** At 6 weeks the fractures were beginning to heal. **D,** The fractures had completely healed at 12 weeks. **E** and **F,** The patient regained complete mobility of both fingers.

tension injury to the distal joint that fractures the dorsal base of the distal phalanx. Surgery is often necessary for these rare injuries because the fracture fragment usually exceeds 50% of the articular surface and the intact portion of the bone is in volar subluxation.[109]

Chronic injuries. Frequently the patient with an injury to the extensor tendon neglects to seek medical attention for weeks and sometimes months after the injury. If the delay is a few weeks, extension splinting should still be used if there is no joint subluxation. In more chronic cases extension splinting has no benefit. If the deformity does not cause disability, no treatment is necessary. However, if the deformity interferes with function and passive extension of the joint remains intact, reconstruction of the terminal extensor tendon can be con-

sidered. Tenotomy of the central extensor tendon at the proximal interphalangeal joint has also been recommended, but such a procedure jeopardizes mobility at a joint where mobility is more important than at the originally injured joint.[20,75] When the distal interphalangeal joint is in chronic subluxation and painful or arthritic changes have developed, arthrodesis is indicated.

Flexor Tendons

Acute injuries. Avulsion of the flexor profundus tendon is the result of violent overstretching of a tendon whose muscle is contracting against resistance. These injuries typically occur in young adult male athletes who participate in sports such as football and rugby in which there is grabbing and clutching of one's opponent. The athlete,

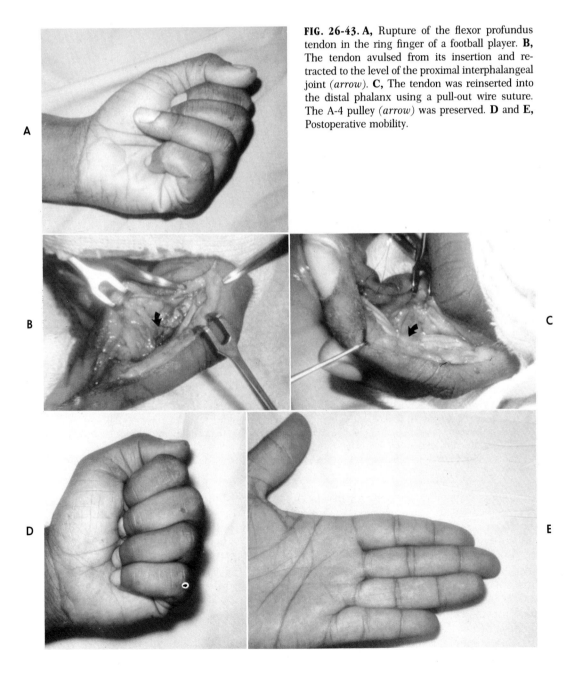

FIG. 26-43. A, Rupture of the flexor profundus tendon in the ring finger of a football player. **B,** The tendon avulsed from its insertion and retracted to the level of the proximal interphalangeal joint *(arrow).* **C,** The tendon was reinserted into the distal phalanx using a pull-out wire suture. The A-4 pulley *(arrow)* was preserved. **D** and **E,** Postoperative mobility.

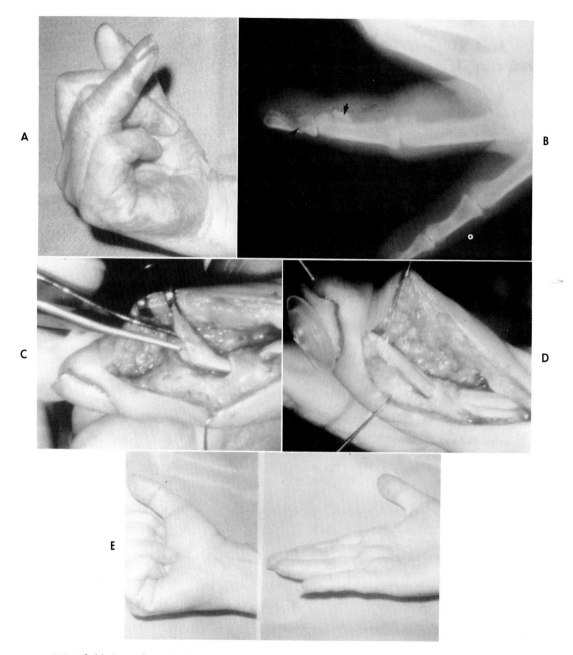

FIG. 26-44. A, Avulsion of the flexor profundus tendon, which also limited flexion at the proximal interphalangeal joint. **B,** Radiographs showed an avulsion fracture *(small arrow)* as well as a fracture of the distal phalanx *(arrow)*. **C,** Surgical forceps grasping the bone fragment with its attached flexor profundus tendon. **D,** The bone fragment and tendon were reattached with a pull-out wire suture, and a Kirschner wire was inserted to stabilize the distal phalanx. **E,** Postoperative mobility.

in an attempt to stop his opponent, forcefully grasps the opponent's jersey. As the opponent struggles to free himself, the injured athlete's finger becomes caught in the jersey and is suddenly extended. Though any finger can be injured in this way, the ring finger is most commonly involved. Various theories concerning the propensity for injury to this finger have been proposed and include the limited independent flexion of the ring finger resulting from the common muscle belly of the profundus,[76] the weakness of the insertion of the profundus into the distal phalanx of the ring finger as compared to the middle

finger,[115] the arrangement of the interconnections between the extensor tendons, the juncturae tendinum, which limit independent extension of the ring finger,[110,111] and that with grasp the finger is "longest" and therefore the most vulnerable to injury.[29] Frequently the seriousness of the injury is not immediately apparent to the athlete. Though there is pain, swelling, and often ecchymoses along the tendon sheath, the athlete sometimes initially is unaware of the loss of flexion at the distal joint. The diagnosis can also be missed by the physician who does not specifically test for function of the

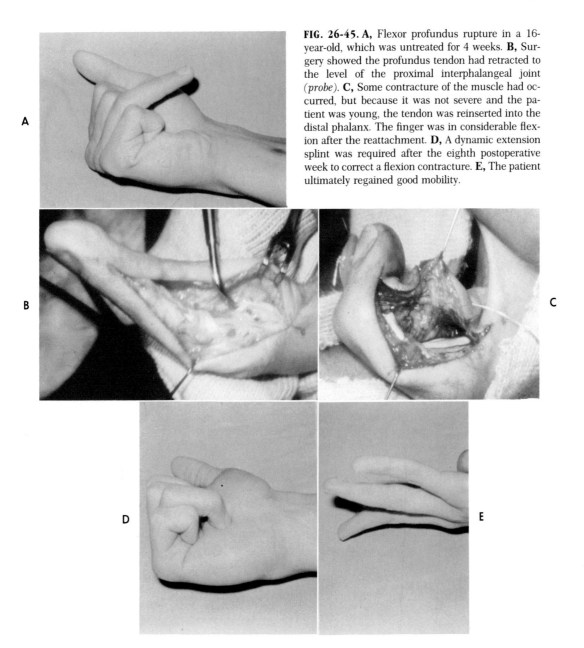

FIG. 26-45. A, Flexor profundus rupture in a 16-year-old, which was untreated for 4 weeks. **B,** Surgery showed the profundus tendon had retracted to the level of the proximal interphalangeal joint (*probe*). **C,** Some contracture of the muscle had occurred, but because it was not severe and the patient was young, the tendon was reinserted into the distal phalanx. The finger was in considerable flexion after the reattachment. **D,** A dynamic extension splint was required after the eighth postoperative week to correct a flexion contracture. **E,** The patient ultimately regained good mobility.

flexor profundus tendon. Radiographs may show a radiopacity if the tendon avulsed with a bone fragment from the base of the distal fragment. The ruptured tendon usually retracts to the level of the proximal interphalangeal flexion crease and can even retract into the palm, where further retraction is prevented by the tethering effect of the lumbrical muscle (Fig. 26-43). If the tendon avulses with a large fragment, the fragment is usually caught at the level of the A-4 pulley, preventing further proximal retraction of the tendon (Fig. 26-44).[109] However, an avulsion associated with a large bone fragment to which the tendon was no longer attached and had retracted to an even more proximal level has been reported.[108] Avulsions associated with comminuted fractures of the distal phalanx have also been reported.[168]

Surgery is necessary for all acute ruptures of the flexor profundus tendon. If there is marked swelling and ecchymoses, the operation should be deferred until the soft tissue reaction to the injury subsides. Elevation and warm soaks hasten the process, and the operation can usually be performed within 1 week. Delaying the surgery for weeks should be avoided because a secondary contracture of the muscle belly develops, precluding the possibility of reinsertion of the tendon.

Chronic injuries. A profundus avulsion that is not diagnosed until weeks after the injury may still be reinserted depending on its level of retraction. The greater the distance of retraction, the greater the contracture of the muscle belly and the less likelihood of success. The ideal situation would be a profundus avulsion that remains in proximity to the distal interphalangeal joint, tethered by an intact vinculum breve. Unfortunately this never occurs, since the vinculum breve always tears with the profundus and the tendon retracts at least to the level of the proximal interphalangeal joint, where it becomes adherent to the two slips of the flexor superficialis tendon. A

tenolysis is necessary to mobilize the profundus and assess the degree of secondary contracture to its muscle belly. The tendon end is grasped with a straight clamp, and traction is placed on it in an attempt to bring it to the base of the distal phalanx. This test should be carried out with the wrist in neutral position and the digit in extension (Fig. 26-45). If the tendon cannot be advanced, it is due to contracture of its muscle. Reinsertion of the tendon under such circumstances might be technically possible by flexing the wrist and fingers enough to relax the muscle-tendon unit; however, this would result in a severe flexion contracture of the digit. If the avulsed profundus has retracted to the base of the digit or into the palm and the injury is of longer standing than a few weeks, a secondary muscle contracture is even more likely. It is difficult to determine the level of tendon retraction before surgery unless the avulsion is accompanied by a bone fragment that is visualized on a lateral radiograph.

Treatment for the chronic case in which repair of the avulsed tendon is no longer possible depends on the degree of functional impairment. For the patient who has normal mobility at the proximal interphalangeal joint and is asymptomatic, no treatment is necessary. If, however, there is volar instability of the distal joint due to the loss of a flexion force on it or the loss of active flexion interferes with grasp, surgery is warranted. The most predictable procedure is an arthrodesis of the distal interphalangeal joint. Resection of the retracted profundus may be indicated at the same time if a tender lump representing the end of the tendon persists in the digit or palm. In certain situations a flexor tendon graft, either as a single[117] or staged[82] procedure can be considered. Tendon graft in the presence of an intact flexor superficialis tendon is a difficult procedure and has the potential to compromise normal mobility at the proximal interphalangeal joint. Therefore the procedure should be reserved for young patients[70,176] or for well-motivated adults, such as musicians, who require active flexion of their distal interphalangeal joint.[110]

Ligament Injuries

Dislocations of the distal interphalangeal joints are far less common than those of the proximal interphalangeal joints. The greater stability at the distal joint is the result of its strong collateral ligaments, the adjacent insertions of the flexor and extensor tendons, and the much shorter lever arm of the distal phalanx.[46] When a dislocation does occur, it is either lateral or dorsal, and it is often compound because of the density of the cutaneous ligaments that firmly anchor the skin to the underlying structures. Reduction can usually be achieved by closed manipulation using digital block anesthesia. If the skin is torn, local debridement, irrigation, and antibiotics are required. Occasionally, when the dislocation is irreducible as a result of entrapment of the volar plate,[143] flexor tendon,[148] or an osteochondral fracture fragment,[182] surgery is required. After reduction by either closed or open measures, the joint is stable. Immobilization need not exceed 2 weeks. Chronic instability is a rare complication.

Fractures

Fractures of the distal phalanges are common and usually result from crushing injuries. Unless the crush is severe, these fractures are rarely displaced, because there are no tendons spanning the bone to deform it. In addition, the phalanx in normally stabilized by the nail dorsally and the fibrous septa in the pulp tissue volarly.[27] Treatment is primarily directed to the soft-tissue component of the injury. A subungal hematoma is often present. If the pain is severe, usually described as pounding or throbbing, it can be quickly relieved by draining the hematoma. The simplest, most effective, and most painless method is using the end of a straightened paper clip, heated by a flame until it is red hot, to burn a hole through the nail. Aseptic technique with preliminary cleansing of the nail is important, because the hole alters any closed fracture of the underlying phalanx into an open one. There may be hemorrhage into the pulp tissue on the volar aspect of the digit tip. If the swelling is severe it can be partially decompressed with multiple puncture wounds made by a needle. A splint is used primarily for symptomatic relief of pain rather than bone stabilization and therefore can be confined to the distal segment of the finger.

In those rare fractures which are displaced, the nail matrix may become interposed between the fracture fragments, resulting in later deformity of the nail and possibly a nonunion. These complications can be avoided by repairing the nail matrix with fine absorbable sutures. Kirschner wire fixation is required only if the soft-tissue support of the bone has been lost.

In the young patient whose epiphyseal plate is still open, acute flexion force on the distal joint is more likely to cause a fracture through the plate than an avulsion of the extensor tendon. Though the injury clinically resembles a drop finger deformity, there is a transverse fracture through the base of the distal phalanx. These are compound injuries because the proximal portion of the nail slips out from under the eponychium and lies superficial to it, preventing reduction. Reduction can usually be accomplished by slightly hyperextending the joint and then replacing the nail under the eponychium.[166,194] In chronic cases it may be necessary to resect the proximal portion of the nail and use internal fixation.

Thumb

CARPOMETACARPAL (TRAPEZIOMETACARPAL) JOINT AREA

Anatomy

The trapeziometacarpal or basal joint of the thumb has often been referred to as a saddle joint because of the configuration of its articular surface, which is concave in its radioulnar dimension and convex in its dorsovolar dimension.[147] The articular surface of the base of the metacarpal has a reciprocal concave-convex configuration, and together the two joint surfaces resemble opposed saddles.[104] If these two saddles had deep congruous surfaces, the joint would be capable of only flexion, extension, abduction, and adduction, but not rotation.

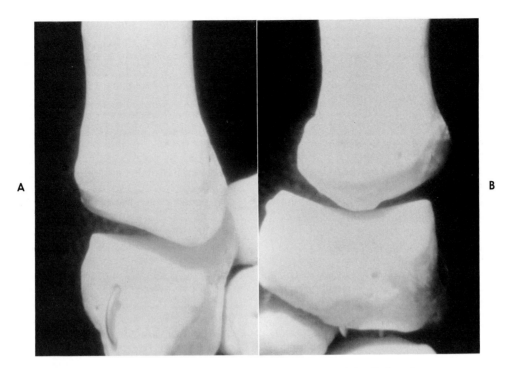

FIG. 26-46. Views of a trapeziometacarpal joint. **A,** Volar. **B,** Dorsal.

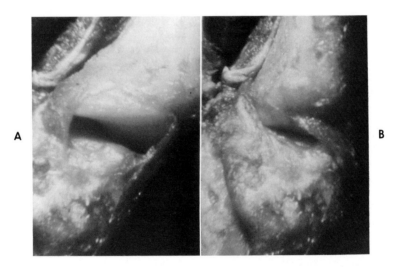

FIG. 26-47. Laxity of the joint capsule permits rotation. **A,** Supination. **B,** Pronation.

The joint would be similar to a western-type saddle, whose deep seat formed by the horn in front and high cantle in the rear permits the rider to move in essentially two planes, forward and backward and side to side. Rotational movements are prevented by the deep contour of the seat and the rider's intimate contact with it. To rotate, the riders must lift themselves off the seat by pressing down with their feet on the stirrups. In the trapeziometacarpal joint the articular surfaces are neither deep nor perfectly congruous (Fig. 26-46). Rather, they resemble an English-type saddle, whose low contours permit the rider not only to move forward and backward and side to side, but also to rotate.

Rotation at the trapeziometacarpal joint, whether pronation or supination, is facilitated not only by the shallow contours of the articular surfaces but also by the laxity of the joint capsule (Fig. 26-47).[160] Pronation or opposition occurs as the longitudinal axis of the metacarpal rotates 20 to 30 degrees from the corresponding axis of the fixed trapezium.[48] Though the joint capsule permits mobility, it also provides for stability. The relative importance of its component ligaments for this function is controversial. At the base of the metacarpal is a prominent beak that, when the joint is in neutral position, faces the distal portion of the ridge of the trapezium. Anchoring these two bony prominences is a stout ligament

referred to by a variety of terms, including the ulnar ligament,[160] anterior oblique ligament,[135] and volar ligament. Volar ligament is probably the most appropriate name because it accurately describes the position of the ligament in its relation to the thumb. Laterally the joint capsule is thin, but dorsally it thickens into the posterior oblique ligament, which together with the volar ligament has an important role in joint stability.[77] In flexion and opposition the volar beak of the metacarpal is in close contact with the trapezium, but in abduction and extension it is slightly elevated and pulls away from the trapezium. Further retraction of the metacarpal is prevented by the volar ligament. The importance of these anatomic features is discussed in the section on treatment for Bennett fractures.

Muscle-Tendon Injuries

Acute closed injuries to the extrinsic tendons or intrinsic muscles are rare at the level of the trapeziometacarpal joint. A chronic strain resulting in de Quervain tenosynovitis at the wrist level can also affect the abductor pollicis longus more distally, causing pain, swelling, and tenderness at its insertion into the base of the first metacarpal.

Ligament Injuries

Acute Injuries

Acute traumatic dislocation of a trapeziometacarpal joint is an unusual injury that has been referred to as a Bennett fracture without a fracture.[132] This may be inaccurate because, though a displaced Bennett fracture is invariably unstable after reduction, a dislocation may be quite stable.[190] Treatment for the dislocation that is stable after reduction is immobilization with a thumb spica cast for several weeks. For dislocations that remain unstable after reduction, there is some controversy concerning the nature of the pathology and treatment. Some believe that the volar ligament is invariably torn,[47] whereas others report that the volar ligament remains intact, but the dorsal capsule is disrupted.[167] Regardless of the particular ligament that is injured, the preferred treatment is reduction followed by stabilization by percutaneous insertion of one or two Kirschner wires, which are maintained for a minimum of 6 weeks. The objective of such treatment is for sufficient scarring to develop at the site of the capsular tear to prevent later joint laxity or instability.

An indication for surgery for the acute injury is if the base of the metacarpal cannot be anatomically reduced, which would indicate interposition of ligamentous tissue.[43] If surgery is required and the volar ligament is found to have been disrupted, repair is difficult if not impossible because of the short length and relative inaccessibility of the ligament. A new ligament must be reconstructed, and the most predictable technique is to use a strip of the flexor carpi radialis tendon.[49] The trapeziometacarpal joint is visualized through a curved incision extending from the ulnar border of the first metacarpal around the base of the thumb into the thenar crease of the palm. Care must be taken to avoid damaging the sensory branches of the radial and musculocutaneous

nerves and the palmar cutaneous branch of the median nerve. The thenar muscles are detached from their origins and mobilized distally. The lateral capsule is incised and the joint surfaces inspected. A drill hole is made in the base of the metacarpal in a dorsal-to-volar direction, with the drill point emerging just distal to the volar beak of the bone. The hole is gradually enlarged using progressively larger drills. The flexor carpi radialis tendon is then exposed through several small transverse incisions along its course in the distal forearm. The tendon is split longitudinally, and one half of its width is divided approximately 6 cm proximal to the wrist flexion crease.

To mobilize and split the tendon in its more distal portion, the sheath covering its passage under the crest of the trapezium must be divided. Care must be taken in splitting the tendon in this location because its distal insertion must be maintained. This part of the operation is facilitated by adequate surgical exposure and by palmar flexion of the wrist, which relaxes the tendon. The detached half of the tendon is then passed through the hole in the metacarpal in a volar-to-dorsal direction. A suture is placed into the end of the tendon, and the suture is passed through the eye of a large curved needle that was inserted into the hole in a retrograde fashion. As the needle is withdrawn, the suture is carried through the hole, and traction on the suture pulls the tendon through the bone. The metacarpal is then reduced and stabilized to the adjacent trapezium with a 0.045 mm nonthreaded Kirschner wire, avoiding spearing the tendon that is running through the bone. The tendon that emerges on the dorsal aspect of the metacarpal is then passed deep to the abductor pollicis longus and sutured to the dorsal and lateral portions of the capsule. It can also be passed around the intact portion of the flexor carpi radialis and back up to the metacarpal and sutured to its periosteum. The thenar muscles are reattached and a plaster splint applied, immobilizing the thumb and wrist. After 4 weeks, the wire is removed and active range of motion exercises are started. These exercises are carried out three to four times daily, the splint being worn at all other times. After an additional week, the splint is discontinued and the frequency of exercises is increased. Active resistive exercises to restore extrinsic and intrinsic muscle strength are begun in the sixth or seventh week.

Chronic Injuries

For acute dislocations that remain unstable after closed reduction and immobilization or for cases of chronic laxity with no secondary arthritic changes, reconstruction of a volar ligament by the same technique described in the previous section is required (Fig. 26-48). If arthritis has developed, arthroplasty is indicated.

Fractures

Fractures of the first metacarpal have two features that distinguish them from fractures of the other metacarpals: (1) their potential to cause an adduction contracture of the web space and (2) the greater importance of maintaining or restoring stability for the trapeziometacarpal joint as compared to the carpometacarpal joints of the fingers.[185] Two important fractures occur at the base

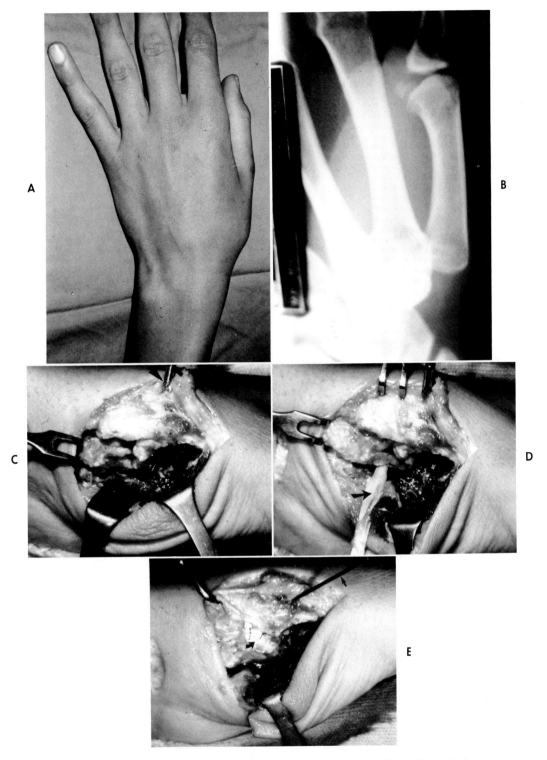

FIG. 26-48. A and **B,** Chronic instability of the trapeziometacarpal joint. The radiograph shows radial subluxation of the metacarpal base with irregularity at its volar beak. **C,** A drill hole was made going from dorsal to volar with the drill tip *(arrow)* emerging near the volar beak. **D,** The flexor carpi radialis tendon *(arrow)* was split for a distance of approximately 6 cm, and one half of its diameter was divided proximally. Its distal insertion was maintained. **E,** The tendon *(arrow)* is passed through the hole in the metacarpal going from volar to dorsal and then brought around to be sutured to the capsule. A Kirschner wire *(arrow)* was inserted to stabilize the trapeziometacarpal joint in its reduced position.   *Continued.*

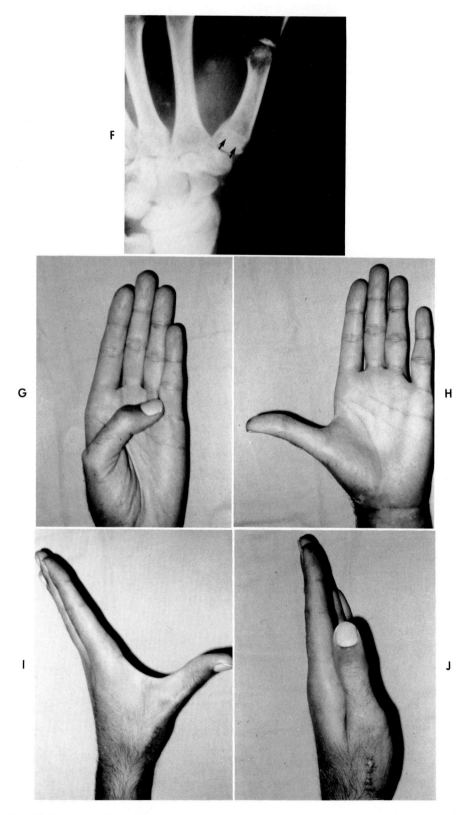

FIG. 26-48, cont'd. F, Postoperative radiograph show the outline of the hole in the base of the metacarpal. **G** to **J,** Stability was restored, and the patient regained complete mobility.

of the first metacarpal, and both are intraarticular: Bennett fractures and Rolando fractures.

Bennett Fractures

In the latter part of the nineteenth century, Edward Bennett described an oblique intraarticular fracture of the first metacarpal.[10] The fracture results in a subluxation or dislocation as the articular surface of the bone splits, separating the main portion of the metacarpal from its volar beak. The beak remains in place by the intact volar ligament, but the metacarpal shaft is displaced radially and dorsally by the pull of the abductor pollicis longus tendon. The dislocation component of the injury is far more important than the size of the volar fragment. If the dislocation is not accurately reduced, malunion with persistent subluxation of the joint occurs, ultimately leading to secondary arthritic changes and significant disability with pain and weakness. A careful radiographic examination to determine the presence of any articular incongruity is therefore the first essential step in the treatment of these fractures. Tomograms may also be required if conventional radiographs do not adequately visualize the articular surfaces of the metacarpal and trapezium.

The nonoperative treatment for a Bennett fracture is either closed manipulation and cast immobilization,[142,149] or closed reduction and Kirschner wire fixation between the first and second metacarpals[89] or across the trapeziometacarpal joint. Stabilization of the joint is accomplished by either inserting the wire at the base of the metacarpal[189] or intramedullarly through the head of the metacarpal and across into the trapezium.[193] Transfixion of the fracture fragment itself has also been proposed,[165] as has skeletal traction.[173] In most cases an accurate reduction can be obtained by manipulation and percutaneous fixation of the joint with one or two Kirschner wires. Transfixion of the small fracture fragment should be avoided because of the risk of causing it to rotate or shift in position as the wire is drilled into it. The method of reduction is essential because the thumb must be held in the position that permits the most accurate alignment of the fracture fragments. As discussed in the section on anatomy, the volar beak of the metacarpal normally pulls away from its contiguous trapezial articular surface with abduction and extension. Therefore placing the thumb in that position to reduce a Bennett fracture has the opposite effect, and the tendency is for the fracture to distract even further. Rather, the metacarpal is

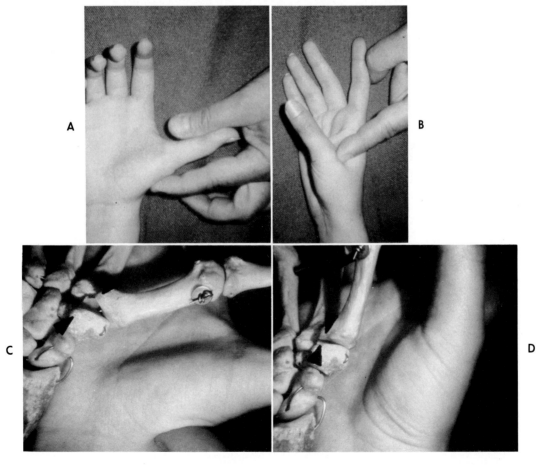

FIG. 26-49. Incorrect and correct methods of reducing a Bennett fracture. **A,** Extension (incorrect). **B,** Pronation (correct). **C,** In extension, the volar beak of the base of the metacarpal is distracted from the trapezium. **D,** In opposition, the articular surfaces of the metacarpal and trapezium are in close contact with each other.

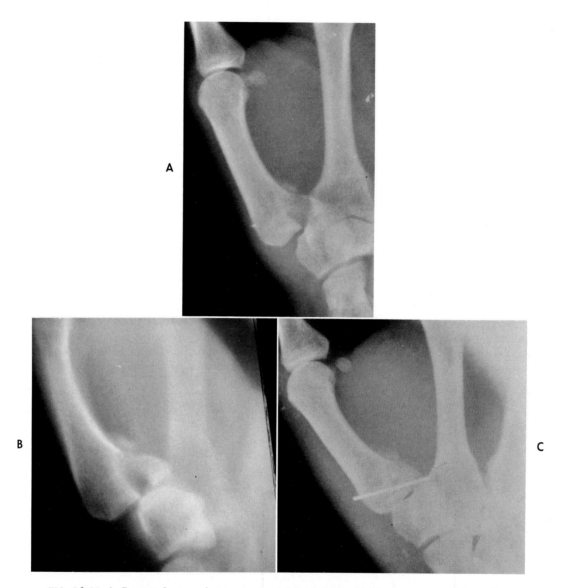

FIG. 26-50. A, Bennett fracture that was untreated for 2 weeks. **B,** Tomograms were obtained to more clearly visualize the incongruity at the fracture site. **C,** An open reduction was required, and the fracture was internally fixed with a Kirschner wire.

held in flexion and opposition because in this position the volar beak of the bone fits snugly into the corresponding surface of the trapezium (Fig. 26-49).[160] If an accurate reduction cannot be obtained and articular incongruity persists, operative reduction is necessary.[62] Internal fixation is usually provided by Kirschner wires, though a small cortical screw can also be used if the fracture fragment is of ample size (Fig. 26-50).

Rolando Fractures

Rolando fracture is another type of intraarticular fracture at the base of the metacarpal. In its classic presentation a Rolando fracture has a T- or Y-shaped configuration. These fractures tend to be more comminuted than Bennett fractures and are therefore usually more serious. When the comminution is severe, skeletal traction may

be the only feasible method of treatment.[63,186] The traction, provided by a single Kirschner wire inserted into the metacarpal in an oblique direction going from distal and ulnar to proximal and radial, exerts two forces of pull on the fracture. One force is longitudinal, which corrects the varus deformity and restores articular congruity. Occasionally these fractures are impacted, and cancellous bone grafting may be required to restore satisfactory reduction.[92]

METACARPAL AREA
Anatomy

Effective hand function depends to a large measure on the ability of the thumb to oppose. The importance of its capacity to face the other fingers was recognized by Hip-

pocrates, who referred to the thumb as the antihand.[195] The anatomic structures responsible for this function include the trapeziometacarpal joint, at which the circumduction movement occurs, and the intrinsic muscles that power this movement. These muscles almost totally encircle the first metacarpal and, except for a narrow area along the dorsal aspect of the bone, form a muscular sleeve for it.

Muscle-Tendon Injuries

Muscle strains are commonly thought to be confined to the larger muscles in the arm and forearm. Such injuries are seen in sports requiring lifting, pushing, throwing, or the use of racquets. These same activities can also affect the intrinsic muscle of the hand, most notably the intrinsics of the thumb. As the demand on these muscles exceeds their ability to function effectively, they fatigue. Such problems may be seen in the individual who forcefully grips the racquet without ever relaxing the grip, even when not hitting the ball. It can also occur in the individual who tightly grips a pen while writing for extended periods and in musicians who practice continuously for many hours. As with any acute strain, cessation of the activity and rest are the essential first steps in treatment. Application of cold compresses may also help to limit soft-tissue swelling. Effective and prompt treatment of the relatively benign acute strain lessens the risk of a chronic condition, in which recovery is more difficult and disability more prolonged.

Fractures

Fractures of the first metacarpal account for 25% of metacarpal fractures, second only to fractures of the fifth metacarpal.[62,146] The vast majority of thumb metacarpal fractures have already been discussed. Extraarticular fractures are usually less problematic, and when they are at the base of the bone they tend to be transversely oriented. Most are radially angulated with the distal fragment adducted and supinated.[27] If the angulation does not exceed 20%, there is rarely any functional impair-

ment because of the wide range of mobility at the adjacent trapeziometacarpal joint. For more severely angulated fractures, reduction is required. This can usually be accomplished by closed measures involving abduction and pronation of the distal fragment. Occasionally the angulation has a greater effect on limiting extension of the thumb rather than its abduction. Some individuals compensate for this problem by hyperextending their metacarpophalangeal joint. Extraarticular fractures can also be obliquely oriented where there is a propensity for shortening. The distal shaft fragment may actually impinge on the dorsoradial margin of the trapezium, which requires open reduction and fixation.[146] In the skeletally immature individual a fracture can involve the proximal metaphyseal epiphyseal plate. They are usually Salter-Harris Type II fractures, which respond well to closed reduction and immobilization.[139]

METACARPOPHALANGEAL JOINT AREA
Anatomy

The metacarpophalangeal joint of the thumb is a condyloid joint, like its counterpart in the fingers, but with important differences. The shape of the head of the first metacarpal is usually less spherical, and its articular surface is wider and flatter with more limited cartilage on its dorsal aspect (Fig. 26-51).[91] There is also greater constancy of the sesamoids in the thumb, which are located in the lateral margins of the volar plate and incorporated into the tendon of the flexor pollicis brevis radially and the adductor pollicis ulnarly. In the fingers the sesamoids are also within the volar plate, but are not associated with the intrinsic muscles.[72] The insertions of the intrinsic muscles in the thumb form thicker and stronger tendinous and aponeurotic expansions on the sides of the joint than is seen in the fingers.[4] This is particularly evident medially, where the adductor muscle and its aponeurosis provide strong support as they span the interval from the volar plate and medial sesamoid to the border of the extensor pollicis longus tendon. Laterally

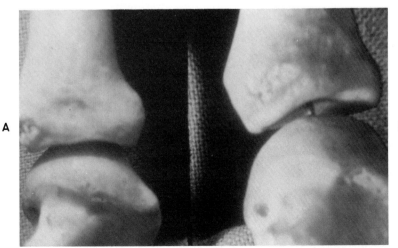

FIG. 26-51. Comparative views of the metacarpophalangeal joints. **A,** Thumb. **B,** Finger.

the support is not as strong where the insertions of the thenar muscles have three components. The flexor pollicis brevis provides two of these components with a deep head insertion into the volar plate and lateral sesamoid, similar to the insertion of the adductor pollicis, and a more superficial insertion on the volar portion of the side of the proximal phalanx. The third component of this lateral expansion is the abductor pollicis brevis, which makes up the most superficial layer and inserts over a broad area more dorsal and distal to the underlying flexor pollicis brevis. Both the adductor and abductor aponeurotic expansions extend dorsally on both sides of the joint and stabilize the extensor pollicis longus in its midline position. This tendon is also stabilized more proximally by radial and ulnar sagittal bands that attach to the volar plate. The extensor pollicis longus, by virtue of its position, is an important extensor of the metacarpophalangeal joint in addition to its more obvious function as the extensor of the interphalangeal joint. The extensor pollicis brevis, which inserts into the base of the proximal phalanx and dorsal capsule, functions only as an extensor of the metacarpophalangeal joint.

The collateral ligaments have two important functions: they provide both lateral stability and dorsal support for the phalanx. Without the dorsal support, the flexors, particularly the intrinsics, no longer function as flexors of the metacarpophalangeal joint. Instead they translocate the phalanx, causing a volar subluxation or dislocation.[169]

The anatomic features of the metacarpophalangeal joint are consistent with its function as a limited hinge. Though the flexion-extension arc varies, including the ability of some individuals to hyperextend the joint, motions are usually more limited than in the metacarpophalangeal joints of the fingers.[35] Abduction and adduction motions are definitely more limited in the metacarpophalangeal joint of the thumb, in which the priority of function is stability rather than mobility.

Tendon Injuries

The most likely tendons to be injured in a closed injury are the extensors. Because the extensor pollicis brevis and extensor pollicis longus are intimately connected with the dorsal capsule and the adductor and abductor aponeurotic expansions, they are usually damaged after a subluxation or dislocation. They are discussed with subluxation and dislocation injuries in the following section.

Ligament Injuries
Dorsal Capsule

Anterior dislocation of the metacarpophalangeal joint is a rare injury that tears the dorsal capsule and the extensor pollicis brevis at its insertion. A concomitant injury to one of the collateral ligaments is common because, rather than the joint being forced in a purely anterior direction, it is commonly deviated anteromedially or anterolaterally.[163] Even a pure flexion injury is likely to cause some damage to the collateral ligaments. If there is any tendency for persistent subluxation after a closed

reduction, it indicates that the dorsal portions of the collateral ligaments have been torn. Surgery is necessary to repair the dorsal capsule. Temporary Kirschner wire fixation of the joint is recommended to protect the repair, because the flexor forces on the joint are more powerful than the extensor forces (Fig. 26-52). If there is also lateral instability as the result of rupture of a collateral ligament, repair of the ligament is also required.

Volar Plate

Acute injuries. Dorsal dislocations are at least 10 times more common than volar dislocations. They result from a hyperextension injury to the joint that tears the volar plate, usually at its proximal attachment.[163] The head of the metacarpal herniates between the intrinsic muscles, which insert into both the radial and ulnar sesamoids. The dislocation is clearly seen on a lateral radiograph, which also aids in determining the location of the tear in the volar plate. If the sesamoids remain close to the dislocated phalanx, the plate must be intact distally but torn proximally. Unlike a volar dislocation, a dorsal dislocation may not be readily reducible by closed measures because the volar plate may be interposed between the dislocated phalanx and the dorsal surface of the metacarpal head. A closed reduction should be attempted and may be successful if carried out properly. Pressure is applied in a distal direction on the base of the dislocated phalanx while the metacarpal is maintained in a flexed and adducted position to relax the intrinsic muscle. If closed reduction is unsuccessful, surgery is necessary to release the entrapped plate. After either closed or operative reduction, a dorsal splint is applied to the digit to prevent complete metacarpophalangeal joint extension but allow for active flexion exercises.

Chronic injuries. Hyperextension at the metacarpophalangeal joint is normally opposed passively by the volar plate and actively by the intrinsic muscles. The flexor pollicis brevis is the most effective intrinsic muscle limiting active hyperextension because of its advantageous line of pull.[178] A distinction must be made between a joint that can actively hyperextend and one that is volarly unstable. The ability to actively hyperextend the metacarpophalangeal joint is not a pathologic condition and can be observed in many individuals. With pressure of the thumb tip against the fingertips or against an object, the hyperextension in a normal thumb disappears, and the joint is stable in slight flexion. With volar instability, however, the joint fails to stabilize during prehension and continues to hyperextend. This is a pathologic condition that may produce a significant disability. Conservative treatment should be tried, including the use of a small dorsal splint to block metacarpophalangeal joint extension and active resistive exercises to strengthen the intrinsic muscles. If these measures fail and the disability is significant, surgery should be considered. An effective procedure is to advance the conjoined tendon of the insertion of the abductor pollicis brevis and flexor pollicis brevis. This technique increases the flexion forces of the muscles on the joint, thereby eliminating the volar instability (Fig. 26-53).[152]

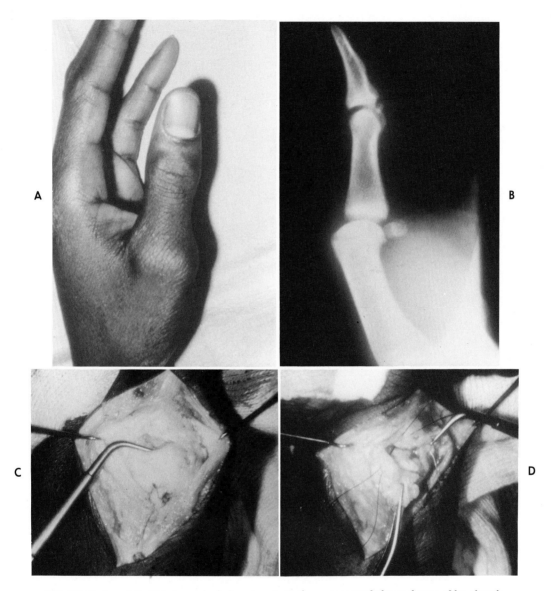

FIG. 26-52. A and **B,** This boxer had chronic pain in the metacarpophalangeal joint of his thumb, which was in volar subluxation. **C** and **D,** At surgery the torn dorsal capsule *(probe)* was repaired with nonabsorbable sutures.

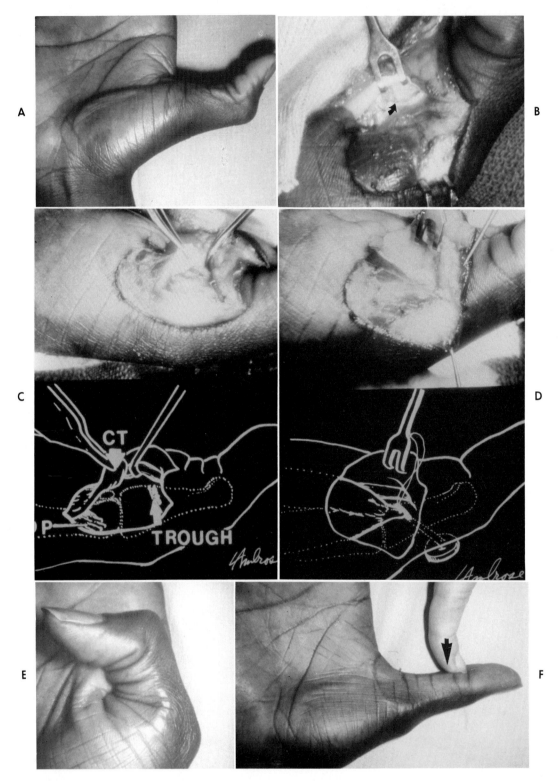

FIG. 26-53. A, Chronic volar instability of the metacarpophalangeal joint in a thumb. **B,** The volar plate is usually intact in these problems, though it is often attenuated. **C,** The conjoined tendon of the abductor pollicis and flexor pollicis brevis is removed, and a trough is made at a more distal level on the phalanx. **D,** The tendon is advanced into the trough. **E** and **F,** Postoperatively, flexion was not impaired, and the previous dorsal instability was corrected.

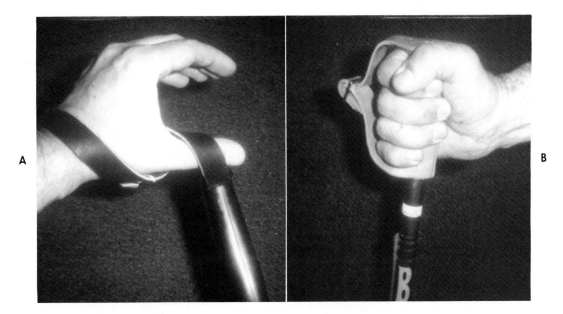

FIG. 26-54. A, The strap on a ski pole may catch around the skier's thumb, pulling it into abduction. **B,** Ski pole with a sword-type grip.

Ulnar Collateral Ligament

Acute injuries. Instability following an injury to the ulnar collateral ligament is common, resulting in a condition often referred to as gamekeeper's thumb. The term does not refer to an acute injury but to a chronic occupational condition that was observed in Scottish gamekeepers.[31] These workers killed hares by placing their thumb and index finger on the animals' heads and hyperextending their necks. The abduction force that this repetitive activity placed on the gamekeeper's thumb gradually weakened the ulnar collateral ligament, resulting in progressive joint instability. Though by common usage and tradition gamekeeper's thumb has indicated an acute as well as a chronic injury to the ligament, a more appropriate term for the acute injury would be skier's thumb because skiing is responsible for most such injuries. It is estimated that between 15% and 25% of all skiing injuries involve the thumb. In 90% of these injuries the damage is to the ulnar collateral ligament of the metacarpophalangeal joint.[52,131] The straps on ski poles have been incriminated as the major cause of these ligament injuries.[137,169] As the skier falls the far end of the pole gets caught in the snow, and the strap, which lies across the palm, pulls the thumb into radial deviation. Poles with sword grips, in which the retention strap is across the dorsum of the hand, should theoretically reduce the incidence of these injuries if the straps are indeed the problem (Fig. 26-54). Unfortunately this has not proved to be the situation; ulnar collateral ligament injuries occur with even greater frequency in skiers using sword grip poles.[131] Apparently, as the palm of the hand strikes the snow, the pole remains wedged in the first web space, resulting in forced abduction of the thumb. The safest poles are those without any grip restraints, because these poles are more likely to fly away from the falling skier. Ulnar collateral ligament injuries

would still occur, but their incidence would be significantly reduced.

The diagnosis and proper classification of the type of ligament sprain depend on a careful examination. The purpose of the examination is to differentiate between the partial injury, in which joint stability has not been compromised, and the third-degree or complete ligament disruption, which results in instability and generally requires surgery. Marked swelling and particularly ecchymoses should alert the examiner to the possibility of a severe ligament injury. The resting attitude of the thumb should be observed and any radial angulation of the joint noted. The area of maximum tenderness should also be determined: whether it is at the insertion of the ligament into the proximal phalanx, where it most commonly disrupts, or proximally at the origin of the ligament on the side of the metacarpal head. Joint stability is best evaluated by stress testing but should always be preceded by conventional radiographs. These are necessary to determine if there is a large, undisplaced intraarticular fracture or an undisplaced epiphyseal injury in the young patient who has not reached skeletal maturity. Obviously stress testing should be avoided in these situations to prevent changing an undisplaced fracture into a displaced one.

A common radiographic finding, best visualized on the posteroanterior view, is a small fracture fragment usually seen at the base of the proximal phalanx. A rarer finding best seen on a lateral view is volar subluxation of the proximal phalanx. When this occurs, there must be a concomitant tear of the dorsal capsule and insertion of the extensor pollicis brevis in addition to a possible tear of one of the collateral ligaments. The fracture fragment usually results from an avulsion injury as the ligament pulls from the bone. If the fragment is attached to the collateral ligament, the distance of its displace-

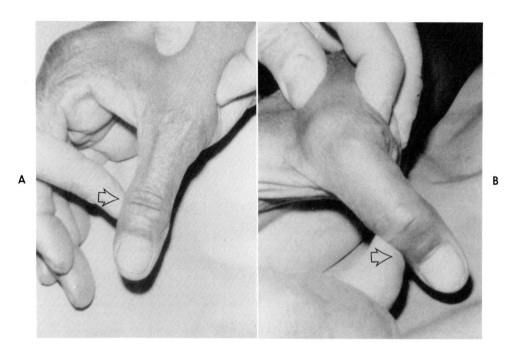

FIG. 26-55. A and **B,** Testing stability of the ulnar collateral ligament in the thumb of a normal individual. In extension the thumb was stable, but in flexion it appeared to be unstable. This was caused by normal laxity of the dorsal capsule at the metacarpophalangeal joint.

ment from the phalanx or metacarpal indicates the distance of displacement of the collateral ligament. If the fragment is displaced, the joint is usually unstable, and surgery is required. Occasionally the fragment may be only minimally displaced, but because it makes up a significant portion of the articular surface, surgery is still necessary. Though a displaced fragment is almost always associated with an unstable joint, a nondisplaced fragment does not necessarily indicate joint stability. It is possible for a ligament to be completely avulsed and displaced from its insertion and yet for an undisplaced fracture fragment to be seen on radiograph. The fragment in such a case is not the result of the avulsion force but rather of a violent shear force as the phalanx comes in contact with the metacarpal head as it realigns itself.[178] Therefore the presence of an undisplaced fragment does not necessarily indicate that the ligament is nondisplaced and the joint is stable.

Special radiographic procedures, including stress radiographs,[84,127] arthrography,[66,159,179] and stress arthrography,[19] have been recommended as useful in determining the severity of ligament damage and the necessity for surgery. Though these examinations undoubtedly provide documentation for obvious pathologic findings, they are by no means infallible and may even be misleading. They should never be used as the sole criterion for surgery. The decision for such treatment depends on the findings of a properly performed stress test.

The technique of carrying out a stress test and interpreting its results is controversial. Opinions vary as to the position in which the metacarpophalangeal joint should be held during the examination. These positions vary from full extension,[137,169] to slight flexion,[127,131] to com-

plete flexion,[145] or even a combination of extension and flexion.[43,47,177] The rationale for holding the joint in full flexion is that the collateral ligaments are maximally tight in this position; therefore any instability indicates a disruption.[18] A practical problem with testing the joint in full flexion is that it may show what appears to be angulation of the joint but is actually axial rotation of the metacarpal at its trapeziometacarpal joint. This occurs because the metacarpal is locked by both collateral ligaments when the metacarpophalangeal joint is in full flexion. Stressing the joint in this position may simply rotate the entire metacarpal. Even if the metacarpal is firmly stabilized and prevented from rotation, rotation can still occur at the metacarpophalangeal joint. This is most likely to occur in individuals who have a large flexion arc at their metacarpophalangeal joint because of a lax dorsal capsule. Again, the joint may appear to be angulating, giving a false positive impression of collateral ligament instability (Fig. 26-55).

The **preferred method of stress testing** is with the joint in full extension. Unlike the metacarpophalangeal joints of fingers, the metacarpophalangeal joint of a thumb must be functionally stable in extension, and it is important to evaluate stability in this position. A possible objection to this method of examination is that a third-degree collateral ligament injury may go unrecognized if the accessory collateral ligament, which is normally taut in extension, is uninjured. This has not proved to be a problem, and a joint that is unstable in extension yet stable in flexion has not been observed. Testing the joint in full extension eliminates rotation of the metacarpal at its trapeziometacarpal joint or rotation of the proximal phalanx at its metacarpophalangeal joint. The ex-

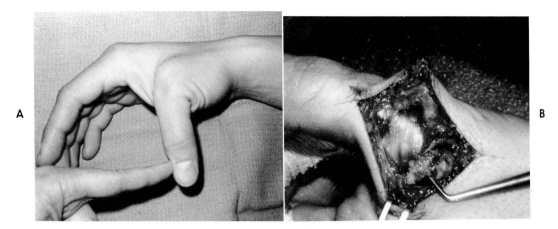

FIG. 26-56. A, Complete instability of the metacarpophalangeal joint with radial stress. **B,** At surgery the distal end of the collateral ligament *(probe)* was seen to be external to the abductor aponeurosis, a classic Stener lesion.

aminer stabilizes the metacarpal with the thumb and index finger of one hand and, with the thumb and index finger of the other hand, grasps the interphalangeal joint, applying force in a radial direction. If there is instability, the joint will angulate. The degree of angulation should be documented. The examiner stresses the joint with one hand and measures the angulation using a goniometer with the other hand. This is done by placing the index finger (right index finger when testing stability of a right thumb) on the radial side of the metacarpal head and stressing the joint with this thumb on the ulnar side of the distal segment. With the other hand, the examiner places a goniometer on the top of the patient's thumb or along its ulnar border to measure the degree of joint angulation. Angulation greater than 30 degrees indicates a third-degree injury.

Occasionally the adductor aponeurosis becomes interposed between the avulsed ligament and its insertion, thereby precluding any possibility of healing with immobilization of the joint as the sole method of treatment. Described by Stener, the lesion that commonly bears his name is the result of a violent abduction injury.[177] The degree of radial angulation of the joint at the time of the trauma must exceed 60 degrees for the proximal edge of the adductor aponeurosis to move distal to the site of the ligament avulsion. When the joint spontaneously realigns itself, the ligament lies external to the aponeurosis. These lesions are usually found in injured thumbs in which there may be angulation in the resting position (Fig. 26-56).

The treatment for a partial ligament injury in which there is no instability is immobilization. If after the first week swelling and tenderness have subsided, the injury must have been a first-degree sprain, and active range of motion exercises are encouraged. If, however, tenderness persists and there is slight joint laxity, the injury was a second-degree sprain, and immobilization should be continued for several additional weeks. Generally, a volar gutter splint is used, although a thumb spica can be substituted.

Conservative splinting has also been recommended for

the acute injury in which there is obvious joint instability. Proponents of this treatment reserve surgery only for cases in which there is later disability or in which the diagnosis of instability is delayed for weeks after injury.[35,137] This rationale for delaying surgery is that not all acutely unstable thumbs will remain painful after a period of immobilization, and that if a later problem develops successful surgery is still possible. However, most physicians do not share this opinion and favor early surgery for the unstable joint. The predictability of primary repair of the ligament to restore stability and reduce the likelihood of later pain, weakness, and secondary arthritis is far greater than when immobilization is used as the primary treatment.* Since a chronically unstable joint can be successfully treated by surgery and insertion of an avulsed ligament is often possible weeks or even months after the injury, one may question the necessity of operating on the acutely unstable thumb. The rationale is simply that it is preferable to repair a ligament than to reconstruct one. Late ligament repair is possible if the ruptured end remains close to its bony insertion. However, if the ligament retracts or folds on itself after injury, the scarring that develops within weeks precludes repair. Late ligament repair would also be impossible for the Stener lesion. Because it is difficult to determine before surgery if the ligament has ruptured in a fashion which would make later repair possible, it is preferable to operate for the acute injury when there is instability. The operation is carried out as soon as the patient's general medical condition and the local wound condition permit. If the thumb is markedly swollen and ecchymotic, it is preferable to delay the operation for several days.

At surgery (Fig. 26-57) a curved incision is made on the ulnar side of the thumb with the apex of the incision at the midaxial line of the metacarpophalangeal joint. Skin flaps are elevated and care taken to identify and protect the sensory branches of the radial nerve. Placement of a retractor around these branches should be avoided, since prolonged retraction during the opera-

---

*References 46, 57, 64, 68, 81, 122, 131, and 177.

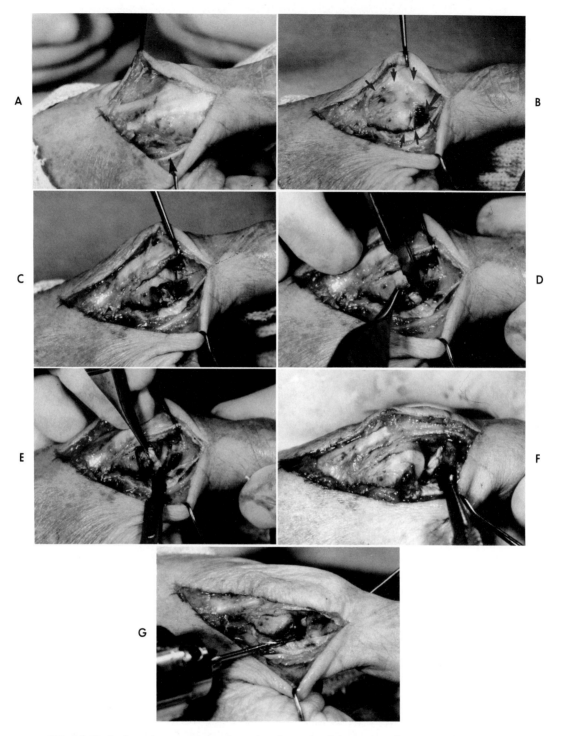

FIG. 26-57. A, Curved incision is made on the ulnar side of the joint, and care must be taken to identify and protect the sensory branches of the radial nerve *(arrow)*. **B,** The hood is incised *(arrow)* to the volar aspect of the extensor tendon. Hemorrhage was noted at the site of the ligament insertion into the phalanx *(large arrow)*. **C,** An incision is made along the dorsal edge of the ligament, retracting the dorsal capsule *(under hook)*. **D** and **E,** Freeing the interval between the ligament and the metacarpal head and releasing the accessory fibers of the collateral ligament may facilitate advancement and reattachment of the ligament. **F,** Dorsal-volar transverse trough is made in the base of the proximal phalanx. **G,** Drill hole is made in the trough, and a Keith needle is inserted.

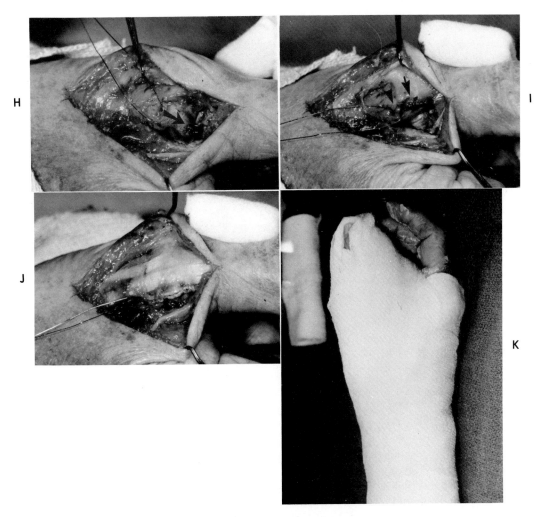

FIG. 26-57, cont'd. H and **I,** The ligament is reinserted using a pull-out wire suture, and padding is placed beneath the button on the radial side of the thumb. **J,** The dorsal capsule is sutured to the dorsal edge of the repaired ligament. **K,** The dorsal hood is repaired. Postoperatively the thumb and wrist are immobilized. A properly applied volar plaster splint is preferable to a thumb spica cast because it is more comfortable for the patient and facilitates changing the bandages.

tion can lead to permanent numbness and dysesthesias. If a Stener lesion is present, the normally well-defined edge of the aponeurosis is obscured by a mass, which represents the retracted and displaced end of the collateral ligament. An incision is made in the aponeurosis along the ulnar edge of the extensor pollicis longus tendon. This permits retraction of the hood further radially, exposing the entire dorsal capsule, which is often torn transversely. The ulnar aspect of the hood is mobilized volarly to visualize the collateral ligament. There is usually some bleeding at the site of the capsular injury or within the joint. An incision is then made along the dorsal edge of the collateral ligament and the dorsal capsule is reflected. The incision should be along the entire length of the ligament, especially to the bony edge of the phalanx. At this point an infolding of the synovial lining, forming a type of meniscal cushion, may be noted. The collateral ligament can now be carefully inspected and

the precise location of the damage determined. In more than 90% of cases, the ligament ruptures at its insertion into the phalanx, but it may also rupture proximally or even within its substance. If the ligament has ruptured distally and folded back on itself, it appears as a ball of tissue against the metacarpal head, and sharp dissection is necessary to unfold it. Freeing the recess between the metacarpal head and the retracted ligament and incising the accessory collateral ligament are helpful to restore length to the ligament before reinsertion.

The most secure method of fixation is to reinsert the ligament directly into the bone. This is accomplished by making a slot on the ulnar side of the phalanx if it is ruptured distally or on the side of the metacarpal head if it is ruptured proximally. A narrow chisel is used for this purpose. The slot must be deep and broad enough to accommodate the ligament. Care must be taken while levering the chisel into the bone not to cause a fracture of

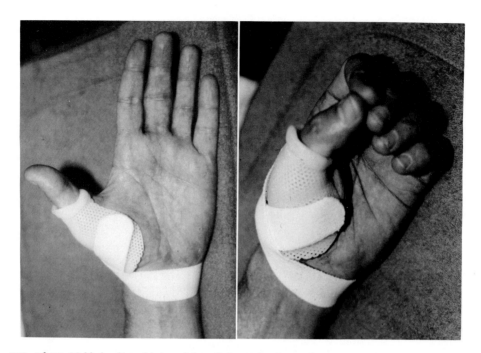

FIG. 26-58. Molded splints fabricated from lightweight thermoplastic materials provide protection for the joint following a first- or second-degree sprain or for the third-degree sprain recovering from surgery. These splints can often be worn while the athlete continues participating in his or her sport, whether it be basketball, gymnastics, hockey, or skiing. In sports such as hockey in which a glove is worn, the splint can be worn underneath.

the articular surface. This can be avoided by starting the slot several millimeters distal to the joint surface. When a fracture fragment accompanies the ruptured ligament, it can be excised before the ligament is reinserted. However, if the fragment makes up more than 15% of the articular surface, it should be reinserted with the ligament.[43] A pull-out wire suture is used. Padding should always be placed beneath the button on the radial side of the thumb to prevent any pressure irritation on the skin. One or two 4-0 nylon mattress sutures are used to reinforce the ligament repair. If the dorsal capsule is torn, and frequently it is torn transversely through its proximal portion, it too is repaired. The incision made in the capsule along the dorsal edge of the ligament is now closed. If there is any tendency for the metacarpophalangeal joint to remain flexed, the sutures between the dorsal capsule and collateral ligament are inserted obliquely to pull the capsule proximally. The joint is now gently stressed to test the efficacy of the repair. The incision in the adductor aponeurosis is also closed with 4-0 nylon mattress sutures. It is unnecessary to transfix the joint with a Kirschner wire routinely. This should be reserved for cases in which there is a concomitant volar subluxation. Postoperatively a volar plaster splint is applied to immobilize the thumb and wrist. After 4 to 5 weeks, the splint is removed several times daily for active range of motion exercises. After an additional week the splint is discontinued and the exercises are increased to an hourly frequency. Ideally, all activities that place the thumb at risk of reinjury should be avoided for another 6 weeks. This delay may be unreasonable for the

professional or serious amateur athlete. If situations warrant, the thumb can be protected by the use of an orthosis. For the athlete who wears a glove, such as the skier or hockey player, a small dorsal gutter splint can be fabricated to fit inside the glove (Fig. 26-58).

Chronic injury. Chronic instability, the true gamekeeper's thumb, is common. It occurs when athletes dismiss their acute injury as trivial and neglect to seek prompt medical attention. Only as their pain persists and they remain unable to grasp effectively do they seek medical attention. As with the acute thumb injury, conventional radiographs are an important part of the examination. If secondary arthritic changes have developed, arthrodesis is the preferred operation. Arthrodesis may also be indicated for the chronically painful thumb, which may not be unstable. This situation is usually encountered in the athlete who reports multiple injuries, none of which was severe enough alone to rupture the ligament but whose cumulative effect has resulted in a diffusely painful and tender joint.

In addition to lateral instability, the extensor pollicis longus tendon may be displaced in a chronic injury because of stretching of the adductor dorsal aponeurotic expansion. The tendon displacement causes an increased extension force on the distal phalanx, resulting in hyperextension of the interphalangeal joint. This condition is similar to the common thumb deformity seen in patients with rheumatoid arthritis.[169]

For unstable joints in which radiographs show no appreciable arthritis, surgical repair of the ligament or some type of soft-tissue reconstruction is warranted. As previ-

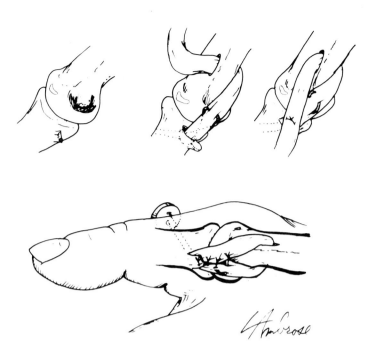

FIG. 26-59. Diagrammatic sequence of reconstruction of a collateral ligament using a tendon graft.

ously stated, a ligament ruptured at either its insertion or origin can often be reinserted into the bone weeks or even months after injury. If reinsertion is possible, it is preferred. If, however, the ligament is found to be irreparable at surgery, joint stability must be restored by another method. Techniques fitting into two categories have been proposed: transferring a tendon to the ulnar side of the metacarpophalangeal joint or reconstructing a new ligament using a tendon graft.[3,177,180] Tendon transfers have included using the extensor indicis proprius,[96] a portion of the abductor pollicis longus,[60] the adductor pollicis,[137] and the extensor pollicis brevis.[162] Proponents for each of these procedures report generally favorable results.

The other surgical option, which is more predictable, is to reconstruct a new ligament using a tendon graft. The technique to be described satisfies the primary objectives of any surgical procedure—it is easily replicable and the predictability of success is high (Fig. 26-59). The surgical approach is identical to that used for the acute injury. The dissection, however, is more difficult because of secondary scarring. This is particularly evident when one is trying to separate the adductor aponeurosis from the underlying dorsal capsule and what remains of the collateral ligament. The dissection should begin distally over the base of the proximal phalanx where the aponeurosis is usually unscarred and easily separable from the underlying phalanx. As the dissection proceeds proximally, there is usually no longer a distinct plane between the hood and joint capsule, and separating the two can be difficult.

After separation is accomplished, the condition of the ligament is evaluated. If scant ligamentous tissue remains, a new ligament should be reconstructed. The palmaris longus tendon is the preferred donor, but in its ab-

sence the plantaris tendon, a toe extensor, or on rare occasions the extensor indicis proprius can be substituted. A drill hole is made in the metacarpal at its head-neck junction, going in a dorsal-to-volar direction. The drill hole, which is to the ulnar side of the bone, is gradually widened with successively larger drill bits. A deep transverse slot is then made on the ulnar side of the base of the phalanx, as used when an avulsed ligament is reinserted. The tendon graft is passed through the hole in the metacarpal. This is accomplished by first passing the suture through one end of the graft, then passing the suture into the eye of a heavy needle that is introduced in a retrograde fashion into the dorsal hole in the metacarpal. The needle is withdrawn, pulling the suture through the hole, and traction on the suture then pulls the tendon through as well. If the tendon is thin, as may be the case when a plantaris tendon is used, it should be folded on itself before being passed through the metacarpal. The tendon emerging from the volar hole is then anchored into the medullary cavity of the proximal phalanx using a pull-out wire suture. The other end of the graft, emerging from the dorsal hole in the metacarpal, is sutured to its other end and to the periosteum on the side of the phalanx with several 4-0 nylon mattress sutures.

Proper placement of the initial suture is important, because if joint stability is not restored the subsequent sutures will be as ineffective as the first. The role of the assistant is important in stabilizing the joint while the sutures are inserted. With one hand the assistant retracts a heavy skin hook that is hooked into the ulnar side of the metacarpal head. Meanwhile the other hand, grasping the distal segment of the thumb, deviates the metacarpophalangeal joint into a correct position. Care must be taken not to overcorrect the joint and deviate it ulnarly, which is possible in loose-jointed individuals. The

limbs of the tendon graft emerging from the volar and dorsal aspects of the metacarpal and converging to the sides of the phalanx form a horizontal V, which approximates the configuration of a normal collateral ligament. The two limbs of the V are then sutured together, which tightens the reconstructed ligament and adds further stability to the joint. If any doubt remains concerning stability, the remaining length of the ligament can be folded back and anchored to the remnant of the collateral ligament on the side of the metacarpal head. Proximal advancement of the dorsal capsule is usually required because chronically unstable joints tend to be flexed or, in some situations, in volar subluxation. Finally, the adductor aponeurosis is closed. If lax, it should be imbricated to add further reinforcement to the reconstructed ligament. Postoperative treatment is the same as for the primarily repaired ligament.

Radial Collateral Ligament

Acute injuries. The radial collateral ligament is injured approximately one tenth as frequently as the ulnar collateral ligament.[30,57,169] The injuries result from adduction force on the joint, usually after a fall or sudden ulnar deviation of the thumb. As with injuries to the ulnar collateral ligament, stress testing is necessary to determine if there is significant joint instability. If there is instability, surgery is necessary. The operative findings vary from those of ulnar collateral ligament rupture, since a Stener lesion never occurs with rupture of a radial collateral ligament. The location of the ligament damage is also not as predictable as with ulnar collateral ligament ruptures, which almost always fail at their distal insertions. A radial collateral ligament tears with equal frequency at either end, where it can be associated with an avulsion fracture. Rarely does it tear in its midsubstance. Repair and postoperative treatment are the same as for the ulnar collateral ligament injury.

Chronic injuries. It is probably more likely that a radial collateral ligament rupture will go unrecognized and become a chronic problem than it is for a similar injury to the ulnar collateral ligament. With radial collateral ligament rupture, pinch and grip strength are not adversely affected because the ulnar collateral ligament, essential for these activities, remains intact. Therefore the athlete rarely seeks medical attention at the time of the injury. However, as acute pain and swelling subside, the athlete notes that the radial side of the metacarpal head remains prominent and tender. In severe cases the proximal phalanx is slightly ulnarly deviated. More important, the athlete experiences pain whenever pressure is applied to the radial side of the thumb, as when pushing open doors, pushing the buttons on some types of door handles, opening lids on large jars, or doing push-ups. Chronic radial collateral ligament injuries can be as disabling as chronic ulnar collateral ligament injuries.

If secondary arthritic changes have developed, arthrodesis is recommended. If no such changes exist, the preferred procedure is reinsertion of the ligament into the bone from which it avulsed. If the ligament cannot be salvaged, a new ligament is reconstructed. A tendon graft is used as in the method described for ulnar collateral

ligament reconstruction. The abductor aponeurosis is closed and, if lax, is imbricated. The tendon of the abductor pollicis brevis, which is partially detached early in the procedure to allow inspection of the ligament damage, can be advanced to add additional lateral support to the joint.

PROXIMAL PHALANGEAL AREA
Anatomy

The anatomic features of the proximal phalangeal area are analogous to the proximal phalangeal area of a finger, where the bone is almost totally ensheathed by the extrinsic and intrinsic muscle systems. The insertions of the intrinsic muscles on both sides of the proximal phalanx in the thumb and their contributions to the adductor and abductor aponeuroses have been described previously.

Tendon Injuries

The problems associated with closed tendon injuries, particularly as they pertain to the dorsal extension expansions, are similar to those encountered in fingers. However, these problems do not have the same deleterious effects on function. Though tendon adherence over the dorsum of the proximal phalanx in a finger limits proximal interphalangeal joint flexion and seriously impairs the function of the finger, similar tendon adherence in a thumb, which limits interphalangeal joint flexion, has only a negligible effect on overall function. Effective pinch and prehension in the thumb are not compromised if the interphalangeal joint is not fixed in extension or hyperextension. This occurs because the mobility of the trapeziometacarpal joint, which is essential to thumb function, remains intact.

Nerve Injuries

Neuropathies of the digital nerves in this area can result from any activity that causes local compression. Similar neuropathies can occur in the fingers, but they are not as common as in the thumb, where the ulnar digital nerve is usually affected. This nerve, which lies in a thin layer of subcutaneous tissue, is particularly vulnerable because of its anatomic position superficial to the ulnar sesamoid. With repetitive local trauma, scarring develops. Mobility of the nerve, which is normally limited by the tethering effect of its branches to the overlying skin, becomes even more limited. Continued repetitive compression causes increasing damage to the nerve. The condition is most commonly encountered in bowlers. It is caused by the constant friction between the thumb and grip hole in the ball.[41] Symptoms include pain, local tenderness, and numbness. On examination, a tender mass can usually be palpated as the digital nerve is rolled under the examiner's finger. Percussion over the mass produces distal paresthesias along the side of the thumb. There is usually a slight sensory deficit in this area as well. In severe and chronic cases, two-point discrimination may be impaired. Treatment consists of cessation of the activity, and in mild cases the symptoms disappear within several weeks. If the athlete decides to continue

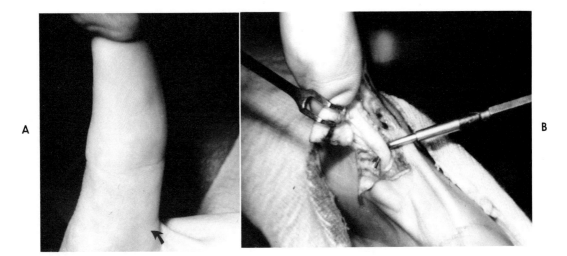

FIG. 26-60. A, Chronic pain and numbness along the ulnar side of a bowler's thumb. The neuro-vascular bundle at the base of the digit (*arrow*) could be rolled under the examiner's digit. **B,** At surgery there was marked thickening of the ulnar digital nerve (*over probe*). An epineurectomy was carried out.

bowling, several changes should be considered, both in delivery technique and in the ball itself, to reduce the risk of recurrence. The bowler should experiment with a three-quarter grip technique, which does not require the entire thumb to be inserted into the ball. If this is unsatisfactory, the hole in the ball can be altered so that the thumb is in greater abduction/extension, which lessens the pressure between the edge of the hole and the ulnar base of the thumb. Contouring the hole may also be of some benefit. In some cases the condition remains resistant to all conservative measures, and tenderness and numbness persist. If the disability becomes unacceptable, surgery is warranted (Fig. 26-60). On exploration the digital nerve appears enlarged and resembles a traumatic neuroma. Unlike the neuroma caused by laceration, it should not be excised. Rather neurolysis with excision of the thickened epineurium is carried out. The results of such treatment are satisfactory, though some permanent sensory deficit may persist in severe and chronic cases.

Fractures

Fractures of the proximal phalanx are similar to those encountered in the fingers. At the distal end of the bone they can be intraarticular, involving one or both condyles, or extraarticular, through the neck of the phalanx. At the proximal end of the phalanx, fractures are also categorized as either intraarticular or extraarticular. Transverse intraarticular fractures are commonly volarly angulated as a result of the pull of the intrinsic muscles. Treatment for any of these fractures is identical to those of a finger.

INTERPHALANGEAL JOINT AREA
Anatomy

The interphalangeal joint is a hinged joint with a wide range of movement in the flexion-extension arc. Not only

is flexion in the range of 90 degrees, but there is also hyperextension to 35 degrees or more. This exceeds the hyperextension seen in any interphalangeal joint of a finger. Structurally the condyles of the proximal phalanx in the thumb are asymmetric with the ulnar condyle being more prominent, wider, and longer in the anteroposterior plane than the radial condyle. The movements of the joint are therefore not through a single axis of rotation; rather, they change, causing the joint to rotate as it flexes. The rotation is toward pronation, which is in concert with the movements of the other joints of the thumb during opposition.[93]

Tendon Injuries

Closed tendon injuries are far less common at the interphalangeal joint of the thumb than at the distal interphalangeal joints of fingers. When they do occur, they usually involve the extensor tendon. As with a drop finger deformity treatment is conservative and involves extension splinting for 6 weeks. Surgery is reserved for the rare chronic case in which the extension lag is so severe that it presents a significant disability.

Ligament Injuries

Though dislocations at the distal interphalangeal joints of fingers may be either dorsal or lateral, dislocations of the interphalangeal joints of the thumbs are almost always dorsal. Lateral dislocations in thumbs are infrequent because of the wider transverse diameter of the condyles of its proximal phalanx, as compared to the transverse diameter of the condyles of the middle phalanx in a finger. In addition, the greater overall mobility of a thumb tends to dissipate a lateral force on its interphalangeal joint, thereby further reducing the likelihood of lateral dislocation.[47]

Dorsal dislocations in thumbs may be compound, as in fingers. The soft tissue over the distal phalanx is firmly anchored by strong, dense skin ligaments and may tear.

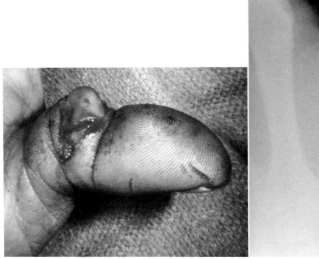
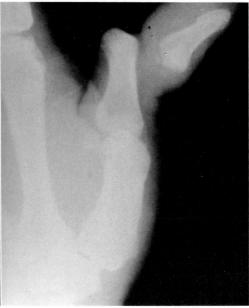

FIG. 26-61. Compound dislocation of the interphalangeal joint of a thumb.

The result is a compound injury as the distal phalanx dislocates. Careful wound lavage is important before reduction of the dislocation. Antibiotic prophylaxis is advisable. Occasionally, the volar plate which remains attached to the distal phalanx, may block the attempted reduction. Surgery may then be necessary. The joint is always stable after reduction, and a dorsal extension block splint is all that is required for several weeks (Fig. 26-61). Chronic instability has not been noted following effective treatment for the acute dislocation.

Fractures

Intraarticular fractures involving the base of the distal phalanx are similar to those encountered in fingers. Treatment is similar as well. One difference in treatment may involve longitudinal fractures, which may be more severe in the thumb. The distal phalanx of a thumb is one third wider than the distal phalanx of a finger, because the pulp stability of the thumb is important for prehension. Because the distal phalanx provides for this stability, widely split or displaced longitudinal fractures may require open reduction and internal fixation.[139]

REFERENCES

1. Abouna JM, Brown H: The treatment of mallet finger: the results on a series of 148 consecutive cases and a review of the literature, *Br J Surg* 55:653, 1968.
2. Admas JP: Correction of chronic dorsal subluxation of the proximal interphalangeal joint by means of a criss-cross volar graft, *J Bone Joint Surg* 41A:111, 1959.
3. Alldred AJ: Rupture of the collateral ligament of the metacarpophalangeal joint of the thumb, *J Bone Joint Surg* 37B:443, 1955.
4. Aubriot JH: The metacarpophalangeal joint of the thumb. In Tubiana R (ed): *The hand,* vol 1, Philadelphia, 1981, WB Saunders.
5. Baldwin LW et al: Metacarpophalangeal joint dislocations of the fingers: a comparison of the pathological anatomy of the index and little finger, *J Bone Joint Surg* 49A:1587, 1967.
6. Barenfeld PA, Weseley MS: Dorsal dislocation of the metacarpophalangeal joint of the index finger treated by late open reduction: a case report, *J Bone Joint Surg* 54A:1311, 1972.
7. Barton NJ: Fractures of the shafts of the phalanges of the hand, *Hand* 11:119, 1979.
8. Barton NJ: Fractures of the phalanges of the hand in children, *Hand* 11:134, 1979.
9. Belsky MR, Easton RG, Lane LB: Closed reduction and internal fixation of the proximal phalangeal fractures, *J Hand Surg* 9A:725, 1984.
10. Bennett EH: On fractures of the metacarpal bone of the thumb, *Br Med J* 2:12, 1986.
11. Blalock HS et al: An instrument designed to help reduce and percutaneously pin fractured phalanges, *J Bone Joint Surg* 57A:792, 1975.
12. Bloem JJAM: The treatment and prognosis of uncomplicated dislocated fractures of the metacarpals and phalanges, *Arch Chir Neerl* 23:55, 1971.
13. Bogumill GP: A morphologic study of the relationship of collateral ligaments to growth plates on the digits, *J Hand Surg* 8:74, 1983.
14. Bohart PG et al: Complex dislocation of the metacarpophalangeal joint: operative reduction by Farabeuf's dorsal incision, *Clin Orthop* 164:208, 1982.
15. Bora JW, Didizian NH: The treatment of injuries to the carpometacarpal joint of the little finger, *J Bone Joint Surg* 56A:1459, 1974.
16. Bosworth DM: Internal splinting of fractures of the fifth metacarpal, *J Bone Joint Surg* 19:826, 1937.
17. Bowers WH: The proximal interphalangeal joint. II. A clinical study of hyperextension, *J Hand Surg* 6:77, 1981.
18. Bowers WH: Sprains and joint injuries in the hand, *Hand Clin* 2:93, 1986.
19. Bowers WH, Hurst LC: Gamekeeper's thumb: evaluation by arthrography and stress roentgenography, *J Bone Joint Surg* 59A:519, 1977.
20. Bowers WH, Hurst LC: Chronic mallet finger: the use of Fowler's central slip release, *J Hand Surg* 3:373, 1978.
21. Bowers WH et al: The proximal interphalangeal joint volar plate. I. An anatomical and biomechanical study, *J Hand Surg* 5:79, 1980.
22. Boyes JH: *Bunnell's surgery of the hand,* ed 5, Philadelphia, 1970, JB Lippincott.
23. Boyes JH, Wilson JN, Smith JW: Flexor tendon ruptures in the forearm and hand, *J Bone Joint Surg* 42:637, 1960.

24. Brewerton DA: A tangential radiographic projection for demonstrating involvement of metacarpal heads in rheumatoid arthritis, *Br J Radiol* 40:233, 1967.
25. Brunet ME, Haddad RJ: Fractures and dislocations of the metacarpals and phalanges, *Clin Sports Med* 5:773, 1986.
26. Burton RI: Extensor tendon: late reconstruction. In Green DP (ed): *Operative hand surgery*, ed 2, New York, 1988, Churchill Livingstone.
27. Burton RI, Eaton RG: Common hand injuries in the athlete, *Orthop Clin North Am* 4:809, 1973.
28. Butt WD: Fractures of the hand: treatment and results, *Can Med Assoc J* 86:815, 1962.
29. Bynum DK, Gilbert JA: Avulsion of the flexor digitorum profundus: anatomic and biomechanical considerations, *J Hand Surg* 13A:222, 1988.
30. Camp RA, Weatherway RJ, Miller EB: Chronic posttraumatic radial instability of the thumb metacarpophalangeal joint, *J Hand Surg* 5:221, 1980.
31. Campbell CS: Gamekeeper's thumb, *J Bone Joint Surg* 37B:148, 1955.
32. Carroll C, Moore JR, Weiland AJ: Posttraumatic ulnar subluxation of the extensor tendons: a reconstructive technique, *J Hand Surg* 12A:227, 1987.
33. Carroll RE, Sinton W, Garcia A: Acute calcium deposits in the hand, *JAMA* 157:422, 1955.
34. Clifford RH: Intra-medullary wire fixation of hand fractures, *Plast Reconstr Surg* 11:366, 1953.
35. Coonrad RW, Goldner JL: A study of the pathological findings and treatment in soft tissue injury of the thumb metacarpophalangeal joint, *J Bone Joint Surg* 50A:439, 1968.
36. Coonrad RW, Pholman MH: Impacted fractures in the proximal portion of the proximal phalanx of the finger, *J Bone Joint Surg* 51A:1291, 1969.
37. Cozzi EP: The proximal interphalangeal joints: a study of the para-articular fibrous structures. In Tubiana R (ed): *The hand*, vol 2, Philadelphia, 1985, WB Saunders.
38. Crawford GP: Screw fixation of the phalanges and metacarpals, *J Bone Joint Surg* 58A:487, 1978.
39. Crawford GP: The molded polyethelene splint for mallet finger deformities, *J Hand Surg* 9A:231, 1984.
40. Dixon GL, Moon NF: Rotational supracondylar fractures of the proximal phalanx in children, *Clin Orthop* 83:151, 1972.
41. Dobyns JH et al: Bowler's thumb: diagnosis and treatment. A review of seventeen cases, *J Bone Joint Surg* 54A:751, 1972.
42. Doyle JR: Extensor tendons: acute injuries. In Green DP (ed): *Operative hand surgery*, ed 2, New York, 1988, Churchill Livingstone.
43. Dray GJ, Eaton RG: Dislocations and ligament injuries in the digits. In Green DP (ed): *Operative hand surgery*, ed 2, New York, 1988, Churchill Livingstone.
44. Dray G, Millender LH, Nalebuff EA: Rupture of the radial collateral ligament of a metacarpophalangeal joint to one of the ulnar three fingers, *J Hand Surg* 4:346, 1979.
45. Dubousset JF: The digital joints. In Tubiana R (ed): *The hand*, vol 1, Philadelphia, 1985, WB Saunders.
46. Eaton RG: *Joint injuries of the hand*, Springfield, Ill, 1971, Charles C Thomas.
47. Eaton RG: Acute and chronic ligamentous injuries of the fingers and thumb. In Tubiana R (ed): *The hand*, vol 2, Philadelphia, 1985, WB Saunders.
48. Eaton RG, Littler JW: A study of the basal joint of the thumb: treatment of its disabilities by fusion, *J Bone Joint Surg* 51A:661, 1969.
49. Eaton RG, Littler JW: Ligament reconstruction for the painful thumb carpometacarpal joint, *J Bone Joint Surg* 55A:1655, 1973.
50. El-Bacha A: The carpometacarpal joints. In Tubiana R (ed): *The hand*, vol 1, Philadelphia, 1981, WB Saunders.
51. Elliott RA: Intrinsics to the extensor mechanism of the hand, *Orthop Clin North Am* 1:335, 1970.
52. Engkvist O, Balkfors B, Lindsjo U: Thumb injuries in downhill skiing, *Int J Sports Med* 3:50, 1982.
53. Faithfull DK: Treatment of chronic instability of the digital joints using a strip of volar plate, *Hand* 13:36, 1981.
54. Flatt AE: *The care of the rheumatoid hand*, St Louis, 1963, Mosby.
55. Flatt AE: *Fractures: care of minor hand injuries*, ed 3, St Louis, 1972, Mosby.
56. Frank G: Injuries of the hand. In Donoghue DH (ed): *Treatment of injuries to athletes*, ed 4, Philadelphia, 1984, WB Saunders.
57. Frank WE, Dobyns JH: Surgical pathology of collateral ligamentous injuries of the thumb, *Clin Orthop* 83:102, 1972.
58. Freeland AE, Jabaley ME, Hughes JE: *Stable fixation of the hand and wrist*, New York, 1986, Springer-Verlag.
59. Froimson AI: Tenosynovitis and tennis elbow. In Green DP (ed): *Operative hand surgery*, ed 2, New York, 1988, Churchill Livingstone.
60. Frykman G, Johansson O: Surgical repair of rupture of the ulnar collateral ligament of the metacarpophalangeal joint of the thumb, *Acta Orthop Scand* 112:58, 1956.
61. Gad P: The anatomy of the volar part of the capsules of the finger joints, *J Bone Joint Surg* 49B:362, 1967.
62. Gedda KO: Studies on Bennett's fracture: anatomy, roentgenology and therapy, *Acta Chir Scand Suppl* 193, 1954.
63. Gelberman RH, Vance RM, Zakaib GS: Fractures at the base of the thumb: treatment with oblique traction, *J Bone Joint Surg* 61A:260, 1979.
64. Gerber C, Senn E, Matter P: Skier's thumb: surgical treatment of recent injuries to the ulnar collateral ligament of the thumb's metacarpophalangeal joint, *Am J Sports Med* 9:171, 1981.
65. Gibson CT, Manske PR: Isolated avulsion of a flexor digitorum superficialis tendon, *J Hand Surg* 12A:601, 1987.
66. Gilbert A, Busy F: The contribution of arthrography to the diagnosis of lesions of the digital ligaments. In Tubiana R (ed): *The hand*, vol 2, Philadelphia, 1985, WB Saunders.
67. Gilbert A et al: Lesions of the volar plates. In Tubiana R (ed): *The hand*, vol 2, Philadelphia, 1985, WB Saunders.
68. Gingrass RP, Fehring B, Matloub H: Intraosseous wiring of complex hand fractures, *Plast Reconstr Surg* 66:383, 1980.
69. Glasgow M, Lloyd GJ: The use of modified AO reduction forceps in percutaneous fracture fixation, *Hand* 13:214, 1981.
70. Goldner JL, Coonrad RW: Tendon grafting of the flexor profundus in the presence of a completely or partially intact flexor sublimis, *J Bone Joint Surg* 51A:527, 1969.
71. Green DP, Rowland SA: Fractures and dislocations in the hand. In Rockwood CA, Green DP (eds): *Fractures*, Philadelphia, 1975, JB Lippincott.
72. Green DP, Terry GC: Complex dislocation of the metacarpophalangeal joint: corrective pathological anatomy, *J Bone Joint Surg* 55A:1480, 1973.
73. Green S, Posner MA: Irreducible dorsal dislocation of the proximal interphalangeal joint, *J Hand Surg* 10A:85, 1985.
74. Gropper PT, Bowen V: Cerclage wiring of metacarpal fractures, *Clin Orthop* 188:203, 1984.
75. Grundberg AB, Reagan DS: Central slip tenotomy for chronic mallet finger deformity, *J Hand Surg* 12A:545, 1987.
76. Gunter GS: Traumatic avulsion of the insertion of the flexor digitorum profundus, *Aust NZ J Surg* 30:1, 1960.
77. Harvey FJ, Bye WD: Bennett's fracture, *Hand* 8:48, 1976.
78. Harvey FJ, Hume KF: Spontaneous recurrent ulnar dislocation of the long extensor tendons of the fingers, *J Hand Surg* 5:492, 1980.
79. Hastings H: *Complex articular fractures of the base of the middle phalanx: treatment by hinged external fixation.* Paper presented at the 42nd annual meeting of the ASSH, San Antonio, 1987.
80. Heim V, Pfeiffer KM: *Small fragment set manual.* Technique recommended by the ASIF group (Ewiss Association for the Study of Internal Fixation), ed 2, New York, 1982, Springer-Verlag.
81. Helm RH: Hand function after injuries to the collateral ligaments of the metacarpophalangeal joint of the thumb, *J Hand Surg* 12B:252, 1987.
82. Honner R: The late management of the isolated lesion of the flexor digitorum profundus tendon, *Hand* 7:171, 1975.

83. Howard LD: Treatment of posttraumatic recurvatum deformities of the proximal interphalangeal joint with occasional locking, but with otherwise free joint mobility. In Cramer LM, Chase RA (eds): *Symposium on the hand,* vol 3, St Louis, 1971, Mosby.

84. Isani A: Small joint injuries requiring surgical treatment, *Orthop Clin North Am* 17:407, 1986.

85. Isani A, Melone CP: Ligamentous injuries of the hand in athletes, *Clin Sports Med* 5:757, 1986.

86. Ishizuki M: Injury to the collateral ligament of the metacarpophalangeal joint of a finger, *J Hand Surg* 13A:444, 1988.

87. Jahss SA: Fractures of the metacarpals: a new method of reduction and immobilization, *J Bone Joint Surg* 20:178, 1938.

88. James JIP: Fractures of the proximal and middle phalanges of the finger, *Acta Orthop Scand* 32:401, 1962.

89. Johnson EC: Fractures of the base of the thumb: a new method of fixation, *JAMA* 126:27, 1944.

90. Johnson FG, Green MH: Another cause of the irreducible dislocation of the proximal interphalangeal joint of a finger: a case report, *J Bone Joint Surg* 48A:542, 1966.

91. Joseph J: Further studies of the metacarpophalangeal and interphalangeal joints of the thumb, *J Anat* 85:221, 1951.

92. Jupiter JB, Silver MA: Fractures of the metacarpals and phalanges. In Chapman MW (ed): *Operative orthopaedics,* vol 2, Philadelphia, 1988, JB Lippincott.

93. Kapandji IA: Biomechanics of the interphalangeal joint of the thumb. In Tubiana R (ed): *The hand,* vol 1, Philadelphia, 1981, WB Saunders.

94. Kaplan EB: Extension deformities of the proximal interphalangeal joints of the finger: an anatomical study, *J Bone Joint Surg* 18:781, 1939.

95. Kaplan EB: Dorsal dislocation of the metacarpophalangeal joint of the index finger, *J Bone Joint Surg* 39A:1081, 1957.

96. Kaplan EB: The pathology and treatment of radial subluxation of the thumb with ulnar displacement of the head of the first metacarpal, *J Bone Joint Surg* 43A:541, 1961.

97. Karthaus RP, van der Werf GJIM: Operative correction of posttraumatic and congenital swanneck deformity: a new technique, *J Hand Surg* 239, 1986.

98. Kelsey JL et al: *Upper extremity disorders: a survey of their frequency and cost in the United States,* St Louis 1980, Mosby.

99. Kettekamp DB, Flatt AE, Moulds R: Traumatic dislocation of the long finger extensor: a clinical, anatomical, and biomechanical study, *J Bone Joint Surg* 53A:229, 1971.

100. Kiefhaber TR, Stern PJ, Grood ES: Lateral stability of the proximal interphalangeal joint, *J Hand Surg* 11A:661, 1986.

101. Kjeldal I: Irreducible compound dorsal dislocation of the proximal interphalangeal joint of a finger, *J Hand Surg* 11B:49, 1986.

102. Kleinert HE, Kasdan ML: Reconstruction of chronically subluxated proximal interphalangeal finger joint, *J Bone Joint Surg* 47A:958, 1965.

103. Kuczynski K: The proximal interphalangeal joint: anatomy and causes of stiffness in the fingers, *J Bone Joint Surg* 50B:656, 1968.

104. Kuczynski K: The thumb and the saddle, *Hand* 7:120, 1975.

105. Landsmeer JMF: Anatomical and functional investigation of the articulations of the human finger, *Acta Anat* 25, 1955.

106. Lane CS: Detecting occult fractures of the metacarpal head: the Brewerton view, *J Hand Surg* 2:131, 1977.

107. Lane CS: Reconstruction of the unstable proximal interphalangeal joint: the double superficialis tenodesis, *J Hand Surg* 3:368, 1978.

108. Langa V, Posner MA: Unusual rupture of a flexor profundus tendon, *J Hand Surg* 11A:227, 1986.

109. Lange RH, Engber WD: Hyperextension mallet finger, *Orthopaedics* 6:1426, 1983.

110. Leddy JP: Flexor tendon: acute injuries. In Green DP (ed): *Operative hand surgery,* ed 2, New York, 1988, Churchill Livingstone.

111. Leddy JP, Packer JT: Avulsion of the profundus insertion in athletes, *J Hand Surg* 2:66, 1977.

112. Leonard MH, Dubracik P: Management of fractured fingers in the child, *Clin Orthop* 73:160, 1970.

113. Lipscomb PR: Management of fractures of the hand, *Am Surg* 29:288, 1963.

114. Lister G: Intraosseous wiring of the digital skeleton, *J Hand Surg* 3:427, 1978.

115. Manske PR, Lesker PA: Avulsion of the ring finger flexor digitorum profundus: an experimental study, *Hand* 10:52, 1978.

116. Massengill MD et al: Mechanical analysis of Kirschner wire fixation in a phalangeal model, *J Hand Surg* 4:351, 1979.

117. McClinton MA, Curtis RM, Wilgis EFS: One hundred tendon grafts for isolated flexor digitorum profundus injuries, *J Hand Surg* 7:224, 1982.

118. McCoy PJ, Winsky AJ: Limbrical loop operation for luxation of the extensor tendons of the hand, *Plast Reconstr Surg* 44:142, 1969.

119. McCue FC: The elbow, wrist and hand. In Kulund D (ed): *The injured athlete,* Philadelphia, 1982, JB Lippincott.

120. McCue FC, Wooten SL: Closed tendon injuries of the hand in athletes, *Clin Sports Med* 4:741, 1986.

121. McCue FC et al: Athletic injuries of the proximal interphalangeal joint requiring surgical treatment, *J Bone Joint Surg* 52A:937, 1970.

122. McCue FC et al: Ulnar collateral ligament injuries of the thumb in athletes, *J Sports Med* 2:70, 1974.

123. McCue FC et al: A pseudo-boutonniere deformity, *Hand* 7:166, 1975.

124. McElfresh EC, Dobyns JH: Intra-articular metacarpal head fractures, *J Hand Surg* 8:383, 1983.

125. McLaughlin HL: Complex "locked" dislocation of the metacarpophalangeal joints, *J Trauma* 5:683, 1965.

126. McMaster PE: Tendon and muscle ruptures: clinical and experimental studies on the causes and location of subcutaneous ruptures, *J Bone Joint Surg* 15:705, 1983.

127. Melone CP: Joint injuries of the fingers and thumb, *Emerg Med Clin North Am* 3:319, 1985.

128. Melone CP: Rigid fixation of phalangeal and metacarpal fractures, *Orthop Clin North Am* 17:424, 1986.

129. Milch H, Green HH: Calcification about the flexor carpi ulnaris tendon, *Arch Surg* 36:600, 1938.

130. Milford L: *The hand,* St. Louis, 1982, Mosby.

131. Miller RJ: Dislocation and fracture dislocations of the metacarpophalangeal joint of the thumb, *Hand Clin* 4:45, 1988.

132. Moberg E, Stener B: Injuries to the ligaments of the thumb and fingers: diagnosis, treatment and prognosis, *Acta Chir Scand* 106:166, 1953.

133. Murakam Y: Irreducible volar dislocation of the proximal interphalangeal joint of the finger, *Hand* 6:87, 1974.

134. Murphy AF, Stark HH: Closed dislocations of the metacarpophalangeal joint of the index finger, *J Bone Joint Surg* 49A:1579, 1967.

135. Napier JR: The form and function of the carpometacarpal joint of the thumb, *J Anat* 89:362, 1955.

136. Neviaser RJ, Wilson JN: Interposition of the extensor tendon resulting in persistent subluxation of the proximal interphalangeal joint of the finger, *Clin Orthop* 8:118, 1972.

137. Neviaser RJ, Wilson JN, Lievano A: Rupture of the ulnar collateral ligament of the thumb (gamekeeper's thumb): correction by dynamic repair, *J Bone Joint Surg* 53A:1357, 1971.

138. Nutter PD: Interposition of sesamoids into metacarpophalangeal dislocations, *J Bone Joint Surg* 22:730, 1940.

139. O'Brien ET: Fractures of the metacarpals and phalanges. In Green DP (ed): *Operative hand surgery,* ed 2, New York, 1988, Churchill Livingstone.

140. Ochiai N et al: Vascular anatomy of flexor tendons. I. Vascular system and blood supply of the profundus tendon in the digital sheath, *J Hand Surg* 4:321, 1979.

141. O'Donoghue DH: *Treatment of injuries to athletes,* Philadelphia, 1970, WB Saunders.

142. Opgrande JD, Westphal SA: Fractures of the hand, *Orthop Clin North Am* 14:779, 1983.

143. Palmar AK, Linscheid RL: Irreducible dorsal dislocation of the distal interphalangeal joint of the finger, *J Hand Surg* 2:406, 1977.

144. Palmar AK, Linscheid RL: Chronic recurrent dislocation of the proximal interphalangeal joint of the finger, *J Hand Surg* 3:95, 1978.

145. Palmar AK, Louis DS: Assessing ulnar instability of the metacarpophalangeal joint of the thumb, *J Hand Surg* 3:542, 1978.
146. Pellegrini UD: Fractures of the base of the thumb, *Hand Clin* 4:87, 1988.
147. Pieron AP: The first carpometacarpal joint. In Tubiana R (ed): *The hand*, vol 1, Philadelphia, 1981, WB Saunders.
148. Pohl AL: Irreducible dislocation of a distal interphalangeal joint, *Br J Plast Surg* 29:227, 1976.
149. Pollen AG: The conservative treatment of Bennett's fracture: subluxation of the thumb metacarpal, *J Bone Joint Surg* 50B:91, 1968.
150. Posner MA: Injuries to the hand and wrist in athletes, *Orthop Clin North Am* 8:593, 1977.
151. Posner MA: Hand and digit injuries. In Scott NW, Nissonson B, Nicholas JA (eds): *Principles of sports medicine*, Baltimore, 1984, Williams & Wilkins.
152. Posner MA, Ambrose L: Intrinsic muscle advancement to treat chronic palmar instability of the metacarpophalangeal joint of the thumb, *J Hand Surg* 13A:110, 1988.
153. Posner MA, Ambrose L: The boxer's knuckle; dorsal capsule rupture of the metacarpophalangeal joint of a finger, *J Hand Surg* 14A:229, 1989.
154. Posner MA, Kaplan EB: Osseous and ligamentous structures. In Spinner M (ed): *Kaplan's functional and surgical anatomy of the hand*, Philadelphia, 1984, JB Lippincott.
155. Posner MA, Wilenski M: Irreducible volar dislocation of the proximal interphalangeal joint of a finger caused by interposition of an intact central slip: a case report, *J Bone Joint Surg* 60A:133, 1978.
156. Pratt DR: Exposing fractures of the proximal phalanx of the finger longitudinally through the dorsal extensor apparatus, *Clin Orthop* 15:22, 1959.
157. Pulvertaft RG: Operative treatment of the injuries of the phalanges and metacarpal bones and their joints. In Fullong R (ed): *Operative surgery*, ed 2, Philadelphia, 1969, JB Lippincott.
158. Redler I, Williams JT: Rupture of a collateral ligament of the proximal interphalangeal joint of the finger: analysis of 18 cases, *J Bone Joint Surg* 49A:322, 1967.
159. Resnick D, Danzig LA: Orthopaedic evaluation of injuries of the first metacarpophalangeal joint: gamekeeper's thumb, *Am J Roentgenol* 126:1046, 1976.
160. Riordan DC, Kaplan EB: The thumb. In Spinner M (ed): *Kaplan's functional and surgical anatomy of the hand*, Philadelphia, 1984, JB Lippincott.
161. Ruby LK: Common hand injuries in the athlete, *Orthop Clin North Am* 33:819, 1980.
162. Sakellarides HT, DeWeese JW: Instability of the metacarpophalangeal joint of the thumb: reconstruction of the collateral ligaments using the extensor pollicis brevis tendon, *J Bone Joint Surg* 58A:106, 1976.
163. Sedel L: Dislocation of the metacarpophalangeal joint. In Tubiana R (ed): *The hand*, vol 2, Philadelphia, 1985, WB Saunders.
164. Sedel L: Dislocation of the carpometacarpal joints. In Tubiana R (ed): *The hand*, vol 2, Philadelphia, 1985, WB Saunders.
165. Segmuller G, Schoneuberger F: Fractures of the hand. In Weber BG, Bruner C, Freuler F (eds): *Treatment of fractures in children and adolescents*, New York, 1980, Springer-Verlag.
166. Seymour N: Juxta-epiphyseal fracture of the terminal phalanx of the finger, *J Bone Joint Surg* 48B:347, 1966.
167. Shah J, Patel M: Dislocation of the carpometacarpal joint of the thumb: a report of four cases, *Clin Orthop* 175:166, 1973.
168. Smith JH: Avulsion of a profundus tendon with simultaneous intraarticular fracture of the distal phalanx: case report, *J Hand Surg* 6:600, 1981.
169. Smith RJ: Post-traumatic instability of the metacarpophalangeal joint of the thumb, *J Bone Joint Surg* 59A:14, 1977.
170. Smith RJ, Kaplan EB: Rheumatoid deformities at the metacarpophalangeal joints of the fingers, *J Bone Joint Surg* 49A:31, 1967.
171. Smith RJ, Peimer CA: Injuries to the metacarpal bones and joints, *Adv Surg* 2:341, 1977.
172. Spinner M, Choi BY: Anterior dislocation of the proximal interphalangeal joint: a case of rupture of the central slip of the extensor mechanism, *J Bone Joint Surg* 52A:1329, 1970.
173. Sponberg O, Thoren L: Bennett's fracture: a new method of treatment with oblique traction, *J Bone Joint Surg* 45B:732, 1963.
174. Stark HH: Troublesome fractures and dislocations of the hand. In American Academy of Orthopedic Surgeons: *Instructional course lectures*, vol 19, St Louis, 1970, Mosby.
175. Stark HH, Boyes JH, Wilson JN: Mallet finger, *J Bone Joint Surg* 44A:1061, 1962.
176. Stark HH et al: Flexor tendon graft through intact superficialis tendon, *J Hand Surg* 2:456, 1977.
177. Stener B: Displacement of the ruptured ulnar collateral ligament of the metacarpophalangeal joint of the thumb: a clinical and anatomical study, *J Bone Joint Surg* 44B:869, 1962.
178. Stener B: Acute injuries to the metacarpophalangeal joint of the thumb. In Tubiana R (ed): *The hand*: vol 2, Philadelphia, 1985, WB Saunders.
179. Stothard J, Caird DM: Experience with arthrography of the first metacarpophalangeal joint, *Hand* 13:257, 1981.
180. Strandell G: Total rupture of the ulnar collateral ligament of the metacarpophalangeal joint of the thumb, *Acta Chir Scand* 118:72, 1959.
181. Strickland JW et al. In Strickland JW, Steichen JB (eds): *Difficult problems in hand surgery*, St Louis, 1982, Mosby, p 126.
182. Stripling WD: Displaced intra-articular osteochondral fracture: cause for irreducible dislocation of the distal interphalangeal joint, *J Hand Surg* 7:77, 1982.
183. Swanson AB: Surgery of the hand in cerebral palsy and the swan neck deformity, *J Bone Joint Surg* 42A:951, 1960.
184. Sweterlitsch PR, Torg JS, Pollack H: Entrapment of a sesamoid on the index metacarpophalangeal joint: report of two cases, *J Bone Joint Surg* 51A:995, 1969.
185. Thiomine JM: The management of recent fractures of the phalanges and metacarpals. In Tubiana R (ed): *The hand*, vol 2, Philadelphia, 1985, WB Saunders.
186. Thoren L: A new method of extension treatment in Bennett's fracture, *Acta Chir Scand* 110:485, 1956.
187. Vanik RK et al: The comparative strengths of internal fixation techniques, *J Hand Surg* 9A:216, 1984.
188. Vom Saal FH: Intramedullary fixation in fractures of the hand and fingers, *J Bone Joint Surg* 35A:5, 1953.
189. Wagner CJ: Methods of treatment of Bennett's fracture-dislocations, *Am J Surg* 80:230, 1950.
190. Watt N, Cooper G: Dislocation of the trapeziometacarpal joint, *J Hand Surg* 12B:242, 1987.
191. Webbe MA, Schneider LH: Mallet fractures, *J Bone Joint Surg* 66A:658, 1984.
192. Wheeldon FT: Recurrent dislocation of extensor tendons, *J Bone Joint Surg* 36B:612, 1954.
193. Wiggins H, Bundens W, Park B: A method of treatment of fracture-dislocations of the first metacarpal bone, *J Bone Joint Surg* 36A:810, 1954.
194. Wood UE: Fractures of the hand in children, *Orthop Clin North Am* 7:527, 1976.
195. Zancolli E: Movements of the thumb: opposition mechanics. In Zancolli E: *Structural and dynamic bases of hand surgery*, ed 2, Philadelphia, 1979, JB Lippincott.

CHAPTER 27 Tendon Injuries of the Hand

Lawrence H. Schneider

The athlete's hand, active in sporting activities, is at risk for specific tendon injuries.[6,35,40] These include injury at both the flexor and extensor insertions at the base of the distal phalanx, as well as the closed extensor injury at the proximal interphalangeal (PIP) joint, which later develops into the boutonnière deformity. These will often appear trivial at the time of injury and yet may produce considerable impairment to the athlete's hand. To avoid a misdiagnosis, which would lead to inadequate treatment, it is necessary to be aware of these lesions.

FLEXOR PROFUNDUS RUPTURE

Avulsion of the profundus flexor from the base of the distal phalanx is a relatively frequent sports injury.* Although football is the sport that seems to produce the majority of these problems, avulsion can occur in almost any sporting activity.[6] The condition is often initially seen as a jamming injury with swelling and pain at the distal interphalangeal (DIP) joint. These findings overshadow the fact that distal joint flexion has been lost. At times with proximal migration of the tendon end, the symptoms may be at the PIP joint. This condition is therefore frequently missed if the trainer or physician is unaware of the usual presentation. Because early and direct repair is generally the best treatment, it is important that the condition be recognized. When missed, and the period for direct repair has been passed, other treatment options are available for the treating surgeon.

Pertinent Anatomy

The flexor digitorum profundus proceeds through the superficialis decussation and finally broadens into a flat tendon that inserts into the proximal third of the palmar aspect of the distal phalanx (Fig. 27-1). The blood vessel containing vinculum breve runs from the dorsal surface of the distal end of the tendon to the distal joint capsule and for a variable distance on to the palmar aspect of the middle phalanx. The profundus tendon is the only flexor of the DIP joint.[44]

Mechanism of Injury

The injury is most often a closed avulsion of the tendon; it occurs when the patient is strongly flexing his or her finger and a sudden extension force is applied to that finger. This happens classically when a tackler in football grasps the jersey of an opponent who pulls forcefully away.[56] While the ring finger is most commonly involved, the reason for this is not entirely clear, and several theories have been advanced. Gunter[20] thought that the ring finger was most frequently involved because of this finger's lack of independent action. He pointed out that the long flexor of the ring finger offers the most resistance to extension when the hand is in a fist position, and therefore it is most likely to rupture at the insertion. Others have supported this belief.[28,29] Wenger[56] had a

---

*References 2, 5, 8, 11, 12, 16, and 41.

571

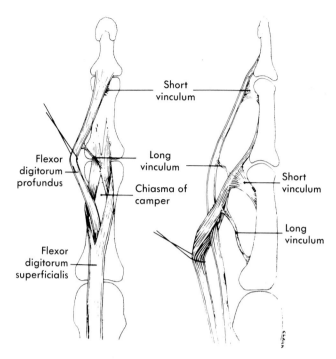

FIG. 27-1. Anatomy of the flexor system. The flexor digitorum profundus passes through the tails of the flexor digitorum superficialis on its way to its insertion on the distal phalanx. At this insertion it is susceptible to avulsion in forceful hyperextension injuries at the distal joint.

similar explanation to Gunter, stating that the most logical explanation is the lack of independent extension of the ring finger when the other digits are tightly flexed. He explained this with photographs. Manske and Lesker[31] tested the breaking strength of the profundus tendon insertion at its attachment to bone. They found that the ring finger profundus insertion was weaker than the insertion of the profundus in adjacent fingers. However, this relative weakness at the attachment is not of a great magnitude and so this theory may offer only a partial explanation.

Examination

The lesion may be a pure avulsion of the flexor tendon from its insertion at the distal phalanx or the tendon can bring along a piece of bone from the distal phalanx.[7] Examination reveals loss of terminal joint flexion and tenderness along the flexor sheath. One can sometimes feel the torn distal end of the tendon and thereby localize it. When the tendon retracts to the palm, a mass is palpable.

The flexor digitorum profundus is the only flexor of the DIP joint, and its avulsion will be obvious when the tip is tested for flexion power. The patient may have proximal swelling at the PIP joint if the tendon has migrated there, or tenderness may be present in the palm in those cases where the proximal end of the tendon has pulled into that area.

Radiographs

Radiographic studies are needed to show whether bone is involved. The significance of these injuries some-

times confuses the unwary examiner. The radiograph may show that a significant segment of bone from the base of the distal phalanx has been avulsed, and this may distract from the nature of the tendon injury. On other occasions, when just a small fragment of bone from the distal phalanx has been avulsed by the tendon, this small piece of bone seen at the level of the PIP joint in the lateral view may lead the examiner to think that this is a minor chip fracture of the PIP joint.

Classification

Early recognition is beneficial, because prompt restitution of the flexor profundus system carries a better prognosis in terms of distal joint flexion.[54] Leddy and Packer[29] presented a classification of these injuries based on the location of the distal end of the tendon.

LEDDY AND PACKER CLASSIFICATION OF AVULSION INJURIES OF THE FLEXOR DIGITORUM PROFUNDUS
Type 1

The tendon end is located in the palm with both vincula ruptured. This type, in my experience, is not often associated with a fracture. Early reattachment of the flexor digitorum profundus is recommended, preferably within the first 2 weeks of injury (Fig. 27-2).

Type 2

In these cases the tendon along with the small bone fragment from the distal phalanx retracts to the level of the PIP joint. The long vinculum remains intact. In these cases a small fragment of bone is seen in the lateral view at the PIP joint, and this gives a clue as to the location of the flexor digitorum profundus (Fig. 27-3). Certainly, early reattachment is indicated, but this lesion is not as emergent a problem as the type

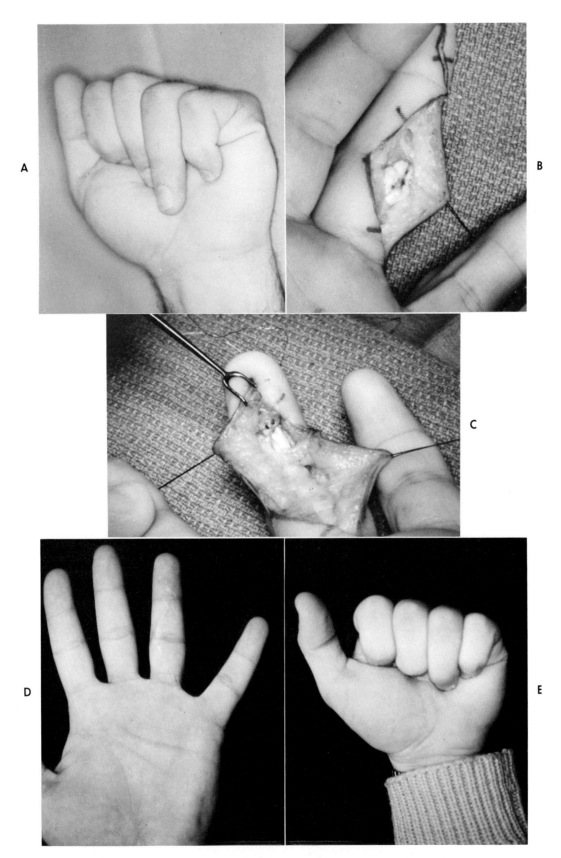

FIG. 27-2. Rupture of the ring finger profundus in a rugby player. **A,** Loss of active flexion is seen at the ring finger 3 days after injury. **B,** Tendon was avulsed from the distal phalanx and was retrievable from the palm—a Type 1 injury. **C,** Reattachment to the distal phalanx was done using the Bunnell technique. **D** and **E,** Range of motion was achieved at 6 months.

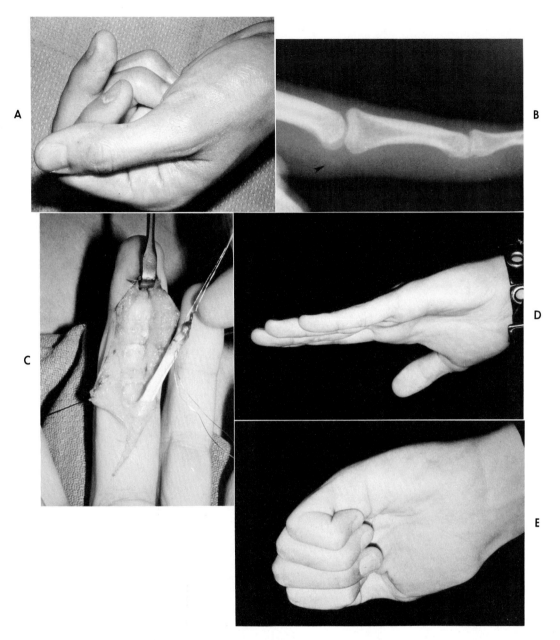

FIG. 27-3. Rupture of the flexor digitorum profundus along with a small bone fragment. **A,** Loss of flexion at the distal joint of the long finger. **B,** Radiograph showed a small bone fragment that was present at the level of the proximal interphalangeal joint—a Type 2 injury. **C,** The tendon is retrieved and is going to be replaced at the distal joint using a Bunnell pull-out technique. **D** and **E,** Range of motion is excellent at 3 months.

1 injury; reattachment can be done up to 4 weeks after injury, with certain reservations as noted below, but rarely beyond that time.

Type 3

This lesion is associated with a large bony fragment. In this instance the fragment, being large, hangs up on the A-4 pulley just proximal to the DIP joint, keeping the tendon out in the finger. Treatment is open reduction and internal fixation, which serves to restore the continuity of the tendon system (Fig. 27-4).

Robins and Dobyns,[42] Smith,[48] and Langa and Posner[26] have recognized a variant of the Type 3 lesion in which not only is the bone fractured but, in addition, the tendon is avulsed from the bony fragment. It would be impossible preoperatively to identify this lesion, which demands both restoration of the joint by open reduction and internal fixation and also a tendon repair. This is a rare injury, and my experience includes just one case in which I used both Kirschner wires and the pull-out wire technique (Fig. 27-5).

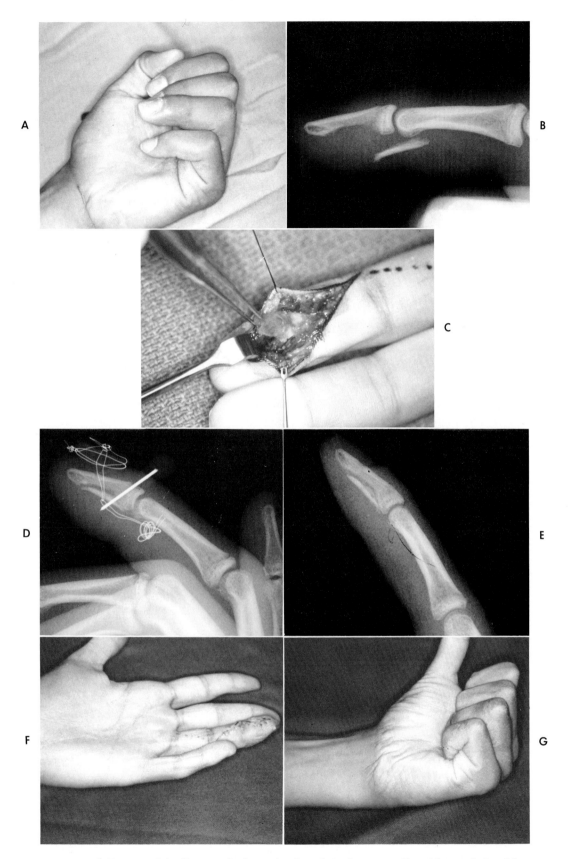

FIG. 27-4. Rupture of the flexor profundus with a large bone fragment—Type 3 lesion. **A,** Painful swelling is seen at the distal joint. This overshadows the loss of distal joint flexion. **B,** Radiograph shows a large fragment that is hung up on the A-4 pulley. There is also a fracture across the base of the phalanx. **C,** The tendon is seen to be attached to the fragment from the distal phalanx. **D,** Reattachment is carried out using a pull-out wire and a Kirschner wire. **E,** After healing, the fragment is held in place by fibrous union. **F and G,** Early range of motion at 4 weeks.

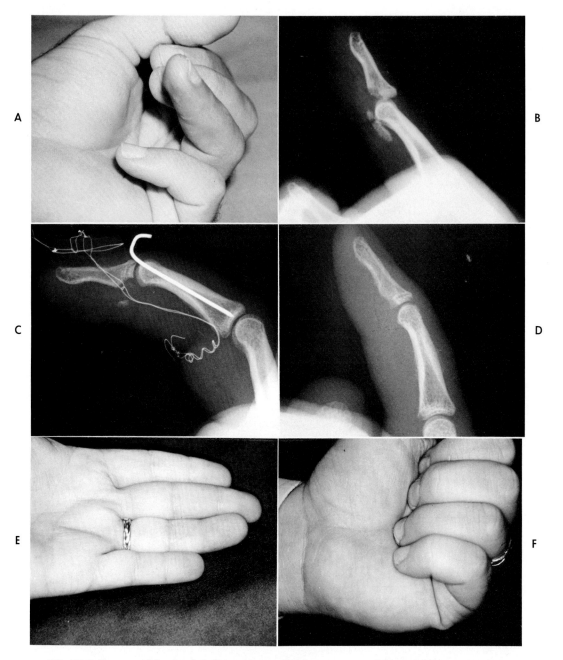

FIG. 27-5. Fracture of the distal phalanx with, in addition, separation of the profundus tendon from the fragment. This finger sustained an avulsive force when caught in the reins of his horse. **A,** Loss of flexion with pain at the distal joint. **B,** The radiograph showed bony avulsion from the base of the distal phalanx and dorsal displacement of the distal phalanx. **C,** On exploration the tendon was found to be separated from the bone fragment. The joint was reduced and stabilized with a Kirschner wire, the bone fragments were discarded, and the tendon was attached directly to the distal phalanx by a pull-out wire. **D,** Radiographic appearance 6 years later. **E and F,** Range of motion at the ring finger at 6 years.

Treatment

Acute Lesions

There is no nonoperative treatment for acute lesions. Splinting the finger for comfort is not unreasonable, but plans should be made for early operative reattachment of the tendon.[39] When recognized early, the reattachment of the tendon end gives the best chance for a good result in terms of distal joint function.

Type 1 lesions. In Type 1 lesions the tendon is retrieved as atraumatically as possible and threaded up the flexor sheath (preserving as much sheath as possible), doing as little damage to that structure as possible. At the distal phalanx the tendon is reattached to bone. The Bunnel tendon-to-bone juncture is best.[44] This should be done early, preferably before 2 weeks have elapsed. If done later, the profundus muscle may contract and

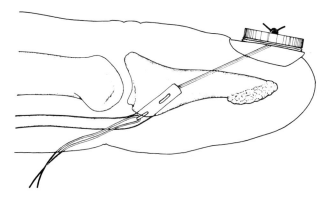

FIG. 27-6. Bunnell technique for reattachment of the flexor profundus to the distal phalanx. (From Schneider LH: *Flexor tendon injuries*, Boston, 1985, Little, Brown.)

shorten. With reattachment the surgeon may find that the finger will be placed in excessive flexion when it is on the operating table. This is recognized by placing the hand flat on the table with the wrist in the neutral position. There is a break in the normal cascade of the fingers. It is a mistake to accept this posture. The surgeon should be prepared preoperatively to abandon the direct repair and either accept the situation or go to tendon grafting or fusion of the joint.

Type 2 lesions. In this lesion the tendon does not pull as proximally as in Type 1 but stays in the finger, so it is not as emergent a procedure. I have reattached these successfully at a later time, again using the Bunnell technique. The pull-out wire in the tendon can incorporate the fracture fragment and be used to pull the fragment into its bed in the distal phalanx.

The reattachment to bone is done using the Bunnell pull-out wire technique (Fig. 27-6). The patient is mobilized early, as in the protected mobilization program.[44] This procedure in these lesions in which the tendon has pulled into the palm is usually performable up to approximately 2 weeks. I have treated a patient in whom the short vinculum of the profundus remained intact and the tendon end had migrated only to the level just proximal to the DIP joint. A patient such as this could probably be treated quite late. Obviously this could not have been predicted before exploration, so the exact time that one can successfully carry out a reattachment is not fixed, and exploration may be needed to make a definitive determination.

Late Lesions

There are patients in whom the initial diagnosis was missed or, as is not uncommon, athletes who elect to defer their treatment when seen at the time of injury. Not infrequently we see an athlete with this lesion past the time that direct repair can be accomplished. Typical is the football player who comes in after the season with loss of distal joint flexion. When passive motion at the DIP joint has been maintained, the choices for treatment include the following.[23,39]

1. *Accepting the lesion as it stands.* This is particularly pertinent for patients who have a fully func-

tional flexor superficialis to motor the PIP joint. Most of the useful arc of motion of the finger has been maintained when the superficialis is fully functional. There is considerable risk to this function if, while the tendon graft is being passed through or around the superficialis decussation, damage is done to this complex area, resulting in adhesion formation and an overall reduction in function. In fingers that are not particularly soft or supple but that show good flexor digitorum superficialis function, it may be justifiable to again offer no treatment. This is particularly true when the distal joint is not hyperextensible.

2. *Stabilization of the tip by fusion or tenodesis.* If the distal joint is unstable, particularly if it tends to hyperextension, fusion can be offered. If damage at the PIP joint results in a flexion contracture at that level, tenolysis and joint release at that joint can be combined with a distal joint fusion without going into more complex procedures. This salvage in which proximal joint function is restored or preserved with stabilization of the distal joint has been referred to as the superficialis finger.[44] At the same sitting one might excise the proximal portion of the flexor digitorum profundus if it is coiled up in the palm and causing a troublesome mass at that location. If at the time of tenolysis of the intact but adherent flexor superficialis a graft for distal joint function has been elected, the staged technique is used.[44]

3. *Tendon graft through the intact flexor superficialis in one or two stages.* This last technique is the only way that motion can be returned to the distal phalanx. Contrary to other opinions, this reconstructive procedure is even better indicated in those in whom the PIP joint is not normal. It is noted that this procedure is done at considerable risk to the function of the finger, and both patient and surgeon should consider the risks when offering this procedure. The patient may opt for one of the more predictable procedures. In my opinion the tendon graft is better indicated in the young and on the ulnar side of the hand (Fig. 27-7). In my experience, which includes 22 palm-to-fingertip one-stage tendon grafts, flexor tenolysis was carried out as a secondary procedure in approximately 50% of cases.[45] Where heavy scarring is found or in those patients who need joint release or tenolysis of the superficialis, then the two-staged tendon reconstruction is indicated.[44]

MALLET FINGER INJURY
Pertinent Anatomy

The distal extensor tendon, formed from contributions from the lateral bands over the middle phalanx, terminates in a central tendon that inserts into the base of the distal phalanx.[53] Some of the fibers of the oblique retinacular ligament also blend into the central tendon and contribute to the extension at the DIP joint. Interruption of this extensor mechanism leads to varying degrees of drooping of the distal phalanx (an extensor lag). In pa-

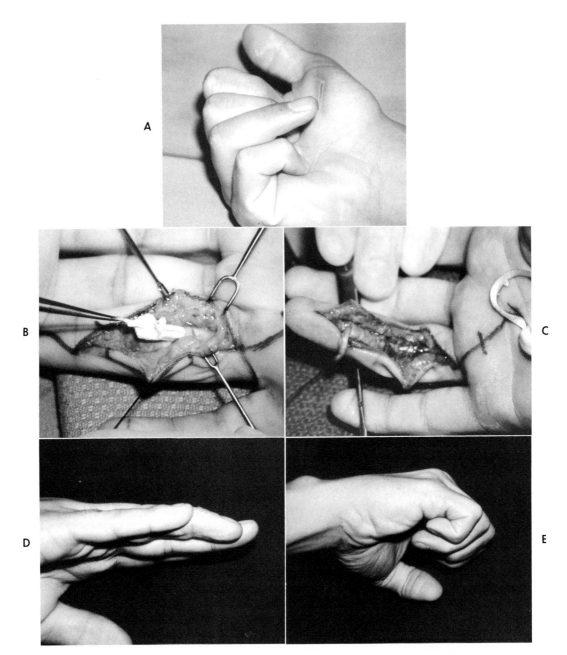

FIG. 27-7. Closed rupture of the flexor digitorum profundus in a 17-year-old football player who reported for treatment 4 months after injury. **A,** Posture of the finger in attempted flexion of the ring finger. **B,** The tendon has been retrieved but is not advanceable to the distal phalanx. **C,** A tendon graft from the palmaris longus is placed within the flexor retinaculum. **D** and **E,** Range of motion returned to the distal interphalangeal joint after 6 months.

tients with hyperextensile PIP joints, the PIP joint tends to adopt a hyperextension posture. This is because with proximal migration of the extensor force more power into extension is placed on the PIP joint. This leads to stretching of the volar supportive structures at the PIP joint. With attempts at extension this problem worsens. The flexor profundus exaggerates the deformity at the DIP with more tension placed in it by the hyperextension at the PIP joint. With time a swan-neck deformity (hyperextension at the PIP joint and flexion at the DIP joint) may result.

Mechanism of Injury

Disruption of the terminal extensor mechanism at the DIP joint produces an extensor lag at that joint.[21,52] This lesion, the mallet finger, which has also been referred to as a baseball finger, is incurred when an object, often a ball, strikes the tip of the extended finger, forcing it suddenly into flexion. This activity tears the extensor mechanism from the base of the distal phalanx. The tendon may be just stretched or attenuated, or torn completely from the bone, resulting in a soft-tissue mallet finger. If the deformity is associated with a fracture in which a

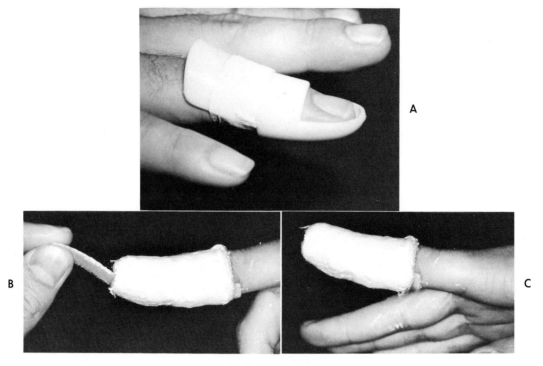

FIG. 27-8. Immobilization devices for mallet fingers. **A,** Plastic splint is comfortable and allows for proximal interphalangeal joint motion. It can additionally be wrapped with tape when the patient is participating in sports. **B** and **C,** Finger cast applied over adherent tape is a reliable form of immobilization.

Types of mallet injuries

- Soft-tissue mallet finger: tendon is stretched, attenuated, or avulsed
- Mallet fracture: tendon is detached with a portion of distal phalanx

fragment of bone comes off from the dorsum of the distal phalanx with the tendon, a mallet fracture is present.

Examination

The patient usually recognizes and points out to the examiner that he or she has lost terminal joint extension. There may be erythema over the dorsum of the joint and some pain with the injury, but there can be remarkably few symptoms. Inability to actively extend the distal phalanx is present to a varying degree. The exact amount of extension loss can be better estimated when compared with an adjacent normal finger, because many patients normally hyperextend at the DIP joint.

Radiographs

Radiographs should be taken to rule out fracture.

Treatment

Acute Soft-Tissue Mallet Injuries

Acute soft-tissue mallet injuries can be treated by well-proven nonoperative methods.[1]

Splints. Many kinds of splints have been recommended; these are applied with the distal joint in extension (Fig. 27-8). One should not force the joint into hyperextension because this risks sloughing of skin on the dorsum of the joint. This treatment requires 6 to 8 weeks of uninterrupted immobilization in extension at the DIP joint. The important point with this treatment is educating the patient to avoid removing the splint to test for healing. If the splint is to be changed, the joint must be kept in full extension. In the past the PIP joint would be included, but this is now known not to be necessary. Inclusion of the more proximal joint may be helpful in the more active or uncooperative patient.

Circular finger castings. The splinting program is difficult to apply in many active athletes and circular finger casting may be a more predictable method of immobilization. In very active or uncooperative patients inclusion of the PIP joint in 45 degrees of flexion in the finger cast will, in addition, help keep the splint from slipping off (Fig. 27-9). The immobilization should not be placed in excessive extension to avoid skin sloughs on the dorsum of the distal joint.

Percutaneous wire fixation. Operative repair is rarely indicated in the acute closed mallet finger. One form of operative treatment is the use of a percutaneous Kirschner wire to fix the DIP joint in extension.[9,10] This is done under metacarpal block of the digital nerves with a single 0.045 Kirschner wire. In the active patient the pin can be cut off beneath the skin and activity allowed (Fig.

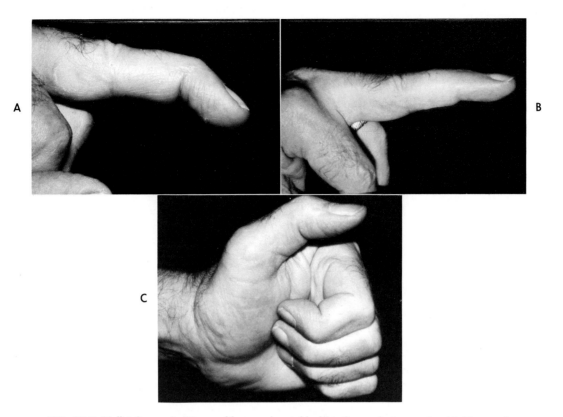

FIG. 27-9. Mallet finger. **A,** 60-year-old man who stubbed his finger playing catch with his grandchild. He had a 45-degree extensor lag at the distal joint. He was treated in a splint, as seen in Fig. 27-8, *A,* for 8 weeks. **B** and **C,** Range of motion achieved at 4 months.

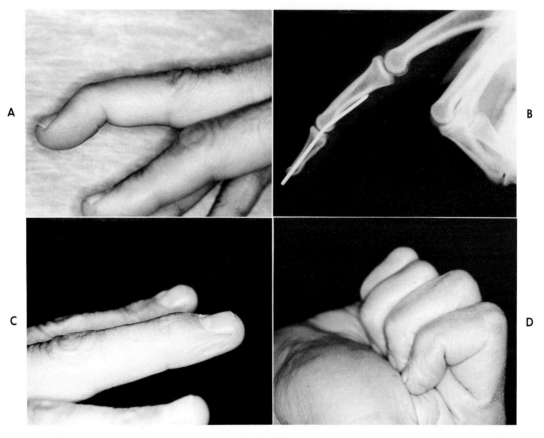

FIG. 27-10. Mallet finger treated by percutaneous Kirschner wire fixation of the distal joint. **A,** Mallet finger in a 50-year-old surgeon. **B,** A 0.62 Kirschner wire was used to transfix the distal interphalangeal joint in extension. The pin was cut off subcutaneously and he resumed activities. It is noted that he inadvertently bent the pin. **C** and **D,** Extension and flexion at 2 years.

27-10). In risk situations the finger should be additionally protected with an external splint.

Open operative repair. Authors have used open operative treatment for the acute soft-tissue mallet finger injury. In my experience these are rarely indicated. Hillman[22] recommended immobilizing the distal joint with a suture placed percutaneously. I see little indication for this procedure.

Chronic Soft-Tissue Mallet Injuries

Not infrequently the mallet injury soft tissue goes untreated and the patient presents for treatment later. This is usually because the significance of the injury was missed or underestimated. Selection of a treatment method is determined individually based on the significance of symptoms and amount of dysfunction present. An array of procedures are available. Judgment is required in their selection, and in fact many of these chronic mallet fingers have little functional impairment and are better left untreated. (A famous professional baseball catcher is said to have had eight untreated mallet fingers and to have done well.)

When treatment is elected there are various options.

Splint application, as in the acute case. It is known that splints may be adequate treatment even for a late mallet finger. A recent paper showed good results in patients who were treated by late splinting 4 to 18 weeks after injury.[38] In fact it is not really known what the outside time period is in which splinting will still effectively correct the problem. The disadvantage of late splinting is the unpredictability of this technique. The advantages of the use of nonoperative treatment in a prolonged long program must be weighed with the fact that many of the operative reconstructive techniques used are also unpredictable.

Surgical reattachment or shortening of the extensor tendon. This usually recovers extension in most cases.[15] The joint needs to be kept extended full time for 6 to 8 weeks and a Kirschner wire is left in place for most of this time. The problem is that most of these, if protected long enough, will restore extension at the price of some flexion loss at the distal joint. In young cooperative patients this can be a reasonable procedure (Fig. 27-11).

Fowler's technique. In this procedure the central slip is released at the PIP joint, which allows the extensor system to more strongly pull distally at the DIP

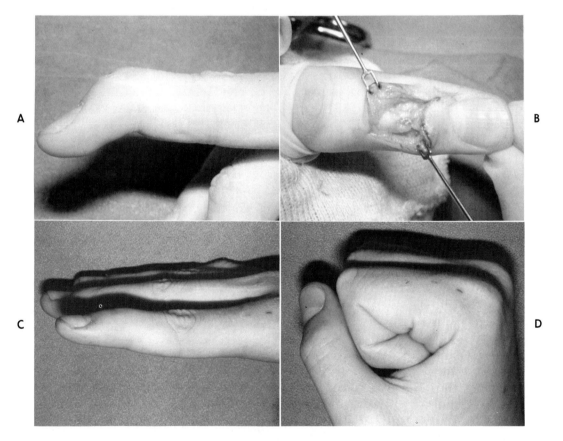

FIG. 27-11. Chronic mallet finger of the index finger in a 16-year-old boy. **A,** This lesion was 5 months old with chronic swelling seen at the dorsum of the joint. **B,** The tendon showed scarring and granulation tissue at the area of disruption. This scarring was excised and the tendon ends were sutured. A Kirschner wire was used to transfix the joint for 6 weeks. **C** and **D,** Excellent recovery at 6 months is seen in these photos.

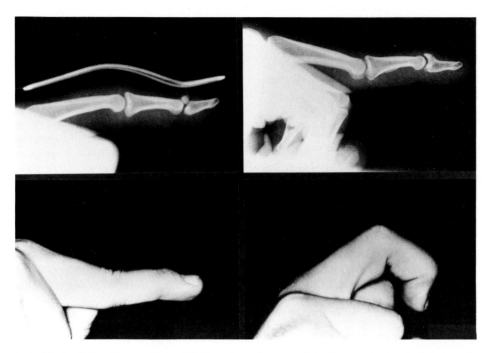

FIG. 27-12. Mallet fracture. *Upper left,* Significant fracture of the base of the distal phalanx with articular surface disruption. Dorsal splinting was shortened to distal to the proximal interphalangeal joint at 2 weeks. The joint was kept in extension uninterrupted for 6 weeks. *Below right and left,* The range of motion achieved at 2 years. *Below right,* Radiograph taken at that time. The patient was asymptomatic. This joint has a remarkable ability to remodel, obviating the need for operative treatment. (From Wehbe MA, Schneider LH: *J Bone Joint Surg* 66A:658, 1984.)

joint, thereby improving extension at that joint.[4,17] This procedure risks the development of a boutonnière deformity.

Tenodermodesis. For late untreated mallet fingers, Iselin, Levame, and Godoy [24] have described a procedure in which the skin and extensor mechanism are excised over the DIP joint in an elliptical fashion. The skin-tendon edges are then reapproximated by three or four nonabsorbable sutures. The aftercare includes splinting for 5 weeks full time and at night for an additional 4 weeks.

Oblique retinacular ligament reconstruction. In this procedure a free tendon graft is inserted along the course of the oblique retinacular ligament from the flexor sheath overlying the proximal phalanx and is distally attached to the terminal extensor tendon. This procedure was described by Thompson, Littler, and Upton[51] and is technically rather complex. It is said to have been simplified by Kleinman and Petersen.[25] I have no experience with this technique.

Fusion. This reliable, predictable procedure is indicated in the patient with painful arthrosis of the joint after failed treatment.

Acute Mallet Fractures

It should be noted that mallet fractures, an injury not infrequently associated with sports, are caused by avulsion of the terminal extensor tendon with a portion of the base of the distal phalanx. Many treatments have been advocated but virtually all of these injuries can be treated by well-proven nonoperative techniques.[46,55] This means uninterrupted splinting of the DIP joint in zero degrees of extension for 6 to 8 weeks. This joint has been seen to remodel despite significant involvement of the articular surface and even with displacement (Fig. 27-12).

Chronic Mallet Fractures

The use of a splint for a patient who is initially seen with this lesion at a late date can still be tried. The cutoff time for splint treatment for untreated injuries is not known.

The chronic untreated mallet fracture can often be accepted by the patient if symptoms are not severe. On one occasion I excised the dorsal bump and reset (shortened) the extensor tendon with some improvement. Fusion of the joint for painful arthrosis is reasonable in symptomatic patients.

Hyperextension Variant of the Mallet Injury

Mention should be made of the hyperextension variant of the mallet injury. Lange and Engber[27] brought our attention to this injury, which was recognized by Bohler.[3] Bohler stated that all mallet fractures did not occur in flexion injuries by avulsion of the bone by the tendon. In the hyperextension variant the base of the distal phalanx is jammed against the head of the middle phalanx, resulting in a major fracture fragment at the dorsal base of the distal phalanx. Lange and Engber[27] re-

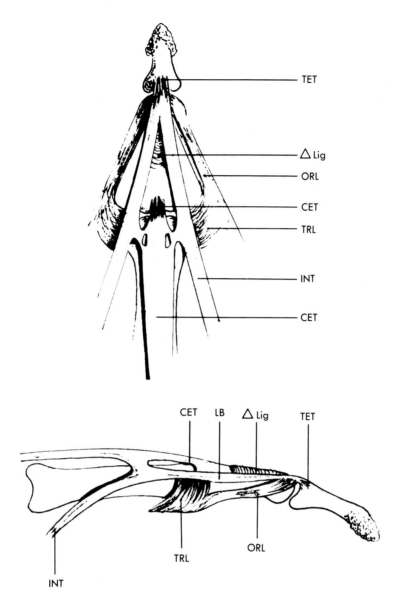

FIG. 27-13. Extensor anatomy. *CET,* Central extensor tendon; *LB,* lateral band; Δ *Lig,* triangular ligament; *TET,* terminal extensor tendon; *INT,* intrinsic tendon; *TRL,* transverse retinacular ligament; *ORL,* oblique retinacular ligament. (From Schneider LH, Smith KL: Boutonniere deformity. In Hunter JM, Schneider LH, Mackin EJ (eds): *Tendon surgery in the hand,* St Louis, 1987, Mosby.)

ported that we should be careful not to hyperextend these injuries in splints because this leads to displacement and possible palmar subluxation of the joint. I believe that this lesion can be treated in the same manner as the usual mallet fracture. Care is taken to splint in minimal flexion or the straight position, but treatment is not really different from that for the mallet fracture sustained in the usual way.

BOUTONNIÈRE DEFORMITY

Disruption of the extensor mechanism at the dorsum of the PIP joint level can lead to a boutonnière (buttonhole) deformity in which there is loss of active extension at the PIP joint and secondary hyperextension at the DIP joint. This deformity can be very disabling to the athlete, and once established it is difficult to treat. The lesion can be caused by an open injury (laceration) to the extensor mechanism at the proximal interphalangeal joint but in the athlete will more often be associated with a closed jamming injury, which forcibly flexes the PIP joint while it is in the extended position.[53]

Pertinent Anatomy (Fig. 27-13)

The extensor hood, also referred to as the extensor or dorsal apparatus, is formed at the metacarpophalangeal joint level by contributions from both the extrinsic extensor systems and the intrinsic tendons.[52] As the exten-

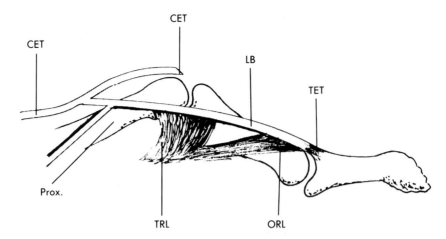

FIG. 27-14. Rupture of the central tendon at the proximal interphalangeal joint starts the process that leads to the boutonnière deformity. *CET,* Central extensor tendon; *LB,* lateral band; *Prox,* proximal phalanx; *TET,* terminal extensor tendon; *INT,* intrinsic tendon; *TRL,* transverse retinacular ligament; *ORL,* oblique retinacular ligament; (From Schneider LH, Smith KL: Boutonnière deformity. In Hunter JM, Schneider LH, Mackin EJ (eds): *Tendon surgery in the hand,* St Louis, 1987, Mosby.)

sor tendon system progresses distally from the hood mechanism, a central slip forms that inserts into the base of the middle phalanx. The extrinsic extensor also contributes two lateral slips that merge with contributions from the intrinsic tendons to form the lateral bands. The major portions of the intrinsic tendons make up these lateral bands while a lesser part goes to the central slip. The lateral bands progress distally and become more dorsal over the middle phalanx and ultimately join each other to insert as the terminal extensor tendon at the base of the distal phalanx. An important ligament over the middle phalanx, the triangular ligament, bridges the two lateral bands and holds these bands in a dorsolateral position. This ligament limits the palmar displacement of these lateral bands in flexion.

Also of importance is the retinacular ligament system. There are two identifiable retinacular ligaments: transverse and oblique. The transverse retinacular ligaments, which insert on the lateral aspect of the lateral bands, serve to prevent the lateral bands from coming dorsally to the midline in extension. The oblique retinacular ligaments run from a palmar position at the proximal phalanx and the flexor sheath and progress dorsally alongside the middle phalanx and finally insert into the distal phalanx alongside the terminal tendon. The retinacular ligaments serve to coordinate movement at the PIP and DIP joints. When the finger normally flexes at the distal joint, the oblique retinacular ligament tightens and tends to flex the proximal joint. The passive extension of the proximal joint also causes extension at the distal joint through these oblique retinacular fibers.

Mechanism of Injury

The mechanism of formation of the boutonnière deformity begins with damage to the central tendon mech-

anism at the PIP joint by a flexion force that is applied while the joint is being extended.[57] The deformity itself is often delayed in appearance especially in the closed athletic injury. At first the patient may be able to actively extend the PIP joint using the lateral bands. With ongoing attempts at function, active flexion of the joint forces the head of the proximal phalanx to "buttonhole" through a defect in the torn or stretched central slip (Fig. 27-14). This subsequently causes stretching or tearing of the triangular ligament and pushes the lateral bands more lateral and palmward. When the lateral bands arrive at a point palmar to the axis of motion of the PIP joint, they become flexors of the joint and are the cause of the deformity. The resulting increased tension in the lateral bands causes increased extensor force to act at the DIP joint, forcing that joint into the extended position. At first the problem is flexible, but with time the transverse retinacular ligaments tighten, holding the now shortened lateral bands below the axis of the PIP joint, and the deformity becomes fixed. Further, the oblique retinacular ligament, with contracture, accentuates the extended position at the distal joint.

Examination

The boutonnière deformity is missed frequently in the acute phase because of its delayed development. The examiner must therefore be alert to the existence and possibility of this lesion. A swollen, painful PIP joint after a sprain or jam should raise suspicion, especially when the swelling and tenderness are noted to be predominantly dorsal at the PIP joint. This joint adopts a position of slight flexion with the DIP joint tending toward extension.[15] The presence of a volar dislocation at the PIP joint should also alert the physician to the boutonnière injury, and after reduction appropriate splinting in the extended position is maintained.

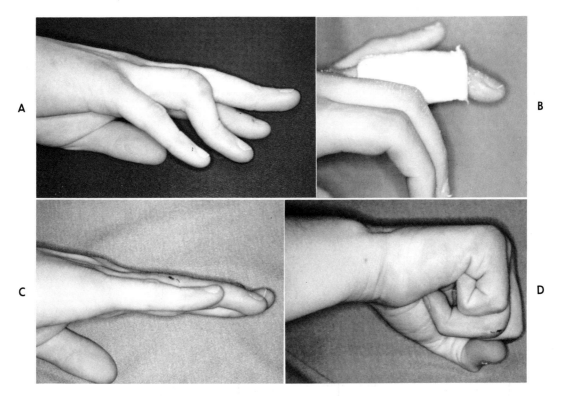

FIG. 27-15. Acute boutonnière deformity in a 15-year-old. The finger is still supple. **A,** Deformity with flexion at the proximal joint and hyperextension at the distal joint. **B,** Finger cast has been applied and the finger will remain in extension at the proximal joint for 6 weeks. The patient is encouraged to flex the distal joint while in the cast. **C** and **D,** Range of motion at 3 months. (From Schneider LH: Injuries to tendons. In Bora FW (ed): *The pediatric upper extremity*, Philadelphia, 1986, WB Saunders.)

Radiographs

Radiographic examination is done to rule out a fracture and may help in the diagnosis of a boutonnière injury if there is a small bone fragment avulsed from the dorsum of the middle phalanx (rare).

Treatment

Acute Boutonnière Deformity

When this injury is recognized, splinting in the extended position at the PIP joint with the DIP joint left free is indicated.[50] The immobilization of the PIP joint in extension should be maintained uninterrupted for 6 to 8 weeks. When the splint is changed, the patient should resist the temptation to test the healing. While the patient is wearing the splint, active and passive flexion of the DIP joint is carried out. This maintains mobility in the distal joint and is believed to help keep the lateral bands up in their dorsolateral position at the middle phalanx. Although all types of dorsal and palmar splints have been used for immobilization of the PIP joint in this problem, I prefer the use of a plaster cylinder cast for the active age group. This is applied in the extended position at the PIP joint. If, because of swelling, full extension cannot be achieved, then the cast is changed weekly until this position is obtained. Six weeks of casting is recommended and then the patient is protected in the ex-

tended position for an additional 2 weeks. In athletic activities an additional 4 to 6 weeks of intermittent splinting is recommended (Fig. 27-15).

Whereas the majority of acute boutonnière injuries can be treated by nonoperative means, a displaced fracture fragment avulsed from the base of the middle phalanx is an indication for open treatment. This is treated by open reduction and internal fixation by Kirschner wires or fine screws if the fragment cannot be reduced by closed means.[53]

Treatment of acute boutonnière injury

- Splint proximal interphalangeal joint in extension
- Leave distal interphalangeal joint free
- Maintain immobilization full time for 6 to 8 weeks
- Protect with splint during athletic activities for an additional 4 to 6 weeks
- Open reduction internal fixation if large displaced fracture of middle phalanx base

---

Under certain conditions where splinting is difficult to use, the application of a transarticular Kirschner wire is indicated for immobilization in the fresh boutonnière deformity. This 0.045-inch pin is driven obliquely across the joint and left in place for 4 to 5 weeks and then splint

protection is maintained for an additional 1 to 2 weeks. While the pin is strong it has been my policy to add a splint for extra protection to the finger for athletic activities.

Early treatment is recommended for this lesion when it is recognized in the acute stage, but the point when closed treatment will not work is really unknown. It is at least 2 months but may even be longer.

Chronic Boutonnière Deformity

Not infrequently these patients present with the deformity at a late date. Treatment differs between those problems that are supple with full range of passive motion and those fixed deformities.

Supple deformities

Nonoperative treatment. Casting is a reasonable method of treatment within 8 weeks of the time of the

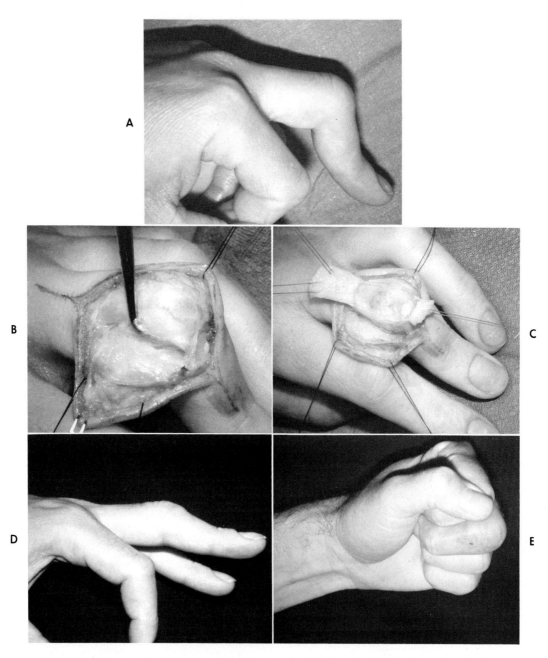

FIG. 27-16. Boutonnière deformity—surgical treatment. **A,** Deformity failed to respond to nonoperative care. **B,** Scarred extensor mechanism at the proximal interphalangeal joint. The probe is showing the transverse retinacular ligament, which is contracted and holding the lateral bands volar to the axis of the joint. These bands are released. **C,** The central tendon is mobilized and will be shortened and reattached to the middle phalanx. **D** and **E,** Range of motion at 8 months.

injury in the supple deformity. Once applied, casting is continued for 8 weeks. Protective splinting is used after this while the patient is being mobilized. Actually the maximal period after injury during which nonoperative treatment could be applied is not known. Souter[50] stated that the 6-week cutoff in his study of Pulvertaft's cases was arbitrary and that closed treatment could probably be initiated even later. This treatment could be applied by either the various splint devices or even a transarticular Kirschner wire.

Operative treatment. It is to be noted that not all patients with this problem need to be treated. A mild deformity that is not worsening (is stable) can often be accepted, since the risks of operative treatment are significant. The problem in treatment here is that extension is relatively easy to regain by surgical treatment but flexion may be difficult to recover postoperatively. An untreated finger with a slight flexion deformity at the PIP joint that flexes fully is more desirable than an operated finger, which is stiff in the extension range. Therefore when an examiner chooses operative repair, the deformity should be significant.

There are many techniques described in the literature. These take widely different approaches but when considering what is known, the reader should view with suspicion those procedures that are based on the tight fixation of the lateral bands over the dorsum of the PIP joint because these prevent the free flexion of that joint and therefore are not successful.

Techniques available include the following:

1. Redistribution of forces at the joints (Littler and Eaton[30])
2. Use of a tendon graft (Nichols[36])
3. Reconstruction using the lateral bands (Matev[32] and Salvi[43])
4. Direct anatomic repair of the central slip (Souter,[50] Elliott,[15] Grundberg,[19] Pardini and others,[37] Smith,[49] Urbaniak and Hayes,[54] and Zancolli.[57])

I prefer the last technique, in which the central slip is reattached to the middle phalanx. Elliot[15] describes this in detail (Fig. 27-16). The lateral bands are mobilized by transsection of the transverse retinacular ligaments and the central slip is mobilized, advanced, and repaired. In the chronic case it is noted that the central slip defect has been filled in with scar tissue, which the surgeon excises before reattachment to the base of the middle phalanx. The amount of central slip to be removed is very little, and it is beneficial to perform this surgery with the patient under local anesthesia so as to better estimate the tension in the repair. The joint is pinned in the extended position to protect the repair. Postoperatively the finger is kept in extension for 6 weeks, 4 with pin protection and 2 more in an extension splint. The recovery period then stresses the recovery of flexion while trying not to lose the regained extension at the PIP joint.

Fixed deformity. When patients have this condition, an attempt can be made to increase joint motion by hand therapy, including range of motion exercises, dynamic splinting, and serial plasters. When these are unsuccessful in recovering passive extension at the PIP joint, this

motion will have to be achieved with a surgical procedure that releases the transverse and oblique retinacular ligaments as part of the mobilization of the lateral bands. This is often sufficient to allow full extension and then the surgeon can proceed to repair the extensor mechanism at the central slip as noted above. It may be necessary, however, in severely fixed cases, to also release the accessory portion of the collateral ligaments or even the volar plate. In advanced articular stiffness, especially where there has been intraarticular damage, it may be necessary to reconstruct the joint using a Swanson implant arthroplasty technique[47] or even to fuse the joint in a useful position. A patient with an implant arthroplasty would be protected by buddy-taping the finger to an adjacent finger for athletic activities.

A procedure that has proved useful in the salvage of the finger with a chronic boutonnière deformity, especially in patients who have difficulty grasping because of the fixed hyperextension at the DIP joint, is the transsection of the terminal extensor tendon at the distal joint. The operation has been credited to Fowler[17] and described by Dolphin.[14] This immediately improves distal joint flexion, and therefore grasp improves, although extension, provided by the oblique retinacular ligament, may be floppy. This procedure is best indicated at the ulnar border of the hand (ring and little fingers) where power grip is important (Fig. 27-17).

Curtis, Reis, and Provost[13] have presented a step-by-step approach to the management of the chronic boutonnière deformity. When surgery is needed it is done in steps modified as the procedure progresses. This approach is very reasonable and should be reviewed by all who treat these lesions.

Pseudoboutonnière Deformity

McCue and colleagues[33,34] have pointed out that some volar plate injuries at the PIP joint that are seen late present with flexion deformities at the PIP joint and an extension posture at the DIP joint that resembles the

---

Pseudoboutonnière deformity

- Results from volar plate injury, not extensor injury
- Flexion deformity at proximal interphalangeal joint like true boutonnière
- Milder distal interphalangeal (DIP) joint extension deformity in pseudoboutonnière
- Acute and passive DIP joint motion possible in pseudoboutonnière
- Calcification and osteophyte formation may occur at volar aspect of distal portion of proximal phalanx

---

boutonniere deformity. It is important to differentiate these lesions from the true boutonnière because the problem is quite different and treatment, by necessity, is different. It is noted, when diagnosing this condition, that the DIP joint extension deformity is not severe and active and passive flexion motion at the DIP joint is pos-

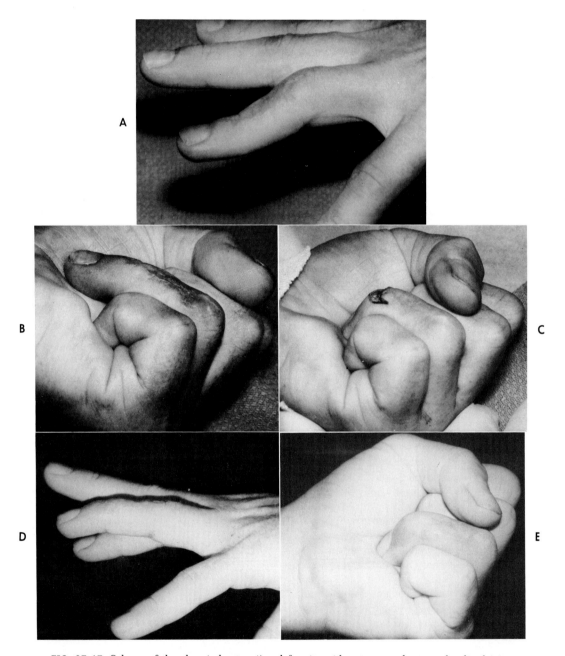

FIG. 27-17. Salvage of the chronic boutonnière deformity with extensor release at the distal joint (Dolphin). **A,** Surgery had been attempted for this deformity. **B,** Patient was most troubled by loss of flexion at the distal joint at his ring finger. This interfered with his power grip. **C,** Transsection of the terminal extensor tendon is done with the patient under local anesthesia. It is seen on the operating table that distal joint flexion is immediately increased. **D,** Posture of the finger in extension at 3 months is improved. **E,** Flexion at 3 months. The finger can now grip.

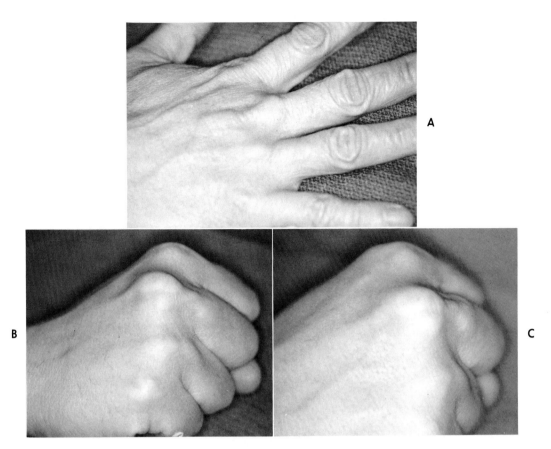

FIG. 27-18. Tendinitis in a karate athlete. **A** to **C,** Nodularity seen at the metacarpophalangeal joint level from frequent punching activity. These masses were asymptomatic.

sible. Another clue is the radiographic appearance of calcification and spurring proximal to the PIP joint at the proximal phalanx. This represents the palmar plate injury and a spontaneous repair reaction. This pseudoboutonnière is a joint lesion and is treatable by operations aimed at release of the palmar plate contracture.

Summary of Boutonnière Treatment

Overall, those experienced in the treatment of the boutonnière deformity will agree that a nonoperative approach is generally preferred in the treatment of this lesion. In mild deformities that persist after conservative therapy, one may elect to accept the problem, since there is considerable risk of increasing the impairment if surgery is unsuccessful. When surgery is elected, there should be careful consideration for the indications and the pathologic condition here. Surgery with the patient under local anesthesia is helpful to evaluate both the problem and the effects of treatment during the procedure. This, combined with aftercare that is closely supervised, is critical if one is to obtain better results with this difficult entity.

HYPERTROPHY OF THE EXTENSOR MECHANISM AT THE METACARPOPHALANGEAL JOINT IN THE KARATE HAND

This condition is seen at the metacarpophalangeal joint level of karate practitioners and presents as a mass that moves with the extensor apparatus. There is a history of repeated striking of the fist against a post as part of the practice routine. The mass represents hypertrophy of the extensor mechanism in response to this trauma and has been called hypertrophic infiltrative tendinitis, the HIT syndrome, by Gardner.[18] Unlike his case, in which surgery was performed, my two patients with this condition were asymptomatic and no treatment was necessary (Fig. 27-18).

REFERENCES
1. Abouna JM, Brown H: The treatment of mallet finger, *Br J Surg* 55:653, 1968.
2. Blazina ME, Lane C: Rupture of the insertion of the flexor digitorum profundus in student athletes, *J Am Coll Health Assoc* 14:248, 1966.
3. Bohler L: Finger fractures. In Bohler L (ed): *The treatment of fractures*, New York, 1956, Grune & Stratton.
4. Bowers WH, Hurst LC: Chronic mallet finger: the use of Fowler's central slip release, *J Hand Surg* 3:373, 1978.

5. Boyes JH, Wilson JN, Smith JW: Flexor tendon ruptures in the forearm and hand, *J Bone Joint Surg* 42A:637, 1960.
6. Burton R, Eaton R: Common hand injuries in the athlete, *Orthop Clin North Am* 4:808, 1973.
7. Buscemi MJ, Page BJ: Flexor digitorum profundus avulsions with associated distal phalanx fractures, *Am J Sports Med* 15:366, 1987.
8. Carroll RE, Match RM: Avulsion of the flexor profundus tendon insertion, *J Trauma* 10:1109, 1979.
9. Casscells SW, Strange TB: Intramedullary wire fixation of mallet-finger, *J Bone Joint Surg* 39A:521, 1957.
10. Casscells SW, Strange TB: Intramedullary-wire fixation of mallet finger, *J Bone Joint Surg* 51A:1018, 1969.
11. Chang WH, Thoms OJ, White WL: Avulsion injury of the long flexor tendons, *Plast Reconstr Surg* 50:260, 1972.
12. Culver JE et al: Avulsions of the profundus and superficialis tendons of the ring finger, *Am J Sports Med* 9:184, 1981.
13. Curtis RM, Reis RL, Provost JM: A staged technique for the repair of the traumatic boutonnière deformity, *J Hand Surg* 8:167, 1983.
14. Dolphin JA: Extensor tenotomy for chronic boutonnière deformity of the finger, *J Bone Joint Surg* 47A:161, 1965.
15. Elliott RA: Injuries to the extensor mechanism of the hand, *Orthop Clin North Am* 1:335, 1970.
16. Fomar RC, Nelson CL, Phalen GS: Ruptures of the flexor tendons in the hands of non-rheumatoid patients, *J Bone Joint Surg* 54A:579, 1972.
17. Fowler SB: Extensor apparatus of the digits, *J Bone Joint Surg* 31B:477, 1949.
18. Gardner RC: Hypertrophic infiltrative tendinitis (Hit syndrome) of the long extensor: the abused karate hand, *JAMA* 211:1009, 1970.
19. Grundberg AB: Anatomic repair of boutonnière deformity, *Clin Orthop* 153:226, 1980.
20. Gunter GS: Traumatic avulsion injuries of the insertion of the flexor digitorum profundus, *Aust N Z J Surg* 30:1, 1960.
21. Hallberg D, Lindholm A: Subcutaneous rupture of the extensor tendon of the distal phalanx of the finger: "mallet finger," *Acta Chir Scand* 119:260, 1960.
22. Hillman FE: New technique for treatment of mallet fingers and fractures of distal phalanx, *JAMA* 161:1135, 1956.
23. Honner R: The late management of isolated lesion of the flexor digitorum profundus tendon, *Hand* 7:171, 1975.
24. Iselin F, Levame J, Godoy J: A simplified technique for treating mallet fingers: tenodermodesis, *J Hand Surg* 2:118, 1977.
25. Kleinman WB, Petersen DP: Oblique retinacular ligament reconstruction for chronic mallet finger deformity, *J Hand Surg* 9A:399, 1984.
26. Langa V, Posner MA: Unusual rupture of a flexor profundus tendon, *J Hand Surg* 11A:227, 1986.
27. Lange RH, Engber WD: Hyperextension mallet finger, *Orthopedics* 6:1426, 1983.
28. Leddy JP: Avulsions of the flexor digitorum profundus, *Hand Clin North Am* 1:77, 1985.
29. Leddy JP, Packer JW: Avulsion of the profundus tendon insertion in athletes, *J Hand Surg* 2:66, 1977.
30. Littler JW, Eaton RG: Redistribution of the forces in the correction of boutonnière deformity, *J Bone Joint Surg* 49A:1267, 1967.
31. Manske PR, Lesker PA: Avulsion of the ring finger flexor digitorum profundus tendon: an experimental study, *Hand* 10:52, 1978.
32. Matev I: Transposition of the lateral bands of the aponeurosis of longstanding "boutonnière deformity" of the fingers, *Br J Plast Surg* 17:281, 1964.
33. McCue FC, Garroway RY: Sports injuries to the hand and wrist. In Schneider RC, Kennedy JC, Plant ML (eds): *Sports injuries*, Baltimore, 1985, Williams & Wilkins.
34. McCue FM et al: Athletic injuries of the proximal interphalangeal joint requiring surgical treatment, *J Bone Joint Surg* 52A:937, 1970.
35. Mosher JF: Flexor and extensor tendon injuries. In Pettrone FA (ed): *AAOS symposium on upper extremity injuries in athletes*, St Louis, 1986, Mosby.
36. Nichols HN: Repair of the extensor tendon insertions in the fingers, *J Bone Joint Surg* 33A:836, 1951.
37. Pardini AG, Sosta RD, Morais MS: Surgical repair of the boutonnière deformity of the fingers, *Hand* 11:87, 1979.
38. Patel MR, Desai SS, Bassini-Lipson, L: Conservative management of chronic mallet finger, *J Hand Surg* 11A:570, 1986.
39. Posch JL, Walker PJ, Miller H: Treatment of ruptured tendons of the hand and wrist, *Am J Surg* 91:669, 1956.
40. Posner MA: Injuries to the hand and wrist in athletes, *Orthop Clin North Am* 8:593, 1977.
41. Reef TC: Avulsions of the flexor digitorum profundus: an athletic injury, *Am J Sports Med* 5:281, 1977.
42. Robins PR, Dobyns JH: Avulsion of the insertion of the flexor digitorum profundus tendon associated with fracture of the distal phalanx. In American Academy of Orthopaedic Surgeons: *Tendon surgery in the hand*, St Louis, 1975, Mosby.
43. Salvi V: Technique for the boutonnière deformity, *Hand* 1:96, 1969.
44. Schneider LH: *Flexor tendon injuries*, Boston, 1985, Little, Brown.
45. Schneider LH: Treatment of isolated flexor digitorum profundus injuries by tendon grafting. In Hunter JM, Schneider LH, Mackin EJ (eds): *Tendon surgery in the hand*, St Louis, 1987, Mosby.
46. Schneider LH: Fractures of the distal phalanx. *Hand Clin North Am* 4:537, 1988.
47. Schneider LH, Smith KL: Boutonnière deformity. In Hunter JM, Schneider LH, Mackin EJ (eds): *Tendon surgery in the hand*, St Louis, 1987, Mosby.
48. Smith JH: Avulsion of the profundus tendon with simultaneous intraarticular fracture of the distal phalanx, *J Hand Surg* 6:600, 1981.
49. Smith RJ: Boutonnière deformity of the fingers, *Bull Hosp Joint Dis* 27:27, 1966.
50. Souter WA: The problem of the boutonnière deformity, *Clin Orthop* 104:116, 1974.
51. Thompson JS, Littler JW, Upton J: The spiral oblique retinacular ligament, *J Hand Surg* 3:482, 1978.
52. Tubiana R, Valentin P: The anatomy or the extensor apparatus of the fingers, *Surg Clin North Am* 44:897, 1964.
53. Tubiana R, Valentin P: The physiology of the extension of the fingers, *Surg Clin North Am* 44:907, 1964.
54. Urbaniak JR, Hayes MG: Chronic boutonnière deformity—an anatomical reconstruction, *J Hand Surg* 6:379, 1981.
55. Wehbe MA, Schneider LH: Mallet fractures, *J Bone Joint Surg* 66A:658, 1984.
56. Wenger DR: Avulsion of the profundus tendon insertion in football players, *Arch Surg* 106:145, 1973.
57. Zancolli E: *Structural and dynamic bases of hand surgery*, ed 2, Philadelphia, 1979, JB Lippincott.

CHAPTER 28

Rehabilitation and Protection of the Hand and Wrist

Vi A. Mayer
Frank C. McCue, III

Interferential current
Neuromuscular stimulation
Point stimulation
Sensory reeducation
Splints
   Static splints
   Dynamic splints
   Precautions
   Materials
   Protective splints
      Metacarpophalangeal joint and wrist
      Thumb
Protective equipment
   Rules
   Prevention

The hand and wrist are vulnerable to injury in almost every sport. Mismanagement from either a medical or a rehabilitation standpoint can result in significant disability and limitation in function. Functional use of hands requires adequate mobility, stability, and sensibility as well as freedom from pain.

All athletic injuries of the hand and wrist should be evaluated by an orthopaedist in a timely manner. To help the athlete avoid a functional residual deficit, we must provide him or her with an early diagnosis, accurate treatment, proper rehabilitation, and protection from reinjury.

Most hand and wrist injuries sustained during athletics are closed injuries involving ligaments, bones, tendons, and neurovascular structures, and these injuries can be treated conservatively. However, when surgical intervention is indicated, it is important that the surgeon be trained in the techniques of hand surgery. Close follow-up is of paramount importance, especially when dealing with young athletes who are impatient about restrictions that may be imposed on them. Their immaturity does not allow them to see the wisdom of compliance. It is helpful to communicate with parents or coaches for support in gaining their cooperation.

CLINICAL EXAMINATION

Clinical examination of the hand is a skill that requires an understanding of functional anatomy of the hand as well as a complete history of the mechanism of injury. A systematic examination should include evaluation of deformity, instability, tenderness, active and passive motion, and edema, as well as nerve and tendon function. Accurate documentation of findings is of great importance. Whenever possible, standardized means of measurements should be used. The **American Society for Surgery of the Hand** (ASSH)[4] and the **American Society of Hand Therapists** (ASHT)[1] have established guidelines for clinical assessment of the hand. Patient treatment is based on the results of a thorough clinical examination as well as on accurate documented measurements.

Hand evaluation

- Deformity
- Instability
- Tenderness
- Motion (active and passive)
- Edema
- Neural function
- Tendon function

Goniometry

A standardized method of measuring and recording joint motion was established by the American Academy of Orthopaedic Surgeons in 1965 (Fig. 28-1).[2] In 1992 the American Society of Hand Therapists built upon the work of previous groups by recommending goniometric placements and the use of positive vs. negative numbers for documenting range of motion measurements. A (−) designates a lack of extension, and a (+) designates hyperextension.[1]

The goniometer size and design should be appropriate to the joint being measured. The circular-bodied goniometers allow lateral placement. Half-circle goniometers allow for lateral, volar, or dorsal placement. The arms of the goniometer must be long enough to allow accurate alignment with long axes of the joints being measured, but not so long that they interfere with motion. Transparent goniometers allow for lateral measurements.[26] Standard goniometers, 7⅞ inches, are used for measuring the wrist and forearm; 6¾-inch goniometers can be adapted by shortening the instrument's arms to 2 inches from the fulcrum for measuring finger joints; 5½-inch stainless steel goniometers are suitable for measuring finger motion.

Electronic and battery-operated goniometers with digital display as well as computer systems are currently available. Their use was not endorsed because of a lack of reliability and validity studies.[1]

Notations should be made as to whether measurements are taken before, during, or after treatment. In most cases joints are measured on the dorsal aspect. However, in the presence of edema or severe joint contracture, lateral placement is preferred.[1] Both active motion (tendon excursion) and passive motion (joint mobility) of flexion and extension should be measured and documented. Limitation of passive motion may be indicative of problems either within the joint itself or of the capsular structures surrounding it. Limitation of active motion may have several causes involving tendons.

Tendinous causes of limited active motion

- Lack of continuity
- Inflammation
- Adherence
- Attenuation
- Sheath constriction

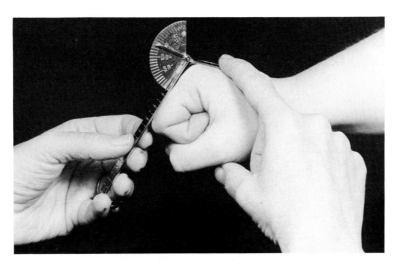

FIG. 28-1. Goniometer designed to measure small joints of the hand.

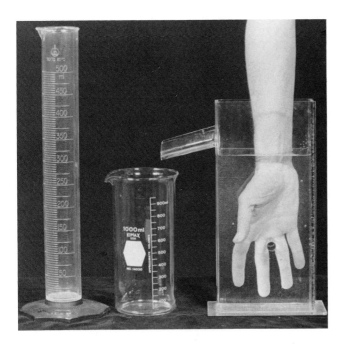

FIG. 28-2. Hand is lowered into the volumeter until the web space between the middle and ring fingers is resting on the dowel. The wrist is held in neutral, then the forearm is aligned with the hand. When used according to instructions, accuracy should be within 10 ml.

Causes may include lack of continuity, inflammation, adherence, attenuation, and constriction of sheath.

Frequent goniometric assessments are helpful in monitoring the effectiveness of a therapeutic program. The therapist should be especially responsive to substantial discrepancies that exist between active and passive motion.

Hand Volume Assessment

Edema is most easily detected on the dorsum of the hand. Bony prominences appear rounded off and there are diminished lines over the joints. Edema on the palmar surface is not as easily detected but is most obvious when flexion exercises are performed. Often, complete motion is not possible because edema is present. Subtle edema may be best observed by doing a comparative examination of the contralateral extremity.

Evaluating volume changes in the hand is necessary to determine the effectiveness of methods of edema control in use. Hand volume may be assessed by several methods. **Circumferential measurements** of the wrist, palm, and fingers are acceptable if they are taken and recorded in a consistent manner using identical bony markings or joint creases. Results should be recorded in centimeters. A more accurate means of assessing edema is possible with the use of a **hand volumeter*** (Fig. 28-2). Its use is based on Archimedes' principle of water displacement.[20] The displaced water is measured in a beaker. Often it is helpful on initial examination to measure the contralateral hand to establish norms for each patient. A comparative study is appropriate only in the absence of appreciable deformity.

Hand volume assessment

■ Circumferential measurements
■ Hand volumeter

Manual Muscle Testing

Manual muscle testing is an effective way of determining the strength of individual muscles. A number of grading systems exist for evaluating muscle strength. The most frequently used is a numerical system devised by Seddon,[88] which grades muscles from 0 to 5 (Table 28-1). Testing should occur only when there is no fear of

---

*Available from Volumeters Unlimited, Idyllwild, Calif, 92349.

TABLE 28-1 Manual muscle testing

Muscle Grade	Range of Motion (ROM)
5 = Normal	Complete ROM against gravity with full resistance
4 = Good	Complete ROM against gravity with some resistance
3 = Fair	Complete ROM against gravity with no resistance
2 = Poor	Complete ROM with gravity eliminated
1 = Trace	Slight contractility with no joint motion
0 = Zero	No evidence of contractility

From Seddon H: *Surgical disorders of peripheral nerves,* ed 2, New York, 1975, Churchill Livingstone.

aggravating the injury. Muscle strength should then be compared with the contralateral extremity.

Criteria for grading muscle strength have recently improved. However, there continues to be some degree of subjective interpretation by the examiner.

Sensibility Testing

Despite the fact that without sensation hand function is tremendously impaired, research into the mechanisms of sensibility has lagged enormously behind research into motor function. Aspects of sensory rehabilitation are often excluded from texts. Seddon[88] and Bowden[16] were among the first to distinguish between academic and functional sensibility recovery in evaluating regeneration. **Academic recovery** is judged in terms of motor and sensory recovery, such as ability to perceive pinprick, touch, and temperature changes, whereas **functional recovery** is judged in terms of the patient's ability to use the hand for functional activities. Tests performed by physicians to evaluate spinal tracts and central nervous system pathways do not correlate with the hand's ability to function (Fig. 28-3).[30] The credit for bringing this differentiation to worldwide attention belongs to Moberg,[70,71] who also spent several decades researching and publishing material on the importance of functional sensory testing.

Because of the vast number of clinical methods available for testing sensibility and the complexity of many tests, a tendency exists to exclude formal testing for sensibility from evaluations of the upper extremity. It is the challenge of the therapist or trainer to choose tests that are practical as well as appropriate to assess patients in the clinical setting. Tests should be administered in a standard manner to eliminate as many variables as possible, thereby allowing follow-up evaluations to be reliably compared.

Weber Two-Point Discrimination

In 1853 Weber described a sensibility test that would provide qualifiable results. He described the use of calipers whose points were held against the skin at different distances apart until the patient was unable to distinguish between two points of contact on the skin with vision occluded.[30]

Moberg[70,71] recognized several limitations of the We-

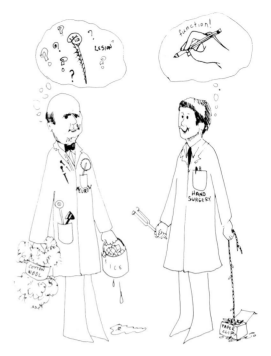

FIG. 28-3. Academic recovery does not equal functional recovery. (From Dellon AL: *Evaluation of sensibility and re-education of sensation in the hand,* Baltimore, 1981, Williams & Wilkins.)

ber test and further refined its use to include the following:

1. Quiet environment
2. Positioning of the tested area to prevent movement
3. Use of a blunt rather than a sharp-tipped instrument
4. Application of least possible pressure, trying not to make the skin blanch

Two-point discrimination is usually measured only in the fingertips. Tables vary from author to author. The American Society for Surgery of the Hand has accepted the following classification: less than 6 mm is normal, 6 to 10 mm is fair, 11 to 15 mm is poor. Rather than referring to charts or tables for normal values, it is advisable to test areas of normal sensation as well as areas thought to have diminished sensation. The results should then be compared to establish normal values for each patient. A review of the literature reveals that the Weber two-point test results leave considerable room for interpretation of normal function.

Moving Two-Point Discrimination

Moving two-point discrimination as described by Dellon[29] adds the variable of motion to the test. Dellon thought that moving two-point discrimination would measure the recovery status of quickly adapting receptors. As a result of his studies, he noted that the improvements in moving two-point discrimination coincided with improvements in patients' functional abilities more frequently than did static two-point discrimination. Moving two-point discrimination is performed similarly to the

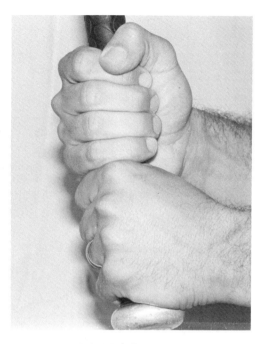

FIG. 28-4. Power grip.

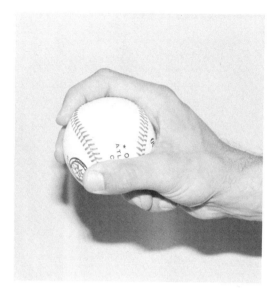

FIG. 28-5. Precision grip.

Grip

Requirements
- Skeletal mobility
- Joint integrity
- Muscle coordination

Stages
- Hand opening
- Closing digits
- Regulating forces

Types
- Power
- Precision

---

two-point discrimination test; however, the stimulus is moved longitudinally rather than merely placed on the skin.

Grip and Pinch Testing
Grip

Various injuries to the hand and wrist can interfere with the athlete's ability to perform activities requiring grip. Grip depends on skeletal mobility, joint integrity, and a combination of contraction and relaxation of the intrinsic and the extrinsic muscle groups. Grip consists of three stages—opening of the hand, closing of the digits to grasp an object, and regulating the force of pressure. Napier[72] divided grip into two types: power and precision.

During **power grip** the wrist is held in dorsiflexion, allowing the long flexors to press the object against the palm. The thumb may be either clasped over the flexed fingers or held tightly against a handle in adduction. Holding a baseball bat is an example of power grip (Fig. 28-4).

Problems that may interfere with maximal power grip include lack of mobility or weakness of the fourth and fifth rays. Limited mobility as well as pain in the carpals and wrist may also play a role in decreased functional grip.

In performing **precision grip** the athlete may hold the wrist in volar flexion or dorsiflexion, and the thumb is opposed to semiflexed fingers. The intrinsic muscles play an important role in required finger motion. Precision grip is required in grasping a baseball (Fig. 28-5).

Before instituting a grip strengthening program, baseline grip strength measurements should be evaluated and recorded. The Jamar hydraulic dynamometer provides an accurate and reliable method of measuring grip strength (Fig. 28-6).[10] The adjustable handle allows an accurate evaluation of overall hand strength. Grip strength is altered by the size of the object being grasped, and therefore readings should be taken in all five grip spans. To measure grip strength, the arm should be held at the side. The elbow should be flexed at 90 degrees with the wrist held in neutral. The therapist/trainer places the dynamometer in the athlete's hand while providing gentle support to the base of the instrument to prevent accidental dropping. The athlete should be instructed to apply a grip force smoothly without rapid wrenching or jerking motions. The therapist/trainer should ensure that substitute patterns are not used. Initially the right and left hand should be tested alternately. The noninvolved extremity may be used for comparison.

In 1954 Bechtol[10] reported the discrepancy in strength between the dominant and nondominant hand to be between 5% and 10%. However, in 1989 Peterson's et al research[79] supported the clinical use of the 10% rule only

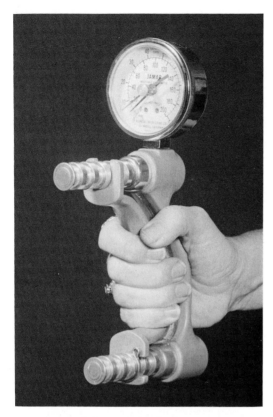

FIG. 28-6. Jamar hydraulic dynamometer.

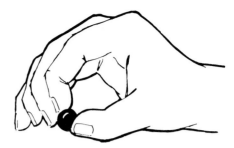

FIG. 28-7. Opposition occurs between the thumb and index finger and is used for picking up small objects. (From Malick MH: *Manual on static hand splinting*, Pittsburgh, 1972, Harmarville Rehabilitation Center.)

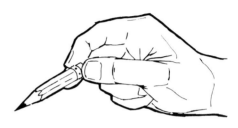

FIG. 28-8. Three-point prehension used to grasp and stabilize large objects most commonly during functional activity. (From Malick MH: *Manual on static hand splinting*, Pittsburgh, 1972, Harmarville Rehabilitation Center.)

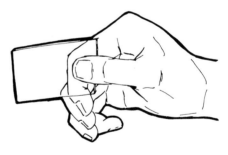

FIG. 28-9. Lateral or key pinch. The most powerful form of pinch. (With permission from Malick MH: *Manual on static hand splinting*, Pittsburgh, 1972, Harmarville Rehabilitation Center.)

for right-handed individuals. They went on to suggest that, when setting goals for left-handed individuals, both hands should be considered of equal strength. Adequate norms for grip strength are not available, although Schmidt and Toews[84] reported that correlations existed between grip strength and height, weight, and age.

Grip strengthening exercises should not be painful. Adequate finger motion should be present before strengthening is initiated. Often it is necessary to start with gentle isometric exercises, gradually increasing effort until pain is no longer a factor. Then the patient progresses to gentle resistance that is gradually increased in graded increments.

Pinch

Opposing the index and middle finger to the thumb is called three-point prehension and is considered to be a weak form of precision grip (Figs. 28-7 and 28-8). Strength and stability are equally important in performing pinch. Adequate thumb function is vital to athletes who perform competitively.

Pressing the thumb against the lateral border of the index finger is termed key, or lateral, pinch and is considered to be a form of power grip (Fig. 28-9).

Pinch may be measured with the use of a commercial pinch gauge. Strengthening exercises to improve pinch may include the use of therapeutic putty, which is available in various graded resistances.

PATHOLOGIC CONDITIONS
Wrist Injuries

The wrist is a complex joint, consisting of 21 separate articulations and a network of ligaments. Nowhere else in the body are so many nerves, tendons, vessels, bones, and ligaments concentrated in such a small area. When a person falls, a great deal of force is absorbed by the wrist, resulting in severe compression.

The frequency of wrist injuries, together with the various possible mechanisms of injury and multiple radiographic views available, makes diagnosis of traumatic wrist injuries difficult (see Chapter 24). To further complicate the problem, obtaining a careful history and phys-

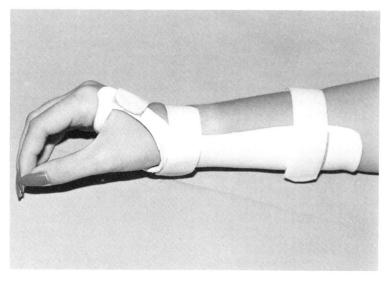

FIG. 28-10. Wrist support splint.

ical examination is not always helpful. Memory for the mechanism of injury may be vague or lost in the excitement of the game. Clinical examination may show generalized tenderness and swelling with pain, as well as limitation of motion in various positions. Despite a lack of a definitive diagnosis, protection should continue as long as symptoms persist (Fig. 28-10). If radiographic studies continue to be normal, symptomatic treatment should occur. If serious problems are passed off as minor and treated inadequately, progressive damage to the joint will occur. Medical treatment and rehabilitation become not only more difficult, but prolonged as well. Return to competition may be delayed or in some situations impossible.

Restoring Mobility

The wrist shows some degree of limitation of motion after being immobilized for a few weeks. The degree of stiffness present increases with age as well as with severity of the injury. Active exercises of the wrist should be started as soon as adequate healing has occurred. In some situations it may be possible to remove the splint only for early active exercises. The protective splint is replaced after exercises. This method of early motion is helpful in preventing further stiffness from occurring in spite of incomplete healing. Limitations in pronation and supination are often overlooked after wrist immobilization. Active forearm exercises should be initiated.

When progress plateaus with the use of active exercises, active assistive exercises should be initiated. Pain should also be a factor in determining when to begin active assistive exercises.

Because of the many articulations present in the wrist, joint mobilization is an effective means of overcoming appreciable limitations of motion. Mobilization refers to any procedure that increases mobility of soft tissue or joints.[49,68,77] Mennell,[68] Kaltenborn,[49] and Paris[77] have

well-established instruction programs for joint mobilization, which is considered a special area of study. It is recommended that therapists and trainers attend a specialized course to become proficient in one of the aforementioned methods.

Before the athlete returns to competition unprotected, a program of progressive resistive exercise should have been a part of the rehabilitation program. Timing of resistive exercise is important. The injury should be well healed, edema should be controlled, and active motion should be substantial and pain free. Providing resistive exercises before adequate healing has occurred will only serve to create tissue reaction and ultimately delay return to competition.

Restoring wrist mobility

- Active exercises
- Active assisted exercises
- Joint mobilization
- Progressive resistance exercises

Restoring Strength

Strength can also be attained by returning the athlete to functional activity. It is psychologically and physically beneficial to allow an athlete to practice partial activity for brief periods as soon as he or she is able to perform comfortably. This is especially helpful in ball handlers. Patients should be monitored carefully for symptoms of overuse. Often they are anxious to return to activity and will overexert if they are not carefully supervised.

Modalities

The wrist is particularly responsive to the use of various modalities. Application of heat before exercise, fol-

lowed by ice after exercise, is often useful to control tissue reaction brought about by exercise.

Hamate Hook Fractures

Hamate hook fractures most often occur in athletes who participate in baseball, golf, tennis, racquetball, and squash.[78] The injury usually occurs when the athlete loses control of the handle of the equipment and the handle strikes the hypothenar area. The fracture occurs with less frequency from direct trauma, such as that which results from a fall.

Resultant patient complaints include a poor grip and wrist pain that is increased by both passive and active dorsiflexion. Symptoms of ulnar nerve impingement or tendinitis of the flexor digitorum profundus of the little finger may also occur. On clinical examination deep pressure produces discomfort over the hook itself.

In an acute nondisplaced fracture conservative methods of treatment include a short gauntlet cast for mobilization and a silicone cast for use during competition when reaction has subsided. Forces on the muscular attachment to the fracture often result in nonunions. If symptoms persist, the displaced hook may be surgically removed. Postoperative therapy consists of application of modalities to improve scar tone and massage to provide desensitization, as well as to improve soft-tissue mobility.

Coban,* a self-adherent disposable elastic bandage, should be wrapped gently over the incision (Fig. 28-11). Its purpose is to provide gentle compression to the area, which reduces edema and also blocks some external stimulation, allowing the athlete to use the hand in a more functional manner at an earlier date.

The use of conventional wraps is not indicated after suture removal because they provide an excessive amount of pressure and block all external stimulation. Active exercises should also be instituted to restore wrist

---

*3M Medical-Surgical Division, St. Paul, MN.

mobility and strength as soft-tissue healing occurs. Return to athletic activity should be gradually instituted and carefully monitored. During the early phase of treatment protecting the area with either padded gloves or equipment is helpful because it allows the athlete to continue sports activities.

Thumb Injuries

The thumb may be considered to have three different functional units: (1) flexion and extension of the metacarpophalangeal (MCP) and interphalangeal (IP) joints, (2) abduction and adduction, and (3) opposition.

Loss of thumb function is said to result in loss of 50% of total hand function. Injuries sustained to the thumb during athletics may include Rolando's fracture, Bennett's fracture-dislocation, metacarpal dislocations and fractures, and collateral ligament sprains.

The remarkable mobility of the thumb is said to result from the function of the carpometacarpal joint.

The MCP joint of the thumb owes its stability to a complex arrangement of ligamentous, capsular, and musculotendinous supporting structures. It is the joint in the hand that is most affected by ligamentous instability. Injury to the ulnar collateral ligament is common in skiers and in ball handlers. Injury to the radial collateral ligament occurs much less frequently. Laxity of the ulnar collateral ligament results in weakness of grasp and pinch, but the radial side of the joint does not receive such stress. Consequently, the functional residual is much less debilitating.

Gamekeeper's Thumb

A complete or partial rupture of the ulnar collateral ligament should be considered as a possible diagnosis in every athletic injury that involves the MCP joint of the thumb. Initially described in 1955 by Campbell,[27] it was called gamekeeper's thumb because of its high incidence among English gamekeepers. At that time the entity was attributed to repetitive trauma to the thumb-index web, which resulted in chronic ligament dysfunction.

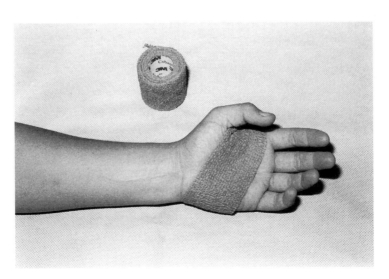

FIG. 28-11. Coban applied after suture removal in hook of hamate rehabilitation.

Today acute ulnar collateral ligamentous injuries are common in sports. Although usually created by forced abduction, torsion in combination with abduction and hyperextension or to a lesser degree a combination of stressed abduction and flexion can be causative factors. In football players the injury may be created by a fall on an outstretched hand or while tackling an opponent. Athletic equipment such as ski poles and lacrosse and hockey sticks also contribute to the high incidence of the injury.

Partial tears to the ulnar collateral ligament respond well to conservative treatment, but complete tears do not; therefore an early determination of the degree of ligamentous disruption is of paramount importance. Diagnosis should be based on a complete history, careful physical examination, and routine radiographs. The history should include the athlete's description of circumstances that led to the injury. The athlete complains of a weakened pinch as well as pain in the first web space.

The main objective of the clinical examination is to evaluate the stability of the joint. Stress testing in abduction creates pain in either partial or complete tears of the ligament. Weakness of pinch between the thumb and the index finger is also present in both complete and partial tears.

To distinguish between complete and partial tears, the MCP joint should be stressed in a flexed as well as in an extended position. To assess individual differences in joint laxity, stability should be compared with the uninvolved MCP joint of the contralateral extremity because stability of the joint varies considerably in the general population. In a complete tear laxity is at least 30 degrees greater than that which is present in the opposite MCP joint.

A partially injured ligament retains its normal anatomic relationship if properly immobilized in a thumb spica cast. The thumb should be positioned in slight adduction to reduce stress on the ligament. The thumb spica should be worn for 3 weeks, at which time it should be replaced by a volar splint. The athlete should be instructed to remove the splint periodically throughout the day to perform active isolated and composite exercises of the thumb and wrist. To restore stability to the joint, protective splinting is continued until 6 weeks from the date of initial treatment.

Indications for surgical intervention of acute ulnar collateral ligamentous injuries include (1) gross clinical instability, (2) interpositional soft-tissue injury, and (3) intraarticular, displaced, or rotated fractures. The postoperative rehabilitation protocol is identical to that for conservative treatment of the injury.

The results of surgical repair of chronic ligamentous injuries are not as good as those receiving acute surgical intervention. The surgical repair of chronic lesions should be performed only at the athlete's request to relieve pain, to improve stability, and to improve thumb-index pinch strength.

The goal of rehabilitation is to preserve or reestablish stability of the thumb. All athletes with thumb injuries should be carefully monitored by the therapist/trainer and referred to the team physician if symptoms persist.

Protective thumb techniques to allow for athletic participation are covered later in this chapter.

Proximal Interphalangeal Joint Injuries

In no instance are early diagnosis, proper medical treatment, and quality rehabilitation more important in preventing residual deformity than in the proximal interphalangeal (PIP) joint. Inadequate long-term protection during practice and competition can lead to reinjury and permanent disability.

The exact number of injuries to PIP joints that occur during athletic activity is unknown. Dislocations are often reduced on the sidelines by the coach or trainer and taped to an adjacent finger. Several weeks later, when the joint remains stiff, swollen, and painful and a contracture begins to ensue, medical attention is usually sought. Occasionally, incorrect diagnosis is made by an inexperienced practitioner. If the condition does not improve or deteriorates in spite of adequate conservative treatment, reexamination or a second medical opinion is advisable.

Proximal interphalangeal joint injuries

- Articular fractures
- Fracture dislocations
- Boutonnière deformities
- Pseudoboutonnière deformities
- Collateral ligament sprains
- Volar plate injuries

Common injuries to PIP joints that occur during athletic activity may include articular fractures, fracture dislocations, boutonnière deformities, pseudoboutonnière deformities, and collateral ligament and volar plate injuries. Splinting guidelines are provided in Table 28-2.

TABLE 28-2 Positioning guidelines for proximal interphalangeal joint injuries

Injury	Joint Position	Splint Surface
Articular fractures	30 degrees flexion	Volar
Fracture-dislocations	Block at 25 degrees flexion; allow full flexion	Dorsal
Boutonnière deformity	Full extension	Volar
Pseudoboutonnière deformity	Full extension	Volar
Collateral ligament injuries		
Mild strain	Functional position	Volar
Incomplete tear	30 degrees flexion	Volar
Volar plate injuries	25 to 30 degrees flexion	Volar or dorsal

From Gieck JH, Mayer V: *Clinics in sports medicine,* Philadelphia, 1986, WB Saunders.

Confusion exists between the boutonnière deformity and the pseudoboutonnière deformity.

Boutonnière Deformity

The boutonnière deformity is the second most common closed tendon injury in athletes. The initial injury is usually caused by blunt trauma over the dorsal aspect of the PIP joint or acute flexion of the joint against active resistance. The classic **boutonnière deformity** consists of hyperextension of the MCP joint, flexion of the PIP joint, and hyperextension of the distal interphalangeal (DIP) joint. The boutonnière deformity is the result of disruption of the central slip of the extensor digitorum communis tendon over the PIP joint.

Early diagnosis is difficult. The complete deformity is not present after acute trauma but develops later if left untreated. Any digital injury that lacks more than 30 degrees of PIP joint extension along with dorsal tenderness directly over the base of the middle phalanx should be treated as an acute tendon rupture. In providing acute care the PIP joint should be splinted in full extension and the DIP joint should be left free to allow active flexion. The position of passive PIP joint extension and active DIP joint flexion serves to relocate the lateral bands to their original anatomic position on the dorsum of the PIP joint. Splints should be worn between 6 and 8 weeks at which time active exercises may be initiated.

When improper diagnosis is made, the finger is often splinted with the PIP joint held in slight flexion for means of comfort. Unfortunately this position leads to further deformity.

In chronic injuries, when a fixed flexion contracture of the PIP joint has developed, static or dynamic splints may be used to gradually reduce the contracture. Many commercial splints are available to reduce flexion contractures of the PIP joint. The choice of splint may depend on the degree of joint contracture as well as the chronicity of the injury. An effective splinting program can make surgical intervention unnecessary even in older neglected cases.

Although numerous surgical procedures have been developed to repair chronic boutonnière deformity, results are not uniformly predictable. Best results are obtained with early diagnosis along with an adequate splinting program.

The player with an acute boutonnière deformity is allowed to participate in athletic activity when he or she is comfortable that adequate protection is available to prevent reinjury. Protective splinting and taping should be worn during athletic activity until complete pain-free motion has been restored.

Pseudoboutonnière Deformity

The **pseudoboutonnière deformity** resembles a classic boutonnière deformity, but is caused by disruption of the volar plate at its proximal membranous portion without disruption of the central slip. The pseudoboutonnière consists of a flexion contracture of the PIP joint, which is more resistant to correction by passive extension than the classic boutonnière, slight hyperextension of the DIP joint, and radiographic evidence of calcification at the proximal attachment of the volar plate.[66] The pseudoboutonnière deformity is usually created by a hyperextension or twisting injury to the PIP joint.

Treatment

When the deformities are treated conservatively, therapeutic measures should consist of dynamic or static splinting exercises, as well as modalities to control pain and edema. Splints should be fabricated so as not to restrict motion of the MCP and DIP joints.

The splint should be worn continuously. Active exercises may be initiated after 6 to 8 weeks. The splint should be worn at all other times until the contracture has been reduced. After that time it may be removed during the day but worn at night to maintain extension. Often increases in mobility and strength of finger flexion result in a loss of extension. Even after correction has been attained, patients should be monitored closely because the deformity may recur.

Chronic pseudoboutonnière deformities are more resistant to splinting programs. Deformities that are fixed in more than 40 degrees of flexion or are disabling to the athlete may require surgical intervention.

Athletic participation is allowed when pain subsides and adequate protective splinting is provided. Protective splinting and taping should be worn during athletic activity until complete pain-free motion has been restored. How early an athlete with PIP joint injury can safely return to play with proper protection is a medical decision. In most instances splints can be fabricated to allow an athlete to return to competition. Buddy tapes do *not* allow adequate protection for painful, swollen joints. Adequate protective splinting should continue until motion is complete and pain free.

Proper management of injuries to the PIP joint can significantly reduce the deformity often seen in athletes who do not receive proper medical care, rehabilitation, or protective splinting.

Distal Interphalangeal Joint Injuries

Injury to the extensor mechanism is one of the most common hand injuries sustained by athletes. The injury occurs when a force, such as a hard-thrown ball, strikes the extended fingertip and forces the distal phalanx into flexion while the extensor mechanism is actively contracting. The distal joint may be passively, but not actively, extended.

Mallet Finger

The most common rupture of the extensor tendon occurs at the insertion into the base of the distal phalanx and is called a **mallet finger.** Most mallet fingers can be treated by conservative methods. Surgical repair of the extensor tendon in the area of the DIP joint is difficult because of a poor blood supply. When the DIP joint is immobilized to treat acute mallet finger, the distal phalanx may be positioned in neutral or slight hyperextension. The degree of hyperextension should not exceed the position at which the dorsal skin begins to blanch. Studies have shown that the degree of hyperextension

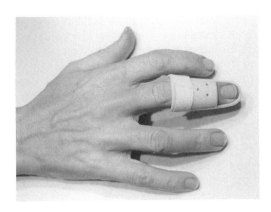

FIG. 28-12. Stack mallet finger splint.

at which skin begins to blanch is widely variable.[82] Crawford[28] obtained satisfactory results in 151 patients with mallet finger with the use of premolded polythene stack splints, which maintain the joint in a neutral position (Fig. 28-12). Metal splints may be placed on the dorsal or volar surface of the digit. Splints should be removed for hand care. When removing the splint, the athlete should be instructed not to allow the distal phalanx to drop into flexion. This may be accomplished by gradually removing the splint while supporting the distal phalanx with the thumb. Splinting should continue for at least 8 weeks, at which time exercises may be initiated to restore mobility. If DIP joint extension decreases at this time, splinting may be renewed on a full- or part-time basis. Protection during athletic activity should continue until mobility has been restored and the joint is pain free. Most mallet finger injuries require protection during play for at least 12 weeks.

Avulsion of the Flexor Digitorum Profundus

Avulsion of the insertion of the profundus tendon of the ring finger is a relatively common athletic injury. Because of the unusual mechanism of injury, the avulsion is commonly referred to as a jersey finger. Typically, when a football player attempts to make a tackle, his fingers grasp the jersey of an opposing player. As the little finger continues to flex and the opposing player pulls away, the ring finger, still caught in the jersey, is extended forcibly while the profundus is maximally contracting. Although the injury may occur in any digit, it is most commonly seen in the ring finger.

Often there is a delay in treatment because neither the nature nor the extent of the injury is immediately recognized. The player may not initially report his injury. Unless the physician is aware of the entity, makes inquiry as to the mechanism of injury, and tests specifically for active flexion of the DIP joint, the injury is not recognized. When the fingers are held in flexion, there is no obvious deformity; lack of active flexion of the DIP joint is erroneously attributed to soft-tissue swelling and tenderness. Radiographs may be helpful in that often a small bony fragment from the distal phalanx is attached to the tendon.

Most physicians agree that primary repair with attachment of the profundus tendon to the distal phalanx is the treatment of choice. The athlete may choose to undergo a delayed surgical repair after the playing season. During this time the athletic trainer should use a therapeutic regimen of modalities and exercises to maintain mobility to all joints of the involved digits. Adequate protection should be provided so as to prevent further injury to the digit during athletic activity.

Delayed surgical procedures are generally more extensive and may require tendon grafting to restore mobility to the distal phalanx. Surgical fusion of the distal phalanx is also an acceptable means of treatment.

The postoperative rehabilitation protocol is similar to that for a flexor tendon repair. Postoperatively a dorsal splint is applied to hold the wrist in slight flexion, the MCPs are positioned in 60 to 70 degrees of flexion, and the PIP and DIP joints are held in relative extension. The splint should be worn continuously for 3 weeks, at which time a rehabilitation program should begin.

Active isolated and composite exercises should be initiated at this time (see blocking exercise instructions on p. 613). Active exercises should be performed gently within pain tolerance, frequently to increase mobility, and through as complete an arc as is possible to prevent tendon adherence. Exercises that are performed once a day during formal therapy are generally not effective in restoring maximum mobility. Exercises should be performed periodically throughout the day with the use of a home program.

During the third through the fifth postoperative week the protective splint should be removed only to perform exercises. During this period the hand and wrist should be maintained in a protected position at all times (Fig. 28-13). To maintain the protected position, the wrist and fingers should not be simultaneously extended. When extending the fingers the wrist should be flexed, and when extending the wrist the fingers should be flexed. Care should also be taken to avoid flexion contractures of the IP joints. If early contracture should occur, gently stretch the joint using active assistive motion while supporting the wrist in flexion to protect the repaired tendon. Protective splinting is maintained until 5 weeks from the date of surgery, at which time light functional use of the hand is encouraged. Heavy use or resistive exercises should not be permitted until 8 weeks from the date of surgery. During the rehabilitation phase the trainer should arrange alternate activities to allow the athlete to maintain cardiovascular conditioning.

When the athlete is cleared for athletic participation, protection should be provided until adequate healing has occurred (8 weeks) and functional motion has been restored.

Flexor tenolysis is an elective surgical procedure that may be performed after primary tendon repair or graft. It may be indicated when, despite appropriate surgery and postoperative therapy with a highly motivated and compliant patient, active range of motion is significantly less than passive range of motion secondary to scar adhesions. Early therapy consisting of frequent active and gentle active assistive exercises is instituted to reduce

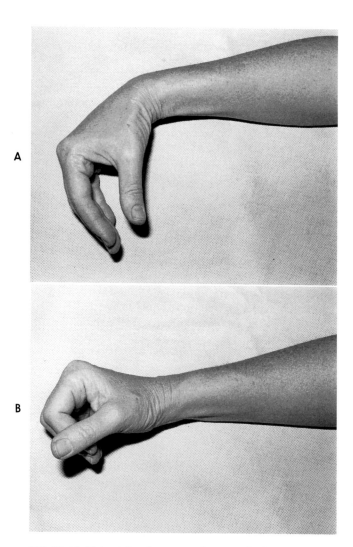

FIG. 28-13. Maintaining the protected position for flexor tendon repair. **A,** Fingers are extended when wrist is flexed. **B,** Fingers are flexed when wrist is extended.

the recurrence of scarring. Carefully monitored postoperative care is required to achieve an optimal goal.

Overuse Syndromes

Overuse injuries occur when too much activity is done over too short a period with inadequate conditioning or improper techniques. Tendinitis and overuse syndromes are common in athletes, and the overall incidence appears to be rising.[80] Of all sports participants, 34% to 50% are injured, and 25% to 50% of these injuries are attributed to overuse.[50] Upper extremity tendinitis and overuse syndromes are most frequently seen in activities that require the hand and wrist to transmit force to an implement, such as in racquet sports and rowing; act as an implement, such as in volleyball and handball; or support the body weight, as in gymnastics. The preparatory weight training required to improve strength and endurance can also readily induce upper extremity overuse syndromes. Early conservative treatment of overuse injuries is best. An essential component in the care of over-

use injuries, and often the most difficult to accept, particularly in competitive athletes, is the concept of relative rest. **Relative rest** is the reduction in the level of imposed stress on the involved area. This allows the body part to recuperate while preventing further damage to the tissue from continued training. Rest ranges from a reduction in training intensity to total abstinence from activity involving the injured part. Arranging alternative activities to maintain the athlete's cardiovascular conditioning without irritating the overuse injury is an important aspect in the management of athletic injuries. As a part of the rehabilitation process, factors that contribute to the cause of the injury, such as improper techniques, equipment, and training, must be addressed to prevent recurrence.

Carpal Tunnel Syndrome

Carpal tunnel syndrome may occur from the repetitive motion or long periods of gripping, throwing, bicycling, and performing repetitive motion with the wrist held in flexion. Symptoms of carpal tunnel syndrome result from irritation or compression of the median nerve at or near the flexor retinaculum. The athlete typically complains of pins and needles, burning sensations, and numbness in the thumb, index, and middle finger as well as being awakened with the hand feeling as if it were asleep. Shaking the hand is helpful in relieving numbness.

Conservative treatment should consist of splinting the wrist in 10 degrees of dorsiflexion, administering nonsteroidal antiinflammatory medications and therapeutic modalities, and ceasing the activity that created the reaction. Treatment should continue until motion is complete and pain free.

If conservative treatment is unsuccessful, the athlete should be referred for medical evaluation. Decompression has been reported to be necessary in several young athletes.[38]

Ulnar Nerve Compression

The ulnar nerve is prone to injury at the wrist because of its vulnerable location in Guyon's canal. The hypothenar area is the void of the protective covering of the palmar fascia. The proximity of the ulnar nerve to the hook of the hamate and the pisiform makes it susceptible to compression with any injuries to these two bony structures.

The condition is characterized by paresthesia of the little finger, as well as half of the ulnar portion of the ring finger. The intrinsic muscle innervated by the ulnar nerve may also be weakened. Occasionally findings are restricted to the deep motor branch of the nerve with atrophy or weakness of the interosseus muscles without evidence of sensory symptoms.

Treatment should include the temporary discontinuation of cycling or racquetball or other athletic activity that may be contributing to the condition. Use of a static splint and nonsteroidal antiinflammatory drugs may also be helpful. Athletic endeavors should not be resumed until symptoms have subsided and causative factors have been evaluated. Either the handlebars or the hypothenar area of gloves may be padded to prevent recurrent symptoms of ulnar nerve compression in cyclists.

In general, upper extremity overuse syndromes in cyclists can be prevented by having an appropriate saddle height, using padded gloves, frequently changing hand positions, not resting on the hands, and strengthening the abdomen muscles through exercise.

In cases resistant to conservative treatment, neurolysis and decompression in Guyon's canal may be indicated.

de Quervain's Disease

de Quervain's disease is the term used to describe stenosing tenosynovitis of the first dorsal compartment of the wrist that involves the abductor pollicis longus and the extensor pollicis brevis sheaths at the radial styloid process. The athlete complains of pain localized to the radial side of the wrist that is aggravated by movement of the thumb. Local tenderness and swelling of the extensor retinaculum of the wrist over the first compartment are present. A module that glides with active motion may also be present.

Although de Quervain's disease is usually the result of overuse, it can also follow a direct blow to the first dorsal compartment or an acute sprained wrist. Activities that require repetitive thumb abduction and extension combined with radial and ulnar wrist movements are thought to contribute to the condition. Occurrence is most common in racquet sports.

With early recognition of the symptoms conservative treatment should be used, consisting of splints, ice, antiinflammatory medications, and cessation of the activity that created the response. The condition should respond quite readily. If symptoms do not subside, the judicious use of a steroid injection may be indicated. In chronic situations surgical intervention may be necessary.

Tendon Injuries

Extensor tenosynovitis. Extensor tenosynovitis, or tendinitis, involves the dorsal extensor retinaculum and the individual extensor dorsal compartments. The condition frequently occurs in lifting and throwing sports. Generally, the condition is treatable through rest, therapeutic modalities, the use of antiinflammatory drugs, and protective splinting or sufficient padding to prevent a recurrence of the condition.

Trigger finger. Trigger fingers result from repetitive trauma along the pulley system at the base of the fingers. Handball players, baseball catchers, gymnasts, and weight lifters may be prone to the condition. Incidence of trigger finger may be decreased by the use of gloves or padding applied to the palmar aspect of the hand. Treatment may include rest, therapeutic modalities, antiinflammatory medications, and corticosteroid injections. Alleviation of the conditions that contribute to the problem may include reviewing handgear worn by the athlete. If symptoms persist despite conservative treatment, surgical release of the A-1 pulley is indicated.

Rehabilitation

Therapeutic heat and cold reduce pain and inflammation and must be applied before an exercise program is initiated. The main goal of rehabilitation is to enable the athlete to resume normal activity when healing is taking place, rather than to allow complete healing before exercise is resumed.[39] Although early motion is important, exercises should only be done in a pain-free range. The longer the immobilization period, the greater the impact disuse atrophy and limited mobility will exhibit. After a therapeutic modality is used, passive exercise consisting of a slow, steady stretch should be initiated for 30 to 60 seconds and repeated several times.

The next progression during the acute stage of overuse injury is strengthening or isometric exercises, which are most effective in the acute stage of treatment. Isometric exercise involves contraction of the muscle, allowing no joint motion. The athlete should only exert force that is comfortable. As healing occurs, the force can be increased. The exercises should be performed with the joint held in various positions for 6 to 10 seconds. The athlete may then progress to using free weights. Progression of the exercise program should be monitored carefully. Resistive exercises in the acute stage of healing aggravate the symptoms. As normal strength returns, exercises to improve endurance are added. The athletic activity that contributed to the injury may be initiated at this time.

An important activity of the practitioner is to review techniques the athlete uses while performing the activity that created the injury. Unless corrected, the injury is apt to recur.

Pitfalls in the rehabilitation of overuse injuries include inadequate rehabilitation time and the return to activity before adequate healing has occurred.

Digital Nerve Injuries

Direct repetitive trauma over the palm and digits, such as is required in many sports, makes digital nerve injuries in the hand a common occurrence. Digital neuromas may also result.

Symptoms may be so severe as to interfere with the athlete's functional ability. Neuromas usually respond to conservative treatment, such as transcutaneous electric nerve stimulation (TENS) and desensitization programs. Evaluating the athlete's equipment is also recommended, since padding or gloves use may help to reduce stress to the painful area.

Bowler's Thumb

Bowler's thumb is a good example of a direct external repetitive force resulting in nerve injury. Most patients complain of paresthesia in the distribution of the ulnar digital nerve, which may be persistent or associated with pressure. Hyperesthesia and tenderness may also be present. Tinel's sign may be present over the nerve. Occasionally two-point discrimination may be altered. Contributing factors to neuroma formation among bowlers may include use of a ball that is too heavy or oversized. Improper bore spread, as well as poor bowling technique, may also contribute to the injury.

At the onset of symptoms many experienced bowlers modify their grip or have the thumbhole of the ball redrilled to alleviate pressure on the ulnar aspect of the thumb. Decreasing the depth of insertion of the thumb into the thumb hole may also help alleviate the problem.

Early recognition and conservative treatment afford

the best opportunity for the correction of bowler's thumb. Surgery is indicated only in severe, resistant cases.

Vascular Injuries

Ischemia of the hand and fingers secondary to repetitive blunt trauma has been labeled the **hypothenar hammer syndrome.**[5,23] Constant trauma to the hypothenar area may cause spasms of the ulnar artery, thromboses, and aneurysms of the hand.[44] The condition has been reported to occur in baseball, karate, rugby, handball, lacrosse, and volleyball. Any athlete who participates in a sport that involves repetitive trauma against the palmar surface of the hand is at risk of developing vascular injuries.[54]

Signs and symptoms of athletes with impending vascular injury include coolness, numbness, cyanosis, paleness, and a positive response to the Allen test.[95] The Allen test can be carried out on a single digit by expressing the blood out of it, occluding both digital arteries, and then releasing the radial digital artery and noting the filling of the digit. The same procedure is carried out on the ulnar digital artery. This procedure independently evaluates the patency of each digital vessel. Athletic trainers can be helpful by providing conservative therapy, reviewing the athlete's techniques, evaluating equipment, and supplying additional protection. Adding padding to the glove can prevent initial digital vessel injury from occurring and possibly prevent added trauma to those athletes already showing digital vessel changes.

An obvious need exists for improvement of the protective gear offered to athletes who perform activities traumatic to the palm and hypothenar area. Studies have reported a correlation between the repetitive trauma to the fingers from catching a ball and the number of years played, frequency of practice, and position played.[54]

Neuromas

Neuromas occur after axonal injury with mechanical disruption of the endoneural myelin barrier. A neuroma of some degree is always produced at the point of injury to a nerve. Not all neuromas are painful. If a neuroma is painful, however, initial treatment should be directed toward **conservative methods of desensitization** rather than toward operative procedures.

Neuromas may be treated with local anesthetic injections. Although results have not been published, TENS has been used for desensitization of painful neuromas for many years. Desensitization techniques used in the treatment of painful neuromas and hyperesthetic scars are similar. Although some neuromas may respond to a program of manual desensitization alone, TENS appears to speed up the process. In the treatment of painful neuroma and hyperesthetic scars, conventional TENS should be used. Electrode placement should be in continuity with the involved nerve, with the distal electrode placed as near the painful site as possible. As the site becomes less painful, the electrode should be placed closer to the neuroma. If conservative treatment is successful, ultimately it should be possible to place the electrode over the neuroma site.

Application of TENS should be followed by a program of manual desensitization. A protocol for manual desensitization developed at the Curtis Hand Center of Baltimore includes a regimented program of various graded stimuli (textures) that progress from moving touch to constant touch and end with percussive stimulation. Each stimulus is performed in a proximal to distal direction, then progresses horizontally from left to right, from right to left, and finally from a distal to a proximal direction. When stimulation in all directions is tolerated, the stimulus or texture is upgraded and training begins at step 1—proximal to distal—and progresses through the various directions and textures as tolerated. The next step of manual desensitization is constant touch, which is reeducated by applying various pressures to the area. The eraser of a pencil or a fingertip may be used as the stimulus. The final stage of desensitization is percussion, which may begin with gentle tapping of a fingertip or the eraser of a pencil.

The staff of the Downey Hand Center of Downey, California, have developed a sensitivity test and kit that is commercially available for testing and treatment of hyperesthesia.[103]

It is important to note that the gradual progression of stimulation is important to the treatment of painful neuromas. Often athletes with hyperesthetic areas are instructed only to perform a percussive type of stimulation. Obviously, compliance to this request is not possible. A successful desensitization program depends on a thorough evaluation and a manual desensitization program that is nonpainful. TENS and injections may also be helpful, although the importance of the physiologic and psychologic bases for manual desensitization cannot be overstressed. Stimulation through functional use is also an important aspect of reeducation.

Painful neuromas that do not respond to conservative treatment should be referred for evaluation for surgical intervention.

Sympathetically Maintained Pain

Sympathetically maintained pain (SMP) syndromes, for example, **reflex sympathetic dystrophy,** are characterized by vasomotor dysfunction, hyperhidrosis, allodynia, burning pain, edema, discoloration, and stiffness in an extremity. They occur after a variety of injuries such as fractures, lacerations, surgical incisions, and soft-tissue injury. Involvement may be limited to one or two digits, or it may be so severe as to involve the entire extremity. The mechanism of injury can be so trivial that the patient may have difficulty recalling the incident that directly precipitated the complaints. There is no known correlation between the severity of the injury and the intensity of the symptoms of SMP, unless the patient suffers a related peripheral nerve injury. The latter patients would most appropriately be diagnosed as having **causalgia,** and because of the associated nerve damage, the syndrome may result in more intractable pain, neurologic deficit and dysfunction, and less successful resolution of symptoms, even with maximal treatment. The pathologic consequences occur in the skin, muscle, blood vessels, and bones of the extremity and can significantly affect its function. Signs and symptoms of the condition occur

in various degrees and may go through changes that can persist for several years if untreated. These include the following:

1. *Edema.* Edematous changes may begin as a pitting type of edema, which eventually becomes brawny and ultimately results in a periarticular thickening of the joints. Ultimately the skin takes on a tight, glossy appearance. Subcutaneous tissue atrophies and progresses until the fingertips become thin and wasted.

2. *Discoloration.* Initial appearance may be pale, erythematous, or cyanotic. Color changes may be paroxysmal and occur in response to ambient temperature changes or stress. Eventually redness develops, especially over the dorsum of the MCP and IP joints, and may progress to include the flexor creases of the hand.

3. *Hyperhidrosis.* Although present in early stages, hyperhidrosis decreases with time. Unusual dryness occurs in later stages.

4. *Allodynia.* Pain to light touch is usually present, causing the patient to hold the extremity in a characteristic protective position, supported by the contralateral hand away from the body.

5. *Hair and nail growth.* Changes in the rate of hair and nail growth may be present. Early in the process these are increased, whereas later the rate of growth decreases. In the atrophic phase hair may be absent and the nails pitted and brittle.

6. *Motor dysfunction.* A syndrome of motor dysfunction, including difficulty initiating movements, stiffness, and tremor, that responds to sympathetic blockade can occur. These motor symptoms may predate painful symptoms by weeks.

7. *Osteoporosis.* Late in the syndrome loss of bone mass and fibrosis of joint capsules become obvious. These findings are especially severe in the absence of an aggressive rehabilitation program initiated early in the course of the disease.

There are no specific diagnostic laboratory tests for SMP, but any test that reflects altered blood flow in the extremity (e.g., thermography or laser Doppler blood flow) supports the diagnosis. Furthermore, in more advanced cases radiographs may show patchy bone thinning of the epiphysis, metacarpals, and phalanges as well as other signs of increased bone turnover. Bone scans have also been used to aid the diagnosis of an SMP syndrome. Unfortunately, these studies do not provide data that are pathognomonic for SMP.

Sympathetic Blocks

Early treatment of SMP syndromes improves the likelihood of symptom resolution. Traditional management has involved serial sympathetic nerve blocks with local anesthetics. Stellate ganglion blocks (for upper extremity or head and neck SMP) or lumbar sympathetic blocks (for lower extremity and pelvic SMP) are administered every 1 to 3 days until symptoms resolve or pain improvement reaches a plateau, usually after 5 to 7 blocks. These techniques result in blockade of sympathetic fibers only. As there is usually no numbness, weakness, or paralysis

associated with proper local anesthetic placement, pain relief is also diagnostic of SMP. Sympatholysis with local anesthetics significantly decreases the characteristic hypersensitivity to light touch (allodynia) and burning pain, an effect that often outlasts the duration of local anesthetic action by several hours to days. Although long-lasting relief may be achieved through the use of neurolytic drugs such as alcohol and phenol, the risk of spillover to somatic nerves is real and can be devastating. As such, these medications should be used under rare circumstances and only after all other therapeutic avenues have been exhausted.

Sympathetic blockade can also be accomplished through other techniques such as brachial plexus and epidural blocks. These alternative injections may be technically easier and better tolerated by some patients and offer a comparable therapeutic response; but they are associated with blockade of somatic nerves, making the diagnosis of SMP more difficult. Intravenous regional (Bier) blocks have also been advocated using local anesthetics in combination with a vasoactive medication such as bretylium or guanethidine. Because of the longer duration of action of bretylium (vs. local anesthetic), these blocks are repeated every 1 to 3 weeks depending on symptoms. Disadvantages include the technical difficulty of finding a vein in a vasospastic extremity and possible nausea and orthostatic hypotension from circulating bretylium after the tourniquet is released.

A few patients with intractable symptoms and good, albeit temporary, relief with local anesthetic block therapy may require a surgical sympathectomy. The advent of thoracoscopy has made this procedure less of a surgical insult. However, symptoms may recur about 6 months after the procedure.

A critical component of the management of SMP is comprehensive physical and occupational therapy to decrease edema and restore mobility. The patient must be

---

Treatment of sympathetically maintained pain

- Stellate ganglion blocks
- Hand rehabilitation
- Transcutaneous electric nerve stimulation
- Medication
- Self-regulation techniques

---

involved in rehabilitation concurrent with and subsequent to the nerve blocks. Therapy may need to be gentle until some degree of pain relief has been achieved from the local anesthetic interventions.

Transcutaneous Electric Nerve Stimulation

TENS as an adjunct has also been shown to be beneficial when the electrodes are placed over the vascular supply to the affected extremity. In this location the stimulation affects sympathetic tone, a change not generally produced by traditional dermatomal stimulation. Maximal therapy would be TENS for 60 minutes, then having the unit in place (if the patient so desires) but turned off for a similar amount of time during waking hours.

TENS may be useful in patients with a low tolerance for nerve blocks or as an initial treatment in mild cases.

Medical Management

Most of the common analgesic medications are of little benefit to the patient with SMP because the primary pain is sympathetically mediated. Even nonsteroidal antiinflammatory drugs may have little effect because the edema associated with the SMP is the result of the alteration in blood flow, not a peripheral inflammatory mechanism. Some use is made of α- and β-adrenergic blocking drugs (e.g., phenoxybenzamine 10 to 40 mg four times a day or propranolol 10 to 40 mg four times a day, respectively) in attempts to manipulate the peripheral circulation and relieve the intense vasoconstriction. Calcium channel blocking drugs (e.g., nifedipine 10 to 20 mg three times a day) have also been used because they produce some vasodilation and may interrupt painful discharges from the injured extremity that serve only to retrigger the exaggerated response in sympathetic tone that results in the clinical syndrome of SMP.

Restoration of comfort without a comprehensive rehabilitation program to restore mobility and decrease edema is inadequate treatment.

Self-Regulation Techniques

Self-regulation techniques include self-hypnosis, biofeedback, and relaxation training. Although these techniques are not appropriate for all patients, selected patients are capable of increasing blood flow to the affected extremity volitionally through one of these modalities. For maximal effect an initial outlay of effort and resources is required (approximately six to eight sessions). In addition, the patient develops greatest facility with the technique if it is practiced regularly.

Rehabilitation

Nowhere in hand rehabilitation is the expression "no pain, no gain" more *inappropriate* than in the treatment of patients with reflex sympathetic dystrophy. A vigorous exercise program is definitely *not* what the doctor should order. Overly zealous, passive exercises performed to the point of pain surely increase the symptoms of dystrophy. Active exercises stopping short of the point of pain are indicated. Short exercise periods of several minutes performed throughout the day are more effective than longer exercise periods performed less frequently. Patients should be informed of the symptoms of overuse to better monitor their exercise program and their level of activity. In selected postoperative cases, controlled joint manipulation may be indicated immediately after successful administration of regional blocks. This procedure may be necessary to reduce tendon and soft-tissue adherence, thereby allowing active motion to occur.

As treatment progresses, a custom-made static thermoplastic splint may be fabricated in a position of comfort to promote relaxation. The splint should gradually be altered until the functional position is obtained. If contractures are present, it may be necessary to ultimately adjust the splint to an intrinsic plus position. The splint should be removed periodically for exercise periods. As hand function improves, wearing time should be decreased. Use of dynamic splints is contraindicated in the acute stage of the condition. They should not be used until edema has subsided and their use does not produce discomfort or an exacerbation of symptoms.

As clinicians, it is important that we be aware of the early symptoms of SMP. It is prudent to refer athletes to the team physician for review if their symptoms appear to be out of proportion to their injury, or if they do not appear to be improving in spite of therapeutic efforts. Early recognition and proper management of the condition produce the best results.

THE OLDER ATHLETE

All older athletes experience some age-related changes. They are generally less flexible and have smaller muscle masses, lower aerobic capacity, and a less adaptable thermoregulatory system.[62,87,97]

Declines in strength have been reported for every muscle group that has been tested, averaging approximately 1% per year after the third decade.[52] The rate of decline appears to vary from muscle group to muscle group and from person to person, which makes characterizing the decline in strength with aging rather difficult. If disease such as osteoarthritis is present, the degree of strength change may be greater than that expected under average conditions.

It appears that continuous resistance exercise training markedly attenuates strength loss with aging but does not eliminate loss altogether.[21,22] The study suggests that a significant portion of the strength loss that occurs with age is a result of disuse.

There are no data to support the concern that athletic participation makes the onset of arthritic joints more likely. What is clear is that injuries incurred during a lifetime of athletics can increase the incidence of arthritis. Most serious athletes suffer from injuries that fall into the overuse category; older athletes are no exception. Older athletes may actually be more prone to this type of injury than younger athletes. However, unlike in younger athletes these injuries are superimposed on an aging musculoskeletal system and recovery may take longer. In older athletes injuries incurred tend to be sports specific.

Golf

Golf is different than most other sports in that almost all of its practitioners play more, rather than less, as they mature. Additional playing time can be satisfying, but it puts players at risk for a number of overuse syndromes directly caused by the motion requirements of golf. The repetitive nature of the activity can exacerbate both preexisting and age-related conditions of the hand and wrist.

Wrist pain in a golfer of any age is encountered frequently. It is almost always on the left side and is probably an overuse syndrome related to repeated extension and radial deviation of the wrist during the swing. Pre-

vention is the best treatment. Attention to proper swing mechanics whereby the golfer works to reduce the wrist extension and radial deviation occurring during the swing usually leads to a resolution of the problem.

Tennis

Older athletes who play tennis regularly seem to fare better than those who play intermittently. Upper extremity strength is valuable to the older tennis player in two ways. With increased strength a player may increase the speed of the racquet head as it contacts the ball, and this translates into power. Power enables the player to hit the ball deeper into the court and to hit the ball more quickly. If combined with control, it allows the player to function better. With advancing age we lose strength and an element of power. The older athlete typically compensates for this decline in strength and power with better control and understanding of the game, which allows him or her to play with more patience.

After an illness or injury there is almost always loss of both strength and flexibility. Regaining strength, endurance, and power requires work. Most athletes try to return to action too quickly. Activity must be resumed gradually at a rate commensurate with the body's physiologic regeneration.

Psychologic Aspects

Older athletes are likely to feel especially threatened by any required change in their activity. Their self-image may be closely connected with their exercise and they may be more willing to live with pain than to alter their established routine. There is need to convince aging athletes that a short-term loss may lead to a long-term gain, to explain the consequences of disregarding symptoms that relate to athletic activity, and to provide specific alternatives. In some cases it may be necessary to replace the competitive aspect of sports with a social component.

One of the most important services the trainer/therapist can provide is to reassure older athletes that, even though they may have developed symptoms of the aging process, these ailments will not stop them from continuing with their athletic activities.

Sports may be the primary avenue through which they derive a sense of self-worth. Such athletes may experience changes in their activity regimen as traumatic. They may persist with activities that are no longer productive in the belief that more effort brings about desired results. In some instances it may be critical for certain individuals to realize that they can no longer be a biker or a runner. It is, however, critical to the patient's well-being that he or she be involved in something, and often this is some type of sport.

Prevention

Injury prevention has always been an integral part of sports medicine. Because even a minor injury can lead to the end of an older athlete's sports participation, prevention is extraordinarily important. Proper equipment selection and use of racquets or clubs, for example, and stretching and training techniques must be encouraged.

DUPUYTREN'S DISEASE

Dupuytren's disease is of genetic origin and occurs primarily in people of northern European origin.[34,35] Clinically it is seen more frequently in males than in females because the disease appears later in women and is less likely to cause a joint contracture that requires treatment. The disease usually appears in the fifth decade in men and somewhat later in women.

Although Dupuytren's disease is progressive, it is not possible to predict how rapidly the disease progresses from the first appearance of a nodule, which is the primary pathologic manifestation of the disease. The initial complaint is usually tenderness over the nodule. The nodule may quickly or slowly enlarge, mature, and then remain quiescent for long periods, often never progressing to the stage of active contracture. In others the initial nodule enlarges, other nodules form, and over a period of months or years tendonlike cords form and are readily palpable in the palm and finger. The MCP joint is most frequently contracted. The PIP joint may be contracted alone or with the MCP joint. Occasionally the DIP joint is contracted.

There is currently no proven nonsurgical method of treatment for Dupuytren's disease. Attempts to use vitamin E, steroid injections, splints, ultrasound, and stretching exercises have been ineffective.

The mere presence of a nodule in the palmar aspect of a digit is not an indication for excision. However, excision may be indicated if a nodule becomes so large that it interferes with hand function. Other indications for surgical intervention include an MCP flexion contracture of 30 degrees or a PIP joint flexion contracture of 15 degrees or more. Web space contractures particularly of the thumb-index web space may also prompt a surgical release in that functional hand use is greatly hampered.

Although many methods of surgical treatment are used today, no one method has been established as superior. Postoperative management techniques also vary. Despite the various surgical and rehabilitation methods that exist, the common goal is to promote wound healing, which minimizes scar tissue and maximizes scar mobility.

It seems only natural to assume that a lump in the palm may have been caused by hand usage. Patients often satisfy their natural curiosity by ascribing the nodule to a pressure point on a machine or even to their golf grip. Studies of large population groups have failed to find any difference between the prevalence of Dupuytren's contracture in manual laborers and office workers.[34,36]

A number of studies of people who have developed Dupuytren's contracture have shown that there is no relationship to handedness.[17,36,66] In a recent study[66] of 812 patients undergoing surgical correction for Dupuytren's contracture 95% were right handed, 5% were left handed, and 1% were ambidextrous. Of this group, 24% showed Dupuytren's contracture in only their right hand, 12% showed involvement only in their left hand, and 64% showed bilateral involvement.[66]

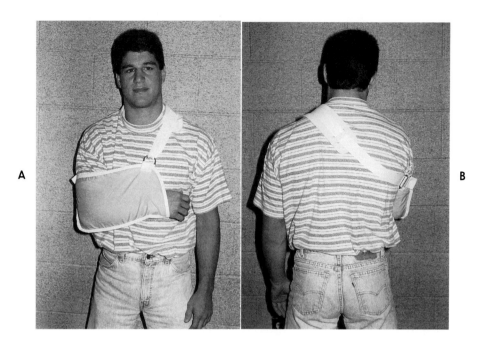

FIG. 28-14. Properly applied sling. **A,** Front. **B,** Back.

TRIGGER FINGER

Idiopathic thickening of the proximal portion of the flexor tendon sheath (A-1 pulley) is the usual cause of trigger finger. Direct pressure on the MCP flexion crease from a racquet or other forcefully grasped tool may serve as a mechanical irritant to incite an inflammatory response.[53,76] Symptoms may run the spectrum from pain, to triggering, to actual locking with active motion. Cortisone injection is recommended as the initial form of treatment. Gloves should be evaluated to ensure that adequate protection (padding) is provided. Occasionally surgical release of the A-1 pulley is necessary and curative.

EDEMA
Prevention of Edema

The prevention and treatment of edema present a constant challenge to trainers and therapists. However, they are critical during all phases of management of the injured hand. If left untreated, edema can be responsible for delaying healing and causing pain, as well as limiting mobility with subsequent compromised functional use. It is a disservice to the athlete if the factors that contribute to the formation of edema are not alleviated immediately after injury occurs. Several factors may contribute to the formation of edema:

1. The hand may be immobilized in a dependent position such as that which occurs from an ill-fitting sling.
2. Painful wrists that are not splinted in dorsiflexion usually drop into palmar flexion.
3. If left unsupported, hands assume a guarded position. The wrist drops into palmar flexion while the MCP and PIP joints assume an extended position.

As edema forms, the longitudinal and the transverse arches are eventually lost because of pressure that is created on the dorsum of the hand. Injured hands should be splinted in a functional position.

4. Attempts are made to hold the extremity in an elevated position for long periods of time without the use of slings or splints. Sling use should be alternated with elevation and active exercises to all uninvolved joints of the extremity.
5. The exercise program for adjacent uninvolved structures may be inadequate.

Elevation

When slings are used, wearing time and proper application should be discussed. The back strap is diagonally positioned so that the weight of the extremity is supported on the opposite shoulder (Fig. 28-14). The elbow and forearm should rest directly on the trough of the sling. The wrist and the midportion of the hand should be supported by the trough of the sling. Allowing the wrist to take on a position of ulnar deviation and palmar flexion will contribute to the formation of edema (Fig. 28-15).

If a sling is used for extended periods of time, the athlete should be instructed to periodically remove the sling and perform active exercises to all uninvolved joints that the sling is immobilizing. Constant use of a sling can result in a shoulder adduction-internal rotation deformity that may eventually develop into a frozen shoulder or shoulder-hand syndrome.

Instruction for elevation while in a supine position should also be provided. Placing the hand anywhere over the trunk while lying down is considered elevation. To increase comfort, it is helpful to support the arm with pillows and therefore promote relaxation. It is best to sup-

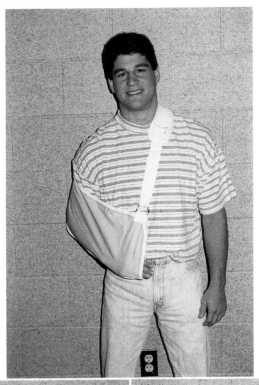

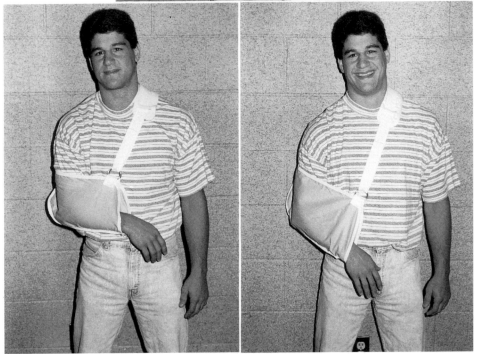

FIG. 28-15. Three common but ineffective methods of sling use.

port the extremity in a comfortable position using pillows of various sizes for support (Fig. 28-16). Providing instruction for awkward positions or asking the athlete to hold the extremity in a specific position while at rest should be avoided.

Splints

Static splints are indicated to provide support, thereby preventing strain of a severely edematous or painful hand and wrist. The splints should be molded in either a func-

tional or intrinsic plus position, depending on diagnosis and clinical examination. When splinting is used for edema control, the use of straps should be discouraged. Use of Coban or an Ace wrap distributes the pressure over a larger area, thereby providing compression to further reduce edema.

Continuous static splinting of an edematous hand can result in joint stiffness. The effects of immobilization may be counteracted by instructing the athlete to remove the splint often during the day to perform active exercises.

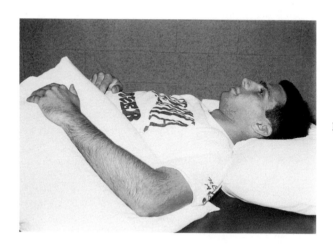

FIG. 28-16. Effective elevation technique—supine position.

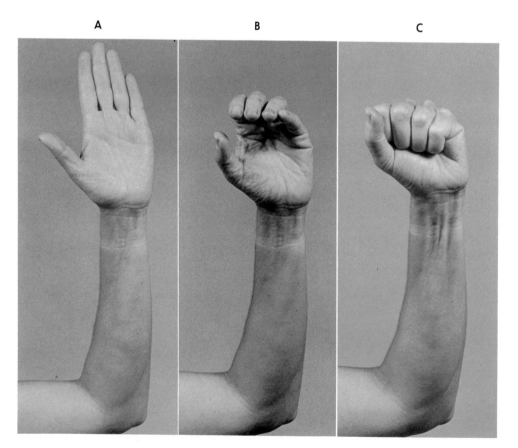

FIG. 28-17. Pumping exercises used for edema reduction. **A,** Starting position. **B,** Mid position. **C,** Maximal position.

Exercise

Short exercise periods performed often are most effective in preventing edema formation. Having the athlete elevate the extremity while performing active pumping types of exercise further enhances edema reduction.

During active movement the blood flow is directly related to the degree of activity in the muscle. Firm fist-making exercise with the extremity elevated should be encouraged periodically throughout the day. Shortened rapid attempts at finger flexion are ineffective. Passive movement produces very little change in blood flow to the limb, though it is helpful in preventing adhesions and maintaining joint mobility. In summary, the only exercise program that is of any consequence in reducing edema is one of *firm, active motion* that takes the digits through as large an arc of motion as comfort allows, performed while the limb is elevated (Fig. 28-17).

Reduction of Edema

One or more of the following techniques may be used to facilitate venous flow, thereby reducing edema in the upper extremity. Instruction provided should be explicit. The athlete should be informed of the consequences of inadequate or total noncompliance. When properly executed, these techniques can do much to reduce edema; however, when carried out poorly they may contribute to an increase in edema.

Constant or Intermittent Compression

Intermittent and constant devices provide an added dimension to rehabilitation of the hand and wrist when they are used for edema control.[42,96] Gentle pressure applied to the digits is effective in improving mobility in extension. An appreciable improvement in flexion after compression can also be observed because of decreased volume throughout the hand.

Constant compression devices such as the Jobst air splint may be used in the following manner.

Preparation. Place stockinette on the portion of the extremity to be placed in the splint.

Position. Position the hand in the air splint so that compression occurs at the fingertips.

Support. Support the extremity on an elevated or inclined surface.

Inflation. Using the airbulb, inflate the splint to tolerance. Initially, it may be necessary to start with gentle pressure and gradually increase it as tolerance increases. The pressure should not be so great as to create throbbing, tingling, or numbness.

Adaptations. If IP joint flexion contractures are present, it may be necessary to place light padding in the palm, thereby reducing painful stress that may occur from forcing the fingers into extension. To increase mobility in finger flexion, the fingers may be loosely taped to encourage composite flexion before being placed in the splint.

Utilization. When the splint for edema control is used with the digits held in extension, it may be left in place for 20 minutes. However, when the splint is used to increase mobility and the fingers are taped in flexion, it must be removed after 10 minutes.

This method of edema control is particularly helpful for use with athletes who are experiencing a moderate degree of edema and do not have regular access to a training room or clinic. Static compression may also be used as an adjunct to intermittent compression as part of a home program in situations where edema is persistent.

Intermittent compression is provided with the use of a compression pump and a pneumatic sleeve. To reduce edema in acute injuries, the external intermittent pressure device increases interstitial pressure, thereby forcing lymphatic fluids back into the venous system. The arm should be elevated on an inclined surface or positioned on pillows at approximately a 30- to 45-degree angle to take advantage of gravity. It is not necessary to check the athlete's blood pressure before compression. Pneumatic sleeves are available for the hand and wrist, as well as for the full arm. In treating injuries of the hand and wrist, the shorter pneumatic sleeve is generally adequate. In treating the upper extremity, 30 to 40 mm Hg provides adequate pressure. The pressure applied should not elicit sensations of throbbing, tingling, or numbness. Various alterations in treatment may be employed when treating acute hand injuries. Small open wounds are not a contraindication to its use; however, these wounds should be covered with a sterile dressing. Felt or foam padding may be used to protect pin sites that are painful to pressure. Padding may also be used to support the palmar surface of the hand if pressure applied to the extended fingers is painful.

Contrary to the belief that more pressure is better, it is not necesary to continually increase the pressure as tolerance improves. Increasing the pressure beyond 40 mm Hg may lead to an increase rather than a reduction in hand volume. After edema is reduced through the use of intermittent compression, the volume loss may be maintained by the use of compression gloves or Coban bandage. Air splints may also be used for maintaining losses as part of a home program.

Massage

Retrograde massage is an important aspect of edema reduction programs involving the hand and wrist. The force of the massage stroke should begin distally and progress proximally. It is beneficial to support the hand on an inclined surface when performing massage. The athlete should be instructed in techniques of retrograde massage so that it may be incorporated into the home program.

Coban is an effective means of reducing edema in the hand. One layer is wrapped proximally to the palm starting at the distal end of the digit. All involved fingers and the palm should be wrapped proximally to the edematous area. The pressure applied should provide adequate compression, but care should be taken to avoid creating a sensation of throbbing, tingling, or numbness.

Two-inch Coban is appropriate for wrapping the palm and forearm; however, the 1-inch width is most practical for wrapping digits. An important feature of Coban is that is does not limit mobility. Coban is also effective when used to secure static finger or hand splints in place. Its use is particularly advantageous in that the use of

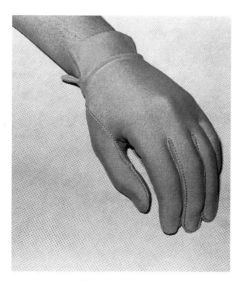

FIG. 28-18. Compression glove.

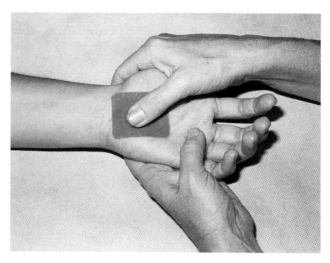

FIG. 28-19. Use of dycem during massage assists in early scar tissue mobilization and desensitization.

strapping or circumferential taping may result in increased edema.

Compression Gloves

Compression gloves provide external pressure that is helpful in maintaining volume loss after treatment (Fig. 28-18). After wearing the gloves, patients often report a decrease in discomfort and increase in functional use of the hand. Many varieties of compression gloves are commercially available. Aris Isotoner Gloves* are available in department stores. One size fits all, and they are available for both men and women. Jobst† produces compression gloves that are available in several sizes. They also make custom edema control garments on request.

Therapeutic Cold

Use of therapeutic heat is contraindicated in treatment of extremities where edema is present. A local effect of therapeutic cold is pain suppression. Cold creates vasoconstriction and is also believed to elevate the pain threshold of sensory nerve fibers, thereby decreasing the degree of pain that is perceived. As a consequence, patients usually experience less pain and guarding and therefore are better able to perform active movement.

A direct application of an ice pack for a 5-minute interval is usually all that a patient will tolerate.

SCAR MANAGEMENT

Deep transverse friction massage, crossing the grain of tightened connective tissue, helps mobilize superficial scar by stretching its adherence to underlying tissue (Fig. 28-19). Heat applied before massage increases the

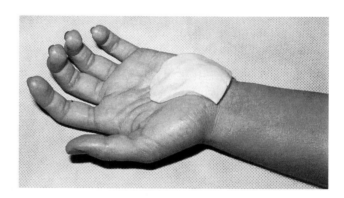

FIG. 28-20. Elastomer pad fabricated to provide compression of scar tissue.

elasticity of the tissues and thus increases the effectiveness of the massage.

Continuous pressure over a superficial scar flattens it and may also help make it softer, more elastic, and more cosmetically acceptable to the patient. The effectiveness of compression has been dramatically demonstrated in its clinical application to hypertrophic scars of burn patients.[57]

In the hand, continuous pressure can be provided with elasticized gloves, such as Isotoner, Coban, elasticized paper bandage, or for firmer and more localized pressure by the use of elastomer, or Spenco* gel sheets (Fig. 28-20).

Elastomer is mixed with a catalyst and spread into the scar. The mixture is then allowed to set, forming an ex-

*Aris Gloves, New York, NY, 10016.
†Jobst Institute, Inc, Toledo, Ohio, 43694.

*Spenco Medical Corporation, Waco, TX.

act mold of the scar and all the skin creases. The durability of the pad is greatly increased if several layers of gauze are placed on the back of the mixture before it has set. If necessary, the pad may be trimmed with scissors once it has set. For best results the pad should be worn constantly if possible, and it is best held in place by a closely fitting splint or Coban wrapping. As the scar matures, new molds must be made to accommodate changes that occur.[57]

Scars in normally mobile areas such as the palm and wrist do not receive adequate compression from elastomer pads alone. The pressure must be applied under a splint that holds the part immobile. With wrist and finger motion the scar moves and stretches and the mold is no longer exact. In these cases Spenco gel sheets (⅛-inch thick) are preferable. Although gel sheets do not conform as exactly to the shape of the scar, they do provide close pressure that is flexible and thereby adaptable to the motion of the scar.

In many instances constant gentle pressure to a hypersensitive area provides relief of symptoms. In these situations compression from a glove or Coban wrap is more helpful than gel sheets.

All athletes requiring surgery of the hand or wrist should be put on a postoperative scar management program. Often the use of gentle massage, compression, and prophylactic desensitization serve to forestall the development of a hypersensitive scar. A hand that has gained adequate mobility may continue to be nonfunctional as a result of a hypersensitive scar. Hypersensitive scars are especially bothersome on the volar aspect of the hand.

EXERCISE

Exercises may be classified in four categories: (1) active, (2) active assistive, (3) passive, and (4) resistive.

Active exercise is the only modality of hand therapy ever shown to be of lasting benefit in the rehabilitation of athletically related hand injuries. Its role, therefore, cannot be overemphasized.[9] Active exercises should be initiated as soon as pain subsides and adequate healing of soft tissue and fractures has occurred. Through active motion it is possible to preserve anatomic structure and tissue nutrition, as well as to prevent adhesions and permit lymphatic drainage.

Active motion must be within pain tolerance. Exercises should be performed gently to avoid tissue reaction but frequently to increase mobility. Tendon adhesions can be avoided with early continuous active exercises aimed at full tendon excursion in both directions. Because active motion plays a primary role in hand therapy, it may be difficult for the practitioner to determine when other types of exercises are indicated.

If passive motion does not exceed active motion, it is necessary to upgrade the exercise program to overcome restriction of joint range. This can be accomplished by several means.

Less tissue reaction occurs when patients are taught to perform active assistive exercises by applying gentle force for short periods several times during the day.

When performing active assistive exercises, patients are more likely to respond to pain and will not incite tissue reactions. As healing occurs, patients should be taught to distinguish between discomfort and pain. Discomfort created by a properly applied force is tolerable and beneficial; *pain is not*. The degree of force and number of repetitions should be altered until no tissue reaction occurs. As further healing occurs, intensity should be increased while tissue reaction is continually monitored.

Purely passive exercises play a small role in hand therapy. Effective alternatives to passive motion, besides active assistive exercise, include joint mobilization and static and dynamic splinting.

If passive motion exceeds active motion in spite of what appears to be an adequate active exercise program, it may be necessary to initiate gentle resistive exercises using a light rubber band to overcome weakness or adherence of tendons. It is important that tension applied is gentle enough to allow motion of the joint.

Active Exercise
Isolated (Blocking) Exercise

Because active exercises play a substantial role in preventing tendon adherence, teaching the athlete to perform active isolated, or blocking, exercises to the flexor digitorum profundus or flexor digitorum sublimus in a timely manner is of utmost importance. The athlete should be instructed to stabilize the joint proximal to the one that is being exercised, using the opposite hand to provide better mechanical advantage (Fig. 28-21). Flexion exercises should be done gently and sustained for 10 seconds, with maximal power stopping just short of pain.

Often the inability to isolate joint motion is caused by muscular cocontraction. To test for cocontraction ask the patient to isolate PIP joint flexion. Place your thumb on the volar aspect of the proximal phalanx of the involved digit. If you feel resistance, the MCP (lumbrical) rather than the PIP (flexor digitorum profundus) joint is being activated.

To overcome cocontraction, various methods of instruction that implement methods of proprioceptive neuromuscular facilitation (PNF) or biofeedback may be used. Possible methods include practicing isolation of an uninvolved DIP joint, flexing all PIP joints simultaneously, and performing bilateral MCP joint flexion exercises over the edge of a tabletop (Fig. 28-22). Many commercial exercise aids are available to assist the therapist. To be effective, devices should support the bone proximal to the joint being exercised to obtain the best mechanical advantage. Devices should also conform to the architecture of the hand by not forcing it into awkward or painful positions (Fig. 28-23).

If motion is still limited, electrical stimulation can be used to redefine the motion, giving the patient a sense of how the muscle contraction feels. When using electric stimulation, a faradic current that produces a tetanus-type contraction should be selected. Electric stimulation should not be used before the fifth postoperative week. Exceptions include doubt about the continuity of a tendon repair or graft.

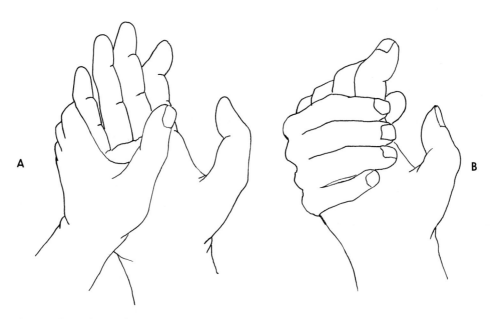

FIG. 28-21. Isolation of active proximal interphalangeal joint motion. **A,** Volar view. **B,** Dorsal view.

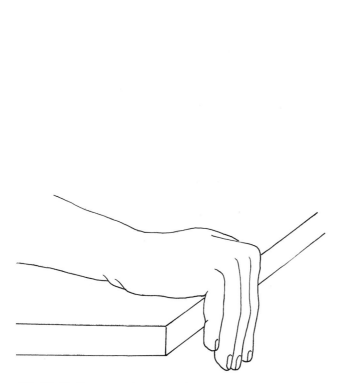

FIG. 28-22. Supporting forearm and wrist on a stationary surface allows for easier active metacarpophalangeal joint isolation.

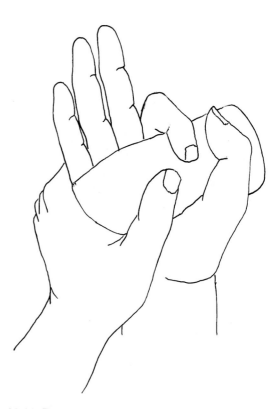

FIG. 28-23. Exercise aids may be necessary to accomplish proper execution of blocking exercises.

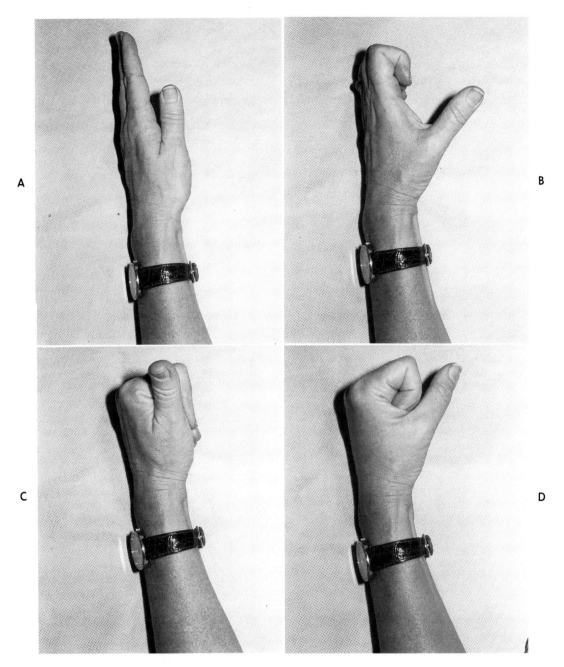

FIG. 28-24. Tendon gliding exercise positions. **A,** Straight starting position. **B,** Hook fist position. **C,** Straight fist position. **D,** Full fisted position.

Tendon Gliding Exercises

Tendon gliding exercises were developed at the Hand Rehabilitation Center in Philadelphia based on a study by Wehbé and Hunter.[100,101] The authors concluded that three different hand positions (hook fist, straight fist, and full fist) produced maximum differential glide between the flexor digitorum profundus, the flexor digitorum sublimus, and surrounding tissues (Fig. 28-24). Maximum excursion of the profundus tendon in relation to the sheath and bone is achieved when making a full fist. Maximum excursion of the superficialis tendon in relation to the sheath and bone is in the straight fist position. The hood position produces maximum differential glide between profundus and superficialis tendons. Initially the exercises are done with the wrist in the neutral position for simplicity. Once the exercises are easily performed, wrist motion may be incorporated in the program to further increase tendon excursion. Tendon adhesions that may result after trauma or surgery or after subacute and chronic synovitis can be prevented or minimized by the use of tendon gliding exercises, which allow each tendon to reach its maximum excursion and

promote differential gliding. They can also improve synovial edema and diffuse hand swelling by mechanically displacing excess interstitial fluid.

Conventional blocking exercises can be used in conjunction with tendon gliding exercises. Blocking exercises can provide isolated gliding of the superficialis or profundus tendon, but these exercises provide markedly reduced excursion because of the restricted joint motion inherent to these maneuvers.

As with any other exercise program, the criteria for the use of differential tendon gliding exercises should be tailored to each athlete's needs. An average program may include 10 repetitions of each exercise twice a day. The usual precautions of exercise programs should be observed. Tendon gliding exercises should be avoided if there is an unstable fracture or until 6 weeks after tendon repair.

Passive Exercise

Clinical experience shows that the benefits of passive motion in the hand are transient at best.[9] Passive motion should be included in a hand therapy program only when active motion is not possible. When passive motion is indicated, the athlete should be instructed to perform the exercises alone. Since pain deters athletes from stressing joints, they are less likely to increase symptoms by overexercising.

Passive exercises have been widely used in the past by physical therapists and have been responsible, in part, for alienating the relationship between physical therapists and the early hand surgeons. Surgeons observed that after physical therapy their patients often appeared to experience increased swelling and decreased mobility, which they attributed to overzealous passive exercises performed by the therapist. Bunnell thought that applying vigorous passive exercises to joints was equivalent to spraining them on a regular basis. He thought the rationale for use of passive motion was unscientific and must be based on comparisons to inanimate objects, such as rusty hinges.[18] As a result of their philosophic differences, early hand surgeons abandoned the use of therapists and personally supervised their patients' rehabilitation. This practice continued until the middle 1970s. By this time many hand surgeons had trained therapists in what they thought were proper atraumatic techniques of hand rehabilitation. As a result of the physicians' efforts, the American Society of Hand Therapists was founded in 1978.

Techniques to improve passive range of motion

- Gentle active assisted exercises
- Static splinting
- Dynamic splinting
- Joint mobilization

Many acceptable methods of improving passive motion in the hand and wrist exist. They include gentle active assistive exercises, static splinting, and slow, deliberate stretching such as that provided by dynamic splints and joint mobilization.

Resistive Exercise

Resistive exercises should be initiated only in the face of pain-free motion. The patient begins with light resistive materials and gradually increases resistance. The therapist continues to monitor for symptoms of tissue reaction as resistance is upgraded.

Monitoring Exercise Programs

Exercises do not have to be painful to be effective. Pain is not gain; it is also not the enemy. Brand[19] describes pain as being the patient's own living cells indicating the limits of the exercise.

Therapists are taught to respect pain. In turn, they must teach patients its significance. Therapists must upgrade rehabilitation programs adequately to make therapeutic gains, but not so rapidly as to create tissue reaction.

As tissues heal, they are able to tolerate stresses that produce discomfort. During this phase it is necessary to help the athlete differentiate between discomfort and pain.

Tissue reactions should be carefully monitored. If increased edema or pain occurs, the therapeutic program should be reviewed and altered accordingly. This is especially important in dealing with individuals who are unable to differentiate between pain and discomfort.

Experience has taught us that compliance with a consistent therapeutic program is superior to an overzealous exercise program performed in a haphazard or inconsistent manner. In the evaluation of a therapeutic program, an apparent lack of progress may be the result of too much rather than too little exercise.

Composite Flexion

Attaining composite flexion, or making a fist, is often the only general clinical impression used in evaluating successful rehabilitation of hand injuries.

However simplistic it may appear, careful attention should be paid to restoring composite finger flexion. Unless contraindicated, all initial home programs should consist of exercises for composite motion as well as isolated joint or blocking motion of the digit. The therapist or trainer should provide instruction to flex digits actively around a cylindric object that is almost within current grasp. When patients are able to grasp the object comfortably, therapists or trainers should instruct them to progress gradually to grasping smaller cylindric objects. This exercise is an excellent means of improving motion, because individuals often relate to grasping the object as an activity rather than as an exercise, and they are generally more spontaneous in their performance. Initially, it may be necessary to instruct the patient to grasp rather than squeeze the object. Patients are often tempted to squeeze before adequate healing has occurred to allow their efforts to be therapeutic.

It may be necessary to augment an active exercise program for obtaining composite finger flexion with the use

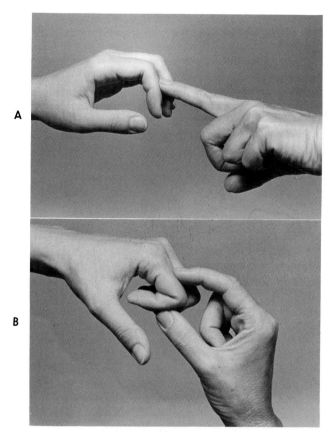

FIG. 28-25. Testing intrinsic tightness.

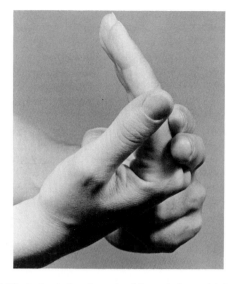

FIG. 28-26. Active isolated proximal interphalangeal joint extension.

continuous 90-degree angle on the digits as improvement occurs. An alternate method of overcoming intrinsic tightness is to use progressive static splinting.

Overcoming intrinsic contracture

- Dynamic splinting
- Serial static splints

---

of a static serial splint. Dynamic splints and flexor gloves are suitable alternatives to splinting.

Intrinsic vs. Capsular Tightness

The test for intrinsic tightness is to place the intrinsics on a stretch by extending the MCP joints while passively flexing the PIP joints. Then the patient relaxes the intrinsics by flexing the MCP joints several degrees while passively flexing the PIP joints. If the PIP joints demonstrate greater passive flexion when the intrinsics are relaxed (flexed MCP joints), intrinsic tightness is present. If the degree of passive PIP joint flexion is unchanged by altering the position of the MCP joints, a joint contracture is present (Fig. 28-25).[46]

Routine therapeutic efforts to improve composite finger flexion are generally not effective in overcoming intrinsic tightness.

Methods of overcoming intrinsic tightness consist of applying a slow, steady force to the middle phalanges while supporting the MCP joints in extension. This is best accomplished by the use of dynamic splinting. A volar base is fabricated on the forearm and wrist, extending distally to support the MCP joints in extension. Individual finger cuffs are attached to the proximal phalanx of each digit. Tension is directed toward the outrigger, which is attached to the base of the splint. The outrigger and cuffs should be altered to maintain a

Maintaining or Restoring Proximal Interphalangeal Joint Extension

Maintaining or restoring PIP joint extension is one of the greatest challenges of rehabilitation. The challenge becomes even greater if measures to preserve extension are not initiated early in the treatment program.

The flexor muscles in the hand are four times stronger than the extensor muscles.[18] Few activities require resistive finger extension. The primary function of the extensor muscles is to move the fingers out of the palm. The functional or working position of the hand involves finger flexion.

It is crucial to the therapy program that extension be evaluated often so that mobility is maintained. Loss of PIP joint extension may occur if splinting is discontinued before adequate soft tissue healing has occurred. It may further be decreased when either substantial gains in flexion are attained or there is increased functional use of the hand.

Isolated PIP joint extension exercises should be a part of all exercise programs involving digits. To perform active isolated PIP joint extension exercises, the patient positions the wrist in a neutral position and stabilizes the MCP joints in maximal flexion by supporting them with the opposite hand. The athlete should be instructed to actively extend the PIP joints (Fig. 28-26).

To further counteract the imbalance, it is often necessary to statically splint the PIP joints in extension. Splints may be worn at night to avoid interfering with functional use and therapeutic programs designed to improve mobility.

HOME PROGRAM

The home program is often considered the most important aspect of hand rehabilitation. Nowhere is its importance greater than in the treatment of athletic injuries.

Injuries sustained by athletes are usually produced by circumstances inherent to their respective sport. When allowed to return to competition, they are exposed to similar recurrent trauma, making reinjury more likely. In the rehabilitation of athletes, our goal is to obtain normal function to the greatest degree possible in the shortest possible time.

Therapists or trainers should provide athletes with adequate instruction so that they are able to carry out all aspects of their programs at home on a daily basis. Instruction should include the use of modalities, exercise aids, splints, and therapeutic exercise. Oral, written, and visual instruction is often required. The symptoms of overuse should also be described so that athletes are able to monitor an appropriate level of activity.

MODALITIES
Therapeutic Heat

Therapeutic heat decreases pain and muscle spasms, reduces joint stiffness, and increases collagen extensibility.

Hydrocollator

Hydrocollators (hot packs) apply moist heat directly to the skin surfaces and have the advantage of being applied while the hand is held in elevation. However, any compromise of peripheral circulation or presence of insensitive digits contraindicates the use of hydrocollators.

Patients should be checked often during treatment to ensure that the intense heat is well tolerated. It is especially important to observe bony prominences and contracted joints for indications of intolerance. Placing weights on hot packs in an attempt to improve finger extension should be discouraged, especially if significant contractures are present.

Hot packs are especially effective when used before wrist exercises.

Whirlpool

Despite the popularity of the whirlpool, it is often used unnecessarily and indiscriminately. Improper use of the whirlpool may not only provide an ineffective modality in some situations, but also the temperature of the water, together with the dependent position of the extremity, often results in increased edema. This technique, used in previous years, has given the whirlpool a bad name. Hand surgery literature is filled with the perils created by the improper use of the whirlpool. Bell and Horton[11] state: "Probably no device deserves more credit for perpetuating hand disability than the whirlpool." The whirlpool can be used in the treatment of hand and wrist injuries if indications, contraindications, and precautions as to its use are employed.

Whirlpool therapy

Proper whirlpool use
- Hand is elevated
- Appropriate temperature

Improper whirlpool use
- Hand is dependent
- Inappropriate temperature

The dependent position can be eliminated by slightly abducting the shoulder and flexing the elbow so that the water level just covers the hand during treatment. Compromising the vascularity of an injured extremity or damaging an insensitive area can be avoided with extremes of hot or cold temperatures. A wide variety of treatment temperatures are cited in the literature.[5,11] Recommended temperatures for providing general whirlpool range from 95° to 105° F for heat, and from 55° to 65° F for cold whirlpool. It is important to note that these statistics are not provided for the treatment of upper extremities. To determine desirable or appropriate water temperatures, it is important to review all information obtained through clinical examination and the available medical information. Hand volume should be observed before and after whirlpool treatment, and water temperature decreased if volume increases. Active exercises are also effective in combating edema if they are performed during whirlpool treatment.

Recommended whirlpool temperatures

- Heat: 95° to 105° F
- Cold: 55° to 65° F

In the treatment of open wounds a disinfectant added to the whirlpool water, together with a clean whirlpool, has been shown to reduce the local bacteria count.[12,72] Following treatment the tank should be drained and thoroughly cleaned. Carefully followed cleaning procedures and periodic cultures are necessary. If cleaning and culturing procedures are not carefully followed, open wounds should not be treated in the whirlpool.

In the absence of open wounds, paraffin or hydrocollator pads along with elevation may be a better method of providing heat before exercise. Whirlpool is not effective when heat is the only desired objective.

Paraffin

The paraffin bath is particularly effective in the rehabilitation of hand and wrist injuries. The advantage of paraffin is that it contours and heats all surfaces, thereby

providing an even heating effect. The presence of oil provides lubrication to dry skin and improves elasticity, making it especially effective as a precursor to massage. Joints can be positioned on a stretch, providing maximal benefit from the heat that is applied to contracting structures. The temperature of 126° F can create skin problems in the face of vascular compromise, neurologic deficits, or early reflex sympathetic dystrophy. Paraffin treatment is also not indicated in individuals with open wounds or exposed internal hardware.

Directions for paraffin application

- Elevate if edema is present.
- Remove all jewelry, and wash and dry hand well.
- With fingers slightly abducted, dip hand and wrist into the bath. Remove quickly and allow to cool. Having started the treatment, maintain constant position of the fingers to maintain heat longer.
- When the paraffin has cooled enough to be comfortable, resume dipping. Continue dipping until you have built up approximately 10 layers of paraffin.
- Cover the hand with clear plastic wrap or a plastic bag. Wrap tightly in a towel to maintain heat.
- Leave the paraffin in place for 20 minutes or as long as the effect of heat is appreciated.
- It is best to dispose of used paraffin.

Fluidotherapy

Fluidotherapy* was introduced as a form of therapeutic heat in 1974.[14] Fluidotherapy is based on the discovery that, in certain hydrodynamic conditions, solid particles can be suspended in air. Essentially, the mixture is similar to a dry whirlpool, which provides massage action and carries heat to body tissues in an effective manner. Because the heat generated is dry (115° to 120° F), temperatures are generally comfortably tolerated. Borrell and his associates[15] have stated that, under these conditions, heat absorbed by the body is four to six times as great as in other forms of hydrotherapy or paraffin treatments. Advantages to this treatment include a decrease in labor and utilities, in that plumbing usage and filling and emptying the apparatus between uses is not indicated. Elevation and active exercises are possible during its use.

Therapeutic Ultrasound

Through the years, various claims have been made concerning the effects of ultrasound. The physical effects that lead to changes must be appreciated if ultrasound is to be used safely and efficiently. Its physical effects, at the levels used therapeutically, can be classified as either primarily thermal or nonthermal.[51,69,93] Thermal effects allow for local tissue heating as a result of absorption. The site and amount of absorption depend on the type of tissue in the path of the beam, the efficiency of the local circulation dissipating the heat, and the fre-

quency of the ultrasound. Nonthermal physiologic changes are caused by cavitation, acoustic streaming, and standing wave formation. Cavitation produces localized damage and formation of free radical formation. Acoustic streaming is the circulatory flow of fluid induced by radiation forces. When the streaming is induced by ultrasound next to a small vibrating object such as a cell or bubble, the movements involved are of microscopic proportion and the process is termed *microstreaming*.[51,93] Standing wave formation is defined as the interaction between the incident and reflected waves between two acoustically different media (e.g., soft tissue and bone).[93]

For diagnoses where heating would not be indicated, nonthermal pulsed ultrasound may be beneficial. Diagnoses such as tendinitis, tenosynovitis, myositis, bursitis, acutely inflamed wounds, and subacute sprains respond better to nonthermal pulsed ultrasound.[69]

Scar tissue management can be enhanced with the use of ultrasound. Heating has been postulated to alter the viscoelastic properties of collagen tissue and collagen molecular bonding, thus facilitating ease of stretch. Deep tissues responsible for decreasing the range of motion at a joint are rich in collagen. Therefore ultrasound is a logically chosen thermal agent to selectively heat these deep structures.[69]

Ultrasound therapy for a wrist or hand injury can be administered using one of three methods[93]: (1) direct coupling, in which the transducer is applied directly to the skin with a gel serving to exclude air between the skin and transducer, (2) water immersion, which is used primarily for treating irregularly shaped areas and in which the transducer should be placed approximately 2.5 cm from the surface of the area being treated, and (3) the bladder method, which uses a water-filled balloon or plastic bag coated with gel; the bladder can conform to irregularly shaped areas, and the transducer is moved over it.

Ultrasound energy has been used to drive antiinflammatory medications (cortisol, dexamethasone, salicylates, hydrocortisone) and local analgesics (lidocaine) through the skin to underlying tissue.[69] The technique to deliver this medication is termed *phonophoresis*.

Low-intensity continuous wave, or pulsed wave, modes have been used in the treatment of acute and chronic wounds to enhance the reparative process. A

Indications and contraindications for therapeutic ultrasound

Indications[37,45,51,69]	Contraindications/precautions
- Tendinitis	- Acute sprains
- Tenosynovitis	- Edematous areas
- Myositis	- Infected wounds
- Bursitis	- Osteomyelitis
- Inflamed wounds	- Epiphyseal plate
- Scar management	
- Contractures	
- Pain	
- Subacute sprains	
- Rheumatoid arthritis	

---

*Fluidotherapy Corporation, 7001 Mullins St., Suite A, Houston, TX 77081.

TABLE 28-3 Transcutaneous electric nerve stimulation (TENS) modes

Mode	Frequency (pps)	Pulse Width (SEC)	Intensity
High TENS	75-150	60	Submotor
Low TENS	2-4	200-300	Contraction
Brief, intense	125-150	150	As strong as tolerable
Burst	50-150 modulated 1-5	75-100	Contraction

number of studies[32,33,37,55] have been reported suggesting that the point at which ultrasound therapy is administered in the course of wound healing is important.

Ultrasound is a useful modality in treating wrist and hand injuries. The frequency, intensity, and duration vary depending on the depth of tissue being treated and the size of area being covered. For superficial healing or tissue treatment a 3-MHz machine is better; however, for deep tissue treatment a 1-MHz machine should be used.

Therapeutic Cold

Therapeutic cold may also be used to decrease pain, muscle spasm, and inflammation. It increases joint stiffness, however, and causes vasoconstriction. Cold is most effective when used immediately after injury and during the acute stage of healing to reduce the effects of edema.

Cold may be used both before and after exercise to reduce resultant edema. Cold is often required after treatment in rehabilitating wrist injuries.

Duration of cold treatments depends on patient tolerance. Icing may be done for 5 to 10 minutes, while cool whirlpool is usually provided for 10 to 20 minutes.

In overuse syndromes cold treatments should be continued until the joint is pain free throughout its range and edema is no longer present. In other diagnoses it is appropriate to progress to the use of heat when edema subsides or when cold is no longer effective as a preexercise modality.

Contrast Therapy

Contrast therapy may be indicated between acute and subacute phases of rehabilitation. In progressing from the use of cold to the use of heat, it may be necessary to bridge the gap between using cold or heat as a precursor to exercise. Contrast therapy consists of alternately submerging the extremity in warm water (102° F) for 2 minutes and then submerging it in cool water (55° to 65° F) for 2 minutes. Beginning with heat, five sessions should take place, always ending in cold.

Electrotherapy

To understand the effect electrotherapy has on a biologic system, a thorough understanding of muscle physiology and neurophysiology is beneficial.[40] The electrotherapy modalities available for the treatment of hand and wrist injuries are (1) high-voltage pulsed stimulation, (2) TENS, (3) low-voltage stimulation, (4) iontophoresis, (5) interferential current, (6) neuromuscular stimulation, and (7) point stimulation.

High-Voltage Pulsed Stimulation

High-voltage pulsed stimulators (HVPSs) are classified by having two distinct specifications: (1) they must be able to transmit a voltage in excess of 100 V, and (2) they must use a twin-peaked monophasic current.[40,93] HVPS with the high voltage and shorter pulse duration allows for deeper penetration of the energy. The shorter pulse width does not allow the capacitance of smaller sensory fibers (C-fibers) to be exceeded, resulting in less cutaneous sensory stimulation. The interpulse interval is much longer than the pulse duration. Because of this there is time for dissipation of the residual ions attracted to the body area; as a result the amount of physiochemical reaction beneath the electrodes is limited.[93] Because of the twin-peaked monophasic waveform, the polarity effect associated with the HVPS is mild in comparison with the effect seen with low-voltage stimulation.

Transcutaneous Electric Nerve Stimulation

TENS is defined as any stimulation in which the current is applied across the skin to stimulate nerve.[40] Various manufacturers have modified the current and the packaging to create a multitude of units, each claiming to elicit unique results. Traditionally, TENS units were designed for their pain relief function. Four modes of application with different parameters have been designed in the attempt to initiate a different pain modulation process (Table 28-3).[40,93]

Low-Voltage Stimulation

A currently less used electrotherapy modality is low-voltage (LV) stimulation. The waveforms associated with LV are faradic (asymmetric biphasic waveform rarely used today), sinusoidal, and galvanic (direct) current. LV delivers voltage up to 150 V.[40] Chemical, thermal, and physiologic events may occur when an electric low-voltage current is applied to the body. Although these responses are desired in several therapeutic situations, if not controlled they can have adverse effects on biologic tissue.[40] Because of the direct current, low voltage, and long pulse duration (1 msec), the LV direct-current stimulator can be used for denervated muscles in which maintaining muscle tone is desired.

Polarity affects the chemical responses from LV direct-current stimulators. Under the positive electrode an acidic reaction occurs, along with a tissue hardening effect and diminished nerve tissue irritability. At the negative electrode is an alkaline reaction in addition to a tissue softening effect and an increase in nerve tissue irritability.[40]

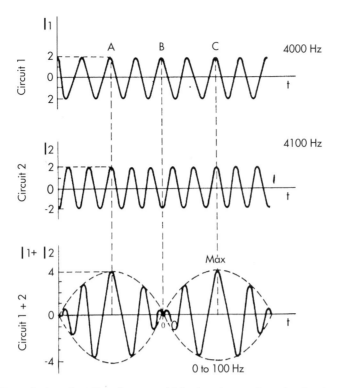

FIG. 28-27. Heterodyning of medium-frequency biphasic pulses produces low-beating interferential current.

Iontophoresis

Iontophoresis is a technique utilizing low-voltage direct current to drive medication into tissues. The electrophoretic principle that like charges repel and unlike charges attract is used with iontophoresis. A number of studies have reported the medications and polarity required to treat certain conditions.[40,92]

Interferential Current

Interferential current is another form of electrotherapy. This unit simultaneously applies two medium-frequency currents to allow a deeper penetration of the stimulation (frequency I = 4000 Hz and frequency II = 4100 Hz, with resultant beat frequency of 1-100 Hz) (Fig. 28-27).[40,93]

Higher frequency currents overcome some of the skin impedance encountered by low-frequency currents but cause minimal or no adverse response in the tissue.

Neuromuscular Stimulation

Neuromuscular stimulation is primarily used to maintain strength and flexibility and to reduce atrophy during healing. Neuromuscular stimulators, due to their parameters, must be used with an innervated muscle; they cannot be used with denervated muscles. To prevent fatigue and maximize strengthening, an interrupted (on-off) mode in current delivery should be used.[40] Several factors make the electrically induced contraction different from the volitional contraction[1]:

- When the muscle is stimulated electrically, all motor units fire in synchrony.
- There is no inhibitory reaction with the electrically induced contraction. Normally the Golgi tendon organ at the musculotendinous insertion reacts to a potentially threatening contraction by reflexively relaxing the muscle. This potentially creates a stronger contraction but removes the normal protective reflex.
- Large nerve fibers are recruited first with electrical stimulation, which is the opposite of what the body prefers to do.
- The frequency of the nerve fiber firing is also affected by electric stimulation. Muscle tetany normally occurs when a nerve fires at a frequency between 25 and 50 pps. Electric stimulators often operate at higher frequencies than those needed to achieve tetany; they thus cause fatigue to occur more rapidly.

Point Stimulation

The use of point stimulation is similar to that of acupuncture except that the points are stimulated with an electric current instead of needles.[40] Monophasic or biphasic current of significant duration is used to stimulate the small C-afferent nerve fibers. This noxious stimulation elicits a pain fiber excitation that prompts a level of pain modulation associated with descending tract inhibition.

■ ■ ■

For all electrotherapy modalities, the site where the electrodes touch the skin serves as a point of conversion between the flow of electrons and the flow of ions within the body's tissues. Properly prepared and placed electrodes increase the efficiency of the electric current while allowing for less discomfort from the treatment.[93] The current, intensity, and type of excitable tissue being stimulated are determined by a combination of electrode size and placement. The size of electrode used inversely affects the density of current; as the size of the electrode decreases, the current density increases.[2] The depth of stimulation and affected tissues stimulated are determined by placement of electrodes. When the electrodes are placed close together, the current flows superficially.[93] As the distance between the electrodes increases, the current penetrates deeper into the tissue. For the most efficient treatment session using any of the aforementioned electrotherapy modalities, knowledge about neurophysiologic and electrophysiologic principles, parameters of specific units, and electrode size and placement guidelines is critical.

Indications and contraindications for electrotherapy

Indications
- Pain
- Edema control
- Tissue healing
- Circulation improvement
- Increase joint mobility
- Scar management
- Muscle spasms
- Muscle reeducation

Contraindications
- Acute infections
- Thrombophlebitic conditions

SENSORY REEDUCATION

Before 1971 poor sensibility following nerve repair was thought to be the result of the surgical procedure. When clinicians observed patients who demonstrated different levels of functional recovery with identical levels of injury and measured clinical sensation (academic recovery), they attributed the variation to motivational factors and persistent use of the extremity.

Dellon[30] postulated that the failure of patients to achieve full recovery of functional sensation in the hand following peripheral nerve injury was related to failure by the patient to achieve full sensory potential.

Their study presented evidence to support the premise that, following nerve injury, patients could be reeducated to correctly interpret, with the cerebral cortex, the profiles of impulses that occur in response to a known peripheral stimulus. A formal sensory reeducation program is based on learning principles of attention, reenforcement, feedback, and memory to improve hand function. The patient can learn to decipher altered messages that are being sent to the brain by nerve fibers that are less populated, smaller, and disorganized when compared to their preinjury state.

Dellon's study demonstrated that the usual pattern of sensation of functional recovery in the hand occurs in the following sequence (Fig. 28-28)[29]:
1. Pain (no longer tested)
2. Vibration of 30 cps (hertz)
3. Moving touch
4. Constant touch
5. Vibration of 256 cps (hertz)

A pain-free hand is necessary before sensory reeducation is undertaken. Painful neuromas, paresthesias, and other painful situations discovered in the initial evaluation should be treated before beginning training. Their specific treatment has been discussed earlier in this chapter.

Dellon[29] has outlined detailed techniques involved in the early and late phase of sensory reeducation.

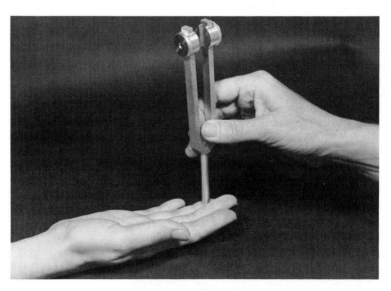

FIG. 28-28. Tuning fork used to test vibratory sense.

SPLINTS

It is not possible to provide optimal hand rehabilitation without using static or dynamic splints. Splints may be protective, supportive, or corrective in design.

Faulty positioning of a limb during either rest or activity could cause deformity if impairment of nerves, muscles, or joints is present. To successfully prevent the development of deformity, we must understand the basic pathologic condition, recognize factors that lead to deformity, and provide appropriate treatment.

Position for static immobilization

- Wrist—30 degrees dorsiflexion
- Metacarpophalangeal joints—70 degrees flexion
- Proximal interphalangeal joints—10 to 20 degrees flexion
- Thumb—Full abduction

Static Splints

When static splinting of the entire extremity is indicated, the hand and wrist should be placed in an intrinsic plus, clam digger, or antideformity position (Fig. 28-29). This preferred position of immobilization preserves the functional length of tissues. The wrist should be placed in approximately 30 degrees of dorsiflexion. The thumb should be placed in full abduction. MCP joints should be positioned in 70 degrees of flexion. PIP joints should be positioned in 10 to 20 degrees of flexion. During periods of immobilization, it is important to preserve the arches of the hand. Volar splints are best and should be fabricated to support the proximal and distal transverse arches, as well as the longitudinal arches.

The intrinsic plus position maintains ligaments of the digital joints under maximal tension, thereby preventing joint contractures. The position also encourages intrinsic tightness; however, tightness can be combated by initiating intrinsic stretching exercises. To stretch intrinsic

muscles passively, the MCP joints are placed in extension while the PIP and DIP joints are flexed (Fig. 28-30).

An alternate position for splinting the hand is in a functional position (Fig. 28-31). The wrist is placed in 30 degrees of dorsiflexion. The MCP joints are flexed in approximately 45 degrees of flexion, while the PIP joints are in 10 to 20 degrees of flexion. The thumb may be placed in opposition or adduction depending on its involvement. Care should be taken to preserve the web space. The functional position is preferred when splinting is indicated to promote relaxation.

Dynamic Splints

Dynamic splints employ traction devices such as rubber bands or springs to alter passive motion of a joint. They may be helpful in accomplishing the following objectives:

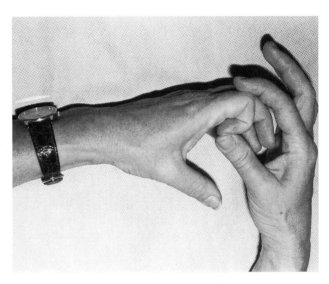

FIG. 28-30. Exercise effective in counteracting tight intrinsic muscles that may result from prolonged immobilization.

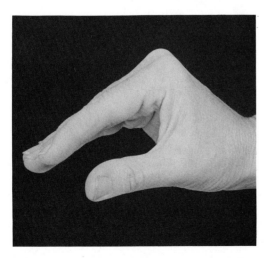

FIG. 28-29. Intrinsic plus-clam digger or antideformity position.

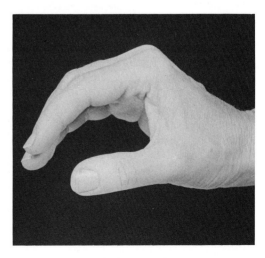

FIG. 28-31. Functional position.

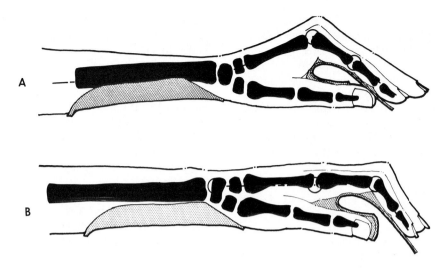

FIG. 28-32. **A,** Properly applied splint. **B,** Improperly applied splint. (From Malick MH: *Manual on dynamic hand splinting with thermoplastic materials,* Pittsburgh, 1974, Harmarville Rehabilitation Center.)

1. Prevention or correction of deformities of the hand or wrist
2. Prevention of joint stiffness by maintaining mobility
3. Strengthening of weak muscles by encouraging proper positioning and assistance
4. Increasing functional capacity of the hand by stabilizing it in a better position for function, to provide mechanical assistance

The philosophy of dynamic splinting is based on the theory of prolonged stretching of tissues, similar to that which is used by orthodontists in the bracing of teeth. The bone proximal to the joint being moved must be stabilized, and the line of pull should be at a right angle to the axis of the bone being affected.[60] The line of pull must be adjusted frequently to maintain the correct direction of pull (90 degrees) as joint motion increases.

Splints should provide adequate stretch without being painful. Patients should be aware of a pulling sensation but not of pain. Rather than prescribing a structured routine, the therapist should instruct the patient to wear the splint until reaching maximal tolerance, at which time the splint should be removed. Wearing time may be relatively short at first but should quickly increase. If wearing time does not progress, the splint should be checked. Lack of effectiveness may be caused by an ill-fitting splint, excessive tension applied to the bands, or in inadequate healing that does not allow tolerance of the forces exerted by the splint. Splinting programs should be supplemented with an exercise program and encouragement of functional use of the extremity.

Dynamic splints provided to improve mobility should not be used for exercising because pulling against the bands strengthens the opposite motion the splint was designed to improve.

Precautions

Splints should be checked often. Ill-fitting splints can contribute to rather than prevent deformity (Fig. 28-32).

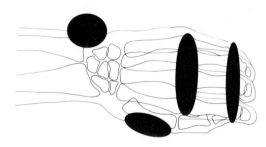

FIG. 28-33. Dorsal view of pressure areas to consider when fabricating splints. (From Malick MH: *Manual on dynamic hand splinting with thermoplastic materials,* Pittsburgh, 1974, Harmarville Rehabilitation Center.)

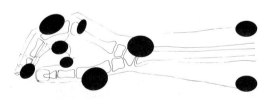

FIG. 28-34. Radial view of pressure areas to consider when fabricating splints. (From Malick MH: *Manual on dynamic hand splinting with thermoplastic materials,* Pittsburgh, 1974, Harmarville Rehabilitation Center.)

Changes in hand volume and improvement in motion necessitate splint alteration. Caution should be taken to avoid creating irritation over bony prominances caused by friction.[59,60] This is especially important when fabricating splints that will be worn during functional use of the extremity. In the hand, pressure areas may occur over the heads of the metacarpals, the pisiform, and the base of the first metacarpal (Fig. 28-33). In the forearm the radial and styloid processes may create similar problems (Fig. 28-34). Eliminating pressure over bony prom-

inences may be done in several ways. Avoiding the area, dispersing pressure over a larger area, or padding are all acceptable means of avoidance. Padding is most often used when protective splints are fabricated for use during athletic activity.

Techniques to eliminate pressure on bony prominences

- Padding
- Avoiding the area
- Dispensing pressure over greater area

Materials

Protective splints for the hand and wrist fabricated from low-temperature thermoplastic materials provide rigid support. The materials have a plastic base and change from a hard state to a malleable state when heat is applied. The reaction of splinting materials to heat varies with the type of material. Temperature extremes in either direction may influence construction techniques. Overheating causes blistering, stretching, and surface irregularities; underheating may produce rough edges and an inequality of pliability.

Splint construction may be influenced by the type of heat used. Some materials require moist heat, whereas others respond to either dry or moist heat. Thickness and rigidity of splinting materials should be considered. Bulky material interferes with dexterity, and thin material may not be strong enough to withstand the pressure placed on it during athletic activity. The use of perforated rather than unperforated splinting material should be considered in the fabrication of protective athletic splints. In our experience several splints made from perforated materials have broken in areas of high stress, making their use inadvisable for protection in sports that require heavy repetitive activity. Splints must be supportive along certain planes of movement but flexible in others.

Soft splints have semirigidity and some pliability and may become more common in the future as we fully understand their desirable properties. Although commercial soft splints enjoy heavy use among recreational athletes, their effectiveness for protection of joints with specific injuries and in contact sports is not well documented in the scientific literature. Soft splints are, however, less apt to create potential injuries to others than rigid splints.

Softcast* is a relatively new casting material used for the fabrication of semirigid athletic protective playing splints. While providing adequate protection for subacute and chronic injuries to the hand and wrist, the end product remains soft and pliable enough to meet the on-field requirements of officials for most sports without the need for additional padding.† The casting material is applied over stockinette. Additional protection may be obtained by incorporating tape moleskin or low-temperature splinting materials into the casting process.[35] Unlike traditional casting materials, Softcast can be either un-

wound or cut with standard bandage scissors. Monovalving and reapplication with Coban or an elastic bandage allow the athlete to apply ice to the involved area.

Protective Splints

When designing protective splints for use in contact sports, the following factors should be considered: Is adequate protection of the injury provided to prevent subsequent injury? Will the athlete be able to compete safely and effectively? Is the splint fabricated from material that is hard and unyielding and could possibly cause injury to opposing players?

The trainer must have basic knowledge of anatomy and kinesiology of the hand, as well as familiarity with the level of skill required of each athlete.

Having access to athletic equipment in the clinic or training room allows a better functional position for immobilization, thereby permitting the athlete to perform all aspects of activity, for example, a baseball player should be able to grasp and release a bat. Having equipment available allows the therapist to immobilize the patient's finger in a compromised position that permits adequate mobility to perform all aspects of the sport (Fig. 28-35).

When fabricating splints, as much length as possible should be maintained for mechanical leverage (Fig. 28-36). Care should be taken not to restrict motion of uninvolved joints. Skin creases created by joints are helpful landmarks to use in designing finger splints (Fig. 28-37).

While at rest the transverse metacarpal arch takes on a concave appearance (Fig. 28-38). When the hand is engaged in functional activities, the arch becomes even more pronounced (Fig. 28-39). The second and third metacarpals are immobile, while the first, fourth, and fifth metacarpals are mobile. Failure to accommodate the transverse metacarpal arch into splints, casts, or protective gear results in decreased dexterity and the need for further joint mobilization when splinting is discontinued (Fig. 28-40).

The longitudinal arch consists of MCP, PIP, and DIP joint flexion. Positioning of the longitudinal arch during splinting is dictated by the medical condition. Possible positions include intrinsic plus, functional position, and optimal position for athletic participation.

Metacarpophalangeal Joint and Wrist

Safe support for the wrist or MCP joint should be circumferential. Fiberglass or silicone casts provide an excellent means of protection. Rules regarding acceptable protective splints vary between states, as well as between professional, college, and high school teams.

If adequately padded, fiberglass or regular casts are allowed. This method provides excellent protection and eliminates the need for changing casts. Another means of protection is the soft or silicone rubber cast. Initially introduced in the 1970s, soft casts are widely used today in both sports medicine and hand clinics.[8]

RTV silicone is available in 1- or 12-lb containers. Because not all casts require 1 lb of silicone, much material is wasted. Buying the larger quantity and dividing it into 4-oz portions may be a reasonable and economical solution to the problem of wasted material (see p. 629).

---

*Scotchcast, 3M Health Care, St. Paul, MN.
†R. Poole, personal communication, 1993.

FIG. 28-35. Protective device molded to allow maximal function.

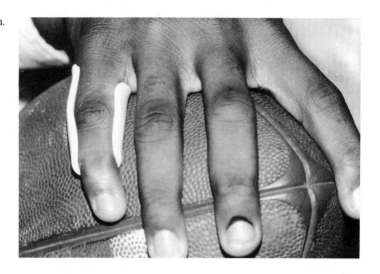

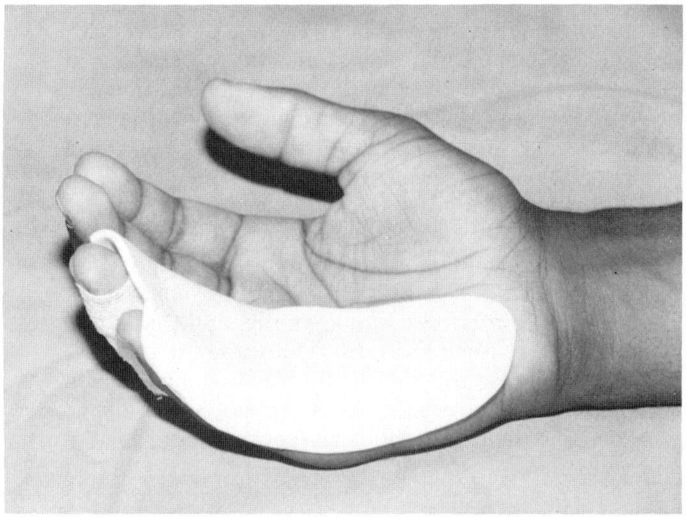

FIG. 28-36. Protection should be of adequate length but should not limit mobility of uninvolved joints.

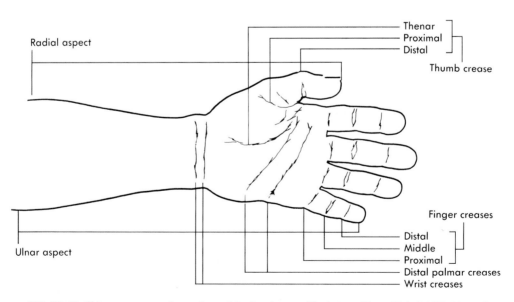

Radial aspect

Thenar
Proximal
Distal

Thumb crease

Ulnar aspect

Finger creases

Distal
Middle
Proximal

Distal palmar creases
Wrist creases

FIG. 28-37. Skin creases on volar surface of the hand created by joints. (From Malick MH: *Manual on static hand splinting*, Pittsburgh, 1972, Harmarville Rehabilitation Center.)

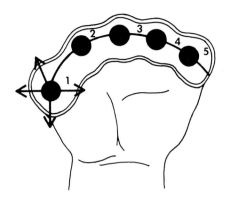

FIG. 28-38. Transverse metacarpal arch at rest. (From Malick MH: *Manual on dynamic hand splinting with thermoplastic materials,* Pittsburgh, 1974, Harmarville Rehabilitation Center.)

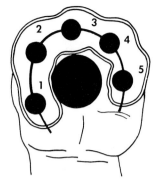

FIG. 28-39. Transverse metacarpal arch during function. (From Malick MH: *Manual on dynamic hand splinting with thermoplastic materials,* Pittsburgh, 1974, Harmarville Rehabilitation Center.)

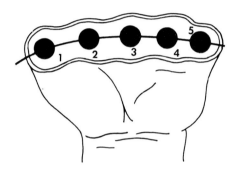

FIG. 28-40. Transverse metacarpal arch, nonfunctional position. (From Malick MH: *Manual on dynamic hand splinting with thermoplastic materials,* Pittsburgh, 1974, Harmarville Rehabilitation Center.)

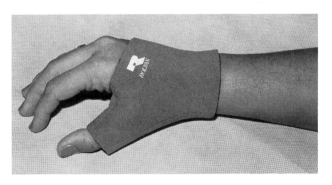

FIG. 28-41. Commercially available soft splint often used by recreational athletes to control thumb pain.

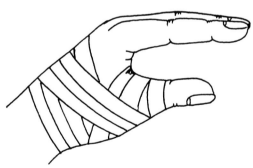
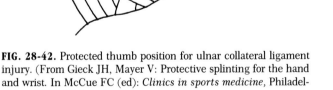

FIG. 28-42. Protected thumb position for ulnar collateral ligament injury. (From Gieck JH, Mayer V: Protective splinting for the hand and wrist. In McCue FC (ed): *Clinics in sports medicine,* Philadelphia, 1986, WB Saunders.)

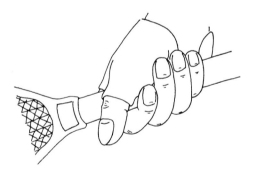

FIG. 28-43. Metacarpophalangeal joint protection. (From Gieck JH, Mayer V: Protective splinting for the hand and wrist. In McCue FC (ed): *Clinics in sports medicine,* Philadelphia, 1986, WB Saunders.)

RTV may be stored in the refrigerator. Larger quantities may be stored in the freezer, which seems to increase its shelf life.

Thumb

When adequate healing has occurred, safe and effective protection should be provided to allow the athlete to return to participation. In designing thumb protection, it is important to consider the diagnosis and the position the athlete plays (Fig. 28-41). Stability is always more important than mobility. The proper position of protection is essential, because protection in an improper position may cause reinjury. When positioning the thumb from ulnar collateral ligament (UCL) injuries, the carpometacarpal (CMC) joint should be slightly flexed and adducted. Protection should prevent extension and abduction, the mechanism that created the initial injury (Fig. 28-42).

Methods of thumb protection may be provided by various means: using low-temperature plastic (Fig. 28-43);

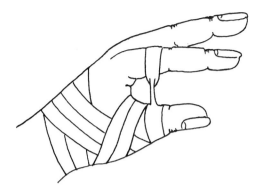

FIG. 28-44. Buddy taping. (From Gieck JH, Mayer V: Protective splinting for the hand and wrist. In McCue FC (ed): *Clinics in sports medicine,* Philadelphia, 1986, WB Saunders.)

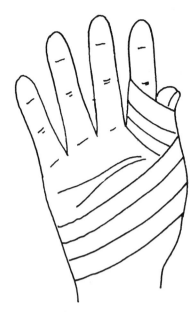

FIG. 28-45. Maximal thumb stability. (From Gieck JH, Mayer V: Protective splinting for the hand and wrist. In McCue FC (ed): *Clinics in sports medicine,* Philadelphia, 1986, WB Saunders.)

taping the index finger to the thumb to provide a buddy type of anchor (Fig. 28-44); or taping the thumb to the hand for stability (Fig. 28-45). Obviously, this method of protection is not suitable for ball handlers.

PROTECTIVE EQUIPMENT

Many types of commercial gloves are available to protect athletes' hand from injury. Such protection should be used whenever it is available. Lacrosse gloves are well designed, since they allow adequate function while providing protection. Most hand injuries in lacrosse players today occur because the player alters or cuts away some of the glove's protection to afford better mobility.

Baseball catchers may add padding to the palms of their mitts to reduce shock and consequently decrease the possibility of developing thromboses or aneurysms of the radial or ulnar arteries.

Skiers should not wear short gloves. Long gloves can protect a skier's wrists from injuries such as cuts, which may occur from the edge of a ski.[61] Children's ski gloves should be checked to ensure that they are long enough to be protective.

It is recommended that long-distance cyclists wear padded gloves. Extra padding in the hypothenar region helps to decrease prolonged pressure from handlebars. Pressure in this area can cause compressure of the ulnar nerve through Guyon's canal. Adaptations may be provided to the athlete's glove or sports equipment to allow practice of skills before having adequate mobility to compete (Fig. 28-46).

Rules

In some cases injuries to the hand and wrist are unavoidable due to the nature of hand involvement dictated by the rules or the environment of the sport. In other cases such injuries point out the need for better protective equipment and training.

In the National Collegiate Athletic Association the rules governing mandatory equipment and equipment use vary by sport.[73] Further variations exist between men's and women's rules, for example, protective gloves

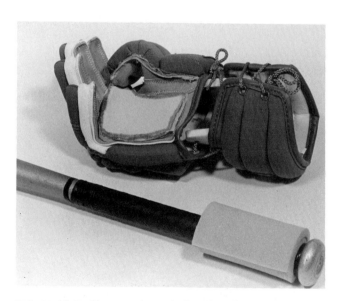

FIG. 28-46. Padding may be applied to the palmar aspect of a lacrosse glove to compensate for limited grasp. A padded bat would better suit a similar need in a baseball player. (From Gieck JH, Mayer V: Protective splinting for the hand and wrist. In McCue FC (ed): *Clinics in sports medicine,* Philadelphia, 1986, WB Saunders.)

are mandatory only in men's lacrosse. Their rules state that "in men's basketball elbow, hand, finger, wrist or forearm guards, casts or braces made of leather, plaster, pliable (soft) plastic, metal or any other hard substance, always shall be declared illegal." In football "hard abrasive or unyielding substances on the hand, wrist, forearm or elbow are prohibited unless covered on all sides with closed-cell foam padding." In wrestling, rules gov-

---

Instructions for fabricating silicone rubber casts[93]

Supplies needed

Tongue blades
Vaseline
4 rolls of Kling* a silicone compound
Scissors
One 2- or 3-inch Ace wrap
Talcum powder
Approximately 1 lb RTV 11 silicone and catalyst

1-inch adhesive tape
Paper towels
Topper sponge gauze strip or 1/16-inch polyform strip
Plastic covering for work surface

Method of fabrication

Divide 1 lb of silicone into four 4-oz containers.
Add 20 drops of catalyst per 4 oz (only mix when needed).
Tape area to be protected.
Cover area of the hand, wrist, and forearm to be supported within the rubber cast with Vaseline to prevent silicone from adhering to skin tape.
Loosely wrap the hand-forearm with enough Kling for 2 layers, then apply prepared silicone with the tongue blade. Smooth out and cover well.
Loosely wrap another two layers of Kling and apply more silicone. At this point internal support is added. We use a strip of polyform to add support to the fracture site, but ½- × 2-inch strips of topper also work well. Impregnate the topper sponge, then put into position.
Continue to wrap Kling—three layers before applying silicone thereafter. Prepare additional silicone as needed. Most splints require 12 to 16 oz of silicone. We suggest using all of the Kling and silicone. Wipe away excess with a paper towel.
After the rubber cast is completed, wrap loosely with a plastic wrap, then the 2- or 3-inch Ace wrap. Do not press or squeeze rubber cast while it is curing.
Curing time is approximately 3 hours.
To remove, cut along ulnar border with bandage scissors.
Trim splint and check fit.
Remove tape, wipe Vaseline off arm with paper towels, then wash with soap and water.
Silicone casts are nonporous and should only be worn during practice and games. The hand and forearm should be dusted with powder before wearing the rubber cast. The cast is held in place with adhesive tape. If worn for more than several hours at a time, the skin may become macerated. Fiberglass or regular hard casts should be worn during the day as well as during practice.

*General Electric Silicone Products Department, Waterford, NY.

---

erning special protective equipment declare that "any mechanical device that does not permit normal movement of the joints and prevents one's opponent from applying normal holds is prohibited."

The National Federation of State High School Associations governs the regulation of mandatory equipment and equipment use of high school athletes. Previously rules did not allow football players to wear any protection on the forearm, wrist or hand that was considered to be hard regardless of how much padding was applied as a covering. Experimentation is being pursued. Currently four state high school leagues allow players to use "special protective equipment made of a hard substance provided all exterior surfaces are covered with closed-cell foam padding no less than one-half inch thick, or an alternative material of the same minimum thickness and similar physical properties is permitted to protect an injury as directed by a physician in writing."* Future rule changes may be forthcoming depending on the statistics gathered by the participating high schools.

Prevention

In most cases the athletic trainer is the first to see hand and wrist injuries incurred during competition or practice. Serious injury and poor results can often be pre-

*Virginia High School League, Inc., Charlottesville, personal communication, 1993.

vented by early recognition and prompt referral to the team physician. The athletes' tendency is usually to disregard hand and wrist injuries. They are usually satisfied with self-taping or padding so long as they can continue to compete.

After a comprehensive evaluation, the physician must determine when treatment must be carried out without creating harmful effects to the athlete's future abilities. Is early treatment mandatory? Are conservative treatment and protection adequate? Is it early or late in the season? Often prompt definitive treatment may allow the athlete to return to play before the season ends. In other situations it may be possible to delay treatment until the end of the season. Adult athletes should be allowed to participate in this decision if a choice exists. Improperly treated injuries of the hand and wrist can result in permanent loss of function.

Because of the significant potential for injury, special attention should be given to protecting athletes' hands from high-speed objects or the external forces that produce contusion or shearing. Gloves and other protective devices should be used whenever possible to prevent injury (Figs. 28-47 to 28-49).

In some sports athletes are allowed to wear their personal preference in glove wear, whereas others are required to wear regulation gloves. Some athletes choose to avoid hand protection because they believe gloves interfere with tactile sensation and flexibility.

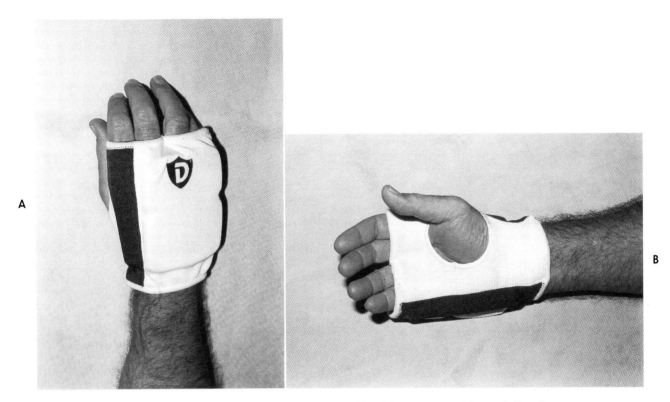

FIG. 28-47. Lineman's glove protects dorsal aspect of hand from contusional forces. **A,** Dorsal view. **B,** Volar view.

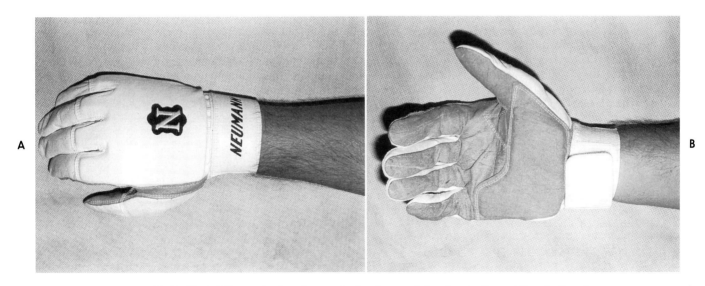

FIG. 28-48. Typical lineman's glove features both palmar and dorsal protective padding. **A,** Dorsal view. **B,** Volar view.

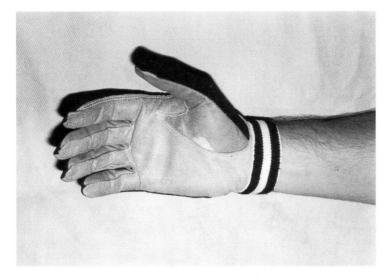

FIG. 28-49. Receiver's glove provides palmar padding and a tacky surface to enhance ball handling.

There is little to be offered in protection against injuries caused by the dynamics of a fall on an outstretched hand or arm. Rules governing the use of hands and arms are constantly being revised, particularly in blocking techniques. The line between the protection of injured parts and protection that allows more vigorous use of the extremity is particularly difficult to draw.

ACKNOWLEDGMENT

The authors gratefully acknowledge Robin Hamill and Gail Hall for their services in preparing discussions on sympathetically maintained pain and electrotherapy, respectively.

REFERENCES

1. Adams L, Green L, Topoozian E: Range of motion in clinical assessment recommendation, ed 2, Chicago, 1992, American Society of Hand Therapists.
2. American Academy of Orthopaedic Surgeons: *Joint motion: method of measuring and recording,* Chicago, 1965, American Academy of Orthopaedic Surgeons.
3. American Society of Hand Therapists: *Clinical assessment recommendations,* Chicago, 1992, American Society of Hand Therapists.
4. American Society for Surgery of the Hand: *The hand—examination and diagnosis,* Aurora, Ill, 1978, American Society for Surgery of the Hand.
5. Arnheim DD: *Modern principles of athletic training,* ed 7, St Louis, 1989, Mosby.
6. Aulicino P: Neurovascular injuries in the hands of athletes, *Hand Clin* 6(3):455, 1990.
7. Baron M et al: Hand function in the elderly: relation to osteoarthritis, *J Rheumatol* 14:4, 1987.
8. Basset FH, Malone T, Gilchrist R: A protective splint of silicone rubber, *Am J Sports Med* 7:358, 1970.
9. Beasley R: Rehabilitation of the hand. In Hunter J et al (eds): *Rehabilitation of the hand,* St Louis, 1978, Mosby.
10. Bechtol CO: Grip test: the use of a dynamometer with adjustable handle spacings, *J Bone Joint Surg* 36A:820, 1954.
11. Bell AT, Horton PG: The use and abuse of hydrotherapy in athletics: a review, *Athl Train* 22(2):115, 1987.
12. Bohannon RW: Whirlpool versus whirlpool and rinse for removal of bacteria from a venous stasis ulcer, *Phys Ther* 62(3):304, 1982.
13. Bonelli S et al: Regional intravenous guanethidine vs stellate ganglion block in reflex sympathetic dystrophies: a randomized trial, *Pain* 16:297, 1983.
14. Borrell RM et al: Fluidotherapy: evaluation of a new heat modality, *Arch Phys Med Rehabil* 58:69, 1977.
15. Borrell RM et al: Comparison of in vivo temperatures produced by hydrotherapy, paraffin wax treatment, and fluidotherapy, *Phys Ther* 69:1273, 1980.
16. Bowden REM: Factors influencing functional recovery. In Seddon HJ (ed): *Peripheral nerve injuries,* London, 1954, Her Majesty's Stationery Printing Office.
17. Boyes JH: Dupuytren's contracture: notes on the age of onset and the relationship to handedness, *Am J Surg* 88:147, 1954.
18. Boyes JH: *Bunnell's surgery of the hand,* ed 5, Philadelphia, 1970, JB Lippincott.
19. Brand PW: *Clinical mechanics of the hand,* St Louis, 1985, Mosby.
20. Brand PW, Wood H: *Hand volumeter instruction sheet,* Carville, La, 1973, U.S. Public Health Service Hospital.
21. Brown M: The well elderly. In Guccione A (ed): *Geriatric physical therapy,* St Louis, 1993, Mosby.
22. Brown M, Coggan A: Is muscle wasting inevitable with aging? *Med Sci Sports Exerc* 22:434, 1990 (abstract).
23. Buchout BC, Warner MA: Digital perfusion of handball players: effects of repeated ball impact on the structures of the hand, *Am J Sports Med* 8(3):206, 1980.
24. Burke ER: Ulnar neuropathy in bicyclists, *Phys Sports Med* 9(4):53, 1981.
25. Cahalan T et al: Biomechanics of the golf swing in players with pathologic conditions of the forearm, wrist, and hand, *Am J Sports Med* 19(3):288, 1991.
26. Cambridge CA: Range of motion measurements of the hand. In Hunter JM et al (eds): *Rehabilitation of the hand,* ed 3, St Louis, 1990, Mosby.
27. Campbell CS: Gamekeepers thumb, *J Bone Joint Surg* 37B:148, 1955.
28. Crawford GP: The molded polythene splint for mallet finger deformities, *J Hand Surg* 9A:231, 1984.
29. Dellon AL: The moving 2 point discrimination test: clinical evaluation of the quickly-adapting fiber receptor system, *J Hand Surg* 3:474, 1978.
30. Dellon AL: *Evaluation of sensibility and re-education of sensation in the hand,* Baltimore, 1981, Williams & Wilkins.

31. Dobyns JH et al: Bowler's thumb: diagnosis and treatment; a review of seventeen cases, *J Bone Joint Surg* 54A:751, 1972.
32. Dyson M, Luke DA: Induction of mast cells degranulation in skin by ultrasound, *IEEFE Trans Ultrason, Ferroelect Freq Control* 33:194, 1986.
33. Dyson M et al: The stimulation of tissue regeneration by means of ultrasound, *Clin Sci* 35:274, 1968.
34. Early PF: Population studies in Dupuytren's contracture, *J Bone Joint Surg* 44B:602, 1962.
35. Farley KL, Sublette JB: Upper extremity semi-rigid support, *J Athletic Training* 27(1):88, 1992.
36. Fisk G: The relationship of manual labor and specific injury to Dupuytren's disease. In Hueston JT, Tubiana R (eds): *Dupuytren's disease,* ed 2, Edinburgh, 1985, Churchill Livingstone.
37. Fyfe MC, Chahl LA: The effect of ultrasound on experimental oedema in rats, *Ultrasound Med Biol* 6:107, 1980.
38. Gibson CT, Manske PR: Carpal tunnel syndrome in the adolescent, *J Hand Surg* 12A(2):279, 1987.
39. Gieck JH, Saliba EN: Application of modalities in overuse syndrome, *Clin Sports Med* 6(2):427, 1987.
40. Gieck JH, Saliba EN: The athletic trainer and rehabilitation. In Kulund D (ed): *The injured athlete,* Philadelphia, 1988, JB Lippincott.
41. Goldstein A: Opioid peptides and endorphins in pituitary and brain, *Science* 193:1081, 1976.
42. Greenberg S, Braun R: Therapeutic uses of the air bag splint for the injured hand, *Am J Occup Ther* 31:38, 1977.
43. Hagberg JM et al: Cardiovascular responses of 70-79 year old men and women to exercise training, *J Appl Physiol* 66:2589, 1989.
44. Ho PK, Dellon AL, Wilgis EFS: True aneurysms of the hand resulting from athletic injury: report of two cases, *Am J Sports Med* 13(2):136, 1985.
45. Hoogland R: *Ultrasound therapy,* ed 2, Delft, Holland, 1989, Enraf-Nonius.
46. Hoppenfeld S: *Physical examination of the spine and extremities,* Norwalk, Conn, 1976, Appleton-Century-Crofts.
47. Hord AH et al: Intravenous regional bretylium and lidocaine for treatment of reflex sympathetic dystrophy: a randomized, double-blind study, *Anesth Analg* 74:818, 1992.
48. Hueston JT, Seyfer AE: Some medicolegal aspects of Dupuytren's contracture, *Hand Clin* 7(4):617, 1991.
49. Kaltenborn F: *Manual therapy for the extremity joints: specialized techniques, tests and joint mobilization,* ed 2, Oslo, Norway, 1976, Olaf Norlis Bokhandel.
50. Kiefhaber TR, Stern P: Upper extremity tendinitis and overuse syndrome in the athlete, *Clin Sports Med* 11(1):39, 1992.
51. Kloth LC, McCulloch JM, Feedar JA: *Wound healing: alternatives in management,* Philadelphia, 1990, FA Davis.
52. Larsson L, Grimby G, Karlsson J: Muscle strength and speed of movement in relation to age and muscle morphology, *J Appl Physiol* 46:451, 1979.
53. Lipscombe PR: Tenosynovitis of the hand and wrist: carpal tunnel syndrome, de Quervain's disease, trigger digit, *Clin Orthop* 13:164, 1959.
54. Lowrey CW et al: Digital vessels trauma from repetitive impact in baseball catchers, *J Hand Surg* 1(3):236, 1976.
55. Lundborg G, Rank F: Experimental intrinsic healing of flexor tendons based upon synovial fluid nutrition, *J Hand Surg* 3:21, 1978.
56. MacKenney RP: A population study of Dupuytren's contracture, *Hand* 15:155, 1983.
57. Malick M: *Manual on static hand splinting,* Pittsburgh, 1970, Harmarville Rehabilitation Center.
58. Malick M: *Manual on dynamic hand splinting with thermoplastic materials,* Pittsburgh, 1974, Harmarville Rehabilitation Center.
59. Malick MH, Carr JA: Flexible elastomer molds in burn scar control, *Am J Occup Ther* 34(9):603, 1980.
60. Malick MH, Carr JA: *Manual on management of the burn patient,* Pittsburgh, 1982, Harmarville Rehabilitation Center, Educational Resource Division.
61. Match RM: Laceration of the median nerve from skiing, *Am J Sports Med* 6:22, 1978.
62. Matheson GO et al: Musculoskeletal injuries associated with physical activity in older adults, *Med Sci Sports Exerc* 21:379, 1989.
63. McCaroll JR: Golf. In Schneider RC, Kennedy JC, Plant ML (eds): *Sports injuries: mechanisms, prevention and treatment,* Baltimore, 1985, Williams & Wilkins.
64. McCaroll JR: Golf: common injuries from a supposedly benign activity, *J Musculoskel Med* 3(5):9, 1986.
65. McCue FC et al: A pseudoboutonnière deformity, *J Br Soc Surg Hand* 7:166, 1975.
66. McFarland RM: Some observations on the epidemiology of Dupuytren's disease. In Hueston JT, Tubiana R (eds): *Dupuytren's disease,* ed 2, Edinburgh, 1985, Churchill Livingstone.
67. Melzak R, Wall PD: Pain mechanism: a new theory, *Science* 150:971, 1965.
68. Mennell J: *Joint pain: diagnosis and treatment using manipulative techniques,* Boston, 1964, Little, Brown.
69. Michlovitz SL: Thermal agents in rehabilitation. Philadelphia, 1990, FA Davis.
70. Moberg E: Objective methods for determining the functional value of sensibility of the hand, *J Bone Joint Surg* 40B:454, 1958.
71. Moberg E: Criticism and study of methods of examining sensibility in the hand, *Neurology* 12:8, 1962.
72. Napier J: The prehensile movements of the human hand, *J Bone Joint Surg* 38B:902, 1956.
73. *NCAA Guide Line—Protective Equipment 4A,* revised June 1991.
74. Nelson RM, Currier DP: *Clinical electrotherapy,* Norwalk, Conn, 1987, Appleton & Lange.
75. Nieder H et al: Reduction of skin bacterial load with use of the therapeutic whirlpool, *Phys Ther* 55(5):482, 1975.
76. Osterman AL, Moskow L, Low DW: Soft tissue injuries of the hand and wrist in racquet sports, *Clin Sports Med* 7(2):329, 1988.
77. Paris S: *Extremity dysfunction and mobilization* (prepublication edition), St Augustine, Fla, 1980, Institute Press.
78. Parker RD et al: Hook of the hamate fractures in athletes, *Am J Sports Med* 14(6):517, 1986.
79. Peterson P et al: Grip strength and hand dominance: challenging the 10% rule, *Am J Occup Ther* 43:444, 1989.
80. Pitner MA: Pathophysiology of overuse injuries in the hand and wrist, *Hand Clin* 6(3):355, 1990.
81. Rayan GM: Stenosing tenosynovitis in bowlers, *Am J Sports Med* 18(2):214, 1990.
82. Rayan GM, Mullins PT: Skin necrosis complicating mallet finger splinting and vascularity of the distal interphalangeal joint overlying skin, *J Hand Surg* 12A(4):548, 1987.
83. Rocco AG et al: A comparison of regional intravenous guanethidine and reserpine in reflex sympathetic dystrophy: a controlled, randomized, double-blind crossover study, *Clin J Pain* 5(3):205, 1989.
84. Schmidt TT, Toews JV: Grip strength as measured by the Jamar dynamometer, *Arch Phys Med Rehabil* 51(6):321, 1970.
85. Schwartzman RJ: Reflex sympathetic dystrophy and causalgia, *Neurol Clin* 10(4):953, 1992.
86. Schwartzman RJ, McLellan TL: Reflex sympathetic dystrophy: a review, *Arch Neurol* 44(5):555, 1987.
87. Seals DR et al: Endurance training in older men and women: cardiovascular responses to exercise, *J Appl Physiol* 57:1024, 1984.
88. Seddon H: *Surgical disorders of peripheral nerves,* ed 2, New York, 1975, Churchill Livingstone.
89. Shiffman L: Effects of aging on hand function, *Am J Occup Ther* 46(9):785, 1992.
90. Smith A: Diagnosis and indications for surgical treatment, *Hand Clin* 7(4):635, 1991.
91. Snyder-Mackler L: The older athlete. In Guccione A (ed): *Geriatric physical therapy,* St Louis, 1993, Mosby.

92. Snyder-Mackler L, Robinson AJ: Clinical electrophysiology: electrotherapy and electrophysiology testing, Baltimore, 1981, William & Wilkins.

93. Starkey C: *Therapeutic modalities for athletic trainers,* Philadelphia, 1993, FA Davis.

94. Stern P: Tendinitis, overuse syndromes, and tendon injuries, *Hand Clin* 6(3):467, 1990.

95. Sugawara M et al: Digital ischemia in baseball players, *Am J Sports Med* 14(4):329, 1986.

96. Vasudevan SV, Melvin JL: Upper extremity edema control: rationale of the techniques, *Am J Occup Ther* 33(8):520, 1979.

97. Wagner JA et al: Heat tolerance and acclimatization to work in the heat in relation to age, *J Appl Physiol* 33:616, 1972.

98. Wehbé MA: Differential tendon gliding in the hand, *J Hand Surg* 9:596, 1984.

99. Wehbé MA: Tendon gliding exercises, *Am J Occup Ther* 41(3):164, 1987.

100. Wehbé MA, Hunter JM: Flexor tendon gliding in the hand. Part I. In vivo excursions, *J Hand Surg* 10A:570, 1985.

101. Wehbé MA, Hunter JM: Flexor tendon gliding in the hand. Part II. Differential gliding, *J Hand Surg* 10A:575, 1985.

102. Wilmarth MA, Nelson SG: Distal sensory latencies of the ulnar nerve in long distance bicyclists: pilot study, *J Sports Phys Ther* 9(11):370, 1988.

103. Yerxa EJ et al: Development of a hand test for use in desensitization of the hypersensitive hand, *Am J Occup Ther* 37(3):176, 1983.

104. Yokota T, Furukawa T, Tsukagoshi H: Motor paresis improved by sympathetic block: a motor form of reflex sympathetic dystrophy? *Arch Neurol* 46:683, 1989.

ADDITIONAL READINGS

Barr N: *The hand: principles and techniques of simple splintmaking in rehabilitation,* London, 1975, Butterworth.

Bergfeld JA et al: Soft playing splint for protection of significant hand and wrist injuries in sports, *Am J Sports Med* 10:293, 1982.

Birrer RB: Sports medicine for the primary care physician, Norwalk, Conn, 1984, Appleton-Century-Crofts.

Black SH: Blisters and torn hands disrupt gymnasts' training, *First Aider* 48(6):10, 1979.

Blazina ME, Lane C: Rupture of the inserter of the flexor digitorum profundus tendon in student athletes, *J Am Coll Health Assoc* 14:248, 1966.

Borrell RM, Henley EJ: Fluidotherapy in a hand clinic, *Arch Phys Med Rehabil* 60:536, 1979.

Cannon N: *Manual of hand splinting,* New York, 1985, Churchill Livingstone.

Carroll RE, Match RM: Avulsion of the profundus tendon insertion, *J Trauma* 10:1109, 1970.

Chang WH, Thoms OJ, White WL: Avulsion injury of the long flexor tendons, *Plast Reconstr Surg* 50:260, 1972.

Cohn BT, Froimson AI: Case report of a rare mallet finger injury, *Orthopedics* 9(4):529, 1986.

Commandre F, Viani JL: The football keeper's thumb, *J Sports Med Phys Fitness* 16(2):121, 1976.

Conn J, Bergan JJ, Bell JL: Hypothenar hammer syndrome posttraumatic digital ischemia, *Surgery* 68:1122, 1970.

Cooney WP: Sports injuries to the upper extremity: how to recognize and deal with some common problems, *Postgrad Med* 76(4):45, 1984.

Culver JE: Instabilities of the wrist, *Clin Sports Med* 5(4):725, 1986.

Culver JE et al: Avulsion of the profundus and superficialis tendons of the ring finger, *Am J Sports Med* 9(3):184, 1981.

Dawson WJ, Pullos N: Baseball injuries to the hand, *Ann Emerg Med* 10(6):302, 1981.

Dellon AL, Jabaley ME: Reeducation of sensation in the hand following nerve suture, *Clin Orthop* 162:75, 1982.

Dobyns JH, Sim FH, Linscheid RL: Sports stress syndromes of the hand and wrist, *Am J Sports Med* 6(5):236, 1978.

Doran GA: Towards preventing reinjury in contact sport, *J Sports Med Phys Fitness* 24(2):90, 1984.

Dunham W et al: Bowler's thumb, *Clin Orthop* 83:99, 1972.

Eckman PB et al: Ulnar neuropathy in bicycle riders, *Arch Neurol* 32:130, 1975.

Ellsasser JC, Stein AH: Management of hand injuries in a professional football team, *Am J Sports Med* 7(3):178, 1979.

Fess E, Phillips C: *Hand splinting: principles and methods,* ed 2, St Louis, 1987, Mosby.

Ganel A, Aharonson Z, Engel J: Gamekeeper's thumb: injuries of the ulnar collateral ligament of the metacarpophalangeal joint, *Br J Sports Med* 14(2/3):92, 1980.

Gerber C, Senn E, Matter F: Skier's thumb: surgical treatment of recent injuries to the ulnar collateral ligament of the thumb's metacarpophalangeal joint, *Am J Sports Med* 9(3):171, 1981.

Gieck J, Buxton BP: Reflex sympathetic dystrophy, *Athl Train* 22(2):120, 1987.

Gieck JH, Mayer V: Protective splinting of the hand and wrist, *Clin Sports Med* 5(4):795, 1986.

Gieck JH, McCue F: Conservative treatment and rehabilitation of athletic injuries to soft tissue of the hand, *J Natl Athl Train Assoc* 318:56, 1971.

Johnson RP: The acutely injured wrist and its residuals, *Clin Orthop* 149:33, 1980.

Kettelkamp DB, Flatt AE, Moulds R: Traumatic dislocation of the long finger extensor tendon: a clinical, anatomical, and biomechanical study, *J Bone Joint Surg* 53A:229, 1971.

Kiel JH: *Basic hand splinting: a pattern designing approach,* Boston, 1983, Little, Brown.

Knight KL: Taping a mallet finger, *Phys Sports Med* 133(11):140, 1985.

Lampe GN: *TENS technology and physiology,* Randolph, Me, 1984, Codman & Shurtleff.

Leach RE: The prevention and rehabilitation of soft tissue injuries, *Int J Sports Med* 3:18, 1982.

Leddy JP, Coyle MP Jr: Injuries of the flexor and extensor tendons, *Prim Care* 7(2):259, 1980.

Leddy JP, Packer JW: Avulsion of the profundus insertion in athletes, *J Hand Surg* 2:66, 1977.

Linscheid RL, Dobyns JH: Athletic injuries of the wrist, *Clin Orthop* 198:141, 1985.

Linscheid RL et al: Traumatic instability of the wrist, *J Bone Joint Surg* 54:1612, 1972.

Lunn PG, Lamb DW: "Rugby finger"—avulsion of profundus of ring finger, *J Hand Surg* 9(1):69, 1984.

Mallach JD: Palmar arch thrombosis, *BMJ* 2:28, 1962.

Martin AF: Ulnar artery thrombosis in the palm, *J Bone Joint Surg* 36B:438, 1954.

Mayer V, Gieck JH: Rehabilitation of hand injuries in athletes, *Clin Sports Med* 5(4):783, 1986.

McCue FC: The elbow, wrist and hand. In Kulund D (ed): *The injured athlete,* Philadelphia, 1982, JB Lippincott.

McCue FC, Abbott JL: The treatment of mallet finger and boutonniere deformities, *Va Med Mon* 94:623, 1966.

McCue FC, Wooten SL: Closed tendon injuries of the hand in athletes, *Clin Sports Med* 5(4):741, 1986.

McCue FC et al: Athletic injuries of the proximal interphalangeal joint requiring surgical treatment, *J Bone Joint Surg* 52A:937, 1970.

McCue FC et al: The coach's finger, *J Sports Med* 2:270, 1974.

McCue FC et al: Ulnar collateral ligament injuries of the thumb in athletes, *J Sports Med* 2:70, 1974.

McCue FC et al: Hand injuries in athletes, *Surg Rounds* 1:8, 1978.

Millander LH, Nalebuff EA, Kadson E: Aneurysms and thrombosis of the ulnar artery in the hand, *Arch Surg* 105:686, 1972.

Moberg E: *Splinting in hand therapy,* New York, 1984, Thieme-Stratton.

Peimer CA, Sullivan DJ, Wild DR: Palmar dislocation of the proximal interphalangeal joint, *J Hand Surg* 9A(1):39, 1984.

Peppard A: Thumb taping, *Phys Sports Med* 10(4):139, 1982.

Primiano GA: Skier's thumb injuries associated with flared ski pole handles, *Am J Sports Med* 13(6):425, 1985.

Primiano GA: Functional cast immobilization of thumb metacarpophalangeal joint injuries, *Am J Sports Med* 14(4):335, 1986.

Reef TC: Avulsion of the flexor digitorum profundus: an athletic injury, *Am J Sports Med* 5(6):281, 1977.

Rothwell AG: The pseudo-boutonniere deformity, *N Z Med J* 89(628):51, 1979.

Ruby LK: Common hand injuries in the athlete, *Orthop Clin North Am* 11(4):819, 1980.

Sakellarides HT: Treatment of recent and old injuries of the ulnar collateral ligament of the MP joint of the thumb, *Am J Sports Med* 6(5):255, 1978.

Spinner M: *Kaplan's functional and surgical anatomy of the hand*, ed 3, Philadelphia, 1984, JB Lippincott.

Stark HH et al: Fracture of the hook of the hamate in athletes, *J Bone Joint Surg* 59A(5):575, 1977.

Toews JV: A grip-strength study among steelworkers, *Arch Phys Med Rehabil* 45(8):413, 1964.

Torres J: Little finger splint, *Am J Occup Ther* 29(4):230, 1975.

Valenza J et al: A clinical study of a new heat modality, *J Am Pod Assoc* 69(7):440, 1979.

Wenger DR: Avulsion of the profundus tendon insertion in football players, *Arch Surg* 106:145, 1973.

Wood MB, Dobyns JH: Sports-related extraarticular wrist syndromes, *Clin Orthop* 202:93, 1986.

Wray RC, Young VL, Holtman B: Proximal interphalangeal joint sprains, *Plast Reconstr Surg* 74(1):101, 1984.

Zemel NP, Stark HH: Fractures and dislocations of the carpal bones, *Clin Sports Med* 5(4):709, 1986.

CHAPTER 29 Athletic Taping and Protective Equipment

Robert C. Reese, Jr.
T. Pepper Burruss
Joseph Patten
Darryl Conway

Soft-tissue injuries to the wrist and hand can be protected with a variety of wrist-taping techniques. Taping is most often used after a mild hyperextension (dorsiflexion) injury. Less commonly, palmar flexion injuries are the basis for wrist taping. In both instances taping is used to limit motion and protect the damaged structures.

WRIST TAPING
Hyperextension Wrist Injury

Wrist extension taping is designed to limit the extension of the wrist and thus protect structures that may be injured after a forced dorsiflexion injury. The goal is to limit wrist extension to a range of motion that is comfortable for the athlete and allows effective participation in sports.

Technique

It is best to apply the tape with the athlete standing and facing the person taping. The athlete's fingers can rest on the taper's chest to provide secure support for the hand and wrist while the tape is being applied. The wrist is held in a neutral to slight dorsiflexion position (Fig. 29-1).

In general, no shaving is required for this technique if underwrap is applied. Occasionally, the area on the forearm at which the anchor strips is placed is shaved to allow better fixation of the anchor strips to the skin. If no underwrap is available and repeated taping is necessary, shaving from the forearm to the hand is indicated. Either way, tape adhesive spray is used.

Underwrap is applied circumferentially from the hand (just proximal to the metacarpophalangeal joints of the fingers) to the midforearm (Fig. 29-2). Anchor strips are applied at the midforearm, over the wrist, and around the hand, just proximal to the metacarpal heads. When the anchor strips are applied along the hand, it is important to have the athlete hold the fingers abducted as far as possible (Fig. 29-3). This prevents tape application with the transverse metacarpal arch in a compressed position. If taping is done with the fingers in a resting or adducted position, pain often occurs during activity in the region of the interosseous muscles between the metacarpals.

Checkreins are most often prepared by creating a butterfly of cloth adhesive tape on a smooth, clean surface. This repeated X configuration of the tape is then applied, centered over the volar aspect of the wrist. The checkreins should extend from the anchor strips proximally to the anchor strips distally, with the center of the butterfly (X) directly on the wrist (Fig. 29-4).

Firm anchoring is achieved by applying tape in a figure-eight pattern over the wrist. The tape is begun at the proximal and radial aspect of the tape job and crossed over to the ulnar side as it is applied on the volar aspect, from distal to proximal. The tape is continued up the dorsum of the hand and around to the radial aspect on the volar surface. Finally, the tape is brought back up proximally to the ulnar side of the forearm. This technique creates a continuous figure eight that incorporates the forearm, wrist, and hand (Fig. 29-5). A series of these

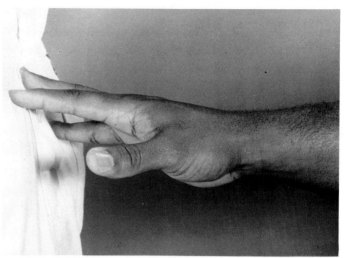

FIG. 29-1. Position for wrist taping. Athlete and taper should be comfortable.

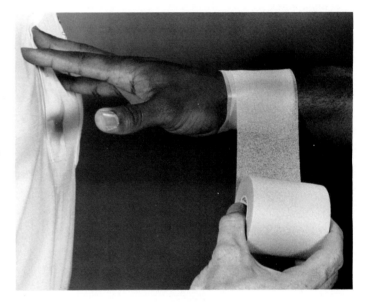

FIG. 29-2. Application of underwrap.

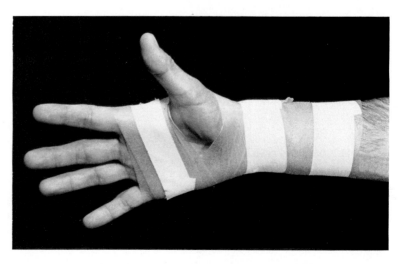

FIG. 29-3. Anchor strips are applied to midforearm, wrist, and hand. Athlete holds fingers wide apart while hand anchor strip is placed.

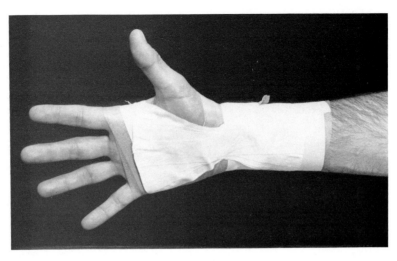

FIG. 29-4. Checkrein butterfly of cloth adhesive tape is fashioned on a smooth, clean surface then applied to volar aspect of wrist.

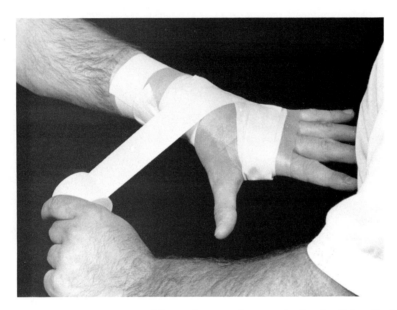

FIG. 29-5. Figure-eight pattern created by winding tape from proximal and radial to distal and ulnar.

figure eights is applied to add strength and bulk to the tape job. These figure-eight strips should not be applied too tightly; this prevents problems with vascular function.

Note that, despite the extensive use of tape, the thumb is entirely free; mobility of the thumb should not be diminished by this technique. If thumb motion is restricted, the tape should be trimmed and removed from the area around the thumb or the entire tape job should be removed and reapplied.

Variations

Tape applied over the wrist contributes to the limitation of the range of wrist motion. If desired, extensive tape buildup can significantly limit wrist motion.

For additional support and strength, crossed **X** strips of moleskin can be applied. These moleskin checkreins contribute to the strength of the tape job without adding as much bulk as repeated cloth adhesive tape strips.

Flexion Wrist Injury

This technique is used when limitation of palmar flexion range of motion is desired after a forced palmar flexion injury.

Technique

The taping technique is essentially the same as for a hyperextension injury, except for the placement of the checkreins and figure-eight strips. The wrist is held in slight dorsiflexion for the tape application. The checkrein

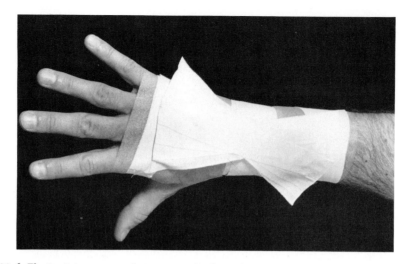

FIG. 29-6. Flexion injury tape technique uses checkrein figure-eight pattern centered on dorsum of wrist.

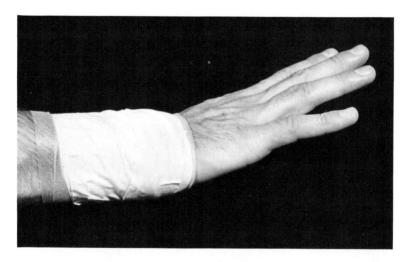

FIG. 29-7. Bulk technique uses repeated circles of tape around the wrist.

X pattern (butterfly) is applied on the dorsal aspect of the wrist. Likewise, the figure-eight pattern is centered over the dorsum of the wrist (Fig. 29-6). This technique limits wrist palmar flexion.

Bulk Wrist Taping

If tape applied to the hand is undesirable or inadvisable, a wrist support with cloth tape can be created that eliminates the hand involvement. This allows the hand to remain untaped but limits overall wrist motion in all planes. An entire roll of 1½-inch tape (15 yd) is used for football linemen.

Technique

The wrist is prepared with underwrap and tape adhesive spray. Cloth adhesive tape is applied circumferentially around the wrist. The tape is applied as a continuous circle and is continued until the desired amount of

wrist restriction is achieved (Fig. 29-7). The bulk of the tape contributes to the limitation of wrist motion and, because of its circumferential nature, limits motion in all directions. An important point to keep in mind when using this technique is that the strength of this technique lies in the amount of tape applied, not in the tightness. If tape is applied too tightly, neurovascular compromise and injury can occur.

Thumb Spica

Following injury to the base of the thumb or metacarpophalangeal area, a mild form of support and protection may be desirable. For example, after healing of a Bennett's fracture, as the athlete returns to participation, protection of the carpometacarpal area may be useful. This taping technique is similar to the fabrication of a thumb spica cast. However, the tape technique is less rigid than the cast and can be applied and removed daily.

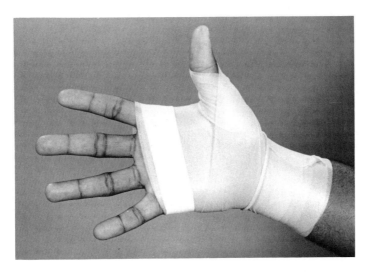

FIG. 29-8. Anchor strips around the metacarpal heads for thumb spica technique.

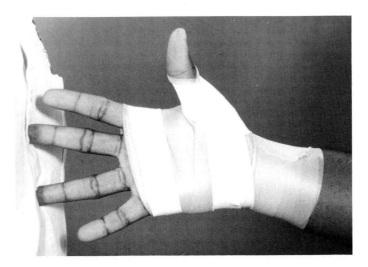

FIG. 29-9. Figure-eight checkreins around the thumb.

Technique

Adhesive spray and underwrap are applied from the forearm, across the wrist, to the hand. The fingers are held abducted to prevent constriction of the metacarpal arch. The thumb is generally held in extended position. However, this position can be varied and the position selected should depend on the examination of the injured region and an appropriate plan to limit specific motions. The position can vary in both the flexion-extension plane and in the abduction-adduction plane. After the thumb has been positioned as indicated, underwrap is applied to the thumb.

Anchor strips of cloth adhesive tape are placed around the metacarpal heads (Fig. 29-8). Figure-eight checkreins are next applied around the thumb and continued over the wrist in a circumferential pattern (Fig. 29-9). These checkreins are varied by reversing the tape direction with each application. The tape direction is dictated by the motion being restricted. The checkreins are anchored with tape extending from the wrist to the thumb, the strip beginning at the forearm and continuing longitudinally to the interphalangeal joint of the thumb (Fig. 29-10). Circumferential loops of tape are applied in a continuous strip to anchor and solidify the tape job. The taping is completed with a figure-eight piece of tape that incorporates the thumb, hand, and wrist.

Variations

A somewhat less bulky form of spica immobilization can be created by initially applying figure eights around the thumb only. This reduces the amount of tape material around the wrist and hand and is appropriate for athletes who require unencumbered thumb movement. However, because of the lack of bulk, the restriction gained and protection afforded are less optimal than with the full tape spica technique. If the wrist needs to be free,

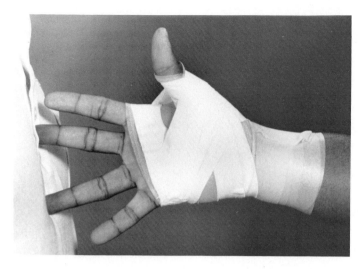

FIG. 29-10. Longitudinal checkreins from wrist to thumb.

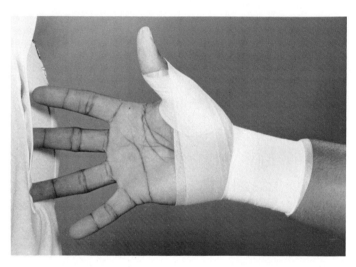

FIG. 29-11. Abbreviated thumb taping technique. Note proximal position of anchor strips.

then more tape can be applied to the thumb in the figure-eight pattern (Fig. 29-9). These extra layers provide bulk to limit motion. When this extra tape is added, it must be borne in mind that tight is not right, but rather it is the bulk that does the job.

Abbreviated Thumb Taping

Athletes who use equipment in their hands, as do football quarterbacks and hockey players, may require a tape application that can limit thumb extension yet allow the wrist to remain mobile. The abbreviated thumb technique is designed for that purpose. It was created by Pinky Newell of Purdue University for use by Bob Griese in a Rose Bowl game.

Technique

Tape adhesive spray and underwrap are applied around the forearm, wrist, and hand. Using 1-inch ad-

hesive cloth tape, a series of two figure eights are applied in opposite directions from the thumb to the wrist. However, the point of application at the wrist is made more proximal than in the usual thumb spica application (Fig. 29-11). This permits greater wrist motion than in the standard thumb spica technique.

Next, a series of abbreviated figure eights are applied, with the thumb positioned just short of the maximum extension desired. This continuous strip should begin on the anchor strip on the wrist, angle up toward the base of the thumb (metacarpophalangeal joint) as if another figure eight were going to be applied. Instead of encircling the thumb, however, the tape is pressed down and redirected to the opposite side of the hand, distal to proximal and around the wrist (Fig. 29-12). The distal point of the tape should be pinched at the redirected angle, so that it adheres to itself, and laid over itself as the next continuous abbreviated figure eight is brought up, over-

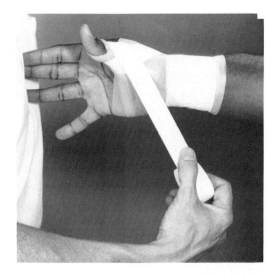

FIG. 29-12. Figure-eight application for abbreviated technique.

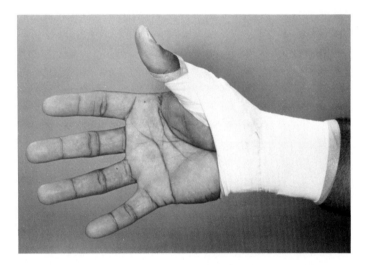

FIG. 29-13. Completed abbreviated tape technique for thumb; palm is left free for grasping.

lapping approximately half the width of tape. This should be continued until the proximal point of the interphalangeal joint of the thumb has been reached. To complete the technique, one final figure eight is laid on, designated more as an anchor strip rather than for support.

By use of this method, in effect, a series of check-reigns preventing extension has been achieved, flexion has not been limited, and the palm is free for grasping (Fig. 29-13).

FINGER TAPING

Injuries to the fingers are quite common in contact sports. A variety of taping techniques are available to support and protect fingers during athletic participation.

Buddy Taping

Buddy taping is used when support of a finger is required but restriction of motion is undesirable. The sup-

port for the injured finger is supplied by an adjacent finger, which acts as a splint. In general, buddy taping is indicated in uncomplicated proximal interphalangeal (PIP) joint injuries and stable, healing fractures of the proximal and middle phalanx. Buddy taping can be done with any two fingers and is easiest to apply when the index, middle, or ring fingers are injured.

Technique

The technique is simple; the injured finger and its adjacent support finger are taped together with circumferential strips centered over the proximal and middle phalanxes (Fig. 29-14). If necessary, the distal phalanxes can be taped together, but occasionally, this is not achievable because of disparities in finger lengths. In this regard, buddy taping of the little and ring fingers is also difficult to fashion because the PIP and distal interphalangeal (DIP) joints are at different levels. With care, however, a satisfactory buddy taping technique can be carried out between any two fingers. Finally, in some in-

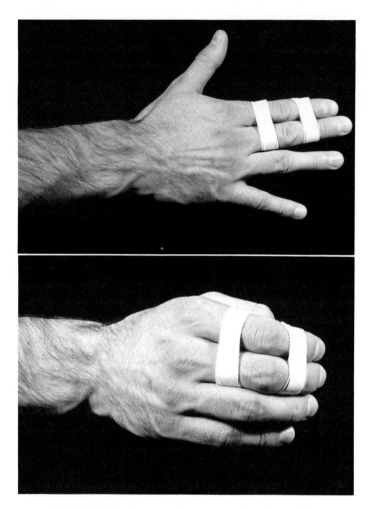

FIG. 29-14. Buddy taping. Taping over joints is avoided.

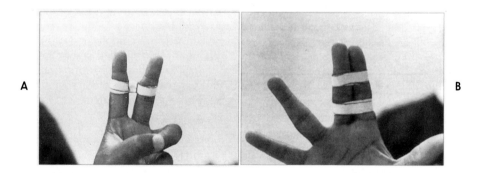

FIG. 29-15. A, Checkreins within the interdigital spaces that result in tape on the palmer aspect of the PIP-DIP joint segment of the fingers. **B,** Buddy taping of the fingers that results in tape on the palmar aspect of the fingers. (From Conway DP, Decker AS: *J Athlet Train* 28[3]:268, 1993.)

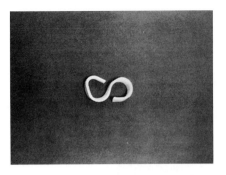

FIG. 29-16. Spencer splint. (From Conway DP, Decker AS: *J Athlet Train* 28[3]:268, 1993.)

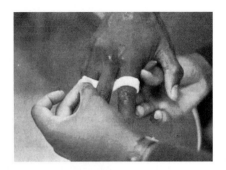

FIG. 29-17. Construction of the Spencer splint on the athlete's finger. (From Conway DP, Decker AS: *J Athlet Train* 28[3]:268, 1993.)

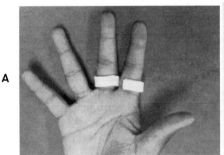 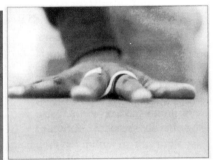

FIG. 29-18. **A,** Palmar view of the Spencer splint. **B,** View of the splint from between the fingers. (From Conway DP, Decker AS: *J Athlet Train* 28[3]:268, 1993.)

stances, thin foam rubber can be applied between the two fingers for added comfort, if necessary.

Metacarpophalangeal Joint Splint

An injury to the metacarpophalangeal joint can cause chronic disability and can pose a serious dilemma to the athletic trainer trying to splint this area without compromising an athlete's gripping, catching, and ball handling abilities or finger dexterity (e.g., basketball players, football centers and backs, soccer goalies, baseball players) (Fig. 29-15). Using a 4½ × ½-inch strip of thermoplastic splinting material (e.g., Orthoplast) arranged in an **S** shape has proven to limit painful abduction of the fingers as well as extension and flexion at the metacarpophalangeal joint (Fig. 29-16). The splint allows for controlled or restricted independent movement of the fingers while eliminating the need for tape distal to the proximal interphalangeal joint and tape anchors on the thenar/hypothenar eminences of the hang, which could impair an athlete's performance. The splint was created by Anthony Decker of the University of Delaware for use on a basketball player.

Technique

Use a paper or cloth tape measure to estimate the length of the thermoplastic material needed. Wrap the tape measure around the fingers in a **S**-shaped pattern starting on the palmar surface of the index finger (Fig. 29-17). Proceed from the palmar surface around the finger to the dorsal surface of the index finger and then through the web space to the palmar surface of the middle digit. Proceed from the palmar surface of the middle finger around to the dorsal surface of the same finger to produce the **S**-shaped pattern. Cut the thermoplastic material to correspond to the length of the tape measure used. The width of the splint should not compromise flexion at the metacarpophalangeal or PIP joints.

Abduct the fingers to a point just before the onset of pain to allow for ample gripping ability and finger dexterity (Fig. 29-18). Heat the splinting material until soft and wrap the pliable material around the desired fingers in a manner identical to that used to measure the piece of splinting material.

After molding the splint, have the athlete hold the hand in cold water, with the splint in place, until the material hardens. After the material has hardened, the trainer may customize the splint by cutting off sharp edges and placing padding or moleskin where desired. The trainer may also tape the splint in a circular or figure-eight pattern using ½-inch tape for added comfort and stability.

The splint may be altered to meet the needs of the in-

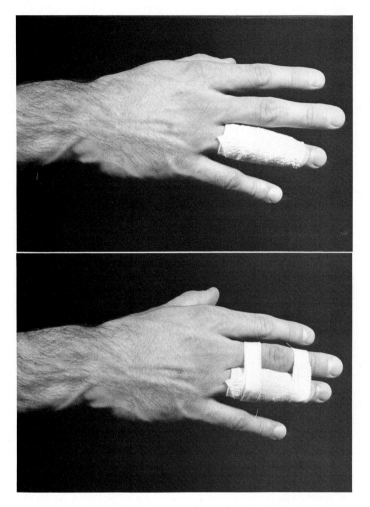

FIG. 29-19. Compression taping for swelling with elastic tape.

jured athlete, depending on the nature of the specific injury. The splint may also be constructed to immobilize two or three metacarpophalangeal joints, depending on the injury; or it may be reinforced using two pieces of thermoplastic material if necessary.

Compression Taping for Swelling

After interphalangeal joint injury, such as a sprain or dislocation, soft-tissue swelling often ensues and further adds to soft-tissue injury, delaying healing and impairing performance. A useful taping technique has been devised to limit swelling and allow continued athletic participation with relatively minimal impedance of the involved finger. This taping technique is used after the injury has been fully evaluated clinically and radiographically, to ascertain that no other more appropriate form of intervention is indicated.

Technique

A layer of underwrap is applied across the injured joint. Circumferential layers of elastic tape are then placed over this (Fig. 29-19). The elastic tape is applied firmly, but not too tightly. A single layer of cloth tape is used over the elastic tape to solidify the tape. The injured

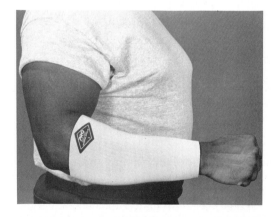

FIG. 29-20. Neoprene sleeves for forearm protection.

finger and an adjacent finger are buddy taped together to provide splinting. At all times the neurovascular function is checked to ensure that compromise is not occurring. A self-adhering compression wrap, such as Coban and cotton wadding, such as Webril, can be substituted

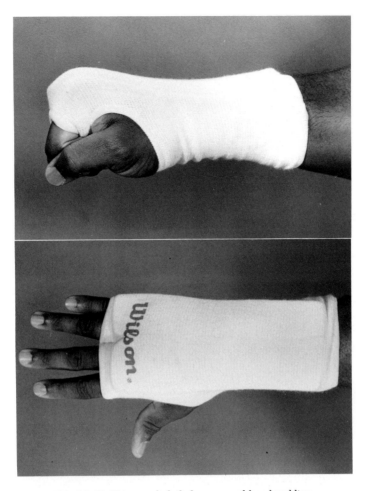

FIG. 29-21. Foam and cloth forearm and hand padding.

for the underwrap and elastic tape, then secured with cloth adhesive tape.

PROTECTIVE EQUIPMENT
Forearm

The forearm is subject to both contusions and abrasions in sports, and several types of equipment are available to protect the athlete from these injuries. Neoprene sleeves are quite popular and serve well as protection for the forearm (Fig. 29-20). Other commercially available pads are generally made from elasticized cloth, incorporating some foam rubber (Fig. 29-21).

Occasionally, a hard shell is desired, as in recovery from a forearm fracture. These can be custom made from thermomoldable plastic and created to protect the appropriate anatomic location desired. It is important that the outside of the hard shell be adequately padded to protect opposing athletes from injury (Fig. 29-22).

Wrist and Hand

Hand protection is generally obtained with the use of specialized gloves. These gloves incorporate special padding, as dictated by the need of the athlete. For exam-

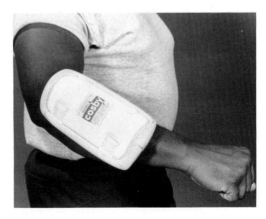

FIG. 29-22. Hard shell can be fabricated for additional forearm protection.

ple, in football, offensive linemen use gloves with padding in the dorsum of the glove, which protects the metacarpophalangeal joints (Fig. 29-23).

Occasionally, a cast can be used to protect an injured area of the wrist or hand during athletic participation.

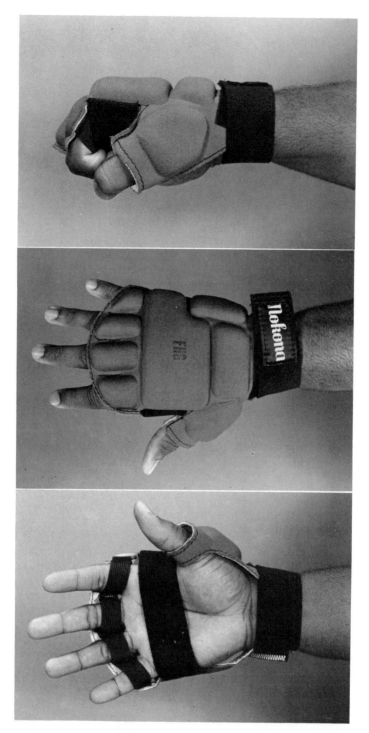

FIG. 29-23. Padded gloves, like these used by football offensive linesmen, are designed to provide protection to dorsum of the hand and metacarpophalangeal region.

These casts are usually made from synthetic cast material, such as fiberglass, and often extend to completely enclose the hand. Adequate padding is required outside the hard shell to protect other athletic participants from injury.

For an additional discussion of specialized equipment used in the rehabilitation of wrist and hand injuries, see Chapter 28.

PART V Skeletally Immature Athletes

CHAPTER 30

Upper Extremity Injuries in the Skeletally Immature Athlete

Jack T. Andrish

Part of the uniqueness of the skeletally immature athlete is the presence of open growth plates (Fig. 30-1). This cartilaginous structure is the vehicle for longitudinal growth via endochondral ossification. Injury to the growth plate carries with it not only reality of consistent and expeditious healing, but also the potential for early or late growth disturbance.

Trauma to the growth plate may be acute or chronic. Acute injury is well recognized and described. Salter and Harris,[67] and more recently Ogden,[52] have written on the subject and have provided classifications for acute growth plate fractures (Fig. 30-2). These injuries, of course, do happen to young athletes, but a more unusual injury is the chronic **stress-related growth plate reaction** that is seen as a result of athletic abuse.[63,66,76,82] The growth plate may be required to withstand several different types and combinations of stress (i.e., tension, compression, shear, and torsion). Within certain physiologic limits, tension or compression may stimulate growth. However, forces beyond these limits retard or stop growth (Fig. 30-3).[52]

The periosteum plays a vital biomechanical role in stabilizing the growth plate. The insertion into the epiphysis is strong, and the periosteum itself is a relatively thick and tough structure. Furthermore, the undulations of the growth plate are thought to help resist displacement by shear stresses. The growth plate is most resistant to tension and least resistant to torsion.[52] Over the metaphysis and diaphysis of long bones the periosteum is loosely attached. This becomes more firmly attached to the growth plate at the perichondrium and, as noted, the epiphysis. Tendons and ligaments tend to insert at the area of the perichondrium. This allows tensile stress to be received by a tensile-responsive structure (i.e., the growth plate). Muscles, on the other hand, tend to originate from the periosteum directly over the metaphysis and diaphysis. This is a loose arrangement with few areas of direct connection to the bone, whereas the tendon insertion into perichondrium carries on into the physeal and epiphyseal cartilage (Fig. 30-4).

Although fractures may occur across the growth plate, more typically at least some component of the injury will be transverse through it. The zone of hypertrophy and the zone of provisional calcification have been most often implicated as the anatomic site of growth plate fractures (Fig. 30-1).[67]

There are other differences between the musculoskeletal systems of immature and mature athletes. First of all, the plasticity of young bone is greater. Bone tends to get stiffer and more brittle with age. Immature epiphyses are also softer than mature calcified bone. This feature also makes the cartilaginous epiphysis susceptible to stress in a different way from the bony epiphysis of the adult. Many of the so-called osteochondroses have their origins in chronic, repetitive trauma to the cartilaginous epiphysis.

Because of the increased plastic behavior of young bone, greenstick fractures are common. Permanent deformation may occur (angular), although most often this

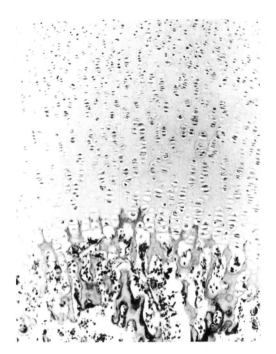

FIG. 30-1. Histology of the growth plate is well recognized. This includes the typical columnar orientation of cells with progressive cellular hypertrophy, provisional calcification, and finally endochondral ossification.

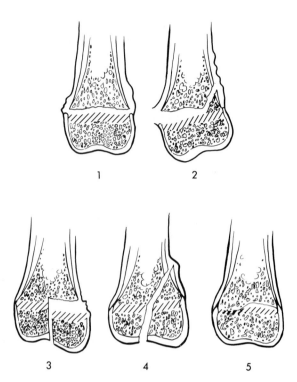

FIG. 30-2. Although other fracture classifications exist, the Salter-Harris classification remains as a practical and popular standard.

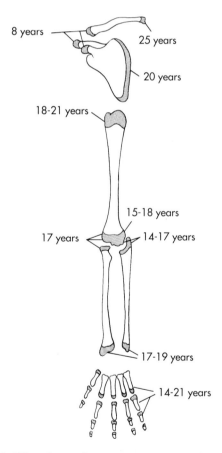

FIG. 30-3. Although significant variations exist in the exact time of growth plate closure, the sequence of closure is generally consistent. (Modified from Ogden JA: *Skeletal injury in the child,* Philadelphia, 1982, Lea & Febiger.)

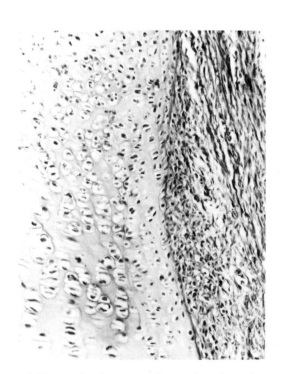

FIG. 30-4. The perichondrium not only provides a physical restraint to the growth plate, but also serves in the transition of tendinous and periosteal attachments extending into the physeal and epiphyseal cartilage.

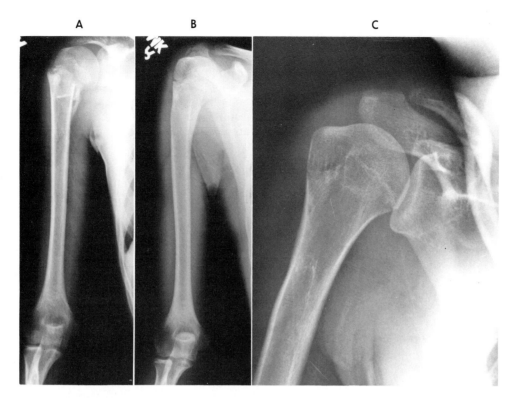

FIG. 30-5. A, This 12-year-old skier sustained a proximal humeral fracture with moderate displacement. **B,** Managed with a sling and swath for 3 weeks, uneventful healing occurred. **C,** Five years later, the bony contour is normal.

deformity is small and fully remodeled during further growth of the bone. Large, angular deformities of long bones may not fully correct themselves, and certainly rotational deformities do not correct themselves with further growth and development (Fig. 30-5).

Just as the epiphyseal ends of growing long bones have special anatomic features related to the cartilage model, secondary ossification, and joint formation, the apophyses also have different features. These growth plates are frequently found on irregularly shaped bone, such as the pelvis, or on metaphyseal areas, such as the tibial tubercle. Although these growth areas generally do not contribute to longitudinal growth, they do contribute to form and usually serve as attachment sites for tendons and ligaments. As in the lower extremities, repetitive traction stress, such as is encountered in organized youth sports, can lead to bony changes resulting from stress-induced apophyseal growth disturbances.[82]

EPIDEMIOLOGY

During a 9-year period from January 1984 to January 1993, 32,080 new sports-related injuries were registered in the Section of Sports Medicine at the Cleveland Clinic Foundation. Of these, 4282 (13.4%) were in young people age 15 and under; 838 (19.6%) of these injuries to young athletes involved the upper extremity. Of course, these figures do not reflect the true incidence or prevalence of upper extremity injuries in youth sports, which surely must be higher.[7,14,16,21] They do, however, repre-

TABLE 30-1 Prevalence of upper extremity injuries in athletes age 15 years and younger

Area of Injury	Percentage (n = 838)
Shoulder	35.7
Acromioclavicular- sternoclavicular	6.9
Upper arm	18.6
Elbow	18.3
Forearm	4.5
Wrist	8.2
Hand	7.8

Data from Cleveland Clinic Foundation, Section of Sports Medicine, 1984 to 1993.

sent the frequency with which they are encountered in a general sports medicine clinic.

A further breakdown of injury prevalence is shown in Table 30-1. From this it can be seen that the region most commonly injured in the upper extremity is the shoulder (42.6%), with the upper arm (18.6%) and the elbow (18.3%) following.

CLINICAL EVALUATION

In a discussion of specific injuries of the upper extremities, the physician must always keep in mind that all is not necessarily what it seems to be when evaluating the skeletally immature athlete. The presence of open growth plates provides additional mechanisms to con-

sider as causes of clinical instability or deformity (acute or chronic). Further, pliable cartilaginous epiphyses provide the opportunity for the development of osteochondroses that may cause joint pain or swelling. Accordingly, radiographic examination of the injured part is mandatory to arrive at a definitive diagnosis. Even then, the radiograph may be misleading. Acute growth plate fractures, nondisplaced, may have radiographs that are initially interpreted as normal, only to demonstrate evidence of fracture 10 to 14 days later when periosteal reaction becomes apparent. Loose bodies may be cartilaginous and radiolucent, later to become calcified and apparent. Osteochondritis dissecans may be purely cystic and easily missed, only to become sclerotic and fragmented at a later time.

The moral to this is that the skeletal system in the child is evolving and undergoing continual change and remodeling. In the diagnosis and management of injuries to children we must always keep this concept of dynamics in mind. Especially in children, the longitudinal evaluation of injuries over time is necessary not only to be able to make the precise diagnosis, but also to better predict the outcome.

SHOULDER
Anatomy

Fig. 30-3 depicts the various epiphyseal centers about the shoulder and their approximate ages at closure. The physician can see that these closures are relatively late; thus many school-age athletes are subject to the peculiarities of injuries to the growth plate. For instance the medial clavicular physis may remain open until age 25 and the proximal humerus until ages 18 to 21. As a physician would expect, the firm periosteal attachments to

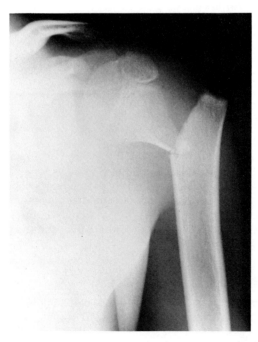

FIG. 30-6. The large metaphyseal component to this Type II growth plate injury is apparent in this 12-year-old boy.

the epiphysis play a major role during the generation of injuries. At the proximal humerus the periosteum has been shown to be thick and tough posteriorly, thus preventing posterior displacement of physeal fracture fragments.[13] Additionally, the rotator cuff attachments onto the physis extend medially onto the metaphysis, further contributing to the characteristic Type II fractures seen in children (Fig. 30-6).

Injury Statistics

In our series 42.6% of injuries to the upper extremity involved the shoulder; I consider the acromioclavicular joint, the clavicle, and the sternoclavicular joint to be part of the shoulder complex as well as the traditional inclusion of the glenohumeral joint. Table 30-2 depicts the most frequent, specific injuries to this area. As can be seen, even in this young age group shoulder instability accounted for the most frequent diagnosis (29.7%), followed closely by problems of the rotator cuff (impingement or strain) (21.1%).

Instability Problems

As with adults, most typically the young athlete with shoulder instability has anterior dislocations or subluxations. The reported incidence of recurrence of symptomatic instability is high. Despite recent reports of success with initial immobilization for 3 to 6 weeks and subsequent rehabilitation, the topic is still controversial.[29] My approach has been to offer 3 to 4 weeks of sling and swath immobilization after the initial reduction, followed by a rehabilitation program that emphasizes rotator cuff strengthening. However, the first recurrence of dislocation is usually a bad sign and should signal an alert to consider surgical repair. Because of open growth plates, young bones, and inconsistent compliance with postoperative regimens, we prefer an operative approach that does not leave metal behind. A standard capsulorrhaphy, such as the Neer capsular shift procedure, should achieve a 95% success rate as measured by prevention of recurrent dislocations.*

The management of subluxation has been similar to that of dislocation except for the initial period of immobilization. It has been my experience that this injury is often more insidious in its presentation and not amena-

---

*References 5, 11, 12, 31, 32, 49, 53, 62, 68, and 80.

TABLE 30-2 Prevalence of injury to the shoulder

Type of Injury	Percentage (n = 299)
Instability	
Possible subluxation	20.7
Possible dislocation	9.0
	29.7
Impingement syndrome	15.7
Rotator cuff strain	5.4
	21.1
Fractures	1.7
Nerve pinch	4.0

Data from Cleveland Clinic Foundation, Section of Sports Medicine, 1984 to 1993.

ble to this early detection and treatment. However, I have had an equally effective (or ineffective) response to rehabilitation programs. Surgical repair may offer generally better results.

Impingement Syndrome

Problems related to inflammation of the rotator cuff are common in the young athlete. This is especially true in the competitive swimmer, in whom this is seen most frequently.[25] Neer[48] has alerted the orthopaedic community to the pathoanatomy of shoulder impingement, and Jobe[35] has defined the relationship of this entity to repetitive microtrauma. This symptom complex of shoulder pain (usually anterior but frequently poorly localized) begins as an inflammatory response of the rotator cuff (and at times the long head of the biceps tendon) to overuse. The accompanying swelling of peritendinous and bursal tissue then becomes subject to impingement with overhead activities.[50] The supraspinatus and the biceps tendon are most often involved with impingement by the coracoacromial arch. With impingement of inflamed structures, continuation of overhead activities, such as in swimming cause self-perpetuation of the cycle (Fig. 30-7). It should also be recognized and remembered that anterior shoulder instability can also produce signs and symptoms of impingement and thus constitute an etiology other than pure overuse. The relocation test has been advocated as one means of differentiating between impingement with and without instability.[37] Subacromial injection of a local anesthetic agent at the time the patient is seen in the office can also help establish the diagnosis of shoulder impingement.

My treatment for this condition is as described by others.[25,35,48,75] As with most overuse syndromes, successful treatment is usually nonoperative and includes activity modification (relative rest), oral antiinflammatory medications, and cryotherapy.

The subsequent management includes a rehabilitation program that emphasizes flexibility and strengthening of the rotator cuff and a gradual return to the sport activity (see Chapter 5).

I have had variable success with operative treatment of the impingement syndrome. For the young person with refractory shoulder pain, subacromial decompres-

sion is advocated.[75] Resection of the coracoacromial ligament alone can be effective in the athlete under age 25.[33] Over this age, acromioplasty is also required. With the development of arthroscopic techniques of subacromial decompression, the subacromial bursa now can be debrided and the coracoacromial ligament can be released without violating the deltoid attachment on the acromion. This has significant implications for rehabilitation. If needed, an arthroscopic acromioplasty can be added. At this time comparative studies of arthroscopic subacromial decompression and open procedures are incomplete. My impression, however, is that the arthroscopic technique offers distinct advantages. Because occult shoulder instability can also mimic the symptoms of impingement,[23,37,61] this must be kept in mind during the formulation of the diagnosis. At the time of arthroscopy an adequate physical examination and a direct look within the glenohumeral joint should be included.[10,78]

Acromioclavicular Injuries and Fractures

Acromioclavicular separations are uncommon in the skeletally immature athlete.[19] When seen, their management is usually no different from that required for the older athlete.[17,22,56,72] An injury unique to the young athlete involves a fracture of the distal clavicle (Fig. 30-8). In effect, this injury is analogous to the metaphyseal fracture seen with growth plate injuries. Usually the coracoclavicular ligaments remain intact and attached to the distal clavicle. Occasionally this deformity may necessitate open reduction and internal fixation with pins placed across the acromioclavicular joint and fracture. However, because considerable remodeling potential exists in children with this injury, some authors advocate nonoperative management regardless of deformity.[19]

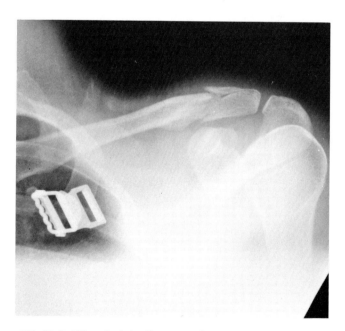

FIG. 30-8. Although skeletally mature, this young athlete sustained a metaphyseal fracture of the distal clavicle, lateral to the coracoclavicular ligaments. Closed management with a Kenny-Howard sling resulted in successful union and prevention of deformity.

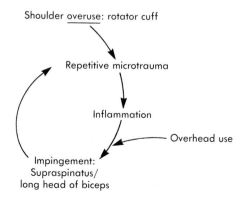

FIG. 30-7. Overuse can result in impingement syndrome. Successful treatment and management are directed toward each phase.

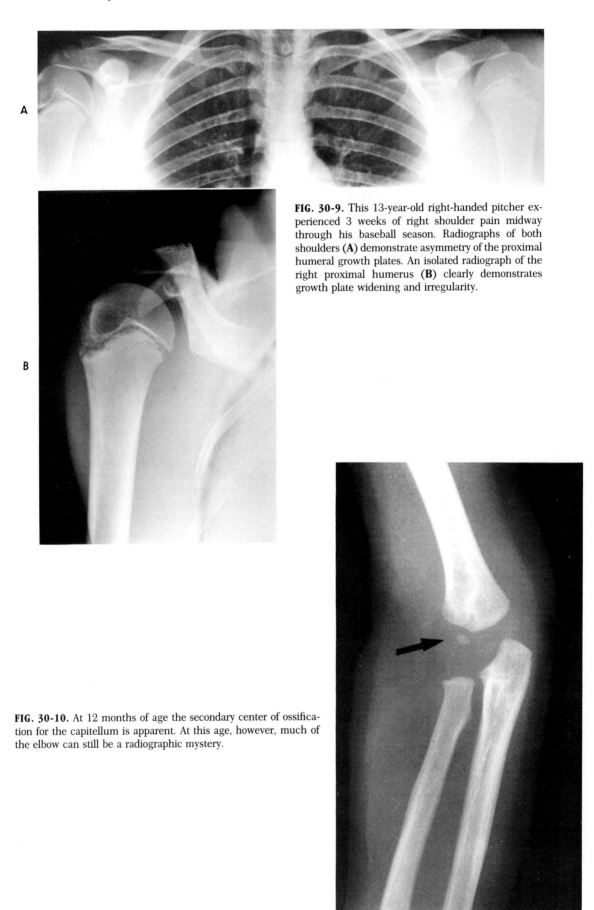

FIG. 30-9. This 13-year-old right-handed pitcher experienced 3 weeks of right shoulder pain midway through his baseball season. Radiographs of both shoulders **(A)** demonstrate asymmetry of the proximal humeral growth plates. An isolated radiograph of the right proximal humerus **(B)** clearly demonstrates growth plate widening and irregularity.

FIG. 30-10. At 12 months of age the secondary center of ossification for the capitellum is apparent. At this age, however, much of the elbow can still be a radiographic mystery.

Little League Shoulder and Elbow

It is, of course, difficult to discuss upper extremity injuries in the skeletally immature athlete without mentioning the entities referred to as little league shoulder and little league elbow. Adams[1] brought attention to this in 1965 with his study of little league baseball pitchers in California. Several studies since then have confirmed its existence but emphasized the lower frequency.[24,27,40,77] Little league shoulder is characterized by pain occurring in a dominant shoulder of a skeletally immature throwing athlete. Radiographs easily demonstrate a widening of the proximal humeral growth plate. This is considered to be either a stress-related change or a subacute Type I growth plate fracture (Fig. 30-9). In either case the treatment is easy: the athlete simply stops throwing for 4 to 6 weeks. Complete healing occurs uniformly and no adverse sequelae result.

ELBOW

Anatomy

Types of injury patterns about the elbow seen in skeletally immature athletes are heavily influenced by age. The distal humerus of the newborn has a single cartilaginous model of the epiphysis. However, by as early as 3 months the ossification center of the capitellum appears (Fig. 30-10). Table 30-3 depicts the sequential times of appearance for the secondary ossification centers about the elbow.[1] It is not unusual for any of these centers of ossification to appear first as two or more foci that later coalesce to become a single bony centrum. The trochlea commonly develops in this manner. Furthermore, this fragmented appearance and development of ossification centers need not be symmetric. Table 30-4

TABLE 30-3 Age of appearance for secondary ossification centers: elbow

	Males	Females
Capitellum	1-2 months	1-6 months
Radial head	3-6 years	3-6 years
Medial epicondyle	5-7 years	3-6 years
Trochlea	8-10 years	7-9 years
Olecranon	8-10 years	8-10 years
Lateral epicondyle	12 years	11 years

Modified from Ogden JA: *Skeletal injury in the child*, Philadelphia, 1982, Lea & Febiger.

TABLE 30-4 Age of fusion for secondary ossification center: elbow

	Males (Years)	Females (Years)
Capitellum	14.5	13
Radial head	16	14
Medial epicondyle	17	14
Trochlea	13	11.5
Olecranon	16	14
Lateral epicondyle	15	12.5

Modified from Pappas AM: *Clin Orthop* 164:30, 1982.

indicates the time of fusion of these ossification centers. Although the sequence of appearance and closure of these ossification centers is consistent, the actual ages involved are variable and most figures quoted in the literature are recognized as being approximations.

Injury Statistics

Of the injuries to the upper extremity that we encountered in the skeletally immature athlete, 18.3% involved the elbow. As expected, the most frequent types of injury were related to overuse (Table 30-5). Fractures accounted for 14.4% of elbow complaints seen in our clinic, and osteochondritis dissecans accounted for 3.2%.

Pappas[54] has provided an excellent review of elbow problems developing in young pitchers. From his experience, injury patterns were distinct and related to stages of development. In childhood, which he defined as terminating with the appearance of all secondary centers of ossification, most problems are related to the secondary ossification centers. Radiographs may demonstrate irregularly shaped or fragmented osseous development. At this stage the problems are usually self-limited if the offending repetitive stress is avoided. Adolescence ends when all ossification centers have fused; problems characteristic of this adolescent period include avulsions, physeal separations, and avascular necrosis.

Little League Elbow

By far the most widely recognized elbow injuries occurring in youth sports are related to throwing—the little league elbow. Numerous studies have analyzed and discussed the pathologic forces generated about the elbow during throwing.[3,13,54] The throwing mechanism consists of three phases: the wind-up or cocking phase, the forward motion or acceleration phase, and the follow-through.[54] Each of these phases places unique force patterns about the elbow.[15,54,79] During the late cocking phase, distraction forces are produced medially, compressive forces are applied laterally, and translational forces exist across the articulation between the olecranon and humerus. These forces neutralize during the acceleration phase. The follow-through produces excessive forces posteriorly throughout the triceps contraction, and compressive and shear forces across the radial capitellar joint with the rapid pronation of the forearm.

Clinical features that have been described in association with the little league elbow[27,40] include flexion contractures and increased valgus carrying angle. Radio-

TABLE 30-5 Prevalence of injury to the elbow

Injury	Percentage (n = 153)
Strain	20.3
Fracture	14.4
Sprain	9.8
Tendinitis	3.9
Osteochondritis dissecans	3.2

Data from Cleveland Clinic Foundation, Section of Sports Medicine, 1984 to 1993.

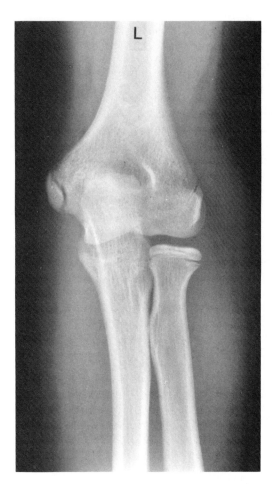

FIG. 30-11. Although hypertrophy of the medial humeral epicondyle can be a normal variant of the dominant upper extremity, widening of the apophysis combined with clinical pain and tenderness can be one characteristic feature of little league elbow.

Clinical findings in little league elbow

- Flexion contracture
- Increased valgus carrying angle

---

graphically, hypertrophy of the medial epicondyle is present but probably represents a normal variant of a dominant extremity. Fragmentation of the trochlea, olecranon, and medial epicondyle can exist, as well as widening of the distance between the medial epicondyle and the humeral metaphysis (Fig. 30-11).

Radiographic findings in little league elbow

- Medial epicondyle hypertrophy or fragmentation
- Trochlear fragmentation
- Olecranon fragmentation
- Widening of distance between medial epicondyle and humeral metaphysis

---

Problems of the radiocapitellar joint are well recognized in the syndrome of elbow pain occurring in young pitchers. Except for the complications and sequelae associated with osteochondritis dissecans, most of the features of the little league elbow are either self-limiting, responding to a simple reprieve from throwing, or are normal anatomic variations that are of no clinical significance.

Osteochondritis Dissecans

The exception to the usual uneventful outcome of well-treated little league elbow is the presence of osteochondritis dissecans of the capitellum, radial head, or both. By no means limited to pitchers, it may be seen in young gymnasts, basketball players, and virtually any active child.[36,57] This condition is believed by some to represent an osteochondrosis not altogether different from Legg-Perthes disease of the hip.[34] Indeed, both represent outcomes of disordered endochondral ossification.[65] Panner's disease of the capitellum may show an identical radiographic picture as well as clinical presentation. Confusion exists as to whether there is any difference between osteochondritis dissecans and Panner's disease.[55] Although Panner's disease may just be a part of the spectrum of osteochondritis dissecans, it is probably better to limit the diagnosis of Panner's disease to children age 10 or younger at the time of onset.

Of the theories that exist to explain the cause,* most relate to avascular necrosis produced on a susceptible epiphysis that receives repetitive compression or shearing forces.[9,47,69] Typically the capitellum may show cystic changes or a radiographic pattern of sclerosis and loose body formation. The radial head may be deformed (Fig. 30-12). Intraarticular findings include softening and fissuring of articular surfaces of the radiocapitellar joint; at times there may be subchondral collapse and bony eburnation. Intraarticular loose bodies are common. They may be osteocartilaginous, as seen in osteochondritis dissecans, or they may be purely cartilaginous, representing by-products of articular surface degeneration.

Treatment of osteochondritis dissecans varies. There is no doubt that some lesions in skeletally immature elbows will heal if provided with the proper environment. This treatment includes a strict avoidance of any throwing and impact loading activities as seen in gymnastics. Pain, tenderness, contracture, and radiographic changes provide objective parameters to judge activity of the disease. Once loose body formation has occurred or healing has been incomplete (as is usually the case) and symptoms persist, surgical intervention is required.[45] Traditionally, this has consisted of an arthrotomy with joint debridement (Fig. 30-13).[6,42] Drilling of the osteochondritis dissecans lesion to stimulate either healing of the loose body within the lesion or fibrocartilaginous filling of a defect has been advocated.[45] This approach may provide relief of pain and mechanical symptoms but usually does not result in much reduction of flexion contracture or development of degenerative arthritis.[6,42] More recently, arthroscopy has been applied to the management

---

*References 2, 8, 38, 39, 41, 47, 54, and 70.

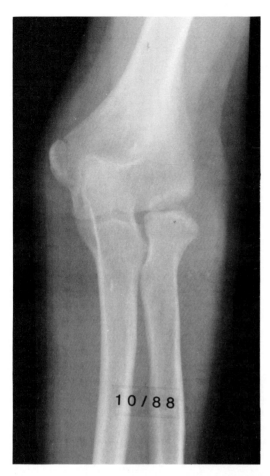

FIG. 30-12. Excessive valgus stress that occurs at the elbow during the act of throwing generates extreme compressive-forces across the radial-capitellar joint. This young pitcher with chronic elbow pain illustrates the typical radiographic features of osteochondritis dissecans. This includes not only cystic and sclerotic changes of the capitellum, but also deformity of the radial head.

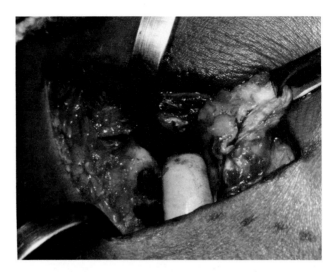

FIG. 30-13. Large osteochondral fragments of the capitellum frequently require debridement. The traditional arthrotomy with removal of loose osteochondral fragments and curettage and drilling of the subchondral bone is frequently required. However, arthroscopic debridement has less morbidity and comparable clinical results.

of this problem.[65] Although the technique of arthroscopy of the elbow is more demanding and certainly has greater potential risk of injuries to neurovascular structures, with attention to detail the procedure is reasonable and the clinical effectiveness of arthroscopic joint debridement and loose body removal makes it rewarding for the surgeon and the young patient alike. It has become my preferred method of surgical management of osteochondritis dissecans of the elbow.

Flexion Contracture

Perhaps no entity involving the young elbow has been more frustrating to manage than the significant flexion contracture. Repetitive hyperextension, as occurs with throwing, can lead to traction injury of the anterior joint capsule, fibrosis, and contracture. Although some degree of flexion contracture may exist in 10%[27,40] of little league pitchers, most contractures are of less than 15 degrees and of little functional significance. Simple rest (i.e., avoiding hard throwing) effects a cure in most instances. However, persistent abuse or the association of osteochondritis dissecans or remote elbow fracture can

result in significant contractures of 30 degrees or more. Treatment initially consists of active range of motion and active assisted range of motion exercises. Throwing is prohibited, as are impact-loading activities. Three months usually provide a reasonable measure of time to judge effectiveness of this rehabilitation program.

An adjunct worth using in refractory cases is the dynamic splinting program, as seen with the Dynasplint.[30] This device applies an extension moment to the elbow with tension adjusted to avoid increasing elbow pain and soreness. It is worn as a nighttime orthosis, as tolerance permits, usually 12 hours per day. My experience has been that these dynamic orthoses can generally reduce the contractures by half of their initial amount over a 3-month period.

Surgical treatment of flexion contractures about the elbow yields unpredictable results. Even young elbows, however, can have osteophytic formation on the olecranon as well as within the olecranon fossa. Loose bodies may also reside in the posterior recess, and with this scenario surgical debridement (open or arthroscopic) of osteophytes and removal of loose bodies can have a significant influence in regaining motion. Postoperative regimens may include continuous passive motion as well as dynamic splints (Fig. 30-14).

Fractures and Dislocations

The most common elbow fracture seen in the young athlete is the **fracture/separation of the medial epicondyle** (Fig. 30-15). This injury is frequently the childhood counterpart of the adult elbow dislocation.[57,73] However, the mechanism need not be a product of violent hyperextension and valgus stress but may also represent an avulsion fracture, as can be seen with throwing and arm wrestling.[28,51] Treatment depends on the amount of displacement and the degree of associated el-

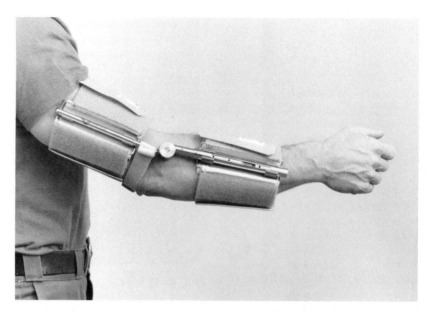

FIG. 30-14. Surprisingly good results with recalcitrant flexion contractures can be achieved with a part-time regimen of dynamic splinting. Application of the Dynasplint is shown.

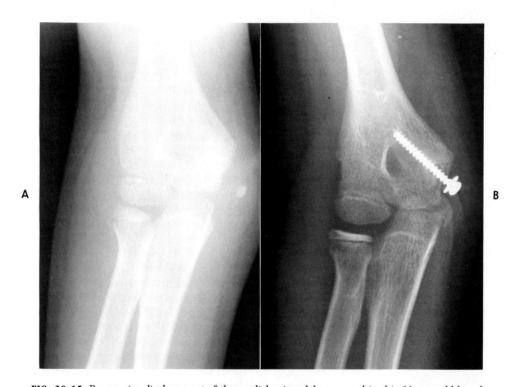

FIG. 30-15. Progressive displacement of the medial epicondyle occurred in this 11-year-old boy despite cast immobilization. **A,** Open reduction was required, and although crossed K-wire fixation is usually adequate. **B,** a screw with a spiked plastic washer was required in this instance.

bow instability. Displacement greater than 5 mm, especially if combined with elbow instability, should direct the surgeon toward an open reduction and internal fixation with either crossed pins or a cannulated screw. Surgical exploration should include identifying the ulnar nerve, which may be intimately involved with and even within the fracture. After the nerve has been identified

and protected, the epicondyle is reduced. If crossed pins are used for fixation, the elbow is immobilized for 3 weeks. If a fixation screw is used, early motion may be encouraged.

In epicondyle fractures that are minimally displaced (less than 5 mm), closed treatment is preferred, that is, a long arm cast for 3 weeks. However, radiographic

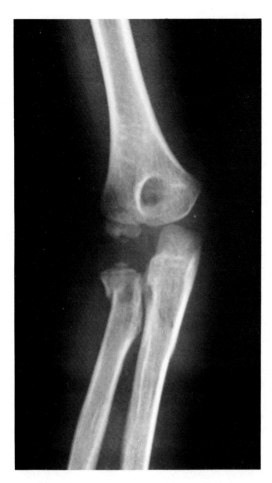

FIG. 30-16. Moderate displacement and angulation, as depicted in this child, is easily remodeled. Angulation of 30 to 40 degrees may be compatible with adequate remodeling and good function.

checks should be made at some point during the first week because the pull of the flexor-pronator musculature can lead to further displacement despite external immobilization. Finally, the same valgus stress combined with hyperextension that injures medial structures can injure lateral structures as well. Most typically, this is to the radial neck in the young athlete but may be to the radial head in the teenager or beyond. The **radial neck fracture** usually does well and is associated with little morbidity. In fact, a good deal of angulation can be accepted before reduction is even necessary (Fig. 30-16).[58] If the child is under 10 years of age, angulation of up to 30 or 40 degrees may be compatible with adequate remodeling and good function. In the child older than 10 years of age, less remodeling potential exists and no more than 15 degrees of angulation should be accepted.[52] Immobilization is carried out for 3 to 4 weeks in angulated radial neck fractures, especially in those requiring open or closed reduction. For minimally angulated fractures, motion may be initiated as soon as comfort allows.

Radial head fractures can be troublesome. Although displacement may be minimal, loss of motion can be significant. If the clinical examination demonstrates good motion, including pronation and supination, closed treatment should be used. A simple sling or posterior splint

for 7 to 10 days, followed by active range of motion activities, is all that is necessary. Further immobilization can lead to excessive stiffness and contracture. However, if the initial displacement is greater than 3 mm or if pronation and supination are limited, open reduction should be performed. Internal fixation with K-wires or small fragment screws is advocated.

Recently, reports have illustrated the occurrence of stress reactions of the immature **olecranon epiphysis** in young gymnasts. These include Osgood-Schlatter–like presentations of apophysitis/tendinitis with radiographic fragmentation of the epiphysis as well as stress fractures of the olecranon physis.[43] Nonunion of olecranon stress fracture has also been described. Although relative rest manages most of these overuse injuries, bone grafting and internal fixation has been required for nonunion.[81]

WRIST AND FOREARM

As the physician might expect, athletic injuries about the wrist unique to the skeletally immature athlete are those involving the growth plate. The distal radius undergoes spontaneous closure of its physis by 17 years in the female and 19 years in the male.[26] As shown in Table 30-1, in our experience 8.2% of injuries to the young upper extremity were to the wrist.

Fractures

Most of the wrist fractures in my study consisted of routine **distal radial fractures,** either metaphyseal, epiphyseal, or both. The common types of tendinitis do occur, but in the skeletally immature athlete an occult underlying stress reaction of bone or growth plate may masquerade as tendinitis. Bone scans are not as routinely helpful here because of the normally increased uptake about the growth plates. However, I still obtain bone scans if my index of suspicion suggests an atypical tendinitis pattern.

Stress-Related Injuries

Several authors have described stress-related injuries of the skeletally immature wrist.[56,76] These have for the most part involved young gymnasts and consisted of radiographic changes compatible with stress-induced changes of the distal radial or distal ulnar growth plates.

Radiographic changes in stress-related wrist injuries

- Widening and irregularity of physis
- Cystic changes
- Haziness of the physis
- Growth plate displacement

These radiographic patterns include widening, irregularity, cystic changes, or haziness of the growth plate.[53] Actual growth plate slippage or fractures of the distal epiphyses have been described.[59]

The mechanism of injury behind these stress-related growth plate changes relates to repetitive hyperextension and rotation, as exemplified by the gymnast practicing a

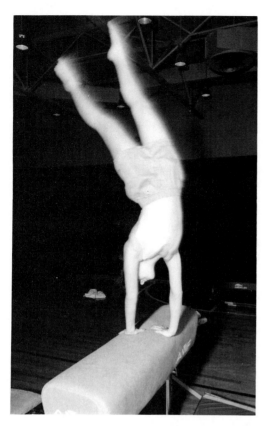

FIG. 30-17. Repetitive impact loading on the extended upper extremity, often combined with rotational forces, have been associated with stress-related growth plate changes of the distal radius and ulna.

TABLE 30-6 Prevalence of injury to the wrist and hand

Injury	Percentage (n = 69)
Wrist	
Fracture	34.8
Sprain	34.8
Contusion	5.8
Hand	
Fracture	41.5
Sprain	7.7
Contusion	1.5

Data from Cleveland Clinic Foundation, Section of Sports Medicine, 1984 to 1993.

twisting vault technique (see Chapter 38).[59] This technique causes the wrist on the side of the twist to go into hyperextension and ulnar deviation (Fig. 30-17). Other activities in gymnastics have been implicated. In particular, the dowel grip used by gymnasts to increase their hook-grip strength has been associated with painful stress-related changes of the distal radial and ulnar growth plates. It is theorized that dependence on this device allows increased tensile forces to be generated across the distal radial and ulnar growth plates, eventually leading to stress injury.[82] As with other overuse injuries in young people, they are self-limiting if allowed time to rest properly.

HAND

Although sprains and dislocations can occur in the young athlete, fractures are the most common event that brings them to the physician's office (Table 30-6).[44] And, as one would expect, these fractures are usually epiphyseal growth plate fractures, which tend to heal rapidly and well with closed reduction and external immobilization alone.[18,44,64] Remodeling of angular deformity of fractures within the plane of motion of the adjacent joint helps further. However, as with adults, rotational deformity does not correct itself and can be especially troublesome in the hand. Finally, because most of these fractures involve the growth plate, the possibility of late de-

formity caused by premature or asymmetric growth arrest must be kept in mind when arranging adequate clinical follow-up.

SUMMARY

The upper extremity is a marvel of engineering design and neuromuscular control, performing a multitude of precise and intricate movements throughout a wide range of motion, yet often sustaining large externally and internally generated forces—a tribute to our evolution. On the other hand, sport tends to push us to our limits of physiologic tolerance, and the young athlete is no exception.[4,20,60,71] Although adult patterns of injury virtually without exception can and do occur in the young, the majority of injury patterns in the young upper extremity are influenced by the existence of a growth plate.[46,74] This structure often represents the weak link in the musculoskeletal system and sustains injury (either chronic or acute) preferentially over ligaments, tendons, or bones. The good news is that the vast majority of these childhood sport trauma injuries will heal well, without sequelae, with relatively simple closed methods of treatment. There are exceptions, however, and we must forever be aware of and alert to these mischievous and at times vicious injury patterns.

Our attention should further be directed not only at the treatment of injury, but also, especially in dealing with youth, on prevention. Careful analysis of the mechanisms of injury and the athletic environments associated with the production of injury patterns continues to provide the knowledge necessary to formulate rational guidelines for the prevention of athletic abuse.

REFERENCES

1. Adams JE: Injury to the throwing arm in the elbow joints of boy baseball players, *Calif Med* 102:127, 1965.
2. Aichroth P: Osteochondral fractures and their relationship to osteochondritis dissecans of the knee: an experimental study in animals, *J Bone Joint Surg* 53B(3):448, 1971.
3. Albright JA et al: Clinical study of baseball pitchers: correlation of injury to the throwing arm with method of delivery, *Am J Sports Med* 6(1):15, 1978.
4. Allen ME: Stress fracture of the humerus: a case study, *Am J Sports Med* 12(3):244, 1984.
5. Arenon JG, Regan K: Decreasing the incidence of recurrence of first time anterior shoulder dislocations with rehabilitation, *Am J Sports Med* 12(4):283, 1984.

6. Bauer M et al: Osteochondritis dissecans of the elbow, *Clin Orthop* 264:156, 1992.
7. Blitzer CM et al: Downhill skiing injuries in children, *Am J Sports Med* 12(2):142, 1984.
8. Campbell CJ, Ranawat CS: Osteochondritis dissecans: the question of etiology, *J Trauma* 6(2):201, 1966.
9. Chan D et al: Chronic stress injuries of the elbow in young gymnasts, *Br J Radiol* 64(768):1113, 1991.
10. Cofield RH, Irving JF: Evaluation and classification of shoulder instability with special reference to examination under anesthesia, *Clin Orthop* 223:32, 1987.
11. Cofield RH, Kavanagh BF, Frassica FJ: Anterior shoulder instability. In AAOS: *Instructional course lectures,* vol 34, St Louis, 1985, Mosby.
12. Cooper RA, Brems JJ: The inferior capsular-shift procedure for multidirectional instability of the shoulder, *J Bone Joint Surg* 74A(10):1516, 1992.
13. Dameron TB, Reibel DB: Fractures involving the proximal humeral epiphyseal plate, *J Bone Joint Surg* 51A(2):289, 1969.
14. DeHaven KE: Elbow problems in the adolescent athlete, *Cleve Clin Q* 42(2):297, 1985.
15. DeHaven KE, Evarts CM: Throwing injuries of the elbow in athletes, *Orthop Clin North Am* 4(3):801, 1973.
16. Devereaux MD, Lachman SM: Athletes attending a sports injury clinic—a review, *Br J Sports Med* 17(4):137, 1983.
17. Dias JJ et al: The conservative treatment of acromioclavicular dislocation: review after five years, *J Bone Joint Surg* 69B(5):719, 1987.
18. Eaton RG: The dangerous chip fracture in athletes. In AAOS: *Instructional course lectures,* vol 34, St Louis, 1985, Mosby.
19. Eidman DK, Siff SJ, Tullos HS: Acromioclavicular lesions in children, *Am J Sports Med* 9(3):150, 1981.
20. Emans JB: Upper extremity injuries in sports. In *Pediatric adolescent sports medicine,* Boston, 1984, Little, Brown.
21. Estwanik JJ et al: Injuries in interscholastic wrestling, *Phys Sports Med* 8(3):111, 1980.
22. Galpin RD, Hawkins RJ, Grainger RW: A comparative analysis of operative versus nonoperative treatment of grade III acromioclavicular separations, *Clin Orthop* 193:150, 1985.
23. Garth WP, Allman FL, Armstrong WS: Occult anterior subluxations of the shoulder in noncontact sports, *Am J Sports Med* 15(6):579, 1987.
24. Grana WA, Rashking A: Pitcher's elbow in adolescents, *Am J Sports Med* 8(5):333, 1980.
25. Greipp JF: Swimmer's shoulder: the influence of flexibility and weight training, *Phys Sports Med* 13(8):92, 1985.
26. Greulich WW, Pyle SI: *Radiographic atlas of skeletal development of the wrist and hand,* Stanford, Calif, and Oxford, England, 1950, Stanford University Press and Oxford University Press.
27. Gugenheim JJ et al: Little league survey: the Houston study, *Am J Sports Med* 4(5):189, 1976.
28. Haw DWM: Avulsion fracture of the medial epicondyle of the elbow in a young javelin thrower: case report, *Br J Sports Med* 15(1):47, 1981.
29. Henry JH, Genung JA: Natural history of glenohumeral dislocation revisited, *Am J Sports Med* 10(3):135, 1982.
30. Hepburn GR, Crivelli KJ: Use of elbow Dynasplint for reduction of elbow flexion contractures: a case study, *J Orthop Sports Med Phys Ther* 5(5):269, 1984.
31. Hovelius L: Anterior dislocation of the shoulder in teenagers and young adults: five year prognosis, *J Bone Joint Surg* 69A(3):393, 1987.
32. Hovelius L et al: Recurrences after initial dislocation of the shoulder: results of a prospective study of treatment, *J Bone Joint Surg* 65A(3):343, 1983.
33. Jackson DW: Chronic rotator cuff impingement in the throwing athlete, *Am J Sports Med* 4(6):231, 1976.
34. Jawish R et al: Osteochondritis dissecans of the humeral capitellum in children, *Eur J Pediatr Surg* 3(2):97, 1993.
35. Jobe FW, Jobe CM: Painful athletic injuries in the shoulder, *Clin Orthop* 173:117, 1983.
36. Koh TJ, Grabiner MD, Weiker GG: Technique and ground reaction forces in the back handspring, *Am J Sports Med* 20(1):61, 1992.

37. Kvitne RS, Jobe FW: The diagnosis and treatment of anterior instability in the throwing athlete, *Clin Orthop* 291:107, 1993.
38. Langenskiold A: Can osteochondritis dissecans arise as a sequel of cartilage fracture in early childhood? An experimental study, *Acta Chir Scand* 109:204, 1955.
39. Langer F, Percy EC: Osteochondritis dissecans and anomalous centres of ossification: a review of 80 lesions in 61 patients, *Can J Surg* 14:208, 1971.
40. Larson RL et al: Little league survey: the Eugene study, *Am J Sports Med* 4(5):201, 1976.
41. Linden B, Telhag H: Osteochondritis dissecans: a histologic and autoradiographic study in man, *Acta Orthop Scand* 48:682, 1977.
42. Maffulli N, Chan D, Aldridge MJ: Derangement of the articular surfaces of the elbow in young gymnasts, *J Pediatr Orthop* 12(3):344, 1992.
43. Maffulli N, Chan D, Aldridge MJ: Overuse injuries of the olecranon in young gymnasts, *J Bone Joint Surg* 74B(2):305, 1992.
44. Markiewitz AD, Andrish JT: Hand and wrist injuries in the preadolescent and adolescent athlete, *Clin Sports Med* 2(1):203, 1992.
45. McManama GB et al: The surgical treatment of osteochondritis of the capitellum, *Am J Sports Med* 13(1):11, 1985.
46. Micheli LJ: Overuse injuries in children's sports: the growth factor, *Orthop Clin North Am* 14(2):337, 1983.
47. Nagura S: The so-called osteochondritis dissecans of Konig, *Clin Orthop* 18:100, 1960.
48. Neer CS: Anterior acromioplasty for the chronic impingement syndrome in the shoulder, *J Bone Joint Surg* 54A(1):41, 1972.
49. Nielsen AB, Nielsen K: The modified Bristow procedure for recurrent anterior dislocation of the shoulder, *Acta Orthop Scand* 53:229, 1982.
50. Norwood LA et al: Anterior shoulder pain in baseball pitchers, *Am J Sports Med* 6(3):103, 1978.
51. Nyska M et al: Avulsion fracture of the medial epicondyle caused by arm wrestling, *Am J Sports Med* 20(3):347, 1992.
52. Ogden JA: *Skeletal injury in the child,* Philadelphia, 1982, Lea & Febiger.
53. Paavolainen P et al: Recurrent anterior dislocation of the shoulder: results of Eden-Hybbinette and Putti-Platt operations, *Acta Orthop Scand* 55:556, 1984.
54. Pappas AM: Elbow problems associated with baseball during childhood and adolescence, *Clin Orthop* 164:30, 1982.
55. Pitt MJ, Sper DP: Imaging of the elbow with an emphasis on trauma, *Radiol Clin North Am* 28(2):293, 1990.
56. Post M: Current concepts in the diagnosis and management of acromioclavicular dislocations, *Clin Orthop* 200:234, 1985.
57. Priest JD, Weise DJ: Elbow injury in women's gymnastics, *Am J Sports Med* 9(5):288, 1981.
58. Rang M: *Children's fractures,* Philadelphia, 1974, JB Lippincott.
59. Read MTF: Stress fractures of the distal radius in adolescent gymnasts, *Br J Sports Med* 15(4):272, 1981.
60. Rettig AC, Beltz HF: Stress fracture in the humerus in an adolescent tennis tournament player, *Am J Sports Med* 13(1):55, 1985.
61. Rowe CR: Recurrent transient anterior subluxation of the shoulder: the "dead arm" syndrome, *Clin Orthop* 223:11, 1987.
62. Rowe CR, Zarins B, Ciullo JV: Recurrent anterior dislocation of the shoulder after surgical repair: apparent causes of failure and treatment, *J Bone Joint Surg* 66A(2):159, 1984.
63. Roy S, Caine D, Singer KM: Stress changes of the distal radial epiphysis in young gymnasts: a report of twenty-one cases and a review of the literature, *Am J Sports Med* 13(5):301, 1985.
64. Ruby LK: Common hand injuries in the athlete, *Clin Sports Med* 2(3):609, 1983.
65. Ruch DS, Poehling GG: Arthroscopic treatment of Panner's disease, *Clin Sports Med* 10(3):629, 1991.
66. Ruggles DL, Peterson HA, Scott SG: Radial growth plate injury in a female gymnast: case study, *Med Sci Sports Exerc* 23(4):393, 1991.
67. Salter RB, Harris WR: Injuries involving the epiphyseal plate, *J Bone Joint Surg* 45A(3):587, 1963.
68. Simonet WT, Cofield RH: Prognosis in anterior shoulder dislocation, *Am J Sports Med* 12(1):19, 1984.

69. Singer KM, Roy SP: Osteochondrosis of the humeral capitellum, *Am J Sports Med* 12(5):351, 1984.
70. Smith AD: Osteochondritis of the knee joint: a report of three cases in one family and a discussion of the etiology and treatment, *J Bone Joint Surg* 42A(2):289, 1960.
71. Sullivan JA: Recurring pain in the pediatric athlete, *Pediatr Clin North Am* 31(5):1097, 1984.
72. Taft TN et al: Dislocation of the acromioclavicular joint: an end-result study, *J Bone Joint Surg* 69A(7):1045, 1987.
73. Teitz CC: Sports medicine concerns in dance and gymnastics, *Pediatr Clin North Am* 29(6):1399, 1982.
74. Tibone JE: Shoulder problems of adolescents: how they differ from those of adults, *Clin Sports Med* 2(2):423, 1983.
75. Tibone JE et al: Shoulder impingement syndrome in athletes treated by an anterior acromioplasty, *Clin Orthop* 198:134, 1985.
76. Tolat AR, Sanderson PL, Stanley JK: The gymnast's wrist: acquired positive ulnar variance following chronic epiphyseal injury, *J Hand Surg* 17B(6):678, 1992.
77. Torg JS, Pollack H, Sweterlitsch P: The effect of competitive pitching on the shoulders and elbows of preadolescent baseball players, *Pediatrics* 49(2):267, 1972.
78. Tulos HS, Bennett JB, Braly WG: Acute shoulder dislocations: factors influencing diagnosis and treatment. In AAOS: *Instructional course lectures,* vol 33, St Louis, 1984, Mosby.
79. Tulos HS, King JW: Lesions of the pitching arm in adolescents, *Clin Orthop* 200:264, 1972.
80. Wagner KT, Lyne ED: Adolescent traumatic dislocations of the shoulder with open epiphyses, *J Pediatr Orthop* 3(1):61, 1983.
81. Wilkerson RD, Johns JC: Nonunion of an olecranon stress fracture in an adolescent gymnast: a case report, *Am J Sports Med* 18(4):432, 1990.
82. Yong-Hing K, Wedge JG, Bowen CVA: Chronic injury to the distal ulnar and radial growth plates in an adolescent gymnast, *J Bone Joint Surg* 70A(7):1087, 1988.

PART VI Neurologic and Vascular Problems

CHAPTER 31   Neurovascular Injuries

George Pianka

Elliott B. Hershman

The spectrum of athletic injuries that involve the upper extremity includes both acute injuries to and chronic conditions of the neurovascular structures. These problems can be difficult to diagnose at times and often are considered only after other, more common athletic injuries are eliminated from diagnostic consideration. Injury to the neurovascular structures, however, should always be considered in the differential diagnosis of an athletic injury. Neurovascular problems can be the primary problem, as in bowler's thumb,[11,63,102] or secondary to other ongoing processes, as with ulnar neuritis[30,35] resulting from chronic valgus instability of the elbow in a throwing athlete. Whether primary or secondary in nature, the neurovascular condition must be addressed to permit safe return to athletics.

Injury to the neurologic system can occur in numerous anatomic locations and create symptoms in the upper extremity. In particular, cervical spine trauma often leads to either peripheral nerve injury at the root level or spinal cord injury in the cervical region.[3] Neck injury must always be considered when athletes describe neurologic symptoms in the upper extremity.[5] The diagnostic approach to differentiating these problems is discussed at length in Chapter 1.

Neurologic problems can arise from injury to the major nerves, as in brachial plexus trauma, or to smaller peripheral nerves, as occurs in carpal tunnel syndrome. The injury level can often be localized from the results of a detailed physical examination. Other diagnostic modalities can be used to confirm or refute the clinician's diagnostic impression. These techniques include nerve conduction studies, electromyography, spinal cord or cortical evoked potentials, magnetic resonance imaging (MRI), and myelography with computerized tomography (CT).

Like neurologic injury, vascular problems can arise in a multitude of sites in the upper extremity. Both arterial and venous injuries can occur, and problems range from injury to the large subclavian vessels to involvement of the significantly smaller ulnar artery. In chronic vascular problems the radiographic evaluation (arteriography or venography) often is an important diagnostic modality because the physical examination can be unrevealing. This is in contrast to acute vascular occlusion, which often manifests dramatic physical findings.

In any of these injuries it is important that the pertinent anatomy be understood so the physical examination is precise and informative. Once an exact diagnosis is

reached, appropriate treatment and counseling can be offered.

ANATOMY
Brachial Plexus

The neurologic elements of the upper extremity originate from the cervical portion of the spinal cord. Cervical roots C5 to C8, as well as thoracic root T1, contribute to the innervation of the upper extremity.

The brachial plexus is formed by the junctions of the ventral rami of the C5 to C8 and T1 spinal nerve roots. Occasionally, there may be a contribution from C4, designated as a prefixed plexus, or less frequently from T2, designated a postfixed plexus. Although observed anatomically, these variations have little clinical significance in most instances. These rami are formed from a dorsal root, which is sensory, and a ventral root, which is motor. The ventral rami lie between the anterior and middle scalene muscles where they share space with the subclavian artery. The plexus continues distally over the first rib and deep to the sternocleidomastoid muscle in the posterior cervical triangle, a region bordered by the trapezius muscle, sternocleidomastoid muscle, and superior border of the clavicle.

The five ventral rami unite just above the clavicle to form three trunks: the upper trunk, consisting of roots C5 and C6; the middle trunk, consisting of root C7; and lower trunk, consisting of roots C8 and T1 (Fig. 31-1). Just below the level of the clavicle, each trunk divides into an anterior and posterior division. These divisions contribute to the formation of three cords.

The posterior divisions from each trunk form the posterior cord, which has contributions from C5, C6, C7, C8, and slightly from T1. The anterior divisions of the upper and middle trunks form the lateral cord, which has contributions from C5, C6, and C7. The anterior division of the lower trunk forms the medial cord, which has contributions from C8 and T1. The three cords, lateral, posterior, and medial, are named in reference to their position relative the axillary artery, running just below the pectoralis minor muscle.

The three cords divide to give five terminal branches to the upper extremity, whereas other branches arise

TABLE 31-1 Major branches of the brachial plexus

Peripheral Nerve	Root Composition	Origin
Long thoracic	C5, C6, C7	Cervical roots
Dorsal scapular	C5	Cervical root
Suprascapular	C5, C6	Upper trunk
Upper subscapular	C5	Posterior cord
Lower subscapular	C5, C6	Posterior cord
Thoracodorsal	C7, C8	Posterior cord
Lateral pectoral	C5, C6, C7	Lateral cord
Medial pectoral	C8, T1	Medial cord
Medial brachial cutaneous	C8, T1	Medial cord
Medial antebrachial cutaneous	C8, T1	Medial cord
Axillary	C5, C6	Posterior cord
Radial	C6, C7, C8	Posterior cord
Median	C5, C6, C7, C8, T1	Medial and lateral cords
Musculocutaneous	C5, C6	Lateral cord
Ulnar	C8, T1	Medial cord

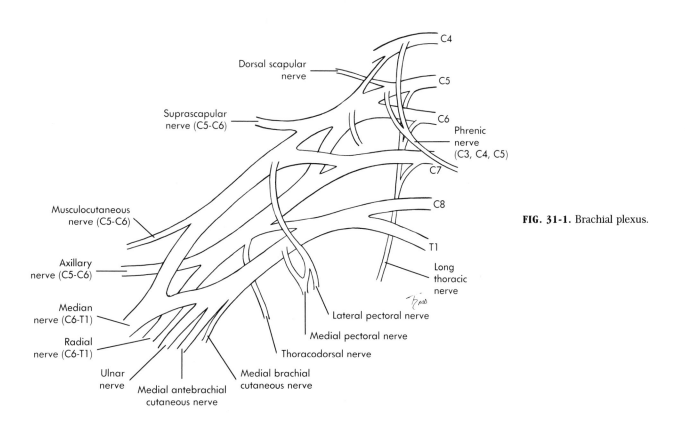

FIG. 31-1. Brachial plexus.

more proximally, either from the cords, trunks, or roots, to supply the shoulder girdle musculature. These branches are summarized in Table 31-1.

The radial nerve is the terminal branch of the posterior cord, the middle trunk, and the C7 ventral ramus. It receives contributions from the upper and lower trunks. The axillary nerve is a branch from the posterior cord, which originates proximal to the radial nerve. Other direct branches from the posterior cord are the thoracodorsal nerve and the upper and lower subscapular nerves.

The ulnar nerve is the terminal branch of the medial cord and lower trunk, arising from the C8 and T1 ventral rami. The medial pectoral nerve and the medial brachial and antebrachial cutaneous branches are also terminal divisions of the medial cord.

The median nerve is formed from continuing portions of the medial and lateral cords. The lateral cord, which arose from the upper and middle trunks, contributes mainly sensory fibers from the ventral rami of C5, C6, and C7. These fibers join with the primarily motor contribution from a branch of the medial cord, originating at the C8 and T1 ventral rami.

The suprascapular nerve is a branch arising from the upper trunk, consisting of the C5 and C6 ventral rami. The C5 ventral ramus sends contributions to the phrenic nerve and provides another branch to form the dorsal scapular nerve. The long thoracic nerve is formed from contributions of the ventral rami of C5, C6, and C7 nerve roots.

Axillary Vessels

The subclavian vessels arise from the aortic arch on the left side and from the innominate (brachiocephalic) artery on the right. The subclavian artery has the transverse scapular artery as a branch and becomes the axillary artery as it crosses the upper border of the first rib. The axillary veins tend to follow the artery and its branches. The brachial plexus is located around the artery. The axillary artery, axillary vein, and brachial plexus travel through the axilla enclosed within the axillary sheath, a fibrous tunnel that is a continuation of the fascia of the neck.

The axillary artery is often described by its relationship to the pectoralis minor: the first segment lies proximal to the pectoralis minor, the second directly behind it, and the third distal to it. There are six main branches arising from the axillary artery—supreme thoracic, thoracoacromial, lateral thoracic, subscapular, anterior humeral circumflex, and posterior humeral circumflex (Fig. 31-2). The axillary artery becomes the bra-

---

Axillary artery branches

- Supreme thoracic
- Thoracoacromial
- Lateral thoracic
- Subscapular
- Anterior humeral circumflex
- Posterior humeral circumflex

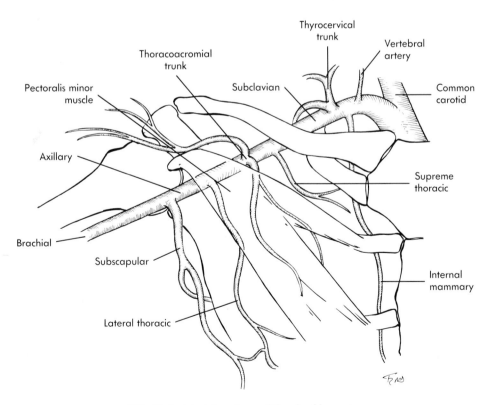

FIG. 31-2. Arterial anatomy of the shoulder region.

chial artery as it crosses the lower border of the teres major.

Arm

The brachial artery continues down the arm along the medial aspect of the biceps. It passes into the elbow region beneath the biceps aponeurosis (lacertus fibrosis).

In the upper arm the radial nerve lies behind the artery, the ulnar nerve is medial to the artery, and the median nerve can be found anterolateral to the artery. The radial nerve continues posterior, winds around the humerus, and continues along the lateral border of the distal humerus. The ulnar nerve becomes more medial as it courses distally, passing through the intermuscular septum to lie posteriorly near the point it crosses the elbow, behind the medial epicondyle.

In the arm the musculocutaneous nerve supplies innervation to the biceps brachii, coracobrachialis, and brachialis muscles. Posteriorly the triceps are innervated by the radial nerve. In addition, the radial nerve provides innervation to the anconeus and brachioradialis muscles. The ulnar and median nerves have no motor branches in the arm, but rather contribute to the forearm, wrist, hand, and fingers with both motor and sensory fibers.

Forearm

The terminal branches of the median, ulnar, and radial nerves provide all of the motor innervation to the muscles of the forearm and hand. The sensory innervation of the forearm and hand is also supplied by these nerves, with the exception of the medial aspect of the proximal forearm (medial antebrachial cutaneous nerve) and varying portions of the mid-to distal lateral forearm (cutaneous portion of the musculocutaneous nerve).

The median nerve lies medial to the brachial artery on the anterior surface of the brachialis at the elbow. It passes with the brachial artery beneath the lacertus fibrosus, then continues between the two heads of the pronator teres. It provides motor control to the pronator teres, flexor carpi radialis, palmaris longus, and flexor digitorum superficialis. The nerve runs between the heads of the flexor digitorum superficialis and continues to the wrist, deep to the flexor digitorum superficialis muscle. An important branch of the median nerve arises about 5 cm below the medial epicondyle. This branch, the anterior interosseous nerve, continues down the forearm on the interosseous membrane and gives motor innervation to the flexor digitorum profundus (index and middle fingers), flexor pollicis longus, and pronator quadratus. The various tissues the median nerve passes through account in large part for the entrapment syndromes that can occur.

The ulnar nerve passes into the forearm between the heads of the flexor carpi ulnaris and continues to the wrist under the cover of this muscle tendon unit. The nerve supplies motor innervation to the flexor carpi ulnaris and the ulnar portion of the flexor digitorum profundus (ring and little fingers).

The radial nerve supplies all the innervation to the extensor aspect of the forearm. After winding posteriorly around the humerus, the nerve comes to lie on the lateral side of the arm. In the region of the elbow, the nerve divides into motor (posterior interosseous) and sensory (superficial radial) branches. The location of this bifurcation is variable and can occur proximal or distal to the elbow.

The majority of the motor supply on the extensor aspect is afforded by the posterior interosseous nerve. This nerve provides innervation to the muscles listed in the accompanying box. The radial nerve or superficial branch generally provides innervation to the extensor carpi radialis longus and/or brevis, but the innervation is variable.

Posterior interosseous nerve-innervated muscles

- Supinator
- Extensor digitorum
- Extensor digiti minimi
- Extensor carpi ulnaris
- Abductor pollicis longus
- Extensor pollicis brevis
- Extensor pollicis longus
- Extensor indicis

The brachial artery divides into two branches, the radial and ulnar arteries. The radial artery passes through the forearm, between the brachioradialis and the flexor carpi radialis. The ulnar artery travels with the ulnar nerve, between the flexor carpi ulnaris and the flexor digitorum profundus.

Wrist and Hand

The median nerve passes through the wrist in the carpal tunnel. Here it lies beneath the transverse carpal ligament (flexor retinaculum). Proximally in the carpal tunnel it is found on the radial side of the superficial flexor tendons, but distally it comes to lie directly beneath the transverse carpal ligament. It gives off the important motor branch to the thenar muscles then continues to branch, providing motor innervation to the first and second lumbricals and sensory innervation to the palmar aspect of the thumb, index finger, middle finger, and radial aspect of the ring finger.

The ulnar nerve passes under the volar carpal ligament in Guyon's canal. It generally divides at about the level of the distal pisiform into its terminal superficial and deep branches. The superficial branch provides sensory innervation to the palmar aspect of the little finger and ulnar aspect of the little finger and ring finger. The deep branch provides motor innervation to the hypothenar muscles, the interosseous muscles, the third and fourth lumbricals, the adductor pollicis, and the deep head of the flexor pollicis brevis.

The superficial radial nerve provides sensory innervation to the dorsum of the hand and radial digits (thumb, index, and middle). Often the dorsum of the ulnar digits has sensory innervation from branches of the dorsal branch of the ulnar nerve.

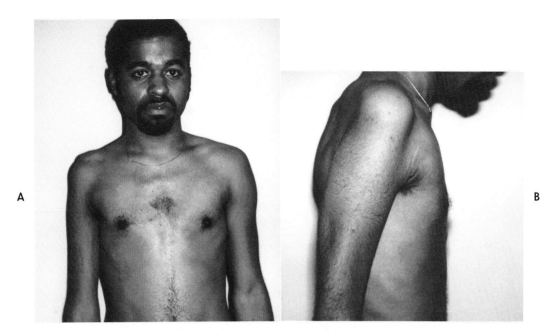

FIG. 31-3. A and **B,** Atrophy can often be used to delineate the region of nerve injury. This lesion has led to atrophy of the right deltoid and biceps, easily noted with careful observation.

The radial artery and ulnar artery each branch to form a deep and superficial component. These branches go on to form the deep and superficial palmar arches. The completeness of these vascular arches is variable, but the deep is more constant than the superficial.

For the reader interested in further discussion of the anatomy of wrist and hand, see Chapter 21 for additional information.

PHYSICAL EXAMINATION

Examination for neurovascular injuries should be part of every routine physical examination. A number of specific features of the neurologic and vascular examinations are important to discuss.

Observation

The patient should be observed carefully, with the trunk and upper extremities disrobed. Subtle areas of atrophy or deformity can be observed in this manner (Fig. 31-3). Discoloration, swelling, and general skin color should be noted because abnormalities may arise in these characteristics with both venous and arterial problems. Any skeletal deformity should be documented.

Joint Evaluation

The active and passive range of motion of the neck, shoulders, elbows, wrists, and hands should be measured. Stability of joints should be evaluated because recurrent instability can result in neurovascular problems.

Motor Examination

The motor evaluation is one of the most important components of the neurologic evaluation. A thorough motor examination can often define the site of a lesion. It is important to differentiate between root level injuries and peripheral nerve injuries, and this can often be done on the basis of the motor examination. The various innervation patterns that can be identified by careful motor examination are outlined in Table 31-2.

When motor function is graded in athletes, it is important to recall the classic muscle grading system.[124] In this system strength is graded as follows:

Grade		Findings
5	Normal (N)	Able to withstand full resistance
4	Good (G)	Able to withstand some resistance
3	Fair (F)	Able to move against gravity
2	Poor (P)	Able to move with gravity eliminated
1	Trace (T)	Able to contract without movement
0	Zero	No evidence of contraction

In athletes, however, strength measurement by manual muscle testing may be difficult because of the tremendous strength of many athletes. Often the examiner cannot overcome an athlete's strength in the injured extremity because of the great strength of the athlete. In this setting, quantifiable strength measurement may be of value. This can be done by using dynamometers, such as Cybex isokinetic equipment, or by using hand-held measuring devices such as the NISMAT—Nicholas Manual Muscle Tester. It must be remembered that strength testing, in general, has limitations resulting from pain and test-subject efforts, so results must be judged in their clinical setting.

TABLE 31-2 Patterns of motor innervation

Root Innervation (Predominant)

C5	C6	C7	C8	T1
Deltoid	Wrist extensors	Triceps	Finger flexors	Hand intrinsics
Biceps		Wrist flexors	Hand intrinsics	
Rhomboids		Finger extensor		
Supraspinatus				
Infraspinatus				

Peripheral Nerve Innervation

Dorsal scapula	*Long thoracic*	*Suprascapular*
Rhomboids	Serratus anterior	Infraspinatus
		Supraspinatus
Thoracodorsal	*Subscapular*	*Lower subscapular*
Latissimus dorsi	Subscapularis	Subscapularis
		Teres major
Medial pectoral	*Lateral pectoral*	*Musculocutaneous*
Pectoralis major	Pectoralis major	Coracobrachialis
Pectoralis minor		Biceps
		Brachialis
Median	*Anterior interosseous*	*Axillary*
Pronator teres	Flexor digitorum profundus	Deltoid
Flexor carpi radialis	(radial half)	Teres minor
Palmaris longus	Flexor pollicis longus	
Flexor digitorum superficialis	Pronator quadratus	
Abductor pollicis brevis		
Opponens pollicis		
Flexor pollicis brevis (superficial)		
Radial two lumbricals		
Radial	*Posterior interosseous*	*Ulnar*
Triceps	Supinator	Flexor carpi ulnaris
Anconeus	Extensor digitorum	Flexor digitorum profundus
Brachioradialis	Extensor digiti minimi	(ulnar half)
Extensor carpi radialis longus and	Extensor carpi ulnaris	Flexor pollicis brevis (deep)
brevis	Abductor pollicis longus	Hypothenar muscles
	Extensor pollicis brevis	Adductor pollicis
	Extensor pollicis longus	Interossei
	Extensor indicis	Ulnar two lumbricals

Reflex Examination

The reflexes of the upper extremity are listed in Table 31-3. Reflexes should be judged in terms of their quality, not just their presence or absence, to determine subtle reflex abnormalities.

Sensory Evaluation

Sensory disturbances can occur in either a dermatomal (root) distribution or in the distribution of peripheral nerves. These are illustrated in Fig. 31-4. If spinal cord lesions are suspected, it is important to evaluate all sensory functions, including light touch, temperature, vibration, position sense, and pain (pinprick).

Vascular Evaluation

Pulses can be evaluated at the wrist for both the radial and ulnar arteries. The Allen test should be performed if vascular injuries are suspected at the wrist. In this test both the radial and ulnar arteries are occluded by the examiner. The patient opens and closes the hand until the hand is blanched. The examiner then releases the pressure on the radial artery and notes the filling of the hand from the radial to the ulnar side. The procedure is then repeated with the examiner releasing the

TABLE 31-3 Upper extremity reflexes

Muscle	Root (Predominant)
Biceps	C5
Brachioradialis	C6
Triceps	C7

ulnar artery initially. Comparisons are made in the patterns of vascular refill.

The brachial artery is easily palpated at the elbow, just medial to the lacertus fibrosus. Obliteration of the pulse implies a vascular problem proximally in the axillary or subclavian region.

Venous tone and patterns should be observed. In axillary vein thrombosis the venous pattern of the involved extremity is increased and the dorsal hand veins do not collapse when raised to the level of the heart (Fig. 31-5).

Adson's test may be helpful in the diagnosis of thoracic outlet syndrome. It is performed by extending the arm and locating the radial pulse. The head is turned to the side being tested. A positive test occurs when the radial pulse is obliterated by the turned head. A modification

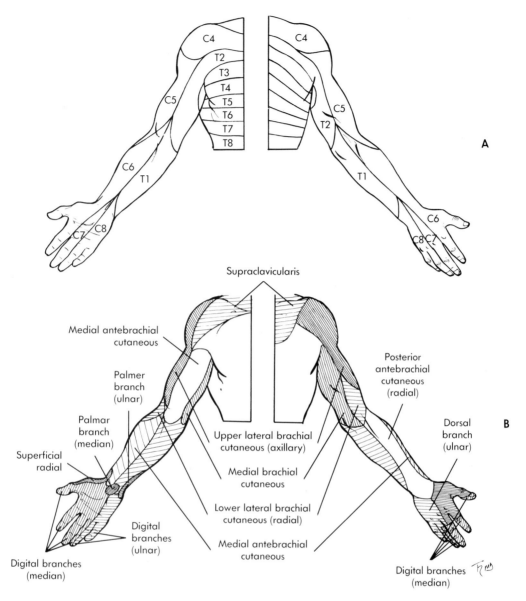

FIG. 31-4. Sensory distribution. **A,** Root dermatomes. **B,** Peripheral nerve distribution.

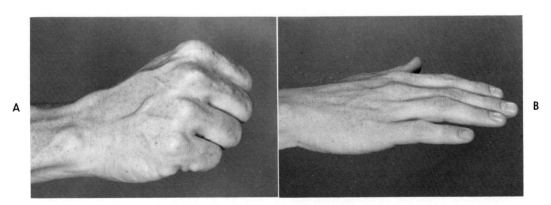

FIG. 31-5. Evaluation of axillary vein patency. **A,** Hand at side, normal prominent venous tone. **B,** Hand at heart level, veins collapse when axillary vein is patent. If appearance of hand is similar to **A,** axillary vein thrombosis is suspected.

of this test has the patient turn the head to the opposite side.[132]

In an examination for a neurologic injury, Tinel's sign should be sought. To elicit Tinel's sign, percussion is performed over a nerve from distal to proximal. The point of maximal pain may represent an entrapment lesion.

ADJUNCTIVE TESTS

The most commonly performed test for evaluation of neurologic injury is electrophysiologic examination. This includes two components—an electromyogram (EMG) and a nerve conduction study (NCS).

An EMG is performed by placing small needles into the muscle being evaluated and observing the nature of the electrical activity in the muscle. Complete denervation leads to absence of total electrical activity. Partial (acute) denervation, indicative of a lesion that has structural integrity of the nerve but functional loss, presents a pattern of fibrillations on the EMG evaluation. These patterns of injury do not generally appear until 2½ to 3 weeks after a neural injury. As healing occurs, these fibrillation potentials disappear, often leaving a pattern of large motor units demonstrated by increased duration and amplitude of the motor units' potentials. This represents sprouting of the intact motor nerves to take over orphaned muscle cells. These large units can be found permanently in the EMG after significant injury, if repair occurs.

The NCS represents direct measurement of nerve conduction throughout the extremity. The measurements are obtained by direct stimulation of the nerve proximally in the extremity and measurement of the time until the impulse reaches a point more distal in the extremity. The standard nerve conduction velocities have been published and are readily available. In addition, the time of conduction across certain regions is also evaluated and compared with the opposite extremity, if uninvolved.

These measurements are known as latency and are typically calculated for the areas across the cubital tunnel (ulnar nerve), carpal tunnel (median nerve), and Guyon's canal (ulnar nerve). Prolonged latency implies a block in nerve conduction in the anatomic region being studied.

For vascular problems invasive testing may be required. Arterial problems are often evaluated with arteriography. If a proximal lesion is suspected, a catheter can be inserted into the femoral artery and advanced to the aortic arch or subclavian artery. Here, contrast injection defines lesions at the subclavian, axillary, and brachial level. Distal lesions can be evaluated similarly or by a brachial contrast injection technique.

On the venous side, venography performed by contrast injection into the hand is indicated if venous occlusion is seriously suspected.

Other more elaborate tests of vascular function include Doppler ultrasound, impedance plethysmography, and vascular phase technetium scanning. These techniques are best used in conjunction with vascular surgeons as part of a comprehensive evaluation.

TABLE 31-4 Correlation of Seddon and Sunderland classification of nerve injuries

Seddon	Sunderland (Degree)				
	First	Second	Third	Fourth	Fifth
Neurapraxia	▓				
Axonotmesis		▓	▓		
Neurotmesis				▓	▓

CLASSIFICATION OF TRAUMATIC NERVE INJURIES

In 1943, Seddon[115,124] described a classification for traumatic nerve injuries. This classification is useful in describing the degree of injury and the potential for recovery. The three classes are as follows:

Neurapraxia—a minimal nerve injury that leads to a temporary, fully reversible nerve conduction block.

Axonotmesis—a moderate injury in which there is interruption of the axons and their myelin sheaths. The endoneural tubes, however, remain intact to guide regeneration.

Neurotmesis—a severe injury in which a nerve is severed completely or destroyed and regeneration cannot occur spontaneously.

Most sports injuries result in either neurapraxia or axonotmesis. However, in moderate athletic trauma, nerves can be injured in such a way that a component of the nerve has a neurotmesis injury, but the majority of injury is usually axonotmesis.[131] Differentiation may be difficult clinically and electrophysiologically. A comparison between the Seddon and Sunderland classification is shown in Table 31-4. The Sunderland classification is more practical and representative of nerve injuries.

SPINAL ACCESSORY NERVE INJURIES

The spinal accessory nerve (eleventh cranial nerve) is the sole motor nerve to the trapezius muscle. The superficial course of this nerve makes it susceptible to injury. The nerve lies in the subcutaneous tissue on the floor of the posterior cervical triangle, bounded by the trapezius, sternocleidomastoid, and clavicle, in its course to innervate the trapezius muscle.[120] Blunt trauma and surgery

---

Sunderland's grades of nerve injury

- Grade I: Interruption of axial conduction, demyelination axons preserved, subtle injury
- Grade II: Axon severed, endoneurium preserved, axons regenerated, full recovery
- Grade III: Endoneurium disrupted, Wallerian degeneration, incomplete recovery (most difficult to assess), most traction injuries
- Grade IV: Perineurium disrupted, neuroma develops, no useful recovery, surgery required
- Grade V: Epineurium disrupted, nerve severed, surgical repair required

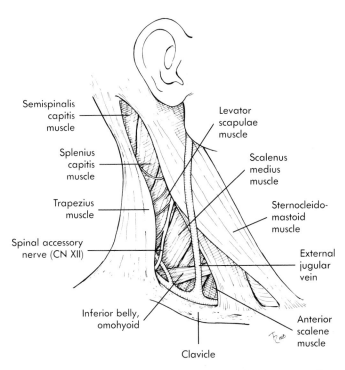

FIG. 31-6. Injury to the spinal accessory nerve can occur from blunt trauma in the region where the nerve crosses the border of the trapezius in the posterior cervical triangle.

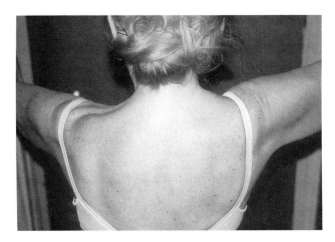

FIG. 31-7. Atrophy of left trapezius muscle.

in the posterior cervical triangle are the two predominant causes of injury to this nerve, resulting in paralysis of the trapezius muscle. This lesion, although uncommon, is painful, deforming, and disabling.

A direct, forceful blow to the neck in the area of the posterior cervical triangle can cause a crushing injury to the nerve where it passes under the upper border of the trapezius (Figs. 31-6 and 31-7). This can be the result of contact between athletes or contact between an athlete and a piece of equipment. Another mechanism is an injury that depresses the shoulder while the head is forced in the opposite direction, resulting in a traction injury to the nerve.[135] Football, lacrosse, and hockey are some of the sports in which this type of injury has occurred.[61,133]

Manifestations of this injury include a dull ache or pain, with drooping of the shoulder and noticeable weakness in arm elevation and abduction. On examination, the patient is unable to shrug the shoulders and shows winging of the scapula when viewed from behind. The sternocleidomastoid muscle is spared. The scapula is rotated downward and displaced laterally as a result of the lack of the suspensory action of the trapezius. This is because of the paralysis of the upper and central portion of the muscle that attaches to the acromion and normally pulls the shoulder upward and inward. The scapula is stabilized on the chest wall by the lower portion of the muscle, and this normal function, which prevents rotation and translation, is lost. The trapezius not only helps suspend the shoulder, but also provides a firm base from which the deltoid muscle acts in elevating the arm. The

pain is thought to be caused by overuse of the levator scapulae and rhomboid muscles and from brachial radiculitis caused by stretching of the brachial plexus.[14]

Initial treatment is conservative. The arm is put into a sling and physical therapy for active and passive exercise is provided to avoid contractures in the arm and shoulder. Paralysis may persist for 3 to 12 months in closed injuries. The function of the trapezius is so vital that even strengthening adjacent muscle groups is inadequate to compensate for the extensive lost functions.

For lesions caused by open trauma or iatrogenic injury, neurolysis and nerve grafting have given variable results, but are generally more successful when performed within 6 months. Intraoperative nerve action potential studies may be done to determine if neurolysis alone is sufficient or whether resection with end-to-end repair or nerve grafts is needed.[33] After 1 year reconstructive procedures, using muscle transfers, are performed to improve shoulder function in isolated injuries,[14] whereas stabilization procedures are preferred for more widespread weakness and neuromuscular disorders.

Dynamic procedures that involve muscle transfers have consisted of transferring the levator scapulae and rhomboid muscles, the Eden-Lange procedure.[14,74] Static fixation of the scapula to the spinous processes has been done using fascia lata grafts.[31]

If the lesion is mild and reversible, athletic participation can be attempted when healing has occurred and dynamic stabilization of the scapula has been achieved through muscle rehabilitation and reeducation. For severe lesions, with little or no functional return, athletic participation is restricted insofar as the involved extremity is concerned.

BRACHIAL PLEXUS PROBLEMS

The brachial plexus is formed by the ventral rami of cervical spinal nerves (C5 through C8 and T1). The nerves then emerge between the anterior and middle

scalene muscles traveling below the sternocleidomastoid muscle and under the clavicle to the axilla. The ventral rami of the fifth and sixth spinal nerves interconnect to form the upper trunk, C7 continues as the middle trunk, and C8 and T1 combine to form the lower trunk. After decussation and reassembly, lateral, posterior, and medial cords are formed from which the terminal nerves to the arm are derived. Knowledge of the brachial plexus and its innervations is essential to proper diagnosis of injuries to this area, in addition to prognostic implications.

Acute Traumatic Injury

Because of its superficial location, surrounding bony structures, and the mobility of the neck and shoulders, the brachial plexus is vulnerable to injury. Traction injuries are found in various contact sports, such as football and wrestling.[4] The majority of information on brachial plexus injuries has come from cases of high-velocity trauma, such as motorcycle accidents.[79,109] Fracture-dislocations of the shoulder may also injure the brachial plexus, whereas dislocations without associated fractures usually injure the axillary nerve more than the brachial plexus. Clavicle fractures and their active callus or hematoma may also cause injury to the brachial plexus or chronic compression. Another example of brachial plexus compression occurs during hiking with heavy backpacks, when the brachial plexus is compressed between the clavicle and first rib by the weight of the pack and the shoulder straps (Fig. 31-8). Injury to the plexus occurs from traction on the nerves from the weight of the pack and from compression of the nerves between the strap and the bony structures. Damage to the brachial plexus may also occur as root avulsions (Fig. 31-9). Cervical nerve root avulsion has a consistently poor prognosis because the nerve cannot be repaired and

does not regenerate. Careful evaluation of brachial plexus injuries is essential to render appropriate treatment and prognosis.

Supraclavicular traction injuries of the brachial plexus have notoriously bad prognoses, probably because of the frequency of root avulsions.[109] In addition to a thorough

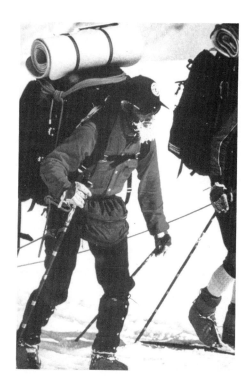

FIG. 31-8. Long periods of direct pressure by the axillary straps of heavy backpack can lead to plexus injury.

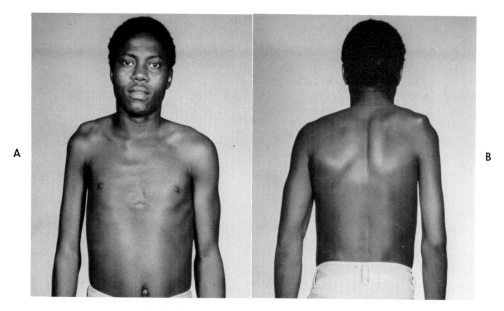

FIG. 31-9. A and **B,** Sandlot football player with C5-C6 root avulsions. Injury occurred when shoulder struck ground and neck was driven to opposite side. Gross atrophy of deltoid biceps and spinati is present. Scapula is winging.

examination, EMG is a helpful adjunct in localizing injuries of the brachial plexus because the paraspinal muscles can be tested and will indicate the severity of nerve damage. Myelography can be used to show root avulsions by demonstrating pseudomeningoceles. Histamine skin testing helps to determine whether the sensory lesion is preganglionic or postganglionic. An absent flare response indicates a postganglionic injury and therefore a more favorable prognosis. Electrodiagnostic testing with sensory nerve action potentials (SNAPs) has replaced the histamine test. A normal SNAP to an anesthetic region implies a poor prognosis because the lesion is preganglionic. Infraclavicular lesions have a relatively good prognosis with a return of motor function in the injured cord or terminal branch.[79,109] Lesions of the upper trunk are more common and have better prognoses than lesions of the lower trunk.[109] Persistent pain in the presence of a brachial plexus injury, regardless of its location, indicates a poor prognosis. The presence of Horner's syndrome is usually a bad prognostic sign in a brachial plexus injury as well.

Knowing the extent of the injury (i.e., neurapraxia, axonotmesis, or neurotmesis and involvement of the cervical spinal roots), one can better anticipate the likelihood of spontaneous improvement or the need for surgery. In closed injuries, without a gross disruption in the brachial plexus, early institution of physical therapy is recommended to prevent contractures. Neurapraxic injuries may take 3 to 4 months to show improvement. The majority of brachial plexus injuries in sports are low-velocity injuries, such as shoulder dislocations, with good prognosis for recovery because the nerves are in continuity and the lesion is either a neurapraxia or a axonotmesis. After 4 months of observation with no improvement and electrophysiologic studies showing continued axonal degeneration, surgery may be indicated to either repair the disruption in the plexus or use cable nerve grafts. In cases of spinal nerve root avulsion, nerve transfer is the only possibility to improve function. Regional nerves, such as the medial pectoral, thoracodorsal, long thoracic, and subscapular, have given the most successful results when used to reinnervate the musculocutaneous and axillary nerve, with an 83.8% rate of overall useful functional recovery. Emphasis is placed on restoring the nerve supply to proximal muscles because effective regeneration of nerves to muscles in the hand rarely occurs in adults. Approximately 2 years are required to obtain the axonal regeneration and return of function. At the end of this period, tendon transfers may be considered to improve the residual muscle function in the arm and shoulder.

Burner Syndrome

Burner syndrome is a specific upper-trunk brachial plexus injury that occurs in contact sports.[12] It is most commonly seen in football and has also been termed upper trunk brachial plexopathy and the stinger syndrome.[98,104]

The brachial plexus consists of contributions of ventral rami of C5 to C8 and T1 roots. Classically, burners involve the C5 and C6 components of the brachial

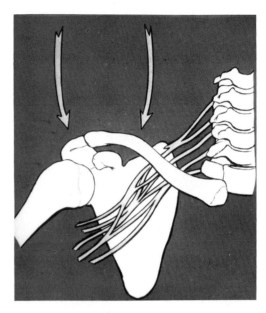

FIG. 31-10. Point of contact in acromioclavicular joint injuries is over acromion (*left arrow*). In burner syndrome impact occurs more medially (*right arrow*).

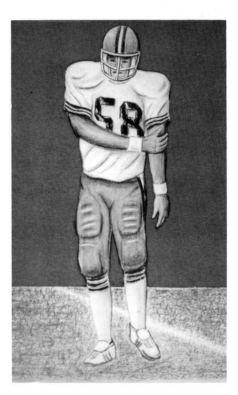

FIG. 31-11. Burner syndrome causes sharp burning pain in shoulder, arm and hand. The athlete may hold the affected arm when leaving the field.

plexus. The injury usually results from a player making head, neck, or shoulder contact with an opposing player.[104] The entire shoulder girdle is depressed in its relation to the neck. This mechanism is similar to the mechanism of an acromioclavicular sprain; however, the point of contact is somewhat different (Fig. 31-10). Other

mechanisms include cervical extension/lateral deviation and direct contact at Erb's point. The player immediately feels a sharp burning pain in the shoulder, radiating into the arm and hand (Fig. 31-11). The pain is described as burning in nature, hence the origin of the descriptive name of this syndrome. The burning is accompanied by weakness of the biceps, spinati, or deltoid muscles, causing weakness in shoulder abduction, external rotation, and elbow flexion. The symptoms usually last for a few minutes, but may persist for 2 weeks or longer. Persistent pain and weakness beyond 2 weeks indicates a more severe injury to the brachial plexus. Clancy, Brand, and Bergfeld[24] have classified these lesions by their clinical features (Table 31-5). Some players experience repeated episodes of burners. Permanent neurologic deficits are, however, rare.

It is important to repeatedly examine athletes who sustain a burner. Often weakness develops in the days or weeks following the injury. Repeated examination identifies those athletes in whom weakness develops in the postinjury period.

There is still some controversy with regard to the exact site and nature of the injury. It is uncertain whether the injury is at the cervical root level,[23] ventral rami, or in the brachial plexus (Table 31-6).[97] Many authors, however, believe the lesion in the true burner syndrome is a traction injury at the upper trunk level.[12,24,104] Other authors have proposed that the injury occurs as the C5 and C6 roots are compressed when the head and neck are extended and laterally flexed to the injured side.[88] Foraminal compression of the roots can be an acute or a chronic problem with this mechanism. A third potential mechanism is a direct blow to the supraclavicular region, causing direct injury to the plexus at Erb's point.

Burners most often are a transitory physiologic block of some or all axons in the involved nerve and would be classified as a neurapraxia by Seddon's classification of nerve injury. Axonotmesis probably does occur in more severe injuries and would coincide with prolonged symptoms weeks from the time of injury. EMG can be helpful in defining the site and extent of the lesion after a period of 3 weeks from the time of the injury. The EMG findings compatible with a brachial plexopathy in a player with burners are fibrillation potentials demonstrated in the upper-trunk–innervated shoulder girdle-musculature (deltoid, biceps, supraspinatus, and infraspinatus) and normal activity in the cervical paraspinal musculature. Often the lesion is mild electrophysiologically, and the site of injury may be difficult to determine.[131] Other studies have found fibrillation potentials in the neck muscles of players with burners consistent with cervical radiculopathy.

TABLE 31-5 Clinical classification of brachial plexus injuries

Grade	Findings
I	Transitory motor/sensory loss; may last minutes to hours; complete recovery within 2 weeks.
II	Significant motor weakness/sensory loss; neurologic examination abnormal at least 2 weeks.
III	Motor and sensory loss at least 1 year's duration.

Modified from Clancy WG, Brand RL, and Bergfeld, JA: *Am J Sports Med* 5:209, 1977.

TABLE 31-6 Burner syndrome

Type	Mechanism	Clinical Findings	Radiographs	Clinical Course
I Traction	Shoulder girdle is depressed. Head may be laterally deviated to contralateral side.	Transient burning pain in upper extremity. No neck symptoms. May develop weakness in C5-C6/upper trunk distribution.	No acute findings.	Often not associated with weakness. Return to play when strength has returned to baseline.
II Direct contact	Compression of the fixed brachial plexus between the shoulder pad and the superior medial scapula when the pad is pushed into the Erb's point.	Transient burning pain in upper extremity. No neck symptoms. May have local tenderness in superclavicular region. A dropped shoulder may occur with repeated injury. Weakness may develop in C5-C6/upper trunk distribution.	No acute findings.	Can reduce incidence by use of interval roll or pad between neck and shoulder pad. Return to play when strength is normal.
III Extension compression	Cervical hyperextension and lateral flexion to the ipsilateral side causing foraminal compression of the nerve roots.	Transient burning pain in upper extremity. Neck pain may be present. Neurologic symptoms may be reproduced by examining the patient supine with the head extended and laterally flexed to the side of the neurologic injury (a variation of Spurling's maneuver.)	Increased incidence of cervical spinal stenosis with a Torg ration <0.8.	Prolonged symptoms. May be associated with repeated clinical episodes. May reduce incidence with posterior and lateral pads. Return to play when strength is normal and athlete is asymptomatic.

EMG and nerve root stimulation studies used in football players have helped delineate the lesion. Findings showed the injury probably results from compression of a fixed brachial plexus between the shoulder pad and the superomedial aspect of the scapular when the pad is pushed into the area of Erb's point, where the brachial plexus is most superficial. A modification of the shoulder pads has decreased the number of stinger injuries in this particular group of athletes.[84,88]

Cervical spine fracture or dislocation may evoke symptoms much like those seen with burners and central cervical spinal cord syndrome.[3,86] Therefore a player with acute burner symptom and symptoms such as neck pain or limitation of motion should be treated as a cervical spine injury because of the similarity in presentation. Radiographs and cervical cord evaluation are negative for acute injury in the burner syndrome. Meyer et al[88] have noted an association between the extension-compression mechanism of injury and cervical spinal stenosis.

Once the diagnosis has been made, the athlete with weakness should be restricted from competition and reexamined on a regular basis. When shoulder strength has returned to normal, participation in athletics can be resumed. Athletes will often use neck rolls, special pads, and extra high shoulder pads to help limit neck motion when they return to football (Fig. 31-12). An interval pad between the neck and shoulder has been shown to be helpful in preventing burners in those athletes with the direct contact mechanism (Fig. 31-12, *B*).[84] All athletes should, however, participate in a neck, shoulder, and upper trunk strengthening program.

The EMG may remain abnormal for years, with large motor unit potentials commonly appearing, so repeat EMG is not often indicated to determine the time for athletic return.[12] Rather, the return to normal strength should be the factor relied on in most situations. Relative strength differences were more accurately discerned with isokinetic strength testing than the manual muscle testing.[114]

Acute Brachial Neuropathy

Acute brachial neuropathy (ABN) is an uncommon cause of shoulder pain and disability. It can, however, present in association with athletic activity and must therefore be included in the differential diagnosis of athletes with shoulder pain.[59] First described among servicemen in the Second New Zealand Expeditionary Force in 1942, it has also been called Parsonage-Turner syndrome, acute brachial radiculitis, and brachial plexus neuropathy.[94]

ABN is a clinical entity of unknown cause characterized by the acute or subacute onset of shoulder pain as-

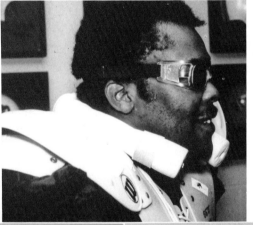

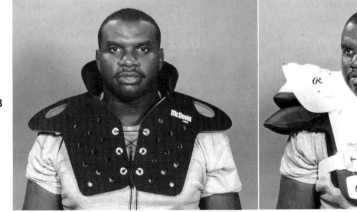

FIG. 31-12. Neck rolls. **A,** Under shoulder pad devices. **B,** Interval pad placed beneath shoulder pads to reduce contact from the medial border of the shoulder pads and the supraclavicular region. **C,** Both pads somewhat limit neck mobility.

sociated with weakness and sometimes with wasting of various forequarter muscles.[127] Involvement is most common in the shoulder and proximal arm. This syndrome can develop in athletes during or following their athletic activity, but the onset cannot usually be related to a specific traumatic event.[59] Characteristically, pain is severe and continues despite cessation of activity. Physical examination often reveals scapular winging, weakness (deltoid, supraspinatus, infraspinatus, biceps, or triceps most commonly), and occasional sensory deficit. EMG usually reveals diffuse plexus involvement and shows fibrillation potentials.

Once the entity is diagnosed, treatment consists of two phases.[59] In Phase 1 support for the affected extremity, rest, and analgesics are indicated. Gentle range of motion exercises are important to maintain joint mobility. Once the severe pain has resolved, the athlete enters Phase 2, or the rehabilitative phase. The entire extremity and upper body require rehabilitation to regain strength in damaged motor units. The need for rehabilitation of all muscles in the upper body must be emphasized because subclinical muscle involvement is common in this entity. Likewise, the trunk-scapula relationship must be considered because serratus anterior and rhomboid involvement frequently occurs.

The issue of returning to sports is difficult to address because the number of athletes reported with this condition is small. Return to participation can generally be considered on a case-by-case basis when individuals have reached a plateau in their strength development, which may take up to 3 years. Athletes should be told at the outset that scapula winging may persist because improvement is generally not observed in this aspect of ABN.[59]

Neurologic Thoracic Outlet Syndrome

Thoracic outlet compression syndrome refers to an uncommon condition in which nerves or vessels or both are compressed in the root of the neck or axilla.[78a] Two clearly defined forms of this condition have been described.[28,34,37] One is a neurologic syndrome that involves the lower trunk of the brachial plexus and is caused by abnormal nerve stretch or compression.[28] Another is a vascular form that involves the subclavian artery and vein and is more common in men than in women.[34,37] Although there are no reports of specific sports causing this problem, athletic activities that involve the use of the upper limbs exacerbate the symptoms.[101] Depending upon the mechanism and level of compression, several disorders are included under the title of thoracic outlet syndrome: cervical rib syndrome, scalenus-anticus syndrome, Wright's hyperabduction syndromes (including pectoralis minor syndrome), and costoclavicular syndrome.*

The coracoid and pectoralis minor act as a fulcrum during shoulder elevation and hyperabduction, such as in swimming, serving, and throwing. The neurovascular structures may be compressed among athletes who repetitively hyperabduct the arm.[122] Shoulder girdle depression in tennis players and pitchers has been de-

scribed to be caused by stretching or microtrauma to the scapular suspensory structures causing compression of the neurovascular structures as they traverse the thoracic outlet.[77,78,99]

The neurologic form of thoracic outlet syndrome often occurs in women of slim build and drooping shoulders. Presenting symptoms include aching pain in the side or back of the neck that extends across the shoulder and down along the inner aspect of the arm and paresthesias in the ulnar aspect of the hand. The sensory findings extend more proximally than an ulnar nerve lesion, whereas the motor findings include thenar and intrinsic muscle weakness and wasting.[28,75,101,108]

Adson's test—palpating the radial pulse with the arm extended while the head is turned toward the affected side, hyperextending the neck—has had a low yield. An important sign has been to reproduce the patient's symptoms by abducting and laterally rotating the arm at the shoulder with a flexed elbow while palpating the pulses at the wrist, Wright's maneuver. The overhead exercise test may elicit symptoms of aching and fatigue in patients with thoracic outlet syndrome after 20 to 30 seconds of rapidly flexing and extending the fingers as the arm is held over head.

Anatomically, an elongated transverse process of C7 and a cervical rib may be found. A fibrous band often extends from the cervical rib to the first thoracic rib, and the lower brachial trunk is stretched and angulated over this band.[108,132] Damage to the C8 and T1 spinal nerves from other causes must be ruled out, such as Pancoast tumor, neurofibromas, cervical spondylosis, cervical disk herniation, carpal tunnel syndrome, and cubital tunnel syndrome.

Evaluation should include cervical spine and chest radiographs. At times, electrophysiologic studies can be useful, and reduced ulnar SNAPs can be recorded.[132] To rule out other diseases that can cause C8 and T1 spinal nerve root pathologic conditions, myelography and computed axial tomography (CAT) scans can also be indicated as part of the workup.

Once the diagnosis of a neurologic thoracic outlet syndrome is made, every effort should be made to manage the patient conservatively.[76] Shoulder muscle exercises are often prescribed, along with local heat and a cervical collar. Surgery should be reserved for persistent symptoms for up to 3 or 4 months unless there is intractable pain, vascular compromise, or neurologic loss.[107] Supraclavicular exploration with division of the fibrous band, if present, is the recommended approach, whereas the transaxillary approach is used for first rib resection.[37,53] The surgical procedure chosen is based on the exact cause for the impingement at the thoracic outlet.[70] While relief of pain is consistent, muscle weakness and wasting do not usually resolve significantly.

Symptoms of neurologic thoracic outlet syndrome

- Aching neck pain
- Radiation into arm, forearm (ulnar side)
- Paresthesias, ulnar aspect of hand
- Intrinsic muscle weakness

---

*References 17, 34, 53, 79, 128, 132, and 134.

AXILLARY VESSEL INJURY
Vascular Thoracic Outlet Syndrome

The vascular form of thoracic outlet syndrome is uncommon. It is characterized by a well-developed cervical rib producing stenosis and poststenotic dilation of the subclavian artery.[34] The subclavian artery is angulated over the cervical rib and further compressed by the scalenus anterior muscle anterior to it.[37] The initial symptoms may vary from intermittent blanching of the hand and fingers as a result of embolization from a thrombus in the subclavian artery to a sudden catastrophic occlusion.

Evaluation should include examination and auscultation of the supraclavicular fossa for the presence of a mass and a bruit. The pulses in the arm may be absent or diminished. The Adson test can be used to reproduce the symptoms by abducting and externally rotating the arm and raising the hand above the head. If the radial pulse disappears, then a lesion of the subclavian artery should be suspected. Unfortunately, this maneuver is of questionable value because up to 80% of healthy people demonstrate a positive test.[132] Another provocative test is to have the patient raise both arms overhead and rapidly open and close the hand; this causes cramping very quickly if vascular thoracic outlet syndrome is present.

The diagnosis is confirmed by angiography, and the treatment is usually first rib resection.[34,107,127] If acute occlusion of the subclavian artery has occurred, then immediate surgery is indicated with first rib resection, removal of the thrombus, and embolectomy.[111] Axillary artery injury has been reported in shoulder dislocation, scapular neck fracture, humeral neck fracture, and clavicle fracture. Examination shows a diminished pulse in the involved extremity; the color and temperature may or may not be decreased, depending on the extent of injury. A difference in the blood pressure between the two limbs can be measured. If a major vascular injury is suspected, an angiogram is mandatory. Vascular repair is performed along with stabilization of an unstable fracture, if present.

Subclavian Vein Thrombosis

Effort thrombosis is a term used to describe a subclavian and axillary vein thrombosis caused by direct or indirect injury to the vein as a result of physical activity.[1] This is a form of thoracic outlet syndrome that accounts for less than 2% of all reported incidents of deep vein thrombosis. This entity has been reported in competitive swimmers[130] and hockey players.[20] Effort thrombosis has important short-term ramifications, such as severe disability and pulmonary embolism, that have been reported to occur in 12% of patients with subclavian vein thrombosis.[7]

The symptoms and disability may persist for a prolonged period in 68% to 75% of cases. Although the majority of cases result from trauma or use of cervical venous catheters, a small portion of the cases are related to various activities that require shoulder abduction.

The clinical presentation of effort thrombosis varies dramatically from intermittent, nonspecific symptoms that consist of a generalized aching of the arm, with a degree of fullness and swelling, to a dramatically swollen, painful arm with dependent rubor. Typically, this oc-

curs in males 15 to 40 years of age, often after a particular physical activity. The symptoms may appear immediately or up to 2 weeks later. The most common symptom noted with time is increased swelling of the arm, which responds to elevation. Swelling may be accompanied by abnormal subcutaneous vein distention, which worsens if the arm is exercised.

A venogram demonstrates occlusion of the axillary and subclavian veins, although the study itself may result in extension of the thrombosis. Doppler studies have been useful in distinguishing intermittent compression from thrombosis. Other noninvasive methods of evaluation include duplex scanning and impedance plethysmography.[73]

The recommended treatment of effort-induced thrombosis is usually conservative. A strict regimen of arm elevation is begun, and the blood is anticoagulated with heparin for 10 days.[85] At that time conversion to warfarin is done to achieve therapeutic levels that prevent extension of the clot and promote recanalization of the vein.

Some of the chronic symptoms noted by patients who have had this entity include easy fatigability of the arm, recurrent swelling, and tightness in the arm. Surgical intervention with thrombectomy may be indicated if a localized thrombus is present to avoid the high risk of chronic symptoms. Surgery is not indicated if an extensive thrombus is present. Chronic symptoms have been reported in 75% of patients treated conservatively. Early clot dissolution with intravenous streptokinase has been achieved with success, provided the clot is less than 2 weeks old.[10]

Other procedures attempted have included decompression of the costoclavicular space and removal of the clavicle or anterior scalene muscle and local fibrinolytic therapy and first rib resection when the clot has resolved.

PERIPHERAL NERVE LESIONS
Shoulder Region
Long Thoracic Nerve

Isolated paralysis of the serratus anterior muscle has been described in a wide variety of sports, including tennis, golf, gymnastics, soccer, bowling, weight lifting, ice hockey, wrestling, archery, basketball, and football.[54] The long thoracic nerve originates from the ventral rami of C5, C6, and C7 cervical nerves and travels beneath the brachial plexus and clavicle over the first rib. The nerve then travels along the lateral aspect of the chest wall to innervate the serratus anterior muscle (Fig. 31-13). Its superficial course and length make it especially vulnerable to injury. Damage to the nerve may be caused by blows to either the shoulder or lateral thoracic wall. Excessive use of the shoulder or prolonged traction, such as in cycling, has been found to cause this nerve injury.

The clinical features include dull ache or pain around the shoulder girdle, a winged scapula, and decreased active shoulder motion.[42,66] Pain may be increased when the head is tilted to the contralateral side or when the ipsilateral arm is raised above the head. Often painless winging of the scapula may be the clinical presentation of someone involved in any of the sports mentioned

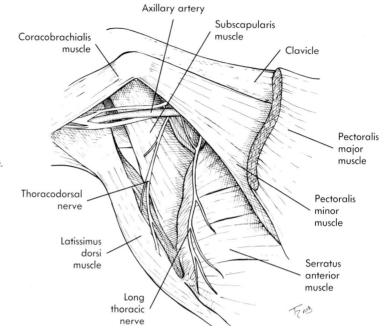

FIG. 31-13. Course of the long thoracic nerve.

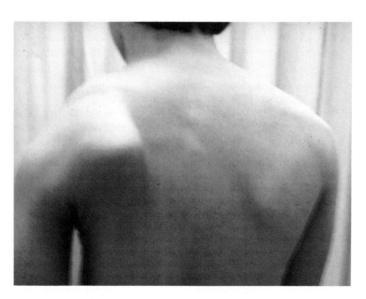

FIG. 31-14. Winging of the left scapula in a weight lifter with injury to the long thoracic nerve.

above. Winging of the scapula is especially prominent during forward pushing, as in push-ups (Fig. 31-14). More severe pain is usually indicative of an acute brachial plexus neuropathy with involvement of other muscles of the arm and shoulder.[59] An idiopathic form of serratus anterior paralysis has been identified. The term *neuralgic amyotrophy* was coined by Parsonage and Turner[94] in 1948 to describe the shoulder girdle syndrome or paralytic brachial neuritis that occasionally may affect only the long thoracic nerve.

The serratus anterior stabilizes the scapula on the posterior thoracic wall, thereby providing a firm point for muscles arising from the scapula to move the arm. The serratus anterior, together with the trapezius and leva-tor scapulae, acts to upwardly rotate the scapula and thus allow greater glenohumeral motion.

Other conditions, such as polymyositis, muscular dystrophy, and cervical spondylosis, must be ruled out.[66] EMG findings of denervation have proved valuable in the diagnosis and prognosis of this injury.

There is no consensus on treatment of this condition, but generally, conservative measures, such as rest from the associated sport and physical therapy, are advised. The prognosis for serratus anterior paralysis is generally good, with recovery occurring up to 2 years after injury.[52]

Return to sports can be considered when the shoulder girdles have symmetric strength parity. The likelihood of complete resolution of scapula winging is low

and should not be used as a criterion for return to athletics.

Suprascapular Nerve

The suprascapular nerve originates from the upper trunk of the brachial plexus and consists of contributions from the fifth and sixth cervical roots. The nerve runs in the posterior triangle of the neck, passing under the body of the omohyoid muscle and anterior border of the trapezius muscle to the scapular notch, where it is firmly fixed in a fibroosseous tunnel. The nerve runs through the scapular notch, which is covered by the transverse scapular ligament, to innervate the supraspinatus mus-

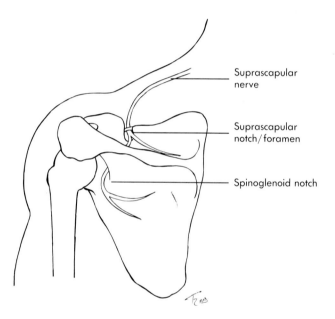

FIG. 31-15. Course of the suprascapular nerve. Entrapment can occur at the suprascapular notch or spinoglenoid notch.

cle, and gives off sensory fibers to the capsular and ligamentous structures of the shoulder and acromioclavicular joint (Fig. 31-15). The majority of reported entrapment neuropathies of the suprascapular nerve have been in the area involving the transverse scapular ligament.[25,55] The nerve then continues around the lateral border of the spine of the scapula, through the spinoglenoid notch, to innervate the infraspinatus muscle. Entrapment here would give symptoms of infraspinatus muscle involvement.

Entrapment of the suprascapular nerve has been associated with traction injuries to the shoulder and with repetitive use of the shoulder.[44] Direct trauma to the shoulder, including shoulder dislocation or fracture, is the most common cause of suprascapular nerve injury.[138]

Activities such as weight lifting, volleyball,[41] and backpacking have been found to cause this rare nerve entrapment syndrome, with trauma from cross-body adduction being implicated in a neurapraxia type of injury to the nerve.[40] Asymptomatic isolated infraspinatus muscle paralysis has been found in volleyball players as a result of cocking of the arm and follow-through while serving.[15,41,89]

Clinical findings include atrophy of the supraspinatus and/or infraspinatus muscles (Fig. 31-16) and poorly localized pain in the posterolateral aspect of the scapula. There is often a loss of strength in abduction and external rotation of the arm.[121] Patients are often evaluated for rotator cuff injury. The diagnosis of suprascapular nerve entrapment should be suspected if the MRI evaluation shows a structurally intact rotator cuff with selective atrophy of the spinatus muscles.[137] Rotator cuff pathologic conditions must be considered in the differential diagnosis in addition to cervical radiculopathy, myopathy, and brachial plexus neuropathy.

Often radiographic, electromyographic, and nerve conduction studies confirm the clinical picture of suprascapular nerve entrapment at the suprascapular or spinogle-

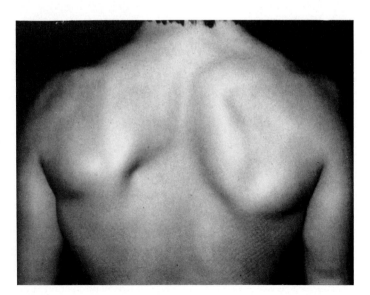

FIG. 31-16. Wrestler with suprascapular nerve injury at suprascapular notch. Observe atrophy of infraspinatus notch and supraspinatus fossa.

noid notch. Conservative therapy with rest, antiinflammatory medication, and physical therapy may be unsuccessful in relieving the symptoms, and surgical decompression may be necessary.[55,125] Explorations of the suprascapular nerve have revealed hypertrophy of the transverse scapular ligament and anomalies of the suprascapular notch. Compression of the spinoglenoid notch has also been identified.[49]

The surgical procedures have ranged from excision of the transverse scapular ligament or spinoglenoid ligament to deepening the suprascapular notch.[45,100] Ganglion cysts often have been found to compress the suprascapular nerve at the notch of the scapula.[62,92,126] The clinical response to decompression of the nerve has varied from no improvement to full restoration of muscle bulk and power and resolution of pain.[55,129]

If return of supraspinatus and infraspinatus function occurs, resumption of participation in athletics can occur. However, since the infraspinatus supplies 90% of the external rotation power of the shoulder and the supraspinatus stabilizes the humeral head in the genoid during elevation, residual weakness will often preclude a safe return to athletics, as the deficits make safe participation difficult to achieve.

Axillary Nerve

The axillary nerve branches from the posterior cord of the brachial plexus and contains fibers from the C5 and C6 nerve roots. The nerve then travels laterally and downward, anterior to the subscapularis muscle, passing just below the shoulder joint and into the quadrilateral space. The axillary nerve next curves around the posterior and lateral portion of the proximal humerus, divides into anterior and posterior branches, and innervates the deltoid and teres minor muscles (Fig. 31-17). A cutane-ous sensory branch of the nerve supplies the lateral aspect of the upper arm.

The usual mechanism of injury to the axillary nerve is trauma, either a direct blow to the shoulder,[13] fracture of the proximal humerus,[16] or a shoulder dislocation, all of which cause stretching of the nerve. Axillary nerve injuries occur in many sports, such as football, wrestling, gymnastics, mountain climbing, and rugby.[9] When the arm is displaced away from the trunk, tension is placed on the nerves. This tension or stretch is most severe for the nerves with the shortest distance from the brachial plexus to their muscle insertion. This would help explain the frequent involvement of the axillary nerve in injuries to the shoulder.

The degree of injury to the axillary nerve can vary. The initial presentation may be weakness in elevation and abduction of the arm, with or without numbness along the lateral aspect of the upper arm. Weakness in abduction may not be readily apparent because the supraspinatus alone may effectively abduct the arm. Wasting of the deltoid muscle subsequently develops (Fig. 31-18). Whenever an axillary nerve injury is considered, one must rule out a posterior cord injury by testing the latissimus dorsi muscle, the nerve of which branches proximal to the axillary nerve, and by testing the muscles innervated by the radial nerve.

Electrophysiologic testing can be used to determine whether there has been a partial or complete axillary nerve injury. If the injury is partial, the treatment is rest, physical therapy, and a sling. Because of the short course of the axillary nerve, some degree of recovery should be expected within 3 months. Surgical intervention is recommended if there is no sign of improvement by 3 to 4 months. Exploration and neurolysis or nerve grafting often gives good results.[43,95] With any form of treatment,

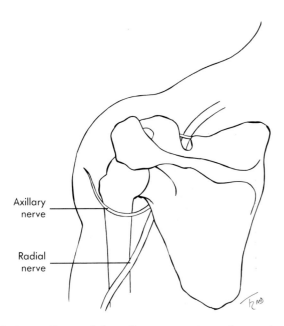

FIG. 31-17. Course of the axillary nerve as it travels posterior to the proximal humerus.

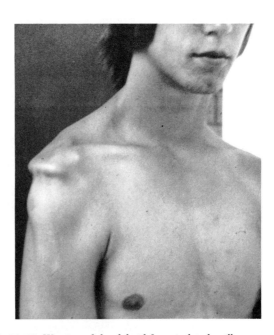

FIG. 31-18. Wasting of the deltoid from isolated axillary nerve injury.

participation in athletics can be resumed when strength parity has been achieved.

Quadrilateral Space Syndrome

The quadrilateral space syndrome involves compression of the posterior humeral circumflex artery and axillary nerve. The quadrilateral space is on the posterior aspect of the shoulder, and its boundaries are the teres minor superiorly, teres major inferiorly, humeral shaft laterally, and the long head of the triceps muscle medially. The axillary nerve and posterior humeral circumflex artery pierce the internervous plane between the teres minor and teres major, supplying the teres minor and deltoid muscles.[21] A sensory branch innervates the skin on the lateral aspect of the upper arm.

Although it is an uncommon syndrome, it has been reported in young people of both sexes.[21] The atypical distribution of pain and paresthesias often results in a delay in diagnosis. The pain is usually intermittent and poorly localized to the anterior aspect of the shoulder. There may be tenderness in the shoulder anteriorly and laterally, often with point tenderness at the insertion of the teres minor. The paresthesias have a nondermatomal distribution in the arm, forearm, and hand. Abduction, elevation, and external rotation of the humerus reproduce or exacerbate the symptoms. There may be a diminished radial pulse with this maneuver leading to an erroneous diagnosis of thoracic outlet syndrome. Selective atrophy of the teres minor muscle has been shown on MRI in several patients, thus helping confirm the diagnosis.[81] Associated nerve compression syndromes such as carpal tunnel syndrome have been reported.[21] Electrophysiologic testing of the deltoid muscle is normal. Cervical spine and other shoulder diseases such as rotator cuff disease must be differentiated because the pain may awaken the patient at night.

A subclavian arteriogram is used to confirm the diagnosis of quadrilateral space syndrome. The arteriogram is performed with the arm at the side initially and then in abduction and external rotation. The dye is followed laterally to the posterior humeral circumflex artery, which is patent when the arm is at the side and may occlude with the arm in 60 degrees or more of abduction and some external rotation. Bilateral arteriograms are not indicated. About 70% of patients with arteriograms showing occlusion of the posterior humeral circumflex artery do not have symptoms severe enough to undergo surgical decompression and live with their discomfort, which may persist.

Surgical decompression of the quadrilateral space is performed by detaching the insertion of the teres minor to the humerus and reflecting it medially, thus removing the superior obstruction of the quadrilateral space. Often one finds tethering fibrous bands overlying the neurovascular bundle. After division of these bands, the arm is brought into 110 degrees abduction and 45 degrees external rotation and the pulse should be palpable in the posterior humeral circumflex vessel. The patient is begun on early active range of motion exercises and then muscle strengthening exercises at three weeks.

Elbow Region
Musculocutaneous Nerve

The musculocutaneous nerve is a mixed motor and sensory peripheral nerve that arises from the lateral cord of the brachial plexus and contains fibers from the C5, C6, and C7 nerve roots. The nerve pierces the coracobrachialis muscle below the coracoid process and travels down the arm between the biceps and brachialis muscles, which it also supplies (Fig. 31-19). The sensory component then continues lateral to the biceps and becomes superficial anterolaterally as it penetrates the deep brachial fascia above the elbow. At this point it becomes the lateral cutaneous nerve of the forearm. In its superficial course, the nerve travels through the antecubital fossa between the median cubital vein and cephalic vein. The anterior division of the nerve supplies sensation to the radial half of the volar aspect of the forearm, whereas the posterior branch supplies the radial third of the dorsal aspect of the forearm.

The presentation of musculocutaneous nerve compression varies according to the site of the lesion.[71] In addition to shoulder dislocations, injury to the nerve proximal to its innervation of the coracobrachialis muscle has been reported to occur in an athlete after throwing a football and in competitive rowing. The findings in such a case consisted of weakness in elbow flexion, atrophy of the brachialis and biceps brachii, a dull ache in the distal forearm with dysesthesias, and absence of re-

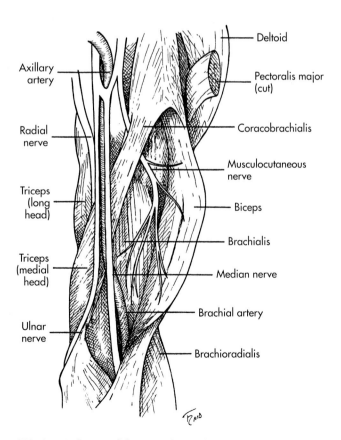

FIG. 31-19. Course of the musculocutaneous nerve in the cutaneous branch of the arm (not shown) continues distally to forearm.

flex in the biceps. Electrophysiologic studies confirmed the location of the lesion. After 4 months, the neurapraxia resolved with resolution of the symptoms.

Weight lifting has also been associated with musculocutaneous neuropathy below the level of the coracobrachialis muscle that manifested painless weakness and atrophy of biceps muscle and dysesthesia in the volar radial forearm. Strenuous exercise was thought to cause either repetitive injury to the nerve by the coracobrachialis muscle or chronic compression as a result of muscle hypertrophy.[18] Cessation of weight lifting resulted in resolution of the symptoms up to 2 months later.

Positioning the arm in abduction, external rotation, and extension while the patient is under general anesthesia has also resulted in musculocutaneous nerve injury.

This syndrome may be confused with a C5 or C6 radioculopathy, brachial plexus injury (especially one involving the lateral cord), and rupture of the biceps tendon. Differentiation is based on careful clinical examination of other muscle groups innervated by the C5 and C6 nerve roots, sensory examination, and electrophysiologic testing.

A **compression syndrome of the lateral cutaneous branch of the musculocutaneous nerve** has also been described.[8,40] Symptoms include pain, paresthesias, dysesthesias, and numbness in the distal volar and dorsal forearm. Pain and tenderness are experienced over the nerve in the anterolateral aspect of the elbow or over the lateral humeral epicondyle and may be caused by compression of the nerve between the biceps aponeurosis and tendon against the fascia of the brachialis mus-

cle. The nerve is relatively fixed in this area, and injury can result from entrapment and compression.

Vigorous exercise consisting of elbow extension and forearm pronation or resisted elbow flexion has been associated with this compression syndrome.[8] Repeated elbow hyperextension, as occurs in backhanding the ball in racquetball and tennis or carrying heavy packages, is also associated with this sensory neuropathy. Occasionally, repeated pronation and supination of the forearm exacerbate the symptoms. Handbag paresthesia is a condition reported to have occurred because of nerve compression caused by the strap of a heavy bag over the antecubital fossa.[56]

Lateral epicondylitis, cervical radiculopathy, brachial plexopathy, median nerve compression, and ruptured biceps brachii should be differentiated on physical examination and electrophysiologic testing.

Initial treatment of compression of the musculocutaneous nerve at the elbow is nonoperative, consisting of rest, restriction of activities, oral antiinflammatory drugs, and the use of slings and posterior splints to prevent full elbow extension and pronation. If symptoms persist beyond 6 to 12 weeks, then injection of steroids and local anesthetic into the musculocutaneous tunnel at the elbow may be attempted.

After approximately 12 weeks of nonoperative therapy, surgical decompression at the elbow is advised. Unlike proximal musculocutaneous nerve compression, which often resolves spontaneously, compression at the elbow persisted in 7 of 11 cases reported by Bassett and Nunley.[8] All of the patients recovered fully after surgical decompression. A triangular wedge of biceps tendon was

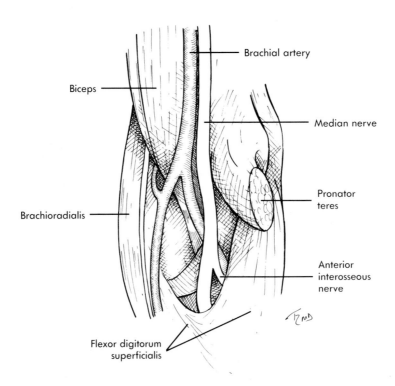

FIG. 31-20. Medial nerve lying medial to the brachial artery. It courses between the heads of the pronator teres and beneath the flexor digitorum superficialis arch—two areas of potential compression.

excised at the level of the lacertus fibrosus, where the tendon was noted to compress the musculocutaneous nerve against the fascia of the brachialis muscle.

Median Nerve

The median nerve is formed by fibers from C5 to C7 spinal nerves from the lateral cord and C8 and T1 fibers from the medial cord. The nerve runs near the brachial artery, toward the elbow on the medial side (Fig. 31-20).

The nerve passes medial to the biceps tendon and brachial artery at the elbow and courses between the superficial and deep head of the pronator teres, where it is often compressed. Another area of compression is under the tendinous insertion of the flexor digitorum superficialis, an area called the sublimis arch. At this level a posterior branch of the median nerve arises—the anterior interosseous nerve. This nerve travels under the sublimis bridge and continues distally between the anterior interosseous membrane and the flexor digitorum profundus muscle.

Pronator teres syndrome in athletes is uncommon but has been reported in baseball players.[6] With today's training programs for development of muscle strength, it is surprising that athletes do not more frequently manifest entrapment from repetitive trauma to the nerves.

Four sites have been identified with entrapment of the median nerve in the elbow region[57,58,67,117,118]:

1. Medial supracondylar process and the ligament of Struthers
2. Lacertus fibrosis
3. Between the two heads of the pronator teres muscle
4. Arch of the flexor digitorum superficialis

The median nerve at these levels carries both motor and sensory fibers to the volar forearm flexors (except for the flexor carpi ulnaris), the medial half of the flexor digitorum profundis, and the median-innervated intrinsics. Therefore both sensory and motor findings may be found. Usually there is an aching pain in the volar forearm over the pronator muscle. The pain is worsened by activity, especially repeated pronation movements with the elbow in extension. Altered sensation is found in the medial innervated thumb and digits. Weakness in finger flexion is uncommon, but, if present, is not limited to interphalangeal joint weakness of the thumb and distal interphalangeal joint weakness of the index finger, as in anterior interosseous syndrome. Often the symptoms can be elicited by resistance to forearm pronation and wrist flexion. Tinel's sign may be positive over the pronator muscle. Electrophysiologic studies may or may not be positive. A positive Phalen wrist flexion test may be positive, and this can cloud the diagnosis.

Pronator syndrome

- Volar proximal forearm pain
- Pain worsened with activity
- Abnormal sensibility in volar thumb, index, and middle fingers
- Finger flexor weakness (variable)
- Tinel's sign over pronator teres

On the basis of clinical findings, a 6-month course of conservative treatment is recommended, provided there are minimal or no motor deficits, once the diagnosis of pronator teres syndrome is made. Cessation of repeated pronation is especially advised.

Exploration of the median nerve at the elbow requires extensive surgery to decompress the four possible sites of compression described above.[67,117,118]

Adequate decompression usually affords relief of symptoms in recalcitrant cases. In resistant cases, transfer of the superficial head of the pronator teres posterior to the median nerve may be necessary.

Anterior Interosseous Nerve

The anterior interosseous nerve is a motor branch of the median nerve that arises at or just above the level of the flexor digitorum superficialis arch. It courses distally to innervate the flexor pollicis longus, flexor digitorum profundus (index and sometimes long finger), and pronator quadratus.

A compression neuropathy is often manifested by proximal forearm pain that is made worse with exercise. There is no sensory disturbance in the forearm or hand. The key clinical findings are weakness or paralysis of the anterior interosseous-nerve–innervated muscles.[60] A typical abnormal pinch attitude can be elicited, consisting of extension of the distal interphalangeal joint of the index finger and interphalangeal joint of the thumb, resulting from weakness of the flexor pollicis longus and flexor digitorum profundus to the index finger.[115]

In about 15% of patients, there may be a Martin-Gruber connection, which transports ulnar fibers in the median nerve to the ulnar nerve in the forearm.[119] If present, entrapment of the anterior interosseous nerve then causes intrinsic muscle paralysis in the hand.

A wide variety of clinical problems can create anterior interosseous nerve syndrome.[38,116,118] Variations in attachment of muscle tendon units, anomalous muscle such as Gantzer's muscle, which is an accessory head of the flexor pollicis longus arising from the medial epicondyle of the humerus, palmaris profundus muscle, enlarged bursae, thrombosed ulnar collateral blood vessels, tumors, or anomalous passage of the radial artery can be the initiating problem. More commonly, fascial bands on the deep head of the pronator teres or a portion of the tendinous origin of the flexor superficialis is responsible for the compression.[116] Careful electrophysiologic testing often can ascertain the site and extent of neural compression.

There are several reports of anterior interosseous neuropathy occurring after excessive forearm exercise, presumably as a result of compression by the muscles through which the nerve travels.[60] Symptoms resolve quickly when the exercise is stopped. A patient with acute shoulder and arm pain who displays signs of an anterior interosseous neuropathy may have an acute brachial plexus neuropathy with involvement of the fascicles going to the anterior interosseous nerve.[103]

Exploration of the anterior interosseous nerve is recommended if spontaneous improvement is not noted in 6 to 8 weeks.

Radial Nerve

The radial nerve consists of nerve fibers from C5 to T1 spinal nerve roots that travel in the posterior cord of the brachial plexus after giving off the thoracodorsal and axillary branches. The nerve travels down the upper arm in the radial groove of the humerus, pierces the lateral intermuscular septum, and enters the anterior compartment of the arm. Above the elbow the nerve innervates the triceps, extensor carpi radialis longus and brevis, and brachioradialis. At the elbow the nerve divides into a motor branch or posterior interosseous nerve and a superficial sensory branch.

Compression syndromes of the radial nerve above the elbow have been reported with sudden forceful contraction of the triceps muscle.[83] The most common cause of high radial nerve palsy is a humeral fracture.[93] Compression of the nerve against the medial side of the humerus occurs in Saturday night palsy, caused by pressure directly over the nerve on the upper arm.[123]

High radial nerve palsies have been described in various sports, including judo, kendo, baseball, mountain climbing, and skiing.[61] Humeral fractures are often associated with many of the palsies. Chronic compression, such as that caused by carrying a heavy backpack, has also caused radial nerve palsies.

Clinical examination is essential to localize the area of injury or compression. In a high radial nerve injury, both motor and sensory deficits are found. The patient is unable to extend the wrist or metacarpophalangeal joints of the hand and has decreased sensation in the first dorsal web space. The triceps is involved only if the injury is proximal to its innervation. On examination a differentiation can be made between radial nerve palsy and posterior interosseous nerve syndrome by noting both radial deviation of the wrist during active wrist dorsiflexion and the lack of sensory findings seen in posterior interosseous nerve syndrome.[117] Proximal lesions, such as in the C7 nerve root or posterior cord of the brachial plexus, can be differentiated by a sensory deficit in the palmar aspect of the third digit and motor abnormalities in the flexor carpi radialis, pronator teres, flexor digitorum superficialis, and flexor pollicis longus. Posterior cord involvement can be demonstrated by deltoid and latissimus dorsi muscle weakness.

EMG and nerve conduction studies can help isolate lesions of the radial nerve.

Prolonged external compression may cause neuronal degeneration requiring several months for recovery.[123] Patients with sleep palsies have almost an 87% chance for full recovery. Radial nerve injuries associated with humeral fractures have a 75% chance of recovering spontaneously, whereas the oblique distal third humeral fracture (Holstein-Lewis) is more controversial, with evidence supporting early exploration because of nerve entrapment in the fracture site.[93]

If the palsy develops after a closed reduction or open reduction and internal fixation, then exploration is often indicated. If no recovery is seen in 8 to 10 weeks, exploration is performed to repair or release the nerve. Tendon transfers may be needed after a year of observation and maintenance of passive motion.

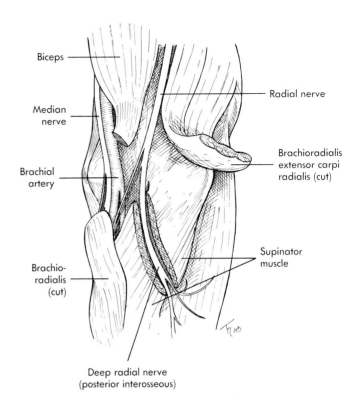

FIG. 31-21. Posterior interosseous nerve travels through the supinator muscle. Compression can occur at the proximal edge of this muscle (arcade of Frohse).

Posterior Interosseous Nerve

The radial nerve divides 3 cm above or below the elbow into a motor branch (posterior interosseous nerve) and a sensory branch (superficial radial nerve). The motor branch lies 1 cm lateral to the biceps tendon over the anterior capsule of the radiohumeral joint and dorsolateral over the radial neck.

The sensory branch usually arises before the motor branch enters the extensor compartment at the radial tunnel, a space lined by the extensor compartment muscles. The posterior interosseous nerve passes through the supinator muscle at an opening called the arcade of Frohse (Fig. 31-21).[82] This arcade is formed by the proximal superficial head of the supinator and has been shown to have a thickened tendinous edge in 30% of patients, thus creating nerve compression.[91]

Four sites of posterior interosseous nerve compression have been identified (Fig. 31-12): (1) fibrous edge of the extensor carpi radialis brevis, (2) arcade of Frohse, (3) fibrous bands attaching the nerve to the radiohumeral joint, and (4) radial recurrent vessels.[118]

Radial tunnel syndrome was first described by Roles and Maudsley[106] in 1972, and it has often been called resistant tennis elbow because inadequate treatment was often rendered as a result of inaccurate diagnosis.

Most patients with posterior interosseous nerve syndrome are not players of racquet sports, but manual workers.[19] Often tennis elbow or lateral epicondylitis may be present along with radial tunnel syndrome.

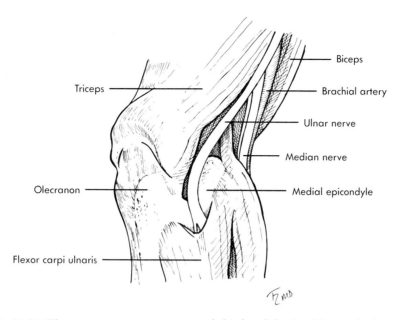

FIG. 31-22. Ulnar nerve entrapment can occur behind medial epicondyle in cubital tunnel.

Compression of the posterior interosseous nerve in the area of the head of the radius manifests itself as an aching pain in the forearm associated with activity.[26] This is due to the presence of some sensory fibers from the joint, muscle, and skin. The pain is usually well localized in the extensor mass below the elbow and may radiate into the dorsal aspect of the wrist.[69] Repetitive wrist flexion and pronation often exacerbate the symptoms. Hand grip may be weak because of the pain of wrist dorsiflexion.

On examination, tenderness is found over the nerve at the radial neck. No tenderness in the lateral epicondyle of the distal humerus is present; this differentiates it from tennis elbow. Resistance to middle finger extension may elicit pain, but this may also be true with tennis elbow. Also, resistance to supination usually elicits the pain. Motor examination is often normal, but some weakness of thumb and finger extension may be found. True paresis has been reported with trauma, such as in Monteggia's fractures, rheumatoid arthritis, or tumors.[80]

Results of electrodiagnostic studies are useful in confirming the lesion, but may prove normal, perhaps because of the intermittent nature of the compression. Other sources of pain in the lateral aspect of the arm include tendinitis, stenosis of the orbicular ligament, tears in the common extensor tendon origin, cervical spine disorders, and radial head injury.

Treatment of spontaneous posterior interosseous nerve palsy is conservative.[26,69,118] The patient is advised to temporarily change activity, use a resting splint, and try a nonsteroidal antiinflammatory drug. If a mass has been detected or the symptoms persist after 6 months of conservative treatment, surgery may be warranted. Weakness is an indication of severe nerve compression, and surgical decompression should be carried out. Results of surgical decompression have been uniformly good, with success rates above 90%.

Ulnar Nerve

The ulnar nerve is the terminal branch of the medial cord of the brachial plexus after the medial cord sends a contribution to the median nerve. In the humerus the nerve lies medial to the axillary artery and brachial artery. At the distal third of the humerus the nerve pierces the medial intermuscular septum and runs along the medial triceps muscle to the groove between the olecranon and medial epicondyle of the humerus. The cubital tunnel lies just behind the medial epicondyle and consists of the ulnar groove, fascial aponeurosis joining the two heads of the flexor carpi ulnaris, and the muscle bellies of these two heads. The nerve courses through the forearm between the flexor digitorum profundus and flexor carpi ulnaris (Fig. 31-22).

The causes of ulnar nerve entrapment in the elbow include the arcade of Struthers, the medial head of the triceps, an anconeus epitrochlearis muscle, the aponeurosis of the flexor carpi ulnaris, osteophytes of the tunnel, ganglia, lipomata, or subluxation of the ulnar nerve. Ulnar nerve entrapment syndrome is a well-documented neuropathy in baseball players, particularly in pitchers.[30,51] Repetitive valgus stress of the elbow is thought to play a key role in the development of this neuropathy in association with valgus instability. Symptoms include pain in the medial aspect of the proximal forearm that may radiate proximally or distally. Paresthesias, dysesthesias, or anesthesia is usually found in the ulnar half of the ring finger and the little finger. If compression is longstanding, findings may include clumsiness and weakness, with wasting of the intrinsic muscles of the hand. Occasionally, weakness in the flexor profundi to the ring and little finger may be detected, although this is more common with ulnar nerve injuries above the elbow. A positive Tinel's sign in the cubital tunnel is a frequent finding, with tingling or shocky sensations traveling proximally and distally. The elbow flexion test, which

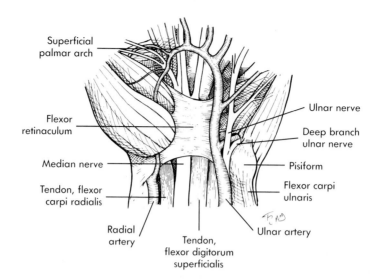

FIG. 31-23. Transverse carpal ligament lies over the median nerve at the carpal tunnel and requires surgical division to relieve symptoms of median nerve compression.

consists of full elbow flexion for 5 minutes, often elicits the symptoms. Electrophysiologic studies generally confirm and localize the site of ulnar nerve entrapment. The physician must carefully exclude disorders of the cervical spinal cord, nerve root, and brachial plexus, such as neurologic thoracic outlet syndrome, which closely resembles ulnar nerve entrapment at the elbow.

Early surgical decompression and submuscular transposition of the ulnar nerve is recommended for baseball players.[29,30,50] Common associated findings at operation include tearing or calcification of the medial collateral ligament. Players often have scarring over the nerve in the ulnar groove. Surgical decompression of the nerve in this group of patients should not be delayed to wait for EMG changes. Injections into the area of the irritated nerve are not recommended. Approximately 60% of the players in one series returned to their preoperative level of play.[30] The prognosis is excellent for isolated nerve involvement without muscle weakness, associated instability, or arthritis of the elbow.[50] During the decompression, the proximal dissection includes resection of the medial intermuscular septum and division of the arcade of Struthers, if one is present.[75] Other procedures used are medial epicondylectomy, decompression, and subcutaneous transposition with a loose fascial sling to prevent a position change of the transposed nerve.[35] The most predictable and effective surgical treatment is an anterior submuscular transposition, also used to treat failed ulnar nerve transpositions.[105] Attention must be paid to the release of the flexor carpi ulnaris aponeurosis, which is thought to play a key role in idiopathic cubital tunnel syndrome.

Wrist

Carpal Tunnel Syndrome

The median nerve enters the hand through the carpal tunnel, which is bordered by the transverse carpal ligament volarly and the wrist bones dorsally. The transverse carpal ligament attaches to the scaphoid and trapezium radially and pisiform and hamate ulnarly. The median nerve shares this space with nine flexor tendons, including the flexor pollicis longus, the flexor digitorum superficialis,[5] and flexor digitorum profundus tendons,[5] all lined by a synovial sheath (Fig. 31-23). The median nerve at this level contains sensory palmar digital branches that innervate three and a half radial digits; a motor branch to the thenar eminence, which innervates the abductor pollicis brevis; opponens pollicis and superficial head of the flexor pollicis brevis; and motor branches to the first and second lumbricals.

Clinical features of carpal tunnel syndrome include paresthesias and pain in the wrist, hand, and three and a half radial digits, especially during sleep. The aching pain may radiate to the elbow or shoulder. With progression of the disease, symptoms occur during the day and can become constant. Patients frequently report stiffness of the fingers in the morning, perhaps caused by swelling around the flexor tendons in the carpal tunnel. Atrophy of the thenar muscles is a late finding in severe carpal tunnel syndrome, but abductor pollicis brevis weakness can often be elicited.[65]

The Phalen wrist flexion test is sensitive for carpal tunnel syndrome, but it may be negative.[96,97] A positive Tinel's sign at the wrist may be elicited in approximately 45% of patients with carpal tunnel syndrome. Two-point discrimination may be abnormal, but vibratory sensory testing is more sensitive in detecting early disease. EMG and nerve conduction studies are important in confirming the diagnosis, although they may be negative in 25% of patients with carpal tunnel syndrome. If a patient describes characteristic paresthesias and demonstrates the appropriate signs, such as a positive Phalen test, there is an 85% certainty of the diagnosis.

Careful clinical examination and electrophysiologic testing can exclude brachial plexus injury, which is one of the problems in the differential diagnosis of carpal tun-

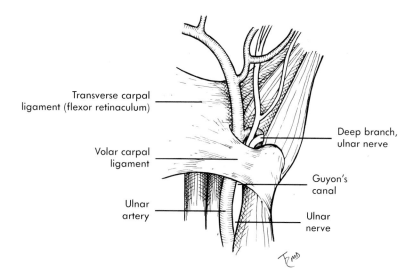

Transverse carpal
ligament (flexor retinaculum)

Volar carpal
ligament

Ulnar
artery

Deep branch,
ulnar nerve

Guyon's
canal

Ulnar
nerve

FIG. 31-24. Anatomy of Guyon's canal.

nel syndrome. Conditions that may be associated with carpal tunnel syndrome include rheumatoid arthritis, thyroid myxedema, acromegaly, multiple myeloma, amyloidosis, diabetes mellitus, pregnancy, local wrist trauma, hemophilia, alcoholism, tumors such as ganglia, lipomas, gout, anomalous muscles in the carpal tunnel, such as palmaris profundus, and thrombosis of a persistent median artery.[48]

Local trauma to the wrist has been found to cause carpal tunnel syndrome in cyclists, throwers, and tennis players. Repeated microtrauma to the contents of the carpal tunnel or prolonged wrist extension in these and other sports may produce mechanical irritation or ischemia in the median nerve, resulting in classic symptoms. Carpal tunnel syndrome has also been known to develop in manual workers, such as jackhammer operators. Flexor tenosynovitis resulting from overuse may be a common cause of median nerve compression in the wrist.

Nonsurgical treatment of carpal tunnel syndrome consists of avoidance of activities that produce symptoms, using a wrist splint in 20 to 25 degrees of dorsiflexion, nonsteroidal antiflammatory medication, and sometimes a cortisone injection into the carpal tunnel.[46] The injection is given 1 cm proximal to the distal wrist flexion crease, between the palmaris longus and flexor carpi radialis tendons. Intratendinous injection may weaken the tendon, causing rupture. Intraneural injection may injure the median nerve irreparably. The majority of patients with carpal tunnel syndrome resulting from repetitive trauma respond to conservative measures.[48] In cases with prolonged symptoms, atrophy, or sensory loss, surgery may be necessary if conservative measures are unsuccessful after 8 to 12 weeks of trial. Division of the transverse carpal ligament has given 90% to 95% of patients good long-term results.[27,47] There is no consensus as to whether tenosynovectomy and internal neurolysis improve results. Complications include failure to fully di-

vide the transverse carpal ligament and injury to the palmar cutaneous branch of the median nerve.

Endoscopic carpal tunnel release remains controversial. Proponents show good early results, whereas critics emphasize the major complications reported with this new technique. There is no consensus on the need for or benefits of a tenosynovectomy and epineurectomy during carpal tunnel release.[2,22,39,90]

Ulnar Nerve

The ulnar nerve at the wrist passes between the pisiform bone and the hook of the hamate through Guyon's canal, the floor of which is the transverse carpal ligament and pisohamate ligament, and the roof of which is the palmar fascia and palmaris brevis muscle (Fig. 31-24). Through the canal pass the superficial terminal branch, supplying sensation to the ulnar palm, little finger, and ulnar half of the ring finger, and the deep terminal branch, which supplies the hypothenar muscles, interossei, third and fourth lumbricals, adductor pollicis brevis, first dorsal interosseous, and a portion of the flexor pollicis brevis.

Compression syndromes at Guyon's canal have been reported as a result of chronic repeated external pressure, ganglia, lipoma, rheumatoid synovial cysts, tumors, anomalous muscles, ununited fractures of the hamate, and ulnar artery aneurysms.[87,113] The most common form of compression occurs at the deep terminal branch distal to the branches supplying the hypothenar muscles, caused by compression between the fibrous origin of the abductor and flexor of the fifth finger and the pisohamate ligament against the hook of the hamate.[113] Symptoms include weakness of all ulnar-innervated muscles of the hand except the hypothenar muscles.[65] This form is found in persons who use tools that press into the palm of their hand and in long-distance cyclists, who experience constant pressure from handlebars, and results in motor weakness and wasting of intrinsic muscles.[36,64]

The second most common site of involvement is the main trunk, both sensory and motor, just proximal to or within Guyon's canal. A less common form of compression can occur more distally, at the superficial terminal branch. This results in a sensory loss only and has been reported with an ununited fracture of the hook of the hamate and an ulnar artery aneurysm caused by trauma.[68]

Investigation should consist of a careful history of work habits, hobbies, and previous injuries, and a careful examination of the wrist and hand should follow.

Electrophysiologic studies help localize the neuropathy to the wrist or hand. Careful examination of the dorsal cutaneous branch of the ulnar nerve can help differentiate between a compression at the level of the wrist and proximally.

Occupational causes for the neuropathy have been found to resolve upon discontinuation of the activity in a large portion of patients. Occasionally, surgical decompression is necessary when no improvement is noted or the symptoms worsen. Touring cyclists often achieve relief of their symptoms by wearing cycling gloves and applying proper padding to the handlebars.[36,64]

Hypothenar Hammer Syndrome

The ulnar artery travels through Guyon's canal, which is bounded by the hook of the hamate laterally, the pisiform bone medially, the transverse carpal ligament dorsally, and the volar carpal ligament on the palmar aspect. The 2-cm segment of the ulnar artery distal to Guyon's canal is very susceptible to trauma since it is relatively superficial, being covered by a thin layer of subcutaneous tissue, palmaris brevis muscle, and skin. Repetitive trauma to the hypothenar portion of the hand may result in signs and symptoms associated with ischemia to the hand and fingers, often exacerbated by exposure to cold (Raynaud's phenomenon). Spasm, thrombosis, and aneurysm formation of the ulnar artery have been found primarily in male laborers who use hammerlike handles, turning valves or using their palms as hammers, hence the term hypothenar hammer syndrome. A history of trauma—acute, chronic, or repetitive—has been reported in all cases. Koga, Seki, and Carol[72] have reported a case involving a female badminton player.

Patients may present with unilateral numbness in the ulnar innervated digits, ischemic pain with pallor, cold intolerance or sensitivity, and a mass in the hypothenar portion of the hand. Signs include a positive Allen test if the ulnar artery is thrombosed, intrinsic muscle cramping during rapid repetitive movement, and a palpable aneurysm if present. Doppler ultrasonography may help make the diagnosis, whereas angiography is seldom needed.

A fracture of the hook of the hamate may be associated with thrombosis of the ulnar artery. Raynaud's disease is differentiated by its bilateral involvement, no history of trauma, and higher incidence in women. Other systemic inflammatory and collagen vascular diseases may be excluded by history, physical examination, and diagnostic testing.

Although sympathetic blocks and sympathectomies have been used, surgical excision of the lesion is the

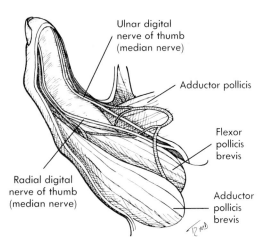

FIG. 31-25. Anatomy of digital nerve of thumbs.

most common and effective form of treatment. Direct ulnar artery repairs and vein graft repairs have been done with about a 50% potency rate but excellent clinical improvement. Urokinase infusion has also been successful in correcting this syndrome.[136]

Hand

Bowler's Thumb

Bowler's thumb is a digital neuropathy of the palmar-ulnar digital nerve that has been described in bowlers and baseball players[11] (Fig. 31-25). The entity is caused by a perineural fibrosis of the ulnar digital nerve of the thumb at the metacarpophalangeal crease as a result of chronic compression and repeated trauma to the nerve from the corner of the thumb hole in the bowling ball.[63]

Often the patient reports a tender nodule at the ulnar metacarpophalangeal crease. A Tinel's sign can usually be elicited.[29] There may also be paresthesias and sensory loss in the distribution of the nerve.

Other causes for compression of the nerve include cysts and tumors from the tendon sheath of the thumb, osteophytes, mucinous cysts, rheumatoid tenosynovitis, schwannomas, or digital neuropathies associated with diabetes mellitus and vascular disorders. Even though the digital nerves are superficial, compression neuropathies are rare.[102]

Upon recognition of an occupation or sports-related neuropathy, protective measures are instituted.[32] A change in the position of the thumb hole may help, or a splint helps resolve the symptoms. Otherwise, cessation of bowling may be necessary. Surgery is rarely indicated, but in the case of unrelieved symptoms, there has been a report that transposing the nerve posterior to the adductor pollicis tendon yields a good result.[11]

REFERENCES

1. Adams JT, Deweese JA: Effort thrombosis of the axillary and subclavian veins, *J Trauma* 11:923, 1971.
2. Agee JM et al: Endoscopic release of the carpal tunnel: a randomized prospective multicenter study, *J Hand Surg* 17A:987, 1992.
3. Albright JP et al: Nonfatal cervical spine injuries in interscholastic football, *JAMA* 236:1243, 1976.

4. Albright JP et al: Head and neck injuries in college football: an eight-year analysis, *Am J Sports Med* 13:147, 1985.
5. Andrich J, Bergfeld JA, Ramo RA: A method for the management of cervical injuries in football: a preliminary report, *Am J Sports Med* 5:89, 1977.
6. Barnes DA, Tullos HS: An analysis of 100 symptomatic baseball players, *Am J Sports Med* 6:62, 1978.
7. Barrett T, Levitt LM: Effort thrombosis of the axillary vein with pulmonary embolism, *JAMA* 146:1412, 1951.
8. Bassett FH, Nunley JA: Compression of the musculocutaneous nerve at the elbow, *J Bone Joint Surg* 64A:1050, 1982.
9. Bateman JE: Nerve injuries about the shoulder in sports, *J Bone Joint Surg* 49A:785, 1967.
10. Becker GJ, Holden RW: Local thrombolytic therapy for subclavian and axillary vein thrombosis, *Radiology* 149:419, 1983.
11. Belsky MR, Millender LH: Bowler's thumb in a baseball player: a case report, *Orthopedics* 3:122, 1980.
12. Bergfeld JA, Hershman EB, Wilbourn AJ: Brachial plexus injury in sports: a five-year followup, *Orthop Trans* 12:743, 1988.
13. Berry H, Bril V: Axillary nerve palsy following blunt trauma to the shoulder region: a clinical and electrophysiological review, *J Neurol Neurosurg Psychiatry* 45:1027, 1982.
14. Bigliani LU, Perez-Sanz JR, Wolfe IN: Treatment of trapezius paralysis, *J Bone Joint Surg* 67A:871, 1985.
15. Black KP, Lombardo JA: Suprascapular nerve injuries with isolated paralysis of the infraspinatus, *Am J Sports Med* 18(3):225, 1990.
16. Blom S, Dahlback LO: Nerve injuries in dislocations of the shoulder joint and fractures of the neck and humerus, *Acta Chir Scand* 136:461, 1970.
17. Bonney G: The scalenus medius band: a contribution to the study of the thoracic outlet syndrome, *J Bone Joint Surg* 47B:268, 1965.
18. Braddom RL, Wolfe C: Musculocutaneous nerve injury after heavy exercise, *Arch Phys Med Rehabil* 59:290, 1978.
19. Bryan FS, Miller LS, Panijayanond P: Spontaneous paralysis of the posterior interosseous nerve: a case report and reviews of the literature, *Clin Orthop* 80:9, 1971.
20. Butsch JL: Subclavian thrombosis following hockey injuries, *Am J Sports Med* 11:448, 1983.
21. Cahill BR, Palmar PE: Quadrilateral space syndrome, *J Hand Surg* 8:65, 1983.
22. Chow JCY: Endoscopic release of carpal ligament, *Arthroscopy* 5:19, 1989.
23. Chrisman OD et al: Lateral flexion neck injuries in athletic competition, *JAMA* 192(7):613, 1965.
24. Clancy WG, Brand RL, Bergfeld JA: Upper trunk brachial plexus injuries in contact sports, *Am J Sports Med* 5:209, 1977.
25. Clein LJ: Supracapsular entrapment neuropathy, *J Neurosurg* 43:337, 1975.
26. Coonrad RW, Hooper WR: Tennis elbow: its cause, natural history, conservative and surgical management, *J Bone Joint Surg* 55A:1177, 1973.
27. Cseuz KA et al: Longterm results of operation for carpal tunnel syndrome, *Mayo Clin Proc* 41:232, 1966.
28. Dale WA: Thoracic outlet compression syndrome: critique in 1982, *Arch Surg* 117:1437, 1982.
29. Dellan AL: Operative technique for submuscular transposition of the ulnar nerve, *Contemp Orthop* 4:17, 1988.
30. DelPizzo W, Jobe FW, Norwood L: Ulnar nerve entrapment syndrome in baseball players, *Am J Sports Med* 5:182, 1977.
31. Dewar FP, Harris RI: Restoration of function of the shoulder following paralysis of the trapezius by fascial sling fixation and transplantation of the levator scapulae, *Ann Surg* 132:1111, 1950.
32. Dobyns JH et al: Bowler's thumb: diagnosis and treatment, *J Bone Joint Surg* 54A:751, 1972.
33. Donner TR, Kline DG: Extracranial spinal accessory nerve injury, *Neurosurgery* 32(6):907, 1993.
34. Eastcott HHG: Reconstruction of the subclavian artery for complications of cervical rib and thoracic outlet syndrome, *Lancet* 2:1243, 1962.
35. Eaton RG, Crowe JF, Parkes JC: Anterior transposition of the

36. Eckman PB, Perlstein G, Altrocchi PH: Ulnar neuropathy in bicycle riders, *Arch Neurol* 32:130, 1975.
37. Falconer MA, Weddell G: Costoclavicular compression to the subclavian artery and vein: relation to the scalenus anticus syndrome, *Lancet* 2:539, 1943.
38. Farber JS, Bryan RS: The anterior interosseous nerve syndrome, *J Bone Joint Surg* 50A:521, 1968.
39. Feinstein P: Endoscopic carpal tunnel release in a community based series, *J Hand Surg* 18A:451, 1993.
40. Felsenthal G et al: Forearm pain secondary to compression syndrome of the lateral cutaneous nerve of the forearm, *Arch Phys Med Rehabil* 65:139, 1984.
41. Ferretti A et al: Suprascapular neuropathy in volleyball players, *J Bone Joint Surg* 69:260, 1987.
42. Foo CL, Swann M: Isolated paralysis of the serratus anterior, *J Bone Joint Surg* 65B:552, 1983.
43. Friedman AH et al: Repair of isolated axillary nerve lesions after infraclavicular brachial plexus injuries: case reports, *Neurosurgery* 27(3):403, 1990.
44. Ganzhorn RW et al: Suprascapular nerve entrapment, *J Bone Joint Surg* 63:492, 1981.
45. Garcia G, McQueen D: Bilateral suprascapular nerve entrapment syndrome, *J Bone Joint Surg* 63A:491, 1981.
46. Gelberman RH, Aronson D, Weisman MH: Carpal tunnel syndrome—results of a prospective trial of steroid injection and splinting, *J Bone Joint Surg* 62A:1181, 1980.
47. Gelberman RH et al: The carpal tunnel syndrome, *J Bone Joint Surg* 63A:380, 1981.
48. Gerstner DL, Omer GE: Peripheral entrapment neuropathies in the upper extremity, *J Musculoskeletal Med* 3:14, 1988.
49. Glennon TP: Isolated injury of the infraspinatus branch of the suprascapular nerve, *Arch Phys Med Rehabil* 73(2):201, 1992.
50. Glousman RE: Ulnar nerve problems in the athlete's elbow, *Clin Sports Med* 9(2):365, 1990.
51. Godshell RW: Traumatic ulnar neuropathy in adolescent baseball pitchers, *J Bone Joint Surg* 53A:359, 1971.
52. Goodman CE, Kenrick MM, Blum MV: Long thoracic nerve palsy: a follow-up study, *Arch Phys Med Rehabil* 56:352, 1975.
53. Graham GC, Lincoln BM: Anterior resection of the first rib for thoracic outlet syndrome, *Am J Surg* 126:803, 1973.
54. Gregg JR, Labosky D, Harty M: Serratus anterior paralysis in the young athlete, *J Bone Joint Surg* 61A:825, 1979.
55. Hadley MN: Suprascapular nerve entrapment, *J Neurosurg* 64:843, 1986.
56. Hale BR: Hand bag paresthesia, *Lancet* 2:470, 1976.
57. Hantz CR et al: The pronator teres syndrome: compressive neuropathy of the median nerve, *J Bone Joint Surg* 63A:885, 1981.
58. Herring S, Nilson K: Introduction to overuse injuries, *Clin Sports Med* 6:225, 1987.
59. Hershman EB, Wilbourn AJ, Bergfeld JA: Acute brachial neuropathy in athletes, *Am J Sports Med* 17(5):655, 1989.
60. Hill NA, Howard FM, Huffer BR: The incomplete anterior interosseous nerve syndrome, *J Hand Surg* 10A:4, 1985.
61. Hirasawa Y, Sakakida K: Sports and peripheral nerve injury, *Am J Sports Med* 11:420, 1983.
62. Hirayama T, Takemitsu Y: Compression of the suprascapular nerve by ganglion at the suprascapular notch, *Clin Orthop* 155:95, 1981.
63. Howell AE, Leach RE: Bowler's thumb: perineural fibrosis of the digital nerve, *J Bone Joint Surg* 52A:379, 1970.
64. Hoyt CS: Ulnar neuropathy in bicycle riders, *Arch Neurol* 33:372, 1976.
65. Hunt JR: The thenar and hypothenar types of neural atrophy of the hand, *Am J Med Sci* 141:224, 1911.
66. Johnson JTH, Kendall HO: Isolated paralysis of the serratus anterior muscle, *J Bone Joint Surg* 37A:567, 1955.
67. Johnson RK, Spinner M, Shrewsbury MM: Median entrapment syndrome in the proximal forearm, *J Hand Surg* 4:48, 1979.
68. Kalisman M, Laborde K, Wolff TW: Ulnar nerve compression secondary to ulnar artery false aneurysm at Guyon's canal, *J Hand Surg* 7:137, 1982.

69. Kaplan PE: Posterior interosseous neuropathies: natural history, *Arch Phys Med Rehabil* 65:339, 1984.
70. Karas SE: Thoracic outlet syndrome, *Clin Sports Med* 9(2):297, 1990.
71. Kim SM, Goodrich JA: Isolated proximal musculocutaneous nerve palsy: case report, *Arch Phys Med Rehabil* 65:735, 1984.
72. Koga Y, Seki T, Carol D: Hypothenar hammer syndrome in a young female badminton player, *Am J Sports Med* 21(6):890, 1993.
73. Kutz JE, Rowland EB Jr: Vascular compression about the shoulder, *Hand Clin* 9(1):131, 1993.
74. Langenskiold A, Ryoppy S: Treatment of paralysis of the trapezius muscles by the Eden-Lange operation, *Acta Orthop Scand* 44:383, 1973.
75. Learmonth JR: Technique for transplantation of the ulnar nerve, *Surg Gynecol Obstet* 75:792, 1942.
76. Leffert RD: Thoracic outlet syndrome. In Omer GE, Spinner M (eds): *Management of peripheral nerve problems*, Philadelphia, 1980, WB Saunders.
77. Leffert RD: Thoracic outlet syndrome and the shoulder, *Clin Sports Med* 2:439, 1983.
78. Leffert RD: TOS, *Hand Clin* 8(2):285, 1992.
78a. Leffert RD: Thoracic outlet syndrome, *J Am Acad Orthop Surg* 2(6):317, 1994.
79. Leffert RD, Seddon H: Infraclavicular brachial plexus injuries, *J Bone Joint Surg* 47B:9, 1965.
80. Lichter RL, Jacobson T: Tardy palsy of the posterior interosseous nerve with a Monteggia fracture, *J Bone Joint Surg* 57A:124, 1975.
81. Linker CS, Helms CA, Fritz RC: Quadrilateral space syndrome: findings at MR imaging, *Radiology* 188(3):675, 1993.
82. Lister GD et al: The radial tunnel syndrome, *J Hand Surg* 4:52, 1979.
83. Lotem M et al: Radial palsy following muscular effort: a nerve compression syndrome possibly related to a fibrous arch of the lateral head of the triceps, *J Bone Joint Surg* 53B:500, 1971.
84. Markey KL, DiBenedetto M, Curl WW: Upper trunk brachial plexopathy: the stinger syndrome, *Am J Sports Med* 21(5):650, 1993.
85. Marks J: Anticoagulation therapy in idiopathic occlusion of the axillary vein, *Br Med J* 1:11, 1956.
86. Maroon JC: "Burning hands" in football, spinal cord injuries, *JAMA* 238:2049, 1977.
87. McCarroll HR: Nerve injuries associated with wrist trauma, *Orthop Clin North Am* 15:279, 1984.
88. Meyer SA et al: Cervical spinal stenosis and stingers in collegiate football players, *Am J Sports Med* 22(2):158, 1994.
89. Montagna P, Colonna S: Suprascapular neuropathy restricted to the infraspinatus muscle in volleyball players, *Acta Neurol Scand* 87(3):248, 1993.
90. Murphy R et al: Major neurovascular complications of endoscopy carpal tunnel release, *J Hand Surg* 19A:114, 1994.
91. Nielsen HO: Posterior interosseous nerve paralysis caused by fibrous band compression at the supinator muscle; a report of 4 cases, *Acta Orthop Scand* 47:304, 1976.
92. Neviaser TJ et al: Suprascapular nerve denervation secondary to attenuation by a ganglionic cyst, *J Bone Joint Surg* 68A:4:627, 1986.
93. Packer JW et al: The humeral fracture with radial nerve palsy: is exploration warranted? *Clin Orthop* 88:34, 1972.
94. Parsonage MJ, Turner JWA: Neuralgic amyotrophy: the shoulder girdle syndrome, *Lancet* 1:973, 1948.
95. Petrucci FS, Morelli A, Raimohdi PL: Axillary nerve injuries: 21 cases treated by nerve graft and neurolysis, *J Hand Surg* 7:271, 1982.
96. Phalen GS: The carpal tunnel syndrome, *J Bone Joint Surg* 48A:211, 1966.
97. Phalen GS, Kendrick JI: Compression neuropathy of the median nerve in the carpal tunnel, *JAMA* 16:524, 1957.
98. Poindexter DP, Johnson EW: Football shoulder and neck injury: a study of the stinger, *Arch Phys Med Rehabil* 65:601, 1984.
99. Priest JD: A physical phenomenon: shoulder depression in athletes, *Sports Care Fit* Mar/April:20, 1989.
100. Rask MR: Suprascapular nerve entrapment: a report of two cases treated by suprascapular notch resection, *Clin Orthop* 134:266, 1978.
101. Rayan GM: Lower trunk brachial plexus compression neuropathy due to cervical rib in young athletes, *Am J Sports Med* 16:77, 1988.
102. Rayan GM, O'Donoghue DH: Ulnar digital compression neuropathy of the thumb caused by splinting, *Clin Orthop* 175:170, 1983.
103. Rennels GD, Ochoa J: Neurologic amyotrophy manifesting as anterior interosseus nerve palsy, *Muscle Nerve* 3:160, 1980.
104. Robertson WC, Eichman PL, Clancy WG: Upper trunk brachial plexopathy in football players, *JAMA* 241:1480, 1979.
105. Rogers MR, Bergfield EG, Aulicino PL: The failed ulnar nerve transposition, *Clin Orthop* 269:193, 1991.
106. Roles NC, Maudsley RH: Radial tunnel syndrome: resistant tennis elbow as a nerve entrapment, *J Bone Joint Surg* 54B:499, 1972.
107. Roos DB: Experience with first rib resection for thoracic outlet syndrome, *Ann Surg* 173:429, 1971.
108. Roos DB: Congenital anomalies associated with thoracic outlet syndrome: anatomy, symptoms, diagnosis, and treatment, *Am J Surg* 132:771, 1976.
109. Rorabeck CH, Harris WR: Factors affecting the prognosis of brachial plexus injuries, *J Bone Surg* 63B:404, 1981.
110. Samardzic M, Grujicie D, Antunovic V: Nerve transfers in brachial plexus traction injuries, *J Neurosurg* 76(2):191, 1992.
111. Sanders RJ, Haug C: Review of arterial thoracic outlet syndrome with a report of five new instances, *Surg Gyn Obstet* 173(5):415, 1991.
112. Schwantzman RJ: Brachial plexus traction injuries, *Hand Clin* 76(2):191, 1992.
113. Shea JD, McClain EJ: Ulnar nerve compression syndromes at and below the wrist, *J Bone Joint Surg* 51A:1095, 1969.
114. Speer KP, Bassett FH III: The prolonged burner syndrome, *Am J Sports Med* 18(6):591, 1990.
115. Spinner M: The functional attitude of the hand afflicted with an anterior interosseous nerve paralysis, *Bull Hosp Joint Dis* 30:21, 1969.
116. Spinner M: The anterior interosseous nerve syndrome with special attention to its variation, *J Bone Joint Surg* 52A:84, 1970.
117. Spinner M: *Injuries to the major branches of the peripheral nerves of the forearm*, Philadelphia, 1978, WB Saunders.
118. Spinner M, Spencer RS: Nerve compression lesions of the upper extremity, *Clin Orthop* 104:46, 1974.
119. Stern PJ, Kutz JE: An unusual variant of the anterior interosseous nerve syndrome, *J Hand Surg* 5:32, 1980.
120. Stewart JD: The brachial plexus. In Stewart JD (ed): *Focal peripheral neuropathies*, New York, 1987, Elsevier.
121. Strohm BR, Brand, Colachis SC Jr: Shoulder joint dysfunction following injury to the suprascapular nerve, *Phys Ther* 45:106, 1965.
122. Strunkel RJ, Garrick JG: Thoracic outlet compression in athletes, *Am J Sports Med* 6:35, 1978.
123. Sunderland S: Traumatic injuries of peripheral nerves: simple compression injuries of the radial nerve, *Brain* 68:5, 1945.
124. Sunderland S: *Nerves and nerve injuries*, ed 2, Edinburgh, 1978, Churchill Livingstone.
125. Swafford AR, Lichtman DH: Suprascapular nerve entrapment—case report, *J Hand Surg* 7:57, 1982.
126. Thompson RC Jr, Schneider W, Kennedy T: Entrapment neuropathy of the inferior branch of the suprascapular nerve by ganglia, *Clin Orthop* 166:185, 1982.
127. Tsairis P, Dyck PJ, Mulder DW: Natural history of brachial plexus neuropathy: report of 99 patients, *Arch Neurol* 27:109, 1972.
128. Urschel HC, Razzuk MA: Management of the thoracic outlet syndrome, *N Engl J Med* 286:1140, 1972.
129. Vastamaki M: *Suprascapular nerve entrapment*, Paper presented at AAOS 54th Annual Meeting, Scientific Program, 1987.
130. Vogel CM, Jensen JE: "Effort" thrombosis of the subclavian

vein in a competitive swimmer, *Am J Sports Med* 13:269, 1985.

131. Wilbourn AJ, Hershman EB, Bergfeld JA: Brachial plexopathies in athletes: the EMG findings, *Muscle Nerve* 9:254, 1986.
132. Wood VE, Twito R, Verska JM: Thoracic outlet syndrome, *Orthop Clin North Am* 19:131, 1988.
133. Woodhead AB: Paralysis of the serratus anterior in a world class marksman, *Am J Sports Med* 13:359, 1985.
134. Wright IS: The neurovascular syndrome produced by hyperabduction of the arms, *Am Heart J* 29:1, 1945.
135. Wright YA: Accessory spinal nerve injury, *Clin Orthop* 108:15, 1975.
136. Yakubov SJ et al: Successful prolonged local infusion of urokinase for the hypothenar hammer syndrome, *Cathet Cardiovasc Diagn* 29(4):301, 1993.
137. Zeiss J et al: MRI and suprascapular neuropathy in a weight lifter, *J Comput Assist Tomogr* 17(2):303, 1993.
138. Zoltan JD: Injury to the suprascapular nerve associated with anterior dislocation of the shoulder: case report and review of the literature, *J Trauma* 19:203, 1979.

PART VII Sport-Specific Injuries

CHAPTER 32   Biomechanics of Throwing

Jacquelin Perry
Ronald E. Glousman

The shoulder and elbow provide highly mobile, dynamic, and forceful coordinated motion. While daily activities depend on the upper extremity for lifting and positioning, athletic endeavors require specific and precise motions with propulsive activity. Interaction between static restraints and the dynamic muscle unit allows for the versatile motion and power that are required in competitive performance.

The extent and directions of motion available at any joint are determined by its bony contours and axes of rotation. Mobility is limited by ligamentous restraints. Both the shoulder and elbow use a two-joint complex to expand the mobility provided.

THE SHOULDER JOINT
Shoulder Motion

Vast three-dimensional mobility is provided by the skeletal characteristics of the shoulder (Fig. 32-1). The humeral articular surface is a superomedially oriented hemisphere (diameter 35 to 55 mm).[43,63] Opposing this is the small, shallow glenoid fossa of the scapula, which has half the contour and one third the surface area.[37] Glenoid area and depth are enlarged by a fibrocartilaginous labrum. This increases the humeral contact areas to 75% vertically and 56% transversely.[68] The effect is enhanced joint stability without impeded mobility from hard bony edges. As a result, the humerus has a wide range of motion in all three planes. Supplementing this is the gliding of the scapula on the thorax as it rotates with the clavicle about the sternal point of origin. The dominance of mobility over stability is even evident in the arm's resting posture.

Shoulder motion patterns

- Elevation
- Rotation—internal-external
- Horizontal flexion and extension

Shoulder mobility is classified by three patterns of motion: elevation, internal-external rotation, and horizontal flexion and extension.

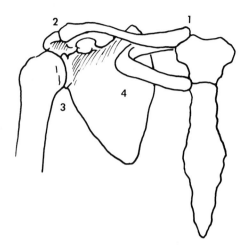

FIG. 32-1. Sites of motion within the shoulder complex. *1,* Sterno-clavicular joint. *2,* Acromioclavicular joint. *3,* Glenohumeral joint. *4,* Scapulothoracic interface. (From Rowe CR: *The shoulder,* New York, 1988, Churchill Livingstone.)

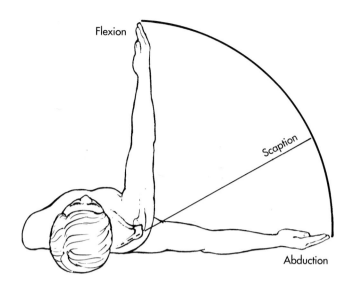

FIG. 32-2. Planes of arm elevation: neutral, flexion, and abduction. (From Rowe CR: *The shoulder,* New York, 1988, Churchill Livingstone.)

Arm Elevation

Raising the arm from the side of the body to its peak overhead position is a theoretical 180-degree arc. Few men (4%) and less than one third of women (28%) actually attain this range. The men's mean range was 167 degrees and the women's 171 degrees.[15,17] These values still display the shoulder as the most mobile joint in the body. Posterior elevation or extension is about 60 degrees.[45]

Arm elevation is a complex action that is best analyzed as three functional modes: planes of motion, scapulohumeral rhythm, and centers of rotation.

Planes of motion. Neutral elevation of the arm occurs in the plane of the scapula (Fig. 32-2). This is angled approximately 30 degrees anterior to the body's coronal plane.[78] Exact alignment is determined by the contour of the thoracic wall on which the scapula rests.

This alignment of the glenoid fossa is matched by 30 degrees retroversion of the head of the humerus on its shaft (measured in relation to the intercondylar line at the elbow) (Fig. 32-3). Hence the glenohumeral joint is designed to follow the plane of the scapula. As the arm is raised in the scapular plane, the path of the humerus is perpendicular to the face of the glenoid; the joint is in neutral alignment. Johnston[34] noted that the inferior capsule remained without torsion only when the humerus was raised in the scapular plane. The term *scaption* has been created to indicate motion in the plane of the scapula.

Flexion is sagittal plane elevation (Fig. 32-2). Placing the arm in this plane includes significant horizontal flexion. Hence the path of the humerus is oblique to the face of the scapula. The inferior joint capsule twists to accommodate this path of arm elevation.[34]

Abduction raises the arm in the coronal plane (Fig. 32-2). This introduces two limitations. An element of horizontal extension is included in the elevation motion. More significant is the potential for impingement of the greater tuberosity against the acromion, since normal

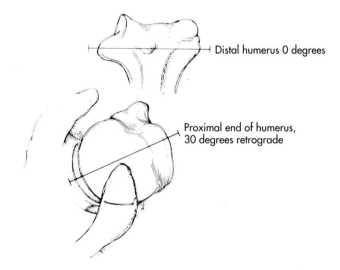

FIG. 32-3. Humeral head retroversion is 30 degrees compared to transverse axis of the elbow. (From Rowe CR: *The shoulder,* New York, 1988, Churchill Livingstone.)

clearance is so minimal that there is no space for tendon thickening. This can be avoided by adding external rotation to the abduction motion.

Differences in the two ranges of motion have necessitated dual testing, because there have been no guidelines for selecting one over the other. The scapular plane represents neutral joint alignment. Clinical experience indicates that it is the simplest path of motion. Patients with limited strength spontaneously choose the scapular plane when asked to raise their arm overhead.

Recent 3-dimensional electrogoniometry and documentation with global coordinates showed that scaption (55-degree plane) was the path of spontaneous shoulder elevation.[54] Scaption also is the plane most used in the activities of daily living.[57] A biomechanical cadaver

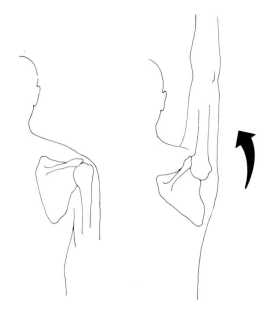

FIG. 32-4. Arm elevation is a combination of scapular and humeral rotation. (From Rowe CR: *The shoulder,* New York, 1988, Churchill Livingstone.)

study[9] found that maximum humeral elevation occurred in a more anterior plane (23 degrees). This difference may relate to in vitro vs. in vivo scapular positioning. The physician can still conclude that testing the scaption range offers the best approximation of maximum arm elevation capability.

Scapulohumeral rhythm. Total arm elevation is the sum of motion at two areas: the glenohumeral joint and the gliding of the scapula on the thorax (Fig. 32-4).[11]

Components of arm elevation

- Glenohumeral motion
- Scapulothoracic motion

At the onset of arm elevation, scapular participation has proved to be highly variable. It may be absent, minimal, or even reversed.[26] This lag in scapular motion persisted through the first 60 degrees of flexion and 30 degrees abduction. Once the scapula started to participate, both segments (humerus and scapula) moved continuously and synchronously. Relative humeral and scapular motion was identified by Inman et al.[26] as a 2:1 ratio. Other investigators have found both higher and lower ratios (2.5:1 to 1.25:1).[15,17,63,68] The average among all

---

Glenohumeral-scapulothoracic rhythm

- 3 degrees of glenohumeral motion for each 2 degrees of scapulothoracic motion
- 2.5:1 to 1.25:1 (humeral:scapular motion)

---

studies is 1.5:1.[77] Hence there are approximately 3 degrees of glenohumeral motion for each 2 degrees occurring at the scapula.[15,17,68]

Instant centers of shoulder motion. Each joint has its own pattern of motion. This is defined by its path of instant centers.

Excursion of the humeral head on the glenoid has been described as both gliding and rolling. Direct radiographic analysis of the glenohumeral joint demonstrated intraarticular displacement to be minimal. At the onset of arm elevation (0 to 30 degrees) Walker[78] found a 3-mm upward shift. This action appears to be correction of arm sag from its dependent position. During the rest of the elevation range, the point of glenohumeral contact remained within 1 mm of the center of the fossa. Hence rolling is not a significant element of shoulder motion.[16,68] Instead, an intact labrum combined with dynamic control keeps the humeral head centered, making gliding of the humeral surface on that of the glenoid fossa the dominant type of motion within the joint.

Serial supine radiographs of multiple posture confirmed the precise centering of the humeral head on the glenoid for all but one position. Maximum extension and external rotation caused notable posterior displacement of the humeral head (4 mm).[19] The presence of terminal transposition also was found in a dynamic cadaver study.[23] Anterior translation accompanied both sagittal flexion and horizontal flexion. Conversely, posterior translation accompanied extension.

Assessment of persons with a painful shoulder showed half of them to have abnormal mechanics.[63] Both humeral head excursion and instant center displacement were increased, with the greater change occurring in excursion.

The scapula was found to follow a more complex path of motion. During its initial setting stage (the first 60 degrees), either there was no motion or the scapula joggled around a center of rotation in the lower part of the blade. Subsequent scapular rotation was grossly centered to the base of the scapular spine until the arm reached 120 degrees. During the final arc the center of rotation shifted to a point near the base of the glenoid. This marked change in instant center location can be related to scapula motion arising first in the sternoclavicular and then the acromioclavicular joints. Clinically, surgeons have found good arm function can be restored despite some compromise in clavicular rotation.[45] Conversely, the clavicle is not an indispensable bone, but its presence adds stability for heavy, overhead arm use.[23]

Scapular rotation also is reflected by the path of the coracoid, while the acromion remains relatively fixed.[78]

Axial Rotation

Internal and external rotation of the arm is a function of the glenohumeral joints. Because of change in relative capsule length, the range varies with arm position (Fig. 32-5). Maximal rotation of approximately 180 degrees is present with the arm at the side of the body (adducted).[7] The larger portion of that range (108 degrees or 60%) is external rotation.[8] Abduction of the arm to 90 degrees reduces the total arc to 120 degrees. Within this range there is more internal than external rotation.[7] At

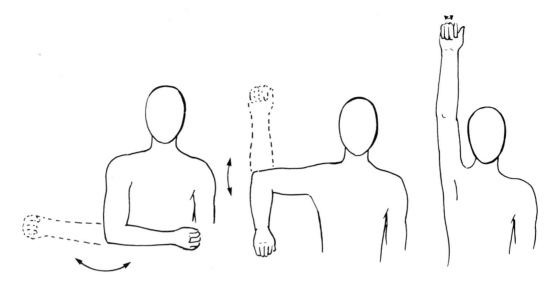

FIG. 32-5. Arm external-internal rotation ranges available with shoulder at 0 degrees, 90 degrees, and full elevation. Relative range indicated by the arcs. (From Rowe CR: *The shoulder,* New York, 1988, Churchill Livingstone.)

peak elevation (by either flexion or abduction), no more than a jog of rotation is possible.

External rotation range with the arm elevated to 90 degrees is critical to throwing. In addition to the level of arm elevation, at least three other factors can modify the resulting range. These are the testing plane, humeral retroversion, and the subject's sex.[38] Testing the 90-degree elevated arm in scaption rather than coronal plane abduction increased the available external rotation by 15 degrees (105 to 120 degrees). Normal retroversion averaged 33 degrees (30 to 35 degrees) in the dominant arm and 26 degrees (22 to 31 degrees) in the nondominant shoulder, a statistically significant difference ($p <$ 0.0010). External rotation greater than 110 degrees was more common with retroversion greater than 35 degrees (59%) compared with 23% with retroversion under 26 degrees. External rotation beyond 120 degrees was always related to increased retroversion. Women averaged 5 degrees more external rotation than men.

Horizontal Flexion and Extension

These motions also have been called horizontal adduction and abduction. Within the normal 180-degree arc only 45 degrees, or 24%, is horizontal extension behind the coronal plane.[8] Most of the motion is glenohumeral. As was true in the scapular plane, the humeral head remains centrally located in the glenoid fossa. The limitation of this motion is the edge of the humeral articular surface. Further effort leads to impingement between the posterior rims of the glenoid fossa and humeral head as wedging replaces gliding.

Shoulder Muscular Control

Raising the arm from its resting position is the basic shoulder motion. Versatility in hand placement or the path of dynamic arm propulsion is accomplished by varying the plane of arm elevation and supplementing the action with horizontal and rotatory motion. This represents a vast number of possible movement combinations. A

simple personal experiment demonstrated that normal selective control is so precise that the arm can be repositioned within 1 degree of the first position. Applying this level of control to the average ranges of shoulder motion indicates that the normal person has the potential to place the hand selectively in 16,000 positions.[55] The fine artist or champion athlete very probably has more precise control and hence a greater number of options available. To allow interpretation of the patterns of muscle control, however, the basic motion patterns are considered separately.

Elevation

Two sources of control are used to raise the arm: the superficial muscle group and the underlying supraspinatus. Within the superficial musculature the deltoid is dominant. Its action is supplemented anteriorly by the clavicular head of the pectoralis major, the coracobrachialis, and the biceps brachii. The exact pattern of muscle action varies with the plane of motion selected.

Selectivity in shoulder control was demonstrated by the simple task of moving the arm through a small conical arc against mild dynamometer resistance. As the arm's direction progressed from medial to upward and lateral the peak muscle action sequentially advanced from the clavicular pectoralis major to the anterior deltoid, the middle deltoid, and last the posterior deltoid. As the arm moved downward, shoulder control shifted from the elevating muscles to depressors (Fig. 32-6).[53]

Deltoid. While the deltoid is a continuous muscular sheet wrapped around the shoulder, it functions as three distinct muscles: anterior, middle, and posterior.

The middle deltoid is dominant: it participates in all arm elevation activities.[73] Supplementing its action are the anterior and posterior heads. They may act synergistically to add an abductor force or assume primary responsibility for arm elevation in their direction (flexion or extension). Hence the pattern of deltoid action varies with the plane of motion used.

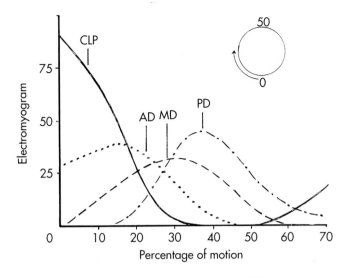

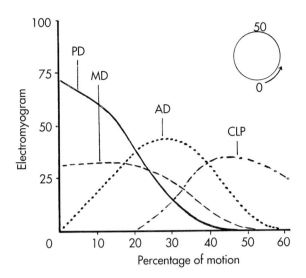

FIG. 32-6. Activation sequence of the humeral elevating muscles during clockwise conical arm movement against 1 kg resistance. *CLP,* Clavicular pectoralis major; *AD,* anterior deltoid; *MD,* middle deltoid; *PD,* posterior deltoid. (Modified from Pearl M et al: *Clin Orthop* 284:116, 1992.)

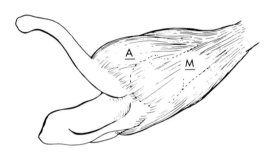

FIG. 32-7. Muscles providing scaption. *A,* Anterior deltoid; *M,* middle deltoid. (From Rowe CR: *The shoulder,* New York, 1988, Churchill Livingstone.)

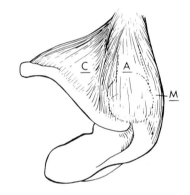

FIG. 32-8. Muscles providing arm flexion (sagittal plane elevation). *C,* Clavicular head of the major; *A,* anterior deltoid; *M,* middle deltoid. (From Rowe CR: *The shoulder,* New York, 1988, Churchill Livingstone.)

Scaption is provided by combined action of the middle and anterior deltoids (Fig. 32-7).[73] Studies using electromyography (EMG) have confirmed the simultaneous action of the anterior and middle deltoids throughout arm elevation.[35] Improved leverage of the anterior deltoid improves its contribution as the arm is raised.

Participation of the posterior deltoid in scapular plane elevation is less consistent. By radiographic analysis an abduction lever was not identified until the arm reached the 90-degree position.[64]

For flexion, the anterior deltoid is the primary muscle. It is assisted by the clavicular pectoralis major, cor-

acobrachialis, and biceps brachii, as well as the middle deltoid (Fig. 32-8). While only the EMG activity of the clavicular pectoralis major has been studied in detail,[26,73] participation by the other muscles has been confirmed. Relative EMG activity of the clavicular pectoralis major and deltoid indicated that these superficial muscles provided about 30% of the arm elevation effort.

Abduction in the coronal plane increases posterior deltoid action at onset of the arc, but the middle and anterior deltoid action remains dominant. (Fig. 32-9)[39]

Hyperextension, or posterior elevation, is dominated by the posterior deltoid. There also is strong participation by the middle deltoid, but the anterior muscle is silent.[73]

Effectiveness of the deltoid muscles depends on their functional fiber length. It is greatest with the arm in the dependent rest period and shortest with full glenohumeral elevation. Anatomically, this represents a 33% reduction in the length of the muscle.[41] Functionally, the

---

Shoulder flexion

Primary motor
- Anterior deltoid

Secondary motors
- Middle deltoid
- Pectoralis major (clavicular head)
- Coracobrachialis
- Biceps brachii

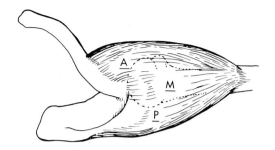

FIG. 32-9. Muscle providing arm abduction (coronal plane elevation). *A,* Anterior deltoid; *M,* middle deltoid; *P,* posterior deltoid. (From Rowe CR: *The shoulder,* New York, 1988, Churchill Livingstone.)

muscle becomes weaker. Such loss of deltoid strength is avoided by scapular rotation.

The deltoid is anatomically capable of initiating, as well as completing, arm elevation independently because of its mass, even though the leverage at 30 degrees is very low.[12] A strenuous effect (about 54% of maximal) would be required, however, with a corresponding limit in endurance.

Biceps brachii. Both the short and long heads of the biceps brachii cross the glenohumeral joint anteriorly and thus have a flexor moment arm. Limitations to its effectiveness result from its distal attachment to the radius; hence it is an elbow muscle. EMG analysis of pitching confirmed that the need for elbow control was the stimulus for biceps action, not humeral elevation. Also, peak activity of the biceps was only 36% of its maximal capacity with a 9 cm^2 cross section and only half of the muscle related to the long head.

The long head of the biceps brachii has an additional role—humeral head stabilization. Between its origin on the superior rim of the glenoid and its passage through the bicipital groove on the humeral shaft, the long head of the biceps lies across the top of the humeral head, parallel to the tendon of the supraspinatus. A cadaver study[40] of humeral head displacement with simulated biceps contractions showed muscle tension in the long head inhibited upward displacement of the humeral head, which otherwise was caused by muscle tension in the short head. A second study[28] demonstrated reduced displacement from an anteriorly directed force when the arm was externally rotated 60 to 90 degrees. This finding is reinforced by a recent biomechanical cadaver study[44] that demonstrated effective stability by the biceps tendon and an efficiency equal to the supraspinatus (0.62 and 0.51, respectively).

Supraspinatus. This muscle is active in all patterns of arm elevation.[26,73] EMG of arm elevation in each of the three basic planes showed an immediate and sustained strong effort (40% of the manual muscle test) by the rotator cuff muscles while the deltoid components increased their intensity in proportion to the demand torque of the arm.[58] Its short leverage (2.2 cm) and modest size (6 cm^2) limit the torque that can be produced, however. Maximal effort (calculated as 98%) could accomplish arm elevation to 30 degrees but not higher. Because this intensity of action would leave no endurance

for a second effort, assistance, not initiation of abduction, is its role.

Deltoid-supraspinatus relationships. Common to all three patterns of arm elevation is combined deltoid and supraspinatus action.[26,27,32,73]

It has been commonly assumed that abduction of the arm is initiated by the supraspinatus and continued by the deltoid.[25] Codman[11] believed that the deltoid could not abduct the arm without the supraspinatus. This interpretation is based on clinical experience with large rotator cuff ruptures. Such a lesion deprives the person of the ability to lift the arm, yet once the arm has been passively raised to the horizontal, the patient can maintain that arm position though strength is reduced.

Three findings contradict the probability that abduction is initiated by the supraspinatus: muscle size, EMG patterns, and cuff mechanics.

The muscle is anatomically too small to lift the arm independently. While it could accomplish the first 30 degrees, a 200% effort would be required to reach the horizontal position. In contrast, the size and leverage of the deltoid would allow the arm to be raised with an effort of 55% of maximum.

Dynamic EMG shows that the middle and anterior deltoids and supraspinatus function synchronously.[27,43] Through such a combined action the calculated intensity of each muscle is 35% of maximal strength. This level of muscular effort would be compatible with long endurance demands.

Measurements of abduction muscle forces using a biomechanical cadaver model confirmed the ability of the supraspinatus to reduce the deltoid demand.[47] Without the supraspinatus, twice as much middle deltoid force was required to center the suspended humeral head in the glenoid, and the force required to elevate the arm was increased 18%. Jiang et al[29] also found that in most positions the moment arm of the supraspinatus equaled or exceeded those of the various deltoid components.

Infraspinatus and subscapularis. In addition to their ability to provide humeral rotation, Inman, Saunders, and Abbott[26] identified these muscles as major contributors to the force couple that facilitates arm elevation. Subsequent studies of normal[67,73] and athletic[3,32] arm function, as well as assessment by axillary and subscapular nerve blocks, questioned the significance of the infraspinatus and subscapularis in arm elevation. The recent study of conical arm motion has provided considerable clarification.[54] With the onset of upward arm motion the rotator cuff muscles sequentially became active (Fig. 32-10). The stimulus would be stretch as the deltoid initiated upward displacement of the humerus. Timing of their peak action paralleled the muscles' relationship to the glenohumeral joint. The anteriorly aligned subscapularis accompanied the flexor onset of a clockwise cone, while the posteriorly aligned infraspinatus became active first with the extension of a counterclockwise cone. In both patterns supraspinatus activity accompanied the upward segment of the arc as a primary elevator.

Electromyographically the infraspinatus is the next most active rotator cuff muscle after the supraspinatus muscle, whereas the subscapularis is more selective.[27,32,33] Because of their potential contribution to gle-

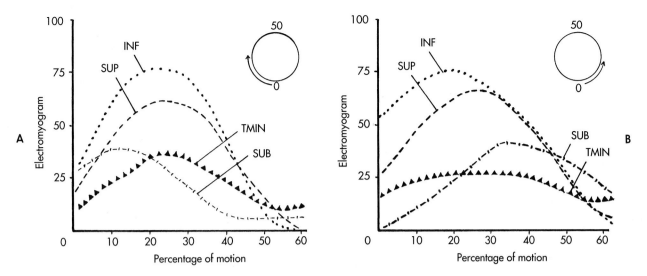

FIG. 32-10. Rotator cuff muscle activation sequence during clockwise (**A**) and counterclockwise (**B**) conical arm movement against 1 kg resistance. *SUB*, Subscapularis; *INF, infraspinatus; SUP,* supraspinatus; *TMIN,* teres minor. (Modified from Pearl M et al: *Clin Orthop* 284:116, 1992.)

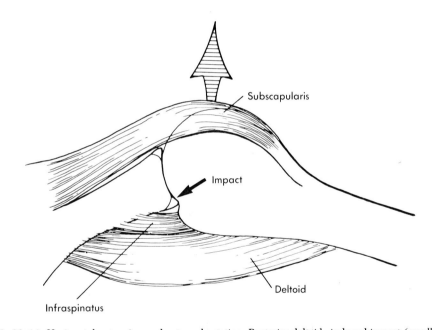

FIG. 32-11. Horizontal extension and external rotation. Posterior deltoid–induced impact (*small arrow*) and anterior shear (*large arrow*) countered by infraspinatus and subscapularis muscle action. (From Rowe CR: *The shoulder,* New York, 1988, Churchill Livingstone.)

nohumeral joint stability, enhancing these muscles' participation in arm elevation is very desirous. Anatomically both muscles have fan-shaped distribution of their fibers. This enables the upper fiber to roughly parallel the alignment of the supraspinatus and thus contribute a similar function. In addition, the lower fibers angle downward to introduce a depressive action. The basic function of these two muscles and the teres minor is humeral rotation on the glenoid.[73]

Infraspinatus activity is stimulated by elevating the arm with some degree of elbow flexion. This introduces an internal rotation torque that must be restrained if hand position is to be preserved. The teres minor would

also participate in this action. EMG studies indicate that the infraspinatus is the more active muscle of this pair.[27,32]

Subscapularis activity relates to its ability to provide internal rotation. Deceleration of external rotation is a common stimulus.[27] It often functions in company with the other internal rotators of the shoulder, such as the pectoralis major, teres major, and latissimus dorsi.

Horizontal Extension and External Rotation

This motion synergy is commonly used to create a propulsive force in sports. It provides the cocking[2,25] phase of pitching,[27,32] throwing,[2] and tennis serve and is also

a significant part of most strokes in swimming.[6,66,72] Both posterior impingement and anterior subluxation are likely complications.

As the middle and anterior deltoids support arm weight, the posterior deltoid increases its activity to draw the humerus backward (horizontal extension) (Fig. 32-11). Two force patterns result: compression and anterior shear.

At the beginning of posterior deltoid action the muscle's line of pull is primarily longitudinal, making compression the major force. Alignment of the muscle tends to concentrate the force at the posterior margins of the humeral head and glenoid fossa. During rapid motion this can be an abrupt and destructive impact of considerable intensity.

The muscle's origin along the length of the scapular spine and insertion at the midhumeral shaft places the posterior deltoid's line of pull a considerable distance behind the glenohumeral joint center. This distance increases as horizontal extension becomes greater. An anterior shear force is induced that increases in intensity as hyperextension proceeds. External rotation accentuates the anterior subluxation tendency by directing the angulated humeral head against the anterior capsule.

Protective forces are available from three rotator cuff muscles: infraspinatus, teres minor, and subscapularis. The infraspinatus is a primary motor for both external rotation and hyperextension. Hence it can reduce the intensity of posterior deltoid action. Also, because it lies adjacent to the joint margin, its actions prevent humeral subluxation. The teres minor, as an external rotator, also reduces the deltoid response.

A dynamic cadaver study[51] of muscle and joint forces demonstrated that during the cocking maneuver the infraspinatus and teres muscles were most effective in reducing the strain on the inferior glenohumeral ligament.

Subscapularis activity at the end of the hyperextension and external rotation effort provides an anterior restraint against humeral displacement. This synergistic sequence is displayed in the EMG analysis of a baseball pitch (Fig. 32-12). The sternal pectoralis major also provides a protective force as its tendon crosses the anterior joint surface when the arm is both hyperextended and externally rotated. Hence initiation of the motion combined with decelerating forces involves a complex synergy and sequence of muscle action.

Internal Rotation and Horizontal Flexion

Acceleration to complete the throwing or propulsive act and then follow-through are performed by the sequence of cocking, acceleration, and follow-through. Muscle activity is stimulated by tension at the end of the cocking phase. EMG recordings show that the major muscle contributing to acceleration is the subscapularis.[27,32] Participation of the sternal pectoralis major and latissimus dorsi was less consistent. The latter muscle was strongly used by professional pitchers, while amateurs called on the pectoralis major.[22] Athletic use of the teres major has not been assessed, but EMG studies of basic arm function identified its action in internal rotation and adduction.[73] This implies that the teres major would be a logical participant in the acceleration to follow-through motion sequence.

During follow-through the weight of the arm creates a distractive force at the shoulder from the pendulous momentum present. The antagonistic action identified in the infraspinatus, teres minor, supraspinatus, and latissimus dorsi[22] acts to decelerate the force and maintain shoulder joint integrity.

Scapulothoracic Articulation

Five muscles directly control the scapula. Functional division of the trapezius into upper, middle, and lower units expands the number to seven. The major and mi-

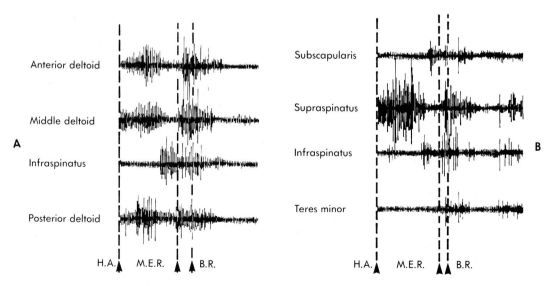

FIG. 32-12. Muscle action during a typical baseball pitch. **A,** Deltoid. **B,** Rotator cuff. Phases of pitching: *H.A.,* hands apart; *M.E.R.,* maximum external rotation; *B.R.,* ball release. (From Rowe CR: *The shoulder,* New York, 1988, Churchill Livingstone.)

nor rhomboids are considered here as one. Hence functional concern revolves around six muscle units: serratus anterior; upper, middle, and lower trapezius; levator scapulae, and rhomboids. Synergistic action of the muscles varies with the scapular motion desired.

Motor controls of the scapula

- Serratus anterior
- Trapezius (upper, middle, and lower)
- Levator scapulae
- Rhomboids

Among the scapula's potential functions, upward rotation in conjunction with arm elevation is the primary clinical concern. The other actions complete the arm's versatility with their significance varying according to the person's occupation or sport.

Although each scapular motion can be performed independently for testing, they normally are an integral component of arm function.

Upward Rotation

Rotation of the scapula is defined by the direction the glenoid moves. Upward rotation is an essential component of arm elevation. Two muscles are recognized as the upward rotators of the scapula: trapezius and serratus anterior. Normally the trapezius and serratus act together, but either also can accomplish scapular rotation independently, though the strength of arm elevation will be less. Independent action by the trapezius is well documented by clinical experience. Isolated loss of the trapezius is a less frequent occurrence. Recent experience with two patients indicated incomplete arm elevation resulting from limited scapular rotation by the serratus. Lack of posterior stabilization allowed the serratus muscle length to be dominated by scapular abduction.

Scapula motion

Upward rotation
- Trapezius
- Serratus anterior

Retraction
- Middle trapezius
- Rhomboids

Protraction
- Serratus anterior

Depression
- Lower trapezius
- Inferior portion of serratus anterior

Within the trapezius, Inman, Saunders, and Abbott[26] found that only the upper segment displayed consistent action in both abduction and flexion. Reduced participation by the lower trapezius in all but the last segment of flexion leaves the scapula free to move anteriorly. These limitations in the contribution of the trapezius to flexion place an added burden on the serratus anterior. This is particularly true in swimming, where maximal upward reach is used to increase one's stroke.

To attain maximal scapular rotation, both the trapezius and serratus anterior must be effective. EMG analysis of swimming demonstrated that the serratus worked at 75% of its maximal muscle test capability.[52] This is too strenuous for a lengthy effort. A similar high level of activity was identified during voluntary arm elevation in all three basic planes, whether the elbow was flexed or extended. Raising the arm to 90 degrees averaged 41% of maximum, while reaching full elevation increased the effort to 66% of maximum. During pitching there also is a short period of serratus activity that exceeds 100% of the manual muscle test. The relative intensity of the serratus consistently was greater than that of the trapezius, which progressed from 34% to 42% maximum. According to Weber's data the two muscles are of equivalent size (12.8 and 12.6 cm^2) and thus should have similar force potentials.[79] The greater effort by the serratus suggests that it is less well developed to meet the functional demands imposed on it. Adequate training is thus particularly significant if one is to lessen the threats of impingement. Maximal overhead reach puts all the muscles in a relatively inefficient situation because of fiber shortening. Activities in flexion reduce the ability of the lower trapezius to contribute, resulting in a higher demand on the serratus. A 75% effort by the serratus cannot be maintained during prolonged swimming sessions, hence better training is indicated.

Retraction (Adduction)

Drawing the scapula back toward the vertebral midline accentuates horizontal extension of the arm. A synonym for this action is scapular adduction. The cocking phase of pitching and pulling relies on such assistance. Several swimming strokes also use this action.

Direct muscle control is provided by the middle trapezius and rhomboids. The latissimus dorsi also retracts the scapula incidental to complete arm extension.

Protraction (Abduction)

Advancement of the scapula anteriorly on the thorax has been called both protraction and scapular abduction (moving away from the vertebral column). The latter term, however, leads to confusion when scapular and humeral motions are considered together. Hence the older term protraction is being adopted again. Protraction is the function of the serratus anterior. There also may be some assistance by the sternal pectoralis major as it horizontally flexes the arm. Follow-through in throwing,[2] pitching,[3] tennis serve, and crawl strokes[11,72] include scapular protraction.

Depression

Descent of the scapula is used to elevate the trunk while the arms are stabilized. The site of arm fixation varies. During gymnastics an overhead bar, ring, or underlying platform is used. Immediate muscular control is provided by the inferior digitations of the serratus anterior and the lower trapezius. Additional force of consid-

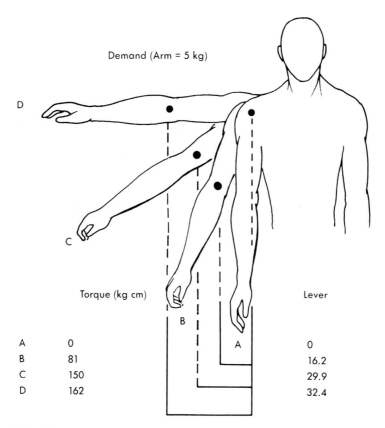

Demand (Arm = 5 kg)

	Torque (kg cm)		Lever
A	0		0
B	81		16.2
C	150		29.9
D	162		32.4

FIG. 32-13. Shoulder torque introduced by arm position. Weight is consistent, but leverage increases with greater elevation. *A* = 0 degrees, *B* = 30 degrees, *C* = 45 degrees, *D* = 90 degrees. (From Rowe CR: *The shoulder,* New York, 1988, Churchill Livingstone.)

erable magnitude is gained from the two large thoraco-humeral muscles: sternal pectoralis major and latissimus dorsi.

Arm Torque

To understand the relationships between arm function and muscle action, some simple rules of mechanics must be appreciated.

Raising the arm from the side of the body moves its center of gravity away from this neutral line. A moment arm (or lever) has been created. This is seen as a demand torque to which the muscles must respond. As arm elevation increases, the functional lever is lengthened, leading to a correspondingly greater torque (Fig. 32-13).

These changes follow the cosine law of trigonometry. The maximal arm lever occurs at 90 degrees elevation. This decreases 71% at the 45-degree position and 50% of maximum with the arm elevated 30 degrees. The significance of these numbers relates to the changing demands arm weight places on the shoulder's abducting musculature.

Flexing the elbow 90 degrees reduces the arm torque 22% because the forearm and hand are opposite the elbow joint. This postural change, however, introduces an internal rotation torque. Hence, while the deltoid demand was lessened, a need for infraspinatus activity was added. Such postural variations can be used in the de-

sign of therapeutic exercises, for performance of a sport, or for basic daily use.

Muscle Forces

Muscles provide the body's active force to create or restrain motion. They function through bony levers. As a result, muscle strength is a torque $(F \times L = T)$, as was arm demand. Both muscle force (F) and lever lengths (L) are modified by joint position.

The maximal force a muscle can produce is proportional to the number of motor cells it contains. These slender fibers (50 μm diameter) are counted indirectly by measuring the muscle's physiologic cross-section. If all the fibers have a longitudinal arrangement, a simple transverse (anatomic) section is sufficient. Pennate muscles have oblique fibers. This means one must count several bundles to attain the perpendicular area of all its fibers, a task that can be done only by detailed anatomic dissection.

Factors in muscle force analysis

- Number of motor cells in muscle
- Type of contraction
- Speed of contraction
- Lever length

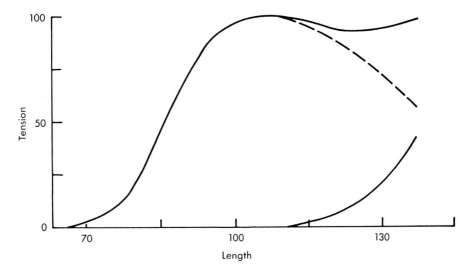

FIG. 32-14. Length tension relationships of muscle. *Top curve,* Total tension; *dotted line,* active tension; *lower curve,* passive tension as muscle is pulled beyond resting length (100%). (From Rowe CR: *The shoulder,* New York, 1988, Churchill Livingstone.)

The type of muscle action is a second strength variable. Isometric contractions provide the basic force. Eccentric action (contraction vs. passive lengthening) has been found to produce the same amount of use.[69] In these two forms of muscle action (isometric and eccentric) the resulting force is a combination of both active and passive tension (Fig. 32-14). The latter arises from the collagenous sheaths enveloping each muscle fiber.[20] Concentric (shortening) contractions lack the advantage of passive tension and thus produce proportionally less force (13% to 20%).[69]

Speed further reduces concentric force. Motion at 214 degrees per second decreases maximal strength by 50%.[56]

Lever length is the final determinant of muscle effectiveness. It varies with joint position. The greater the perpendicular distance between the muscle's line of pull and the fulcrum of motion, the more effective is the muscle's force.

At the onset of arm elevation in the scapular plane only the middle deltoid has an effective lever. Abduction to 60 degrees increases the muscle's leverage by 60%. It then remains relatively stable. The anterior deltoid, with much of its origin on the clavicle, starts with an insignificant abduction lever, but rapid and continual arm elevation moves a greater proportion of the muscle lateral to the joint center. By 90 degrees it has surpassed that of the middle deltoid. In the resting position the origin of the posterior deltoid on the scapular spine places most of the muscle mass medial to the shoulder joint center. This alignment does not significantly improve until the arm has abducted 120 degrees. These improvements in mechanical leverage counter the effects of shortened muscle fiber (sarcomere) length. They also accommodate the increase in arm demand so that elevation strength is maintained. In contrast, lever length for the supraspinatus remains fairly constant throughout the range of arm elevation. This means there is no leverage advantage available to compensate for the reduction in

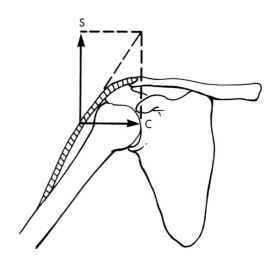

FIG. 32-15. Joint forces induced by muscle action (middle deltoid is the model). C, Compression (perpendicular to plane of joint); S, shear (parallel to joint). (From Rowe CR: *The shoulder,* New York, 1988, Churchill Livingstone.)

muscle fiber length. Consequently, the supraspinatus becomes progressively less effective.

Shoulder Joint Forces

As muscles act to control the arm, they create forces within the joint. These forces are classified by their alignment to the joint surface as either compression or shear (Fig. 32-15). Those directed toward the center of the joint (i.e., perpendicular to the plane of the glenoid fossa) are called compression. Shear forces are parallel to the joint surface.[64]

The line of pull of most shoulder muscles is oblique to the plane of the glenoid fossa. As a result, both compression and shear forces accompany muscle action. The compressive forces contribute to joint stability as they drive the humeral head into the glenoid socket. In con-

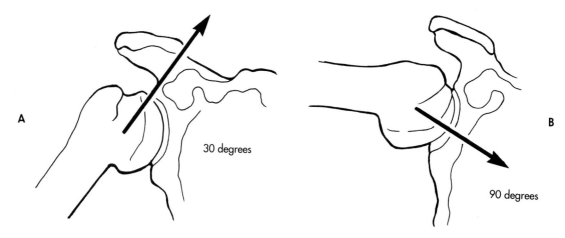

FIG. 32-16. Direction of the joint forces with shoulder in 30-degree **(A)** and 90-degree **(B)** scapular abduction. (From Rowe CR: *The shoulder,* New York, 1988, Churchill Livingstone.)

trast, shear forces threaten the stabilizing tissues by the sliding strains created. The magnitude of the forces is determined by the intensity of muscle action. The amounts of shear and compression vary as the muscle's alignment changes.

During arm function the forces within the shoulder joint are related to two major muscle groups: deltoid and rotator cuff. They differ markedly in their patterns of compression and shear.

In addition to differing in their direction of pull, the muscles also vary significantly in size with moderately different fiber lengths and relatively similar moment arms. These factors make the subscapularis the strongest rotator cuff muscle (53% of the total capability). In sequence the others are infraspinatus (23%), supraspinatus (14%), and teres minor (10%).[36]

Deltoid

The deltoid changes from a vertical to horizontal muscle as the arm is elevated. This alters the relative dominance of shear and compression force produced. During scapular plane abduction, the force patterns of the anterior and posterior components are similar to that of the middle head. With the arm at rest, the middle deltoid's line of pull is 27 degrees to the glenoid face. As a result, at the initiation of abduction, the dominant direction of deltoid pull is vertical, creating significant upward shear (89% of the muscle's total force vs. a compression value of 45%) (Fig. 32-16). Further elevation progressively makes the muscle's line of pull more horizontal. Shear is reduced and compression increased. Above 60 degrees abduction, compression exceeds shear.

Rotator Cuff

Force patterns of the rotator cuff muscle contrast sharply with the deltoid. Their dominant directions are horizontal and downward. The supraspinatus is basically horizontal (Fig. 32-17). As a result, compression is the dominant joint force generated. There is a much smaller vertical shear, equaling 34% of the muscle force.

All three of the other rotator cuff muscles have a mean downward alignment (Fig. 32-18). While their precise di-

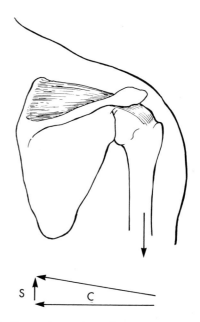

FIG. 32-17. Supraspinatus joint forces, compression dominant. (From Rowe CR: *The shoulder,* New York, 1988, Churchill Livingstone.)

rection has not been measured, it approximates 45 degrees for the infraspinatus and subscapularis and 55 degrees for the teres minor.[56] Their inferior shear force (71% to 82%) would counteract that of the deltoid. Inman[26] noted that during routine arm elevation the deltoid and rotator cuff contracted synchronously. He called this action the shoulder-force couple with the upward and downward forces in balance (Fig. 32-19). Inman also postulated that arm abduction could not occur without rotator cuff coordination.

The combined effect of such muscle action was calculated by Inman, Saunders, and Abbott[26] as creating a shoulder joint compression force equaling body weight. These authors also found that peak joint force occurred at 90 degrees, whereas maximal shear was at the 60-degree position.

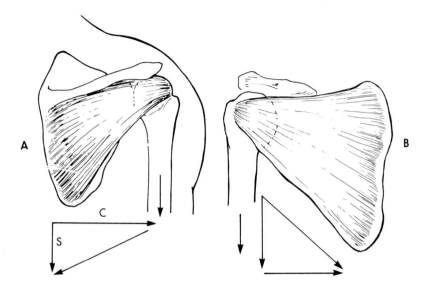

FIG. 32-18. Depressor muscles of the rotator cuff: shear force is strong and downward. **A,** Infraspinatus. **B,** Subscapularis. *S,* Shear; *C,* compression. (From Rowe CR: *The shoulder,* New York, 1988, Churchill Livingstone.)

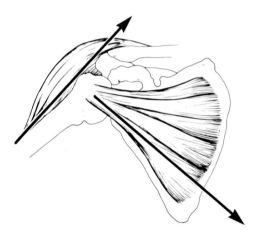

FIG. 32-19. Inman force couple between deltoid and depressor muscles in the rotator cuff. (From Rowe CR: *The shoulder,* New York, 1988, Churchill Livingstone.)

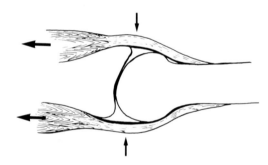

FIG. 32-20. Rotator cuff muscle action creates compressive and encircling shear forces to stabilize the humeral head of the glenoid fossa. (From Rowe CR: *The shoulder,* New York, 1988, Churchill Livingstone.)

Biceps Role in Rotator Cuff Tears

The role of the biceps at the shoulder has been controversial.[5,18] EMG analysis during pitching demonstrated that the biceps functions predominate at the elbow rather than at the shoulder during throwing.[74] The similarity of the biceps and brachialis firing patterns supported this finding. Biceps activity correlated with motion, occurring as the elbow flexed during late cocking and as the elbow decelerated during follow-through. The heads of the triceps worked together, also correlating with elbow motion.

The biceps does make a small functional contribution to the shoulder during abduction and flexion when the arm is externally rotated and supinated.[5,18] Evaluation of the lateral biceps (long head) action in shoulders with rotator cuff tears revealed that the muscle may be a sig-

nificant contributor to both flexion and abduction in the compromised shoulder.[74] This was supported by the significantly increased activity of the lateral biceps during shoulder flexion and abduction with a torn rotator cuff. Before this study a consistent intraoperative finding had been an enlarged biceps tendon in association with a major rotator cuff tear. The increase in EMG activity along with the observed enlargement of biceps tendon width would implicate a use-induced hypertrophy of the tendon. Therefore it is suggested that the practice of sacrificing the interscapular portion of the biceps tendon for grafting material or tenodesis during rotator cuff repair should be examined more discriminately.

Dynamic Shoulder Stability

As identified by the muscle force pattern at the shoulder, the function of the rotator cuff is to reduce the shearing strain introduced by deltoid action. Contouring of the tendons around the humeral head adds a direct restraining force.

Muscle action transforms the tissue into straighter, tense bands (Fig. 32-20). Both compression and shear forces are created to stabilize the humeral head on the glenoid. The favorable balance between compression and shear force makes shoulder elevation to 90 degrees the optimal position of joint stability.

THE ELBOW
Elbow Mobility

The elbow is limited by bony constraints, joint geometry, capsule, ligaments, and muscles. Normal elbow hinge motion includes 5 degrees of hyperextension and 150 degrees of flexion. Axial rotation of the radius about the ulna averages 130 degrees (75 degrees of pronation and supination to 55 degrees). Elbow extension is limited by four factors. Two are skeletal impingement between the forearm and the humerus (i.e., the radial head against the anterior capitellum) and impact of the coronoid process against the trochlea. Two other limitations relate to the soft tissue. These include tension of the anterior capsule and the musculature. The range of forearm rotation occurring at the elbow also is modified by the soft tissues.[1] Total rotation from supination to pronation in the intact arm is around 130 degrees. When the muscles are removed from a cadaver, the range increases to 190 degrees, and when the ligaments are cut, the range increases to 210 degrees.[1]

Instant Centers of Elbow Motion

The axis of elbow flexion and extension passes through the trochlea. The instant center of rotation occurs within a 2- to 3-mm zone at the center of the trochlea.[49] The axis of rotation is internally rotated 3 to 8 degrees relative to the plane of the epicondyles, and its perpendicular axis has a lateral opening angle of 4 to 8 degrees relative to the long axis of the humerus.[1]

The carrying angle that is formed by the long axes of the humerus and ulna in the frontal plane averages 10 to 15 degrees in men and 15 to 20 degrees in females. Because the trochlea is not orthogonal to the humerus, the carrying angle changes, being greatest at full extension and diminishing during flexion.

The longitudinal axis of forearm rotation or supination-pronation runs proximally from the distal end of the ulnar center to the center of the radial head. The ulna remains fixed with the radius rotating over the ulnar shaft during pronation and supination.

Movement of the elbow joint occurs about two basic planes, the transverse and longitudinal axis. Isometric muscle contraction often occurs to maintain or check the position of the elbow in space as the limb is moved at the shoulder.

Elbow Muscle Control
Flexion

There are three primary elbow flexor muscles: brachialis, biceps, and brachioradialis. Being superficial, mobile, and large, the biceps brachii is most conspicuous. The biceps, by inserting on the radius, acts first as a supinator and then flexes the elbow. With the forearm pronated, the biceps is less effective because its functional

---

> **Elbow flexors**
> - Brachialis
> - Biceps brachii
> - Brachioradialis

leverage is less. The biceps also acts to decelerate elbow extension.

The brachialis, which lies deep to the biceps, is of similar size. Its more pennate form leads to a greater physiologic cross-section (45%), which compensates for the shorter lever length. The insertion of the brachialis on the ulna makes the actions of this elbow flexor independent of forearm position.

Brachioradialis action also is sensitive to forearm rotation but in a reverse relationship. Supination laterally displaces the muscle so that its flexion capability is much reduced. Conversely, middle position and pronation put the brachioradialis in a very favorable flexor position on the anterior surface of the joint. While its leverage is good, the muscle is small (36% of the biceps).

The pronator teres as well as the finger and wrist flexors and extensors have limited elbow flexion capability.

Extension

The medial head of the triceps and anconeus are most active during elbow extension with the lateral and long head of the triceps supplementing the extension force.[75] There is increased activity of the triceps with increasing elbow flexion resulting from its secondary action as a decelerator and from an increasing stretch reflex.

> **Elbow extensors**
> - Triceps
> - Anconeus

Forces

Muscles create the force needed to lift the arm and move it from one position to another. Incidental to that action, forces are created within the joint. Some contribute to stability while others threaten joint integrity. The balance of joint forces depends on arm position and the pattern of responding muscles.

The forces created within the elbow joint depend on the joint position. This is because the line of action of the arm muscles changes during flexion and extension. The maximal elbow flexion strength occurs at 90 degrees with decreasing force during extension. Because the flexor muscles have such a poor mechanical advantage with the elbow in relative extension, the isometric forces have to be greatest in this position. Flexor muscle action introduces a posterosuperior compressive force across the distal humerus.

Elbow Stability

Unlike the unconstrained glenohumeral joint, the elbow is one of the most stable joints secondary to its bony

interlocking anatomy. Stability is enhanced and supported by the static soft tissue stabilizers.

The radial collateral ligament lies on the axis of rotation and therefore is taut throughout elbow motion. In contrast, the ulnar collateral ligament components are taut during different positions of elbow motion.[1]

During extension varus stress is shared between the bony anatomy and lateral collateral ligament complex. Valgus stress is shared between the bony anatomy and medial collateral ligament (anterior component). During flexion the bony anatomy provides the majority of varus stability, whereas the medial collateral ligament provides the majority of stability to valgus stress.

ATHLETIC SHOULDER FUNCTION

Athletic injuries to the shoulder are common. It was observed that athletes often had selective weakness of specific rotator cuff muscles rather than generalized muscle impairment. This led investigators to question whether Inman's conclusions regarding single plane motion and analysis could be applied to sport-specific activities.[21,32,33]

The basis of the difference found during athletic endeavors was one of functional demand. Casual elevation of the arm in any of the basic planes presents a prolonged three-dimensional challenge to stabilize the arm in space. Consequently, the humeral rotator muscles act in synchrony with the deltoid, which is raising the arm. The EMG data have demonstrated that the rapid and precise motion patterns characterizing the individual sports stimulate more selective muscle action as well as specific periods of great intensity.

The concept of the separate and independent action of the deltoid and rotator cuff helped to explain selective muscle weakness seen in the throwing athlete. Therefore a specific rehabilitation program to individually strengthen the rotator cuff muscles in the throwing athlete was devised.[50] This program has remained in effect for both prevention and rehabilitation, and it is used by both amateur and professional athletes.

While each sport has its own phasic pattern, there is also a commonality among them.[56] With the exception of swimming, each arm cycle begins with a gentle approach to the appropriate starting position. Subsequently, the shoulder structures are cocked to provide a tense, highly forceful unit ready for an accelerated release.[75] Once the critical effect has been accomplished, the muscles respond to decelerate the limb so that residual force will not cause injury. In this sequence baseball pitching provides the clearest model, but the same pattern is evident in the other sports under different phasic terms.

Throwing
Phases of Throwing Motion

During a baseball pitch the deltoid is responsible for arm elevation with active forward flexion and abduction of the humerus.[2,26] In most sports only a moderate level of muscle effort is required. The exceptions are high activity in swimming and the tennis backhand stroke. The baseball pitch has been divided into five stages described as follows (Fig. 32-21).

STAGE I

Windup or preparation stage, ending when the ball leaves the gloved hand.

STAGE II

Early cocking stage, a period of shoulder abduction and external rotation, that begins as the ball is released from the nondominant hand and terminates with foot-ground contact.

STAGE III

Late cocking stage, arm function continuing until maximal external rotation at the shoulder is attained.

STAGE IV

Acceleration stage, starts with internal rotation of the humerus and ends with ball release.

STAGE V

Follow-through stage, starts with ball release and ends when all the motion is complete.

All heads of the deltoid (anterior, middle, and posterior) experience peak activity in early cocking when the arm is elevated to 95 degrees. Subsequently, in late cocking, the activity of the deltoid diminishes as the rotator cuff muscles increase their action. This sequential pattern of muscle activity, beginning with the deltoid and

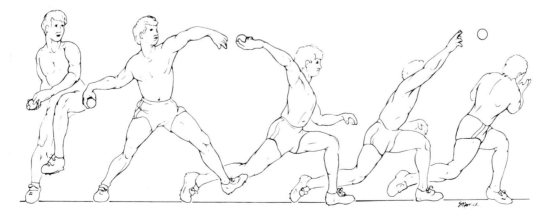

FIG. 32-21. Phases of the pitch, from left to right: wind-up, early cocking, late cocking, acceleration, follow-through.

ending with the rotator cuff, contradicts the obligatory synergy proposed by Inman. It also emphasizes and demonstrates the importance of the rotator cuff in throwing. In addition to providing rotational motions, the muscle's compressive force contributes to joint stability, enabling the shoulder to remain abducted despite reduced deltoid action.[13,14]

The supraspinatus has been thought to play an important role in humeral abduction. Its action in pitching demonstrates peak activity in late cocking when the arm already is abducted and most prone to subluxation.[76] The supraspinatus contributes to the stability of the joint by drawing the humeral head toward the glenoid.[42,64] This correlates with the compressive force pattern Poppen[64] noted at the glenohumeral joint in abduction. The markedly greater use of the supraspinatus muscle by the amateur pitchers compared to the professionals is a strong endorsement for preliminary conditioning.[22] Fatigue from overuse could readily subject the amateurs to shoulder injury. As the athlete becomes proficient, efficient and economical use of the muscles takes place, preventing overuse and injury.

The infraspinatus and teres minor are responsible for external rotation of the shoulder.[4,42] Their action contributes to stability by drawing the head toward the glenoid fossa. The activity patterns are similar for both muscles, with peak activity in late cocking and follow-through. Their intense effort provides 70 degrees of external rotation in less than 0.03 second.[14]

The subscapularis has its peak activity in late cocking and acceleration. By contracting eccentrically it protects the anterior joint, which is under extreme tension.[13] It then continues to function as an internal rotator to help carry the arm across the chest during acceleration and follow-through.[30]

Professional throwing athletes demonstrate selective use of the individual rotator cuff muscles.[22] The professional pitchers are able to use the subscapularis muscle exclusively among the rotator cuff muscles during the acceleration phase of pitching. This is in contrast to the amateurs, who tend to use all the rotator cuff and biceps muscles. The proper, coordinated motion of the trunk, shoulder, and elbow by the professional renders the supraspinatus, infraspinatus, teres minor, and biceps unnecessary for acceleration. Repetitive activities such as pitching can lead to muscle strains and tendinitis.[65] Overuse syndromes may occur earlier and more often in the athlete who uses the muscle unnecessarily. Efficient muscle use, learned through training, may improve endurance and avoid an injury that is secondary to overuse.

The pectoralis major and latissimus dorsi function together to act as internal rotators and eccentrically contract to protect the joint along with the subscapularis during late cocking.[33] Further increase of their activity during acceleration indicates that intense internal rotation and forceful arm depression provide the principal propulsive force.

The serratus anterior controls the scapula to provide a stable glenoid to serve as a secure platform for the humeral head.[4,26] This provides a stable platform with which the humeral head articulates. Serratus anterior activity is important for both upward and scapular protraction during late cocking. This allows the scapula to keep pace with the humerus, which is horizontally flexing and externally rotating. The relatively low level of trapezius activity during the cocking and acceleration phases implies that this muscle primarily provides supplementary scapular stabilization to enhance the rotational action of the serratus anterior during pitching. During follow-through the adductive action of the trapezius serves to decelerate scapular protraction.

Throwing Shoulder with Impingement

Analysis of the shoulder in throwers with subacromial impingement demonstrates discrepancies in the pattern of muscle use between the impingers and normals.[48] During late cocking, deltoid activity continues in the impingers while decreasing in the normals. A lower level of supraspinatus action renders it less able to assist the deltoid during cocking. Presumably this dynamic imbalance results from supraspinatus inhibition to reduce tension on an injured tendon.

The internal rotators (subscapularis, pectoralis major, and latissimus dorsi) and serratus anterior also have dramatic differences during both early and late cocking in the impinged shoulders. Their reduced activity may contribute to increased external rotation, superior humeral migration, and impaired scapular rotation, which would predispose or aggravate the impingement syndrome.

The data provide evidence that the neuromuscular differences seen may account for the initial or persistent impingement problems in the throwing athlete. Complete reconditioning and retraining of these muscles must be accomplished as part of a preventive or rehabilitative program.

Throwing Shoulder with Instability

Evaluation of the patients with an isolated diagnosis of glenohumeral instability reveals differences from the normals.[21] The increased activity of the biceps during acceleration with instability is mild, but it could represent a compensatory mechanism to help stabilize the humeral head against the glenoid. This is consistent with the difference occurring in late cocking and acceleration when the arm is most prone to subluxation.

The mild enhancement of supraspinatus activity throughout cocking and acceleration may help to stabilize the joint in the instability patient by drawing the humeral head toward the glenoid.

The pectoralis major, subscapularis, and latissimus dorsi all demonstrate marked decreased activity during the pitch in patients with instability. Inhibition of the synergistic activity of these muscles allows for persistent or accentuated external rotation. This neuromuscular difference is postulated to be a factor in producing or maintaining chronic anterior instability.

Decreased serratus anterior activity in the instability patient diminishes horizontal protraction of the scapula, which normally begins during late cocking. Early fatigue of the serratus anterior will then add to the stress on the anterior restraints.

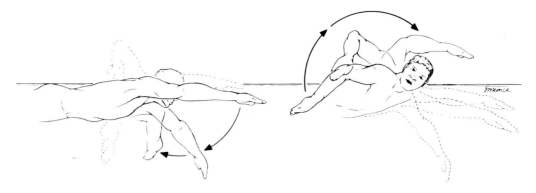

FIG. 32-22. Phases of the freestyle stroke, from left to right: pull-through, recovery.

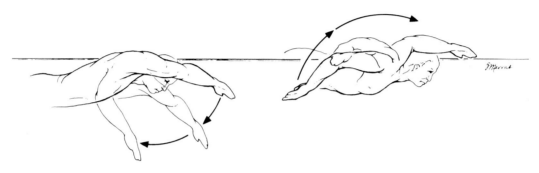

FIG. 32-23. Phases of the butterfly stroke, from left to right: pull-through, recovery.

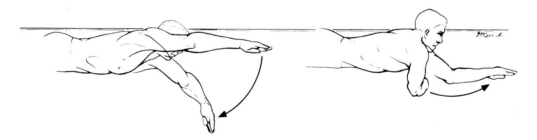

FIG. 32-24. Phases of the breaststroke, from left to right: pull-through, recovery.

As part of a conservative or postsurgical rehabilitative program, the thrower with subluxation should strengthen and retrain the muscles about the shoulder. Data have been provided to support the internal rotators and scapular protractors as key points of focus in patients with instability.

Upon careful clinical evaluation of throwing athletes with impingement findings, many were found to have underlying anterior instability. Clinically, we found that when both entities were present, the instability problem had to be addressed primarily or the symptoms persisted (see Chapter 33).

Swimming

The swimming strokes are broken down into the pull-through and recovery phases as described by Richard-son, Jobe, and Collins (Figs. 32-22 to 32-24).[66] EMG studies of shoulder activity during swimming also emphasize the importance and motion specificity of the rotator cuff.

During the recovery phase there is intense cuff muscle activity as the supraspinatus and subscapularis, and to a lesser extent the infraspinatus, assist the three heads of the deltoid to lift and advance the arm in preparation for the next pull-through.[60] Also vigorously active are the rhomboid and upper trapezius to retract the scapula. The abduction and extension of the arm in swimming can be likened to the cocking phase of throwing, but there also is significant internal rotation. This position places the arm at risk for subacromial impingement.[24] The final forward reach after the hand has entered the water also threatens impingement.

During pull-through the teres minor exhibits an intense external rotation effort to restrain the internal rotation component of the pectoralis major and latissimus dorsi as they pull the body forward. These large muscles provide the propulsive power similar to the acceleration phase of throwing. The serratus anterior is continuously active as it contributes scapular protraction in pull-through for both forward reach and propulsion and then in recovery allows the acromion to rotate away from the humerus at the beginning of the stroke. While the early dry land study indicated a nearly maximum level of effort in recovery,[52] our recent underwater data[61] identified less intense but more continuous serratus anterior action throughout the stroke. If over the course of a number of cycles this muscle fatigues, scapular rotation may not coincide with humeral abduction and impingement may precipitate. The other muscle threatened with fatigue is the subscapularis. It also shows continuous and usually vigorous action throughout the stroke. During the butterfly stroke the pattern of muscle action is very similar to that of the freestyle, with the addition of more intense infraspinatus and supraspinatus action. These swimming studies have indicated that particular attention must be paid to the rotator cuff and serratus anterior in an effort to decrease the common problem of swimmer's shoulder impingement syndrome.[10]

The Painful Shoulder in Swimmers

Freestyle swimming with a painful shoulder results in significantly reduced activity of several muscles while others increase their actions to provide compensatory function. These functional modifications can be correlated with the observed stroke errors.[70] A more lateral hand entry relates to the reduced middle and anterior deltoid action in terminal forward reach, creating a foreshortened stroke. Excess rhomboid action, a mild increase in the infraspinatus, and reduced serratus activity suggest preparation for an early hand exit. The dropped elbow in recovery is consistent with the anterior deltoid's significant decrease in intensity and the lack of the usually strong subscapularis burst at that time. These findings imply that the athletes who continue to swim with a painful shoulder have found the most expedient ways to avoid aggravating impingement.

Similar maneuvers to avoid impingement are seen in the butterfly stroke, though the individual muscle actions are different.[62] Wider hand entry is consistent with the increased posterior deltoid action. The reduction in activity of the scapular rotators (upper trapezius, serratus anterior) and key cuff muscles (supraspinatus, teres minor) are signs of reduced terminal reach. The patterns of altered muscular action provide guidelines as to the stressful motions to be accommodated.

Tennis

The tennis serve is divided into five categories corresponding to the baseball pitch (Fig. 32-25).[46]

Both the forehand and backhand ground strokes are divided into three stages (Figs. 32-26 and 32-27):

STAGE I

Racquet preparation stage begins with shoulder turn, ending with the initiation of weight transfer to the front foot.

STAGE II

Acceleration stage initiates with weight transfer to the front foot accompanied by forward racquet movement, culminating at ball impact.

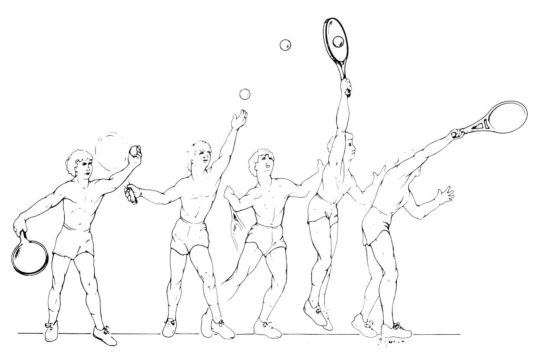

FIG. 32-25. Phases of the tennis serve, from left to right: wind-up, early cocking, late cocking, acceleration, follow-through. (From Morris M et al: *Am J Sports Med* 17[2], 1989.)

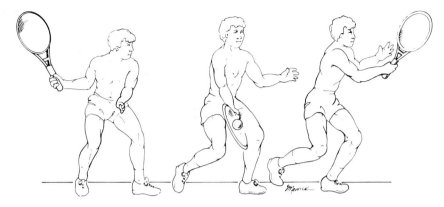

FIG. 32-26. Phases of the tennis forehand, from left to right: preparation, acceleration, follow-through. (From Morris M et al: *Am J Sports Med* 17[2], 1989.)

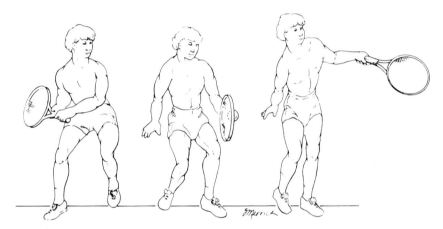

FIG. 32-27. Phases of the tennis backhand, from left to right: preparation, acceleration, follow-through. (From Morris M et al: *Am J Sports Med* 17[2], 1989.)

STAGE III

Follow-through stage begins at ball impact and ends with completion of the stroke.

The tennis serve requires a complex sequence of muscle activity with phases similar to those observed in baseball pitching. Compared to pitching, deltoid muscle function is low during cocking because abduction is contributed to by trunk rotation. The tennis serve acceleration and follow-through phases demonstrate muscle patterns and activity that are similar to those observed in throwing.

The tennis serve is very similar to the overhead throw, and thus a conditioning program as outlined for pitchers may be used for tennis players. Emphasis should be placed on the rotator cuff and serratus anterior.

Analysis of the forehand ground stroke reveals a similar passive windup sequence. Again, trunk rotation provides a force for shoulder motion. In follow-through there is a marked decrease in activity among the accelerating muscles and a concomitant increase in the external rotators responsible for deceleration. The backhand ground stroke is similar in concept but opposite in muscle activity to the forehand. Follow-through demonstrates deceleration with increased activity of the internal rotators.

Golf

Shoulder activity during a right-handed golf swing was evaluated.[30]

The phases of the golf swing are divided as follows (Fig. 32-28):

TAKE-AWAY

This phase begins with the initiation of motion in the address position to the end of the backswing.

FORWARD SWING

Phase lasting from the end of the backswing until the club becomes horizontal.

ACCELERATION

Phase lasting from the point at which the club is horizontal until ball contact.

FOLLOW-THROUGH

Phase lasting from ball contact until the end of motion.

Analysis of the golf swing reveals a different pattern of action in its four phases.[30] Relative quiescence of the deltoid and supraspinatus and dominance of rotator cuff muscle activity was observed.[31] This may be explained by the limited elevation of the arm in the golf swings

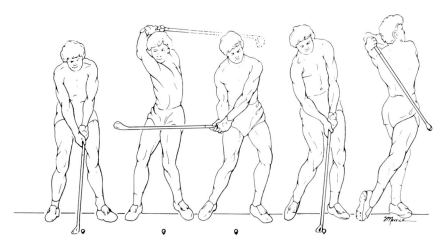

FIG. 32-28. Phases of the golf swing, from left to right: take-away, forward swing, early acceleration, late acceleration, follow-through. (Modified from Jobe FW: *Am J Sports Med* 17[6], 1989.)

compared to pitching, swimming, and tennis. Again, rotator cuff activity is seen to be dictated by motion demands and not in obligatory synergy with the deltoid. The subscapularis is more active than any other muscle throughout the swing. In addition, infraspinatus action is prominent on the right but minor on the left.[59] The latissimus dorsi and pectoralis major provided power bilaterally and showed marked activity during acceleration. As part of a training program, the golf player should emphasize the rotator cuff, pectoralis major, and latissimus dorsi in both arms.

ATHLETIC ELBOW FUNCTION
Throwing

Analysis of the muscles about the elbow during a pitch includes the extensor digitorum communis (EDC), brachioradialis, flexor carpi radialis (FCR), flexor digitorum superficialis (FDS), extensor carpi radialis longus (ECRL), extensor carpi radialis brevis (ECRB), pronator teres, and supinator.[71]

The windup or preparation phase has relatively low activity in all groups as the forearm is slightly pronated and flexed and the wrist extended. Muscle activity is highest in the EDC, ECRB, and pronator teres. There is little difference between the fast ball and the curve.

Early cocking is terminated as the front foot touches the ground and the hand and ball are positioned back as far as possible. The elbow is flexed, the wrist and metacarpophalangeal joints extended, and the forearm slightly pronated. Muscle activity is of moderate intensity in the wrist extensors (ECRB and ECRL), metacarpophalangeal extensors (EDC), brachioradialis, and pronator teres when a fast ball is thrown. Activity is markedly lower in the brachioradialis when a curve ball is thrown, suggesting that less elbow flexion is required for its delivery.

Late cocking is terminated by maximal humeral external rotation and 90 degrees of abduction. The wrist is extended, the elbow flexed, and the forearm pronated to 90 degrees with increased forearm pronation when the fast ball is thrown. There is an increased activity in the wrist extensors and supinator when the curve ball is thrown. This suggests that with the curve ball the ball is positioned differently in the hand, and the forearm is slightly more supinated.

Acceleration is an explosive, short stage. The elbow is extended and the wrist and metacarpophalangeal joints are flexed to propel the ball forward. The difference between the fast ball and curve is most apparent at acceleration because the ECRL and ECRB activity is higher with the curve ball. This probably is a reflection of the different posture necessary at the release point of the curve.

Follow-through is terminated by maximal pronation of the forearm as the humerus is internally rotated and adducted across the chest. The wrist extensors again demonstrate more activity when the curve ball is thrown.

The results show low to moderate activity in all muscles during all phases of the pitch. The function is more likely positioning to accept the transfer of energy from the larger trunk and girdle structures. The most notable difference between the fast ball and the curve ball is an increase in the ECRL and ECRB activity during late cocking, acceleration, and follow-through of the curve as compared to the fast ball. This probably is a reflection of the different posture necessary at the release point of a curve.

Tennis

Analysis of elbow function in tennis players reveals predominant activity of the wrist extensors in all strokes.

The muscles include the biceps, triceps, brachialis, EDC, ECRL, ECRB, pronator teres, and FCR.

The ground strokes are divided into four phases.

PHASE I

This phase is racquet preparation, which begins with the first motion of the backswing and ends with the first forward motion of the racquet.

PHASE II

This phase is acceleration, which begins with forward racquet movement and ends with ball contact.

PHASES III AND IV

These phases are follow-through, which begins with the ball contact and ends with completion of the stroke. Phase III is early follow-through, which is the first 25% of the time in the phase, and phase IV is late follow-through, which is the last 75% of the time.

The serve was divided into the following six phases:

PHASE I

This phase is wind-up, which begins with the first motion of the racquet and until ball release from the nonracquet hand.

PHASES II AND III

These phases are cocking that initiates with ball release and continues to the point of maximal external rotation in the serving shoulder. Phase II is early cocking, which is the first 75% of the time, and phase III is late cocking, which is the last 25% of the time.

PHASE IV

This phase is acceleration, and it starts with forward motion of the arm and continues until ball contact.

PHASES V AND VI

These phases are follow-through, beginning with ball contact and continuing until completion of the stroke. Early follow-through (Phase V) is the first 25% of the time in the phase, and late follow-through (Phase VI) is the last 75% of the time.

During the ground strokes, the muscles appear to stabilize the arm as a rigid extension of the racquet. The racquet-arm unit then accepts the transfer of energy from the shoulder and trunk as they rotate and as body weight shift occurs.

The muscles at the elbow act to control elbow flexion and extension, forearm rotation, and the four motions of the wrist (flexion, extension, radial, and ulnar deviation).

The triceps and brachialis function only to control the elbow hinge. They show low to moderate activity throughout the ground strokes. This implies that the muscles have a positioning function and that the inherent stability of the elbow joint provides the resistance against the forces of the stroke.

The biceps has two functions: to perform flexion at the elbow and to control forearm rotation. The biceps shows low to moderate activity during the ground strokes except for an increase in activity during forehand acceleration and early follow-through. Brachialis activity remained low during these phases. This implies that in addition to its role in positioning the elbow in flexion, the biceps was serving to stabilize forearm rotation.

The pronator teres shows increased activity during forehand acceleration. This synergistic activity with the biceps appears to stabilize the forearm against rotation.

Wrist and grip stability are found in a position of extension and radial deviation. The highest elbow activity during the ground strokes is in the muscles that control the wrist. The radial wrist extensors, ECRB and ECRL, are active in both strokes.

The EDC also shows high activity during the back-hand where resistance of the flexor moment, brought on by acceleration and ball contact, is required.

The role of the muscles about the elbow is different during the serve than during the ground strokes. Instead of acting as an extension of the racquet, their role is to act much like the springs of a catapult, cocking the racquet and then contributing to its acceleration forward.

During the cocking of the racquet, the primary muscle action relates to wrist control. The ECRB, EDC, and ECRL all show high activity. The elbow and forearm positions are achieved passively at the elbow by shoulder position and gravity.

During acceleration the primary site of muscle action was found to be at the elbow and forearm. The triceps shows its only phase of high activity in any stroke as it provides power by extending the elbow. The increased activity of the pronator teres provides position and power at the forearm.

The biceps shows a significant increase in activity in late follow-through. Its action appears to be deceleration of the supination/extension movement brought on in the acceleration phase.

The major function during ground strokes is stabilization of the elbow, forearm, and wrist with major activity at the wrist. During the serve the muscles' function is to produce movement at three sites: the elbow, forearm, and wrist. From this motion cocking and acceleration of the racquet are obtained.

Power in the serve comes from increased activity in the triceps and pronator teres. The predominant activity of the wrist extensors in all the strokes may be one cause for their frequent injury.

SUMMARY

The muscles of the shoulder and elbow act according to their mechanical qualities and are function or sport specific. Separating the professional from the amateur athlete further refines this principle and demonstrates that individual muscles of the rotator cuff act independently.

Evaluation of the different sports reveals that, while the rotator cuff function is important in all, the emphasis and role of the individual muscles vary. The importance of serratus anterior muscle activity to stabilize and protract the scapula is a consistent finding. At the elbow, the major demand is placed on the muscles controlling the wrist. Thus it is critical to understand the demands placed upon the upper extremity in a particular sport or activity to treat pathologic conditions.

REFERENCES

1. An K, Moorey B: Biomechanics of the elbow. In Morrey B (ed): *The elbow and its disorders*, Philadelphia, 1985, WB Saunders.
2. Atwater AE: Biomechanics of overarm throwing movements and of throwing injuries, *Exerc Sport Sci Rev* 7:43, 1979.
3. Basmajian JV, Bazant FJ: Factors preventing downward dislocation of the adducted shoulder joint, *J Bone Joint Surg* 41A:1182, 1959.
4. Basmajian JV, Deluca CJ: *Muscles alive: their functions revealed by electromyography*, Baltimore, 1985, Williams & Wilkins.

PHASE II

This phase is acceleration, which begins with forward racquet movement and ends with ball contact.

PHASES III AND IV

These phases are follow-through, which begins with the ball contact and ends with completion of the stroke. Phase III is early follow-through, which is the first 25% of the time in the phase, and phase IV is late follow-through, which is the last 75% of the time.

The serve was divided into the following six phases:

PHASE I

This phase is wind-up, which begins with the first motion of the racquet and until ball release from the nonracquet hand.

PHASES II AND III

These phases are cocking that initiates with ball release and continues to the point of maximal external rotation in the serving shoulder. Phase II is early cocking, which is the first 75% of the time, and phase III is late cocking, which is the last 25% of the time.

PHASE IV

This phase is acceleration, and it starts with forward motion of the arm and continues until ball contact.

PHASES V AND VI

These phases are follow-through, beginning with ball contact and continuing until completion of the stroke. Early follow-through (Phase V) is the first 25% of the time in the phase, and late follow-through (Phase VI) is the last 75% of the time.

During the ground strokes, the muscles appear to stabilize the arm as a rigid extension of the racquet. The racquet-arm unit then accepts the transfer of energy from the shoulder and trunk as they rotate and as body weight shift occurs.

The muscles at the elbow act to control elbow flexion and extension, forearm rotation, and the four motions of the wrist (flexion, extension, radial, and ulnar deviation).

The triceps and brachialis function only to control the elbow hinge. They show low to moderate activity throughout the ground strokes. This implies that the muscles have a positioning function and that the inherent stability of the elbow joint provides the resistance against the forces of the stroke.

The biceps has two functions: to perform flexion at the elbow and to control forearm rotation. The biceps shows low to moderate activity during the ground strokes except for an increase in activity during forehand acceleration and early follow-through. Brachialis activity remained low during these phases. This implies that in addition to its role in positioning the elbow in flexion, the biceps was serving to stabilize forearm rotation.

The pronator teres shows increased activity during forehand acceleration. This synergistic activity with the biceps appears to stabilize the forearm against rotation.

Wrist and grip stability are found in a position of extension and radial deviation. The highest elbow activity during the ground strokes is in the muscles that control the wrist. The radial wrist extensors, ECRB and ECRL, are active in both strokes.

The EDC also shows high activity during the back-

hand where resistance of the flexor moment, brought on by acceleration and ball contact, is required.

The role of the muscles about the elbow is different during the serve than during the ground strokes. Instead of acting as an extension of the racquet, their role is to act much like the springs of a catapult, cocking the racquet and then contributing to its acceleration forward.

During the cocking of the racquet, the primary muscle action relates to wrist control. The ECRB, EDC, and ECRL all show high activity. The elbow and forearm positions are achieved passively at the elbow by shoulder position and gravity.

During acceleration the primary site of muscle action was found to be at the elbow and forearm. The triceps shows its only phase of high activity in any stroke as it provides power by extending the elbow. The increased activity of the pronator teres provides position and power at the forearm.

The biceps shows a significant increase in activity in late follow-through. Its action appears to be deceleration of the supination/extension movement brought on in the acceleration phase.

The major function during ground strokes is stabilization of the elbow, forearm, and wrist with major activity at the wrist. During the serve the muscles' function is to produce movement at three sites: the elbow, forearm, and wrist. From this motion cocking and acceleration of the racquet are obtained.

Power in the serve comes from increased activity in the triceps and pronator teres. The predominant activity of the wrist extensors in all the strokes may be one cause for their frequent injury.

SUMMARY

The muscles of the shoulder and elbow act according to their mechanical qualities and are function or sport specific. Separating the professional from the amateur athlete further refines this principle and demonstrates that individual muscles of the rotator cuff act independently.

Evaluation of the different sports reveals that, while the rotator cuff function is important in all, the emphasis and role of the individual muscles vary. The importance of serratus anterior muscle activity to stabilize and protract the scapula is a consistent finding. At the elbow, the major demand is placed on the muscles controlling the wrist. Thus it is critical to understand the demands placed upon the upper extremity in a particular sport or activity to treat pathologic conditions.

REFERENCES

1. An K, Moorey B: Biomechanics of the elbow. In Morrey B (ed): *The elbow and its disorders*, Philadelphia, 1985, WB Saunders.
2. Atwater AE: Biomechanics of overarm throwing movements and of throwing injuries, *Exerc Sport Sci Rev* 7:43, 1979.
3. Basmajian JV, Bazant FJ: Factors preventing downward dislocation of the adducted shoulder joint, *J Bone Joint Surg* 41A:1182, 1959.
4. Basmajian JV, Deluca CJ: *Muscles alive: their functions revealed by electromyography*, Baltimore, 1985, Williams & Wilkins.

5. Basmajian JV, Latif A: Integrated actions and functions of the chief flexors of the elbow: a detailed electromyographic analysis, *J Bone Joint Surg* 39A:1106, 1957.

6. Batterman C: Mechanics of the crawl arm stroke, *Swimming World* 7:4, 1966.

7. Bechtol CO: Biomechanics of the shoulder, *Clin Orthop* 146:37, 1980.

8. Boone DC, Azen SP: Normal range of motion in joints in male subjects, *J Bone Joint Surg* 61A:756, 1979.

9. Browne AD et al: Glenohumeral elevation: a three-dimensional study, *Orthop Trans* 14(2):402, 1990.

10. Clancy WG: Shoulder problems in overhand overuse sports, *Am J Sports Med* 7:138, 1979.

11. Codman EA: *The shoulder*. Brooklyn, 1934, G Miller.

12. Colachis SC, Jr, Strohm BR, Brecher VL: Effects of axillary nerve block on muscle force in the upper extremity, *Arch Phys Med Rehabil* 50:647, 1969.

13. Digiovine NM et al: An electromyographic analysis of the upper extremity in pitching, *J Shoulder Elbow Surg* 1(1):15, 1992.

14. Dillman CJ, Fleisis OS, Andrews JR: Biomechanics of pitching with an emphasis upon shoulder kinematics, *J Sports Phys Ther* 18(2):402, 1993.

15. Doody SG, Freedman L, Waterland JC: Shoulder movements during abduction in the scapular plane, *Arch Phys Med Rehabil* 51:595, 1970.

16. Dvir Z, Berne N: The shoulder complex in elevation of the arm: a mechanism approach, *J Biomech* 11:219, 1978.

17. Freedman L, Munro RR: Abduction of the arm in the scapular plane: scapular and glenohumeral movements, *J Bone Joint Surg* 48A:1503, 1966.

18. Furlani J: Electromyographic study of the biceps brachii in movements of the glenohumeral joint, *Acta Anat* 96:270, 1976.

19. Galinat BJ et al: Normal and abnormal mechanics of the glenohumeral joint in the coronal plane, *Orthop Trans* 11:553, 1987.

20. Garfin SR et al: Role of fascia in maintenance of muscle tension and pressure, *J Appl Physiol* 51(2):317, 1981.

21. Glousman RE et al: Dynamic EMG analysis of the throwing shoulder with glenohumeral instability, *J Bone Joint Surg* 70A:220, 1988.

22. Gowan ID et al: A comparative EMG analysis of the shoulder during pitching: professional vs. amateur pitchers, *Am J Sports Med* 15:586, 1987.

23. Harryman DT et al: Translation of the humeral head on the glenoid with glenohumeral motion, *Orthop Trans* 14:595, 1990.

24. Hawkins RJ, Hobeika PE: Impingement syndrome in the athletic shoulder. Symposium on injuries to the shoulder in the athlete, *Clin Sports Med* 2:391, 1983.

25. Hollingshead WH: *Anatomy for surgeons*, vol 3, The back and limbs, New York, 1958, Hoeber-Harper.

26. Inman VT, Saunders JB de CM, Abbott LC: Observations on the function of the shoulder joint, *J Bone Joint Surg* 26:1, 1944.

27. Inman VT, Saunders JB de CM: Observations on the function of the clavicle, *Calif Med* 65:158, 1946.

28. Itoi E et al: Stabilizing function of the biceps in stable and unstable shoulders, *J Bone Joint Surg* 75B(4):546, 1993.

29. Jiang CC et al: Muscle excursion measurements and moment arm determination in rotator cuff muscles, *Orthop Trans* 12(2):486, 1988.

30. Jobe FW, Moynes DR, Antonelli DJ: Rotator cuff function during a golf swing, *Am J Sports Med* 14:388, 1986.

31. Jobe FW, Perry J, Pink M: Electromyographic shoulder activity in men and women professional golfers, *Am J Sports Med* 17(6):782, 1989.

32. Jobe FW et al: An EMG analysis of the shoulder in throwing and pitching: a preliminary report, *Am J Sports Med* 11:3, 1983.

33. Jobe FW et al: An EMG analysis of the shoulder in pitching: a second report, *Am J Sports Med* 12:218, 1984.

34. Johnston TB: The movements of the shoulder joint, *Br J Surg* 25:252, 1937.

35. Jones DW Jr: *The role of shoulder muscles in the control of humeral position (an electromyography study)*, Master's thesis, Cleveland, 1970, Case Western Reserve University.

36. Keating JF et al: The relative strength of the rotator cuff muscles: a cadaver study, *J Bone Joint Surg* 75B(10):137, 1993.

37. Kent BE: Functional anatomy of the shoulder complex, *Phys Ther* 51:867, 1971.

38. Kronberg M, Bronstrom LA, Soderlund V: Retroversion of the humeral head in the normal shoulder and its relationship to the normal range of motion, *Clin Orthop* 253:113, 1990.

39. Kronberg M, Nemeth G, Bronstrom LA: Muscle activity and coordination in the normal shoulder: an electromyography study, *Clin Orthop* 257:76, 1990.

40. Kumar VP, Satku K, Balasubramaniam P: The role of the long head of the biceps brachii in the stabilization of the head of the humerus, *Clin Orthop* 244:172, 1989.

41. Lucas DB: Biomechanics of the shoulder joint, *Arch Surg* 107:425, 1973.

42. MacCowaill MA, Basmajian JV: *Muscles and movements: a basis for human kinesiology*, New York, 1977, Robert Krieger.

43. Maki S, Gruen T: Anthropometric study of the glenohumeral joint, vol 1, *Transactions of the 22nd Annual Meeting of the American Orthopaedic Research Society,* 1976.

44. Malicky DM et al: Anterior glenohumeral stabilization efficiency in a biomechanical model combining ligamentous and muscular restraints, *Transactions of the 39th Annual Meeting of the Orthopaedic Research Society,* 1993.

45. Matsen FA III: Biomechanics of the shoulder. In Frankel VH, Nordin M (eds): *Basic biomechanics of the skeletal system*, Philadelphia, 1980, Lea & Febiger.

46. McCormick J et al: *An EMG analysis of shoulder function in tennis players*. Unpublished study, Biomechanics Laboratory, Centinela Hospital, Inglewood, Calif, 1985.

47. McMahon PJ et al: Muscle forces for glenohumeral abduction in the scapular plane in a simulated supraspinatus tear. *Orthop Trans* 17(2):430, 1993.

48. Miller L et al: *EMG analysis of shoulders in throwers with subacromial impingement*. Unpublished study, Biomechanics Laboratory, Centinela Hospital, Inglewood, Calif, 1985.

49. Morrey B, Chao E: Passive motion of the elbow joint, *J Bone Joint Surg* 58A:501, 1976.

50. Moynes DR: Prevention of injury to the shoulder through exercises and therapy: symposium on injuries to the shoulder in the athlete, *Clin Sports Med* 2:413, 1983.

51. Mutschler TA et al: Stability of the glenohumeral joint: a dynamic model, *Orthop Trans* 10(2):322, 1986.

52. Nuber GW et al: Fine wire electromyography analysis of muscles of the shoulder during swimming, *Am J Sports Med* 14:7, 1986.

53. Pearl ML et al: An electromyographic analysis of the shoulder during cones and planes of arm motion, *Clin Orthop* 284:116, 1992.

54. Pearl ML et al: A system for describing positions of the humerus relative to the thorax and its use in the presentation of several functionally important arm positions, *J Shoulder Elbow Surg* 1:113, 1992.

55. Perry J: Normal upper extremity kinesiology, *Phys Ther* 58:265, 1978.

56. Perry J: Anatomy and biomechanics of the shoulder in throwing, swimming, gymnastics and tennis: symposium on injuries to the shoulder in the athlete, *Clin Sports Med* 2:247, 1983.

57. Perry J: Shoulder function for the activities of daily living. In Matsen FA, Fu FH (eds): *The shoulder: a balance of mobility and stability*, Rosemont, Ill, 1993, American Academy of Orthopaedic Surgeons.

58. Perry J, Barnes G, Merson J: Normal electromyographic values of six shoulder muscles during free motion, *Orthop Trans* 3(2):322, 1979.

59. Pink M, Jobe FW, Perry J: Electromyographic analysis of the shoulder during the golf swing, *Am J Sports Med* 18(2):137, 1990.

60. Pink M et al: The normal shoulder during freestyle swimming: an electromyographic cinemagraphic study of twelve muscles, *Am J Sports Med* 19(6):569, 1991.

61. Pink M et al: The normal shoulder during the butterfly stroke, *Clin Orthop* 288:48, 1993.

62. Pink M et al: The painful shoulder during the butterfly stroke, *Clin Orthop* 288:48, 1993.

63. Poppen NK, Walker PS: Normal and abnormal motion of the shoulder, *J Bone Joint Surg* 58A:195, 1976.

64. Poppen NK, Walker PS: Forces at the glenohumeral joint in abduction, *Clin Orthop* 136:165, 1978.

65. Richardson AB: Overuse syndromes in baseball, tennis, gymnastics and swimming: symposium on injuries of the shoulder in the athlete, *Clin Sports Med* 2:379, 1983.
66. Richardson AB, Jobe FW, Collins HR: The shoulder in competitive swimming, *Am J Sports Med* 81:159, 1980.
67. Saha AK: *Theory of shoulder mechanism: descriptive and applied,* Springfield, Ill, 1961, Charles C Thomas.
68. Saha AK: Mechanics of elevation of glenohumeral joint: its application in rehabilitation of flail shoulder in upper brachial plexus injuries and poliomyelitis and in replacement of the upper humerus by prosthesis, *Acta Orthop Scand* 44:668, 1973.
69. Schmidt GL: Biomechanical analysis of knee flexion and extension, *J Biomech* 6:79, 1973.
70. Scovazzo ML et al: The painful shoulder during freestyle swimming, *Am J Sports Med* 19(6):571, 1991.
71. Sisto D et al: An electromyographic analysis of the elbow in pitching, *Am J Sports Med* 15:260, 1987.
72. Slater-Hammel AT: An action current study of contraction-movement relationships in the tennis stroke, *Res Q* 20:424, 1949.
73. Sugahara R: Electromyographic study of shoulder movements, *Jpn J Rehabil Med* 11:41, 1974.
74. Ting A et al: *EMG analysis of lateral biceps muscle action in shoulders with rotator cuff tears,* Unpublished study, Biomechanics Laboratory, Centinela Hospital, Inglewood, Calif, 1986.
75. Travill AA: Electromyographic study of the extensor apparatus of the forearm, *Anat Rec* 144:373, 1962.
76. Turkel SJ et al: Stabilizing mechanisms preventing anterior dislocation of the glenohumeral joint, *J Bone Joint Surg* 63A:1208, 1981.
77. Wadsworth TG: *The elbow,* New York, 1982, Churchill Livingstone.
78. Walker PS: *Human joints and their artificial replacements,* Springfield, Ill, 1977, Charles C Thomas.
79. Weber EF: *Ueber die Langenverhaltnisse der Fleischfasen der Muskeln im allgemeinen,* Berlin, 1851, Ber Verh K Sach Ges Wissensch.

CHAPTER 33

Diagnosis and Treatment of Shoulder Injuries in Throwers

Ralph A. Gambardella
Frank W. Jobe

A wide variety of injuries can afflict the shoulder girdle in baseball.[24,54] The throwing athlete places unusually high demands on the shoulder joint. This joint is the link in transferring force generated from the trunk to the arm and thereby imparting speed to the baseball. The shoulder is greatly adapted to this function by the multiple planes of motion (i.e., scapular, sagittal, and coronal) available to it. However, these large degrees of freedom also make this joint more susceptible to injury.

Many injuries in the shoulder girdle are caused by the repetitious act of throwing and are therefore considered overuse problems rather than acute injuries.[40] Because overuse problems are more associated with the repetition of the throwing act, it is understandable that the majority of problems are going to afflict the pitcher rather than a player in a different position. Although this chapter focuses on many of these overuse problems created by the act of throwing, it is important to remember that shoulder injuries also occur as a result of direct contact and acute injury associated with that type of contact. Acute anterior shoulder dislocations as well as recurrent shoulder subluxation problems have been known to occur as a result of head-first sliding, with the arm caught in an abducted and externally rotated position. In addition, acromioclavicular joint separation can easily occur with blows to the superior aspect of the shoulder girdle as outfielders crash into walls and barriers while attempting to catch fly balls.

There are five basic classifications of shoulder injuries involving the throwing athlete. The first is the subacromial space complex of injuries and involves impingement syndromes, rotator cuff tendinitis, bicipital tendinitis, and subdeltoid bursitis. The second classification is glenohumeral instability and includes both anterior and posterior subluxation or dislocation problems as well as labrum injuries[33]; by far the most common problem is that of anterior subluxation. Acromioclavicular joint problems, neurovascular entrapment syndromes, and injuries to the physis in adolescents round out the more common overuse syndromes that occur in the throwing athlete. It is important to remember that instability often causes problems with the subacromial space and therefore the first two classifications often coexist.

The most critical problem confronting the clinician is

the realization that the various types of shoulder injuries can be present in combination. The clinician must identify and address each particular problem to successfully treat the injured athlete. In many throwers it is not unusual to have rotator cuff tendinitis, anterior subluxation, and a labral injury. Therefore it is of paramount importance to obtain a detailed history and perform a comprehensive physical examination. The advent of new techniques, such as gadolinium-enhanced magnetic resonance imaging (MRI) and arthroscopy, has illuminated our understanding of these complex problems, allowing the physician to make a more accurate diagnosis.[2,29] It is only with an accurate diagnosis that a successful treatment and rehabilitation program can be outlined for the athlete.

Classification of shoulder throwing injuries

- Subacromial space problems
- Glenohumeral instability
- Acromioclavicular problems
- Neurovascular entrapment syndromes
- Physeal injuries

FUNCTIONAL ANATOMY

The shoulder girdle is made up of four functional joints. They are the glenohumeral joint, the acromioclavicular joint, the sternoclavicular joint, and the scapulothoracic complex. Whereas normal motion in most humans would allow for 160 degrees of forward flexion and abduction, the throwing athlete often exhibits increased shoulder motion and in particular *increased external rotation* in the abducted plane. Shoulder abduction occurs as a combination of both glenohumeral and scapulothoracic motion in a 2:1 ratio. Although this ratio may differ in throwers, large deviations from this ratio caused by fatigue or injury place additional demands on the ligamentous structures as well as the muscle tendon units.

The glenohumeral joint is a very unstable joint, and the stability in the joint is enhanced anteriorly by the gle-

noid and humeral head retroversion. In addition, stability both anteriorly and posteriorly is enhanced by the glenoid labrum and fibrous structures that increase the coverage of the humeral head, thereby enhancing the stability in all planes. Of particular importance are the capsular reinforcements, which have been described as the glenohumeral ligaments of the shoulder. In the throwing athlete the importance of the inferior glenohumeral ligament in the prevention of anterior and anteroinferior instability has now been well documented. The rotator cuff adds support and restraint to the glenohumeral joint and is of particular importance with the follow-through phase of the throwing mechanism. Finally, the biceps tendon also has a role as a humeral head depressor and, in addition, in throwing has been shown to be an important decelerator of the forearm.

The subacromial space is a fixed space containing the subdeltoid bursa and loose fibroconnective tissue. This space is bounded superiorly by the undersurface of the acromion, inferiorly by the superior border of the rotator cuff, laterally by the deltoid, and medially by the coracoacromial ligament. Alterations in the subacromial space caused by osteophyte formation along the undersurface of the acromion, thickening of the rotator cuff or subdeltoid bursa, or alterations of the coracoacromial ligament can all cause problems to the shoulder in the throwing athlete.

THROWING MECHANICS

The throwing mechanism has been divided into five phases: (1) windup, (2) early cocking, (3) late cocking, (4) acceleration, and (5) follow-through (Fig. 33-1).[28,34] Highest stresses on the anterior and inferior capsular structures occur during Phase 3, when maximal abduction and external rotation are attained.[37] In addition, high stresses are imparted to posterior capsular structures during Phase 5. These large stresses are counterbalanced by intense periods of muscle activity by the shoulder girdle muscles.[11]

Peak muscle activity is measured in percentages of manual muscle strength tests (MMT) with 100% MMT

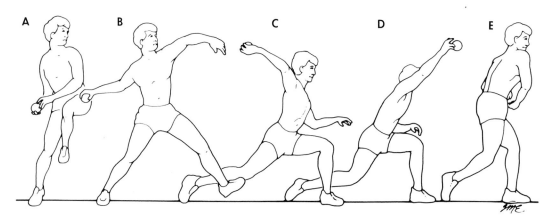

FIG. 33-1. Mechanics of throwing. **A,** Windup. **B,** Early cocking. **C,** Late cocking. **D,** Acceleration. **E,** Follow-through.

being the peak 1-second electromyographic signal during an MMT. During the baseball pitch the deltoid exhibits peak activity in early cocking (42% MMT) with a second peak occurring at follow-through (43% MMT).[26,27] Supraspinatus peak activity (45% MMT) occurs at late cocking, with a less intense peak at follow-through. The supraspinatus contributes to joint stability by compressing the humeral head toward the glenoid.

The subscapularis is most active (115% MMT) in late cocking, when the shoulder is in maximal external rotation and again in deceleration as the arm is internally rotated (151% MMT).[30]

MECHANISM OF INJURY: IMPINGEMENT VS. INSTABILITY

Although there appear to be patients who are seen clinically as either pure impingers or pure subluxators, most appear with symptoms and physical findings indicative of both problems. In the throwing athlete the primary event is probably anterior subluxation or instability. This occurs associated with the terminal stage of windup when the shoulder is abducted and maximally rotated. With the repetition of the throwing act, the high stresses generated on the anterior capsule during Phase 3 lead to stretching of the anterior capsule and, in particular, the inferior glenohumeral ligament (Fig. 33-2). As this complex stretches and flattens, shoulder subluxation begins to occur. Whether this primary instability is caused solely by mechanical breakdown or is a result of rotator cuff muscle fatigue and imbalance is unknown. However, this early instability initiates a cascade of events leading to both impingement and labral problems.

As instability progresses, abnormal demands are placed on the rotator cuff. Alterations in force are generated at the joint level, and an abnormal firing sequence of the shoulder girdle muscles occurs, particularly because of an imbalance in the scapular rotators (e.g., serratus, and rhomboids), which are overworking and fir-

ing out of sequence in an effort to keep the humeral head in the glenoid. The inability of the muscles to act in synchrony leads to chronic irritation of the rotator cuff and in particular the supraspinatus as it passes under the acromion and coracoacromial arch during Phases 3 and 4 of the throwing act. In addition, the supraspinatus is overworking in an attempt to stabilize the subluxating humeral head.[14] It does this by acting as a humeral head depressor. This may explain the greater electromyographic maximal activity seen in the supraspinatus with amateur pitchers than that seen in the professional thrower.[15]

Impingement of the rotator cuff can be divided into external and internal impingement. External or subacromial mechanical impingement can result in subdeltoid bursitis, rotator cuff tendinitis, and bicipital tendinitis. This irritation may result in thickening of the cuff and "in substance" changes in the rotator cuff, as can be seen with MRI scanning. However, as instability progresses, internal impingement occurs. Internal impingement consists of undersurface, or joint side, partial tearing of the supraspinatus or infraspinatus. With the shoulder in full abduction and external rotation (Phase 3), the undersurface of the rotator cuff impinges against the posterosuperior labrum. This results in fraying and partial tearing of both the labrum and cuff in those areas. This internal impingement differs from the external impingement of the rotator cuff that occurs as a result of narrowing of the subacromial space. This type of internal impingement is secondary to anterior instability and can be identified arthroscopically but requires visualizing the cuff and posterosuperior labrum with the arm moved into the fully abducted and externally rotated position. This internal impingement is not seen in the stable shoulder.

Another finding in the joint often seen arthroscopically is a roughened area of articular cartilage on the humeral head that is smaller and posterior to the normal location of the classic Hill-Sachs lesion. Whereas the Hill-Sachs humeral defect is thought to be secondary to an anterior

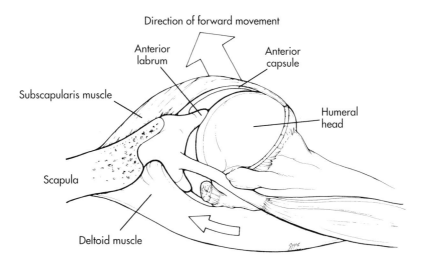

FIG. 33-2. Phase three of the throwing motion. Highest stresses are placed on the anterior and inferior capsule and labrum.

dislocation,[19] chondromalacic changes seen just inferior to the bare area are most likely caused by levering posteriorly against the posterior glenoid in anterior humeral head subluxation.

Instability may be associated with anterior labral thinning and attenuation of the inferior glenohumeral ligament. However, as instability progresses to recurring dislocation, frank tearing of the anterior labrium and the classic Bankhart lesion can occur.[5]

DIAGNOSIS
History

The clinical history becomes extremely important in the diagnosis of shoulder injury in the athlete because it gives the astute clinician important clues necessary to make the appropriate diagnosis.[53] A detailed history becomes extremely important when physical examination shows signs of both impingement and instability.

First, it is important to determine whether the onset of the problem occurred acutely with one particular throw or whether there was an accumulation and gradual onset of symptoms associated with the repetitive act of throwing. Although many athletes may try to attribute their problem to one particular game or event, it is important to quiz the patient in an effort to determine if there were other subtle symptoms or problems that may have led to the onset of what the patient may often think is an acute injury. For example, on questioning, many throwers may state that before noticing the onset of pain with each throw they experienced shoulder soreness or stiffness after activity for several weeks.

Consequences of subacromial impingement

- Subdeltoid bursitis
- Rotator cuff tendinitis
- Bicipital tendinitis

The location of the pain both anatomically and by particular phase of throwing is also important.[23,32] Many patients with anterior subluxation experience pain posteriorly in Phase 3 of throwing with the arm at 90 degrees of external rotation. This position corresponds with the anatomic findings of internal impingement in the anteriorly unstable thrower.

Pain with full forward flexion is common in impingement. Pain with forward flexion across the chest seen in Phase 5 of throwing can indicate an acromioclavicular joint problem. Many throwers who are experiencing anterior subluxation describe a feeling of weakness, giving way, or a dead arm, especially in Phase 3. Attempts should also be made to elicit symptoms of clicking, which may be mechanical in nature, as seen in a bucket-handle labrum tear.

Pain radiation from the neck to the shoulder or pain associated with neck range of motion may indicate a cervical problem. In addition, pain radiation below the elbow, especially with unrelated elbow pathologic findings,

is often seen in cervical radiculopathy. Associated sensory or motor deficits should also be noted.

The history of how the athlete's problem has been treated is important in trying to determine an appropriate course of action. This is especially true because many of these patients have been seen and treated for several weeks by primary care physicians before evaluation. Response to rest, oral antiinflammatory medication, and physical therapy should be recorded. Of paramount importance is to determine exactly what has been done in terms of physical therapy. Often therapy may have consisted only of the use of modalities such as ice, ultrasound, and heat rather than a comprehensive rotator cuff exercising program. This information is important in determining whether and when surgical intervention is indicated.

Finally, remember that shoulder pain that is not activity related may also be secondary to malignancy (Pancoast's tumor) or neurovascular syndromes or referred from cardiac or diaphragmatic problems.

Physical Examination

A complete physical examination consists of inspection, palpation, recording range of motion and muscle strength, and an assessment of joint stability. The examination should begin with a visual inspection of the upper torso, which can be accomplished only if all the patient's clothing above the waist is removed.

Inspection

Whereas most physicians have been taught to look for symmetry, this may be misleading when inspecting an athlete's shoulder. This is because throwing athletes typically exhibit hypertrophy of the shoulder girdle musculature. This hypertrophy can also make palpation of underlying structures more difficult. However, generalized hypertrophy also enhances recognition of specific muscle wasting, as seen with more chronic problems involving specific neurologic deficits. An example would be the wasting of the supraspinatus and infraspinatus muscles seen as a result of suprascapular nerve entrapment. Visualization of the acromioclavicular joint may detect prominences consistent with previous acromioclavicular joint separation or injury.

Palpation

After inspection, palpation of anatomic landmarks should be performed to elicit areas of tenderness. Anterior structures that can be palpated include the acromioclavicular joint, coracoid process, biceps tendon, and anterior capsule. The biceps is often best palpated with the patient supine and the arm held by the examiner to relax the deltoid. In this position the tendon becomes a subcutaneous structure and even in normal patients palpation may be mildly uncomfortable. In these instances comparison with the contralateral shoulder can be helpful. In the supine position the anterior capsule can also be palpated. The insertion of the supraspinatus into the greater tuberosity can be palpated just inferior to the anterolateral tip of the acromion. With the patient standing with the hand in an anatomic position (palm forward)

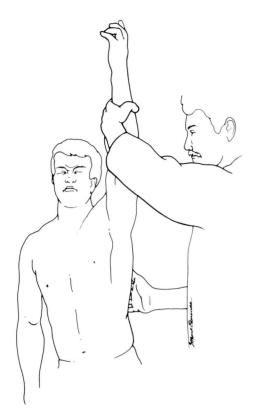

FIG. 33-3. Impingement sign. Pain with full forward flexion.

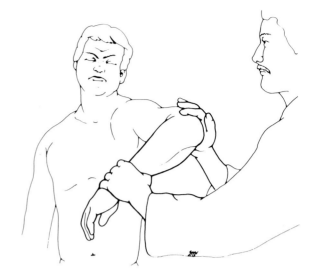

FIG. 33-4. Hawkins sign. Pain with forward flexion and internal rotation.

the supraspinatus insertion into the greater tuberosity sits just inferior to the lateral tip of the acromion. Posterior structures that can be palpated for tenderness include the vertebral border of the scapula with its associated rhomboid muscles, posterior capsule, and teres minor. The latter two structures are best palpated with the patient prone. Tenderness along the trapezius and paracervical musculature may be seen in athletes with associated cervical problems.

Range of Motion

Evaluation of shoulder range of motion should consist of recording forward flexion, abduction, abduction/external rotation, internal rotation, forward flexion across the chest, and extension. Throwing athletes normally exhibit an increase in external rotation with a concomitant decrease in internal rotation when compared with the contralateral shoulder. When the physician examines abduction, visualization of the scapula from the posterior aspect is important. Incongruent and uneven scapulothoracic motion may be the earliest sign in athletes with glenohumeral instability. Pain elicited in the fully forward flexed position has been described as a positive **impingement test** (Fig. 33-3). This finding can also be demonstrated by first stabilizing the scapula and then allowing forward flexion and internal rotation of the humerus to bring the supraspinatus under the coracoacromial ligament complex as described by Hawkins and Hobeika (Fig. 33-4).[18] Horizontal adduction across the chest should be evaluated for tightness of posterior cap-

sular structures and may also elicit discomfort in the acromioclavicular joint indicative of acromioclavicular joint arthrosis.

Strength Evaluation

Muscle strength can be evaluated usually by manual motor testing, although more specific evaluation with the assistance of isokinetic testing may also be indicated. The supraspinatus test is performed by applying manual resistance while the shoulder is abducted 90 degrees and forward flexed 30 degrees and with the athlete's thumbs pointing toward the floor (i.e., forearm internally rotated) (Fig. 33-5). This test may be recorded as positive for eliciting pain only or for pain and weakness and as such may be helpful in the detection of rotator cuff tears. Weakness of the serratus anterior muscle can be elicited by having the patient do a push-up against the wall and observing for winging of the scapula.

Stability Evaluation

Glenohumeral instability is best examined with the patient supine. Patient cooperation is extremely important in terms of allowing the muscles about the shoulder girdle to relax to allow examination of the underlying capsular structures. The **apprehension test** is performed with the patient supine and the arm abducted 90 degrees and maximally externally rotated. In this position patients with recurrent anterior dislocation problems exhibit immediate apprehension and try to prevent the examiner from bringing the arm into this position. These patients also complain of pain along the anterior capsule with the shoulder in this position. However, patients who are having a problem with anterior subluxation and, in particular, the throwing athlete exhibit a different response to the apprehension test. In the thrower whose shoulder is in mild anterior subluxation, the maximally abducted and externally rotated position often produces discomfort but not apprehension. Pain typically is elic-

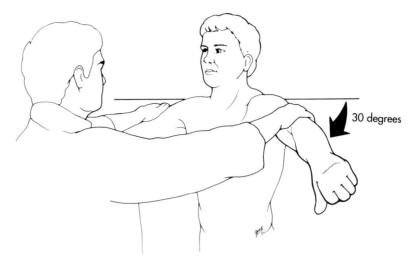

FIG. 33-5. Supraspinatus test. Arms abducted 90 degrees, forward flexed 30 degrees, and internally rotated 180 degrees (thumbs pointing to floor). Manual resistance causes pain or weakness or both.

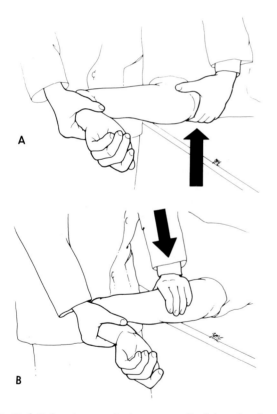

FIG. 33-6. Relocation test. **A,** Arm maximally abducted and externally rotated; patient complains of pain. **B,** Arm maximally abducted and externally rotated with force directed posteriorly; patient's pain eliminated.

ited posteriorly. This is internal impingement and may be indicative of undersurface rotator cuff tears and labral damage.

A **relocation test** can then be performed to confirm this diagnosis. The relocation test is done by first performing the apprehension maneuver and then repeating the same maneuver with a posteriorly directed force generated along the shaft of the humerus using the examiner's hand in an effort to eliminate the anterior subluxation (Fig. 33-6). With the humeral head now being held in place with the force being generated posteriorly as the arm is brought into an abducted and externally rotated position, the patient has no pain. In this position, with a posterior force applied, the internal impingement has been eliminated.

Subtle degrees of anterior and posterior instability can also be evaluated with the patient's shoulder in a supine position. With the humeral head held between the thumb anteriorly and fingers posteriorly, the examiner can apply forces anteriorly or posteriorly to elicit capsular laxity. In addition, labral injuries, and in particular superior labrum anterior-posterior (SLAP) lesions, may be detected by adding an axial load along the shaft of the humerus. As the head is then directed posteriorly with the addition of this compressive force, a palpable and sometimes audible click can be elicited supportive of a posterior labral tear.

Radiographic Examination

Routine radiographic views of the shoulder should include a true anteroposterior (AP) view as well as views in internal and external rotation, a transaxillary lateral view, and a scapular notch view. The scapular notch view has been found to be particularly helpful in evaluating possible impingement because the various anatomic variants in the acromion can be identified.

CONDITIONING AND REHABILITATION

A comprehensive conditioning program is required by the athlete who desires optimal performance. This program must include flexibility, strengthening, and endurance activities. The athlete who is involved in throwing activities must, in addition to general conditioning, perform sport-specific upper extremity and endurance exercises.[35]

The **warm-up period** is important because it allows increased efficiency of body functions by raising body temperatures. This can be done by performing jogging or cycling type of activities. In addition, the shoulder can benefit from local application of heat in the form of hot packs, whirlpool, and so on before stretching during the warm-up period because this may enhance blood flow to the shoulder. In the thrower, shoulder **stretching exercises** should be limited to those involving the posterior capsule. This is because the throwing shoulder normally has an increased range of external rotation in the abducted plane. Anterior stretching, particularly in the abducted position, may further damage an already attenuated capsule and should be avoided. It is not unusual for a thrower to have limited internal rotation, and posterior capsular stretching is important in preventing injury.

Strengthening of the shoulder girdle musculature is important both for maintenance and as part of a rehabilitation program after injury. Strengthening of the deltoid and rotator cuff muscles is mandatory, but it has become increasingly important to also exercise the scapular stabilizers (i.e., serratus, rhomboids, teres major, latissimus, and trapezius). Progressive isotonic and isokinetic exercises are done to achieve maximal performance levels.

All conditioning programs should include a **cool-down period** after activity (i.e., throwing). This often takes the form of cryotherapy with application of ice to the shoulder for 10 to 15 minutes and may be accompanied by elevation or massage or both. The application of cold results in decreased blood flow to deeper structures and reduction of metabolic activity. This is believed to reduce swelling and further degradation of inflamed tissues.

A successful rehabilitation program for the athlete's shoulder must be individualized to the player's problem.[25] Many factors, such as severity and chronicity of the problem as well as expected performance levels, must be assessed to determine length of rehabilitation. All successful therapy programs must also be integrated with a progressive throwing program to return the athlete to preinjury status. Our **rehabilitation program** consists of three phases. Phase 1 involves the use of modalities to reduce pain, inflammation, and edema. This is followed by a range of motion program placing only minimal stress on the involved structures. Phase 2 involves specific stretching of tightened capsular structures and isotonic strengthening activities.

Phase 3 involves progressive strengthening and includes isokinetic exercises. During this phase the athlete can begin a progressive shoulder throwing program, advancing back to preinjury status with the addition of maintenance stretching and strengthening exercises. The time frame involved must be individualized and needs to be continually reviewed and revised jointly by the athlete, trainer, therapist, and physician.

IMPINGEMENT SYNDROMES

Shoulder impingement is common in the throwing athlete.[9,18,22] Anatomically, this syndrome involves the subacromial complex, consisting of the undersurface of the acromion, subdeltoid bursa, coracoacromial ligament, rotator cuff, and biceps tendon. The rotator cuff and long head of the biceps act as humeral head depressors, preventing humeral head migration with subsequent mechanical impingement occurring against the bony roof and coracoacromial ligament. The subdeltoid bursa normally allows smooth gliding with glenohumeral motion. As the arm is abducted from 80 to 125 degrees, the greater tuberosity comes close to the anterior acromion.

Pathophysiology

A simple imbalance of the rotator cuff with relative weakness of the supraspinatus allows the vertical force of the deltoid to produce more of a compressive force as the arm is abducted. This can establish subdeltoid bursal thickening and further supraspinatus irritation. The area of the supraspinatus involved has been described by Rathbun and Macnab[38] as an area of relative hypovascularity, and further irritation, thickening, and fibrosis can occur. In addition, inflammation of the long head of the biceps tendon can occur as it passes through the groove as this critical area again passes beneath the coracoacromial arch. Therefore supraspinatus tendinitis and bicipital tenosynovitis can occur independently of one another or in combination.

Impingement leading to rotator cuff disease can occur along two separate pathways. The three-stage impingement classification described by Neer[31] delineates the pathway of the general population where aging may produce rotator cuff injury irrespective of throwing athletes. In Stage 1 edema and hemorrhage of the rotator cuff (particularly the supraspinatus) occur. This progresses with repeated trauma to Stage 2 changes of thickening and fibrosis. Stages 1 and 2 are both reversible. However, further deterioration results in Stage 3 changes with osseous degeneration and eventual tear formation. The second classification delineates the pathway of rotator cuff disease seen in the younger athletic throwing population. These athletes typically have internal impingement, which is secondary to primary anterior glenohumeral instability. Remember that in the thrower both external and internal impingement can be present. This is specific to the thrower and is initiated by underlying primary anterior glenohumeral instability.

History

The athlete with impingement syndrome often has a history of a painful arc of motion. In particular, abduction from 80 to 125 degrees with the arm internally rotated reproduces symptoms. Most patients describe pain as sharp and activity related. As in most inflammatory processes, pain usually increases after activity. Some patients may also complain of night pain, especially when sleeping with the arms overhead. Depending on which structures are inflamed, slight differences in history can be noted. Patients with bicipital tenosynovitis complain of pain in the anterior quadrant of the shoulder, especially along the bicipital groove. This pain occurs often just before ball release (end of Phase 4). Athletes with supraspinatus tendinitis tend to localize pain deeper in the shoulder or laterally at the deltoid.

Physical Examination

Visual inspection of shoulder abduction usually reveals asynchrony when viewed posteriorly. The scapulothoracic incongruent motion is the athlete's subtle attempt to reposition the humeral head beneath the acromion in an effort to clear the inflamed tissues. This can also lead to scapulothoracic bursitis.[44] Atrophy of the supraspinatus or infraspinatus may or may not be seen. A painful arc of motion can be elicited with abduction from 60 to 125 degrees. Tenderness can be palpated over the supraspinatus at the greater tuberosity (just lateral to the acromion) or biceps tendon if the groove is involved. A positive impingement test either in the forward flexed position (Neer) or in 90 degrees of forward flexion with the humerus internally rotated (Hawkins) is usually present. The isolated supraspinatus test may be positive for either reproducing pain or for eliciting both pain and weakness. In pure external or subacromial space impingement syndromes there are no physical findings suggestive of glenohumeral instability, but in the thrower subtle instability should always be suspected.

Treatment

Nonoperative Treatment

Over 90% of all impingement syndromes respond to conservative management.[25,31] This takes the form of a physical therapy program of rotator cuff strengthening exercises in combination with the use of nonsteroidal oral antiinflammatory agents. Injection of corticosteroids should be used sparingly and only in combination with an ongoing exercise program because they have been shown to reduce tensile strength and may lead to further osseous deposition. The physical therapy program should be individualized. Strengthening of the supraspinatus, infraspinatus, and teres minor are performed based on the primary structures involved as determined by physical examination. We recommend that all rotator cuff exercises be performed with the arm at the side to prevent further irritation of these inflamed structures. Exercises for the scapular rotators (i.e., serratus, rhomboids, and teres major) should also be performed to help regain scapulothoracic congruent motion. The use of ultrasound, in particular phonophoresis, can complement a therapy program. Phonophoresis can be especially effective in bicipital tenosynovitis.

Operative Treatment

When conservative management has failed, surgical options have traditionally included isolated coracoacromial ligament resection or anterior acromioplasty.[16,36] Although these procedures have produced good results overall, Tibone[46] reported poor results after acromioplasty in the throwing athlete. Although both procedures can now be done arthroscopically, there is no reason to believe results will improve. The reason for this is that in the thrower glenohumeral instability often is present. Under these circumstances the impingement is more likely to be internal impingement with undersurface rotator cuff tears and labral injury. Subacromial space surgery usually does not eliminate this pathologic condition. The humeral head can continue to migrate and thereby compress the rotator cuff because of capsular laxity. It is therefore of primary importance when contemplating a surgical decompression of the subacromial space that glenohumeral instability is ruled out as a diagnosis. This often necessitates a diagnostic shoulder arthroscopy before performing acromioplasty. Stage 3 changes require open surgical repair.[47]

GLENOHUMERAL INSTABILITY

Recurrent anterior subluxation of the shoulder is the single most important problem in the throwing athlete, and the diagnosis can be the most difficult to make.[41] In the 1950s and 1960s, Rowe and Zarins,[42] like Blazina and Saltzman,[6] started to report on throwers with a **dead arm syndrome** and associated this with transient subluxation. Others have subsequently shown that severe stresses are placed on the anterior capsular structures during Phase 3 of throwing, which can result not only in injury to the capsule leading to instability, but also in injury to the labrum. The key restraint in Phase 3, in which the arm is maximally abducted and externally rotated, is the anterior inferior glenohumeral ligament, as shown by Turkel and associates[49] and more recently by Warren.[50,51] The insertion of this ligament into the labrum is often the site of tearing.

History

The common complaint of the athlete with anterior subluxation is that the shoulder feels as if it were dead in the cocking position. Few throwers may actually be aware that the shoulder is slipping or popping, but many can describe only vague complaints of feeling that something is not right in the shoulder. Much more commonly, sharp pain or weakness or both may be the only symptoms with which the athlete presents.[13] Clicking or popping may be present and may indicate the presence of associated labrum tears.

Location of the athlete's pain can also be misleading. Athletes with moderately severe anterior instability complain of pain *anteriorly* along the glenohumeral joint in the late cocking phase of pitching. In these patients the apprehension test is almost uniformly positive. Also up to 40% of these patients, according to Rowe and Zarins,[42] had radiographic evidence of Hill-Sachs lesions and, in addition, changes noted along the glenoid rim. However, in the athlete who has only mild anterior glenohumeral instability, the presenting symptom may be only pain, and, in fact, the pain felt in the cocking phase is usually *posterior* rather than anterior. Patients do not complain of giving way or slippage but may complain of symptoms consistent with an impingement.

The posterior pain is secondary to inflammation within the cuff and to possible undersurface rotator cuff tears and labral fraying. These symptoms correlate well with the internal impingement findings at the time of arthroscopy. Additionally, posterior pain may be secondary to traction of the posterior structures as the arm moves from the late cocking position and begins to accelerate. Howell et al[21] have shown that in the maximally abducted and externally rotated position the center of the humeral

head is approximately 4 mm posterior to the center of the glenoid and as the arm then forward flexes and rotates in acceleration, the humeral head glides anteriorly, producing sheer stress on the glenoid and the labrum. One should remember also that increased laxity results in diminished clearance for structures under the coracoacromial arc, and the athlete will then have impingement symptoms.

Physical Examination

Shoulder motion should be carefully assessed, because often patients with evidence of anterior subluxation have a loss of external rotation in the maximally abducted position. A positive apprehension sign in this position is present in the thrower with moderate to severe subluxation; however, it is usually absent in more mild cases of instability. In the presence of mild instability, the patient may exhibit a positive relocation sign as described earlier. Tenderness may be palpated posteriorly along the glenohumeral capsule, and tenderness may also be elicited along the insertion of the supraspinatus. A positive impingement test and other physical findings consistent with impingement may often be present.

Physical findings in instability

- Loss of external rotation in abducted positions
- Apprehension sign
- Relocation sign of Jobe
- Anterior or posterior glenohumeral capsular tenderness
- Supraspinatus tenderness

Radiographic Evaluation

Radiographic evaluation may be helpful in patients with anterior instability. Again, in the more severe cases of instability, plain radiographs, including a true AP view of the shoulder, a West Point axillary view, and Stryker notch views, have been helpful in detecting the presence of Hill-Sachs lesions. However, in athletes with mild or moderate anterior instability, routine radiographs, sophisticated CT scans with and without contrast, and MRI techniques have been helpful. Gadolinium-enhanced MRI has been especially useful in detecting labral tears.

Operating Room Evaluation

Examination with the patient under anesthesia and diagnostic shoulder arthroscopy are often necessary to confirm the diagnosis. At the time of arthroscopic evaluation the anterior subluxation of the humeral head can be seen and demonstrated in the abducted and externally rotated position. Abnormalities of the anterior labrum are often present. These labral changes may consist of flattening and thinning anteriorly with an absence of the normal anterior inferior glenohumeral ligament or may consist of actual tears in the labrum as described in the classic Bankhart lesion. Bucket-handle tears or flap tears may occur. In a few of these patients simple arthroscopic resection of the labrum tear may improve symptoms,[1] but this does not alter the instability, and many of these athletes go on to develop recurrent problems with throwing. Therefore athletes must be cautioned that arthroscopic labral resection alone usually does not allow the thrower to return to throwing. As a result of the impingement syndrome that may be present secondarily, associated arthroscopic findings may include fraying of the posterior labrum and of the supraspinatus portion of the rotator cuff.[3] Andrews and associates[4] have further identified a series of glenoid labrum tears related to the long head of the biceps. In their series the majority of tears were located over the anterosuperior portion of the glenoid labrum near the origin of the tendon of the long head of the biceps into the glenoid. Snyder has identified SLAP lesions, which can also occur in conjunction with instability. In general, one should be cautioned that, despite the presence of arthroscopic findings consistent with impingement, the initiating event is usually that of anterior glenohumeral instability.

Arthroscopic findings in instability

- Anterior subluxation of humeral head
- Flattening and thinning of anterior labrum
- Labral tears
- Attenuation of inferior glenohumeral ligament

Treatment

The treatment of the majority of patients with mild anterior subluxation revolves around a well-supervised shoulder rehabilitation program done in conjunction with a physical therapist. This program will be successful only if the athlete stops throwing completely during this period of rehabilitation. Selection of the proper exercise program will vary with each patient, but the importance of exercising scapular rotators, the serratus anterior, as well as the rotator cuff musculature is now being realized. Rehabilitation also is not complete without a supervised gradual return to throwing with attention to proper throwing mechanics.

Nonoperative Treatment

The rehabilitation program consists of three phases. In Phase 1 range of motion exercises are performed, but care is taken to avoid undue stress to the anterior capsule. This is accomplished by performing exercises with the shoulder in the scapular plane. External rotation exercises are done with the arm by the side and limited to 45 degrees. External rotation, internal rotation, abduction, flexion, and extension exercises are performed using rubber tubing and progressing to free weights. Mobilization of the posterior capsule is also important.

In Phase 2 emphasis on eccentric strengthening is begun and isokinetic strengthening and endurance training are started. Again, these exercises are done with the arm at the side.

In Phase 3 stress is gradually applied to the anterior capsule by allowing isokinetic internal rotation and external rotation exercises to be performed with advancing degrees of shoulder abduction. When strength and en-

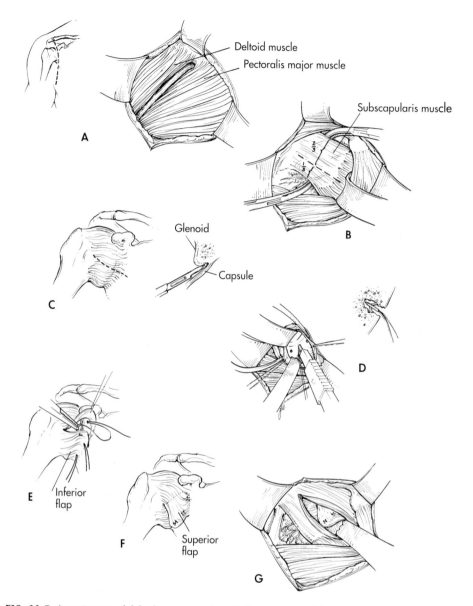

FIG. 33-7. Anterior capsulolabral reconstruction. **A,** Skin incision, deltopectoral groove. **B,** Subscapularis split. **C,** Capsular incision. **D,** Holes placed in glenoid from the 3 o'clock to the 5 o'clock positions. **E,** Inferior flap advanced superiorly. **F,** Superior flap advanced inferiorly. **G,** Flaps tied into place.

durance testing demonstrates 80% of function compared to the uninvolved side, then sport-specific activities such as a progressive throwing program can be initiated.

Operative Treatment

The surgical treatment of moderate and severe anterior glenohumeral instability has centered around repair of the Bankhart lesion when present and various anterior capsular reconstructive procedures.[7,20,43,48] Although these procedures have generally met with uniform success, the ability of the professional thrower to return to his or her previous level of activity has been dismal. Because of these inconsistent results in the professional thrower the **anterior capsulolabral reconstruction** was devised. The goal of this surgical proce-

dure is to reconstruct the anterior inferior glenohumeral ligament complex with minimal disruption of anatomic structures, thereby allowing both reinforcement of the anterior capsule and early return of full motion so necessary for the pitcher's successful return.

Anterior capsulolabral reconstruction (Fig. 33-7)

Surgical technique. An 8- to 10-cm axillary incision is made beginning 1 cm inferior to the tip of the coracoid. The deltopectoral groove is identified and split, retracting the cephalic vein laterally. The conjoined tendon is retracted medially. The subscapularis is then split in line with its fibers along the lower one fifth of its width. This is done to preserve as much neurovascularity of the muscle as possible. With the anterior capsule now exposed, a splitting incision is made, reflecting the capsule off the

glenoid side both superiorly and inferiorly. If the capsule is redundant inferiorly, then the inferior flap should be carefully reflected from the glenoid down to the most inferior portion. This must be done with the utmost caution to prevent damage to the axillary neurovascular structures. Three drill holes are then placed along the anterior glenoid from the 3 o'clock to the 5 o'clock position. Next the inferior flap is pulled superiorly and sutured along the anterior glenoid, recreating the anterior inferior glenohumeral ligament and labrum. This is done using nonabsorbable No. 1 Ethibond suture attached via Mitek suture anchors. The superior flap is then sutured in position, reinforcing the anterior capsule.

There are several important technical points to remember in performing this procedure. First, it is mandatory to recreate the anterior inferior glenohumeral ligament and thereby provide a new labral soft-tissue bumper. Second, it is important to cause minimal disruption of normal anatomy. This means that the subscapularis must be split rather than completely resected, as in the classic Bankhart repair. Exposure may be limited medially by the intact coracobrachialis.

Postoperative rehabilitation. Postoperatively the patient is immobilized in an abduction splint at approximately 90 degrees of abduction and 45 degrees of external rotation for 2 weeks. During this time the splint may be removed to allow the shoulder to adduct and to allow passive abduction. In addition, active elbow range of motion is encouraged, as are forearm strengthening activities such as squeezing a softball. Isometric exercises may also be performed during this period.

At 2 weeks the patient is no longer required to use the abduction splint and the patient is started on a progressive active and passive range of motion program with emphasis placed on protecting the anterior repair. Active external rotation with the arm by the side and the elbow flexed 90 degrees can also be performed with the use of rubber tubing. Shoulder shrugs and supraspinatus strengthening activities can be begun at this time. At 6 weeks shoulder flexion strengthening exercises may be added, as well as the use of the upper body ergometer for endurance training. By 8 weeks the patient should have regained a full range of motion. Resistive exercises are continued and isokinetic strengthening activities can begin in the third and fourth months but should be done with faster speed and in a position of flexion to protect the anterior joint capsule.

At 4 months isokinetic strengthening may begin for flexion and abduction, and training at slower speeds may be initiated. Progressive strengthening activities should be performed with emphasis on eccentric modes. At 4 to 5 months after surgery isokinetic testing may be performed. If the isokinetic testing shows 80% or above compared to the other involved shoulder, then a progressive shoulder throwing program can be initiated. As the shoulder throwing program is initiated, it is important to continue strength, flexibility, and endurance training.

The throwing program usually requires approximately 3 months to perform. This program involves progressive tossing of a ball with increasing distance and duration, initially on an alternate-day program and then progress-

ing to a throwing-2-days, resting-1-day sequence. When the athlete returns to the mound the throw should be at half speed, emphasizing accuracy and technique. The athlete then progresses from half speed to three-fourths speed, with eventual return to a normal pitching regimen. It is this smooth progression from one phase to another under close supervision that determines when an athlete can actually return to full competition. The time frame involved is variable and must be individualized to the athlete's need and condition of the shoulder. Rapid progression from one phase to the next without adequate rest and reassessment by the athlete, therapist, and physician will only result in delays, complications, and ultimate failure. Usually 1 year or more of rest is necessary before the athlete can compete.

Throwing program

- Alternate day, light tossing
- Throw 2 days and rest 1 day
- Half speed from mound
- Three-fourths speed from mound
- Full return

ACROMIOCLAVICULAR JOINT PROBLEMS

The acromioclavicular joint provides support for the upper portion of the shoulder. The articulation is not a direct one, because a disk of fibrocartilage is present between the two bones. The joint is stabilized primarily by the coracoclavicular ligament. However, the forward and backward motion of the distal clavicle is further controlled by the coracoacromial ligament, whose importance in throwing has previously been discussed.

Abduction and external rotation of the shoulder cannot occur without axial rotation of the clavicle, which produces sheer forces at the acromioclavicular joint. In addition, the follow-through phase of throwing is associated with positioning the arm in a degree of forward flexion across the chest. This produces high compression forces at the acromioclavicular joint as well. Accumulation of these stresses in the throwing athlete results in degenerative changes in the fibrocartilaginous disk, as well as on the articular surfaces of the joint.

History and Physical Examination

The athlete typically experiences pain at the acromioclavicular joint associated with phase 3 (late cocking) or phase 5 (follow-through) of the throwing motion. Pain is usually sharp and very specific. Associated bicipital symptoms are common.

Physical examination reveals tenderness to palpation at the acromioclavicular joint, usually anteriorly. Forward flexion at shoulder level across the chest reproduces symptoms. Remember that the acromioclavicular joint symptoms may exist with impingement as well. Degenerative changes may be seen radiographically, with sclerosis and lytic irregularities often noted in the distal

clavicle. Degenerative bone spurs may also be present on either side of the joint inferiorly. Interestingly, no correlation has been found between the degree of degenerative changes and symptoms.

Treatment

Mild symptoms may respond to rest, oral antiinflammatory agents, and a mobilization program. Bathing the acromioclavicular joint with a corticosteroid solution may also reverse acute symptoms and provide long-lasting relief. In athletes whose condition does not respond to nonoperative management, surgical resection of the distal clavicle has provided good relief.[8] Distal clavicle resection can be accomplished either arthroscopically or with open techniques.

The amount of bone resected is critical, because the clavicle provides attachment for both shoulder girdle musculature (deltoid and pectoralis) and ligamentous structures (coracoclavicular ligament). The proper amount of bone resection should still retain maximal length with these attachments and yet provide complete clearance in the remaining joint to prevent impingement throughout a complete range of motion of the shoulder. Laboratory studies undertaken have shown weakness of muscles in the surgically treated patient. Functionally, throwers have been able to return to their previous level of activities without problems.

NEUROVASCULAR ENTRAPMENT SYNDROMES

Neurovascular entrapment syndromes are relatively rare in the thrower, but when they occur they may cause significant loss of function and may end the athlete's career. These syndromes can be further divided into those involving the thoracic outlet, those involving the suprascapular nerve, and those involving the quadrilateral space.

Thoracic Outlet Syndrome

Thoracic outlet problems in the thrower can be manifested by various nonspecific complaints and often confusing and vague physical signs.[45] Athletes may complain of diffuse muscle aching or easy fatigability. Pain and paresthesias involving the neck or entire upper extremity may be present. Complaints of weakness, numbness, tingling, and temperature changes, as well as nocturnal complaints, are all possible.

Physical examination should include Adson's test and the hyperabduction maneuver of Wright and Lipscomb,[52] as well as the costoclavicular maneuver described by Baker and Thorberry. Radiographs may indicate the presence of cervical ribs. Electromyographic studies, including nerve conduction velocity studies, and vascular studies may be necessary to make a definitive diagnosis.

Many thoracic outlet problems can be relieved with nonoperative management emphasizing proper posture, as well as shoulder girdle muscle strengthening. Axillary artery occlusion and venous thrombosis may require anticoagulants or surgery.[52] Surgical release of the anterior scalene muscles and cervical rib excision have also been described as treatment for thoracic outlet problems not improved by more conservative management.

Suprascapular Nerve Entrapment

The suprascapular nerve is a motor nerve originating from roots C5 and C6 and passing to the upper border of the scapula, where it then passes through the scapular notch covered by the transverse scapular ligament. It is at this level that the supraspinatus muscle is innervated. The nerve then passes around the neck of the scapular spine before providing innervation to the infraspinatus muscle. It is at this point where entrapment usually occurs in the thrower and appears as an isolated infraspiratus atrophy.

Athletes may be seen with vague posterior or posterolateral shoulder pain. Because the supraspinatus and infraspinatus are not functioning properly, other problems, such as rotator cuff tendinitis, bicipital tenosynovitis, and bursitis, may also be present. On physical examination one should observe wasting of either the infraspinatus alone or in combination with the supraspinatus, depending on the level of entrapment.

Treatment must include a period of rest from throwing in an effort to relieve further irritation to the nerve. Often, rest in combination with a flexibility and strengthening program for the atrophied rotator cuff muscles as well as the scapular rotators is all that is necessary. In cases of long-term entrapment with significant atrophy, surgical release at either level may be performed, but these procedures have not enjoyed much success in our experience. Interestingly, there are pitchers who have been able to continue throwing even at a professional level despite chronic wasting of the infraspinatus musculature from long-standing entrapment problems. This is because during normal throwing the infraspiratus only functions at 30% MMT. If the athlete can restrengthen the remaining infraspiratus muscle despite entrapment, he will be able to throw at preinjury levels.

Quadrilateral Space Syndrome

The quadrilateral space is formed superiorly by the teres minor, inferiorly the teres major, medially by the long head of the triceps, and laterally by the neck of the humerus. Through this space pass the posterior circumflex vessels and the axillary nerve. Compression of these structures can occur in the abducted externally rotated position of the arm, which is seen in the terminal cocking phase of throwing. Fibrous bands can also be present in this space, which can further entrap these structures. The thrower is seen with nonspecific shoulder pain and only occasionally with paresthesias. The symptoms appear to coincide with Phase 3 of the throwing motion when the arm is maximally abducted and externally rotated.[39] As such, patients may note symptoms only associated with a particularly hard throw. Physical examination of the shoulder is normal, although again this problem may coexist with other more common shoulder disorders. Tenderness directly over the quadrilateral space often is present but may be confused with the tenderness seen in this area with the more common teres minor tendinitis. Electromyography is usually negative, al-

though rarely a mild denervation pattern may be seen in the deltoid. The diagnosis is confirmed by subclavian arteriography at which time the posterior circumflex artery can be seen to occlude with humeral abduction and external rotation.

In patients who remain symptomatic, surgical decompression through a posterior shoulder approach has been effective. This is a rare entity and only a few cases in throwers exist, but surgical decompression has been successful in the throwers treated.

ADOLESCENT INJURIES

Adolescent shoulder injuries occur via the same basic mechanisms as in the adult, but the physeal growth plate changes the types of injuries seen. Capsular structures about the shoulder joint have greater strength than the epiphyseal plate; therefore the plate becomes the most vulnerable spot for injury. There are several growth plates about the shoulder including those of the acromion, coracoid, proximal humerus, and glenoid, with many of the growth plates staying open beyond the age of 18 years.

Little League Shoulder

Little league shoulder is a term coined by Dotter[12]; it is manifested by shoulder pain in the throwing athlete associated with throwing activities. Pain is usually about the shoulder and deltoid in a nonspecific pattern and is worse after activity and especially after hard throwing. Physical examination is usually normal with the exception of palpable tenderness over the proximal humerus physis. Patients may also exhibit signs of impingement.

The diagnosis can usually be made with the aid of radiographs that reveal widening of the proximal epiphyseal plate of the humerus.[10] Often, comparison radiographs of the opposite limb are necessary. Callus bone formation may subsequently occur secondary to periosteal reaction. It is felt that this physeal fracture occurs because of the relative weakness of the zone of hypertrophy in the physis, which is subject to both sheer and torque as the shoulder moves from abduction and external rotation to internal rotation as one goes from Phase 2 to Phase 5 of pitching.[17] The athlete will respond to a period of rest, allowing this stress fracture to heal, and the athlete can return to playing without problems as long as attention is paid to conditioning and the prevention of overuse.

Other injuries in the adolescent include those seen in the adult, such as impingement and instability problems.

REFERENCES

1. Andrews JR, Carson W: The arthroscopic treatment of glenoid labrum tears in the throwing athlete, *Orthop Trans* 8:44, 1984.
2. Andrews JR et al: Arthroscopy of the shoulder: technique and normal anatomy, *Am J Sports Med* 12:1, 1984.
3. Andrews JR et al: Arthroscopy of the shoulder in the management of partial tears of the rotator cuff: a preliminary report, *Arthroscopy* 1:117, 1985.
4. Andrews JR et al: Glenoid labrum tears related to long head of the biceps, *Am J Sports Med* 13:337, 1985.
5. Bankart ASB: The pathology and treatment of recurrent dislocation of the shoulder joint, *Br J Surg* 26:23, 1939.
6. Blazina ME, Saltzman JS: Recurrent anterior subluxation of the shoulder in athletes—a distinct entity, *J Bone Joint Surg* 51A:1037, 1969.
7. Bost F, Inman V: The pathologic changes in recurrent dislocation of shoulder: a report of Bankart's operative procedure, *J Bone Joint Surg* 24:595, 1942.
8. Cahill BR: Osteolysis of the distal part of the clavicle in male athletes, *J Bone Joint Surg* 64:1053, 1982.
9. Cahill BR: Understanding shoulder pain. In AAOS: *Instructional course lectures,* vol 34, St Louis, 1985, Mosby.
10. Cahill BR et al: Little league shoulder, *J Sports Med* 2:150, 1974.
11. Cain PR et al: Anterior stability of the glenohumeral joint: a dynamic model, *Am J Sports Med* 15:144, 1987.
12. Dotter WE: Little leaguer's shoulder: a fracture of the proximal epiphyseal cartilage of the humerus due to baseball pitching, *Guth Clin Bull* 23:68, 1953.
13. Garth WP et al: Occult anterior subluxations of the shoulder in noncontact sports, *Am J Sports Med* 15:579, 1987.
14. Glousman et al: Diagnostic electromyographic analysis of the throwing shoulder with glenohumeral instability, *J Bone Joint Surg* 70A:220, 1988.
15. Gowan ID et al: A comparative electromyographic analysis of the shoulder during pitching: professional versus amateur pitchers, *Am J Sports Med* 15:586, 1987.
16. Ha'eri G, Wiley AM: Shoulder impingement syndrome: results of operative release, *Clin Orthop* 168:128, 1982.
17. Hansen NM: Epiphyseal changes in the proximal humerus of an adolescent baseball pitcher, *Am J Sports Med* 10:380, 1982.
18. Hawkins RJ, Hobeika PE: Impingement syndrome in the athletic shoulder, *Clin Sports Med* 2:391, 1983.
19. Hill HA, Sachs MD: The grooved defect of the humeral head: a frequently unrecognized complication of dislocation of the shoulder joint, *Radiology* 35:690, 1940.
20. Hill JA et al: The modified Bristow-Helfet procedure for recurrent anterior shoulder subluxations and dislocations, *Am J Sports Med* 9:283, 1981.
21. Howell SM et al: Normal and abnormal mechanics of the glenohumeral joint in the horizontal plane, *J Bone Joint Surg* 70A:227, 1988.
22. Jackson DW: Chronic rotator cuff impingement in the throwing athlete, *Am J Sports Med* 4:231, 1976.
23. Jobe CM, Jobe FW: Painful athletic injuries of the shoulder, *Clin Orthop* 173:117, 1983.
24. Jobe FW: Thrower problems, *Sports Med* 7:139, 1979.
25. Jobe FW, Moynes DR: Delineation of diagnostic criteria and a rehabilitation program for rotator cuff injuries, *Am J Sports Med* 10:336, 1982.
26. Jobe FW et al: An EMG analysis of the shoulder in throwing and pitching, *Am J Sports Med* 11:3, 1983.
27. Jobe FW et al: An EMG analysis of the shoulder in pitching: a second report, *Am J Sports Med* 12:218, 1984.
28. King JW et al: Analysis of the pitching arm of the professional baseball pitcher, *Clin Orthop* 67:116, 1979.
29. Lombardo SJ: Arthroscopy of the shoulder, *Clin Sports Med* 2:309, 1983.
30. Moynes DR et al: Electromyography and motion analysis of the upper extremity in sports, *Phys Ther* 6:1905, 1986.
31. Neer CS: Anterior acromioplasty for the chronic impingement syndrome in the shoulder: a preliminary report, *J Bone Joint Surg* 54A:41, 1972.
32. Norwood LA et al: Anterior shoulder pain in baseball pitchers, *Am J Sports Med* 6:103, 1978.
33. Pappas AM et al: Symptomatic shoulder instability due to lesions of the glenoid labrum, *Am J Sports Med* 11:279, 1983.
34. Pappas AM et al: Biomechanics of baseball pitching: a preliminary report, *Am J Sports Med* 13:216, 1985.
35. Pappas AM et al: Rehabilitation of the pitching shoulder, *Am J Sports Med* 13:223, 1985.
36. Penny JN, Welsh RP: Shoulder impingement syndromes in athletes and their surgical management, *Am J Sports Med* 9:11, 1981.
37. Perry J: Anatomy and biomechanics of the shoulder in throwing, swimming, gymnastics and tennis, *Clin Sports Med* 2:247, 1983.

38. Rathbun JB, Macnab I: The microvascular pattern of the rotator cuff, *J Bone Joint Surg* 52B:540, 1970.
39. Redler MR et al: Quadrilateral space syndrome in a throwing athlete, *Am J Sports Med* 14:511, 1986.
40. Richardson AB: Overuse syndromes in baseball, tennis, gymnastics and swimming, *Clin Sports Med* 2:379, 1983.
41. Rockwood CA: Subluxation of the shoulder: the classification, diagnosis and treatment, *Orthop Trans* 4:306, 1980.
42. Rowe CR, Zarins B: Recurrent transient subluxation of the shoulder, *J Bone Joint Surg* 63A:863, 1981.
43. Rowe CR et al: The Bankart procedure: a long-term end-result study, *J Bone Joint Surg* 60A:1, 1978.
44. Sisto DJ, Jobe FW: The operative treatment of scapulothoracic bursitis in professional pitchers, *Am J Sports Med* 14:192, 1986.
45. Strukel RJ et al: Thoracic outlet compression in athletes, *Am J Sports Med* 6:35, 1978.
46. Tibone JE: Shoulder impingement syndrome in athletes treated with an anterior acromioplasty, *Clin Orthop* 188:134, 1985.
47. Tibone JE et al: Surgical treatment of tears of the rotator cuff in athletes, *J Bone Joint Surg* 68A:887, 1986.
48. Torg JS et al: A modified Bristow-Helfet-May procedure for recurrent dislocation and subluxation of the shoulder: report of two hundred and twelve cases, *J Bone Joint Surg* 69A:904, 1987.
49. Turkel SJ et al: Stabilizing mechanisms preventing anterior dislocation of the glenohumeral joint, *J Bone Joint Surg* 63A:1208, 1981.
50. Warren RF: Subluxation of the shoulder in athletes, *Clin Sports Med* 2:339, 1983.
51. Warren RF: Instability of shoulder in throwing sports. In AAOS: *Instructional course lectures,* vol 34, St Louis, 1985 Mosby.
52. Wright RS, Lipscomb AB: Acute occlusion of the subclavian vein in an athlete: diagnosis, etiology and surgical management, *J Sports Med* 2:343, 1975.
53. Yocum LA: Assessing the shoulder: history, physical examination, differential diagnosis, and special tests, *Clin Sports Med* 2:281, 1983.
54. Zarins B et al: *Injuries to the throwing arm,* Philadelphia, 1985, WB Saunders.

CHAPTER 34

Prevention and Rehabilitation of Shoulder Injuries in Throwing Athletes

Karen M. Griffin

Christina Bonci

Beth Sloane

Anatomic and biomechanical considerations

Mechanics of throwing

Prevention in baseball

Injury assessment, initial treatment, and rehabilitation
    Proprioceptive neuromuscular facilitation
    Progressive functional rehabilitation and return to
       throwing

The upper extremity is the primary site of acute and chronic injuries from throwing. The volatile action of the throwing mechanism places high stresses and demands on the shoulder and elbow. As a result, shoulder and elbow problems are common among throwers from atraumatic intrinsic forces from the physiologic overload of the repetitive high-frequency, high-velocity demand on the upper extremity. The foundation for which the coordinated sequence of throwing occurs is the structural integrity and functional dynamics of the shoulder joint. A dysfunctional shoulder is one that has lost the delicately balanced relationship between mobility and stability. For rehabilitation programs to have influence on restoring and maintaining this relationship, the physician must incorporate pertinent anatomic and biomechanical considerations of the throwing shoulder before selecting rehabilitation activities.

ANATOMIC AND BIOMECHANICAL CONSIDERATIONS

The athlete's shoulder is truly complex given the rehabilitation parameters involved in regaining normal osteokinematics and neuromuscular function at a competitive status. The shoulder is composed of four joints that work together as a single unit: the sternoclavicular, the acromioclavicular, the scapulothoracic, and the glenohumeral. Motor control is established through the contraction and relaxation of the many muscles that surround the various joints. Fifteen muscles provide scapular motion, nine muscles provide glenohumeral motion, and six muscles support the scapula on the thorax.[10] According to Inman, Saunders, and Abbott,[11] who studied the function of the shoulder joint, maintaining the rhythm of smooth and coordinated motion requires intact joints and the preservation of strength and power in the muscles that move them.

This statement has broad implications for the glenohumeral joint. Static and dynamic control of the joint depends on the stabilizing effects of the ligamentous, capsular structures and of the muscles. There is individual variation in the composition and strength of these stabilizers, thereby influencing the degree of effective restraint.[9]

The fibrous tissue structures of the shoulder, consisting of the anterior capsular ligaments (specifically the inferior glenohumeral ligament, which exists as a local thickening of the shoulder capsule, and the glenoid labrum, which exists as a hoop of pliable tissue attached to the peripheral edge of the saucerlike glenoid cavity), all provide limited static anterior reinforcement. The subscapularis tendon also deserves mention as a static stabilizer because of its insertion into the shoulder joint capsule and lesser tubercle of the humerus. However, it has been documented that the ability of this tendon to act as an effective buttress in preventing anterior humeral head subluxation decreases with abduction. When the arm is abducted above 90 degrees, the tendon undergoes a positional shift to a more superior location, where it no longer provides coverage for the inferior portion of the humeral head, thus compromising its stabilizing effects.[37] The shoulder joint's inherent lack of static restraints, coupled with its three-dimensional mobility from a ball and socket configuration, forces it to rely heavily on dynamic control or the almost perfect synergism of the muscles that cross the joint.

The thrower relies heavily on the dynamic effect of the rotator cuff for joint compression. Saha[33] described this dynamic rotator cuff effect as a steering mechanism

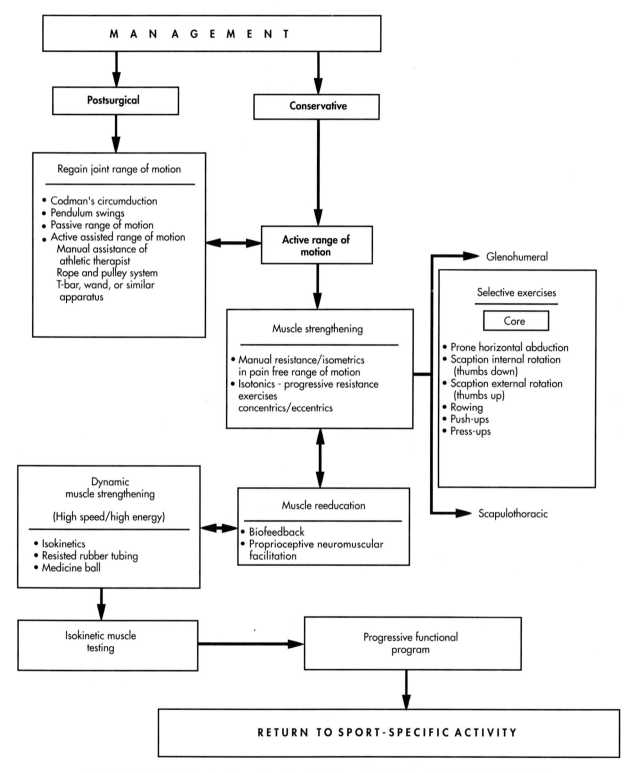

FIG. 34-1. Rehabilitation algorithm. (From Bonci C, Sloane B, Middleton K: *J Sports Rehabil* 1:146, 1992.)

functioning to position the humeral head on the glenoid. Through action of the steering muscles, in particular the supraspinatus and the infraspinatus, the instantaneous center of rotation of the glenohumeral joint is maintained when the 90-degree abducted arm achieves a position of maximal external rotation and then forcefully accelerates from external to internal rotation.[38]

The functional considerations of the glenohumeral joint must not override the importance of addressing those of the scapulothoracic articulation, which is often neglected in rehabilitation programs. The scapular protractors, the serratus anterior, and the scapular retractors, composed of the middle trapezius and the major and minor rhomboids, counterbalance one another to maintain proper scapulothoracic angular relationship. During arm elevation the serratus anterior's primary function is to permit the scapular inferior angle to externally rotate.[32] This action is critical for enhancing joint stability by maintaining the glenoid fossa in optimal position to receive the humeral head. Inferior scapular abduction also preserves length and tension properties of the deltoid muscle and removes the acromion from the path of the elevating humerus.[7,8,27]

Retraining and restoring scapular positioning to accompany the humerus in the execution of overarm skills help facilitate appropriate functioning of the rotator cuff muscles that are responsible for activating and stabilizing the glenohumeral joint. This should not be overlooked in the design of rehabilitation programs. By virtue of the synchronous contraction of the rotator cuff muscles, the humeral head is pressed into the glenoid fossa, locking it into a position that provides a secure scapulohumeral link for upper extremity function.[29] It follows then that restoring and maintaining this relationship of the humeral head relative to the glenoid fossa are key to preserving joint stability.

With a better understanding of functional anatomic and joint biomechanical principles of the throwing athlete, the potential to design rehabilitation strategies that have a more profound influence on mobility and dynamic stability of the glenohumeral joint cannot be underestimated. An algorithm (Fig. 34-1) has been developed for ease of application of these principles into various stages of rehabilitation.[5] Emphasis is placed on selective exercises geared to promote maximum recruitment of muscles affecting the coordinated rhythm of the glenohumeral and scapulothoracic joints as well as techniques to facilitate muscle reeducation. Whether the management is surgical or conservative, the athlete enters the rehabilitation sequence at some point along the algorithm as his or her pathologic state dictates.

MECHANICS OF THROWING

Injuries to the upper extremity caused by the throwing motion in sports have stimulated progressive research and analysis. High-speed cinematography and dynamic electromyography (EMG) with computer-assisted analysis have allowed study of the complex throwing act. The mechanics of baseball pitching have been described by Tullos and King,[37] Jobe et al,[13,14] Pappas,[26] McLeod,[23] King, Bielsford, and Tullos,[19] and Prentice and Cooma.[30]

McLeod[23] described the pitching mechanism as an act divided into five phases: wind-up, cocking, acceleration, release and deceleration, and follow-through. Important in the consideration of the mechanical analysis of the movement of the arm is the involvement of the entire body. The **wind-up** is a balance phase that prepares the pitcher for the proper body alignment and weight shift to lead into the cocking phase. In this phase kinetic energy is stored and the pitchers have the opportunity to "hide" the ball from the batters. During the wind-up the opposite knee is lifted upward and the body placed in a position so that all segments of the body (legs, hips, trunk, and arms) contribute to the throw.

Cocking is the next phase that applies tension on the accelerator muscles. The opposite leg is extended forward and planted just left of midline of the path to the plate. The hips follow, internally rotating to provide maximal thrust. At this point the arm is abducted and in extreme external rotation, and the shoulder and trunk progress forward to provide extrinsic loading to the pitching arm.

Forward movement of the ball occurs in the **acceleration** phase. The body continues its forward motion and the pectoralis major and latissimus dorsi fire to horizontally adduct and internally rotate the arm. The arm drags behind as tremendous force is applied. During this acceleration a considerable extension force is placed on the elbow joint.

The **deceleration** phase is stated to be two times greater than acceleration forces.[14] The humerus has a high rate of internal rotation during the deceleration phase. The rotator cuff musculature is instrumental in decelerating the motion of the arm and stabilizing the humerus in the glenoid cavity. In the **follow-through** phase there is a stretch of the rotator cuff and a reduction of tension on the posterior shoulder structure.

The rapid acceleration and deceleration forces that occur often predispose the throwing arm to injury.[2] The forces involved in each phase may lead to injuries that may be musculotendinous, articular, capsular, or neural. The muscle activation pattern of the shoulder during each phase of throwing was outlined in studies by Jobe et al.[13-15] The supraspinatus, infraspinatus, teres minor, subscapularis, and anterior, middle, and posterior portions of the deltoid muscle were observed in five pitchers. An acceleration phase of 0.1 second was noted; next came a follow-through phase in which there were significant muscular contractions of all the muscle groups to decelerate the arm. In the later EMG study the activities of the pectoralis major, biceps, triceps, latissimus dorsi, serratus anterior, and brachialis muscles were examined. Large rotational torques are produced in the humerus with each phase of the throw.[22]

Other throwing sports such as fast-pitch softball, football, javelin, and water polo require special consideration because of the differences in technique and the weight of the projectile to be thrown over a given distance. The increased popularity of women's fast-pitch softball has encouraged initial high-speed cinematography and bio-

mechanical analysis of the fast pitch. Main objectives for proper mechanics of the fast pitch have been described by Kempf[18] for the pitcher to maintain natural motion with the throw and to use effective power line positioning, good weight shift, and the total body during phases of the pitch.

Wick et al[40] explained that throwing a football places different demands on the elbow and shoulder girdle than does throwing a baseball. Comparison of throwing a football and throwing a baseball reveals that the football is heavier, the wind-up in throwing a football is less than a baseball, the forward fling is shorter, and the follow-through is in a different arc and is not as powerful.[3] Patterns of throwing in water polo are similar to those of baseball, with a positioning phase, a wind-up, a throw, and a follow-through. Rollins et al[31] described specific modifications in water polo. The initial stance includes holding the ball out of the water, positioning the opposite arm in front for balance, and an eggbeater motion of the legs to maintain position. The windup includes cocking of the throwing arm, vertical upward push with the kick leg, ball push-off, and a pull with the opposite or steadying arm. During the moment before throwing the ipsilateral hip is abducted, and the contralateral hip is flexed. Greater elbow flexion and external humeral rotation are related to increased ball velocity.

PREVENTION IN BASEBALL

Bad habits of throwing are often developed at a young age during early participation in any given sport. Little League players who are anxious and enthusiastic about their sport are often encouraged to increase the frequency of throwing with less emphasis on the quality of throwing if there is little knowledgeable instruction available. Set patterns of faulty throwing mechanics become set kinetics for the individual. Proper body mechanics are of primary importance in avoiding injury from repetitive high-velocity throwing. Effective coaches concentrate on proper pitching technique for an individual thrower who experiences chronic arm problems. Biomechanical analysis with the use of high-speed cinematography can detect problem points during the throwing act. This is also a valuable tool in the rehabilitative phase so that once a player overcomes an injury, faulty mechanics can be corrected to prevent reinjury. Knowledgeable pitching coaches can readily see a mistake leading to the breakdown of mechanics. Points that are stressed when identifying errors in the mechanics of pitching are (1) to avoid overextending the arm and shoulder, (2) to avoid overextending the planted leg, and (3) to point the planted leg in the proper direction to avoid opening up or staying closed too long, causing a compensation of the body in the delivery of the throw.[34] The shoulder is abducted 90 degrees with proper pitching motion. With the overhead, three-quarter, or sidearm delivery the body lean, or trunk side flexion, as well as elbow flexion differs; however, the shoulder remains at 90 degrees of abduction. If the throwing arm is abducted to a much greater degree than this, impingement problems are likely. The throwing act that is mechanically sound less-

ens the chance of injury and promotes an increased longevity of the thrower in his or her sport.

To promote increased longevity of the throwing athlete, the athlete may participate in a year-round conditioning and off-season throwing program. This is a period when overstressed areas of the body have a chance to recover and readapt to the demands placed on it during the season. Incorporating a maintenance program is important if an injury has occurred and the arm has been rehabilitated during the season. This period also allows for a total body strengthening and conditioning program as well as specific skill acquisition and training. Specific shoulder exercises performed during the off-season may mimic some of the core exercises. Additionally important during this time is that the athlete is working on trunk and lower extremity strength, power, and endurance. Individualizing the program depending on the physician's assessment of the athlete should give particular emphasis to deficit or problem areas.

INJURY ASSESSMENT, INITIAL TREATMENT, AND REHABILITATION

Differential diagnosis of the throwing shoulder provides the sports therapist with valuable information in regard to specific structures implicated. Injury to the rotator cuff has been attributed to eccentric overloading with its role of deceleration of the arm during the throwing act, its association with impingement of the subacromial structures between the head of the humerus and the coracoacromial arch, and stresses occurring to the musculature with glenohumeral joint instability. Associated injury of the biceps tendon and glenoid labrum, traction injuries to the head of the humerus and scapula, and degenerative changes of the inferior surface of the acromion are often noted.[1]

For the young athlete Jobe and Pink[16] proposed an instability continuum in which the overuse and potential to stretch stabilizing structures lead to asynchronous muscle firing and subsequent subluxation with secondary impingement and rotator cuff injury. Emphasis is made that surgical intervention to the rotator cuff alone treats one isolated aspect but does not address the primary instability problem. The injured young throwing athlete is considered unstable until proven otherwise.

Evaluation of the throwing athlete should include a detailed subjective assessment. The sports therapist should determine the athlete's primary subjective complaint and functional limitation. The objective assessment should include active and passive range of motion, resisted strength tests, and accessory motion tests to ascertain glenohumeral stability. The initial treatment plan should be appropriate to the assessed injury's nature, severity, and irritability, and its stage in occurrence and repair should be determined by the athlete's presenting signs and symptoms.[22] An eclectic approach of treatment and rehabilitative techniques allows the physician to formulate the best program according to the unique deficiencies of each athlete. Treatment appropriate for a stage of acute inflammation and pain may be Grade I or II oscillating mobilization for pain modulation; active rest by

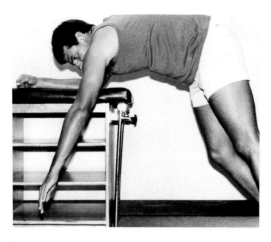

FIG. 34-2. Circumduction exercises help stimulate mechanoreceptors of the joint to decrease shoulder pain.

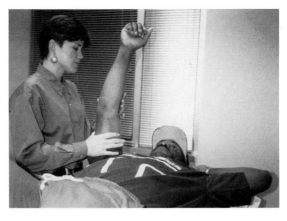

FIG. 34-3. Exercise of isometric cocontractions for joint stabilization.

avoiding aggravating activities that provoke pain but beginning pain-free arc motion of shoulder pendulum and swings (Fig. 34-2); passive or active assisted range of motion in supine position; a selection of modalities to decrease pain and control inflammation; and the physician's selection of a nonsteroidal antiinflammatory medication.

A progression of active assisted and active range of motion is initiated with the sports therapist being acutely aware of the integrity of the involved shoulder. Initially flexion and abduction may be limited to 90 degrees to avoid irritating the shoulder and external rotation performed at 45 degrees abduction with precautions of not overstretching the anterior joint capsule. Athlete education of postural awareness and correction and position modification to avoid impingement are additionally important. Pool exercises for upper extremity range of motion may be beneficial as well as pool running and other exercises for the lower extremity and trunk to prevent deconditioning. Other land conditioning may be progressed if it does not aggravate the involved shoulder. A normal return to active range of motion precedes strengthening exercises.

Strength progression likewise should be advanced depending on the assessment of the athlete's signs and symptoms. Isometric exercises are performed without osteokinematic movement and therefore can be used in early phases of rehabilitation to increase static muscular strength without causing an increase in joint irritation. The athlete may begin isometric exercise at submaximal effort to maximal resistance and progress at incremental multiangled positions. Dynamic joint stability is promoted via isometric work of cocontractions of the shoulder girdle musculature through manual resistance (Fig. 34-3). This manual contact open-chain proprioceptive activity may progress from low forces applied slowly, and as the shoulder improves, the joint may be challenged to respond to high forces applied rapidly and randomly.

Resisted isotonic exercise for the rotator cuff may be initiated with low resistance and high repetitions, be per-

formed in patterns that isolate specific rotator cuff muscles (Fig. 34-4), and then progress to functional patterns required for throwing. From EMG studies, Blackburn, McLeod, and White[4] advocated positioning in the prone position with the shoulder in horizontal abduction and the arm externally rotated and abducted to 100 degrees or prone external rotation with the shoulder at 90 degrees of abduction and the elbow flexed to 90 degrees for maximal recruitment of supraspinatus; increased recruitment of the infraspinatus in prone horizontal abduction with arm externally rotated and abducted to 90 degrees; and positioning for strengthening of the teres minor in prone shoulder extension with the arm abducted to the side of the body and externally rotated. Additional EMG studies performed by Jobe and Pink[16] identified three exercises as significant and consistent to the muscles responsible for humeral motion: scaption internal rotation (Fig. 34-5), prone horizontal abduction in external rotation, and press-ups (Fig. 34-6). Four exercises were shown to provide increased recruitment of muscles responsible for scapular rotation: scaption external rotation, rowing, push-ups (Fig. 34-7), and press-ups. These exercises are identified as the core or rehabilitation programs and can be performed to strengthen the rotator cuff and scapular musculature concentrically and eccentrically.

The ongoing challenge throughout the rehabilitation process is that of regaining the critical balance of shoulder joint stability and mobility. Muscle imbalances about the shoulder girdle should be addressed by including stretching of the tight muscles and strengthening of the weak muscles. It is important for the athlete to regain normal throwing motion and flexibility needed for the throwing action provided that the soft-tissue structures are not compromised by an increase in laxity of the shoulder joint (Fig. 34-8). Flexibility is important for the throwing arm because the arm is propelled through an arc of motion limited to the range of passive mobility. Inflexibility of the posterior musculature assessed by end range feel in horizontal adduction and internal rotation creates increased stress to the posterior shoulder structures on follow-through. Stretching in positions of inter-

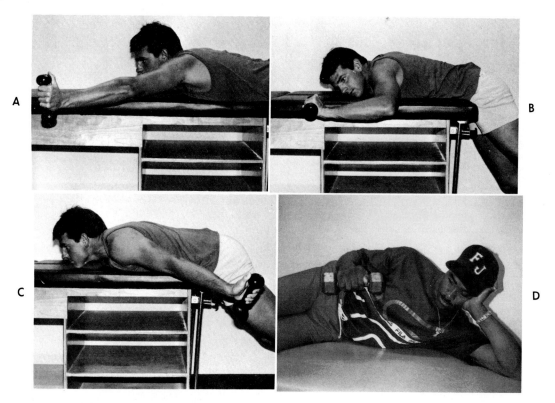

FIG. 34-4. Optimal positions for exercising rotator cuff. **A,** Prone horizontal abduction at 100 degrees with arm in externally rotated position. **B,** Prone external rotation strengthening position. **C,** Prone extension with arm in external rotated position. **D,** Side-lying external rotation as an alternate position.

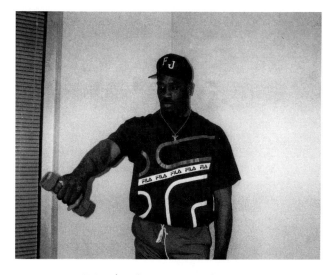

FIG. 34-5. Scaption internal rotation.

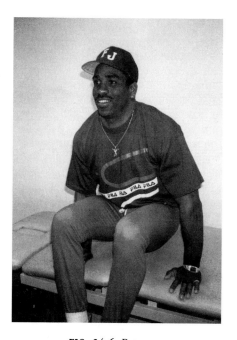

FIG. 34-6. Press-up.

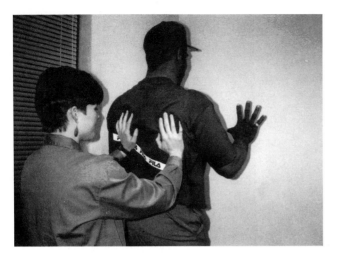

FIG. 34-7. Facilitated wall push-up.

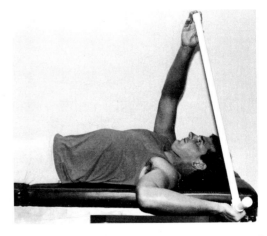

FIG. 34-8. Supine external rotation may be used if joint tightness is assessed.

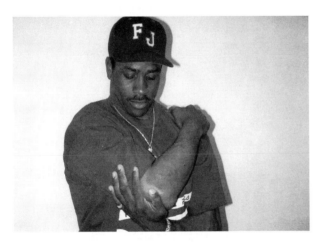

FIG. 34-9. Horizontal adduction stretch.

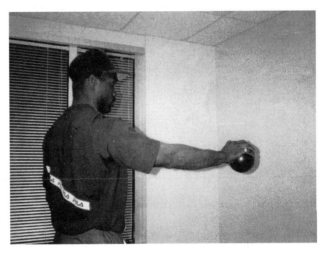

FIG. 34-10. Plyoball writing, a proximal stability for distal mobility exercise.

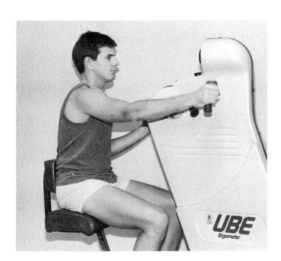

FIG. 34-11. Cybex upper body ergometer for shoulder girdle endurance and strengthening.

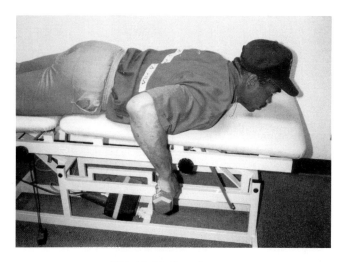

FIG. 34-12. Posterior row.

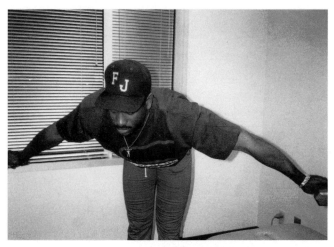

FIG. 34-13. Horizontal abduction.

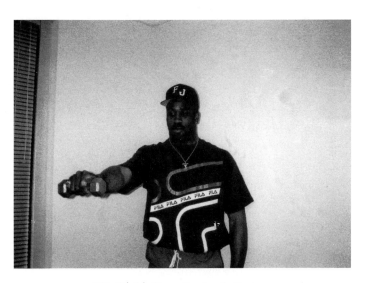

FIG. 34-14. Strengthening in flexion.

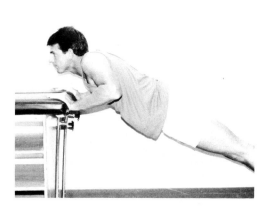

FIG. 34-15. Modified push-up.

nal rotation and horizontal adduction is encouraged for maintaining posterior flexibility (Fig. 34-9).

Strengthening of the scapular muscles provides a stable base for the scapulohumeral muscles to work on—proximal stability for distal mobility (Fig. 34-10). An exercise modality that may be used to encourage shoulder girdle endurance and strengthening is an upper body ergometer (Fig. 34-11). Strengthening the trapezius, levator scapulae, rhomboids, pectoralis minor, and serratus anterior in the early phases of the rehabilitation program is stressed. The posterior row (Fig. 34-12), horizontal abduction (Fig. 34-13), flexion (Fig. 34-14), shoulder shrug, press-ups (Fig. 34-15), and push-ups are excellent for strength progression of the scapular rotators. The deltoid, latissumus dorsi, and pectoralis major are strengthened with exercises of horizontal abduction with humeral external rotation, press-ups, and scaption. Weight-bearing closed-chain exercises promote dynamic stability with proprioceptive input to increase awareness of joint position through muscular cocontraction, weight shifting, and rhythmic stabilization (Fig. 34-16).

Proprioceptive Neuromuscular Facilitation

Proprioceptive neuromuscular facilitation (PNF) is a rehabilitative method that incorporates individual muscle contractions into a pattern of muscular activity or mass movement. This concept was originally developed by Kabat[17] in the 1950s and later was adapted further by Knott and Voss.[20] The technique employs spiral/diagonal movement patterns that adhere closely to normal functional patterns of movement. Each diagonal has two patterns that are antagonistic to each other.

Advocates of PNF claim that superior results are achieved through the use of facilitation techniques as compared with more traditional approaches. Facilitation techniques such as stretch, traction, approximation, irradiation, manual contacts, verbal commands, and maximal resistance are used throughout the range of motion

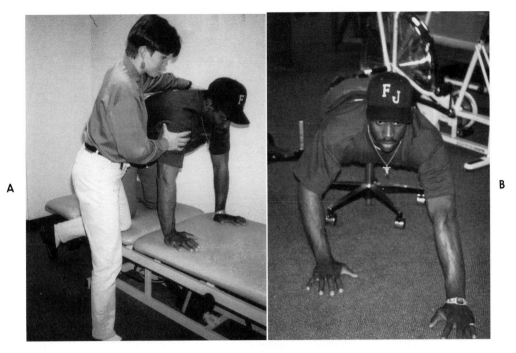

FIG. 34-16. A, Weight-bearing stability challenged in all-fours position. **B,** Stool walks.

in a spiral/diagonal movement pattern for functional performance or isometrically for joint stabilization.[35] The sports therapist determines the degree of range, rate, and volitional control produced by the injured athlete during the specific PNF patterns. Facilitation techniques are coupled with the athlete's voluntary effort to promote response of the agonist and relaxation of the antagonist.[39] Manual contact or hand placement provides a sensory input to the agonistic muscles and is important in promoting the correct muscular activity or providing security to the injured body part. Pressure is applied to the muscle belly or tendon or to the joint itself. It is important that therapists use the correct manual contact and position themselves in the correct diagonal with the direction of the movement. This allows them to properly and smoothly move with the athlete's movements to promote the correct action.

Maximal stretch of the muscles is used initially to facilitate the muscular contraction. This initial stretch is the application of the basic physiologic principle that a greater force is produced after a muscle has been maximally lengthened. Norton and Sahrmann[25] confirmed this commonly accepted principle. They found that greater muscular activity is created when a passive stretch or manual resistance is applied to a muscle at the same time that a voluntary contraction is performed. The stretch reflex can also be initiated by taking the body part past the point of tension by applying a quick stretch at the maximal length of the muscle. The application of a maximal stretch to a muscle can be beneficial in eliciting a motor response but should be used with caution in postinjury or postoperative conditions that may be contraindicated.

Maximal resistance plays a major role in PNF patterns. It has been found to elicit a greater muscular contraction by raising the motor response to threshold level and by recruiting more motor units.[17,18] The resistance can be graded to demand maximal effort throughout the full range of motion or to allow for an isometric contraction. Maximal resistance can also be used to provide overflow (irradiation) from stronger to weaker muscles or to the contralateral extremity.[28] It is evident from observation and analysis of overhead throwing and striking skills that these athletic skill patterns follow closely the basic PNF spiral/diagonal patterns of the shoulder developed by Knott and Voss.[20]

The wind-up phase of the pitching motion involves some internal rotation of the shoulder, followed by external rotation in the cocking phase, and finally completing the motion in the final phase of ball release with internal rotation and adduction. When examining the PNF spiral and diagonal pattern of no. 2 (D2) flexion, the physician finds that it corresponds with the wind-up and cocking phase in the throw. It involves a sequential movement of flexion, abduction, and external rotation. The D2 extension pattern of extension, adduction, and internal rotation correlates closely to the final follow-through phase. Adaptations of these two D2 patterns allow for closer replication of overhead throwing. This can be done by starting with the D2 flexion pattern and adding elbow flexion and finger flexion, followed by the D2 extension with elbow extension patterns (Fig. 34-17).

Although the advantages of PNF outweigh the disadvantages, one drawback to this technique is that it is time consuming and requires the direct hands-on attention of a therapist. In the more advanced stages of the rehabil-

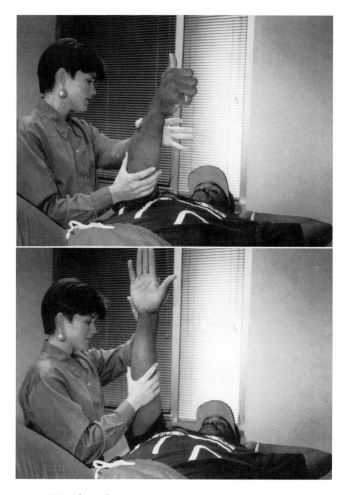

FIG. 34-17. Proprioceptive neuromuscular facilitation.

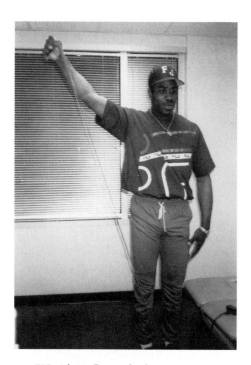

FIG. 34-18. Resisted tubing exercises.

itation program, alternative methods for resistance in PNF patterns can be used to augment the normal hands-on methods. PNF patterns can easily be adapted to resisted rubber tubing (Fig. 34-18), pulley weights, or free weights and therefore do not require the direct attention of the therapist.

PNF patterns and techniques are invaluable to the rehabilitation process and should play an integral role in returning an athlete to normal functional levels. Through the use of angular movement, facilitative input, specifically emphasized resistance, and proper adaptation of PNF techniques, an athlete has the greatest chance for successful return to a normal level of activity.

Progressive Functional Rehabilitation and Return to Throwing

Additional proprioceptive work may be progressed with the use of weighted plyometric balls during stretch-shortening exercise to acquire proper timing and coordination of muscle activity. This principle of eccentric-concentric coupling challenges the body's proprioceptors to facilitate an increased muscle recruitment over a minimal period of time. The rehabilitative challenge lies in incorporating activities to simulate the high-speed ac-

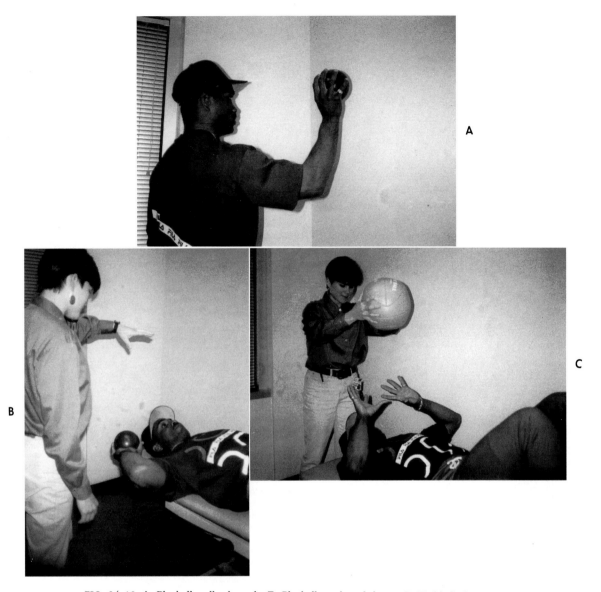

FIG. 34-19. A, Plyoball wall rebounds. **B,** Plyoball catch and throw. **C,** Mediball chest pass.

tions and high-energy loads that are characteristic of the throwing act. In advanced phases of rehabilitation high-energy strengthening exercises may also include isokinetics, medicine ball activities, and an inertia unit. Isokinetics may be used to decrease reciprocal innervation time of agonist and antagonist muscles and provide maximal resistance through a velocity spectrum. The athlete should regain quick explosive reactions that are controlled and efficient. Plyometric drills of medicine ball throws and eccentric exercise emphasis with an inertia unit may provide means of addressing this challenge (Fig. 34-19).

These activities are limited, however, because resultant speeds and motion fall short of replicating the act of throwing in its entirety. Thus a return to throwing should start with rehearsal of the throwing motion to regain proper mechanics involving the entire body; once re-

gained, speed of movement can be increased. Return-to-throwing programs give emphasis to total body warm-up and stretching, proper mechanics, and progression through graduated throwing distances.[21,24] Konin, Axe, and Courson[21] outlined an interval throwing program for football quarterbacks. A baseball interval throwing program modified by Medich[24] (Fig. 34-20) recommends the "crow-hop" (hop, skip, and throw) method to discourage flat-footed tossing from the beginning.

The goal, after injury to the throwing athlete, is that of returning to an optimal preinjury status. The progression of treatment and rehabilitation depends on the athlete's signs and symptoms and response to the selected intervention.[6] Rehabilitation includes restoring normal glenohumeral and scapulothoracic motion needed for throwing, strength progression of the rotator cuff and scapular muscles, postural awareness and correction,

45° Phase

Step 1 A. Warm-up throwing
        B. 45° (25 throws)
        C. Rest 15 minutes
        D. Warm-up throwing
        E. 45° (25 throws)

Step 2 A. Warm-up throwing
        B. 45° (25 throws)
        C. Rest 10 minutes
        D. Warm-up throwing
        E. 45° (25 throws)
        F. Rest 10 minutes
        G. Warm-up throwing
        H. 45° (25 throws)

60° Phase

Step 3 A. Warm-up throwing
        B. 60° (25 throws)
        C. Rest 15 minutes
        D. Warm-up throwing
        E. 60° (25 throws)

Step 4 A. Warm-up throwing
        B. 60° (25 throws)
        C. Rest 10 minutes
        D. Warm-up throwing
        E. 60° (25 throws)
        F. Rest 10 minutes
        G. Warm-up throwing
        H. 60° (25 throws)

90° Phase

Step 5 A. Warm-up throwing
        B. 90° (25 throws)
        C. Rest 15 minutes
        D. Warm-up throwing
        E. 90° (25 throws)

Step 6 A. Warm-up throwing
        B. 90° (25 throws)

        C. Rest 10 minutes
        D. Warm-up throwing
        E. 90° (25 throws)
        F. Rest 10 minutes
        G. Warm-up throwing
        H. 90° (25 throws)

120° Phase

Step 7 A. Warm-up throwing
        B. 120° (25 throws)
        C. Rest 15 minutes
        D. Warm-up throwing
        E. 120° (25 throws)

Step 8 A. Warm-up throwing
        B. 120° (25 throws)
        C. Rest 10 minutes
        D. Warm-up throwing
        E. 120° (25 throws)
        F. Rest 10 minutes
        G. Warm-up throwing
        H. 120° (25 throws)

150° Phase

Step 9 A. Warm-up throwing
        B. 150° (25 throws)
        C. Rest 15 minutes
        D. Warm-up throwing
        E. 150° (25 throws)

Step 10 A. Warm-up throwing
        B. 150° (25 throws)
        C. Rest 10 minutes
        D. Warm-up throwing
        E. 150° (25 throws)
        F. Rest 10 minutes
        G. Warm-up throwing
        H. 150° (25 throws)

180° Phase

Step 11 A. Warm-up throwing
        B. 180° (25 throws)
        C. Rest 15 minutes
        D. Warm-up throwing
        E. 180° (25 throws)

Step 12 A. Warm-up throwing
        B. 180° (25 throws)
        C. Rest 10 minutes
        D. Warm-up throwing
        E. 180° (25 throws)
        F. Rest 10 minutes
        G. Warm-up throwing
        H. 180° (25 throws)

Step 13 A. Warm-up throwing
        B. 180° (25 throws)
        C. Rest 10 minutes
        D. Warm-up throwing
        E. 180° (25 throws)
        F. Rest 10 minutes
        G. Warm-up throwing
        H. 180° (50 throws)

Step 14 Begin throwing off the mound with monitoring from pitching coach or return to respective position with throwing velocity gradually increased to game competition levels.

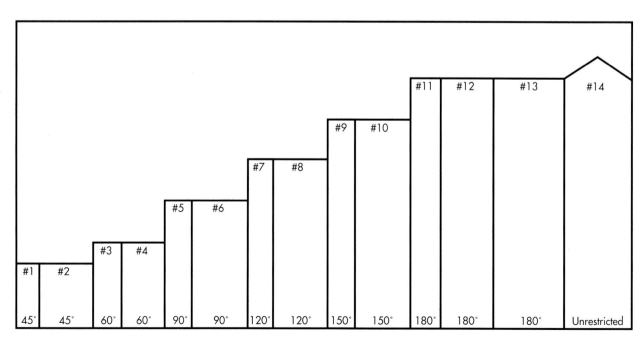

FIG. 34-20. Baseball interval throwing program. (From Medich G: *Sports Med Update* 2:1, 1987.)

correction of muscle imbalances, restoring joint proprioception and dynamic stabilization, conditioning for the entire body, and a gradual progressive return to throwing.[12,36]

REFERENCES

1. Andrews JR, Carson WG: Glenoid labrum tears related to the long head of the biceps, *Am J Sports Med* 13:337, 1985.
2. Andrews JR, McLeod WD: Mechanisms of shoulder injuries, *Phys Ther* 66:1906, 1966.
3. Axe MJ: *Comparison of baseball and football throwing,* Paper presented at Injuries to the Throwing Arm Conference, Phoenix, 1985.
4. Blackburn TA, McLeod WD, White B: EMG analysis of posterior rotator cuff exercises, *J Nat Athl Train Assoc* 25:40, 1990.
5. Bonci C, Sloane B, Middleton K: Nonsurgical/surgical rehabilitation of the unstable shoulder, *J Sports Rehabil* 1:150, 1992.
6. Coleman AE, Axe MJ, Andrews JR: Performance profile-directed simulated game: an objective functional evaluation for baseball pitchers, *J Orthop Sports Phys Ther* 9:101, 1987.
7. Doody S, Freedman L, Waterland J: Shoulder movements during abduction in the scapula plane, *Arch Phys Med Rehabil* 51:595, 1970.
8. Freedman L, Munro R: Abduction of the arm in the scapular plane: scapular and glenohumeral movements, *J Bone Joint Surg* 48A:1503, 1966.
9. Garth WP, Allman FL, Armstrong WS: Occult anterior subluxations of the shoulder in the non-contact sports, *Am J Sports Med* 15:579, 1987.
10. Hughston JC: Functional anatomy of the shoulder. In Andrews JR, Carson WG (eds): *Injuries to the throwing arm,* Philadelphia, 1985, WB Saunders.
11. Inman VT, Saunders M, Abbott LC: Observations on the function of the shoulder joint, *J Bone Joint Surg* 26:1, 1944.
12. Jobe FW, Moynes DR: Delineation of diagnostic criteria in a rehabilitation program for rotator cuff injuries, *Am J Sports Med* 10:336, 1982.
13. Jobe FW et al: EMG analysis of the shoulder in throwing and pitching: a preliminary report, *Am J Sports Med* 11:3, 1983.
14. Jobe FW et al: EMG analysis of the shoulder in pitching: a second report, *Am J Sports Med* 12:218, 1984.
15. Jobe FW et al: Electromyography and motion analysis of the upper extremity in sports, *Phys Ther* 66:1905, 1986.
16. Jobe FW, Pink M: Shoulder injuries in the athlete: the instability continuum and treatment, *J Hand Ther,* Apr-June:69, 1991.
17. Kabat H: Proprioceptive facilitation in therapeutic exercise: In Lichts E (ed): *Therapeutic exercise,* New Haven, 1965, Elizabeth Lichtl.
18. Kempf C: *Injuries around the diamond,* Paper presented at Spring Sports Medicine Conference, Nashville, 1994.
19. King JW, Bielsford JH, Tullos HS: Analysis of the pitching arm of the professional baseball pitcher, *Clin Orthop* 67:116, 1969.
20. Knott M, Voss DE: *Proprioceptive neuromuscular facilitation: patterns and techniques,* New York, 1956, Harper & Row.
21. Konin J, Axe M, Courson R: Interval throwing program for quarterbacks, *J Sports Rehabil* 1:3, 1993.
22. Maitland GD: *Peripheral manipulation,* London, 1977, Butterworth.
23. McLeod WD: The pitching mechanism. In Zarins B, Andrew JR, Carson WG (eds): *Injuries to the throwing arm,* Philadelphia, 1985, WB Saunders.
24. Medich G: *The interval throwing program, Sports Med Update* 2:1, 1987.
25. Norton BJ, Sahrmann SA: Reflex and voluntary electromyographic activity in patients with hemiparesis, *Phys Ther* 58:951, 1978.
26. Pappas AM: Biomechanics of baseball pitching, *Am J Sports Med* 13:216, 1985.
27. Perry J: Anatomy and biomechanics of the shoulder in throwing, swimming, gymnastics, and tennis, *Clin Sports Med* 2:247, 1983.
28. Pink M: Contralateral effects of upper extremity proprioceptive neuromuscular facilitation patterns, *Phys Ther* 61:1158, 1981.
29. Poppen NK, Walker PS: Normal and abnormal motion of the shoulder, *J Bone Joint Surg* 58A:195, 1976.
30. Prentice WE, Cooma E: The use of proprioceptive neuromuscular facilitation techniques in the rehabilitation of sports-related injury, *Phys Ther* 21:26, 1986.
31. Rollins J et al: Water polo injuries to the upper extremity. In Zarins B, Andrews J, Carson WG (eds): *Injuries to the throwing arm,* Philadelphia, 1985, WB Saunders.
32. Saal JA: Rehabilitation of throwing and tennis-related shoulder injuries. In Saal JA (ed): *Rehabilitation of sports injuries: state of the art reviews,* Philadelphia, 1987, Hanley and Belfus.
33. Saha AK: *Theory of shoulder mechanism,* Springfield, Ill, 1961, Charles C Thomas.
34. Sain J, Andrews JR: Proper pitching techniques. In Zarins B, Andrews JR, Carson WG (eds): *Injuries to the throwing arm,* Philadelphia, 1985, WB Saunders.
35. Svendsen DA, Matyas TA: Facilitation of the isometric voluntary contraction with traction, *Am J Phys Med* 62:27, 1983.
36. Townsend H et al: Electromyographic analysis of the glenohumeral muscles during a baseball rehabilitation program, *J Sports Med* 19:3, 1991.
37. Tullos HS, King JW: Throwing mechanism in sports, *Orthop Clin North Am* 4:709, 1973.
38. Turkel SJ et al: Stabilizing mechanisms preventing anterior dislocation of the glenohumeral joint, *J Bone Joint Surg* 63A:1208, 1981.
39. Voss DE, Ionta MK, Myers BJ: *Proprioceptive neuromuscular facilitation patterns and techniques,* Philadelphia, 1985, Harper & Row.
40. Wick H et al: A kinematic comparison between baseball pitching and football passing, *Sports Med Update* 6(2):13, 1991.

CHAPTER 35

Evaluation, Treatment, and Prevention of Elbow Injuries in Throwing Athletes

James R. Andrews
Scott P. Schemmel
James A. Whiteside
Laura A. Timmerman

The uninjured elbow in the throwing athlete works as a finely tuned articulation to deliver the final momentum to the forearm, hand, and eventually to the object being thrown with great acceleration. The injured elbow in the throwing athlete can present with symptoms of pain, tenderness, swelling, and limitation of motion, all in response to repetitive valgus vector forces and stresses. When impaired, the elbow responds very much like the shoulder in that momentary prolapse and pain during acceleration and at release point prevent the thrower from achieving both normal velocity and control.

The elbow joint is unique in that it allows for flexion and extension because of the ulnar hinge relationship with the humerus and rotation because of the radiocapitellar and radioulnar articulations. To understand the pathophysiologic etiology of elbow problems in throwers, including pitchers, quarterbacks, and javelin throwers, one must visualize the mechanics of throwing motion, which has been extensively studied in baseball pitchers. Thus the baseball pitcher serves as an excellent clinical model for the study of other throwers.

BIOMECHANICS

A thorough understanding of elbow joint biomechanics is essential for any physician involved in the treatment of the throwing athlete. This knowledge, combined with a comprehensive grasp of elbow anatomy, serves as the cornerstone for the diagnosis and treatment of elbow injuries.

Slocum[51] was one of the first to classify throwing injuries into medial tension and lateral compression phenomena. Numerous articles that followed confirmed and expanded on this concept. Essentially, all pathologic conditions of the elbow resulting from the repetitive act of throwing can be related to the excessive tensile and compressive forces that are generated about this joint. Throughout this chapter, as evaluation, treatment, and prevention of elbow injuries are discussed, understanding of the biomechanical concepts serves as a reference framework.

Throwing athletes, regardless of their specific sport, suffer similar injuries to the elbow. The pathophysiology of these injuries has been best described in baseball play-

ers generally and pitchers specifically. Analysis of the pitching mechanism allows for the most comprehensive understanding of throwing mechanics. This mechanism consists of several phases: wind-up, cocking, acceleration, deceleration, and follow-through.[29,33,59]

Wind-Up

The first phase of the pitching mechanism is the wind-up. In this phase the pitcher prepares for delivery of the ball by assuming correct body posture and balance. Initially, both feet are planted. The weight is then shifted back on to the ipsilateral leg with the contralateral leg brought up into a tucked position with the hip and knee flexed to about 90 degrees. The hips and shoulders are externally rotated 90 degrees or greater to the intended line of the throw. The elbow is flexed, the forearm pronated, and the wrist extended. During this preparatory phase there is little activity in any of the muscle groups about the elbow or in the forearm (Fig. 35-1, *A*).[50]

Cocking

The wind-up phase is followed by the cocking phase, which as the name implies involves positioning, or cocking, the body, arm, and ball in such a manner to provide the optimum acceleration for ball delivery. The contralateral leg is extended out of its tucked up position and planted out in front of the body. This initiates internal rotation of the previously externally rotated pelvis and is followed by internal rotation of the shoulder and a forward thrusting of the chest. The humerus is brought up into a 90-degree abducted position and is maximally externally rotated. The elbow is flexed approximately 90 degrees, and the wrist and metacarpophalangeal joints are extended.[50] The forearm is slightly pronated initially and is fully pronated by the end of this phase for a fast ball, though less so for a curve ball. Electromyographic (EMG) studies and high-speed motion analysis indicate that minor changes in forearm rotation as well as in wrist and finger position are the primary determinants of the spin placed on the ball during the delivery of the pitch.[50] This concept was recognized by astute pitching coaches long before technical analysis was possible.[45] These minor changes are in contrast to the highly improbable proposed active pronation or supination of the forearm during the high-speed event of ball acceleration and release.[1,44] By assuming the cocking posture, the hand and ball are positioned far behind the arm and body. This allows for extrinsic tension to be applied to those muscle groups that will be used subsequently to accelerate the ball in the next phase. In the terminal stage of cocking, the shoulder and chest smoothly move forward, with the hand and ball left behind, thus maximally increasing the extrinsic muscle tension already developed.

The muscle activity about the elbow during the cocking phase is moderately intense.[50] Principal muscles involved in assuming the position include the wrist extensors, the metacarpophalangeal joint extensors, and the brachioradialis and pronator teres. A curve ball requires less activity in the brachioradialis and pronator teres than does a fast ball; however, a curve ball requires more supinator and wrist extensor activity than does a fast ball.[50]

Five phases of pitching

- Wind-up
- Cocking
- Acceleration
- Deceleration
- Follow-through

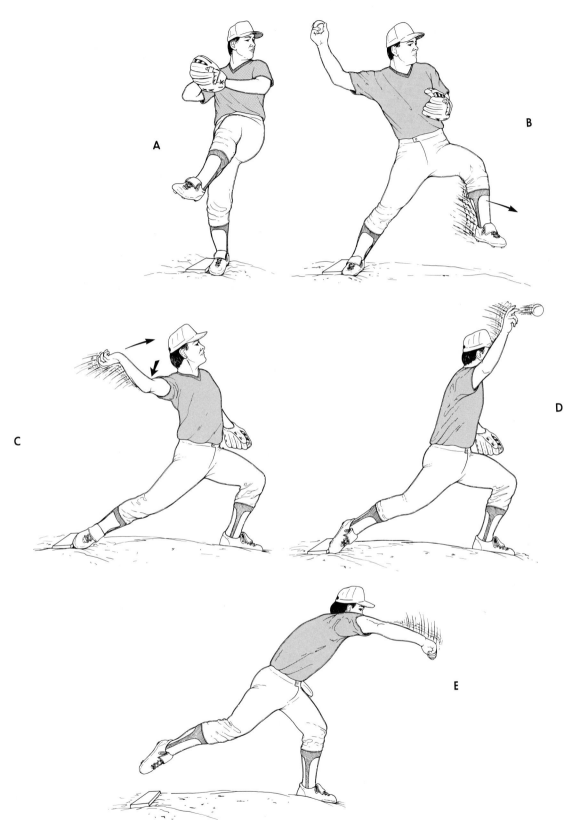

FIG. 35-1. Five phases of pitching. **A,** Wind-up phase. **B,** Cocking phase. **C,** Acceleration phase. **D,** Deceleration and ball release phase. **E,** Follow-through phase.

Interpretation of these variances for the different pitches is being evaluated on an ongoing basis.[6] Decreased EMG activity in the brachioradialis does not necessarily indicate less elbow flexion for a curve ball. It simply reflects less flexion force with no dependence on elbow angle. The fine technical differences in muscle use and joint positioning with the delivery of various pitches and throwing techniques will be fully delineated only after further integration of EMG studies and high-speed motion analysis (Fig. 35-1, *B*).

Muscle activity and pitch selection

- Curve ball: more supinator and wrist extensor activity
- Fast ball: more brachioradialis and pronator teres activity

---

Acceleration

The acceleration phase is that component of the pitching mechanism that occurs between the cocking phase and ball release. Acceleration refers specifically to the forces that are imparted to the ball and not the various arm segments during the phase. The trunk and, at times, the humerus go through deceleration phases during acceleration of the ball. Over the course of approximately 50 to 80 msec the ball is accelerated from a stationary position to a speed in excess of 80 miles per hour.[33] This first involves the transfer of momentum generated within the body of the pitcher as he moves forward through this phase. This momentum is transferred in a whiplike fashion sequentially from the trunk to the shoulder, the humerus, the elbow, and the forearm. Finally, the momentum is imparted to the hand and ball as the release point is approached.

The forward motion at the chest and shoulder that was present at the termination of the cocking phase is stopped, and the pitcher moves his trunk forward as he transfers his weight onto the forward-planted contralateral foot and leg. This allows for an orderly transfer of the anterior momentum from the legs to the trunk and into the shoulder. At the same time, during the first half of this acceleration phase, the anterior muscles, primarily the pectoralis and subscapularis, contract to accelerate the humerus anteriorly along a horizontal plane. Also the shoulder internal rotators, subscapularis, latissimus dorsi, and teres major contract to start the internal rotation of the humerus. Thus at this point in the acceleration phase tremendous forward forces are generated in the humerus. The forearm, hand, and ball, however, are essentially left behind. This results in the elbow being placed in a position of extreme valgus, generating significant tensile forces across the medial side of the elbow joint and compressive loads at the lateral side of the joint.

At the halfway point of this phase the rate of adduction of the humerus is decreased by imposition of a deceleration from the teres minor, infraspinatus, and supraspinatus muscles. As the humerus decelerates, it allows for a transfer of momentum to the forearm, thus adding to the rate of internal rotation and further accel-

erating the ball. As the forearm and wrist accelerate, the centrifugal force generated begins to impose an extension force across the elbow joint. If left unprotected at this point, the elbow would rapidly and forcibly hyperextend. However, the rate of extension is regulated by the active participation of the elbow flexors, particularly the biceps and the brachialis muscles. At this point in the acceleration phase a large degree of torque is present at the elbow joint and is coupled with a high rate of extension, both of which combine to cause relatively high shear forces to be imposed on the articular cartilage. It is these shear stresses that can initiate articular surface degeneration in the joint.

As the release point is approached, the forearm, hand, and ball are accelerated to their maximum velocity, which occurs at the end of the acceleration phase. The grip on the ball is loosened, and over the next 6 to 10 msec the ball leaves the hand.[33] Because of the high rate of forearm internal rotation and elbow extension, the hand will rotate down off the ball, and, through proper positioning of the fingers, the pitcher can impart the desired spin. This is called the release point, and from this moment on the relative arm motion must be decelerated (Fig. 35-1, *C*).

Deceleration

The momentum developed throughout the acceleration phase results in an outward force on the arm of approximately 300 pounds as the deceleration phase is entered.[33] This 300-pound force must be opposed through active muscle contraction to maintain some appositional stability of the glenohumeral joint and to oppose the forward motion of the shoulder. In addition to the distracting force on the glenohumeral joint, the internal rotation forces in the humerus generated through the acceleration phase must be opposed. The external rotators of the shoulder, as well as the posterior deltoid, contract to stop the arm. The deceleration forces are significantly large and act over a very short duration, making them difficult to measure, but in general the deceleration torques generated about the shoulder are greater than those of the acceleration phase.[33]

In summary, the forces that must be counteracted through deceleration include humeral internal rotation, glenohumeral distraction, and elbow extension. Essentially all the shoulder muscles contract violently at this point; in addition, large muscle groups, particularly the biceps, brachialis, and brachioradialis, contract in an attempt to slow elbow extension velocity. If the elbow extension velocity is not decelerated entirely, hyperextension injuries common to the elbow can occur. Additionally, if the elbow extension is decelerated too rapidly, the extremely high flexion forces required can overstress the long head of the biceps muscle and its tendon (Fig. 35-1, *D*).

Follow-Through

Finally, in the follow-through phase of throwing, the body moves forward with the arm, reducing the distraction forces applied to the shoulder and relieving the tension generated in the rotator cuff muscles. As the shoulder, trunk, and ipsilateral leg move forward in the follow-

through, the pitcher is able to maintain his balance and position himself for his next action or reaction.

Although the pitching mechanism has been observed and analyzed by many authors over the last 25 years, only recently has the specific muscle activity occurring about the elbow during the various phases of pitching been identified. Recent EMG analysis, combined with high-speed photography carried out by Sisto et al,[50] has increased our understanding of the muscle forces generated about the elbow during the throwing act. Measurable muscle activities about the elbow have been shown to be only mild to moderate throughout all phases of pitching. It appears that the muscles act to position the elbow and forearm into a posture that allows maximum transfer of the energy and momentum developed by the large muscles of the shoulder girdle and trunk. Rapid, forceful contraction of the muscles about the joint as a means of enhancing ball delivery does not seem to occur. In addition, forceful contractions of muscles about the joint as a means of altering ball delivery (i.e., as with a curve ball) do not seem to occur. Rather, ball grip, combined with minor changes in muscle activity levels that allow for an alteration in elbow and wrist positioning before ball release, appears to be all that is necessary to generate the desired changes in ball delivery that are seen with different types of pitches.

Pitch selection mechanics

- Ball grip affects pitch type
- Forceful muscle contraction to alter joint movement *does not* occur

---

It has been often theorized that forceful firing of the flexor-pronator mass to promote rapid forearm pronation and wrist flexion contributes to medial elbow morbidity.[1] This has been associated particularly with little league elbow as well as pathologic changes in pitchers who compete at higher levels. However, recent EMG studies (discussed previously), combined with our knowledge of forces generated across the throwing elbow biomechanically, lead us to believe that medial elbow morbidity is less likely to be caused by forceful, active contraction of the flexor-pronator muscle group mass and more likely to be secondary to significant passive distraction generated across the elbow during the acceleration phase of throwing. The wrist and hand musculature are very important in determining the type of pitch. However, it is difficult to study these structures with EMG and motion analysis because of the close proximity of the structures and the extremely rapid speeds of the pitching motion.

FUNCTIONAL ANATOMY

The anatomy of the elbow should be studied with respect to the stability it offers in resistance to large valgus and extension forces generated by the act of throwing. The ulnar collateral ligament has been shown to be the primary stabilizer of the elbow.[36,47,60] Secondary stabilizers are both bony and soft-tissue structures.[36] Bony

contributions include the articulations of the olecranon, olecranon fossa complex, and the radial head and capitellum. The secondary soft-tissue stabilizer is primarily the forearm flexor-pronator muscle mass arising from the medial epicondyle of the humerus. Rather than simply noting where these structures exist relative to one another, it is important to understand how they function to stabilize the joint against the previously noted forces.

Elbow stability

Primary
- Ulnar collateral ligament

Secondary
- Bony articulations: olecranon, olecranon fossa complex, radial head, and capitellum
- Soft tissue: flexor-pronator muscle group

Osseous Structures
Humeroulnar Articulation

The humeroulnar joint provides for elbow flexion and extension. The humeral contribution consists of the trochlea, the coronoid fossa anteriorly, and the olecranon fossa posteriorly. The trochlea is covered by hyaline cartilage over a 330-degree arch, and it projects anteriorly from the shaft of the humerus at an angle of approximately 30 degrees. In the AP plane the trochlea has a 6-degree valgus slope, which, along with the proximal ulna, determines the carrying angle at the elbow. A 3- to 5-degree internal rotation of the trochlea with respect to the epicondylar line has been described.[35] It appears to result in a 5-degree external rotation of the ulna in terminal extension and a 5-degree internal rotation in initiating flexion from full extension. The ulna's contribution to this joint consists of the following: (1) the trochlear notch for articulation with the trochlea, (2) the olecranon process for articulation with the olecranon fossa, and (3) the coronoid process for articulation with its corresponding fossa in the humerus. The trochlear notch has a 30-degree posterior inclination that corresponds with the 30-degree anterior rotation of the distal humerus. This configuration allows for up to 150 degrees of flexion through the humeroulnar articulation.

In the throwing athlete it is not the hyaline cartilage–covered trochlea or the trochlear notch that serves as the primary site of bony pathologic change. Unlike the articular surfaces of the radius and the capitellum, the articular surfaces of the trochlea and trochlear notch rarely serve as the source of condylar defects, chondromalacia, or articular loose bodies. Rather the olecranon process, the corresponding olecranon fossa, and, to a lesser extent, the coronoid fossa are affected.[2,62] These frequently mentioned valgus stresses are stabilized in a secondary manner by the olecranon within the olecranon fossa over the last 30 degrees of extension. These valgus stresses result in the abutment of the medial aspect of the olecranon process against the medial olecranon fossa. Hyperextension forces cause straight posterior and posterolateral abutment of the olecranon in the olecranon fossa, leading to subsequent osteophyte formation in these ar-

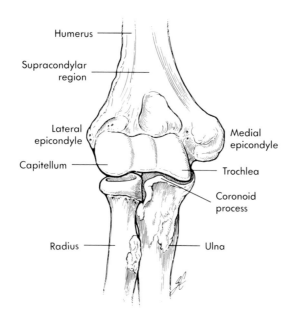

FIG. 35-2. Frontal view of elbow, showing the large coronoid fossa, smaller radial fossa, and trochlea medial to the capitellum.

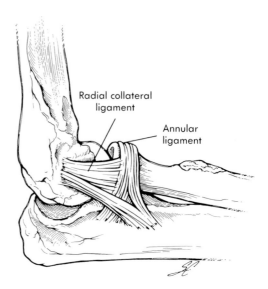

FIG. 35-3. Radial collateral ligament is often less well defined surgically than anatomically.

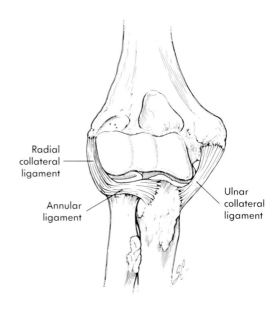

FIG. 35-4. Frontal view reveals distal attachment of the ulnar collateral ligament to the medial margin of the coronoid process and a portion of the radial collateral ligament/annular ligament complex attachment to the lateral margin of the ulna.

eas. These changes are discussed further under posterior injuries. Anteriorly, abutment of the coronoid process within the coronoid fossa can result in osteophyte formation on the coronoid process or within the fossa itself (Fig. 35-2).

Radiocapitellar Articulation

Unlike the trochlear ulnar articulation, the radiocapitellar joint is essentially unconstrained. The capitellum is hemispheric and covered by hyaline cartilage. The radial head, with its hyaline cartilage surface, is concave and articulates with the capitellum. It is free to rotate about the capitellum in pronation and supination. Rotation can be completed through an arch of 160 to 170 degrees. As with the trochlear ulnar joint, radiocapitellar joint pathologic change is determined by the force patterns developed in the throwing elbow. The radiocapitellar joint is a site of compression loads and serves as a secondary stabilizer to these valgus forces.[36,47] Articular cartilage changes, including dramatic chondral defects, can be found in both the radial head articular cartilage and in that of the capitellum.

Proximal Radioulnar Articulation

The proximal radioulnar articulation consists of the radial head, the annular ligament, and the radial notch of the ulna. Contact of this articulation covers only one fifth of the radial head at any one time, with the annular ligament providing the remainder of coverage and support to this joint. The radioulnar joint is a very infrequent source of bony pathologic change in the throwing elbow.

Ligamentous Structures

The ligamentous anatomy about the elbow reflects the dominant forces that occur at this joint, not only in the act of throwing but also in its everyday use at work and at home. For most activities, primary stresses placed across the elbow are in a valgus direction with varus stresses to the elbow being infrequent.[35]

Radial (Lateral) Collateral Ligament

These types of stresses are reflected in the phylogenetic development of the radial collateral ligament, which varies in size and course from individual to individual (Fig. 35-3).

The radial collateral ligament originates from the lateral epicondyle and inserts primarily into the annular ligament around the radius, where a few nonfunctional fibers also attach to the radial notch of the ulna (Fig. 35-4). This ligament does not perform the function of a true

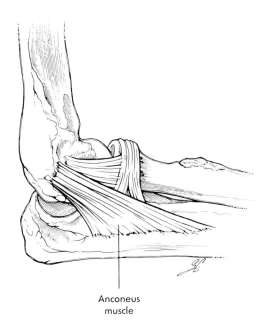

FIG. 35-5. Anconeus muscle acts as a secondary support structure to the radial collateral ligament.

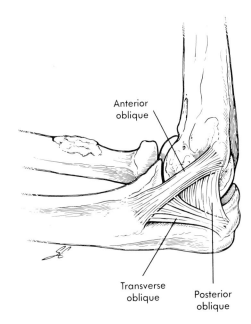

FIG. 35-6. Normal anatomic alignment of the three components of the ulnar collateral ligament.

ligament with bone-to-bone attachments. However, the anconeus muscle, with its origin just posterior to that of the radial collateral ligament on the lateral epicondyle of the humerus, inserts onto the radial border of the ulna and assumes the function of a dynamic collateral ligament attaching bone to bone. Thus the anconeus appears to aid in elbow stabilization against a varus stress (Fig. 35-5).[60] The radial collateral ligament structure has been shown to be important in resisting not only varus stress, but also posterolateral pivotal stresses to the elbow.[42]

Radial collateral ligament

- Origin: lateral epicondyle
- Insertion: annular ligament; radial notch of ulna
- Supplements: anconeus muscle
- Function: weak stabilizer against varus stress, posterolateral stability

---

Ulnar (Medial) Collateral Ligament

In contrast, the ulnar (medial) collateral ligament is a well-defined and consistent structure that would be more aptly considered as a ligamentous complex. It consists of an anterior oblique component that originates from the undersurface of the medial epicondyle of the humerus and inserts into the ulna just posterior to the coronoid process on the sublime tubercle. The posterior oblique component arises from the same point and passes posterior and distal and inserts into the ulnar surface of the midolecranon. A less well developed transverse ligament courses from the insertion of the posterior oblique to the insertion of the anterior oblique bundle and deepens the trochlear notch of the ulna.

The anterior oblique ligament is taut in both flexion and extension. It does not lie on the axis of elbow flexion, but, because of its rectangular shape, its anterior fibers are taut in extension while its posterior fibers become taut in flexion.[47] Thus, as a whole, the anterior oblique component is taut throughout the full range of motion. Conversely, the posterior oblique segment of this ligament is taut only in flexion and is slack in extension. Sectioning of the posterior oblique ligament does not alter the stability of the elbow to valgus stress if the anterior oblique ligament is intact. Furthermore, sectioning of the anterior oblique ligament results in elbow instability even when the posterior oblique component is intact.[47] The transverse oblique ligament represents essentially a thickening of the joint capsule and plays no real role in joint stability (Fig. 35-6).

Histology studies of the ulnar collateral ligament showed that the anterior bundle is composed of two layers.[54] A deep substantial layer of collagen fibrils is within the capsular walls of tissue. External to this deep layer is a thin superficial layer. In the posterior bundle only one inner layer exists within the capsular walls. There were two destined and separate anterior and posterior bundles. The histology of the ligament corresponded to the clinical findings of an undersurface tear of the anterior bundle.

The ulnar collateral ligament is the cornerstone of the throwing elbow, and its importance and that of the anterior oblique fibers in the stabilization of this joint

---

Ulnar collateral ligament components

- Anterior oblique
- Posterior oblique
- Transverse

---

against the forces incurred in throwing cannot be over-emphasized. The incompetence of this structure, acute or chronic, is the initiator for much of the morbidity associated with the throwing elbow.

Musculotendinous Structures

The remaining structures about the elbow—the musculotendinous insertions and origins and the major nerves and vessels—will not be exhaustively covered here because they are well known to the surgeon. Some of this anatomy is reviewed elsewhere in this chapter during presentation of nerve entrapment syndromes about the elbow. There are, however, some pertinent anatomic entities that deserve discussion.

Flexors

The flexors of the elbow joint—the brachialis, biceps, brachioradialis—are not commonly involved in the generation of symptoms at the elbow. Their role in elbow deceleration is essential in the throwing act, and it is through this mechanism that they are subject to repetitive forces that may result in symptoms. The most common musculotendinous unit about the elbow involved in throwing that demonstrates pathologic change is that of the superficial flexor-pronator group. This muscle group, which takes its tendinous origin from the medial epicondyle, consists of the flexor carpi radialis, flexor digitorum sublimis, pronator teres, palmaris longus, and flexor carpi ulnaris muscles. This common flexor-pronator muscle mass serves as a dynamic secondary stabilizer of the elbow against valgus forces. As such, the forces that produce pathologic changes within this structure are primarily tensile ones.[14,26]

Extensors

On the lateral side of the elbow the brachioradialis, extensor carpi radialis longus and brevis, and a portion of the common extensor tendons originate from the distal humerus. As noted earlier, the brachioradialis serves as a flexor of the elbow, and in the throwing athlete its importance lies in its deceleration of elbow extension that occurs during the throwing act. The extensor carpi radialis longus and brevis are important because they relate to the lateral epicondylitis phenomenon that occurs in many athletes.[14,26,38]

Growth and Ossification Centers

In little league and adolescent elbows the yet unfused secondary center of ossification of the medial epicondyle is subject to the same valgus forces as in the mature athlete; as a result, separation or fragmentation of this growth center can occur.[1,13] It is not within the scope of this chapter to fully review the development of the secondary centers of ossification about the elbow.[23] Briefly, however, it is important to note that the capitellum, trochlear, and lateral epicondylar growth centers unite into one common growth center before their union with the distal humerus. The capitellar growth center first appears at approximately 1 year of age; the trochlear and lateral epicondylar growth centers appear around age 10. These three centers fuse together at approximately 13 years in the female and 15 years in the male and subse-

quently unite to the distal humerus at approximately 16 years of age in both sexes. The trochlear growth cartilage rises from two separate secondary ossification centers, which should not be mistaken for fragmentation of this growth cartilage during this time. The medial epicondylar growth center's appearance and time of ultimate union with the humerus are the most variable. It usually appears between the ages of 7 and 8 in the female and 8 and 9 in the male. It is the last of the growth centers to fuse to the distal humerus, doing so at approximately age 14 in the female and 18 in the male. In comparison with the other growth centers about the distal humerus, it is more strongly subjected to repetitive tensile loads accompanying the throwing act than are the other growth centers. As such, it is the growth center that is most predisposed to injury in throwing sports.[1,44] Finally, the radial head growth center appears in the female and male at approximately ages 6 and 7, and fusion occurs at ages 14 and 16, respectively.

Neuroanatomy

Although tardy ulnar nerve palsy and ulnar neuritis as related to the throwing elbow are discussed under nerve lesions, a detailed understanding of the course of the nerve and its anatomic relationships at the elbow is imperative.[23] In the arm the ulnar nerve pierces the medial intermuscular septum, passes from the anterior to the posterior compartment of the arm, and lies on the front of the medial head of the triceps muscle. The superior ulnar collateral artery passes with the ulnar nerve behind the medial epicondyle. The nerve enters the forearm after passing posterior to the epicondyle and dives between the two heads of origin of the flexor carpi ulnaris muscle that arise from the ulna and humerus. The lateral bed of the ulnar nerve as it passes behind the medial epicondyle directly overlies the medial aspect of the olecranon and the olecranon tip. It is important to realize this close approximation in differentiating the various causes of ulnar neuritis in the throwing elbow. In addition to these classic causes of ulnar nerve pathologic change in the elbow (which are well described in many textbooks), it is important to understand that pathologic changes that take place on the medial border of the olecranon, as well as its tip, can have a direct effect on the ulnar nerve.

PHYSICAL EXAMINATION

The ancient medical dictum that obtaining a factual chronicle of events surrounding an injury is essential to a successful diagnosis holds great truth in the care of the throwing athlete with elbow problems. It is not sufficient just to know the general area of involvement and that pitching aggravates the problem. Rather, the history must produce specifically *what* the problem is—pain and its characteristics and/or restriction of motion and disability. Then, as clearly as can be noted, the history must produce *where* the primary location of this symptom complex is, *when* it was first observed, and *when* it became a limiting factor. The mechanisms that precipitated the problem need to be determined. *How* did it happen? Was the onset acute or insidious, in only one phase

of throwing, or after changing playing position, training, or technique? In addition to basic information of age, length of time in sport, and level of sports participation, the projected timetable of the athlete should be documented (e.g., red-shirted this season, need to report for winter league, and so on) to fashion a treatment regimen that is suitable for all concerned within the bounds of judicious, expert care.

Inspection

This initial phase of examination requires exposure of the trunk and arms in a comfortable, unobstructed setting to evaluate the neck, shoulder, and upper arm as subtle sites of pathologic change that can affect the elbow. A measurable exercise-induced muscular hypertrophy is often noted in the triceps, biceps, and extensor and flexor forearm muscles bilaterally as a result of weight training. However, unilateral hypertrophy is usually noted in the sport-dominant arm. In the anatomic, extended position, the pitching arm may appear longer and bigger and may have a carrying angle of 10 to 15 degrees greater than the nondominant arm. Confirmation of variances, if needed, can be made radiographically.

Common throwing arm changes

- Unilateral muscle hypertrophy (triceps, biceps, forearm flexors, and forearm extensors)
- Increased carrying angle
- Flexion contracture

Visualization

Visualization of the exposed skin about the elbow may contribute to the diagnosis by allowing for the detection of the following: (1) areas of contusion or ecchymoses, (2) redness caused by cellulitis, (3) scarring secondary to healed burns or surgery, (4) blanching from vascular insufficiency, (5) petechiae from platelet deficiencies, (6) eczematoid or psoriatic rashes, and (7) rheumatoid nodules. Further information can be obtained by noting uneven surface contours resulting from bulging as in olecranon bursitis, posterior dislocation, or a depression in the antecubital space as a result of rupture of the bicipital tendon from its insertion on the radius.

Range of Motion

Range of motion about the elbow is measured in flexion/extension and pronation/supination. Ordinarily, except in congenital laxity and Marfan's syndrome, the elbow extends only to 0 degrees and flexes to about 150 degrees or less if impeded by increased muscle mass. Hyperextension of the elbow, though common in gymnasts, is rare in throwers. Instead, incomplete extension (flexion contracture) tends to occur and often is asymptomatic. This flexion contracture can result from either capsular sprain, flexor muscle mass strain anteriorly, or intraarticular loose bodies, whereas the inability to completely flex indicates triceps strain, capsular tightness, or loose bodies.

Possible causes of elbow flexion contracture

- Repetitive capsular sprain
- Flexor muscle strain
- Intraarticular loose bodies

Pronation and supination should allow for about 150 degrees of forearm rotation. Failure to do so may reflect radiocapitellar osteochondritis, loose bodies, or motor nerve entrapment with resulting biceps, pronator teres, pronator quadratus, and supinator muscle paresis. Others include causes of decreased range of motion, edema and other swelling as a result of muscle fatigue, and increased forearm fascial compartment pressure resulting from overuse.

Palpation

The skin about the elbow should be palpated to evaluate temperature and sensation. Inflammation may cause an increase in temperature. When contracted, forearm muscles should produce a firm, even tone without localized herniation of a fascial defect or a ganglion. Brachial artery pulsation should be palpated, and deep tendon reflexes of the biceps, triceps, and brachioradialis muscles should be obtained by percussion.

Deep palpation about the elbow may reveal sites of unreported tenderness resulting from traction osteophyte formation on the medial side of the humeral ulnar joint, or swelling adjacent to the head of the radius caused by increased intracapsular pressure, or in the distal, medial area of the humerus from an anomalous supracondylar process.

The course of the ulnar collateral ligament anterior bundle should be carefully palpated. Tenderness at the medial epicondyle insertion, or more commonly at the distal ulnar insertion, can indicate a ligament injury. The course of the ulnar nerve should also be palpated and a Tinel's test performed. It is essential to compare tenderness to palpation to the normal elbow, since tenderness may be present solely due to the examination itself. For completeness, palpation is systematically carried out over the medial, anterior, lateral, and posterior aspects of the elbow to determine the specific areas of pain and/or limited motion.

Stability

Integrity of elbow function depends on the ligamentous structures medially, laterally, and anteroposteriorly. Medially, there is a well-developed ulnar collateral ligament (medial collateral ligament) that is divided into three portions: (1) the all-important anterior oblique, (2) the less important posterior oblique, and (3) the functionally unimportant transverse oblique ligament. Because of its unique positioning, the anterior oblique ligament is taut throughout the full range of motion and is the prime stabilizer on the medial side against valgus stress during acceleration and deceleration phases of pitching. The posterior oblique ligament is taut only in flexion and plays a secondary role in medial stability, as does the ra-

diocapitellar joint laterally, which acts as a buttress to guard against extreme valgus deformation.

To test for **medial stability,** the elbow is stressed by placing a valgus pressure on the distal forearm held at 20 to 30 degrees of flexion, a position that allows for disengagement of the olecranon from its fossa. The medial opening is determined and compared to that of the uninvolved side. The examiner should stand with the involved arm between his or her arm and body, and then place both hands at the elbow. The examiner can then apply the stress by shifting the body while palpating the ulnohumeral joint. Varus stress can also be applied to evaluate varus stability. The patient can also be placed supine, with the arm abducted 90 degrees and the elbow visualized directly. Stressing can then be performed with the humerus locked in external rotation. This position allows for easier visualization of the ulnohumeral joint and the ulnar nerve.

On the lateral aspect of the elbow some stability is maintained by the radial collateral ligament that arises from the lateral epicondyle and is inserted into the annular ligament about the proximal radius. Significant additional support comes from the extensor muscle mass and the anconeus muscle that inserts on the ulna.

Anterior stability depends very little on the integrity of the trochlear-olecranon complex. Instead, control of anterior displacement relies especially on the ulnar collateral ligament, the anterior capsule, and, to a lesser extent, the radial collateral ligament. There are no ligaments to control posterior displacement. Proper alignment, then, depends on the anterior capsule and the abutment of the radial head and the coronoid process of the ulna against the adjacent humerus.

Further stability is obtained by muscular competency and interaction of the three primary flexors of the elbow (the biceps, the brachialis, and the brachioradialis muscles), the primary extensor (the triceps muscle), the pronators (the pronator teres and pronator quadratus muscles), and the supinator and the biceps muscles. Together with the medial flexor and lateral extensor forearm muscle groups, muscular stability is added to the principal ligamentous support. In the throwing athlete the dynamic contraction of the muscles about the elbow most likely is a major contribution to elbow stability.

Localization of Pain

The elbow is most vulnerable to soft tissue injury by the production of a considerable valgus stress in the phases of cocking, acceleration, and deceleration of the pitching motion. The soft-tissue injury consists of microscopic tearing, fluid, and inflammatory cell accumulation, resulting in acute pain. Chronic pain and limitation of motion result from repeated bleeding insults to the stressed area, which attempts to heal by inflammation, followed by fibrous scarring, and later by calcification. Localization of the most painful site requires identification of the underlying anatomy.

Medial

Using the medial epicondyle as a landmark, palpation for tenderness is begun locally and then distally over the flexor-pronator muscle tendinous mass. This area most commonly is subject to fatigue, with microtears caused by excessive valgus tensile forces that scar and result in flexion contractures.

Deep to the flexor muscle mass the anterior oblique portion of the ulnar collateral ligament is a frequent source of ligamentous sprains caused by chronic stress. Its integrity is determined by performing the valgus stress test of the forearm with the elbow slightly flexed. The posterior oblique ligament lies posterior and inferior to the medial epicondyle and is less commonly involved in medial traction injuries. Medial discomfort can also be elicited by percussion over the ulnar nerve above, in, and below the ulnar groove. The combination of flexor muscle mass strain, ulnar collateral ligament sprain, and ulnar neuritis is frequently encountered because all three can be produced by the same valgus stress forces.

Other sources of medial pain are as follows: (1) medial epicondylitis caused by injury of the tendinous origin of the flexor-pronator muscle mass, (2) avulsion fractures of the medial epicondylar ossification center, often occurring in young pitchers, (3) ulnar traction spurs arising from the coronoid process of the ulna and the medial epicondyle of the humerus, and (4) osteochondral loose bodies.

Sources of medial elbow pain

- Flexor-pronator tendon origin inflammation
- Anterior oblique portion of ulnar collateral ligament sprain
- Ulnar neuritis
- Avulsion fractures
- Osteochondral loose bodies
- Traction spurs (coronoid process or medial epicondyle)
- Flexor-pronator muscle strain

Lateral

Laterally the site of pain may be located at the lateral epicondyle, denoting overload tendinitis of the common extensors, but it is predominantly located at the extensor carpi radialis brevis. Although more commonly noted in racquet sports (tennis elbow), lateral epicondylitis does occur after prolonged pitching with fatigue, a condition that allows for excessive forearm pronation and wrist flexion after release in the deceleration motion phase. True extensor musculature strains are infrequent and tend to occur in the poorly conditioned or older batting and throwing athlete.

Sources of lateral elbow pain

- Lateral epicondylitis
- Radiocapitellar impingement/degeneration
- Posterior interosseous nerve entrapment

When valgus stress occurs medially, compression of the radiocapitellar articulation occurs laterally, resulting in osteochondrosis (Panner's disease) in the young ath-

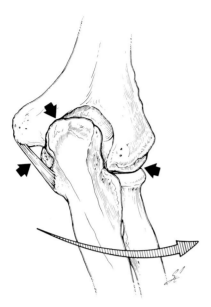

FIG. 35-7. Posterior view of elbow, illustrating the three major sites of trauma in valgus extension overload stress.

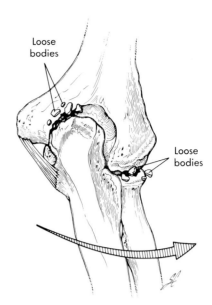

FIG. 35-8. Posterior view of the elbow reveals stretching of the ulnar collateral ligament and osteophyte formation as a result of chronic valgus extension overload stress.

lete and articular fragmentation and bony overgrowth in the capitellum and radial head in the mature athlete. Progression to loose body formation does occur. Therefore careful palpation of the area proximal to the radial head needs to be performed.

Tenderness about the supinator muscle suggests compression entrapment of the posterior interosseous branch of the radial nerve. Increased proximal tenderness can indicate injury to the radial nerve (radial tunnel syndrome). If fullness deep to the anconeus muscle and posterior to the lateral epicondyle is noted, hemarthrosis of an acute injury or effusion of a chronic irritation is a probability.

Posterior

Valgus stress in throwing produces a shearing force posteriorly in the olecranon fossa that initiates formation of spurs, osteophytes, and loose bodies and later leads to degenerative changes, all of which may be tender to palpation (Figs. 35-7 and 35-8). Extension overload (extensor valgus overload syndrome) in the deceleration and follow-through phases can produce localized pain and tenderness by impingement of the olecranon on the posteromedial aspect of the olecranon fossa. To test for valgus extension overload–produced pain, the partially flexed and supinated forearm is brought into a valgus position and then forcefully extended to abut the olecranon and its medial fossa to reproduce symptoms that may be difficult to localize otherwise. A positive valgus extension overload test produces pain with the maneuver. Acute, forceful hyperextension of the elbow can result in avulsion fractures of the tip of the olecranon, whereas chronic overuse tends to produce triceps tendinitis, which may lead to contracture. Direct posterior trauma

---

Sources of posterior elbow pain

- Loose bodies
- Degenerative changes of the olecranon and olecranon fossa
- Triceps tendinitis
- Olecranon avulsion
- Olecranon bursitis

---

can produce characteristic swelling of olecranon bursitis, which may become very painful when infected. Loose bodies need to be sought in the posterior compartment medially and laterally.

Anterior

The location of anterior elbow pain is not limited to the antecubital fossa where bicipital tendon strains and avulsions are encountered. Hypertrophied muscles of the medial forearm wrist flexors, the lateral elbow flexors, and the brachioradialis can become swollen and tender from fatigue after exercising. Muscle hypertrophy and exercise-induced edema can create a syndrome of anteromedial pain secondary to increased pressure within the fascial planes of the forearm. Diffuse anterior elbow tenderness can be attributed to anterior capsulitis, which is seen after an incidental hyperextension injury but usually not with repetitive throwing. Although mostly anteromedial in location, vague postexertional discomfort can be a finding in the pronator teres syndrome as a result of entrapment of the median nerve at the level of the pronator teres. When this occurs, typically, parethesias of the thumb and index finger are also noted.

Sources of anterior elbow pain

- Biceps strain/avulsion
- Flexor-pronator exertional compartment syndrome
- Pronator syndrome
- Anterior capsulitis

RADIOGRAPHIC EVALUATION

Accurate interpretation of radiographic studies performed on the throwing elbow requires both a comprehensive knowledge of the broad spectrum of afflictions that are possible at this joint and a thorough physical examination. As a result of extensive overlap in the various clinical entities occurring within the region of the elbow, radiographs, stress studies, arthrograms, and CT arthrography often play an important role in determining the working diagnosis and subsequent treatment (see Chapter 14). Radiographs alone, without careful correlation with physical findings, can be a source of misinformation rather than an aid to diagnosis.[46]

Standard Views

The initial radiographic evaluation of the injured elbow in the throwing athlete should consist of an AP radiograph comprising a 90-degree flexed lateral view and two oblique views. An axial radiograph, which is taken with the elbow flexed to 110 degrees, the arm lying on the cassette, and the beam angled 45 degrees to the ulna, should also be obtained (Fig. 35-9). This allows for the best view of the olecranon as it articulates with the trochlea and puts the medial aspect of the olecranon in profile. Of note in most skeletally mature elbows in high-caliber pitchers is the generalized humeral hypertrophy that is present (Fig. 35-10). This was initially described

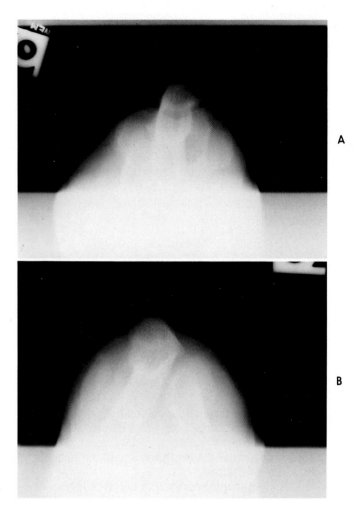

FIG. 35-9. Normal axial views of immature (**A**) and mature (**B**) elbow.

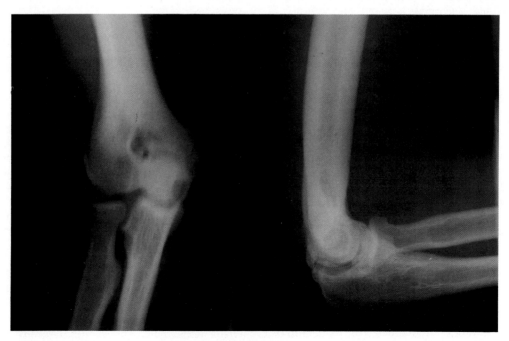

FIG. 35-10. Humeral hypertrophy of the dominant arm is a common finding in throwing athletes. Note also posterior compartment pathologic change.

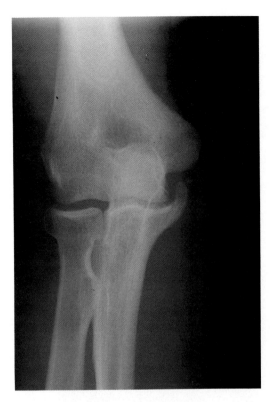

FIG. 35-11. Traction spurring in a professional pitcher of the medial coronoid with calcification of the ligament.

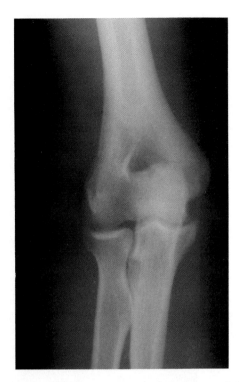

FIG. 35-12. Traction spurring of proximal ulna at site of ulnar collateral ligament insertion with kissing lesion of trochlea. Note calcification in the substance of the ligament.

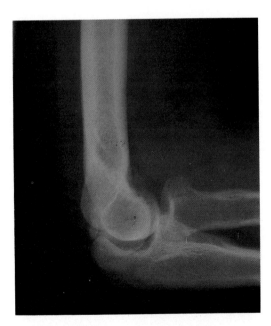

FIG. 35-13. Calcification in the anterior capsule of a baseball pitcher. Note the posterior compartment loose body.

in tennis players by Jones et al[28] and noted also in baseball players by Jobe and Newber.[26] Because this finding represents an adaptive change of exercise, it is not felt to be pathologic or directly responsible for any other pathologic conditions occurring about the elbow.

Medial

Because the medial elbow is subjected to tensile loads during throwing, the bony pathologic changes identified on radiographs are directly related to this phenomenon. In the youngster whose growth centers are fully present but not yet fused, the medial epicondyle can show various effects of the applied forces. These changes include fragmentation and accelerated growth of the epicondyle and, on occasion, the frank separation and subsequent displacement of the epicondyle through the growth apophysis.[13,32,44] Comparison radiographs may be helpful in fully delineating the magnitude of these changes. As the elbow matures, the separation can be more peripheral and not involve the entire epicondyle.[44,64] In the fully mature skeleton, smaller avulsion fragments can also occur directly off the epicondyle.

On routine views radiopaque densities may be identified in the ulnar collateral ligament. These densities represent calcifications and later ossifications within the tendon substance that occur in advanced stages of the overuse pathology spectrum. Traction spurring may also be seen on the proximal medial ulna at the site of the medial collateral ligament insertion (Fig. 35-11).[9,11,18,24,51] This may be accompanied by a kissing lesion from the inferior medial surface of the trochlea (Fig. 35-12).

Anterior

Anteriorly in the elbow, any spurring of the coronoid process should be noted on a lateral radiograph, as should any calcification occurring in the anterior capsule

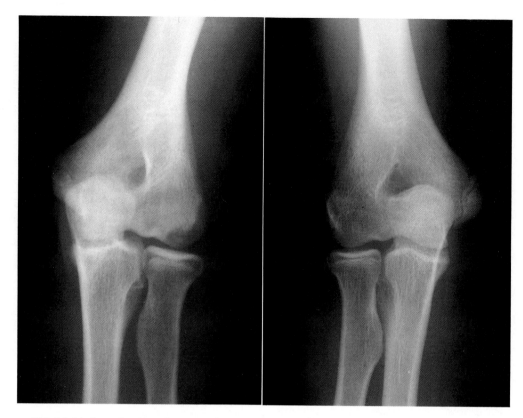

FIG. 35-14. Osteochondritis dissecans of capitellum and radial head hypertrophy in 15-year-old right-handed pitcher. Normal left side for comparison.

or tendinous insertions of the elbow flexors (Fig. 35-13). These calcifications can occur as the result of tension injuries developing in those structures during elbow deceleration.[24,51]

Lateral

Laterally the compressive and shear forces to which the radius and capitellum are exposed lead to characteristic radiographic findings.[49] These findings primarily consist of osteochondritis dissecans of the capitellum, radial head hypertrophy, and occasionally an osteochondral defect or fracture from the capitellum or radial head (Fig. 35-14).[1,2,26,29,44] Further elaboration on the cause of these changes is covered later in this chapter. Osteochondral fragmentation of the capitellum and radial head hypertrophy are ominous signs for competitive athletes.[9,24,57] In the osteochondritic lesion a portion of the capitellum shows irregular ossification and rarefaction within a crater. This crater may have a sclerotic rim, and a loose body may be noted. The lateral radiograph shows flattening of the capitellum.[64] The lucencies in the capitellum may be seen better on oblique views and arthrotomograms (Fig. 35-15). More recently, CT arthrography has been helpful in identifying these lesions in the capitellum as well as in locating any intraarticular loose bodies.[2]

Posterior

Posteriorly the olecranon and the olecranon fossa are the sites of bony pathologic changes. The compressive

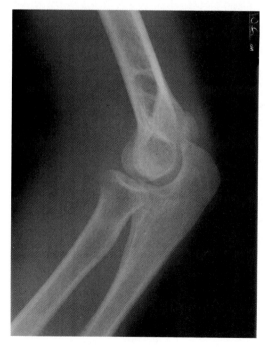

FIG. 35-15. Osteochondritis of capitellum in 13-year-old female basketball player seen only on oblique view with forearm supination.

loads generated between the medial wall of the fossa and the corresponding medial tip of the olecranon result in degenerative changes and osteophytes.[24,29] This so-called valgus extension overload syndrome is a manifestation of combined valgus and compressive forces developing in the throwing elbow.[62] The posterior osteophyte, thus formed, can be fractured off and serve as a source of loose bodies.[24,26,29] These osteophytes are best identified on the axial view as described earlier.[62] Straight posterior osteophytes are more readily apparent and often can be identified on a routine flexed lateral view.[48,49]

Magnetic Resonance Imaging

As the technique of magnetic resonance imaging (MRI) is refined, the studies relative to the thrower's elbow are improving. MRI has been shown to be useful in evaluating osteochondritis dissecans, olecranon osteophytes, biceps tendon ruptures, triceps tears, and ulnar collateral ligament injuries.[37] MRI is also useful in evaluating ulnar collateral ligament injuries in baseball players.[34] We have reported on the use of CT arthrogram and MRI in the evaluation of ulnar collateral ligament injuries.[56] We noted that the MRI was useful for full-thickness tears of the ligament, but was less sensitive in detecting partial injuries. A current study at our institution (ASMI) is examining the usefulness of MRI with intraarticular contrast, and preliminary results suggest the saline MRI is accurate in delineating partial injuries to the ulnar collateral ligament.

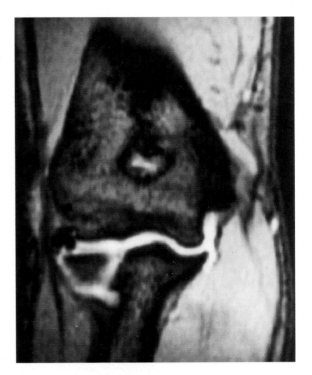

FIG. 35-16. Saline magnetic resonance image. (From Timmerman LA, Schwartz ML, Andrews JR: *Am J Sports Med* 22(1):26, 1994.)

INJURIES

A distinction can be made between injuries of the elbow in the throwing athlete and the throwing injuries of the elbow. Throwing injuries of the elbow refer to the overuse syndromes that occur as a result of repetitive stresses incurred in structures about the elbow as a result of throwing over many months or years. Although the clinical manifestations of a throwing athlete's symptoms may be acute at onset, essentially all of these injuries are the result of pathologic changes occurring at the subclinical level over various periods. The cumulative pathologic changes occurring in the anatomic structures about the joint eventually exceed the body's ability to repair or compensate for them, thus resulting in presentation of the athlete to the trainer or the physician with his or her symptoms. These overuse injuries differ from acute, traumatic injuries to the elbow that result from a single injury or episode. These traumatic injuries refer specifically to accidents or injuries not caused by the act of throwing itself that the throwing athlete may incur to his dominant elbow in the course of his athletic event or during daily living. An example of this injury might include an acute rupture of the ulnar collateral ligament caused by a valgus force resulting from an attempt to tag out a runner on a base path. Another example might be an asymptomatic subluxing ulnar nerve that suffers a direct blow when it is in its subluxed position on the medial epicondyle, or a posterior dislocation of the elbow in an athlete that may or may not be related to his athletic participation. Although these types of injuries can occur in the general population, their presentation in the dom-

inant elbow of a throwing athlete requires special consideration if these individuals are to continue to participate at a high level of competition.

Naturally, success in the treatment of the throwing athlete's elbow is closely correlated with the accuracy of the diagnosis. Diagnostic acumen, in turn, depends on a thorough knowledge of those factors already discussed in this chapter—biomechanics, anatomy, and radiography, combined with a thorough examination.

In discussing the various clinical entities about the elbow, it is convenient to group the lesions into medial, lateral, posterior, and anterior injuries. These areas can be further subdivided into bony vs. soft-tissue injuries or combinations thereof; even further subdivision into the skeletally mature or immature athlete is also helpful. However, because of unique considerations, the immature elbow is discussed separately in this chapter.

Medial Elbow Injuries
Ulnar Collateral Ligament Injury (Noncontact)

Ulnar collateral ligament rupture in the throwing athlete often presents as an acute event of moderate to severe medial elbow pain that occurs specifically during the act of throwing. It is often accompanied by a pop heard by the athlete. It is not uncommon for the injury to occur on a cold day following inadequate warm-up. The athlete complains of acute medial elbow pain and may have concomitant signs of ulnar nerve irritation. Medial elbow ecchymosis may be found on examination. When a history similar to this is obtained, until proved otherwise, the diagnosis must be torn ulnar collateral lig-

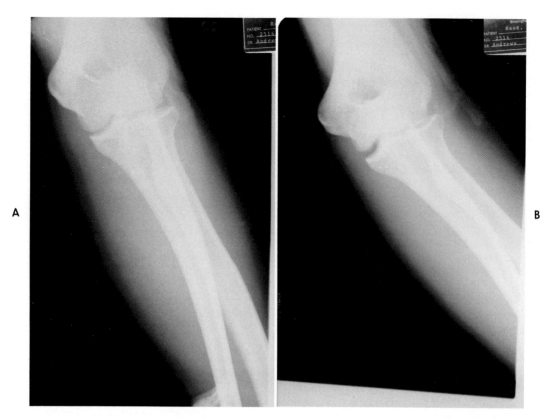

FIG. 35-17. A, Anteroposterior radiography of the elbow before stressing. **B,** The elbow after a valgus stress is applied. Note the widened medial joint space.

Findings in acute ulnar collateral ligament injury

- Moderate to severe medial elbow pain
- Onset during throwing
- Pop felt or heard by athlete
- Medial elbow ecchymosis
- Ulnar nerve symptoms
- Positive elbow arthrogram (complete tears)
- Positive gravity stress test (under anesthesia)

---

ament. A high index of suspicion of a tear is paramount for the prompt diagnosis and initiation of treatment for this injury.

In the acutely injured thrower the physical examination for instability can be inhibited by muscular spasm and pain. The close proximity of the various anatomic structures (namely, the flexor-pronator flexor mass, the ulnar collateral ligament, the ulnar nerve, and the medial olecranon fossa and process) makes differentiation by palpation very difficult. The **gravity stress test** has been described as a means of determining medial elbow instability.[47,63] This test is carried out by having the patient lie in a supine position on a table in the radiology suite. The patient's involved arm is abducted 90 degrees at the shoulder and is maximally externally rotated. The elbow is flexed approximately 20 degrees to clear the olecranon from its fossa. The force of gravity opens the medial elbow in the face of instability. An AP radiograph is obtained, and any opening of the medial elbow is de-

termined (Fig. 35-17). Unfortunately, regional or general anesthesia is often required to complete the gravity stress test without too much patient discomfort. Therefore this test cannot always be used to determine the integrity of the ulnar collateral ligament before an anesthetic is administered. We have found an **elbow arthrogram** to be very helpful in determining the status of the ulnar collateral ligament. It has been our experience that an elbow arthrogram showing leakage of dye through the medial joint capsule indicates not only a tear of the capsule itself but also a tear in the anterior oblique fibers of the ulnar collateral ligament and is thus consistent with medial elbow instability (Fig. 35-18). This arthrographic finding has been confirmed by the gravity stress test and under direct observation in those individuals who have undergone subsequent examination under anesthesia and surgical repair.

For the last several years we have found the CT arthrogram to be useful in evaluating the integrity of the medial capsule. At times it detects a contrast leak that may be missed on the AP radiograph view of the elbow with contrast. With rotation the contrast leak may overlie the joint.

In addition, the contrast may leak down the ulnar insertion, corresponding to an undersurface tear of the ulnar collateral ligament (Fig. 35-19).[55] The contrast can also leak proximally, although anatomic studies have shown that there is a small potential space under the medial epicondyle between the anterior bundle and the humerus. In contrast, the distal ulnar insertion of the an-

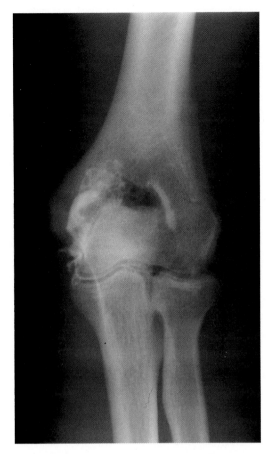

FIG. 35-18. Positive arthrogram demonstrates dye leakage from the medial joint. Close anatomic relationship of the ulnar collateral ligament and medial joint capsule results in their concomitant injury.

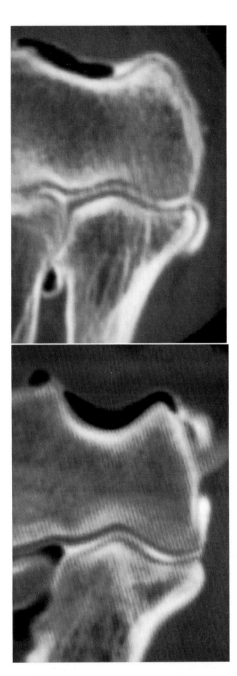

FIG. 35-19. T-sign on computed tomography arthrogram. (From Timmerman LA, Andrews JR: *Am J Sports Med* 22(1):33, 1994.)

terior bundle is within 1 mm of the articular margin. When the contrast leaks distally, it corresponds to a T sign.[55]

We have found that the presence of contrast is the useful feature of the imaging study. Saline or gallium contrast MRI can serve the same purpose in delineating the ligament and the attachment. MRI without the contrast is less sensitive in detecting partial tears.[56]

Although the athlete may perceive of this injury as a singular episode, in reality the pathologic processes occurring within the ligament structure have been chronically at work. These progressive destructive changes can occur in overuse syndromes when activity is not abated. These changes include edema and inflammation initially, followed by fibrotic scar formation within the ligamentous structure, and finally calcification and in some cases ossification of this scar tissue. Because these pathologically altered tissues cannot serve the function of the ulnar collateral ligament in its resistance to the repetitively applied valgus forces, the ligament ultimately fails. In some cases only minimal stress, rather than throwing the "high hard one," leads to final rupture. Almost all patients with acute ulnar collateral ligament injuries have a history of pain and tenderness over the medial aspect of the elbow—pain that was associated with throwing for months or years before the acute episode.

Many have had corticosteroid injections into the medial aspect of the elbow in an attempt to alleviate these symptoms, and this may play some role in the ultimate weakening and failure of the ulnar collateral ligament.[25,40,53]

Acute ulnar collateral ligament insufficiency in the throwing athlete, if left untreated, almost universally results in chronic ulnar collateral ligament insufficiency. In the report on the reconstruction of the ulnar collateral ligament in athletes by Jobe, Stark, and Lombardo,[27] the first 16 patients included eight who had a history of rupture occurring as a sudden catastrophic event. On

FIG. 35-20. Three views of tearing of the anterior oblique portion of the ulnar collateral ligament. **A,** Midsubstance. **B,** At the medial epicondyle. **C,** At its insertion into the ulna.

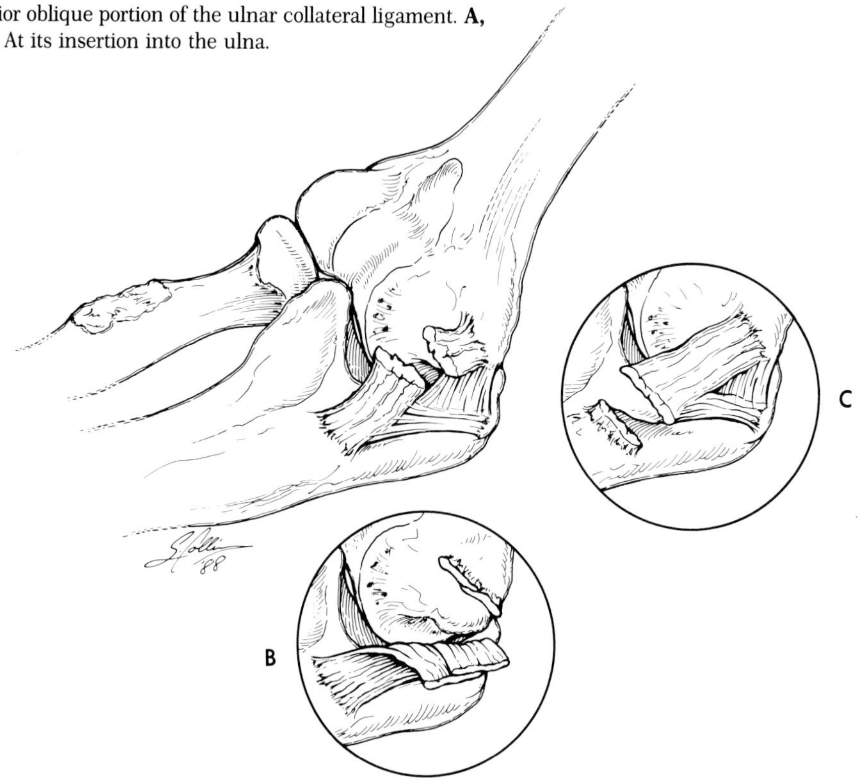

clinical examination these patients had valgus instability as determined by a positive gravity medial stress test. All elected to undergo a period of rehabilitation in an attempt to avoid surgery, but because all conservative measures were ineffective, after an average of 7 months after injury all of the patients chose to have effective ulnar collateral ligament reconstruction.

As noted previously, a ruptured ulnar collateral ligament in the throwing athlete does not commonly occur in normal healthy tissue, even if it presents as an acute injury. However, this injury pattern can and does occur in teenage throwers who experience a singular acute and complete tear of their anterior oblique fibers. Typically, at the time of surgery, the ligament is found to have torn through normal tissue or to have avulsed off its origin or insertion (Fig. 35-20). In these cases direct repair is an appropriate option. In the adult athlete most of the ligaments are found at the time of surgery to be attenuated and scarified, making primary repair difficult if not contraindicated. In these instances the surgeon must be prepared to reconstruct the ligament in the same manner in which such reconstruction is performed in repairing chronic ligamentous insufficiency.

Primary repair. The medial aspect of the elbow is approached through a curvilinear incision centered just anterior to the medial epicondyle. As the incision is deepened through the subcutaneous tissue, the medial antebrachial cutaneous nerve should be identified and protected throughout the remainder of the procedure. The ulnar nerve should be identified proximal to the cubital tunnel, and its courses should be traced to the two heads of the flexor carpi ulnaris. Care should be taken in the initial identification of the nerve to ensure that it has not undergone an anterior dislocation directly into the operative field. The ulnar nerve should be decompressed and routinely transposed. The interval between the forearm flexor mass and the ulnar insertion is found distally. The ligament can then be exposed without taking down the flexor mass.

With reflection of this muscle mass, the underlying ulnar collateral ligament will be exposed and identified. Usually the anterior oblique band of the ulnar collateral ligament, as well as capsular tissue both anterior and posterior to this band, is completely disrupted. In many cases midsubstance tears of the ligament do not occur; instead avulsion injuries off of either the medial epicondylar origin or at the insertion point into the medial aspect of the coronoid process of the ulna are present. In the skeletally immature we have seen avulsion of the ligament with a bony fragment usually from the medial epicondyle, and one case of avulsion distally of the sublime tubercle with the ulnar collateral ligament attached.

If the tendon appears healthy, a midsubstance tear of the anterior oblique band is repaired with a 2-0 Ticron suture or a similar nonabsorbable suture, and the capsule is then repaired with an absorbable suture. If the anterior oblique ligament is disrupted through an avulsion injury from either the humerus or the ulna, it can be repaired back to this bony structure through drill holes. With an acute injury augmentation may be necessary in addition to the primary repair of the ligament. (This is described in the following section on chronic ulnar collateral ligament insufficiency.)

Postoperatively the patient is splinted for 10 days in

90 degrees of elbow flexion. At this point a functional brace, which allows elbow flexion from 30 to 60 degrees, is applied. Over the next 5 weeks the brace is removed three times a day for range of motion exercises, with the goal being full range of motion by 6 weeks. At 6 weeks postoperatively progressive resistance exercises are initiated and continued through the twelfth week. At this point functional activities, including a well-supervised and controlled interval throwing program, are started. This program is completed on an individual basis over a 1- to 3-month period. A return to competitive throwing is thus accomplished at 4 to 6 months postoperatively. It is our opinion that prompt repair of this injury and proper postoperative rehabilitation allow the throwing athlete the best chance for return to his or her previous level of activity.

Chronic Ulnar Collateral Ligament Insufficiency

The pathologic processes of the overuse syndrome can result in progressive attenuation of the ulnar collateral ligament. This stretching out of the structure leads to ligamentous insufficiency even in the absence of a singular catastrophic episode of ligament failure. However, in most cases there is a history of medial elbow problems. Some athletes report a previous severe injury, suggestive of acute ligament rupture, which was not diagnosed or where definitive treatment was not carried out. Typically, these athletes present later with the same clinical findings as throwers with progressively attenuated ligaments: tenderness over the medial aspect of the elbow, posteromedial pain, and radiographic changes consistent with valgus extension overload.[26,62]

Jobe, Stark, and Lombardo[27] have described reconstruction of the ulnar collateral ligament using autogenous tendon grafts in an attempt to allow for a return of the throwing athlete to a previous level of competition. Using this technique, 10 of 16 throwing athletes successfully returned to their previous level of throwing capability, and one athlete was able to return only to a lower level of throwing capability.

In a more recent report from the same institution, Conway et al[17] reported the results after ulnar collateral ligament reconstruction or repair for treatment of medial instability in throwing athletes. They noted that 68% of the patients who underwent reconstruction returned to the previous level of participation. The ability to return to play was slightly less successful in the direct repair group, with only 50% achieving the previous level of play.

Schwab et al[47] have also described good results with a procedure for osteotomy of the medial epicondyle with transfer to a proximal and anterior position on the humerus in the reconstruction of a chronically lax ulnar collateral ligament. This may be problematic in a throwing athlete because the isometry of the ligament is altered, and motion may be difficult to obtain.

Ligament reconstruction. The surgical technique for ulnar collateral ligament reconstruction uses the same approach as that previously described for primary repair. The flexor-pronator muscle mass is reflected off the medial epicondyle, beginning distally and reflecting this

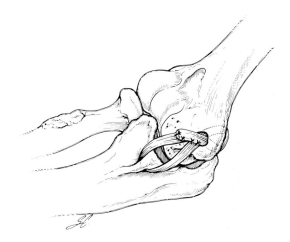

FIG. 35-21. Example of figure-eight reconstruction of chronic ulnar collateral ligament insufficiency using an autogenous tendon graft.

structure in an anterior and proximal direction. This dissection is completed when there is adequate exposure of the entire ulnar collateral ligament from origin to insertion. The ulnar nerve is mobilized proximally from the medial intermuscular septum in the arm and is freed distally to where it enters the interval between the two heads of the flexor carpi ulnaris. The firm edge of the intermuscular septum is excised to prevent ulnar nerve irritation after the transposition.

The anterior oblique and the posterior oblique bundles should be identified and inspected. A 3.2-mm drill bit is used to develop osseous tunnels in both the distal humerus and proximal ulna. Entrance to these tunnels should correspond to the point of origin of the ligament from the medial epicondyle and point of insertion of the anterior oblique fibers to the proximal ulna. The palmaris longus is the preferred tendon for reconstruction; however, in its absence, either the plantaris or a toe extensor tendon is suitable. If placed correctly, some part of the reconstructed tendon should be taut throughout the full range of motion without acting as a tether either to full flexion or to extension. The ulnar nerve is transposed anteriorly in the subcutaneous fashion. The nerve is stabilized in this position by two nonconstricting fascial slings formed from the flexor muscle fascia (Fig. 35-21).

Postoperatively for 1 week gentle range of motion in a hinged brace is started at 30 to 90 degrees, progressing to 0 to 110 degrees by week 4. The brace is discontinued after 6 weeks, with motion at 0 to 130 degrees. After 1 week light active progressive resistance exercises are initiated for the shoulder and elbow. At 4 weeks resistance is increased, with gradual progression to maximum resistance being reached at 4 months. At this point functional activities, including a well-supervised and controlled interval throwing program, may be initiated. Patients return to throwing activities at 6 to 12 months based on individual progress.

The surgical technique and postoperative regimen are further described in the works of Jobe, Stark, and Lom-

bardo,[27] Conway et al,[17] Schwab et al,[47] and Woods and Tullos.[63]

Medial Epicondylar Fracture

Like most injuries on the medial aspect of the elbow in the throwing athlete, medial epicondylar fractures, although occurring acutely, are a result of chronic tensile overload. The forces applied to the medial epicondyle through both the ulnar collateral ligament and the origin of the flexor-pronator muscle mass result in adaptive changes within the epicondyle. These changes include the overgrowth of the medial epicondylar apophysis in the adolescent, as well as its occasional fragmentation, which is noted in the section on little league elbow.[13,32,44] These same forces no doubt exist throughout the baseball pitcher's career, and, when they exceed the body's ability to adapt or repair itself, these fractures occur.[2,9,26,29]

The medial epicondylar apophysis is the last of the growth centers about the distal humerus to fuse with the metaphysis; it occurs at around age 14 in females and as late as age 17 in males.[23] Most medial epicondylar fractures in individuals in this age group penetrate the apophyseal growth plate, with the entire fragment being displaced. The fragment includes the origin of the flexor-pronator muscle and may or may not include the attachment of the ulnar collateral ligament. We have seen com-

plete avulsions of the medial epicondyle where the fracture does not include the ulnar collateral ligament (Fig. 35-22). The ulnar collateral ligament attaches to the base of the medial epicondyle and in some cases is spared in regard to this specific type of injury. Regardless of its degree of displacement, in the throwing athlete it should

---

Medial epicondylar avulsion fracture

- Anatomic reduction in the throwing athlete
- No displacement acceptable

---

be anatomically reduced and secured internally with K-wires or an interfragmentary screw (Fig. 35-23). Although minimal and even moderate displacement of the medial epicondylar apophysis would be clinically acceptable for some individuals, the resulting laxity of the ulnar collateral ligament in the throwing athlete could be disabling in the individual's sport. In addition, epicondylar apophyseal displacement can alter the relationship of the ulnar collateral ligament to the elbow joint axis of rotation. Subsequent tethering of the joint by the ligament can result in loss of flexion and extension. What appears as minimal displacement on an AP radiograph can be significant on the lateral view because the fragment often displaces in the anteroposterior plane. Both the AP and lateral radiographs need to be carefully inspected.

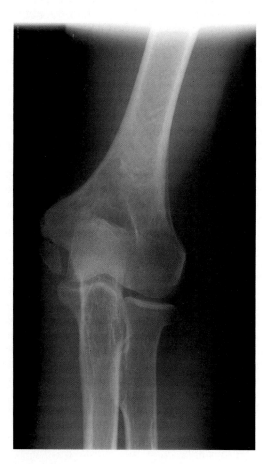

FIG. 35-22. Fracture in a youth through the growth plate of the medial epicondyle with minimal medial instability.

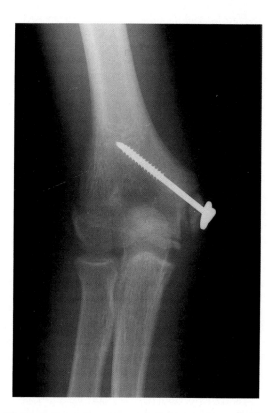

FIG. 35-23. Postoperative radiograph demonstrating reduction and fixation of medial epicondylar Salter I fracture by interfragmentary screw.

In the skeletally mature elbow the medial epicondylar fracture is less frequently a large fragment but more often a smaller bony lesion, which in some cases can even be comminuted or fragmented[2,44] (Fig. 35-24). This, however, does not ensure that the ulnar collateral ligament's origin on the medial epicondyle remains intact or that the ulnar collateral ligament has not failed in its midsubstance.[12,63] It is extremely important in the face of a medial epicondylar fracture, regardless of its size or its relative displacement, to determine the integrity of the ulnar collateral ligament. This can be quite difficult in the case of an acute injury in which muscular pain and spasm cause the patient to guard the elbow. An elbow arthrogram or a contrast MRI, as described in the section on ulnar collateral ligament injury, is also indicated in this circumstance to establish the competence of this ligament.

Any throwing athlete who shows ulnar collateral ligament incompetence of the throwing elbow requires open repair or reconstruction of this structure.[27,63] The surgical technique and postoperative treatment of these patients are described under the section on isolated ulnar collateral ligament repairs. Treatment of the accompanying medial epicondyle fracture depends on its size and comminution. The fracture fragment can be reduced and fixed to the distal humerus; if it is small or fragmented, it can be excised at the time of ulnar collateral ligament reconstruction. Berkley, Bennett, and Woods[12] have observed that medial epicondylar fracture fragments that involve the ulnar collateral ligament must be anatomically reduced, since even small degrees of rotational displacement can result in a functional lengthening of the ulnar collateral ligament and subsequent instability in the throwing elbow.

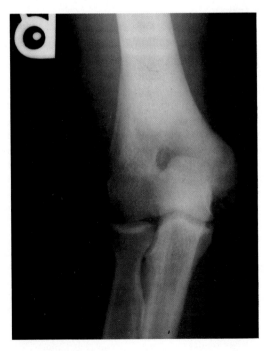

FIG. 35-24. Chronic avulsion fragmentation of the medial epicondyle in a professional baseball pitcher. Although currently asymptomatic, this player had a history of intermittent medial elbow pain.

Substantial medial epicondyle fractures occur in some instances without ulnar collateral ligament involvement. There seems to be a paucity of attention in the current literature to the treatment of these fractures. Berkley, Bennett, and Woods[12] have suggested that stable, nondisplaced fractures should be immobilized at 90 degrees of flexion for 3 to 4 weeks, with subsequent actively protected range of motion. Fractures that are displaced more than 1 cm in elbows that are stable to valgus stress should be treated with open reduction and internal fixation. Jobe and Newber[26] have stated that any such fracture displaced more than 2 mm should be reduced, and our clinical experience leads us to agree.

Muscle and Tendon Injuries

Flexor-pronator strain. Slocum[51] noted that the fibers of the flexor-pronator muscle group were particularly susceptible to overloading because of valgus strain of the arm during the act of throwing. He thought that this muscle group underwent a state of temporary myostatic contracture secondary to fatigue and that this prevented its return to normal resting length. If the individual athlete continued to throw despite these myostatic contractures, microscopic tears would take place within the muscle substance and would result in secondary fibrosis and a permanent loss of elbow extension. King, Brelsford, and Tullos[29] in their description of physical findings in the professional baseball pitcher, noted not only hypertrophy of the dominant upper extremity musculature from the shoulder through the forearm but also the now commonly recognized flexion contractures at the elbow present in these high-caliber pitchers. Over 50% of the pitchers examined showed fixed deformities in flexion at the elbow. They also noted valgus deformities of the elbow as a second common finding occurring in approximately 30% of the pitchers. Elbow flexion contractures have been identified in pitchers as young as those participating in Little League. Two major studies evaluating little leaguer's elbow show a 12% and 5% prevalence of elbow flexion contractures in these young athletes.[22,32] These percentages undoubtedly increase as the pitchers continue their careers and expose their medial muscle groups to this chronic repetitive tensile loading. Despite the prevalence of flexion contractures in high-level pitching, an elbow flexion contracture in a young pitcher with a sore medial elbow should *not* be disregarded. As noted by Slocum,[51] early elbow flexion contractures are a result of myostatic muscle activity and spasm. With appropriate rest and abstinence from throwing, this can be a reversible physical finding. The goal should be to limit the extent of pathologic change and its subsequent cumulative effect on the medial flexor-pronator muscle group.

> Flexion contracture in growing athletes must not be ignored!

Flexor-pronator complete tear. Acute, complete, or extensive tearing of the belly of the flexor-pronator muscle is believed to be a rare lesion (Fig. 35-25). In an analysis of 100 symptomatic baseball players conducted by

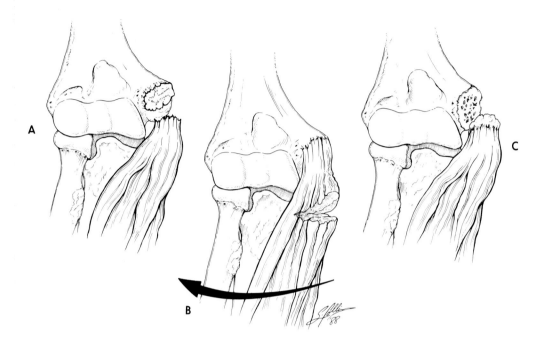

FIG. 35-25. Flexor-pronator muscle mass under valgus stress may tear away from its origin on the medial epicondyle **(A)**, tear in midsubstance **(B)**, or avulse adjacent bone from its origin **(C)**.

Barnes and Tullos,[9] only two cases of flexor forearm muscle rupture were identified. Primary operative muscle repairs were unsuccessful. The postoperative rehabilitation period was lengthy, and the players were never able to return to an effective asymptomatic level of throwing. Fortunately, lesser degrees of pronator muscle mass strain are symptomatic for a short period of time and respond to a protocol of physical therapy combined with icing. Occasionally, ossification occurs within the muscle belly near its origin. This is seldom symptomatic, but if it does prove to be painful it can be excised without injury to the underlying joint capsule or ulnar collateral ligament.

Medial epicondylitis. Because of repetitive tensile forces applied to the flexor-pronator muscle mass, medial epicondylitis is a frequent finding in the throwing athlete. The tensile forces generated in the throwing act primarily exert their pull directly at the flexor-pronator origin from the medial epicondyle; thus tenderness develops at this insertional point. Similar to that for minor muscle belly injuries, these symptoms should respond to a physical therapy program combined with an eccentric stretching and strengthening protocol, as outlined in the rehabilitation section of this chapter (see p. 773). If conservative treatment fails, open elliptical excision of the degenerated tissue is indicated, with careful repair of the defect in the medial flexor mass.

Traction spurs. One additional lesion that is amenable to surgical intervention is a traction spur, which can develop on the ulna just medial to the ulnar coronoid process, immediately adjacent to or associated with the ulnar collateral ligament.[11,18,24,44] This traction spurring or calcific mass can develop either independently of the ulnar collateral ligament or within the substance of the ligament itself. Should the traction spur or calcific mass

prove to be painful, it can be excised through an incision in the flexor-pronator muscle; great care should be taken to identify and protect the ulnar collateral ligament insertion into the ulna.[11,18,24] The physician must be sure that the integrity of this ligament remains intact and that removal of the spur does not subsequently result in medial elbow instability. If this occurs, augmentation of the ligament with a tendon autograft may be necessary.

Nerve Injury

Considerable attention is paid to medial traction and lateral compression forces as primary causes of pathologic states of the elbow in the throwing athlete. Often, however, repetitive throwing motion and the consequences of medially and laterally applied forces concurrently produce subtle neuropathies that mimic other injuries. About the elbow, the ulnar, medial, radial, and musculocutaneous nerves are exposed to direct trauma and are indirectly susceptible to inflammation as the result of the following: (1) local tight fibrous tissue and muscular hypertrophy; (2) anomalous muscles; (3) anatomic, vascular, and neural variations; (4) bony irregularities; and (5) abnormally lax or tight connective tissue.

Factors in nerve injury

- Muscular hypertrophy
- Fibrous bands
- Anomalous muscle
- Anatomic, vascular, or neural variations
- Bone irregularity
- Lax or tight connective tissue

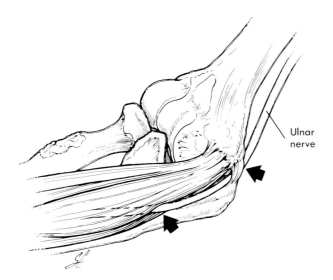

FIG. 35-26. Two common sites of ulnar nerve compression: proximally at the cubital tunnel and distally between the two heads of the flexor carpi ulnaris.

Ulnar Nerve

The ulnar nerve, the continuation of the medial cord of the brachial plexus in the middle of the arm, pierces the medial intramuscular septum, passes alongside or deep to fibers of the medial head of the triceps muscle, and is located in a superficial groove (ulnar sulcus) between the olecranon and the medial epicondyle. Without giving off branches proximal to the elbow, the ulnar nerve enters the forearm between the humeral and ulnar heads of the flexor carpi ulnaris muscle. A thickening of this fibrous connection (arcuate ligament of the cubital tunnel) between the two heads causes a compression entrapment and, along with the arcade of Struthers in the distal arm and the ulnar groove of the medial epicondyle, is a common site for ulnar neuritis (Fig. 35-26). Near the elbow motor innervation is given off to the flexor carpi ulnaris and the ulnar half of the flexor digitorum profundus muscles. Repetitive, overhand throwing tends to accentuate normal stretching of the ulnar nerve, especially during the cocking phase of flexion and external rotation and in the acceleration phase with valgus stress on the ulnar collateral ligament. During these motions, which result in increased traction, any mechanical tethering of the ulnar nerve along its course can cause a friction type of neural dysfunction, i.e., medial epicondylar separations, ulnar traction spurs, and irregularities in the ulnar groove. More commonly, with flexion friction ulnar neuritis is the result of recurrent subluxation or infrequent dislocation of the ulnar nerve out of the ulnar sulcus or groove. Although occurring normally in 16% of the general population, subluxation of the ulnar nerve is noted especially in congenitally lax throwing athletes.[15] Individually, either hypertrophy of forearm flexor musculature or increased forearm fascial compartment pressure can compress the ulnar nerve, especially in the region of the arcuate ligament. The medial head of the triceps and anomalous anconeus epitrochlearis muscles can also hypertrophy and locally entrap the ulnar nerve.

The indecorous-sounding **tardy ulnar nerve neuritis syndrome** is a late developing traumatic ulnar neuropathy that can occur in pitchers and is usually reported years after compression injuries caused by epicondylar fractures and constriction of fibrous bands between the heads of the extensor carpi ulnaris muscle.

Initially the athlete complains of posteromedial elbow pain and intermittent parethesias in the fourth and fifth fingers, aggravated by throwing but improved by rest. Sensory deficits may be noted in the ulnar half of the ring finger, little finger, palmar hypothenar area, and specifically in the dorsoulnar aspect of the hand. Clinical signs of muscular weakness are late findings. Variation of neural anastomoses with the median nerve (Martin-Gruber) makes hand and finger configuration deficits difficult to interpret. The laboratory finding of decreased ulnar nerve EMG activity and velocity may lag behind symptoms and a positive Tinel's sign.

Median Nerve

Medial and lateral roots from the brachial plexus unite to form the median nerve. The nerve accompanies the brachial artery down the arm and courses under the supracondylar process (if present) and the infrequently present ligament of Struthers—without giving off branches—to lie medially at the elbow, deep to the bicipital fascia and superficial to the brachialis muscle. The median nerve enters the forearm between the two heads of the pronator teres and gives motor branches to the pronator teres, flexor carpi radialis, palmaris longus, and flexor digitorum superficialis muscles. Arising from the

---

Potential sites of median nerve compression

- Anomalous suprascapular and posterior humeral circumflex arteries
- Ligament of Struthers
- Lacertus fibrosis
- Pronator teres
- Flexor digitorum superficialis arch

---

median nerve distal to the level of the epicondyles is the pure motor branch, the anterior interosseous nerve. The anterior interosseous nerve then passes through the forearm and innervates the flexor pollicis longus, the medial half of the flexor digitorum profundus, and the pronator quadratus. The main branch of the median nerve continues deep to the tendinous origin of the flexor digitorum superficialis and eventually enters the carpal tunnel at the wrist. Entrapment, which produces compression, friction, or increased traction, can occur from muscle hypertrophy and anatomic variations when there is repetitive throwing. In the shoulder infrequently the median nerve can be divided by anomalous suprascapular and posterior humeral circumflex arteries, a condition that results in neurologic deficits in the hand. More important, there are several sites of median nerve involvement about the elbow. Infrequently fractures about the supracondylar area and the aberrant ligament of Struthers from the anterior medial supracondylar process can occur, causing inflammation. In the proximal forearm

the median nerve can be constricted by the terminal fibers of the biceps tendon (lacertus fibrosis); by, in, or under the hypertrophied pronator teres; and by the thickened flexor digitorum superficialis arch (flexor superficialis bridge).

Pronator teres syndrome is caused by repetitive athletic pronation movements, forced gripping, or direct trauma, which cause compression of the median nerve at the pronator teres level and to a lesser extent by entrapment in the lacterus fibrosis or at the flexor superficialis bridge. Symptoms may vary, but characteristically there are vague postexertional pains in the proximal volar aspect of the forearm, together with paresthesia of the thumb, index, and long fingers. Also found are a negative Phalen test (wrist flexion that does not produce median nerve hand involvement), late occurring weakness in the medial-innervated intrinsic muscles and sensory changes in the hand, and normal function of extrinsic muscles innervated by the anterior interosseous nerve. Because EMG nerve studies may not be diagnostic, clinical maneuvers can enhance symptoms. Resisted pronation of the flexed elbow at 90 degrees with progression to full extension intensifies pain in the proximal forearm because of compression of the median nerve at the level of the pronator teres. Resisted supination with the elbow flexed heightens forearm discomfort because of compression at the lacertus fibrosis, and resisted flexion of the long finger magnifies volar symptoms because of compression at the flexor digitorum superficialis arch.

The **anterior interosseous nerve syndrome** can occur with the pronator teres syndrome in athletic overuse situations and in crush injuries. In the throwing athlete who complains of poor mechanical function of the thumb, index, and long fingers, a presumptive diagnosis of anterior interosseous nerve syndrome can be made from the position of the thumb and index finger in a pinch maneuver. The distal phalanx of the index finger is hyperextended with hyperflexion of the proximal interphalangeal joint. The thumb assumes a position of hyperextension of the interphalangeal joint and hyperflexion of the metacarpophalangeal joint. In addition, the area of pulp contact of the thumb with the finger is more proximal. These attitudes are the result of lack of function of the long flexors of the thumb and index fingers. The weakness of the pronator quadratus can be determined by comparing the amount of resisted forceful supination of the forearm in the flexed position with that in the extended position. There are no cutaneous sensory fibers to evaluate in the anterior interosseous nerve. Congenital soft-tissue variations and Martin-Gruber anastomoses with the ulnar nerve tend to complicate the determination of the site of primary pathologic change.

Radial Nerve

As the largest branch of the brachial plexus, the radial nerve is the continuation of the posterior cord. The radial nerve winds posterior to the humerus and comes to lie anteriorly. In the arm it supplies the three heads of the triceps, the anconeus muscles, and the sensory nerves to the arm and forearm. Having reached the lateral side of the arm, the radial nerve pierces the lateral

intramuscular septum and runs between the brachialis and brachioradialis muscles. In the distal third of the arm it innervates the brachioradialis and the extensor carpi radialis longus muscles. Usually at the level of the radiocapitellar joint of the elbow the radial nerve bifurcates into a superficial and a deep branch. After giving off a motor branch to the extensor carpi radialis brevis muscle, the superficial branch of the radial nerve continues distally in the forearm to supply sensation over the radiodorsal area of the hand, thumb, index finger, long finger, and one half of the ring finger.

The deep branch of the radial nerve at the elbow is the posterior interosseous nerve. It passes between the two heads of the supinator, deep to the arcade of Frohse, into the supinator muscle, which it innervates. Distally the posterior interosseous nerve supplies a superficial group of muscles, including the extensor digitorum communis, extensor digiti quinti, extensor carpi ulnaris, and a deep group of muscles: the abductor pollicis longus, extensor pollicis longus and brevis, and the extensor indicis proprius.

Areas of compression of the radial nerve about the elbow can occur around the lateral epicondyle and in the radial tunnel, which extends from the radial head to the supinator muscle. Such areas of entrapment at times may be the result of Monteggia-type dislocations or fractures of the radius and a congenital fibrous band located anterior to the radial head, anomalous radial recurrent vessels, and the hypertrophied external carpi radialis brevis muscle. However, the most common site of compression is either the posterior interosseous branch or the radial nerve as it enters the arcade of Frohse, which is a fibrous thickening of the supinator muscle, or the hypertrophied muscle itself. Compression at this level produces motor dysfunction but no cutaneous sensory deficits comparable to the purely motor anterior interosseous nerve counterpart. Forearm muscle hypertrophy, repetitive, forceful elbow motion, wrist flexion and extension, and congenital variations in the throwing athlete cause entrapment, increased traction, and friction.

The athlete may present with deep aching of the extensor muscle mass after throwing or batting or after direct trauma to the lateral elbow. If injury occurs to the radial nerve before deep branching, sensory paresthesia along the superficial radial nerve distribution may be noted. If the insult to the radial nerve at this level is severe, there may be inability to extend the wrist and fingers; sensory deficits in the thumb, index, and long fingers, and loss of brachioradialis muscle function. High involvement of the posterior interosseous nerve may yield only loss of extension at the metacarpophalangeal joints of the thumb and fingers.

Analogous to tardy ulnar nerve syndrome, **tardy posterior interosseous nerve syndrome** with symptoms occurring years after the initial injury is now a recognized entity.

Anterior lateral elbow pain can be enhanced clinically by resisted supination of the forearm with the elbow in full extension. This provocative maneuver compresses the supinator muscle. Lidocaine injection into the radial tunnel is diagnostic of radial nerve injury if the extensor

pain is relieved and posterior interosseous nerve palsy results.

In the differential diagnosis of lateral elbow pain, systemic disease such as diabetes, periarteritis nodosa, and heavy metal poisoning need to be considered along with lateral epicondylitis and tennis elbow.

Musculocutaneous Nerve

Often overlooked on the lateral aspect of the elbow and forearm is the contribution of the musculocutaneous nerve that is formed from the splitting of the lateral cord of the brachial plexus. It pierces and innervates the coracobrachialis and courses between the brachialis and the biceps muscles to the lateral side of the arm. The musculocutaneous nerve exits the deep fascia lateral to the biceps at the elbow and continues into the forearm as a lateral antebrachial cutaneous nerve distally to the thenar eminence. The biceps and the greater part of the brachialis muscles are supplied by the motor branches of the musculocutaneous nerve.

Entrapment of the musculocutaneous nerve can occur at the level of the bicipital aponeurosis, resulting from repetitive forceful pronation of the forearm and extension of the elbow in the deceleration phase of throwing after ball release. Also the nerve is susceptible to direct trauma and the pressure of muscle hypertrophy as are the other nerves about the elbow.

A vague description of discomfort over the lateral antebrachial cutaneous nerve distribution in the forearm is often the initial complaint of the athlete. There may be palpable tenderness anteriorly, and local pressure over the bicipital aponeurosis may magnify symptoms. Not to be disregarded is the role of the biceps and brachialis muscles in controlling elbow extension in the deceleration phase of throwing. It is imperative to test the strength of flexion of the forearm in a pitcher with control problems to rule out musculocutaneous nerve entrapment.

Medical Treatment of Soft-Tissue Injuries

Rest is the medical treatment most often prescribed for soft-tissue injuries about the elbow caused by repetitive throwing. Actually, rest for the throwing athlete means refraining from the offending throwing action and, after diagnosis, institution of supervised, therapeutic exercise (passive, active, and resisted). Except when casting for fractures and splinting for postsurgical cases, immobilization is considered an enemy of the elbow. Medical treatment is directed toward safely and effectively restoring full range of motion, developing muscular strength and endurance, and attaining previous levels of flexibility and proficiency while maintaining cardiovascular fitness and total body well-being. Methods and modalities of treatment have changed over the years, but basic principles of therapy have persisted. After supportive measures, formal medical treatment for inflammation resulting from sprains, strains, contusions, and surgery about the elbow essentially is implementation of a formal rehabilitation program. The inflammatory reactive process can develop from direct trauma, but more often it results from repetitive, excessive stress placed on ligamentous,

muscular, articular, or nervous tissue; this produces microtrauma, edema, weakness, tightness, limited motion, and pain. Should throwing continue, ligamentous injury, nerve irritation, and muscular imbalance become apparent, and abnormal biomechanics ensue, often initiating new symptoms. This disuse cycle is obviated by judiciously adhering to the guideline of not working through undiagnosed pain.

The primary treatment for elbow pain is **cryotherapy.** Ice in a ziplock bag or a commercial ice pack is applied directly to the involved area and held in place with an elastic wrap for 20 to 30 minutes. A sling may be needed for comfort. Heat is to be avoided early because, although comforting, it produces local swelling, whereas ice produces local anesthesia that permits motion and reduces swelling and edema.

As part of the clinical assessment, the degree of elbow (1) flexion/extension, (2) forearm pronation/supination, and (3) the valgus carrying angle are measured. Flexion contracture, increased carrying angle, and incomplete supination are frequently encountered in athletes who have been throwing for several years. An estimate of medial and lateral stability as compared to the uninvolved arm is noted in response to stress with the elbow flexed at 20 to 30 degrees to free the olecranon from its fossa.

Motion

Once the pathologic condition is ascertained, a patient-specific aggressive therapeutic exercise program is devised with the goal of expediently returning the athlete to action within the propriety of sound medical judgment. The principal idea in the rehabilitation or treatment scheme (the terms are essentially interchangeable) is to restore range of motion. The foundation of this protocol is simple: slow **passive stretching,** followed by **active stretching** through the available range of motion, using pain as a guide. These motions should be held for 6 to 10 seconds and done in sets of 10 to 12, repeating them at least three times a day. **Proprioceptive neuromuscular facilitation (PNF)** is also used to regain range of motion. PNF depends on proprioceptor stimulation of the muscle when it is maximally stretched and then completely shortened in the functional position. The technique requires substantial knowledge and should be employed initially by professional therapists and trainers.

Flexibility about a joint refers to ease of movement through the range of motion. Ordinarily after injury, as the range of motion returns to normal, the ability to bend or extend with facility follows. Although range of motion and flexibility are not synonymous, they must be congruous. For the athlete, flexibility implies the propitious use of full range of motion.

Strength

The second principle in therapeutic exercise is to restore strength, which is known to be measurably decreased within 48 hours after injury and the beginning of inactivity. Strength, the power to resist a force, is defined as static (isometric) when there is no joint movement and dynamic (isotonic) when motion ensues. To

produce strength, muscles contract and shorten concentrically and lengthen against resistance eccentrically. The prime example is the biceps brachialis group that flexes the elbow in the wind-up phase (concentric contraction) and acts to resist elongation in elbow extension (eccentric contraction) during the deceleration phase of throwing.

Concentric and eccentric muscular contractions play equally significant roles in athletic endeavors, a fact not to be overlooked in rehabilitation protocols. In various training modes, overflow from concentric strength training gains to eccentric strength training gains, and vice versa, does occur.[20] Uniquely, eccentric contractions require lower muscular energy per unit of tension than do concentric contractions. Also, because of both noncontractile and contractile tissue working in elongation, eccentric muscles contract at approximately 36% greater mean tension than can be achieved concentrically. In general, using eccentric (negative) rehabilitation techniques offers an alternative to conventional concentric (positive) methods; however, each has a precise functional significance. As mentioned, the eccentric action of the biceps brachialis musculature in controlling deceleration must be intricately meshed with concentric muscular action in acceleration to provide the trajectory and velocity components of performance. Therefore, once adequate range of motion and flexibility are achieved, therapeutic exercise must be directed toward enhancing sport-specific functional activities.

There are three main types of muscle-strengthening exercises. **Isometric exercise** is performed by contracting muscle groups without associated joint movement. This technique requires two-thirds maximum effort held for 6 seconds in multiple sets of 10. Isometric exercise is most efficacious in early rehabilitation before full range of motion is restored and when insufficient strength may prevent use of other equipment.

Isotonic exercise typically is performed with free weights and is characterized by variable speed and fixed weight. Based on the DeLorme principle, weight is lifted six to ten times until fatigue occurs. Over time, muscle strength increases, and more weight is added to overload the muscles. This is referred to as progressive resistance exercise (PRE) and is the gold standard of muscle-strengthening programs. In contrast to maintenance programs, isotonic exercises are performed daily by the injured athlete.

Isokinetic exercise is characterized by fixed speed and accommodative resistance as exhibited in the Orthotron and Cybex equipment. These machines provide equivalent resistance to that which the athlete exerts through the entire range of motion. The advantage over isotonic exercise is that slow speed isokinetic exercise (60 degrees per second) stimulates muscle strength at more functional levels.

Variable resistance equipment, like Nautilus, now is in vogue in fitness centers, health spas, and high school, college, and professional team training rooms. To use these machines, the athlete must produce near maximum force through the available range of motion. For colleges the weight room with free weights, power racks, and Nautilus-like machines serves as a recruiting tool.

However, unless properly instructed in the use of these machines, athletes may sustain musculoskeletal injuries from improper use. Also, the progression from specific therapeutic exercises to freelance weight training after injury should be done only with the knowledge and direction of the physician/therapist/trainer team.

Manual resistance can be used to produce isometric or isokinetic exercise. Although not truly consistent in the amount of resistance, manual resistance, whether self-imposed or one-on-one, can be easily adapted to the use of specific muscle groups.

Modalities

Physical therapy modalities are useful adjuncts to exercise therapy. Electrical stimulation of muscles can be advantageous early as a countermeasure to pain and later in rehabilitation for reeducation of muscular contraction. The use of heat, in the form of hydrocollator packs (150° to 160° F), warm whirlpools (105° to 110° F), paraffin baths, and ultrasound should be considered after the acute phase of injury when muscle spasm occurs and increased flexibility and range of motion are needed to return to functional activity.

Modalities used in elbow rehabilitation

- Electrical stimulation
- Cryotherapy
- Heat
- Ultrasound

Caution, however, is suggested when using the many modalities now available. Just as the physician must carefully individualize aggressive therapeutic exercise, the proper and successful use of rehabilitative modalities rests on the expertise of skilled professional therapists and trainers.

Exertional Compartment Syndromes

Exertional compartment syndromes rarely occur in the throwing athlete. Despite numerous professional athletes involved in throwing who have very well developed flexor-pronator muscle groups, there are no extensive studies in the literature on this problem. Bennett[11] reported a syndrome in which a pitcher was unable to continue throwing for more than two or three innings because of marked pain and swelling over the flexor-pronator muscle group. On examination, he found this athlete to have distinct fullness over the pronator teres. He described a compartment release that consisted of a cruciate division of the fascia of the flexor-pronator muscle group, which provided relief of these symptoms. On close evaluation of his report, however, it appears that he may have been referring to a pronator teres syndrome with proximal forearm pain secondary to compression of the median nerve; this seems likely because he specifically implicates the lacertus fibrosis and the proximal fascial arcade of the flexor digitorum sublimis. If in doubt, these lesions could be differentiated and confirmed on the basis of nerve conduction studies or compartment

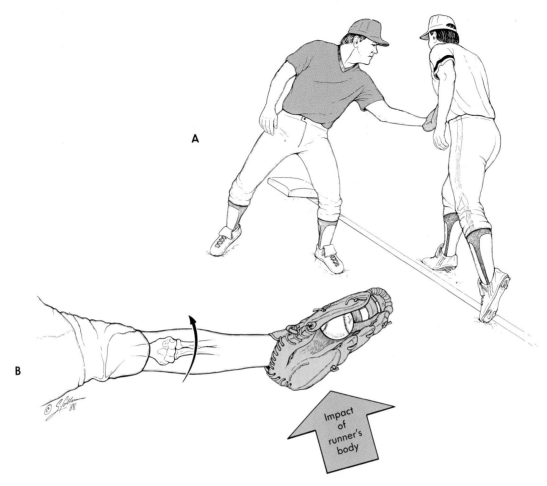

FIG. 35-27. A, Example of a forceful valgus stress applied to the ulnar collateral ligament of the extended elbow. **B,** Close-up, composite drawing of first baseman's glove and bony anatomy of the elbow and the production of valgus traction medially and compression laterally.

pressures, with appropriate treatment being directed to the lesion once the diagnosis has been established.

Acute Traumatic Injuries to the Medial Elbow
Ulnar Collateral Ligament Rupture

Contact injuries. Ulnar collateral ligament rupture differs from the rupture of the isolated ulnar collateral ligament resulting from overuse (noncontact) in the throwing athlete. The contact injury occurs when the forearm and elbow are forced into marked valgus deviation by a single applied force or blow (contact), as in the football quarterback whose forearm is hit during cocking, acceleration, or at release of the ball while attempting a pass. It has also been described in baseball infielders who ex-

tend the arm to tag a passing runner whose body force exerts a marked valgus overload on the infielder's medial elbow (Fig. 35-27).[39]

Regardless of the causing mechanism, this is a serious injury for any throwing athlete, as there is evidence that absence of a functional ulnar collateral ligament adversely affects throwing performance.[27] This diagnosis must be specifically ruled out by appropriate tests, including the elbow arthrogram and a gravity stress test, if possible. If the diagnosis is confirmed, surgical intervention is indicated.

The surgical approach for this lesion is similar to that described for ulnar collateral ligament repair (see p. 766). The associated pathologic state at surgery may differ from patient to patient when this ligament has been ruptured by a singular traumatic event. Whether there is additional anatomic disruption depends on the degree of force applied to the medial aspect of the elbow. This includes flexor-pronator origin avulsions, intramuscular disruption, and disruption of the soft tissues, all of which stabilize the ulnar nerve within the cubital tunnel.[39] Care must be taken to immediately identify the ulnar nerve above the level of the elbow and to trace it into the

---

Mechanisms of ulnar collateral ligament injury

- Noncontact: acute injury (pitching)
- Noncontact: chronic injury (pitching)
- Contact: acute injury (football)
- Associated with posterior elbow dislocation

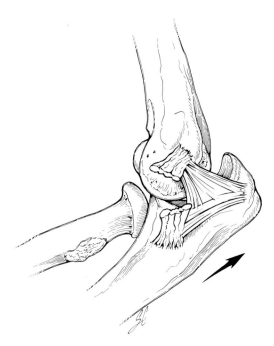

FIG. 35-28. Posterior dislocation of the elbow after midsubstance tear of the anterior oblique portion of the ulnar collateral ligament.

area of ecchymosis and tissue disruption to ensure that it has not been displaced directly into the surgical field. In any event, the ulnar nerve should be decompressed and transposed because leaving it in its anatomic location will result in excessive fibrosis developing about the nerve. The flexor-pronator muscle mass is reapproximated to the medial epicondyle through drill holes. The results of repairing the ulnar collateral ligament acutely warrant using this approach rather than reconstructing the ligament using a free autogenous graft.[39]

Elbow dislocation. Elbow dislocations have been treated successfully by reduction, limited immobilization, and early range of motion therapy. In most cases only minor sequelae usually result from this standard form of treatment. There is, however, a reported 9% to 14% incidence of recurrent elbow dislocation following a posterior fracture-dislocation.[61] This recurrent dislocation appears to be caused by the instability that results from disruption of the ulnar collateral ligament at the time of the initial dislocation (Fig. 35-28).

Tullos et al[60] have shown that the anterior oblique ligament band of the ulnar collateral ligament was torn in 34 of 37 patients in whom a posterior elbow dislocation had occurred earlier. Disruption of this ligament was diagnosed by a positive stress test and confirmed at the time of acute surgical repair following initial dislocation. With this high rate of ulnar collateral ligament injury associated with posterior elbow dislocations, it is imperative to test for the integrity of the ulnar collateral ligament in any patient, particularly the throwing athlete. Should the throwing athlete suffer this injury in the dominant arm, acute repair of the ligament following reduction of the dislocation is indicated if the athlete desires the best chance for return to his or her previous level of throwing activity.

Ulnar Nerve Contusion

The section of this chapter that deals with nerve entrapment syndromes about the elbow describes the clinical presentation and subsequent management of irritation of the ulnar nerve caused by compressive and tensile forces occurring about the nerve and associated with the act of throwing. However, the athlete can incur an injury to the ulnar nerve independently of these irritating forces. This refers specifically to a direct blow being applied to the ulnar nerve while it is subluxed from its posterior position in the cubital tunnel anterior to the medial epicondyle. In this position the nerve is unprotected and can be injured directly rather than indirectly, as occurs in the repetitive act of throwing.

Recurrent dislocation of the ulnar nerve as the elbow is moved through a range of motion has been identified in up to 16% of the general population. The nerve may either sublux onto the medial epicondyle or completely dislocate anterior to the medial epicondyle. Childress[16] found that those nerves that subluxed on the medial epicondyle but did not translocate anterior to it were at greater risk of direct injury, whereas the completely dislocating ulnar nerve was at increased risk for friction neuritis.

A direct blow to the ulnar nerve in its subluxed position is acutely painful and may be the initiating factor in a chronic ulnar nerve irritation. The initial injury should be treated with rest, ice, and a gradually increasing mobilization as the acute episode subsides. As far as possible or as appropriate in the athlete's sport, protective padding should be used; if recurrent ulnar neuritis develops as a result of this initial injury, formal anterior transposition of the nerve is indicated.

Lateral Elbow Injuries
Bony Injuries

Slocum's list[51] of lateral compression injuries of the elbow resulting from baseball pitching are as follows: traumatic osteochondritis dissecans, fracture of the capitellum, and traumatic arthritis. The first of these, osteochondritis dissecans, is discussed in depth in that part of this chapter concerned with the skeletally immature elbow in the throwing athlete. As described by Slocum, the forces at work on the outer side of the elbow include compression caused by valgus overload, rotational forces resulting from pronation and supination of the forearm, and extension forces that are applied during the deceleration phase of the throwing act. Much of the literature that concerns lateral elbow problems in the throwing athlete refers specifically to the skeletally immature elbow. It is noteworthy that there is an absence of reports identifying bony lateral lesions as a significant source of pathologic change in mature throwing athletes.

Lateral compression injuries

- Traumatic osteochondritis dissecans
- Fracture of the capitellum
- Traumatic arthritis

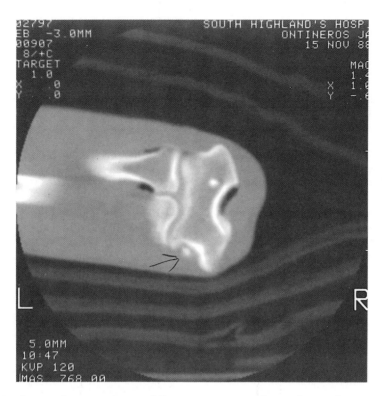

FIG. 35-29. Computed tomography scan following air-contrast arthrography reveals a tear in the capsule on the ulnar aspect of a right elbow.

An analysis of 100 symptomatic baseball players by Barnes and Tullos[9] included 50 elbow injuries, of which 11 were symptomatic secondary to loose bodies, only one of which originated from the radiocapitellar articulation. Indelicato et al[24] reported on 25 professional baseball players who underwent a reconstructive surgical procedure on their dominant elbow. None of the players in the study had any radiographic evidence of lateral compartment disease. In 20 of the 25, good results were obtained; however, in two of the five with unsatisfactory results, loose bodies were removed from the posterior compartment, and the radiohumeral joint was visualized at that time. Significant articular degeneration in the radiohumeral joint was noted in these two cases.

This is not to say that radiocapitellar lesions do not occur or have not been reported. We have evaluated the radiographs of 65 professional baseball pitchers participating at various levels of competition ranging from class A baseball to the major leagues.[46] These pitchers were randomly selected and radiographically evaluated, using a routine throwers' series of radiographs (previously described) as part of their preseason physical evaluation. Interestingly, in none of these radiographic evaluations were any capitellar or radial head injuries identified. We cannot conclude that radiocapitellar lesions occur only in the adolescent or skeletally immature throwing athlete, but we think the infrequency of capitellar and radial head injuries in skeletally mature athletes may be because athletes who incur such injuries during their career are unable to continue to compete. These individuals, therefore, are victims of the natural selection process in high-

caliber throwing. Slocum[51] believed that the predominance of the lateral elbow injury in the skeletally immature thrower may be because of increased ligamentous laxity about the elbow in this age group and the smaller surface area of articulation between the capitellum and radius, resulting in greater stress concentration on these joint surfaces.

When chondral defects are noted in the skeletally mature pitching elbow, they can arise from either the radial head articular cartilage or the capitellum. In some cases, these chondral defects can be quite large, with both osseous and cartilaginous components affected, whereas in other cases they are small osseous lesions or strictly cartilaginous loose bodies not identified on conventional radiographs.[2]

Chondromalacia of the capitellum and accompanying classically described softening, fibrillations, and fractures have been identified arthroscopically. Use of CT arthrography or MRI (Fig. 35-29), which is now routinely employed in the evaluation of a high-caliber throwing athlete with elbow pain, helps delineate any lateral compartment changes. A definitive diagnosis is best accomplished through arthroscopic visualization of the radiocapitellar articulation.[4] As discussed in a later section on that topic, elbow arthroscopy has become a safe and effective technique in both the evaluation and treatment of elbow injuries of the throwing athlete. It allows for complete inspection of the joint, including the radiocapitellar articulation. Previously, when open techniques were used to treat other lesions in the throwing athlete, this articulation was not well visualized. Thus the integ-

rity of the radiocapitellar joint was not confirmed, and the pathologic change within this articulation contributing to unsatisfactory results was only speculative.

In the skeletally mature elbow, chondral lesions and loose bodies can be safely removed, in most cases through an arthroscopic approach.[4] Despite their origin from the radiocapitellar articular surfaces, these loose bodies can often be found lying in the posterolateral compartment of the elbow. Thus it is necessary to carry out a complete evaluation of an elbow during arthroscopy regardless of the presenting or obvious complaints and radiographic findings. In the skeletally mature elbow debridement of the articular defects is carried out to promote a fibrocartilaginous healing response. It does not seem to be advantageous to pin back osteocartilaginous loose fragments from these joint surfaces. The surgical technique for the arthroscopic treatment of these injuries is further delineated under the section on elbow arthroscopy.

Soft-Tissue Injuries

Tendinitis on the lateral aspect of the elbow in the throwing athlete is uncommon. In the general population, lateral epicondylitis occurs seven times more frequently than medial epicondylitis and is a common presenting complaint in racquet sports.[38] Lateral epicondylitis occurring in the throwing athlete is an overuse-type syndrome, more likely related to forearm and wrist biomechanics than to valgus-related stresses applied directly across the elbow. The lateral elbow pain of tendinitis must be differentiated from that of radial tunnel syndrome, which also is a rare finding in throwing athletes.

The treatment for this condition remains essentially a nonsurgical one. Physical therapy plays a major role and should include ice massage with wrist extensor and flexor stretching; in addition, an eccentric reconditioning program should be used as described in the rehabilitation section of this chapter. Recalcitrant cases may require surgical release of the extensor carpi radialis brevis.

Posterior Elbow Lesions

Lesions in the posterior elbow, specifically at the olecranon and olecranon fossa, are probably the most common type of injury in the throwing athlete. Fortunately, most reports in the literature, combined with our personal experience, indicate that these lesions are not only amenable to surgical treatment but also are ones in which the athlete has a good chance of returning to his or her previous levels of throwing.[9,11,24] In Barnes and Tullos' study[9] of 100 symptomatic baseball players, 50 of whom had elbow injuries, 10 of the 50 had posterior compartment bodies that were removed surgically, resulting in all 10 of them returning to their previous level of throwing. In a review of 25 cases of correctable elbow lesions in professional baseball players, Indelicato et al[24] reported that 14 of 25 underwent surgical removal of loose bodies from the posterior compartment, yielding complete satisfaction in 12 of 14 cases.

We have completed a review[8] of 72 professional baseball players who underwent elbow surgery. Posterome-

dial osteophytes of the olecranon were the most common diagnoses, occurring in 65% of the cases. The reoperation rate after arthroscopic excision of a posteromedial osteophyte from the olecranon was 29% with a second debridement required. The integrity of the ulnar collateral ligament must be carefully evaluated at the time of osteophyte removal, and after the removal of this buttress the valgus stress on the ligament may be increased. We noted that in 25% of the patients requiring reoperation after osteophyte excision, an ulnar collateral ligament reconstruction was also performed.

Bony Injuries

Valgus extension overload conditions. Except for triceps tendinitis (discussed later), posterior elbow pathologic change is primarily bony in nature. With the exception of a rare traction-induced stress fracture of the olecranon tip, these bony injuries are believed to result from the rapid and forceful extension and valgus forces applied to the elbow in the late acceleration and complete deceleration phases of throwing.[29] It should be recalled that, as the forearm and wrist accelerate through the later stages of the acceleration phase of throwing, the centrifugal force that is generated begins to impose an extension force across the elbow joint. At this point in the acceleration phase a large degree of torque and a high rate of extension are present at the elbow joint. These two forces combine to cause a relatively high shear force to be imposed on the articular cartilage of the posteromedial olecranon and, more particularly, on the corresponding medial wall of the olecranon fossa. This is known as valgus extension overload.[62] Any valgus instability, even if minor, leads to further abutment of the posteromedial olecranon against the olecranon fossa. In addition, the tip of the olecranon process impinges into the olecranon fossa in the posterior aspect of the humerus, and repetitive impingements can cause osteophytic bone formation directly at the tip of the olecranon and in the fossa itself. Thus both the tip and the posteromedial aspect of the olecranon can serve as sites of bony osteophytes that may subsequently fracture and become the source of loose bodies. Osteophyte and loose body formation can also arise in the olecranon fossa itself. If not specifically sought out, posteromedial corner osteophytes are sometimes overlooked. These osteophytes are the result of valgus extension overload (as noted previously). They can be delineated by the axial view taken as part of the routine radiographic study (Fig. 35-30). The osteophytes not only serve as a source of loose bodies, but also, because of the nature of their position, can result in friction irritation on the undersurface of the ulnar nerve as it passes directly over the posteromedial portion of the joint while it rests in the cubital tunnel. Forced extension of the elbow during physical examination can produce complaints of posterior elbow pain caused by straight posterior osteophytes. However, the posteromedial osteophytes of the valgus extension overload syndrome may not be symptomatic unless a valgus component to the extension is added. With the valgus force applied to the forearm as the elbow is brought into extension, the patient's symptoms relative to these osteophytes can be reproduced.

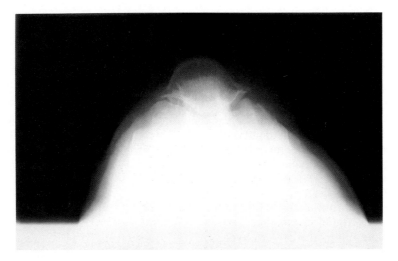

FIG. 35-30. Axial view demonstrates significant posterior osteophytes both medially and laterally.

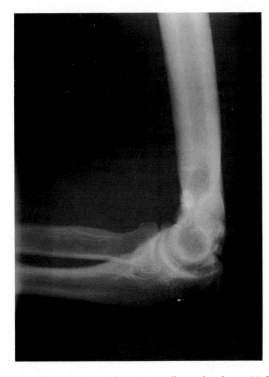

FIG. 35-31. Posterior osteophytes are well visualized on a 90-degree flexion lateral view. This osteophyte has fractured away from the olecranon tip.

The treatment of posterior elbow pain in the presence of posterior and posteromedial osteophytes is initially conservative (Fig. 35-31). Attempts are made through rest, ice, and various physical therapy modalities to alleviate the thrower's symptoms to a point where he or she can return to the preinjury activity. However, if symptoms persist despite these measures, surgical intervention is indicated. We have found arthroscopic excision of osteophytes and removal of loose bodies to be a successful and reproducible technique for the treatment of these lesions.[7] Occasionally with the valgus extension overload syndrome, purely cartilaginous hypertrophy is noted in the posteromedial aspect of the olecranon fossa complex. Although these lesions are not seen radiographically, at the time of arthroscopy they can be readily identified and removed. Using the arthroscopic techniques, thorough debridement of the posterior compartment is achieved. More exacting removal of the offending pathologic tissue is possible through arthroscopic techniques than with open surgery. This allows for maximum retention of bone to act as a secondary stabilizer against the valgus forces of the throwing act. Although the operative procedure does not alter the repetitive forces that initiated the development of the pathologic condition, it does offer the competitive athlete a chance to return to his or her previous level of throwing, symptomatically improved, but with the knowledge that the changes as well as the symptoms may recur. Postoperative care for arthroscopic debridement of the posterior compartment includes a posterior splint for 2 to 3 days, followed by range of motion activities and a stretching and strengthening program once range of motion has been achieved. In general, throwing athletes are able to resume their previous activity approximately 6 to 8 weeks postoperatively.

Fractures. Fractures of the olecranon include avulsions of the tip of the olecranon caused by acute traction through the insertion of the triceps tendon and stress fractures caused by repetitive extensor action.[11,18,41,51] The avulsion injuries can be treated symptomatically with immobilization; however, if they prove to be persistently painful despite conservative treatment, they may require surgical excision. The rare olecranon stress fracture may also require surgical intervention when painful. Often asymptomatic, actively throwing athletes have been identified with the lesion on routine evaluation.

Soft-Tissue Conditions

Triceps tendinitis. Triceps tendinitis, although occurring less frequently than medial epicondylitis or lateral epicondylitis, is seen on occasion.[14,26,51] It, like the other tendinitis problems of the elbow, should respond to rest and proper physical therapy modalities (outlined in the rehabilitation section of this chapter). However, like

other forms of tendinitis, it may be slow to respond and may prove to be frustrating for both the treating physician and the athlete who wishes to return promptly to his or her previous asymptomatic level of activity.

Anterior Elbow Lesions

Most anterior elbow problems in the throwing athlete are soft tissue in nature. Those lesions, affecting the anterior aspect of the elbow, include biceps tendinitis and anterior capsular strain accompanied by periosteal reaction and bony hypertrophy or spur formation. Hypertrophy of the coronoid process is also seen (Fig. 35-32). The biceps tendon is exposed to large eccentric loads during the deceleration phase of the throwing act.[33] With the brachioradialis and brachialis, the biceps tendon serves to decelerate the elbow to prevent marked, forced hyperextension secondary to the tremendous centrifugal forces generated at ball release. Preseason conditioning should include an eccentric biceps strengthening program to train this musculotendinous unit to perform in the manner expected of it during the throwing act. Rest, physical therapy modalities, and stretching and strengthening programs are prescribed for bicipital tendinitis. Both the anterior joint capsule and the brachialis insertion on the anterior aspect of the elbow are exposed to these same tensile forces during elbow extension and may also become symptomatic. With repetitive elbow flexion, bony anterior elbow lesions arise from the abutment of the coronoid process into the coronoid fossa. Osteophyte formation and loose body generation can occur from either surface. If symptomatic, these lesions are amenable to arthroscopic excision.

THE SKELETALLY IMMATURE THROWING ATHLETE

The degree of skeletal maturity of the athlete's elbow is determined radiographically by correlating chronologic age with the appearance and fusion of the secondary centers of ossification of the distal humerus, olecranon, and radial head. Although there may be variability in development because of genetic, nutritional, and hormonal factors, maturation usually proceeds in an orderly, predictable fashion. Comparable application of acute or repetitive trauma sufficient to produce pathologic changes at one age may yield different clinical and radiologic findings at another age. For the immature athlete, intrinsically it is bone age that determines the characteristic changes that the trauma of throwing produces. Extrinsically the causes of change are force, caliber, frequency, and the biomechanics of throwing. In the young athlete, as in the more mature one, the five different phases of throwing produce equivalent shearing and compressive forces laterally and traction forces medially. Also, full or hyperforced extension produces increased pressure posteriorly and stretching anteriorly.

Repetitive microtrauma produces progressive physiologic changes in soft and bony tissue that can become painful, ultimately compromising strength and motion. Potentially the most injurious component of throwing in the immature elbow occurs during the early acceleration

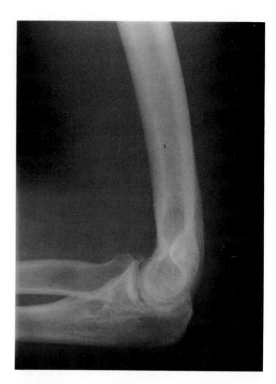

FIG. 35-32. Note the spurring of the coronoid process and subtle reactive changes at the coronoid fossa as a result of abutment by the spur.

phase when the forward-moving shoulder imparts a valgus stress on the trailing elbow. This valgus stress imparts a medial pull or stretch on the soft tissue structures and their bony attachments and a compression with shearing of the capitellum laterally on the radial head. In the follow-through phase, as the valgus elbow extends, increased pressure is exerted on the posteromedial olecranon as it impinges the olecranon fossa. These forces inflict different sequelae at arbitrarily selected but convenient subdivisions of immaturity. This multiplicity of information has led to confusion of the nomenclature and classification of pathologic states in the elbow in the immature athlete. In contradistinction to the shoulder, where little league shoulder is described by Dottier[19] as one entity (epiphyseal fracture of the proximal humerus), several pathologic conditions are loosely combined under the umbrella of little league elbow.

Medial Problems

First brought to medical attention by Brogdon and Crowe,[13] little league elbow is seen radiographically as cortical thickening, medial epicondylar enlargement, fragmentation, beaking, and separation in response to overuse. Clinically called medial epicondylitis, little league elbow occurs predominately between ages 9 and 12 and, when recognized and treated early, seldom becomes debilitating. Technically, the entity is classified as a **medial traction apophysitis,** since throwing produces tension stress force across the epiphyseal plate in an area of bone that does not contribute to humeral length and that, at this age, is extracapsular.

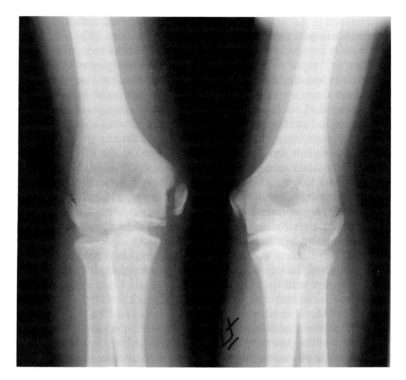

FIG. 35-33. Salter I medial epicondylar fracture through the apophysis in a 12-year-old right-handed shortstop. Injury occurred with a hard throw to first base. Left arm for comparison.

Radiographic findings in little league elbow

- Cortical thickening
- Medial epicondylar enlargement, fragmentation, or beaking
- Separation of the medial epicondyle

In addition to the flexor-pronator muscle group, the medial apophysis gives origin to the two major stabilizing portions of the ulnar collateral ligament: (1) the anterior oblique band, which is taut both in flexion and extension, and (2) the posterior band, which is taut in flexion only. Medial stability is often overlooked if the elbow is not tested clinically by active stressing or passively by the radiographic gravity medial stress technique. Traction medial apophysitis during throwing clinically produces medial tenderness and swelling, decreased extension, and localized pain on valgus stressing. Aggravation of symptoms is noted on resisted flexion/extension and pronation of the wrist. Radiographically, with continued throwing despite medial symptoms, greater irregularity of the epiphyseal plate develops, along with increased displacement of the apophysis. Subsequently, or with a forceful throw, significant avulsion occurs, which usually displaces the apophysis distally (Fig. 35-33). However, the fragment, often accompanied by a small piece of metaphyseal bone, may migrate into the joint or become attached to the coronoid process. True avulsion is indicated when the injured elbow has 5 mm or more of displacement compared to the uninvolved elbow. Reapproximation is needed, yet some controversy still exists as to whether surgical replacement yields better results than conservative methods. Nevertheless, an incarcerated joint fragment requires manipulation or extraction.

Fusion of secondary centers of ossification of the medial epicondyle occurs last in the distal humerus. As maturation continues, confusion may develop on discerning an avulsion fracture if irregularity and fragmentation of the ossification center normally occur. Once fused, avulsion of a fragment or of the entire epicondyle can occur as a result of a single throw in a player with a heavy throwing history. Fibrous nonunion does result and may be painful. Ectopic bone, traction osteophytes, and spurring are evidence of sustained trauma and are seen concurrently with increased valgus deformity.

Repetitive traction stress forces in the skeletally more mature young adult may produce inflammation at the origin of the flexor-pronator muscle–epicondylar interface, resulting in microscopic or macroscopic avulsion of the musculotendinous insertion. Less frequently, tearing of the proximal muscle fibers is found. Such strains and muscular avulsions are clinically indiscernible, with differentiation being merely didactic.

As in the mature athlete, ulnar neuropathy in the young athlete can result from traction produced in the throwing motion, irritation from subluxation out of the ulnar groove, or compression from fascial adhesions secondary to lateral avulsion fractures. The incidence of ulnar nerve involvement increases with maturity of the thrower and the number and velocity of the throws.

Lateral Problems

The major throwing-related trauma that can occur to an immature athlete's elbow laterally centers around the capitellum. In a 1929 study, Panner[43] reported on three children (ages 7, 10, and 10) with a capitellar pathologic condition similar to osteochondritis dissecans but without loose body formation. Believing that such a pathologic condition was accident related, he concluded that, although trauma might be the incidental cause, another essential factor must exist for the disease to develop, yet he had no assurance as to what that factor was. He believed that the entity now commonly known as osteochondrosis of the capitellum, or Panner's disease, was comparable to the pathologic change associated with Osgood-Schlatter's, Koehler's, and Calvé-Perthes' diseases. In osteochondrosis typically there is rarefaction and blurring of the structures, initially leading to diminished size and fuzziness of the edges of the ossification center. The clinical symptoms are mild, and there is no corpora libera formation. Recovery is slow but complete.

The lateral epicondyle is subject to far less pathologic change in the immature elbow than the medial epicondyle, primarily because of the nature of the throwing motion. However, in the follow-through phase sufficient forceful extension traction is produced to occasionally cause avulsion of the lateral apophysis along with a fragment of the condyle, the origin of the extensor muscles of the forearm and wrist, and the radial collateral ligament. Clinically the findings may mimic an extension-type supracondylar fracture. Caution is indicated in making a radiologic diagnosis of avulsion of the lateral apophysis in the young athlete because there is normally a separation of the ossification center and the metaphysis of the humerus in youth.

Woodward[64] reported Mayo Clinic experience of capitellar lesions, two thirds of which were baseball pitching–initiated symptoms occurring between the ages of 9 and 15 years. In that report irregular ossification and rarefaction with a crater formation were noted along with flattening of the capitellum and loose body formation. His radiographic diagnosis was osteochondritis dissecans with some familiar and constitutional tendencies. Woodward distinguished osteochondritis dissecans from the osteochondrosis of Panner. The latter is noted at an earlier age, involves the whole ossification center of the capitellum, forms no loose bodies, and requires only conservative treatment. Woodward reported that, after surgical removal of loose bodies (when needed) in osteochondritis dissecans, the prognosis for the return to normal function was good.

Adams' study[1] clearly demonstrated that, in addition to the recognized entity of medial apophysitis, little league elbow occasionally involved osteochondritis of the capitellum and the head of the radius. Guggenheim et al,[22] however, failed to recognize radiographic evidence of aseptic necrosis of the capitellum or the radial head in his study of 595 little league pitchers. Ellman,[21] Tullos and King,[58] and Larson et al[32] concluded that conditions described as osteochondrosis or osteochondritis dissecans both result from compression forces that develop during throwing as a secondary component of medial valgus stress. In 1930 Kirby[30] reported on two pitchers (ages 19 and 24) in whom he found lateral foreign bodies that were pieces of cartilage chipped from the head of the radius as the head was "brought backward suddenly with great force against the condyle of the humerus."

Since Koonig,[31] in 1889, coined the term *osteochondritis dissecans* to mean a dissected piece of articular cartilage (in the knee), its etiology has been depicted as hereditary, vascular, or traumatic.

A possible clarification of this picture was presented by Singer and Roy,[49] who concluded that osteochondrosis and osteochondritis dissecans are stages of the same entity with different bone ages at onset and that the level of activity is responsible for the variable radiographic findings. They postulated that early trauma resulted in vascular supply disruption and further damage, which by the age of 13 or 14 progressed to loose body formation and secondary changes in the radial head, followed ultimately by arthritic degeneration.

It is not the intent here to ignore polarization of opinions regarding the cause and subsequent pathologic state of the medial and lateral compartment of the elbow as a result of throwing. Instead, it seems prudent to agree that the classic definition of Brogdon and Crowe[13] of medial epicondylitis (apophysitis) be reserved for the term little league elbow and, to avoid confusion, lesions (lateral, posterior, and anterior), whether osteochondrosis or osteochondritis dissecans, be considered as secondary entities. Also there should be agreement that, compared to medial lesions, lateral lesions present at an older age, occur less frequently, and may have debilitating long-lasting consequences.

Posterior Problems

The posterior oblique portion of the ulnar collateral ligament, which distally is attached to the medial olecranon, is taut in flexion and lax in extension. The radial collateral ligament laterally attaches to the annular ligament and not to the radius. Combined, these two ligaments provide only minimal stability for the immature elbow joint. This leaves the posterior elbow particularly vulnerable to exertional trauma. In 1941 Bennett[10,11] was the first to recognize that the mechanics of throwing could produce stress sufficient to result in cartilaginous changes of the olecranon and the adjacent humerus. Wilson et al[62] and Andrews[2] showed that in the early acceleration phase of pitching excessive valgus stress is applied to the elbow, causing wedging of the olecranon into the olecranon fossa and the formation of posteromedial osteophytes and loose bodies.

During the follow-through phase of throwing, impingement more posterior on the olecranon tip can occur. More important, however, in this phase the forceful contraction of the triceps occurs with stress being applied to its insertion into the olecranon.

Radiographic findings depend on bone development at the time of repetitive stress. Early there is noted irregular ossification of the secondary centers and traction ap-

ophysitis. Later, avulsion fractures occur with loose body formation. There may be nonunion of the secondary ossification centers and lack of fusion between the ossified center and the olecranon. In the young adult, major or minor avulsions of the triceps tendon at the olecranon insertion may develop, especially in athletes with hypertrophied musculature. Heterotropic bone formation may occur at that level and may limit extension.

Anterior Problems

The anterior capsule of the immature elbow is susceptible to hyperextension stress as seen in young pitchers with generalized laxity, poor strength, and improper mechanics. Symptoms of capsulitis may be masked by concurrent tenderness of the distal biceps, brachialis, and flexor group muscles.

Anteriorly, early radiographic changes are trochlear hypertrophy accompanied by subtle changes in the ossification centers. Subsequently, osteochondritis of the trochlea is noted and is followed by loose body formation. Trochlear osteophytes may develop later. Coronoid osteophyte formation, after ossification is complete in males

at about age 13, is caused by the repetitive anterior hyperextension stress of throwing.

Treatment

The treatment of elbow injuries in the immature athlete begins with an understanding of the developmental bony anatomy. Pappas[44] has observed that during childhood most throwing problems are related to the development of secondary epiphyses in the medial epicondyle, trochlea, capitellum, and olecranon. Characteristically these lesions can be self-limiting once throwing is eliminated. Once pain free, gradual return to baseball is permitted after the athlete completes rehabilitation techniques to improve strength and flexibility.

As secondary ossification centers fuse, fragmentation, avulsions, and physeal separations occur. Partial immobilization is necessary and each situation must be individualized for possible surgical intervention. Pappas[44] noted that the capitellum is particularly susceptible to avascular necrosis and compression deformation leading to loose body formation. Surgical removal of osteocartilaginous fragments is recommended only as a means of

TABLE 35-1 Summary of findings in the medial, lateral, posterior, and anterior elbow in the immature athlete

Children 7 to 10 Years	Little League 9 to 12 Years	Pony League 13 to 14 Years	High School 15 to 18 Years	College/Professional 19+ Years
Medial				
Increased cortical thickening of humerus Hypertrophy of arm muscles	Fragmentation, beaking, separation, hypertrophy, asymmetry, and increased density of medial epicondylar epiphysis (Brogdon and Crowe[13]) (classic little league elbow) Ulnar neuropathy	Avulsion and *fatigue* Fracture of medial epicondylar epiphysis	Avulsion fracture of entire medial epicondyle Fracture fragment of medial epicondyle Valgus deformity	Nonunion of medial epicondyle to humerus Ectopic bone formation Traction osteophytes and spurs Avulsion of flexor-pronator muscles at origin
Lateral				
Osteochondrosis of capitellum (Panner[43])	Early osteochondritis of capitellum Apophyseal separation and fragmentation of lateral epicondyle	Erosion, deformity, and osteochondritis dissecans of capitellum Deformity, hypertrophy, and osteochondritis of head of radius Premature closure of radial head epiphysis	Overgrowth of radial head Radiocapitellar joint incongruity	Osteochondritis dissecans and avulsion fracture of radial head (Kirby[30]) (baseball pitcher's elbow) Loose bodies Degenerative arthritic changes Flexion contractures
Posterior				
Triceps hypertrophy	Osteochondritis and hypertrophy of olecranon Irregular ossification of secondary centers of ossification olecranon	Traction apophysitis Avulsion fracture of olecranon	Nonunion of secondary centers of ossification and olecranon Nonunion of olecranon physis Posteromedial osteophytes, spurs, and loose body formation	Avulsion of triceps at insertion Hypertrophic bone formation at triceps insertion Degenerative arthritic changes
Anterior				
	Trochlear hypertrophy Subtle changes in ossification centers of trochlea	Osteochondritis of trochlea	Osteochondritis dissecans; osteophytes of trochlea Loose bodies Coronoid osteophyte formation	Degenerative arthritis changes

restoring range of motion. Often lesions of the capitellum are found to be refractory to treatment, leading to disability.

Avulsion of secondary centers may require surgical repair because some result in painful nonunion. Nevertheless, for the immature athlete stress reactions medially, compression forces laterally, impingement posteriorly, and stretching anteriorly are rehabilitated in a generic fashion just as in the mature athlete. Patience is paramount (Table 35-1).

ARTHROSCOPY OF THE ELBOW

Arthroscopy has proved to be a very useful adjuvant in the diagnosis and treatment of elbow injuries in the throwing athlete. It has helped us gain a more thorough understanding of the diverse pathologic changes that can occur within the symptomatic throwing elbow. Accurate diagnoses are often difficult because of the close anatomic relationship in the elbow area of structures involved in throwing injuries and the amount of overlap in their clinical presentation when injured. Although most of the problems occurring about the elbow result from overuse and involve soft tissue, the ability to identify or rule out specific intraarticular cartilaginous and osteocartilaginous entities is very valuable. Previous reports in the literature have noted the difficulty in determining the reasons for unsatisfactory results when open operative intervention has been carried out for a seemingly symptomatic lesion.[24] When possible and appropriate, combining an arthroscopic examination of the elbow joint with any elbow procedure in the throwing athlete allows us to fully document the status of all compartments and joint surfaces. This enables us to develop a more accurate diagnosis and prognosis for the individual patient and serves as a means by which we can more accurately assess the results of our surgery.

Indications

Current indications for elbow arthroscopy include the treatment of most intraarticular elbow pathologic states previously treated through arthrotomy.[3,4,7] For the throwing athlete, this would consist of debridement of any acute, traumatic, chondral, or osteochondral lesions, including treatment of osteochondritis dissecans when indicated by the patient's symptoms and age. Anterior osteophytes in the region of the coronoid process impinging in the coronoid fossa or any hypertrophy of the coronoid process can be debrided. In addition, posterior osteophytes, either those found directly posterior on the tip of the olecranon or those found classically with valgus extension overload can also be addressed. Loose bodies, from whatever source, are optimally treated by arthroscopic extraction (Fig. 35-34). Loose body extraction is the procedure for which arthroscopy is most commonly and successfully used in the treatment of the throwing athlete. Valgus instability due to ulnar collateral ligament injury can be evaluated (Fig. 35-35). In addition to these indications, arthroscopic evaluation of the elbow should

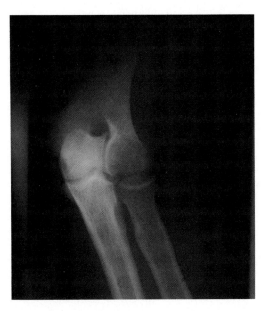

FIG. 35-34. Loose bodies can be found in any area of the elbow joint and are one of the primary indications for elbow arthroscopy.

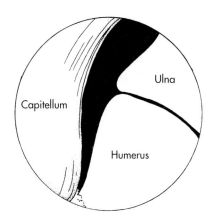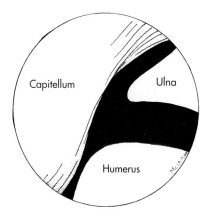

FIG. 35-35. Valgus stress test.

be completed in any throwing athlete in whom a definitive diagnosis for persistently disabling pain has not been made, and it should also be completed as part of the workup and treatment in any athlete undergoing elbow surgery for a soft-tissue problem (such as anterior transposition for ulnar neuritis or removal of extraarticular painful bony deposits) in whom the diagnosis is unclear.

Indications for arthroscopy in throwers

- Evaluation of valgus instability
- Debridement of chondral or osteochondral injuries
- Loose body removal
- Osteophyte debridement (coronoid fossa/process, olecranon fossa/process)
- Diagnostic dilemma

Surgical Technique

The patient is placed on a standard surgical table with the forearm and wrist supported in a wrist gauntlet that is connected to an overhead pulley system suspended from the end of the table. The shoulder is abducted to 90 degrees, allowing the entire arm to extend over the side of the table. With the elbow at 90 degrees of flexion, excellent access to both medial and lateral aspects of the elbow can be achieved. The elbow can be extended as necessary for the posterior portal placement, which is commonly done with the elbow at 30 degrees short of full extension. Full pronation and supination of the forearm are possible.

Positioning of the arm in this manner not only allows for excellent access but also, because of the 90 degrees of elbow flexion, enhances protection of the neurovascular structures in the antecubital fossa. The important neurovascular structures running across the front of the elbow (median nerve, brachial artery, and radial nerve) are relaxed in this position and are more easily displaced away from the direct operating field as the various portals are made and instruments are introduced. For excellent control of bleeding without obstruction to the operating field, a tourniquet is placed as far proximally as possible on the arm during elbow arthroscopies.

After routine sterile prep and drape, the procedure is initiated by first identifying the bony landmarks about the elbow. These include the medial and lateral epicondyle, radial head, and the tip of the olecranon. Using these palpable bony structures as landmarks and keeping in mind the underlying soft-tissue anatomy, standard arthroscopic portals can be established in a reproducible and safe method. These portals include the anterolateral, anteromedial, straight lateral, posterolateral, and posterior sites, which are usually established in this sequence.[3,4,7]

More than any other joint, the elbow requires predistention to allow for safe and effective penetration of the capsule. With joint distention the vital structures are further pushed away from the joint, and the tough anterior capsule is tensed to allow for penetration with the tro-

car. Predistention is accomplished by directing an 18-gauge spinal needle into the joint through the lateral soft spot directly over the anconeus muscle. Saline is introduced from a 40-ml syringe, and backflow is confirmed.

Portals

Anterolateral Portal

The anterolateral portal is located approximately 3 cm distal and 1 cm anterior to the lateral epicondyle. This portal is just anterior to the radial head at the joint line. Following predistention, a no. 11 surgical scalpel is used to make a small incision through the skin only. The blunt trocar is then directed toward the center of the joint and penetrates the deep fascia overlying the extensor carpi radialis brevis. The lateral antebrachial cutaneous nerve passes approximately 1 cm lateral and posterior to this portal.

The deep branch of the radial nerve before penetrating the supinator muscle is approximately 1 cm anterior and medial to this portal. The superficial branch of the radial nerve is slightly more medial.

Via this portal the arthroscopic anatomy best visualized is on the medial aspect of the elbow anteriorly. This includes the coronoid process and coronoid fossa. The medial joint capsule is well seen and through it hemorrhage in the ulnar collateral ligament is sometimes noted. Visualization of the radiocapitellar interface via this portal is limited.

Anteromedial Portal

The anteromedial portal is established approximately 2 cm distal and 2 cm anterior to the medial epicondyle. As with the anterolateral portal, when the trocar is introduced into the elbow, it should be directed toward the middle of the joint. The trocar penetrates the deep fascia overlying the tendinous portion of the pronator teres muscle. The median nerve is located approximately 1 cm lateral to this portal. Before arthroscopic evaluation of any elbow, a complete history and examination for previous elbow surgery, in general, and ulnar nerve transposition, in particular, should be completed. It is not uncommon for baseball pitchers to have had a previous ulnar nerve transposition. If a nerve transfer has been done, an anteromedial portal should not be established. The brachial artery is just lateral to the median nerve and farther away from the instruments. The medial antebrachial cutaneous nerve is 1 cm medial to this site. This portal allows excellent visualization of the radiocapitellar joint.

Straight Lateral Portal

The straight lateral portal is placed through the lateral soft spot of the elbow. This soft spot is bordered by the capitellum, trochlear notch of the ulna, and head of the radius. It is the area in which elbow aspiration is commonly done. Introduction of a trocar into the elbow from this portal penetrates the deep fascia over the anconeus muscle. As previously described, an 18-gauge needle is initially placed into this portal site for predistention of the elbow joint. Later, a formal portal is made at this site for

the introduction of the arthroscope and visualization of the underlying bony anatomy, including the trochlea and trochlear notch. It is important to visualize this articulation at the time of elbow arthroscopy to determine the presence of any loose bodies or fragments between these joint surfaces. The arthroscope can be directed from this portal into the posterior elbow.

Posterolateral Portal

The posterolateral portal is located in line with the lateral epicondylar ridge, approximately 3 cm proximal to the olecranon tip. This point is located on the lateral edge of the triceps tendon. With the arthroscope in the straight lateral portal and the lens directed posteriorly, an 18-gauge spinal needle is placed into the posterior elbow compartment under direct arthroscopic visualization. The skin portal is made, and the trocar and sheath are then directed toward the olecranon fossa. This portal can be used in conjunction with the straight posterior portal and the straight lateral portal for visualization and instrumentation of the posterior aspect of the elbow.

Straight Posterior Portal

The posterior portal is placed proximal to the tip of the olecranon in the midline of the triceps. Correct proximal-to-distal placement is determined once the offending pathologic condition has been arthroscopically identified. An 18-gauge spinal needle penetrates the triceps fascia and is directed toward the pathologic area. Once the needle is arthroscopically identified, a small skin incision is made at the point of needle entry and the trocar and sleeve are inserted, following the same path as the needle. This path usually is approximately 3 cm proximal to the tip of the olecranon. The arm should be placed 30 degrees short of full extension at the elbow before marking this portal and introducing a trocar. This arm position is maintained while working in the posterior elbow. The posterior portal sheath perforates the deep fascia of the triceps as it is directed toward the olecranon fossa. The ulnar nerve lies at least 2 cm medial to the portal site. Directly through this portal the olecranon tip, the posterior aspect of the trochlea, and the olecranon fossa can be visualized. This portal serves as access for instrumentation into the posterior joint, while visualization is accomplished with the arthroscope in the posterolateral portal.

Operative Technique

Arthroscopic evaluation is not complete until all intraarticular structures have been visualized. A minimum of three portals (the anterolateral, straight lateral, and posterolateral) are necessary to complete this task. Valgus instability can be evaluated initially with the arthroscope in the anterolateral portal. The opening of the ulnohumeral joint in response to valgus stress can be evaluated.

To perform this valgus stress test, the arm is placed in approximately 70 degrees of flexion, because this is where the most instability is noted after sectioning the ligament,[52] and this position allows room for the arthro-

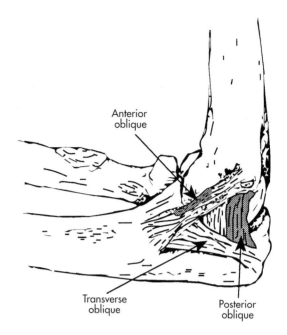

FIG. 35-36. Portion of ligament visualized arthroscopically. (From Timmerman LA, Andrews JR: *Am J Sports Med,* 22(5):667, 1994.)

scope to visualize the medial wall. The humerus is stabilized, and a valgus stress is applied to the forearm. Normally there is no opening (or a very small amount) in the ulnohumeral joint space. If there is more than 2 or 3 mm of opening in this space to valgus stress, ulnar collateral ligament injury should be considered (Fig. 35-36).[54] We have reported on the arthroscopic anatomy of the ulnar collateral ligament. Only the anterior 20% to 30% of the anterior bundle and the posterior 30% to 50% of the posterior bundle are visualized at arthroscopy. Significant tears of this ligament might not be seen, but the secondary valgus instability due to the ligament injury can be seen. If a medial reconstruction is planned, the medial portal is avoided.

The establishment of additional portals is determined by the individual pathologic condition present. In reviewing the appropriate portal selection for various procedures within the elbow joint, certain points should be remembered. Radiocapitellar chondromalacia or loose fragments are best visualized through the anteromedial portal with instrumentation through the anterolateral portal. Coronoid fossa and coronoid process osteophytes are visualized with the arthroscope through the anterolateral portal and are instrumented through the anteromedial portal. The straight lateral portal is employed for inspection of the trochlea of the humerus and its articulation with the trochlear notch for identification of any loose bodies within this area. The arthroscope is introduced through this portal into the posterior compartment to aid in the establishment of the posterolateral portal. However, the posterior and posterolateral portals into the olec-

ranon fossa are best used for posterior compartment visualization, with instrumentation occurring through the corresponding unoccupied portal. With this technique the osteophytes at the tip of the olecranon, the posterior medial olecranon, and olecranon fossa changes can be visualized and excised.

By following the previously discussed guidelines and by maintaining a conscious appreciation of the course of the underlying anatomic structures, reproducible, safe evaluation and treatment of intraarticular elbow pathologic states in the throwing athlete can be accomplished.

REFERENCES

1. Adams JE: Injury to the throwing arm, *Cal Med* 102(2):127, 1965.
2. Andrews JR: Bony injuries about the elbow. In AAOS: *Instructional course lectures*, vol 34, St Louis, 1985, Mosby.
3. Andrews JR, Angelo RL: Elbow arthroscopy. In Wadsworth TG (ed): *The elbow*, ed 2, New York, 1988, Churchill Livingstone.
4. Andrews JR, Carson WG: Arthroscopy of the elbow. In Zarins B, Andrews J, Carson WG (eds): *Injuries to the throwing arm*, Philadelphia, 1985, WB Saunders.
5. Reference deleted in proofs.
6. Andrews JR, McLeod WD: Work in progress.
7. Andrews JR, St Pierre RK, Carson WG: Arthroscopy of the elbow, *Clin Sports Med* 5(4):653, 1986.
8. Andrews JR, Timmerman LA: *Outcome of elbow surgery in professional baseball players*, Paper presented at the American Academy of Orthopaedic Surgeons Specialty Day, Feb 1994, New Orleans.
9. Barnes DA, Tullos HS: An analysis of 100 symptomatic baseball players, *Am J Sports Med* 6(2):62, 1978.
10. Bennett GE: Shoulder and elbow lesions of the professional baseball pitcher, *JAMA* 117:510, 1941.
11. Bennett GE: Elbow and shoulder lesions of baseball players, *Am J Surg* 98:484, 1959.
12. Berkeley ME, Bennett GE, Woods GW: Surgical management of acute and chronic elbow problems. In Zarins B, Andrews J, Carson WG (eds): *Injuries to the throwing arm*, Philadelphia, 1985, WB Saunders.
13. Brogdon BG, Crowe NE: Little leaguer's elbow, USAF Hospital, Lackland Air Force Base, Texas Department of Radiology 83(4):671, 1960.
14. Cabrera JM, McCue FC III: Nonosseous athletic injuries of the elbow, forearm and hand, *Clin Sports Med* 5(4):681, 1986.
15. Childress HM: Recurrent ulnar nerve dislocation at the elbow, *J Bone Joint Surg* 38A:978, 1956.
16. Childress HM: Recurrent ulnar nerve dislocation at the elbow, *Clin Orthop* 108:168, 1975.
17. Conway JE et al: Medial instability of the elbow in throwing athletes, *J Bone Joint Surg* 74A(1):67, 1992.
18. DeHaven KE, Evarts CM: Throwing injuries of the elbow in athletes, *Orthop Clin North Am* 4(3):801, 1973.
19. Dottier WE: Little leaguer's shoulder: fracture of proximal epiphyseal cartilage of humerus due to baseball pitching, *Guthrie Clin Bull* 23:68, 1953.
20. Ellenbecker TS, Davies GJ, Rowenski MJ: Concentric versus eccentric isokinetic strengthening of the rotator cuff, *Am J Sports Med* 16(1):64, 1988.
21. Ellman H: Osteochondrosis of the radial head, *J Bone Joint Surg* 54A:1960, 1975.
22. Guggenheim JJ et al: Little league survey: the Hughston study, *Am J Sports Med* 4(5):189, 1976.
23. Hollinshead WH: *Anatomy for surgeons: the back and limbs*, vol 3, Philadelphia, 1982, Harper & Row.
24. Indelicato PA et al: Correctable elbow lesions in professional baseball players: a review of 25 cases, *Am J Sports Med* 7(1):72, 1979.
25. Ismail Am, Balakrishnan R, Rajakumar MD: Rupture of patella ligament after steroid infiltration, *J Bone Joint Surg* 51B:503, 1969.
26. Jobe FW, Newber G: Throwing injuries of the elbow, *Clin Sports Med* 5(4):621, 1986.
27. Jobe FW, Stark H, Lombardo SJ: Reconstruction of the ulnar collateral ligament in athletes, *J Bone Joint Surg* 68A(8):1158, 1986.
28. Jones HH et al: Humeral hypertrophy in response to exercise, *J Bone Joint Surg* 59A(2):204, 1977.
29. King JW, Brelsford HJ, Tullos HS: Analysis of the pitching arm of the professional baseball pitcher, *Clin Orthop* 67:116, 1969.
30. Kirby FJ: Foreign bodies in the elbow joint, *JAMA* 95:404, 1930.
31. Koonig F: *Lehrbuchder Allgemeine Chirugic fur Aerzten and Studirende*, Berlin, 1889 A Hirschwald.
32. Larson RL et al: Little league survey: the Eugene study, *Am J Sports Med* (4)5:201.
33. McLeod WD: The pitching mechanism. In Zarins B, Andrews J, and Carson WG (eds): *Injuries to the throwing arm*, Philadelphia, 1985, WB Saunders.
34. Mirowitz SA, London SL: Ulnar collateral ligament injury in baseball pitchers: MR imaging evaluation, *Radiology* 185(2):5573, 1992.
35. Morrey BF (ed): *The elbow and its disorders*, Philadelphia, 1985, WB Saunders.
36. Morrey BF, An KN: Articular and ligamentous contributions to the stability of the elbow joint, *Am J Sports Med* 11:315, 1983.
37. Murphy BJ: MR imaging of the elbow, *Radiology* 184(2):525, 1992.
38. Nirshl RP: Tennis elbow, *Orthop Clin North Am* 3(4):787, 1973.
39. Norwood LA, Shook JA, Andrews JR: Acute medial elbow ruptures, *Am J Sports Med* 9(1):16, 1981.
40. Noyes FR, Grood ES: Effect of intra-articular corticosteroids on ligament properties: a biomechanical and histological study in rhesus knees. *Clin Orthop* 123:197, 1977.
41. Nuber GW, Diment MT: Olecranon stress fractures in throwers, *Clin Orthop* 278:58, 1992.
42. O'Driscoll SW, Bell DF, Morrey BF: Posterolateral rotatory instability of the elbow, *J Bone Joint Surg* 73A:440, 1991.
43. Panner HJ: A peculiar affectation of the capitellum humeri resembling Calve-Perthes' disease of the hip, *Acta Radiol* 10(3):234, 1929.
44. Pappas WM: Elbow problems associated with baseball during childhood and adolescence, *Clin Orthop* 164:30, 1982.
45. Sain J: Proper pitching techniques. In Zarins B, Andrews J, Carson WG (eds): *Injuries to the throwing arm*, Philadelphia, 1985, WB Saunders.
46. Schemmel SP et al: Radiographic changes in the asymptomatic professional baseball player (manuscript in preparation).
47. Schwab GH et al: Biomechanics of elbow instability: the role of the medial collateral ligament, *Clin Orthop* 146:42, 1980.
48. Singer KM: Radiographic evaluation of the throwing elbow. In Zarins B, Andrews J, Carson WG (eds): *Injuries to the throwing arm*, Philadelphia, 1985, WB Saunders.
49. Singer KM, Roy SP: Osteochondrosis of the humeral capitellum, *Am J Sports Med* 12:351, 1984.
50. Sisto DJ et al: An electromyographic analysis of the elbow in pitching, *Am J Sports Med* 15(3):211, 1987.
51. Slocum DB: Classification of elbow injuries from baseball pitching, *Texas Med* 64:48, 1968.
52. Sojbjerg JO, Ovensen J, Neilsen S: Experimental elbow instability after transection of the medial collateral ligament, *Clin Orthop* 218:186, 1987.
53. Sweetnam R: Corticosteroid arthropathy and tendon rupture, *J Bone Joint Surg* 51B:397, 1969 (editorial).
54. Timmerman LA, Andrews JR: Histology and arthroscopic anatomy of the ulnar collateral ligament of the elbow, *Am J Sports Med* 22(5):667, 1994.
55. Timmerman LA, Andrews JR: Undersurface tears of the ulnar collateral ligament in baseball players: a newly recognized lesion, *Am J Sports Med* 22(1):33, 1994.
56. Timmerman LA, Schwartz ML, Andrews JR: Preoperative evaluation of the ulnar collateral ligament by magnetic resonance imaging and computed tomography arthrography: evaluation in 25 baseball players with surgical confirmation, *Am J Sports Med* 22(1):26, 1994.

57. Tivnon MC, Anzel SH, Waugh TR: Surgical management of osteochondritis dissecans of the capitellum, *Am J Sports Med* 4:121, 1976.
58. Tullos HS, King JW: Lesions of the pitching arm in adolescents, *JAMA* 220:264, 1972.
59. Tullos HS, King JW: Throwing mechanism in sports, *Orthop Clin North Am* 4(3):709, 1973.
60. Tullos HS et al: Adult elbow dislocations: mechanism of instability. In Anderson LD (ed): *Instructional course lectures,* St Louis, 1986, Mosby.
61. Wheeler DK, Linscheid RL: Fracture-dislocation of the elbow, *Clin Orthop* 50, 1967.
62. Wilson FD et al: Valgus extension overload in the pitching elbow, *Am J Sports Med* 11(2):83, 1983.
63. Woods EW, Tullos HS: Elbow instability and medial epicondyle fractures, *Am J Sports Med* 5(1):23, 1977.
64. Woodward AH, Bianco AJ: Osteochondritis dissecans of the elbow, *Clin Orthop* 110:35, 1975.

CHAPTER 36   Tennis Injuries

Robert P. Nirschl

Racquet and throwing sports are common producers of overuse injuries. Tennis, a complex neurophysiologic sport, involves the actions of running, catching, hitting, and throwing in many body segments. Although tennis injuries commonly occur in the upper extremity, the experience at the Virginia Sportsmedicine Institute reveals a higher incidence in the lower extremities and trunk. In addition, recreational athletes often have preexisting deficiencies or abnormalities such as arthritic changes and muscular weakness, which are vulnerable to sport abuse.

Overall, my experience reveals a 50% split between upper and lower extremity problems. Lateral tennis elbow, shoulder tendinosis (supraspinatus), medial tennis elbow, ulnar nerve dysfunction (Zone 3 medial epicondylar groove compression), and ulnar side wrist problems (triangular fibrocartilage complex [TFCC] and distal radioulnar joint) are the most common problems in the upper extremity. More common lower extremity problems include ankle sprains, knee maladies (patellofemoral joint, meniscal, and tendinosis problems are most common), lower leg overuse in association with pronated feet (shin splints, plantar fasciitis, Achilles tendinosis, fatigue, and strain), and muscle tendon strains or pulls (gastrocnemius, Achilles, quadriceps, hamstrings, and thigh adductors). Trunk problems, including abdominal muscle strain, lumbar strain, rhomboid and levator scapular strain, lumbar disk syndrome, and aggravation of cervical and lumbar osteoarthritis, are also not unusual. This chapter is directed to upper extremity problems. In general, lower extremity injury solutions are similar to the treatment protocols used in other running sports, although some variations are needed concerning shoe wear, conditioning, tennis sport techniques, and equipment.

Common upper extremity tennis injuries

- Lateral tennis elbow tendinosis
- Shoulder tendinosis
- Medial tennis elbow tendinosis
- Ulnar nerve dysfunction
- Triangular fibrocartilage complex and collateral ligament injury (wrist)
- Distal radioulnar joint dysfunction

ETIOLOGY OF SHOULDER AND ELBOW TENDINOSIS

Many variables have been suggested or identified concerning tendinosis injury. It should be noted that the term *tendinosis* has been substituted for the term *tendinitis*. This is because histologic evaluation of surgically removed tendon overuse tissue fails to reveal inflammatory cells. It is my opinion that the pathoanatomy of tendon overuse reflects a degenerative, rather than an in-

flammatory, process. My observations, and those of others,[10,17,21,22] include the following:

1. Overuse (play exceeding three times per week), poor technique, and improper use of equipment
2. Ages 35 to 55 are most common for tennis elbow and shoulder tendinosis
3. Constitutional factors (mesenchymal syndrome, gout estrogen deficiency, and hereditary mechanical issues)
4. Inadequate conditioning (lower and upper extremities)
5. Postural deficiencies (thoracic kyphosis with tight shoulder adductors and internal rotators)

A survey of professional tennis instructors reveals that their major frustrations in teaching include students who use tennis as a conditioning tool, poor racquet preparation, and the perception that tennis is primarily an upper body sport.[2,4] These conceptual errors are common injury producers.

Variables contributing to tendinosis

- Overuse, poor technique, and improper use of equipment
- Age
- Constitutional factors
- Inadequate conditioning
- Postural deficiencies

PATHOLOGIC CONSIDERATIONS IN SHOULDER TENDINOSIS AND LATERAL AND MEDIAL TENNIS ELBOW

Common Misconceptions

The concepts of pathologic change concerning these common tendinosis problems are often misunderstood. In my opinion, traditional surgical approaches have perpetrated continuing confusion.

Lateral Tennis Elbow

The traditional surgical concepts (tendon release[11] and the Bosworth procedure[5]) concentrate the surgical effort on the extensor aponeurosis, orbicular ligament, and lateral joint soft tissues. Transverse incisions of these tissues have obscured the origin of the extensor brevis, thereby negating accurate identification of the true pathoanatomy.

Medial Tennis Elbow

Muscle slide by transverse incision obscures pathologic changes in the medial epicondylar origin of the pronator teres and flexor carpi radialis. Excess release also harms normal tissue and increases the potential for dynamic valgus instability.

Rotator Cuff Tendinosis

The concept of primary impingement has focused on the volume of the coracoacromial arch. Surgical techniques (acromioplasty and release of coracoacromial ligament) have tended to distract from the identification and treatment of the primary pathologic problem in the rotator cuff (usually supraspinatus).

Spectrum of Tendinosis

A diagnosis of tendinosis alone is not in itself sufficient to organize an adequate treatment plan. The spectrum of pathologic change in tendinosis is substantially varied. The basic pathologic categories for repetitive microtrauma include the following:

1. Chemical inflammation only (changes are temporary without permanent tissue change)
2. Pathologic alteration: angiofibroblastic degeneration (modifiable but not reversible to normal tissue)
3. Angiofibroblastic degeneration (tendinosis) and rupture
4. Associated changes: fibrosis, soft (hydroxyapatite) calcification, hard (bony exostosis) calcification, iatrogenic cortisone alteration, adjacent tissue involvement

The basic categories for tendon macrotrauma include (1) partial mechanical dissociation with partial continuity and (2) complete mechanical disassociation (i.e., no continuity). It is worth noting that angiofibroblastic tendinosis is not noted histologically in sudden violent macrotrauma Stage II to an otherwise normal tendon.

Tendinosis stages

Stage I:	Chemical inflammation only
Stage II:	Pathologic alteration—angiofibroblastic degeneration (tendinosis)
Stage III:	Angiofibroblastic degeneration and rupture

It is commonly accepted that the pathologic pattern of chronic tendinosis is etiologically based on repetitive mechanical microtrauma (tendon dissociation), with the resultant tissue being the product of the healing reaction. Because angiofibroblastic changes are not commonly noted after major macrotrauma (for example, Achilles rupture), other explanations must be sought. In my opinion, angiofibroblastic change is a degenerative process rather than a reparative process. Goldie[8] has previously reported similar changes but did comment on the process. A likely cause of this degeneration is anoxia and infarct secondary to vascular compromise.[14,23] Rupture through angiofibroblastic tissue with secondary fibrosis is also common. Combinations of mechanical dissociation from macrotrauma and tissue degeneration of microtrauma are also possible; one concept is not mutually exclusive of the other. Overall, however, the common problems referenced (shoulder tendinosis and tennis elbow) are characteristically chronic tendinosis from repetitive overuse microtrauma.

With such a wide variability in the pathologic spectrum, it is quite clear that the treatment plan must be individualized to the specifics of pathologic change for consistent success.

CONCEPTS OF TENDON OVERUSE

The basic mechanical processes of tendon overuse are (1) intrinsic—tendon stress from intrinsically produced tensile forces, primarily repetitive muscle contractile tension, (2) extrinsic, either compression (abrasion or impingement) or stretch (secondary to forces outside the musculotendonous unit), or (3) combinations.

Tendinosis common to racquet and throwing sports characteristically occurs by intrinsic overload. In analysis of tennis elbow with reference to tennis mechanics, intrinsic overload with superimposed extrinsic overload (e.g., ball impact) seems most likely.

SECONDARY ROLE OF IMPINGEMENT IN SHOULDER TENDINOSIS

The supraspinatus is subject to major repetitive intrinsic overload in the cocking, acceleration, and follow-through phases of the tennis serve and in the overhead stroke. Young athletes in other sports, such as swimming and throwing, have similar intrinsic overload.[1] Objective evidence of coracoacromial arch stenosis is commonly lacking, further supporting the observation that intrinsic overload is likely the key factor in the etiology of rotator cuff tendinosis from athletic activities. As reported by Neer,[15] in older age groups subacromial changes may ultimately occur, but in my opinion, this phenomenon is more likely secondary to upward humeral migration with reactionary changes occurring via secondary impingement.

In my observation, tennis-induced shoulder tendinosis most commonly occurs in the supraspinatus tendon by intrinsic overload during the serve and overhead strokes. The primary factors in progressive sequencing appear to be the following:

1. Eccentric loading of the supraspinatus tendon during the acceleration and follow-through phases of the tennis serve and in overhead or throwing motions
2. Fatigue progressing to physiologic weakness and chemical inflammation
3. Vascular compromise, permanent tendon change (angiofibroblastic degeneration) with occasional progression to rupture (partial or complete); pathologic change results in expansion of both physiologic and structural weakness
4. Loss of humeral head control and upward humeral migration; the rotator cuff is a key stabilizer in humeral head control
5. Labral damage (for example, degeneration with or without detachment)
6. Secondary impingement in the coracoacromial arch
   a. Subdeltoid bursitis
   b. Humeral greater tuberosity exostosis formation or erosion, subacromial exostosis, and coracoacromial ligament traction spur
   c. Mechanical dissociation of cuff (for example, rupture or Nirschl Stage III)
7. Acromioclavicular osteoarthritis commonly noted after the fifth decade; may occur independent of rotator tendinosis but is commonly associated

In young athletes participating in racquet sports, swimming, and throwing, major fibrosis and bony exostosis are the exceptions. In the sixth and seventh decades in recreational athletes, associated subacromial changes occur but these are still the minority (25% in my experience). This finding is supported by the classic 1972 report of Neer[15] in which only 25% of patients were noted to have subacromial changes but also in association with full-thickness cuff ruptures. Older recreational athletes are more likely to sustain full-thickness rotator cuff tears, and major upward humeral migration is common in this situation.

On the basis of present clinical observations, the concept of primary impingement as advanced by Neer is unlikely in the majority of cases. At most, Bigliani's report[3] on cadaver dissections would support coracoacromial arch compromising acromial variation of 40%. My surgical observation in partial-thickness rotator cuff disease notes a subacromial compromise of approximately 10% (uncommon before the fifth decade). Although an occasional patient may have an acromial variant sufficient enough to cause primary impingement, I conclude that the majority of cases of rotator cuff tendinosis (certainly in the younger racquet sport group) are caused primarily by intrinsic musculotendinous overload, just as in tendinosis of other body areas. This conclusion is also supported by the successful clinical response of the majority of rotator cuff cases to rehabilitative exercise (i.e., a change in the acromial bony anatomy is not achieved by exercise). Treatment should be directed at the etiology of the intrinsic musculotendinous overload.

DIAGNOSTIC KEYS

The keys to the diagnosis of tendinosis are well recognized by most physicians. Signs of local palpable tenderness and pain on specific stress to the musculotendinous unit in question are major diagnostic aids. Classic historical onset of pain in anatomic patterns following multiple repetitions solidifies the diagnosis.

Laboratory aids include sonography, magnetic resonance imaging (MRI), computerized axial tomography (CAT) scan, arthrogram, and routine radiographs in individualized circumstances.

With reference to the shoulder, the following points seem appropriate.

1. A positive impingement sign does not imply that impingement is the cause of symptoms (for example, pinching a tender Achilles tendon does not imply that pinching is the causative factor). The clinician should confirm the diagnosis by seeking a positive supraspinatus stress test.
2. The large majority of shoulder tendinosis problems do not reflect a full-thickness tear. A normal arthrogram therefore does not imply the absence of major pathologic change.
3. Major weakness of surrounding scapular muscles and thoracic muscles is common. Tendinosis and muscle strain of these groups are often present and should be identified.

TREATMENT CONCEPTS

The healing response after injury follows a basic sequence: (1) inflammatory exudation or hemorrhage, (2) cellular invasion, (3) collagen and ground substance production, and (4) maturation and strengthening.

The basic concepts for the treatment of tendinosis are designed to control or enhance these aspects of the biologic healing response. Implementation of these concepts takes the following form[6,16,17,19]: (1) relief of pain and chemical inflammation, (2) promotion of healing, (3) promotion of general fitness, (4) control of force loads, and (5) surgery as needed.

Treatment stages

- Relief of pain and chemical inflammation
- Promotion of healing
- Promotion of general fitness
- Control of force loads
- Surgery as needed

These concepts are germane to all sports injuries. Each sport, however, is unique, and the individualized variations in specific implementations are numerous.

Relief of Pain and Chemical Inflammation

My treatment protocol incorporates the principles of protection, rest, ice, compression, elevation, medication, and modalities (PRICEMM). It is designed to minimize any harmful excesses of inflammatory exudation, hemorrhage, and diminished oxygen perfusion.

It should be noted that rest is defined as absence of abuse, not absence of activity. Antiinflammatory medication is helpful regarding inflammation and exudation, but it does not provide a stimulus for cellular response and maturation and must therefore be used only in the perspective of a larger treatment plan. With reference to the modalities of physical therapy, the most helpful modality in my experience, other than ice and heat, is high-voltage electric stimulation.[18]

Promotion of Healing

The goal in this category is to enhance the proliferative invasion of vascular elements and fibroblasts, followed by collagen deposition and ultimate maturation. This is accomplished by (1) central aerobics and general conditioning exercise and (2) absence of abuse.

Promotion of healing techniques

- Rehabilitative exercise
- High-voltage electric stimulation
- Central aerobics and general conditioning exercise
- Absence of abuse

The initiation of these programs occurs after chemical inflammation and pain control are secure (usually 1 to 3 weeks for tennis elbow and shoulder tendinosis).

Rehabilitative exercise often involves the use of multiple resistance systems in proper sequence. The con-

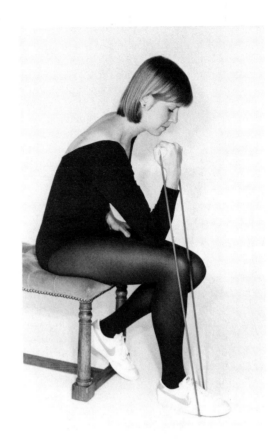

FIG. 36-1. Isoflex muscle resistance exercises. Elastic tension cord exercises of varying resistances in proper sequence with isometric, isotonic, and isokinetic techniques are important to the rehabilitative effort. (From Nirschl R: Muscle and tendon trauma: tennis elbow. In Morrey BF [ed]: *The elbow and its disorders*, Philadelphia, 1985, WB Saunders.)

cepts of endurance training are used (namely, many repetitions and low resistance). The resistance systems include water, calisthenics, isometrics, isotonics (weight resistance), isoflex (elastic tension cord resistance), and isokinetics (hydraulic resistance).[24]

Each resistance system has its own characteristic and must be properly sequenced for maximal effect (Fig. 36-1). High-voltage electric simulation is theorized to duplicate some aspects of the piezoelectric effect. Central aerobics exercise increases general blood supply and therefore probably enhances peripheral oxygen perfusion.

General Body Conditioning

General body conditioning offers many advantages in enhancing rehabilitation for specific body part injury:
1. Central and peripheral aerobics, providing the opportunity for increased regional perfusion
2. Neurophysiologic synergy and overflow, providing minimization of weakness of adjacent uninjured tissue (domino effect)
3. Fat and weight control

It is the goal, therefore, to offer a maintenance or enhancement program for body fitness and also provide an additional stimulus for the healing of injured tissue.

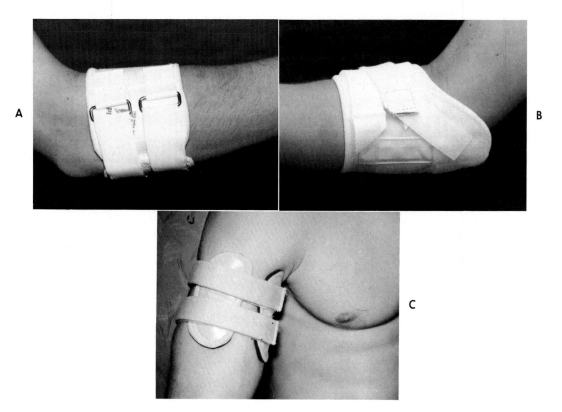

FIG. 36-2. A, Lateral counterforce elbow brace. Counterforce bracing it used to decrease pain and control abusive force overloads. Adequate design includes multiple tension straps and wide bracing for full patient control. Curved contours allow accurate fit to key areas in the conically shaped extremities. **B,** Medial counterforce elbow brace. Medial protection adds extra support for the common flexor origin. **C,** Biceps counterforce brace. Counterforce support of the biceps has subjective relief of activity-related rotator cuff pain in some patients. (Courtesy Medical Sports Inc., Arlington, Va.)

Control of Force Loads

In addition to tissue improvement, it is highly appropriate to minimize or eliminate potential injury-producing abusive force loads during rehabilitation, at the time of sports return, or during activities of daily living. The basic concepts for implementation are (1) counterforce bracing, (2) improved sports technique, (3) control of activity duration and frequency, and (4) use of proper equipment.

Bracing

Counterforce control of intrinsic overload of the elbow and shoulder tendons is appropriate (Fig. 36-2). The counterforce concept of constraining key muscle groups while maintaining muscle balance has proved quite helpful. Elbow counterforce bracing has been noted by Groppel and Nirschl[9] to decrease elbow angular acceleration and decrease electromyographic (EMG) muscle activity. Blatz[4] has reported on counterforce bracing of the biceps for shoulder tendinosis. I have also noted some anecdotal success in relief of activity-related rotator cuff pain by use of a biceps counterforce brace.

Improved Sports Technique

Certain activities allow a variety of techniques to accomplish certain goals. Inadequate tennis techniques concentrate abusive force loads to the upper extremity (especially medial lateral elbow). Those techniques that place priority on lower body participation have proved to be effective in decreasing the potential for injury (Figs. 36-3 and 36-4).

Control of Intensity and Duration of Activity

Abusive training techniques commonly result in injury.

Use of Proper Equipment

The tennis racquet plays a large role in force loads. Much research needs to be done in this area. Present clinical observation suggests that a midsize (90 to 100 square inches of hitting zone) graphite composite lightweight medium flex racquet offers the best protection.

Good quality synthetic string with string tension at the racquet manufacturer's recommended low range for the specific racquet in question seems best to control abusive force loads.

Appropriate grip size has been correlated with the hand size. Use of the anthropometric hand measurement of the ring finger I described initially in 1973 has worked well (Fig. 36-5).[17]

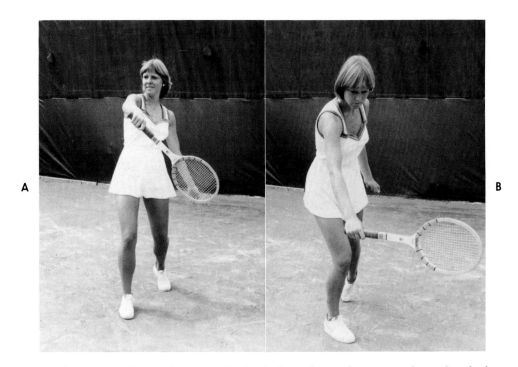

FIG. 36-3. A, Faulty backhand tennis stroke. Poor body weight transfer increases abusive force loads to the vulnerable forearm muscle groups. **B,** Quality backhand tennis stroke. Proper lower body and shoulder action protects forearm muscle groups.

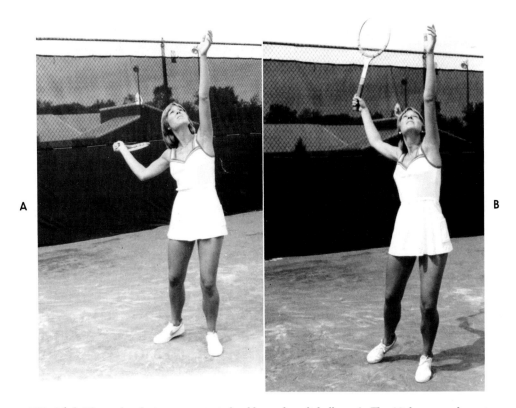

FIG. 36-4. Elevated technique to protect shoulder and medial elbow. **A,** The 90-degree-angle position is most derogatory because the shoulder shear forces are greatest in this case. In addition, forces on the medial elbow are greater. Therefore this position increases the chances of injury to both the shoulder and medial elbow. **B,** High arm elevations are more protective to the shoulder tendon cuff (shoulder scapular elevation releases the tight coracoacromial canal and diminishes rotator cuff shear forces). Higher elevations also diminish medial elbow force load. (From Nirschl R, Sobel J: *Tennis elbow prevention and treatment,* Arlington, Va., 1994, Medical Sports Publishing.)

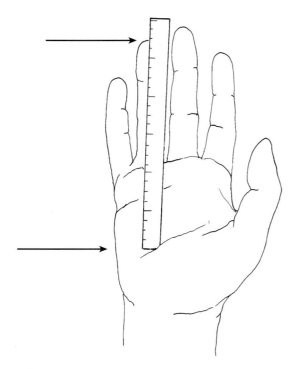

FIG. 36-5. Hand size measurement to determine proper grip handle size. Measurement of the ring finger along the radial border from the proximal palmar crease to the ring finger tip is a good technique for determining proper grip handle size. (From Nirschl RP, Sobol J: *Tennis elbow: prevention and treatment,* Arlington, Va., 1994, Medical Sports Publishing.)

SURGICAL CONSIDERATIONS
Indications for Surgery

If rehabilitation is unsuccessful or if the damage on clinical evaluation of the acute injury eliminates rehabilitation as a viable approach, surgical intervention is considered. For this topic, shoulder tendinosis and tennis elbow are discussed.

The criteria for surgery for any chronic tendinosis is basically an inability to heal or to mature pathologic tissue (for example, angiofibroblastic degeneration [tendinosis], fibrosis, calcification, iatrogenic cortisone changes, or combinations) by nonsurgical methods. The following are clinical guidelines for surgical selection:

1. Failed quality rehabilitative program (In my observation, most rehabilitative programs are of poor quality)
2. Altered quality of life
3. Constant pain or rest pain
4. Objective laboratory changes (radiograph, arthrogram, MRI, or sonogram)
5. Persistent weakness, atrophy, and dysfunction

A quality rehabilitation program, of course, includes the concepts of chemical inflammation control, promotion of healing, general conditioning, and control of abusive forces. In most instances patients referred to me for surgery have not had a quality rehabilitation program. In these circumstances a trial of the full rehabilitation program is prescribed before a final consideration for surgery.

In the event surgery is undertaken, the hallmarks of good surgical concept and technique include the following:

1. Identification of the symptoms causing the pathologic change
2. Resection of the pathologic tissue
3. Tendon closure by repair of circumambient adjacent normal tissue
4. Protection of normal tissue (for example, avoidance of excessive tissue dissection)
5. Appropriate postoperative rehabilitation

To implement these principles, specific techniques have been developed.

Concepts of Shoulder Surgery

As noted in the section on the secondary role of impingement, my conclusion is that restoring health to the rotator cuff is the highest priority. Enlarging the coracoacromial arch is appropriate with proper indication but does not ensure healing of the rotator cuff. In my view the traditional acromioplasty is unnecessarily punishing to normal structures (for example, the acromion, deltoid, and coracoacromial ligament) without benefit to the stated goal of restoring health to the injured rotator cuff.[7,15]

The concept of individualization of surgery cannot be overemphasized. No one technique will ever suffice for each situation but must be adapted to the findings. The usual rotator cuff pathologic findings that I have noted at surgery are from two basic groups: (1) partial-thickness rotator cuff tendinosis and (2) full-thickness rupture.

The critical zone of supraspinatus angiofibroblastic degeneration occurs just lateral to the bicipital groove, extending from the humeral head greater tuberosity proximally 2 inches. Erosions, calcification, and fibrosis are common associated cuff findings. Additional adjacent findings are as follows:

1. The coracoacromial ligament is invariably normal in appearance. Occasional traction spurs occur at the acromial attachment (anteromedial acromion).
2. Acromioclavicular osteoarthritis is present in approximately 75% of patients age 50 years and older.
3. Greater tuberosity exostosis or erosion is present in approximately 25% of patients age 50 years and older.
4. Biceps tendon alteration occurs in approximately 10% of patients after age 50. Biceps rupture is unusual but does occur on occasion.
5. Identifiable subacromial exostosis, coracoacromial ligament traction spurs, or anterior acromial hook variants are present in approximately 10% of patients with partial-thickness tears and 25% with full-thickness tears.
6. Anterosuperior labrum tears or degeneration occurs in 90% of throwing sport and racquet sport athletes who have partial-thickness rotator cuff tendinosis as noted in my series of cases diagnosed by arthroscopic investigation. Supraspinatus labral instability patterns (SLIPs) as described by Guidi and Nirschl[10a] demonstrate a common association between rotator cuff disease and glenohumeral instability.

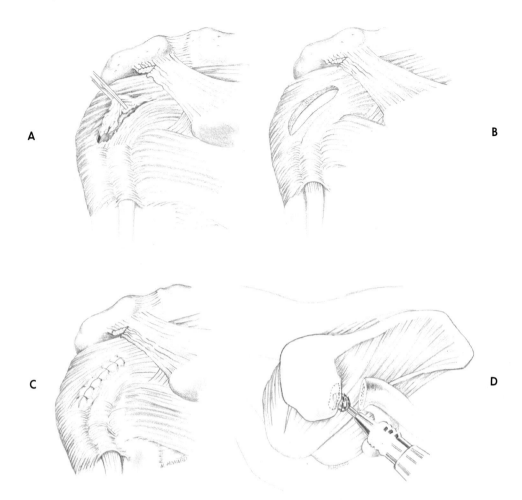

FIG. 36-6. Principles of open rotator cuff surgery. **A,** Identification of tendon showing tear or major pathologic change. Excision of pathologic tendinosis to freshen edges. Removal of pathologic tissue enhances pain relief and healing. **B,** Prepared tendon ready for repair. If exposure is needed or a small coracoacromial ligament traction spur is present at the anteromedial edge of the acromion, a small anterior ligament is released and the traction spur is removed. The deltoid is not harmed, and a full acromioplasty is neither necessary nor recommended to avoid iatrogenic harm. **C,** Repair of relatively small longitudinal tear. In layer tears or tears with retraction from the greater tuberosity, reattachment by multiple suture through bone or bone anchor is recommended. **D,** Acromioclavicular osteoarthritis or more major subacromial exostosis. In cases with clearly identifiable subacromial exostosis (less than 25% in my experience) or acromioclavicular osteoarthritis, partial abrasion acromioplasty or resection of the acromioclavicular joint as indicated is undertaken. The deltoid origin is always preserved. Even in these cases a segment of the coracoacromial ligament is preserved.

The surgical treatment as noted varies, depending on the findings. If surgical selection has been correct (via clinical examination, radiograph, sonogram, arthrogram, CAT scan, MRI, or diagnostic arthroscopy), the patient will have supraspinatus angiofibroblastic degeneration with or without varying degrees of erosion, fibrosis, or rupture. In the prearthroscopic era full-thickness elliptic resection of the pathologic tissue was performed with tendon closure for partial thickness primary intrinsic overload tendinosis.[18] This technique is still used on occasion but in large part has been supplanted by arthroscopic techniques for partial-thickness tendinosis (Fig. 36-6).

In my opinion the coracoacromial ligament is an important structure, functioning as a passive constraint to upward humeral migration. The ligament is therefore not resected unless major tightness is present or exposure is needed. The front 30% edge of the coracoacromial ligament is released if a traction spur or subacromial exostosis is present at the anteromedial edge of the subacromion. Even in cases of major rotator cuff rupture requiring acromioclavicular joint resection (for exposure or osteoarthritis), some segment of the ligament is retained.

Open Technique

To protect normal tissues, such as the deltoid, the incision is placed at the level of the acromioclavicular joint and directly parallel to the fibers of the deltoid. Under no routine circumstances is the deltoid incised from its origin on the acromion (Fig. 36-6).

If additional pathologic changes are present, these are treated as indicated:

1. Resection of the acromioclavicular joint for osteoarthritis.
2. Resection of the greater humeral tuberosity bony exostosis.
3. Resection of pathologic bursal tissue but retention of normal bursal tissue.
4. Removal or smoothing of the underside of the acromion by abrasion technique. It is unnecessary and, in my opinion, undesirable (via harm to deltoid origin) to use the traditional acromioplasty technique. The traditional technique increases postoperative morbidity and delays rehabilitation. Overall, supplemental surgery for the acromioclavicular joint, greater tuberosity and subdeltoid bursa is relatively common, but the necessity of any type of acromial surgery is, in my experience, 25% for full-thickness and 10% for partial-thickness cuff disease.
5. Resection of any pathologic segment of the long head of biceps. It is unnecessary in most instances to expand the surgery by tethering the biceps in the groove. This concept offers no advantage, increases postoperative morbidity, and delays rehabilitation. If full biceps rupture has occurred, only debridement is undertaken unless the circumstance is unusual. Biceps surgery was indicated in approximately 5% of patients in my surgical series.
6. If major rotator cuff rupture is of such magnitude as to compromise repair, an autogenous patch graft (iliotibial band) is indicated. Currently, for rotator cuff tears greater than 5 cm, a patch graft offers increased security of repair and is undertaken if the primary repair is frail but full cuff coverage of the humeral head must be achieved for the graft to revascularize.
7. Massive unrepairable tears are debrided only. This offers pain relief, but function (strength, endurance, and active motion arcs) remain compromised to varying degrees. Function in these circumstances can, however, be surprisingly good for activities of daily living. An autogenous or allograft fails in unrepairable cases (the humeral head is left uncovered in the primary repair attempt) and is therefore not recommended.

Author's Preferred Technique—Arthroscopic and Open

My current surgical approach for rotator cuff tendinosis with particular reference to racquet, throwing, and swimming sport athletes is heavily based in arthroscopic technology. Arthroscopic approaches are utilized for diagnostic, as well as definitive, operative intervention. Basic indications for surgery include a failed quality rehabilitative program and unacceptable quality of life, which includes athletic performance.

As noted, the variation in pathoanatomic presentation is substantial. It is critical to address each abnormality with the priorities dedicated to rotator cuff tendinosis and glenohumeral instability, if present. Statistically, important considerations also include clearance of bursitis for a clear arthroscopic look at the acromioclavicular joint,

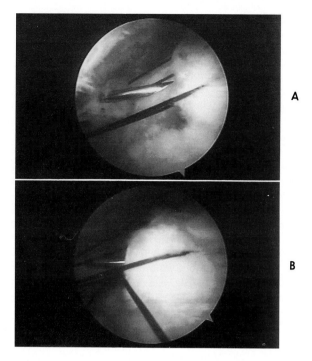

FIG. 36-7. Arthroscopic repair of rotator cuff rupture. **A,** Sutures in edge of cuff. Needle over cuff defect with entry over greater tuberosity. **B,** Mobilized cuff pulled over defect awaiting final fixation.

as well as the subacromion and coracoacromial arch side of the rotator cuff, especially at its insertion into the greater tuberosity (i.e., critical zone).

All shoulders are viewed arthroscopically, even those with known full-thickness tears, since these shoulders often have major glenohumeral changes including chondromalacia, loose bodies, bicipital tendinitis or rupture, labral tears and capsular insufficiency, and synovitis. Whether full-thickness tears or partial-thickness cuff tendinosis, these abnormalities are attended to by arthroscopic debridement or arthroscopic repair via biodegradable tack or multiple suture transglenoid capsular repair. I prefer to use the lateral decubitus position with 10 to 15 pounds of traction. It is rare to require more than two portals.

In cases of partial-thickness cuff tendinosis, debridement of the cuff is undertaken. The majority of changes are on the glenohumeral side, primarily the critical zone of the supraspinatus but occasionally extending to the infraspinatus. Careful inspection of the coracoacromial arch side of the cuff is also undertaken with bursectomy and cuff debridement (not common) as indicated. Abnormal presentation of the acromioclavicular joint, coracoacromial ligament, and subacromial area are also debrided as indicated (approximately 10%).

In full-thickness tears glenohumeral pathology is attended to in a similar fashion. Depending on circumstances, small tears (2 cm or less) that have not retracted or are freely mobile may be attended to by arthroscopic fixation into the humeral head with biodegradable tacks (Fig. 36-7). The cuff is mobilized to the greater tuberos-

ity first and captured by the tack fixation into the trough of the tuberosity.

Large or retracted tears are approached by open technique. The patient is rolled from lateral position to a supine semi–beach chair position and redraped (usually in less than 3 minutes), and the open procedure proceeds. A small deltoid, minisplit incision starting at the acromioclavicular joint (usually less than 4 cm) suffices in most instances. Under no circumstances is the deltoid released from the acromion, since this is unnecessary and harmful. Full open repair is best accomplished by anchor into bone with either bone anchors or suture placement through drill holes placed in the bone.

About 25% of cases with full-thickness tears can be expected to demonstrate acromioclavicular osteoarthritis or subacromial exostosis/coracoacromial traction spurs. In these instances open techniques for resection of the acromioclavicular joint and removal of spurs is undertaken. Care is taken to preserve the integrity of the coracoacromial ligament in all cases.

Postoperative Protocol

A. Partial-thickness tendinosis—arthroscopic
1. Outpatient surgery
2. Sling 1 to 2 days
3. Initiate high-voltage electrical stimulation plus active and passive motion exercises 2 or 3 days postoperatively; no restrictions regarding motion
4. Resistance exercises to patient comfort start 7 to 10 days postoperatively
5. Gradual return to racquet sports in 4 to 6 weeks; play to win in 3 to 4 months
B. Associated repair of anterior glenohumeral instability (labrum or capsule)
1. Outpatient Surgery
2. a. Daytime sling and swath 5 to 7 days
   b. Nighttime sling and swath 3 to 4 weeks
3. Motion restricted for 3½ weeks as follows:
   a. External rotation to neutral
   b. Abduction to 30 degrees
   c. Extension to neutral
   d. No other restrictions of motion
4. Electric stimulation and other motions as previously mentioned
5. Gradual return to racquet sports after 8 weeks; play to win in 5 to 6 months
C. Full-thickness tear with fixation of cuff into bone
1. Outpatient surgery
2. Sling 4 to 5 days
3. Electrical simulation plus active assisted motion in 2 or 3 days. No active abduction for 4 to 8 weeks, depending on magnitude and direction of tear and quality of repair and tissues. In frail repair rehabilitation is aided by autogenous tendon graft (donor iliotibial band).
4. Gradual return to racquet sports when patient is capable of comfortable full active abduction (usually 3 to 4 months). Play to win when abductor power is equal to noninjured arm (usually 6 to 9 months).

Note: In tears of less than 3 cm, 75% of active range is often present. Full functional power return varies depending on quality of tissue and repair. Controlled return to tennis is usually initiated at 2 months. If the quality of the remaining tissue is good and the repair is firm, full return to racquet sports is usual. Tears that do not allow repair of normal tendon to normal tendon have a prognosis for diminishing return. Early results with the autogenous tendon patch graft are encouraging for improved prognosis in those patients who have compromised quality of tendon tissue.

Tennis Elbow

The etiologic factors and pathologic changes discussed for shoulder tendinosis are likewise germane to lateral and medial tennis elbow. Intrinsic musculotendinous overload results in the same sequences of pathologic change. The activities of tennis most likely to initiate difficulty are the backhand stroke for the lateral elbow and the serve and late forehand stroke for the medial elbow.

The usual pathologic sequence for tendon change is (1) chemical inflammation, (2) progression to angiofibroblastic degeneration, and (3) progression to (partial or total) rupture.

Tendon degeneration sequence

Stage I: Chemical inflammation
Stage II: Angiofibroblastic degeneration (tendinosis)
Stage III: Tendinosis with rupture (partial or total)

Lateral Tennis Elbow

In patients in our surgical series who had demonstrated pathologic change (98%), the extensor carpi radialis brevis was involved in 100% of cases; the anterior edge extensor aponeurosis (finger extensors) in 35% (in no surgical case of lateral tennis elbow [over 750 cases] have I ever observed a total involvement of the extensor communis); the bony exostosis of the lateral epicondyle in 20%; and the radial nerve in less than 1%. Partial rupture of the extensor brevis tendon was noted in approximately 15% of our surgical series. Combinations of pathologic conditions are not unusual.

Medial Tennis Elbow

In patients who had surgically demonstrated pathologic change (93%), the pronator teres and flexor carpi radialis were involved in 100% of our series, and the flexor carpi ulnaris in 10%. Partial rupture of tendons was noted in 3%.

Associated medial elbow abnormalities (surgical cases—racquet sports). Ulnar nerve dysfunction occurred in 60% of our surgical series; medial collateral ligament sprain in 2%; osteocartilaginous loose bodies in 1%; and triceps tendinitis in 1%. In baseball pitchers the associated abnormalities of ulnar nerve dysfunction, medial collateral ligament sprain, osteocartilaginous loose bodies, and triceps tendinitis are statistically higher.[12,13,25,26]

Author's Surgical Indications

Surgical indications for tennis elbow are similar to those discussed for shoulder tendinosis. Again, the tech-

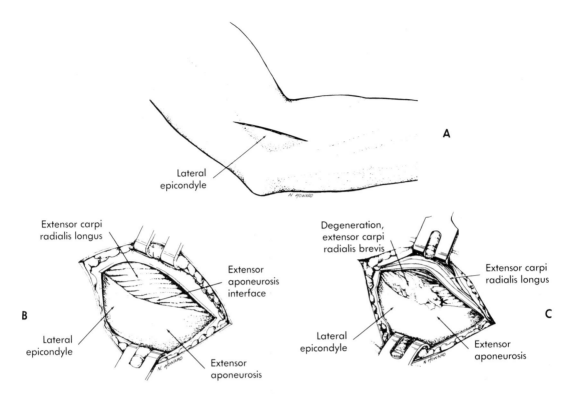

FIG. 36-8. Surgical technique for lateral tennis elbow tendinitis. **A,** Incision is slightly anterior to lateral epicondyle and extends from the level of the radial head to 1 inch proximal to the lateral epicondyle. **B,** Interface between extensor carpi radialis longus and extensor aponeurosis is identified. **C,** Extensor carpi radialis longus is retracted anteriorly and origin of extensor carpi radialis brevis comes into view. The normal origin includes some attachment of the brevis to the anterior edge of the extensor aponeurosis as well as the anterior lateral epicondyle and distal anterior lateral condylar ridge. If surgical indications are correct, changes of grayish edematous tendon alteration (tendinosis) should be visible without the use of optical assistance. (From Nirschl R: *Clin Sports Med* 7[2], 1988.)   *(Continued.)*

nique must be individualized to the circumstance. The basic concept is to identify pathologic change, resect abnormal tissue, and repair adjacent healthy tissue. Harm to normal structures is avoided (e.g., tendon releases, orbicular ligament or synovial fringe incision). The goal of surgery is not tendon release but resection of pathologic tissue. Who would release the Achilles tendon as a primary treatment for Achilles tendinosis?

Lateral tennis elbow. The incision extends from 1 inch proximal and just anterior to the lateral epicondyle to the level of the radial head. The interface between the extensor longus and extensor aponeurosis is identified, and a splitting incision is made between. The extensor longus is retracted anteriorly, bringing the extensor brevis origin into view. The brevis origin normally attaches to the underside anterior edge of the aponeurosis distal to the epicondyle, at the anterior ridge of the epicondyle, and to the distal humeral ridge. In the properly selected case a dull, grayish edematous tissue is noticed instead of the normal glistening tendon.[20]

This pathologic tissue often encompasses the entire origin of the extensor brevis to the level of the lateral joint line. In approximately 35% of cases, pathologic change is noticed in the anterior underside of the extensor apo-

neurosis; this is also removed. If pathologic changes occur in the extensor aponeurosis, it is unusual to have an area greater than 15% involved. Calcific exostosis of the lateral epicondyle is present in 20% of the cases. If these changes are observed, the anterior aspect of the extensor aponeurosis is partially peeled off the lateral epicondyle, and the bony exostosis is removed.

A small longitudinal opening may be made in the synovium anterior to the radial collateral ligament for inspection of the lateral compartment. In the classic case it is rare to find any changes in the lateral joint compartment, synovial fringe, or orbicular ligament, and I do not routinely inspect the joint unless the clinical presentation suggests an additional intraarticular problem.

Two or three drill holes are placed through the lateral condyle bone to the cancellous level to enhance vascular supply. The extensor brevis maintains some soft-tissue attachments to the orbicular ligament and extensor at the level of the radial head; thus minimal brevis retraction takes place. It is unnecessary therefore to suture the remaining brevis to retain proper mechanical length. This finding is pertinent to the retaining of normal strength after healing has occurred (Fig. 36-8).

Medial tennis elbow. The surgical concepts for medial

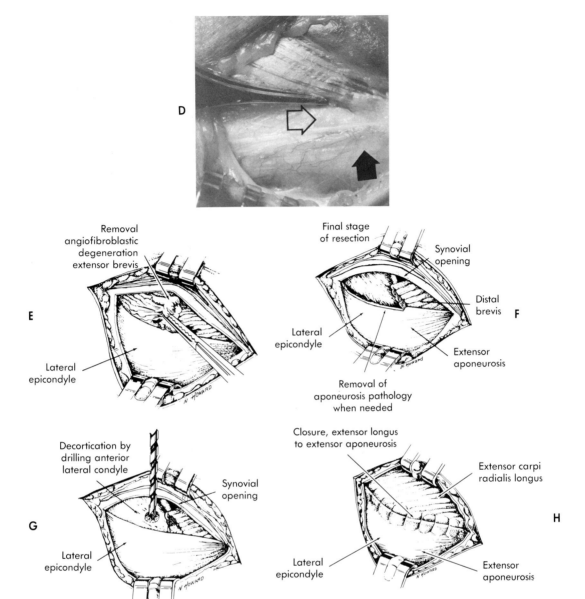

FIG. 36-8, cont'd. D, Gross visual appearance of angiofibroblastic change. Dark arrows identify normal tendon appearance of inferior edge of extensor carpi radialis longus. Open arrow identifies grayish homogeneous changes in extensor brevis characteristic of angiofibroblastic hyperplasia. **E,** Removal of angiofibroblastic degeneration of extensor brevis. In the typical case the extensor aponeurosis and lateral epicondyle are not disturbed. **F,** Final stage of angiofibroblastic resection. All pathologic tissue is removed. In approximately 35% of cases some alteration is noted in the anterior edge of the extensor aponeurosis. The pathologic change is removed if present. A small opening in the synovium is made to inspect the lateral compartment, but it is rare to identify any pathologic changes. **G,** Vascular enhancement. To enhance vascular supply, three holes are drilled through the cortical bone of the anterior lateral condyle to cancellous bone level. **H,** Repair. The extensor longus is now firmly repaired to the anterior margin of the extensor aponeurosis. Because the extensor brevis is still attached to the underside of the extensor longus, it is unnecessary to suture the distal brevis. Note that a firm attachment of the extensor aponeurosis to the lateral epicondyle is maintained at all times.

tennis elbow are the same as those for the lateral (i.e., excision of angiofibroblastic tendinosis tissue without harm to normal structures). In addition, ulnar nerve dysfunction may be an associated problem, and surgical treatment may be required to resolve this difficulty as well.

The majority of pathologic changes are present in the origin of the pronator teres and flexor carpi radialis close to their attachment to the medial epicondyle.[19] Pathologic change in the flexor carpi ulnaris also occurs occasionally. On rare occasion, rupture into the medial joint

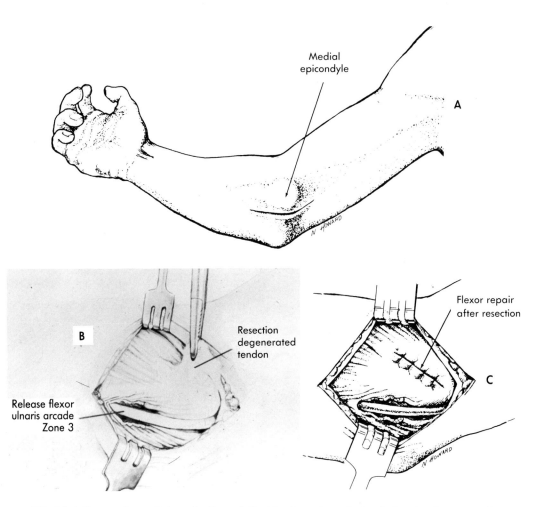

FIG. 36-9. Surgery for medial tennis elbow. **A,** Incision is made as depicted. Care is taken to avoid harm to the sensory cutaneous nerve just anterior to the medial epicondyle. **B,** Resection of angiofibroblastic degeneration. The angiofibroblastic changes are usually in the origin of the pronator teres and flexor carpi radialis. The pathologic tissue is removed in longitudinal and elliptic fashion, leaving attachments of normal tissue intact. If dysfunction of the ulnar nerve has been noted clinically, decompression of the ulnar nerve in Zone 3 of the medial epicondylar groove is done. If specific indications for ulnar nerve transfer are present, anterior subcutaneous transfer is undertaken. **C,** Medial epicondylar attachments of normal tissue are not disturbed. (From Nirschl R: Muscle and tendon trauma: tennis elbow. In Morrey BF [ed]: *The elbow and its disorders,* Philadelphia, 1985, WB Saunders.)

with secondary pseudobursal formation has been observed.

The incision is longitudinal, approximately 3 inches long, and parallels the medial epicondylar groove starting approximately 1 inch proximal and just posterior to the medial epicondyle. Care is taken to avoid the medial antebrachial cutaneous nerve just distal and anterolateral to the epicondyle. Exposure of the common flexor origin tendon is easily attained by skin retraction anterolaterally. A thin muscle layer may mask the pathologic changes of the tendon underneath. It is important to have a clear understanding of the patient's primary area of tenderness before the anesthetic is given because this area precisely locates the location of pathologic change.

A longitudinal incision is made in the tendon origins at the prime area of tenderness, extending from the tip of the medial epicondyle distally for about 2 inches. The tendons are spread, and the lesion comes clearly into

view if the surgical indications are correct. All excision of pathologic tissue is performed longitudinally and elliptically, including resection to the joint in the occasional case. All normal tissue attachments of the medial epicondyle are left intact. (*Caution:* The common flexor origin is a key medial stabilizer, and indiscriminate release of normal tendon attachment can lead to medial instability.) The resulting elliptic dead space is then closed with absorbable suture (usually 0-1 size) (Fig. 36-9).

Ulnar Nerve

So that a logical treatment sequence is established, the medial epicondylar groove is divided into three zones: Zone 1, proximal to the medial epicondyle; Zone 2, at the medial epicondyle; and Zone 3, distal to the medial epicondyle.[20] Overall, nerve dysfunction usually occurs by either compression or tension forces. The majority of ulnar nerve symptoms in the racquet sports occur by

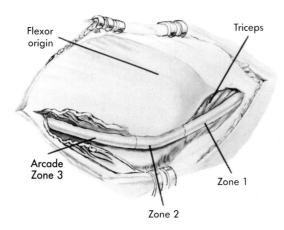

FIG. 36-10. Medial epicondyle ulnar nerve zones. The most common ulnar nerve clinical problem in the racquet sport athlete is compression in Zone 3. Surgical decompression is the treatment of choice in those patients. Specific criteria for ulnar nerve transfer are as noted in the text. (From Nirschl R: Muscle and tendon trauma: tennis elbow. In Morrey BF [ed]: *The elbow and its disorders*, Philadelphia, 1985, WB Saunders.)

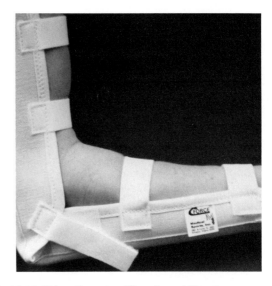

FIG. 36-11. Velcro Fastening Elbow Immobilizer increases patient comfort and enhances the rehabilitative effort. (Courtesy Medical Sports, Inc., Arlington, Va.)

compression in Zone 3. Compression from osteophytic spurs, loose bodies, or rheumatoid synovitis can occur in Zone 2, and Zone 1 compression may be caused by a tight medial intermuscular septum.

Tension forces can occur with a subluxating or dislocating ulnar nerve (either congenital, traumatic, or iatrogenic), skeletal valgus (usually from fracture malunion), or medial ligament rupture with secondary dynamic valgus instability (common in throwers). A hostile scar environment from prior disease, trauma, or surgery may result in combinations of compression and tension.

What I currently consider indications for anterior ulnar nerve transfer are dysfunctions, primarily secondary to tension problems, including the following: (1) nerve subluxation or dislocation from the epicondylar groove, (2) skeletal valgus, (3) dynamic valgus ligamentous instability, (4) unresolvable hostile environment, and (5) necessity of surgical exposure to the medial elbow compartment.

In my experience 60% of racquet sport patients operated on for medial tennis elbow have symptoms reflective of ulnar nerve dysfunction. In most instances the offending problem is compression dysfunction at Zone 3 of the medial epicondylar groove. Decompression of this zone by release of the flexor ulnaris arcade generally resolves the symptoms. If the indications for ulnar nerve transfer are present, transfer is undertaken. My preference is anterior subcutaneous transfer with easy relaxed angles. Release of the proximal motor branch with a small amount of flexor ulnaris muscle aids in the attainment of a relaxed angle distally (Fig. 36-10).

Posterior Tennis Elbow

Triceps tendinosis as an isolated entity is relatively uncommon. It is more often associated with posterior compartment osteoarthritis, osteocartilaginous loose bodies, and medial tennis elbow. Surgical intervention is quite

straightforward, with a longitudinal incision in the triceps tendon usually at or close to its olecranon attachment. Elliptic excision of the angiofibroblastic changes, as in the medial tennis elbow approach, is undertaken.

Postoperative Care

For lateral, medial, and posterior tennis elbow the postoperative course is similar. The elbow is fully protected at 90 degrees for 2 days in a counterforce elbow immobilizer. The immobilizer is light and allows active use of the wrist, hand, and shoulder as the patient's tolerance permits (Fig. 36-11). Partial protection is utilized for another 5 days. Motion exercises are started the third postoperative day.

Limbering exercises are continued for 2 to 3 weeks, followed by strength and endurance resistance exercises, usually starting at 3 weeks after surgery. Strength resistance exercises included isometrics, isotonics, isoflex, and isokinetics in proper sequence and intensity. Resistance exercise is continued until full strength returns. Full strength in the dominant arm is approximately 10% greater than in the nondominant arm in the average person and 20% greater in the competitive racquet and throwing sport athletes. Usually full strength return requires on average 4½ months for lateral and 5½ months for medial tennis elbow. Although full racquet and throwing sport competitive activity is not recommended until full strength returns, modified sport technique patterns are often initiated starting at 6 weeks after surgery.

Results

Our experience with the described elbow surgical techniques encompasses approximately 900 cases. Of these, 85% experienced complete pain relief, 12% experience partial pain relief with or without mild strength deficits but improved over the preoperative condition, and 3% of patients experienced no pain relief or strength improvements. None of the failure group were noted to

have increased pain or strength deficits secondary to surgery.

Complications have been unusual, with the exception that 0.6% had temporary superficial infection, and 1% of patients have noticed a loss of extension of up to 5 degrees.

SUMMARY

Tennis is both a lower and an upper body sport. Upper extremity injuries of shoulder tendinosis and tennis elbow tendinosis are common.

Quality rehabilitation for shoulder tendinosis and tennis elbow tendinosis includes relief of pain, promotion of healing, a general fitness program, and control of abusive overloads. If rehabilitation fails and proper indications are present, surgical correction is highly effective for resolution of symptoms and return to tennis.

REFERENCES

1. Andrews JR: Personal communication, February 1987.
2. Andrews JR, Carson WG, Ortega K: Arthroscopy of the shoulder: technique and normal anatomy, *Am J Sports Med* 12:1, 1984.
3. Bigliani L: Analysis of acromial variations, *Orthop Trans* 10:216, 1986.
4. Blatz D: Personal communication, March 1986.
5. Bosworth DH: The role of the orbicular ligament in tennis elbow, *J Bone Joint Surg* 37A:427, 1955.
6. Curwin S, Stanish WD: *Tendonitis: its etiology and treatment,* Lexington, Mass, 1984, The Collamore Press.
7. Ellman H: *Arthroscopic decompression of the subacromial space,* Paper presented to the annual meeting of the American Academy of Orthopaedic Surgeons, San Francisco, January 1987.
8. Goldie I: Epicondylitis lateralis humeri: a pathological study, *Acta Chir Scand* (suppl) 339:69, 1964.
9. Groppel J, Nirschl RP: A biomedical and EMG analysis of the effects of counter-force braces on the tennis player, *Am J Sports Med* 14:195, 1986.
10. Gruchow HW, Pelltier D: An epidemiologic study of tennis elbow, *Am J Sports Med* 7:234, 1979.
10a. Guidi E, Nirschl R: Supraspinatus labral instability pattern in rotator cuff disease. Presented to ADSSH annual meeting, Sun Valley, Idaho, July 1993.
11. Hohmann G: Das wesen und die behandlung des sogenannten tennisellen bogens, *Munch Med Wochenschr* 80:250, 1933.
12. Indelicato PA et al: Correctable elbow lesions in professional baseball players: a review of 25 cases, *Am J Sports Med* 7:72, 1979.
13. Jobe FW: Thrower problems, *Sports Med* 78:139, 1979.
14. Mosley HF, Goldie I: The arterial patterns of the rotator cuff, *J Bone Joint Surg* 45B:780, 1963.
15. Neer CS: Anterior acromioplasty for the chronic impingement syndrome in the shoulder: a preliminary report, *J Bone Joint Surg* 54A:41, 1972.
16. Nirschl RP: Tennis elbow, *Orthop Clin North Am* 4:787, 1973.
17. Nirschl RP: *Arm care,* Arlington, Va, 1983, Medical Sports Publishing.
18. Nirschl RP: Shoulder tendonitis. In Pettrone FA (ed): *AAOS symposium on upper extremity injuries in athletes,* St Louis, 1986, Mosby.
19. Nirschl RP: Soft-tissue injuries about the elbow, *Clin Sports Med* 5:637, 1986.
20. Nirschl RP, Pettrone FA: Tennis elbow: the surgical treatment of lateral epicondylitis, *J Bone Joint Surg* 61A:832, 1979.
21. Priest JD, Braden J, Gerbierich JG: The elbow and tennis. Part I, *Phys Sport* 9(4):80, 1980.
22. Priest JD, Braden J, Gerbierich JG: The elbow and tennis. Part II, *Phys Sport Med* 8(1):77, 1980.
23. Rathbun JB, MacNab T: The microvascular patterns of the rotator cuff, *J Bone Joint Surg* 52B:540, 1970.
24. Sobel J, Nirschl RP: Conservative treatment of tennis elbow, *Phys Sports Med* 9:42, 1981.
25. Wilson FD et al: Valgus overload in the pitching arm, *Am J Sports Med* 11(2):83, 1983.
26. Woods GW, Tullos HS, King JW: The throwing arm: elbow joint injuries, *Am J Sports Med* 1:43, 1973.

CHAPTER 37

Prevention and Rehabilitation of Racquet Sports Injuries

Janet Sobel
Frank A. Pettrone
Robert P. Nirschl

FACTORS IN INJURY

A survey[29] conducted among teaching tennis professionals about their major frustrations with their students revealed a number of factors that these professionals consider as frequent causes of injury among tennis players. The most commonly observed problems include:

    Students using tennis as a means of achieving cardiovascular and/or musculoskeletal fitness

    Getting the racquet back too late as a result of poor timing, poor conditioning, or poor appreciation of the sport's mechanics

    The common misperception of tennis as an upper body sport

It is interesting that these same three errors are among the leading factors contributing to injury in tennis players.

Using Tennis to Get in Shape

Tennis, to a greater extent than many other sports, requires full body involvement and is based on a **link system** of force transfer: from the legs, through the trunk, into the arms, to the racquet. Failure or error in timing, strength, or form at any link along the way is likely to invite injury to a more distal link in the progression.[15]

So often today people are deciding to start a conditioning program, and tennis looks like an attractive avenue. Unfortunately, novices often bring onto the court some combination of old injuries that were never adequately rehabilitated, day-to-day posturally induced muscle weakness and flexibility deficits, poor cardiovascular condition, and a generally slow-moving body. The injuries that result are often products of these inadequacies. Treating upper extremity injuries incurred in racquet sports must therefore involve a close and thorough evaluation of the individual's overall fitness level. An injury prevention program must also address these issues.

History of Prior Injury

All too often, when a patient presents with an arm injury, the focus of attention is the arm and the remainder of the body is neglected. As a result, true etiologies are overlooked and go uncorrected. Despite subsequent rehabilitation of the arm injury, the player is plagued with injury after return to playing. For example, an old high school knee injury that was not adequately restored may well alter a player's timing, agility, and power. The body compensates for this deficiency during a match, setting up the shoulder, elbow, or wrist for potential injury. Whenever a player has an arm injury, particularly when there is no other apparent etiology, the player's injury history needs to be extensively reviewed.

Perception of Tennis as an Upper Body Sport

As previously mentioned, proper tennis mechanics involve using the body as a link system. Quality stroke mechanics in any shot obtains power from quick footwork, knee action from flexion to extension, trunk rotation, forward weight transfer, and full shoulder motion. Control is derived from hitting with a firm elbow and wrist (Fig. 37-1). Faulty strokes move the lower body minimally and use the arm as the primary power source. When the upper body is repeatedly used for power, it becomes vulnerable to overuse injury. This is the most common etiology of arm injury.

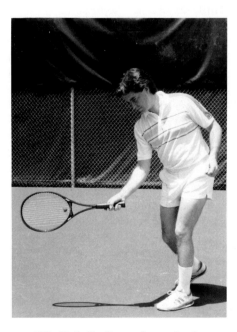

FIG. 37-1. Quality stroke mechanics.

Inadequate Stroke Preparation

Getting the racquet back too late is often a result of poor understanding of the mechanics of the sport or slowness in getting to the ball on time. It inevitably results in improper swing techniques: late strokes, using the forearm muscles as the primary power source, and hitting the ball with excessive wrist action.

Heredity and Physical Variables

Some individuals are more likely to sustain overuse injuries, regardless of the quality of stroke mechanics, based on certain aspects of their physical makeup. These factors, with respect to the upper extremity in the racquet sports, include:

- *Individual variations in anatomic design:* Increased carrying angle at the medial aspect of the elbow is a factor to consider in susceptibility to medial tennis elbow. Acromial slope may be a factor in vulnerability to shoulder rotator cuff tendinosis and wear-and-tear changes.
- *Chemical makeup:* Hormonal variation in women as a result of gynecologic factors (hysterectomy, menopause) may make them more susceptible to tendinosis.[22] Certain individuals' tissue quality is less capable of withstanding higher force loads and is less efficient at healing.
- *Age:* Upper extremity injuries are seen with much higher frequency in 35- to 55-year-old players.[25,35]

Postural Considerations

Postural maladaptations caused by daily activities play an enormous role in the vulnerability to injuries to the shoulder and elbow in the racquet sports. The typical desk worker's posture has exaggerated anteroposterior spinal curves, with the head forward. The muscle imbalances that commonly result include weak abdominal and scapulothoracic muscles and tight pelvic, lower back, and anterior shoulder muscles. Tennis imposes similar maladaptations respective to the shoulder.

It becomes virtually impossible for the muscles to overcome their imposed inadequacies when called on to do so during tennis. Tight pelvic muscles do not allow the needed excursion of trunk rotation and extension. Tightness across the anterior area of the shoulder protracts the scapulae and prevents the needed range for good form in overheads and serves. Weak upper back muscles are inadequate scapula retractors and rotators and often necessitate overload of the arm and forearm to generate power. The head-forward position places undue overload on the cervical structures, predisposing to a myriad of neck problems. Resultant nerve irritation may lead to weakness of the scapular and arm muscles.

If we do not address and correct these maladaptations, perpetration of inefficient energy use, unnecessary strain on all body parts, and injury susceptibility are the results.

Equipment and Environment

Certain racquet characteristics play a significant role in upper extremity injury in tennis. The market has opened up a multitude of options in size, shape, materials, and stringing of tennis racquets. Prevention or rehabilitation of a player's injury should include a discussion of the racquet currently being used by the athlete.

Racquet evaluation should include the following questions:

What racquet are you now using, and how long have you been playing with that racquet?

So often a player's injury (especially at the elbow) dates to within 1 month after starting to play with a new racquet. Either the racquet itself may not be a good one for the player's arm, or the arm cannot adjust to the differences.

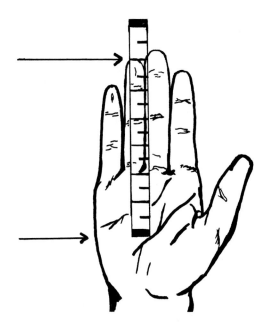

FIG. 37-2. Nirschl technique for proper handle size: measure from proximal palmar crease to the top of the ring finger. Place ruler between long and ring fingers.

Racquet evaluation

- Length of time using racquet
- Racquet material
- Racquet head size
- String tension
- Grip size

What is the racquet material?

Racquet material is not likely to significantly affect the shoulder or wrist. However, the introduction of metal racquets created an epidemic of tennis elbow injuries because of their poor vibration-absorbing nature. A study of 534 players in China found an incidence of tennis elbow highest with aluminum racquets (62%) or twice as high as with any other material. This same study found one and one-half times the injury rate with medium-weight racquets than with lightweight ones.[34] Graphite composites are currently considered to be the best in terms of torsion and vibration control and thus the most protective against tennis elbow. More flexible racquets seem best, especially with the new wide-body designs.

What racquet head size are you using?

The oversized racquets have enormous appeal for many older people, beginners, and those who have problems getting to the ball quickly. Unfortunately, this larger head size makes the arm susceptible to injury because of the torque effect on shots hit off-center. The midsize racquet (95 to 110 square inches) is preferable when considering injury avoidance in the upper extremity.

What is the string tension?

Higher stringing tension generally offers more control but increases the torque and vibration in the arm. Our recommendation for injury prevention is to stay at the lower end of the manufacturer's recommendation.

What is the size of the grip?

It is remarkable how few recreational players know what the measurement of their racquet's grip is or whether it is appropriate. The general advice by the salesperson is to use what is comfortable. Sometimes players use whatever grip size is available in the desired racquet. The result may be poor play and unnecessary injury. A grip too small lessens control and sets the stage for excessive wrist motion. A grip too large also compromises racquet control. A good measure of grip size[24] is given in Fig. 37-2.

Guidelines for racquet selection for nontournament players in terms of arm protection against abusive force overloads are given in the box. All these factors need to be addressed as part of a patient's treatment for an upper extremity injury. Furthermore, to fully evaluate and offer meaningful help to avoid reinjury, the possible causative factors in the patient's game should be identified. Regardless of the quality or extensiveness of the rehabilitation, reinjury is inevitable if the player repeats the same faulty patterns that created the initial injury. Because it is unrealistic to get out with every patient and analyze technique, we have found it helpful to refer to teaching professionals who can correct poor technique.

Guidelines for racquet selection by nontournament players

- Head size: midsize
- Material: graphite composite (medium flex)
- Handle: size as measured
- Weight: well-balanced, light
- Stringing material: synthetic nylon (restring every 6 months)
- String tension: lowest range of manufacturer's recommendation

---

MECHANISMS OF INJURY

Elbow

Lateral Tennis Elbow

By far the most common upper extremity tennis injury is lateral tennis elbow, an overuse tendinosis of the extensor tendons (primarily the extensor carpi radialis brevis). In the inexperienced player this is often a result of a faulty backhand (e.g., the ball is hit with the front of the shoulder up and the power source is the forearm muscles) (Fig. 37-3). A two-handed backhand is far more protective and should be considered for these players (Fig. 37-4). A study by Giangarra et al[14] comparing forearm muscle activity in the two-handed and one-handed strokes, which found only minor differences in muscle activity, led the authors to identify the contribution of the second arm as a provider of motion control. A late forehand with resulting wrist snap to bring the racquet head perpendicular to the ball is another factor in poor technique.

Highly skilled players are vulnerable to lateral tennis elbow in their serve: the ball is often hit with full power and speed with the forearm in full pronation and wrist snap, thus increasing the load on the already taut extensor tendons.[32] The frequency and intensity of the tournament level player's schedule enhance the overload effect, because there is often limited time between matches for recovery or rest.

Biomechanical factors in lateral tennis elbow

- Faulty backhand using wrist extensors for power
- Late forehand with wrist snap and pronation
- Serve with forceful forearm pronation and wrist snap

Medial Tennis Elbow

Medial tennis elbow occurs with one fifth the frequency in the racquet sports as does lateral tennis elbow. In the inexperienced player medial tennis elbow is often

a result of the late forehand with its resultant wrist snap to bring the racquet head forward quickly. These players also may improperly try to impart topspin on the ball by pronating over it, again overloading the medial tissues.

Medial tennis elbow can also result from quality serve and overhead motions. In the back-scratch and early acceleration positions there is tremendous valgus stress on the medial tissues. These structures are susceptible to injury as the racquet head accelerates upward to full impact with forearm pronation and, finally, wrist snap. This combination of valgus stretch, pronation, and wrist snap with the high repetition and intensity of the competitive player may lead to medial overload. Medial tennis elbow may be associated with ulnar nerve compression and dysfunction.

Posterior Tennis Elbow

Triceps tendinosis is rare in the racquet sports but may result from sharply extending the elbow excessively, primarily in the serve but sometimes with improper forehand or backhand ground strokes. A more common problem is olecranon compartment osteoarthritis.

Shoulder: Rotator Cuff Tendinosis

The rotator cuff is subject to injury in the well-executed tennis serve and overhead smash and sometimes in the high backhand volley. The rotator cuff is responsible for creating external rotation in the serve and for maintaining the position of the humeral head in the glenoid. In the follow-through the posterior components of the rotator cuff are eccentrically loaded to decelerate the arm. If the rotator cuff strength is inadequate to handle arm deceleration, it may be susceptible to intrinsic tendon overload.[1] The rotator cuff is vulnerable also in the highly skilled player by virtue of the sport-induced muscle imbalance in and of itself: the strength ratio of external rotators to internal rotators tends to be quite low (65%), and these muscles have difficulty overcoming the powerful upward pull of the deltoid on the humeral head

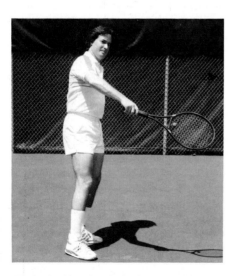

FIG. 37-3. Faulty backhand with the front shoulder up using forearm muscles for power and excessive wrist action.

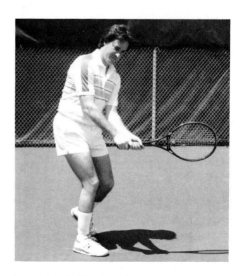

FIG. 37-4. Two-handed backhand protects the extensor tendons.

MECHANISMS OF INJURY
Elbow
Lateral Tennis Elbow

By far the most common upper extremity tennis injury is lateral tennis elbow, an overuse tendinosis of the extensor tendons (primarily the extensor carpi radialis brevis). In the inexperienced player this is often a result of a faulty backhand (e.g., the ball is hit with the front of the shoulder up and the power source is the forearm muscles) (Fig. 37-3). A two-handed backhand is far more protective and should be considered for these players (Fig. 37-4). A study by Giangarra et al[14] comparing forearm muscle activity in the two-handed and one-handed strokes, which found only minor differences in muscle activity, led the authors to identify the contribution of the second arm as a provider of motion control. A late forehand with resulting wrist snap to bring the racquet head perpendicular to the ball is another factor in poor technique.

Highly skilled players are vulnerable to lateral tennis elbow in their serve: the ball is often hit with full power and speed with the forearm in full pronation and wrist snap, thus increasing the load on the already taut extensor tendons.[32] The frequency and intensity of the tournament level player's schedule enhance the overload effect, because there is often limited time between matches for recovery or rest.

Biomechanical factors in lateral tennis elbow

- Faulty backhand using wrist extensors for power
- Late forehand with wrist snap and pronation
- Serve with forceful forearm pronation and wrist snap

Medial Tennis Elbow

Medial tennis elbow occurs with one fifth the frequency in the racquet sports as does lateral tennis elbow. In the inexperienced player medial tennis elbow is often

a result of the late forehand with its resultant wrist snap to bring the racquet head forward quickly. These players also may improperly try to impart topspin on the ball by pronating over it, again overloading the medial tissues.

Medial tennis elbow can also result from quality serve and overhead motions. In the back-scratch and early acceleration positions there is tremendous valgus stress on the medial tissues. These structures are susceptible to injury as the racquet head accelerates upward to full impact with forearm pronation and, finally, wrist snap. This combination of valgus stretch, pronation, and wrist snap with the high repetition and intensity of the competitive player may lead to medial overload. Medial tennis elbow may be associated with ulnar nerve compression and dysfunction.

Posterior Tennis Elbow

Triceps tendinosis is rare in the racquet sports but may result from sharply extending the elbow excessively, primarily in the serve but sometimes with improper forehand or backhand ground strokes. A more common problem is olecranon compartment osteoarthritis.

Shoulder: Rotator Cuff Tendinosis

The rotator cuff is subject to injury in the well-executed tennis serve and overhead smash and sometimes in the high backhand volley. The rotator cuff is responsible for creating external rotation in the serve and for maintaining the position of the humeral head in the glenoid. In the follow-through the posterior components of the rotator cuff are eccentrically loaded to decelerate the arm. If the rotator cuff strength is inadequate to handle arm deceleration, it may be susceptible to intrinsic tendon overload.[1] The rotator cuff is vulnerable also in the highly skilled player by virtue of the sport-induced muscle imbalance in and of itself: the strength ratio of external rotators to internal rotators tends to be quite low (65%), and these muscles have difficulty overcoming the powerful upward pull of the deltoid on the humeral head

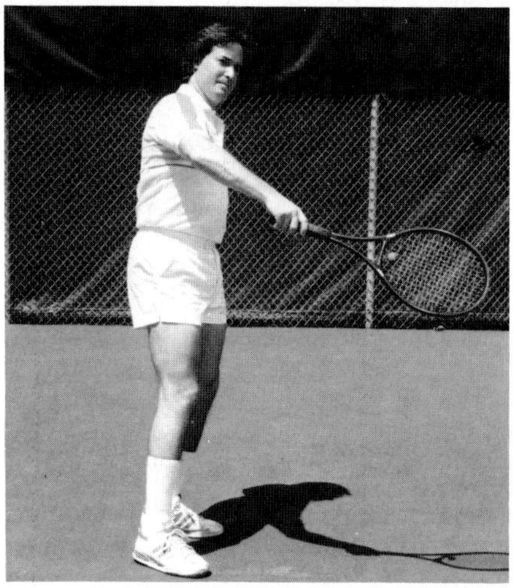

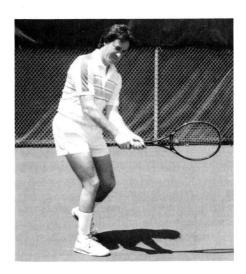

FIG. 37-3. Faulty backhand with the front shoulder up using forearm muscles for power and excessive wrist action.

FIG. 37-4. Two-handed backhand protects the extensor tendons.

when the arm is raised as well as the enormous forces of the internal rotators pulling the arm forward in acceleration and follow-through. Scapular muscle deficiencies are also common in tennis players, thereby providing an inadequate platform to support the rotator cuff.

Incorrect use of excessive forearm pronation to generate topspin can result in increased eccentric load to the posterior cuff in its effort to decelerate arm pronation and its subsequent effect of internally rotating the humerus.[12] This relationship has also been noted in the tennis serve.[32]

In a faulty serve with inadequate shoulder elevation, the shoulder structure may also be subject to excessive coracoacromial friction. The faulty serve is often characterized by inadequate knee extension and lower back action with the pelvis parallel to the net, a twisting arm, and inadequate arm elevation at impact. The key technique to protect the shoulder tissues is high elevation above the horizontal to full extension at impact. In the older population arthritic changes may develop in the shoulder complex. Grinding the soft tissues against these changes by rotation in the range of 90 degrees of abduction can lead to further problems. It is especially important to check the rotator cuff strength in all players because an inadequate asymptomatic rotator cuff may allow excessive displacement of the humeral head with resultant added wear and tear. A vicious cycle may result:

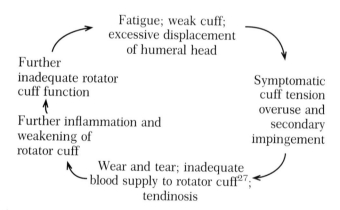

Improving the blood supply, nutrition, and strength to the cuff, as well as improving performance, can help break the cycle and lessen or eliminate the rate or extent of the changes.

Scapula

The scapular muscle groups are often weakened by constant eccentric stretch overuse in the serve and tennis overhead. In addition to contributing to rotator cuff tendinosis, the scapular muscles may become injured independently. The levator scapulae and rhomboids often become symptomatic with tendinosis or myositis, respectively.

Bursitis may occur at the inferior angle of the scapula with poor lower body and trunk mechanics in the serve: inadequate pelvic rotation and back movement may lead to excessive shoulder movement in the cocking position, with resultant friction at the bursa. Bursitis may also occur at the superior angle of the scapula.

Forearm

Forearm injuries are rarely seen in the racquet sports and are therefore considered only briefly. **Pronator teres syndrome,** in which the player complains of volar forearm pain after playing, can result from forceful repetitious pronation with tight gripping. Symptoms may involve the median nerve and are reproduced by gripping tightly with resisted pronation from the elbow at 90 degrees to full extension. **Compression of the dorsal branch of the radial nerve** along its path may result in an aching pain over the extensor mass in the proximal aspect of the forearm with possible distal radiation or paresthesias along the radial nerve. The player is likely to experience tenderness approximately four fingerbreadths distal to the lateral epicondyle over the supinator. Myositis of the extensor muscles is occasionally noted at the distal musculotendinous junction.

Wrist

Wrist **ulnar collateral ligament sprain** may result from exaggerating laying the wrist back. This is an error beginners often make in taking their instructors too literally. Cocking the wrist back rigidly at ball impact is a weak position for the wrist and allows no pliability for shock absorption, leaving the ulnar collateral ligament vulnerable at ball impact. The quality position puts the wrist at its greatest mechanical advantage: this is the position of anatomic strength, or the handshake position.

Lack of wrist firmness during play can be injurious to the distal aspect of the radioulnar joint, where pronation and supination occur. This may be seen on late ground strokes with a floppy wrist, ending with supination or pronation in the follow-through, or with excessive wrist roll, resulting in a synovitis at this joint. Injury to the triangular fibrocartilage complex may also occur secondary to similar etiologies. Tendinosis and subluxation of the extensor carpi ulnaris, is also noted in tennis. On the radial side of the wrist, radiocarpal synovitis has been noted. Grip size, stroke technique, and forearm muscle strength need to be addressed in players with these problems.

REHABILITATION PRINCIPLES

After upper extremity injury, all parts of the upper body kinetic chain must be recognized. A comprehensive rehabilitation program includes the following components:
1. Comprehensive evaluation
2. Relief of pain and inflammation
3. Protection against abuse in sports and activities of daily living
4. Promotion of healing by rehabilitation exercise to the injured part and conditioning to the adjacent part
5. Maintenance or enhancement of overall fitness level
6. Sport-specific exercise and restoration of functional performance
7. Return to sports

Pain and Inflammation Relief

The hallmark of the phase of pain and inflammation relief is represented by the acronym **PRICEMM:**

Protect the injured part against further damage. This implies avoiding motions that stress or compromise the injured tissue.

Rest in this context means avoiding further abusive overload, not absence of activity. In fact, we encourage the player to maintain as high an activity level as possible while staying away from those activities that may further aggravate the injured part. Absolute rest (e.g., immobilization) should be avoided if medically reasonable. Although it undoubtedly helps to eliminate abuse, absolute rest also encourages atrophy, deconditions tissue, lessens vascular supply to the area because of reduced demand, and is detrimental to the healing process. To determine the appropriate type and level of activity, pain offers the best guide. Reproducing the pain that prompted seeking medical attention should be interpreted as interfering with the needed rest of the injured part.

Ice is indicated as long as the signs of inflammation persist, which may mean throughout all rehabilitation and sports return. It encourages local vasoconstriction, lessens the inflammatory response, slows local metabolism, and helps to relieve pain and muscle spasm through counterirritation and slowed nerve conduction velocity.

Compress and **Elevate** if appropriate to assist venous return and minimize swelling.

Medications and Modalities: It has been our experience that a brief early course of antiinflammatory medications in conjunction with therapeutic modalities helps to speed the rehabilitation process.

NOTE: It has also been our experience that an arm that has had several cortisone injections is significantly more difficult to rehabilitate. If at all possible, cortisone injections should be used only with the following guidelines:

1. Avoid cortisone injection directly into tendon.
2. No more than three injections in the same location.
3. The primary indication for injection is when pain is so intense that it compromises compliance with the rehabilitation exercise program and/or significantly compromises activities of daily living, and nonsteroidal, antiinflammatory drugs are ineffective.
4. A 7-day rest period is recommended after injection before resumption of the exercise program.

Useful modalities for upper extremity injuries

- Electric stimulation
- Ultrasound
- Ice
- Heat

Modality Specifics

We have found certain physical therapy modalities to be most effective.

High-voltage electric stimulation (HVES) is effective in pain reduction, enhancing circulation, quieting muscle spasm, and decreasing swelling and inflammation. Continuous stimulation with a high pulse rate (at least 100 pps) for 20 to 40 minutes is recommended for these goals. HVES also can be very effective in muscle reeducation and lessening muscle disuse atrophy postoperatively. For these goals the stimulation parameters would differ. Furthermore, HVES may play a role in stimulating the body's biologic healing process by virtue of the electric current itself. In recent years, several new stimulators have been introduced such as interferential and neuroprobe. Since the supportive data on each are sparse, it is up to the users and patients to determine which is most effective for the specific need.

Ultrasound is a deep-heating modality in which sound waves are absorbed by the tissue, producing heat as well as nonthermal effects resulting from a vibration of tissue. It is thought to increase cell membrane permeability, resulting in better transport of metabolic products. It may help enhance connective tissue extensibility by enhancing collagen fiber separation. Ultrasound is thus very good before exercise because it makes the tissue more susceptible to remodeling by tensile forces. It is also quite effective in managing muscle spasm. It is of questionable value over bony areas because bone picks up sound waves, causing an intense deep pain and making it difficult to achieve a therapeutic dosage. Ultrasound should not be used over the growth lines of children and adolescents.

Phonophoresis uses the ultrasound to drive whole molecules of an antiinflammatory medication (usually steroids) through the skin into the inflamed tissues. Great caution must be used if the medium is a steroid, however, because of its potentially dangerous effects. Steroids have been found to lessen collagen and ground substance production and decrease the tensile strength of tendons, and they may lead to failure of weight-bearing tissue under stress. In our opinion the potential benefits of phonophoresis cannot justify its use in view of these dangers, especially where cortisone injections have already been tried.

Transverse friction massage is considered by many to be an effective way of increasing circulation to tissue and lessening excessive or abnormal scar tissue formation. The area is massaged deeply across the direction of its fibers. It can be very painful and should probably be saved for situations of chronic tissue damage where the goal is to bring the tissue to an acute, more manageable state.[4,7] There is no experimental or clinical research available at this time that substantiates the value of transverse friction massage.

Heat applications promote vascular supply to an area and may help with muscle relaxation. In inflamed tissue, however, heat may cause further swelling.

Ice is an immensely useful tool when pain and evidence of chemical inflammation (swelling, heat, tenderness, pain) are present. Vasoconstriction, swelling control, and pain and spasm relief commonly occur with ice therapy. PRICEMM duration and the rest period vary, based on the severity and nature of the problem and the individual's needs. All too often the athlete misinterprets the pain and inflammation relief gained from the rest period as a sign that he or she can return to play, and then immediately on return the pain reinitiates. The reason is clear: absence from abusive activity generally relieves

pain but fails to effect a cure. Steps must be taken to rehabilitate the injured part (e.g., restore the quality of the tissue and condition it for the demands of the sport).

Promotion of Healing and Rehabilitative Exercises

We continue to protect against abusive overload and minimize inflammation, often by continuing ice, electrical stimulation, and protective activity, with superimposed rehabilitative exercise. The ice, electrical stimulation, and sometimes antiinflammatory medicines are helpful as needed to minimize pain and inflammation through the exercise period and allow for more effective work on rehabilitative exercises. The goals of these early exercises are to enhance oxygenation and tissue nutrition, to prevent or minimize neurophysiologic reflex inhibition (thus minimizing unnecessary atrophy), to align collagen fibers along the lines of stress and inhibit excessive scar formation, and to stimulate the joint mechanoreceptors, all while protecting the healing fibers against excess stress or reinjury.[8] These exercises involve very low–intensity, submaximal effort and progress gradually and methodically, primarily based on our knowledge of biologic healing time factors and the patient's pain. As the exercises progress, the goals become reconditioning and restoration of strength, endurance, and flexibility for functional performance.

Several studies in the past 15 years point to the necessity of rehabilitation exercises after injury. A study by Cruchow and Pelletier[6] in 1979 found that tennis players who had not had resistance training had an increased incidence of tennis elbow complaints. Furthermore, tennis players who exercised after tennis elbow had a 31% recurrence vs. a 41% recurrence of those who did not exercise.

Throughout this effort, we need to address the individual's overall fitness level, including aerobic and anaerobic capacity, coordination and agility, correction of lingering deficits from old injuries, and overall strength, endurance, and flexibility of other body parts. Particular attention should be paid to the following:

Lower body strength, agility, and mobility; strength throughout a flexible motion range of the gluteals, abdominals, and balancing of the agonist/antagonist muscle groups throughout the lower body

Correcting postural faults in daily life that promote injurious imbalances (e.g., functional dorsal kyphosis, scapular protraction, head forward) resulting in overload of neck structures, strength/weakening of scapular stabilizers, tightness of the anterior chest wall, and excessive lateral scapular slide

Restoration of balanced strength and flexibility of force-couple relationships, to establish the normal interplay of stability and mobility among the dynamic components of the shoulder joint complex: scapular stabilization and dynamic control of the scapulothoracic musculature, as described by Wilk and Arrigo,[34] is essential to long-term success

Identification and correction of weakness and/or muscle imbalances throughout the upper quarter, including the neck, scapulothoracic area, shoulder, elbow, wrist, and hand

Exercise forms superimposed to challenge and stimulate the neuromuscular potential: additionally, each weak muscle isolated, disallowing compensation (e.g., external rotation, wrist extension); but this must be interplayed with combined motion patterns for specific functional movement

The goal is to create a functional, balanced upper quarter that is conditioned to meet the demands of tennis and daily life. This involves a thorough evaluation of mobility and strength, isolating each muscle group and joint motion (both accessory and active). Once the weaknesses and imbalances are identified, injury-specific rehabilitation involves a background conditioning program with specific emphasis on rehabilitation exercises to correct the weaknesses. Throughout rehabilitation, pain guidelines must be clearly explained to the patient. Many athletes have a "no pain, no gain" attitude, and unless the difference between rehabilitation and sport exercise is defined by the practitioner, there is great risk of additional injury. It has been our experience that acceptable and nonacceptable pain can be identified and differentiated as follows:

Pain that decreases with continued activity is acceptable.

Pain that increases with continued activity is unacceptable.

Activity that reproduces the localized pain symptoms for which the athlete sought attention is unacceptable.

Generalized muscle soreness throughout the muscle-tendon unit is acceptable.

Pain that is relieved after postexercise icing is acceptable.

Pain that lasts 4 hours or more after exercise is unacceptable.

Using these simple guidelines enables maximum effectiveness and efficiency of the rehabilitation effort.

It has been our experience that no one form of strengthening exercise can possibly answer all the needs of a quality rehabilitation effort. Thus the exercise program invariably involves overlapping of isometrics, isotonics, rubber tubing exercises (Isoflex, Medical Sports, Arlington, Va.), and isokinetics for strengthening and endurance work. Flexibility is generally done manually. Its sequencing and intensity are highly specific to the part of the body and the nature of the tissue. Thus flexibility is discussed individually with each body part.

Isometrics are helpful early in rehabilitation because they can effectively decrease swelling (through the pumping action of the muscle), they do not irritate the joint because there is no motion, and they prevent neural dissociation (the muscle contractions stimulate the mechanoreceptor system).[10] We begin with multiangle isometrics in limited motion arcs at submaximal intensity, progressing to maximal intensity isometrics in the shortened, middle, and lengthened positions. These can be done throughout the day; a good general guideline is the rule of 10s: 10 repetitions, 10 seconds hold per repetition, 10 times per day. The 10-second hold involves a 2-second increase in forces, a 6-second hold, followed by a 2-second decrease. This gradient increase and decrease in force production, as specified by Davies and Ellenbecker,[9] maximizes effectiveness through minimizing pain and joint capsule stress. If a particular angle is painful, it can be worked around, with the patient taking ad-

vantage of the overflow of benefits to 15 degrees on either side of the exercise angle.[19]

Midrange isotonics begin on a daily basis with very high repetitions (e.g., two to three sets of 15 to 20 repetitions) and no weight, progressing to full range and then gradually increasing the weight and decreasing the repetitions, with the eventual goal of a strength-training regimen performed two or three times per week. To start, then, the goal is to mold the fiber alignment along the lines of stress and to prepare the damaged tissue to effectively handle the greater loads to come. Such an isotonic program stimulates the body's own biologic healing and allows for early controlled eccentric loading. The advantages of eccentric loading in rehabilitating overuse injuries are (1) it creates less compressive forces across the joint; (2) it may offer greater tendon loading[30]; and (3) it makes the muscles work as they will need to in the sport. Many of the loads to the upper extremity musculotendinous units in the racquet sports are eccentric ones (e.g., the wrist extensors and posterior rotator cuff, and the scapular stabilizers, in the serve). Their inadequacy against the multiple repetitions of eccentric loads throughout their range of motion is a major factor in their high injury rate.

Once the exercises can be done with 1.4 kg (3 pounds), **Isoflex,** or rubber tubing, exercises are initiated and done on alternate days with the isotonics. The progression variables here are the repetitions, range of motion, rate of exercise, and placement of the anchor end of the tubing for resistance intensity. Once slow-motion repetitions are mastered, timed high-speed endurance bouts follow. The Isoflex and isotonic programs complement each other well in that we can alternate endurance and strength training. Whereas isotonics generally work best in the muscle's midrange, Isoflex works the end range and is more conducive to eccentric emphasis. This is particularly effective in training the stabilizing or decelerator muscle groups (e.g., the scapular retractors, posterior rotator cuff, biceps).

Once good control of the injured part through a reasonable range of motion is demonstrated, **isokinetics** are initiated.[26] The available variables in isokinetic exercises are range, speed, intensity of effort, and duration. We start with short bouts, limited range, and submaximal effort in the middle speeds, working toward full motion arc endurance bouts throughout a velocity spectrum, with emphasis on the higher speeds. These take the best advantage of what isokinetics have to offer: most racquet sport movements occur at higher speeds. In following the specific adaptation to imposed demands (SAID) principle[33] of neurophysiologic patterning, we need to exercise appropriately to prepare for the sport's demands. Higher speed exercise is likely to impose fewer compression forces on the joint, since fewer fibers can be recruited and thus less torque can be generated.

Concentric and eccentric exercises must be included, preferably in all the strengthening modes (with the exception of isometric). Particular emphasis should be placed on eccentric loading of those muscle groups on which tennis places high decelerative demands (e.g., the scapular rotators, posterior rotator cuff, biceps, and wrist

extensors). In a 6-week study on college tennis players by Ellenbecker et al[13] on concentric and eccentric isokinetic rotator cuff training, statistically significant strength improvements were found in concentric and eccentric strength, but no improvements were found in maximum serving velocity in the eccentrically trained group. The concentrically trained group did show improvement in maximum serving velocity. Although the role of eccentric training in tennis performance is not clear, its role in injury prevention is more evident.

Although the upper extremity functions in an open kinetic chain in tennis, closed kinetic chain exercise is needed to enhance dynamic scapulothoracic stabilization and to effectively stimulate agonist-antagonist cocontraction throughout the arm.

The principles and techniques of **proprioceptive neuromuscular facilitation (PNF)**[20] are applicable with all of the above forms as well as with the manual resistance of a partner, therapist, or coach. These exercises place specific demands on the neuromuscular mechanism through stimulation of the proprioceptors to elicit a specific desired response. Three motion components (flexion-extension, abduction-adduction, and internal-external rotation) combine to form a diagonal pattern: antagonistic movement patterns comprise the two movements of each diagonal. The components are selected to create movement patterns of facilitation that will work muscles from their fully lengthened to their shortened state. Techniques of rhythmic stabilization, and rapid reversal are effective for challenging dynamic neuromuscular control.[20]

An excellent overall upper body exercise form is **cycling with the arms.** This can be performed using either a specifically designed upper body exerciser (UBE, Lumex Corp., Ronkonkoma, NY) or sitting on the floor behind a stationary bicycle, pedaling with the arms. Low-resistance, high-speed endurance bouts or sprint workouts can be developed based on the individual's needs.

Sport-Specific Exercise and Functional Performance Training

The need for exercises per se is completed once the following criteria are met: (1) full pain-free range of motion; (2) strength and endurance tests demonstrate adequate balance of muscles around the joint and normal strength of the injured tissue.

Full restoration of strength and mobility is critical before sport-specific exercises and return to play. If strength and mobility are not restored, we can safely assume that the deficits will persist and may predispose the player to future problems. Once rehabilitation is completed, we can address the specific demands of the sport with emphasis on coordinated interaction of antagonists and supporting muscles, agility, skill, and speed drills, plyometrics, and performance training. At this time it is hoped that the preinjured status of the rest of the body has been maintained or enhanced and that deficits elsewhere that may have set the stage for the injury have been effectively addressed. On return to sports the player should be offered some specific guidelines to deal with future problems. A sense of how to interpret the body's

warning signals and when and how to respond gives the player some control over minimizing the likelihood of furthering an injury. Using a pain scale such as the following can be helpful[3,23]*:

Phase I: Soreness after activity, usually gone in 24 hours

Phase II: Mild soreness and stiffness before activity, which disappears once warmed up; mild soreness after activity

Phase III: Stiffness before and mild pain during activity but not enough to alter activity

Phase IV: Pain during play that alters ability to perform

Phase V: Constant pain, even at rest

Whenever possible, return to sport is controlled by manipulating the variables of duration, frequency, types of strokes, and intensity of competition. By interplaying and progressing these components methodically, any injury-promoting factors can be identified and addressed. The player begins with stroke production drills without a ball, with emphasis on proper form and mechanics. If that is well tolerated, the player hits a foam ball, which is followed by short bouts on the court using ground strokes. Increasing time on the court is then alternated with introducing more challenging strokes until full-duration play with all strokes is tolerated. Finally, he or she can return to competitive play. The rehabilitation exercises should be continued three times per week through sport return until well after the player is fully back and asymptomatic.

Commitment to an ongoing conditioning program to offset the imbalances imposed by tennis and to maintain the tissues' ability to adapt to the demands of the sport is essential to minimize future injury potential.

INJURY-SPECIFIC REHABILITATION

Application of the above principles to the most common tennis injuries needs to be highly individualized for each patient. This is based on the findings of a thorough evaluation. Tennis-specific subjective evaluation must include all aspects of tennis activity, injury history, and daily activities. Initial objective evaluation must include observation of posture and alignment and dominant to nondominant differences (e.g., scapular slide,[18] muscle hypertrophy, and atrophy).

Ranges of motion and flexibility are evaluated with particular attention to tightness of internal rotation and the inferior posterior capsule, glenohumeral joint play and stability testing; pectoral and latissimus tightness; and elbow flexion contracture. Integrity of the static stabilizers (e.g., capsular ligaments), joint stability, and impingement tests are addressed.

Strength of all scapulothoracic, shoulder, elbow, wrist, and grip muscles is assessed. The common weaknesses found in many tennis players include the scapular retractors, lower trapezius, serratus anterior, supraspinatus,

shoulder external rotators, biceps, wrist extensors, and grip. Isolated weakness of a muscle group, agonist/antagonist ratios, and force couple interactions throughout the arm must be identified and normalized. The emphasis must be on total arm strengthening and comprehensive upper quarter dynamic balance.

Once these are restored, functional testing in preparation for sports return may include isokinetic concentric and eccentric tests for isolated motion peak torque, work, agonist/antagonist ratios, plyometric performance drills, and functional movement pattern strength and endurance. The following discussion presents guidelines based on what has been most successful in our experience and is in no way intended to be a formula. In fact, we are most successful using this only as a basic framework for modifications based on the patient's input and feedback. It is constantly reevaluated and altered to achieve our goals as efficiently and thoroughly as possible; and with each patient the process is different.

Lateral Tennis Elbow

Lateral tennis elbow generally is manifested by extreme tenderness just anterior and distal to the lateral epicondyle (extensor carpi radialis brevis) and weakness and/or pain with stress testing, wrist extension, third finger extension, and grip. Occasionally supination is involved. Symptoms are intensified when testing is done with the elbow straight because the tissues are further stressed in this position.

Rehabilitation should follow these guidelines:

Avoid actions or activities of daily living that reproduce the lateral elbow pain. This often includes shaking hands, picking up a coffee cup, excessive computer use, and turning a key. In tennis some players may be able to continue easy hitting, but the backhand must be avoided.

Wear a counterforce brace for any activities that are potentially abusive (e.g., extensive writing or typing, hand shaking, occupational stresses, needlework). The brace is worn during exercises and return to play.

Heat, electric stimulation, and ice are the modalities we have found most effective. Usually four to six sessions over 2 or 3 weeks are sufficient.

It has been our experience that transverse function massage is not only painful and unnecessary but may result in iatrogenic synovitis, which presents a great conservative care challenge.

Exercises begin with daily repetitions (no weight) of wrist extension, pronation, and supination and elbow flexion within pain-free motion arcs. Full range exercises and weight are added on to tolerance until 1.4 kg (3 pounds) is comfortable, at which time alternate-day Isoflex exercises begin (five repetitions to start). The Isoflex exercises are wrist extension, pronation, supination, and radial and ulnar deviation. At this time, the isotonic exercises are performed with the arm straight and unsupported, placing greater stress on the extensors.

Instruct the patient to squeeze a tennis ball and open the fingers against the resistance of a rubber band several times throughout the day. These exercises are done

---

*Phases I and II are usually self-limiting and respond to antiinflammatory measures. Phase III requires activity modification and antiinflammatory measures. If ignored, it is likely to worsen. Phases IV and V require medical attention, major activity modifications, and full rehabilitation.

first with the elbow bent at the side and progress over time until they can be done with the arm out straight.

Isokinetic exercises begin concentrically with submaximal effort, avoiding motion extremes, in the moderate-speed range (90 degrees to 180 degrees per second). These can be initiated early if these guidelines are adhered to by the patient. Progression variables include full motion, full effort, full velocity spectrum from 60 degrees to 300 degrees per second.[26] Early 5-second bouts are progressed to 20-second bouts. Eccentric isokinetic exercises should begin in the passive mode and progress to eccentric mode based on the patient's tolerance. Ellenbecker's study[11] on the total arm strength isokinetic profile of 22 highly skilled tennis players demonstrated a dramatic drop in wrist extensor single repetition work output at 300 degrees per second, creating a marked agonist/antagonist imbalance. This motion can effectively be emphasized, once tolerated, with eccentric work. Starting at slower speed (30 degrees to 90 degrees per second), the patient may progress with time to higher speeds if tolerated. Because the eccentric isokinetic physiologic overflow seems to cover a greater range than in concentric isokinetics, a velocity spectrum program might cover 30-degree per second increments.[8]

Arm cycling and leg work are done for strength and agility.

Flexibility exercises to the wrist are added last, once the arm is relatively pain free. We have found that early stretching of damaged tendons delays healing and slows the rehabilitative effort. The strength exercises are done through the fullest possible pain-free motion arcs, but flexibility exercises per se are done last.

Grip testing: the dominant arm should test out approximately 20% to 25% stronger than the nondominant arm. Tests should be done with the elbow bent and straight.

Isokinetic testing at 60 degrees per second should demonstrate certain relationships:
Dominant arm 15% to 25% higher than nondominant (recreational players show less difference, tournament players more difference).

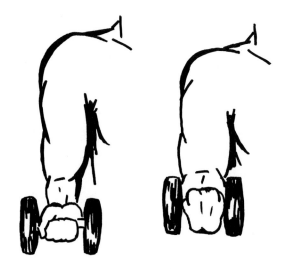

FIG. 37-5. Wrist flexion.

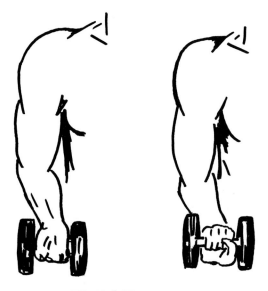

FIG. 37-6. Wrist extension.

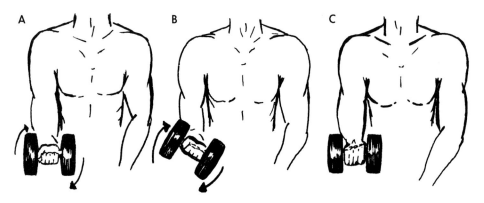

FIG. 37-7. Pronation-supination. **A,** Full supination. **B,** Supinated pronation. **C,** Full pronation.

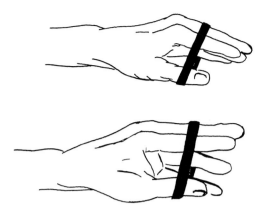

FIG. 37-8. Rubber band for finger extensors.

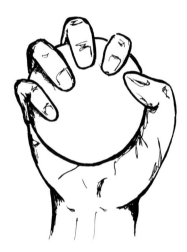

FIG. 37-9. Tennis ball squeeze.

Flexors strongest group, then pronators, then supinators, with extensors weakest; extensors should be 60% to 70% of flexors; supinators should be 80% to 90% of pronators.

Progressive sports return: Following the concepts of a gradual methodical progressive return, a program such as the following is recommended[24]:

15 minutes, forehand only
30 minutes, forehand only
30 minutes, forehand and backhand (two-handed)
45 minutes, forehand and backhand
45 minutes, all strokes
Serve
Full play
Competitive play

Medial Tennis Elbow

Medial tennis elbow is manifested by tenderness over the medial epicondyle and may or may not involve ulnar nerve symptoms, as well as pain and/or weakness on wrist flexion, finger flexion, grip, and pronation.

Activities involving tight gripping, strengthening exercises with the wrist fully extended (e.g., Nautilus biceps curls, push-ups), and fly machines should be avoided.

Exercises are as with lateral tennis elbow but include wrist flexion (Figs. 37-5 to 37-9). Sports return should follow a progression such as the following[24]:

15 minutes, backhand and lobs
30 minutes, backhand and lobs
30 minutes, backhand, lobs, and forehand (no topspin)
45 minutes, backhand, lobs, and forehand
45 minutes, all strokes
Serve
Full play
Competition*

Rotator Cuff Tendinosis

Shoulder rotator cuff tendinosis often is manifested by:

Shoulder pain that is aggravated in activities of daily living by lying on that side (thus compromising vascular supply to the supraspinatus)[27]; holding the arm in the 90- to 110-degree range (e.g., driving with arm on back of seat); and hyperextension with internal rotation (e.g., putting on a coat or putting a wallet away, reaching back, overhead).

Visible wasting of the cuff muscles around the scapula as compared with the uninvolved side. Since the injury most commonly occurs in the dominant shoulder, the atrophy is particularly dramatic.

Altered scapulohumeral rhythm in arm elevation.

Pain and/or weakness on supraspinatus testing in the "empty can" position as described by Jobe and Moynes[17]; prone horizontal abduction in full external rotation as described by Blackburn[2]; shoulder rotator testing with the patient prone and shoulder abducted to 90 degrees; lower trapezius testing prone.

Positive impingement and/or joint laxity tests.[1]

The rehabilitation program should include:

Avoiding activities with the arm fully overhead or hyperextended with internal rotation or adducted across the chest at 90 degrees; avoiding sleeping on the involved side.

Electric stimulation, ultrasound, heat, and ice as needed.

Postural correction: the slumped posture itself tends to collapse the shoulder joint so that there is less freedom of movement. With inflammation present, the effects become even worse, sometimes carrying over to the other tissues. Furthermore, the slumped posture creates a detrimental muscle imbalance as discussed on p. 811. Thus emphasis on good posture throughout the player's day is critical to rotator cuff tendinosis resolution and avoidance of recurrence.

Early flexibility exercises. Unlike with other areas of tendinosis, we begin these immediately to the shoulder, because shoulder flexibility exercises do not stretch (and therefore irritate) the injured tissue. The purposes of these exercises are to maintain full motion

---

*Late strokes must be avoided throughout.

arcs for strengthening exercises, to prevent capsular adhesions, and to correct the muscle imbalances of poor posture. These include pendulum exercises with a cuff weight, PNF diagonals and techniques, gentle mobilization if needed, and passive static and dynamic stretching to restore normal internal rotation, horizontal adduction and elevation.

A tight posterior capsule may result in anterior humeral head translation in external rotation and in elevation, creating or perpetuating the continuum of shoulder impingement and instability as described by Jobe.[16] Pectoral and latissimus stretching is essential to allow needed scapular retraction. Stretches at this time must avoid anterior humeral head translation, until joint stability is restored.

Rehabilitation exercises of the rotator cuff muscles in a protected position. The cuff weaknesses must be corrected first to avoid further abnormal joint mechanics and further damage. Rehabilitation exercises are given in the box on p. 818. These exercises are selected because of their high-activity effect on the rotator cuff muscles as well as their protective nature.[17,21]

Rehabilitation exercises are done with high repetitions and low weight. Cybex standing internal-external rotations in the scapular plane are started early in the treatment at submaximal midspeed bouts (60 to 180 degrees per second), progressing to high-speed duration bouts (180 degrees to 300+ degrees per second). External rotator muscle strength must be emphasized because their weakness as a rule is the greatest muscle imbalance at the shoulder and at the same time the demands on them (concentric and eccentric) in swinging are enormous. At the same time, subscapularis strength is needed for support of the anterior capsule.

Once manual muscle testing of each of the rotator cuff muscles in their independent action is normal, we begin shoulder conditioning exercises that presuppose the integrity of the cuff and stress the combined interplay of the dynamic components of the shoulder joint complex (e.g., military press, PNF diagonals

through increasing motion arcs, triceps press, prone internal-external rotations, prone overhead lifts, and horizontal lifts, push-ups and press-ups with a plus).

Upper body cycling, starting with the seat high, can be initiated immediately (Fig. 37-10). As the integrity of the rotator cuff improves, the seat can be lowered to work the shoulder in higher degrees of elevation. Throughout this exercise emphasis must be placed on active muscle control of the scapulothoracic stabilizers. The patient's attention to good posture and scapular movement greatly enhances the value of this workout.

Force-couple balancing of the scapulothoracic group and strengthening of the muscles that create the normal scapulohumeral rhythm provide the needed base for desirable glenohumeral overhead motion. These include the upper and lower trapezius; trapezius and serratus anterior; serratus anterior, trapezius and rhomboids; rotator cuff and deltoid.[29]

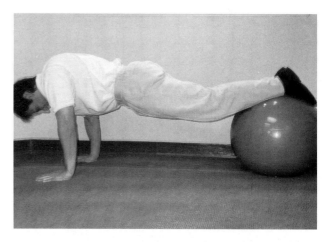

FIG. 37-11. Closed kinetic chain stabilization exercise with physioball.

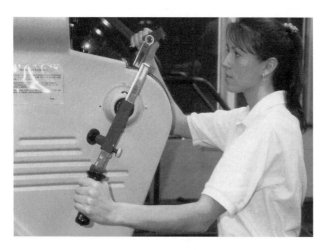

FIG. 37-10. Upper body ergometer.

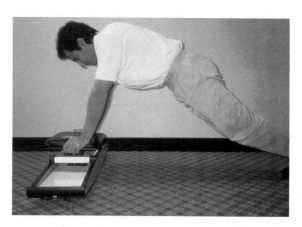

FIG. 37-12. Closed kinetic chain endurance exercise with Profitter.

Closed kinetic chain exercises are employed to enhance dynamic scapulothoracic stabilization capabilities. These may begin with balancing in quadriped position, then challenge is added with manual resistance using rhythmic stabilization and rapid reversal techniques in PNF diagonals.[20] Further progression includes these techniques in the plantigrade and tripod positions. Balancing with or without manual resistance with arms increasingly further apart and push-ups on a physioball very effectively stimulate agonist/antagonist co-contraction of the upper quarter muscle groups (Fig. 37-11). Upper extremity Profitter and Stairmaster workouts stimulate dynamic endurance of the stabilizers (Fig. 37-12).

Functional training. Once normal strength and mobility balance of the upper quarter are restored, stretch-shortening exercises, or plyometrics, are integrated to maximize the neuromuscular potential for explosive activity. Using 2- to 4-pound medicine balls with a rebound system (Plyopack, Shape Medical Systems, San Bruno, Calif.) allows the athlete to work at different heights and levels of challenge. A progression may be developed from the chest pass, to a two-handed soccer overhead throw, then a two-handed chest pass, then side-to-side throws (Fig. 37-13). Plyometric push-ups against the wall, table, and floor can be done independently or against manual resistance. Tubing resistance can advance to biceps curls, 90/90 (with the leg, shoulder, and elbow at 90-degree angles) rotations, and PNF diagonals into endurance plyometric training. A comprehensive tennis-specific plyometric program is detailed by Chu.[5]

Criteria for return to play include:

Full pain-free motion arcs that meet the demands of the sport

An isokinetic test that demonstrates normal strength, normal torque curve shapes, and adequate balance of agonist-antagonist muscle relationships

Graduated return to play with a progression such as[24]:

15 minutes, forehands
30 minutes, forehand and backhand
45 minutes, forehand and backhand
45 minutes, all strokes
Serve
Full play
Competition

Technique modifications as needed

Continued ice after play and continuing the exercises on a maintenance program

A detailed interval tennis program is described in depth by Ellenbecker.[12]

INJURY PREVENTION PROGRAM

A supplemental program for any sport is designed to contribute to the prevention of injuries and enhance performance. Many factors need to be addressed in designing a preventive program.

Specificity of Training

Address the specific needs of the individual as determined by injury history, current fitness level, level of sports participation, and specific tests of his or her strength, flexibility, and endurance. Thus sports preparation may well involve any or all of these categories of exercise:

Rehabilitative exercise: to stimulate healing of injured or vulnerable tissue and return it to its normal state

Conditioning exercise: to get in shape, improving the performance ability of a normal body part

Sports exercise: to enhance skill level, with progressive competition

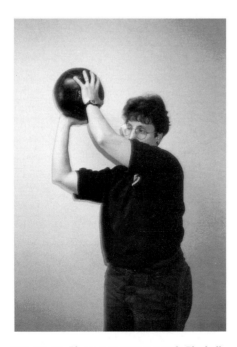

FIG. 37-13. Plyometric training with Plyoball.

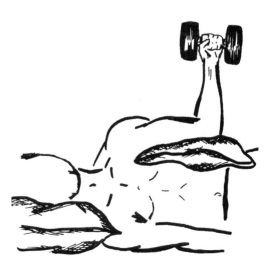

FIG. 37-14. Side-lying external rotation.

Basic rehabilitation exercises for rotator cuff muscles

Side-lying internal rotation

Exercise benefits:	Subscapularis, infraspinatus, teres minor
Starting position:	Lie on involved side, involved arm in front of body at side, elbow bent 90 degrees.
Exercise action:	Slowly rotate arm inward toward abdomen, then slowly rotate back out again.

Side-lying external rotation (Fig. 37-14)

Exercise benefits:	Infraspinatus, teres minor, subscapularis
Starting position:	Lie on good side; hold involved elbow bent to 90 degrees with pillow between arm and side.* Involved hand holds weight on stomach.
Exercise action:	Holding elbow close to side, externally rotate arm so that hand points to ceiling. Hold 2 seconds, and then slowly lower.

Empty can (Fig. 37-15)

Exercise benefits:	Supraspinatus
Starting position:	Sitting or standing, raise arm out to side and forward 30 degrees in front of body (arm parallel to floor). Internally rotate shoulders so that thumb points down as in emptying a can.
Exercise action:	Keeping elbow straight, slowly lower arm to thumb at waist level. Hold 2 seconds, and then raise to starting height.

Note: If painful, begin by doing these with thumb pointing up.

Prone horizontal abduction (Fig. 37-16) (airplanes)

Exercise benefits:	Rhomboids, middle trapezius, supraspinatus, deltoid
Starting position:	Lie on bench on stomach with involved arm hanging to floor, thumb pointing toward ceiling, hand at eye level.†
Exercise action:	Raise arm out to side as high as you can to plane of body. Slowly lower.

Biceps curls

Exercise benefits:	Biceps
Starting position:	Stand with arm at side, weight in hand.
Exercise action:	Bend elbow, bringing hand to shoulder. Slowly lower.

*The pillow is necessary to avoid wringing out the vascular supply when the arm is fully internally rotated.[31]
†An electromyographic study done by Blackburn et al[2] found this position to elicit the greatest overall activity in the posterior rotator cuff.

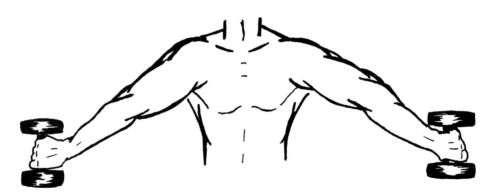

FIG. 37-15. Empty can.

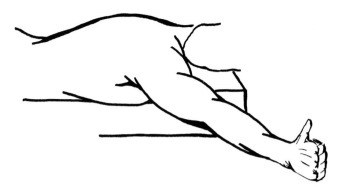

FIG. 37-16. Prone horizontal abduction.

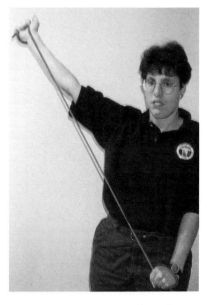

FIG. 37-17. Isoflex, or rubber tubing.

The goal here is to get the player in shape for the sport, that is, to prepare him or her for maximal performance participation and to minimize injury risk.

General Fitness Level

Overcome the imbalances created by the individual's daily activities and fill in the fitness gaps. Never has the significance of well-rounded physical fitness been appreciated as it is now. True physical fitness includes a well-balanced integration of musculoskeletal strength, flexibility, and endurance, neuromuscular and cardiovascular efficiency, good nutrition, and weight control. Unfortunately, no one sport does all this, and supplemental work is needed to create a fully conditioned, healthy athlete. Tennis as a sport encompasses substantial body involvement and therefore promotes reasonably, but not totally, balanced development of muscular strength, flexibility, and endurance. Furthermore, tennis stimulates coordinated eye-hand skills, agility, and reaction times. The effects in the area of cardiovascular and respiratory (aerobic) training are limited, however, because of brief activity bursts separated by long, minimal-activity intervals. Recommended aerobic supplements to choose from are walking, jogging, and running, Stairmaster, Profitter training, bicycling, swimming, Nordic track or cross-country skiing, aerobics classes, and rowing. For the athlete to enhance the current level, the chosen activity would have to be done maintaining the target heart rate, four or five times per week, 30 minutes at a time.

Strength Program

The most common strength deficits in most people are:
- Legs: hip flexors, hamstrings, and groin, especially in their extreme motion limits; ankle dorsiflexors and evertors
- Trunk: lower and upper abdominals
- Arms: shoulder external rotators and flexors, triceps, wrist extensors, grip

Thus a supplemental strength program for a tennis player should first test the individual for weaknesses in these areas and then include exercises for the following as dictated by their tests:

Gluteals, hamstrings (e.g., curls, crunches, hyperextensions, squats)

Abductors and adductors

Gastrocnemius muscles, dorsiflexors and evertors of the ankle

Abdominals (e.g., bicycle, reverse curls, crunches, crunch-twisting)

Scapular stabilizers (e.g., press-ups with a plus, rowing, prone overhead lifts in external rotation, military press)

Rotator cuff (e.g., internal and external rotations, scaption, prone horizontal abduction in external rotation)

Triceps (e.g., French curl, overhead press)

Wrist extensors

Finger extensors (e.g., work against a rubber band)

Grip (e.g., squeeze a tennis ball)

Guidelines for an isotonic free-weight program would be:

Two sets of 12 to 15 repetitions; increase by 1 kg (2 pounds) once this is comfortable for three consecutive exercise sessions

2 seconds to raise, 2 seconds to hold, 3 seconds to lower

Full motion arcs

For players who travel a lot, we recommend an Isoflex, or rubber tubing, program, such as that given in the box on p. 820 (Fig. 37-17).

Flexibility Program
Goals

The goals of flexibility exercises for tennis are[28]:

Injury prevention during sports participation. All the motion demands that may be encountered on the court must be met comfortably beforehand to avoid getting into unmanageable positions while playing. Equally as important is strength throughout the motion extremes.

Overcoming the imbalances imposed by the sport. Tennis is actually one of the better sports in terms of challenging all the body parts in their motion extremes.

Isoflex exercise program

Military press

Exercise benefits: Trapezius, supraspinatus, deltoid

Starting position: Anchor loop with nonexercise hand on abdomen. Exercise hand holds loop at shoulder height, palm facing away from body.

Exercise action: Raise arm to overhead position. Slowly lower arm.

Horizontal abduction with outward rotation (airplanes)

Exercise benefits: Supraspinatus, rhomboids, posterior deltoid, middle trapezius

Starting position: Tubing anchored with nonexercise hand on nonexercise shoulder. Exercise arm held out at eye level, thumb pointing back and elbow straight.

Exercise action: Pull tubing backward, behind plane of body.

PNF D$_2$

Exercise benefits: Trapezius, supraspinatus, infraspinatus, middle deltoid

Starting position: Stand with loop anchored on nonexercise hip. Exercise hand and thumb on that hip.

Exercise action: Turn thumb outward, bringing arm up and out to overhead position, halfway between head and shoulder.

Shoulder external rotation

Exercise benefits: External shoulder rotators (infraspinatus and teres minor)

Starting position: Stand with feet comfortably spread. Hold Isoflex handle in exercise hand, waist high, with loop in other hand on hip.

Exercise action: Keeping exercise elbow at side, place firm tension on Isoflex by pulling handle away from exercise hip with exercise hand. Slowly externally rotate handle outward as far as possible.

Shoulder internal rotation

Exercise benefits: Anterior deltoid, pectoralis, teres major, latissimus dorsi, subscapularis

Starting position: Loop Isoflex around doorknob. Stand to the left of the door. Hold Isoflex handle in right hand just to side of right hip.

Exercise action: Place firm tension on Isoflex by moving further from the doorknob if necessary. Pull handle away from right hip with right hand. Now, slowly internally rotate handle inward as far as possible.

Extensor wrist curl

Exercise benefits: Forearm extensors

Starting position: Sit in chair and place Isoflex under right foot. Hold handle in right hand, palm down. Support forearm on thigh with wrist and hand extended beyond knee.

Exercise action: From wrist-down position, slowly raise hand and bend wrist backward as far as possible.

Flexor wrist curl

Exercise benefits: Forearm flexors

Starting position: Sit in chair and place Isoflex under right foot. Hold handle in right hand, palm up. Support forearm on thigh with wrist and hand extended just beyond knee.

Exercise action: From wrist-back position, slowly curl wrist up.

Trunk twist

Exercise benefits: Quadratus (back flank muscles); oblique abdominals

Starting position: Stand on Isoflex loop with right foot. Hold Isoflex handle in right hand with right arm extended down right side.

Exercise action: Lift Isoflex handle up and out to right side approximately 15 cm (6 inches) while bending from the waist as far to the left as possible. Slowly twist the trunk to the left and backward as far as possible. Hold for 3 seconds. Relax and return to starting position. Repeat to the opposite side.

Back extension

Exercise benefits: Midline, paralumbar muscles; quadratus lumborum

Starting position: Hold Isoflex in front of body so handle is between both feet. Bend forward approximately 90 degrees (less if you are unable to bend to 90 degrees). Grasp either side of loop with hands. NOTE: The lower the loop is grasped, the greater the exercise efficiency.

Exercise action: Holding firmly to Isoflex loop, slowly uncurl back to full starting position. Hold for 3 seconds. Relax and return to starting position.

Isoflex exercise program—cont'd

Hip flexion
Exercise benefits: Iliopsoas, rectus femoris, sartorius; quadriceps
Starting position: Secure Isoflex anchor strap to right ankle with attach zone
                                       facing forward. Stand with left foot on Isoflex with handle
                                       to outside of foot. Pull right leg forward until mild tension
                                       occurs.
Exercise action: Holding knee straight and ankle up, pull right leg forward and
                                       up as far as possible.

Ankle plantar flexion
Exercise benefits: Calf muscles
Starting position: Secure Isoflex anchor on right foot with attach zone on the
                                       bottom of the foot. Sit on floor with knee straight. Hold Isof-
                                       lex handle in both hands at waist level.
Exercise action: Pull foot and ankle up as far as possible. Firmly holding Isof-
                                       lex handle, point toe and ankle down as far as possible.

Ankle dorsiflexion
Exercise benefits: Ankle dorsiflexor
Starting position: Secure Isoflex anchor strap on right foot with the attach zone
                                       on top of foot. Place Isoflex loop under chair leg; sit on floor
                                       away from chair until mild tension on Isoflex occurs.
Exercise action: Slowly pull toes and ankle up as far as possible.

Flexibility exercise program

- Supine hamstring stretch for hamstring and calf muscles
- Supine hip twist for hip rotators, abductors, lower back
- Alternate knee-to-chest for lower back, gluteals, hip rotators
- Sitting groin stretch for groin, inner thigh
- Sitting figure-4 stretch for hamstrings, lower back, Achilles tendon
- Spinal twist for spinal muscles, hips
- Quadriceps stork stretch for iliopsoas, quadriceps
- Standing adductor lunge for groin
- Trunk side bend for iliotibial band
- Wall stretch for gastrocnemius, soleus
- Triceps overhead stretch for inferior capsule
- Horizontal adduction stretch for posterior area of shoulder; emphasize holding shoulder blade near spine
- Forearm stretch for wrist flexors and extensors

Dynamic stretches for tennis

- Swing the racquet in controlled but full motion arcs.
- Reach arms up alternately (as if climbing a ladder at the highest rungs).
- Holding a racquet with hands overhead, bend side to side.
- Hold a racquet behind your back with arm fully overhead, elbow fully bent (back-scratch position as in serve). Racquet handle is held by dominant arm, and nondominant arm grabs the head. Pull the head down, thus stretching the inferior capsule of the dominant arm.
- Punch across body with arms at shoulder height.
- In forward-bent position, knees bent and legs wide apart, lunge from side to side.
- Holding a racquet, rotate trunk, twisting side-to-side with arms at shoulder level and then overhead.

Supplemental exercise program

Area for improvement	Exercise
Serve and overheads	Pullover, row, press-ups with a plus, triceps, French curl, shoulder flexion-extension, rotator cuff
Grip strength and racquet control	Forearm muscles, wrist extensors, tennis ball squeeze
Court movement and acceleration	Quadriceps, gluteals, hamstrings, abductors, adductors, gastrocnemius, soleus, squats

---

Good form. The player with good form avoids compensating for an area of inflexibility with excessive motion in another body part.

Lessening the work effort by the antagonist.

Common flexibility deficits in most people include:

Legs: gastrocnemius, hamstrings, iliotibial band, soleus, adductors

Trunk: lower back, pectorals

Arms: anterior area of shoulder, shoulder flexors, wrist extensors

A recommended flexibility program for anyone should be based on findings on the following tests:

1. Shoulder internal rotators, pectorals
2. Shoulder inferior and posterior joint capsule
3. Wrist flexors (should be 90 degrees) and extensors (should be 80 degrees)

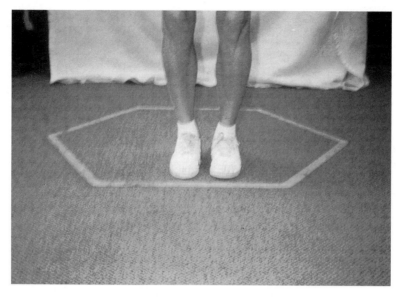

FIG. 37-18. Hexagon drill.

4. Hamstrings (These are best tested lying on the back with the hip of the test leg bent 90 degrees so that the thigh is perpendicular to floor. Normal hamstring flexibility allows the knee to be straightened fully so that the whole leg is straight and perpendicular to floor.)
5. Hip flexors (Thomas test)
6. Long sitting toe touch for lower back, hamstrings, gastrocnemius, and soleus
7. Iliotibial band

Exercises

The exercise program given in the box is designed to meet the goals discussed above for tennis. These should be done only after a proper warm-up. It is not necessary to do all the exercises; select those that are appropriate as determined from testing.* In each exercise the following procedure should be advised:
Stretch as far as you can, going just short of pain.
Then inhale deeply and as you exhale, stretch a bit farther, still without pain.
Hold this fully stretched position for 20 seconds, breathing easily.
Relax.
Repeat this procedure three times for each stretch.
In addition to the static stretching, dynamic stretching (see the box, middle right, on p. 821) is very effective after warming up and before playing. In a controlled manner, with exaggerated but flowing motions, the part is actively moved through the motion extremes. The mo-

---

*NOTE: A highly individualized evaluation is essential to determine where functional deficits exist. A number of misconceptions and much time have been wasted from the lack of specificity and vagueness of many exercise programs.

To enhance specific tennis skills, a supplemental exercise program (see the box, bottom left, on p. 821) should include exercises specific to the demands of the sport.[31]

Agility and tennis drills

Agility drills
Run the lines sideways (first within singles, then between doubles lines), touching down at each side.
Jump rope.
Do side-to-side jumps over 20- to 30-cm (8- to 12-inch) blocks.
Use balance board.
Hexagon drills (Fig. 37-18)

Tennis drills
Hit the ball, with player and ball staying in the alley (Fig. 37-19).
Practice ball toss alongside a pole, tossing the ball parallel to the pole.
Instructor hits while the player is running forward. Player must split step and go in either direction.

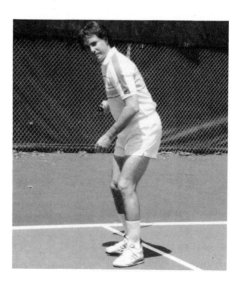

FIG. 37-19. Agility drills.

tions of the sport are mimicked but without the stresses of impact or weight bearing.

Finally, agility and tennis drills (see the box on p. 822) should be included. In general, a teaching tennis professional is the best resource on such drills.

SUMMARY

Racquet sport injuries are rarely seen in isolation. Injury is often present before the athlete actually recognizes its signs. As a result, tissue overload and compensation extend over the entire kinetic chain. Injury rehabilitation is based on thorough evaluation and knowledge of the specific role of the injured part in the kinetic chain. The findings are applied to a comprehensive program of total upper quarter balanced strength and mobility and subsequent functional performance training. Any factors that affect the dynamic interplay of the structures must be addressed. The athlete must recognize and incorporate the need for an ongoing conditioning program to meet the sport demands as well as to overcome the imbalances created by sport participation. We can look forward to gains in our knowledge as we combine scientific research with patient interaction.

REFERENCES

1. Andrews JR, Kupferman SP, Dillman CJ: Labral tears in throwing and racquet sports, *Clin Sports Med* 10:901, 1991.
2. Blackburn TA et al: EMG analysis of posterior rotator cuff exercises, *Athl Training* 25:40, 1990.
3. Blazina HE et al: Jumper's knee, *Orthop Clin North Am* 412:665, 1973.
4. Chamberlain G: Cyriax's friction massage: a review, *J Orthop Sports Phys Ther* 4(1):16, 1982.
5. Chu D: *Power tennis training,* Champagne, Ill, 1995, Human Kinetics.
6. Cruchow HW, Pelletier D: An epidemiologic study of tennis elbow, *Am J Sports Med* 7:234, 1979.
7. Cyriax J: *Textbook of orthopaedic medicine,* vol 1, Baltimore, 1969, Williams & Wilkins.
8. Davies G: *A compendium of isokinetics in clinical usage and rehabilitation techniques,* ed 4, Onolaska, Wis, 1992, S&S.
9. Davies G, Ellenbecker T: *Orthopedic physical therapy home study course 93-1: total arm strength rehabilitation for shoulder and elbow overuse injuries,* APTA Orthopedic Section, 1993.
10. deAndrade JR et al: Joint distension and reflex muscle inhibition in the knee, *J Bone Joint Surg* 47A:313, 1965.
11. Ellenbecker T: A total arm strength isokinetic profile of highly skilled tennis players, *Isokinet Exerc Sci* 2:1, 1992.
12. Ellenbecker T: Rehabilitation of shoulder and elbow injuries in tennis, *Clin Sports Med* 14:1, 1993.
13. Ellenbecker T, Davies G, Rowinski M: Concentric vs. eccentric strengthening of the rotator cuff, *Am J Sports Med* 16:64, 1988.
14. Giangarra CE et al: Electromyographic and cinematographic analysis of elbow function in tennis players using single and double strokes, *Am J Sports Med* 21:394, 1993.
15. Groppel J: *Tennis for advanced players,* Champaign, Ill, 1984, Human Kinetics.
16. Jobe FW, Kvitne RS: Shoulder pain in the overhand or throwing athlete: the relationship of anterior instability and rotator cuff impingement, *Orthop Rev* 18:963, 1989.
17. Jobe F, Moynes D: Delineation of diagnostic criteria and rehabilitation program for rotator cuff injuries, *Am J Sports Med* 10:336, 1982.
18. Kibler WB: Role of the scapula in the overhead throwing motion, *Contemp Orthop* 22:525, 1991.
19. Knapik JJ et al: Angular specificity and test mode specificity of isometric and isokinetic strength training, *J Orthop Sports Phys Ther* 4:2, 1983.
20. Knott M, Voss D: *Proprioceptive neuromuscular facilitation,* New York, 1968, Harper & Row.
21. Moseley JB et al: EMG analysis of the scapular muscles during a shoulder rehabilitation program, *Am J Sports Med* 20:128, 1992.
22. Nirschl R: Mesenchymal syndrome, *Va Med Monthly* 96:659, 1969.
23. Nirschl R: Tennis elbow, *Orthop Clin North Am* 4(3):787, 1973.
24. Nirschl R: *Arm care,* Arlington, Va, 1983, Medical Sports Publishing.
25. Nirschl R, Pettrone F: Tennis elbow, *J Bone Joint Surg* 61A:832, 1979.
26. Quillen WS: Application of isokinetic exercises in rehabilitation, In Davies G (ed): *A compendium of isokinetics in clinical usage,* LaCrosse, Wisc, 1984, S & S.
27. Rathburn J, McNab J: The microvascular pattern of the rotator cuff, *J Bone Joint Surg* 52B:540, 1970.
28. Sobel J: *Supplemental exercises for throwing, swimming, gymnastics,* Paper presented at AAOS symposium on upper extremity injuries in athletes, Washington, DC, 1984.
29. Sobel J: Shoulder rehabilitation—rotator cuff disease. In Pettrone F (ed): *Athletic injuries of the shoulder,* New York, 1995, McGraw-Hill.
30. Stanish W: *Tendinitis: its etiology and treatment,* Lexington, Mass, 1984, Collamore Press.
31. Stone W, Kroll W: *Sports conditioning and weight training,* ed 2, Boston, 1986, Allyn & Bacon.
32. VanGheluwe B, DeRuysscher I, Craenhals J: Pronation and endrotation of the racket arm in a tennis serve. In Jonsson B (ed): *Biomechanics X-B,* Champagne, Ill, 1987, Human Kinetics.
33. Wallis EL, Logan GA: *Body conditioning through exercise,* Englewood Cliffs, NJ, 1964, Prentice-Hall.
34. Wilk K, Arrigo C: Current concepts in the rehabilitation of the athletic shoulder, *J Sports Phys Ther* 18(1):365, 1993.
35. Yang and Peng: *J Formosan Med Assoc,* 1984.

CHAPTER 38 Upper Extremity Gymnastic Injuries

Garron G. Weiker

Since Charles Froland introduced gymnastics to the Harvard College program in 1825, the United States has seen a continued and steady growth of participation in the sport. In recent years, probably because of extensive television coverage of Olympic competition, the number of gymnastic participants has grown in exponential proportions. There are no readily available accurate figures of the number of participants, but conservative estimates[13,42,50] place the number at over 600,000 in more than 2000 private clubs across the nation. In addition, there are many gymnasts participating in high school, intercollegiate, and privately owned membership gyms.

The actual number and distribution of injuries within the sport is not well defined despite the efforts of several authors in recent years.* In club gymnastics an injury incidence of 11.9 in 100 participants over the course of a 9-month period was noted. Of these, 12.5% of the overuse problems and 20% of acute injuries involved the upper extremity. More than 50% of the injuries involved the upper extremity in the small number of males seen in this study (Fig. 38-1). A review of women's intercollegiate gymnastics noted an injury rate of 94% (66 of 70 gymnastics-competing seasons) in which 20 of the 66 reported injuries involved the upper extremity. Of these 26, 10 involved the supraspinatus tendon, four involved the wrist, and four involved the elbow.[45]

Meeusen and Borms[34] pooled data from numerous gymnastic studies in an effort to develop a comprehensive review of injuries in gymnastics. They demonstrated a wide variance of injury rate, ranging from over 90% to only 2.4%. That number is based on the number of injuries per 100 gymnasts per year. The incidence and distribution varied immensely among studies. Acute injury vs. overuse injury varied from a low of 44% acute to a high of 88% acute. Injuries of the upper extremity accounted for 25% to 30% of injuries seen in most of the studies they reviewed. These wide variations and results undoubtedly reflect to some extent the populations studied and the training centers in which they were studied. There are obviously major differences between the injuries of beginning casual gymnasts and those of the elite-level international competitors. Then we must factor in the wide variation in quality of coaching and facilities. I speculate that the variances also reflect a wide variation

---

*References 6, 12, 18, 34, 45, and 49.

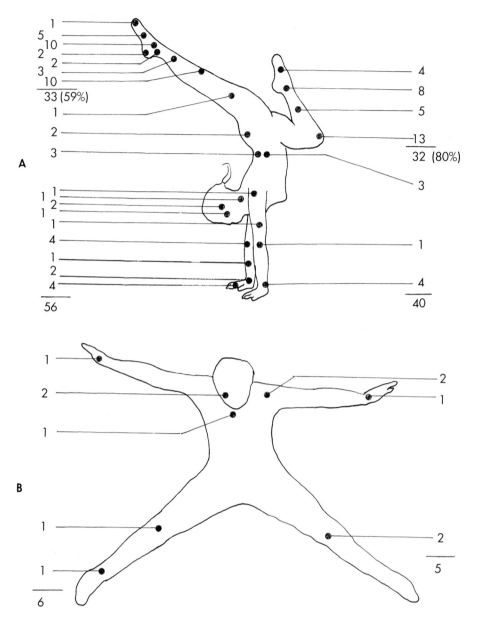

FIG. 38-1. Overuse injuries (*right*) and acute injuries (*left*) in 9 months of club gymnastics. **A,** Female. **B,** Male. (From Weiker GG: *Clin Sports Med* 4(1):39, 1985.)

in quality of data retrieved by various investigators, as well as methodology used.

Despite the major variations seen within these injury incident studies and the complex, confusing picture they paint, there are several principles that can be gleaned from them. Gymnastics does indeed lead to injuries. However, it seems to be at an acceptable rate when compared with other sports.[54] The injury patterns are somewhat unique to this sport, but they do follow their own patterns, and once an individual becomes familiar with the sport and its related problems, it should be no more confusing than caring for any other group of athletes. Finally, any physician who is going to care for entry-level gymnasts must make the effort to become familiar with

the sport, the apparati, the psychology of the sport, and the unique medical problems associated with the sport, as well as the unique requirements for successful return to competition after injury.

Evaluation of gymnastics problems is complicated by the extreme variability of experience and exposure. Male and female competitors participate in different events as well as different numbers of events. The age of participation ranges from 2 years to the mid-20s, and the level of activity varies from "bouncing babies" programs to elite international competition. Coaching varies from physical education majors assigned to coach school gymnastics to highly qualified full-time professionals. Facilities vary from temporarily assembled mats and equip-

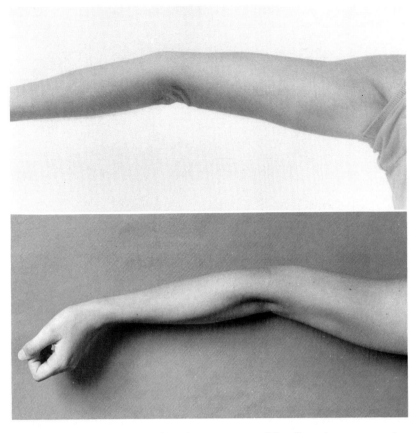

FIG. 38-2. Examples of physiologic hyperextension of the elbows in two gymnasts.

ment to permanent built-in practice and competition areas within the major private clubs.[17] Care of athletes also varies extensively, from programs with affiliated physicians who have a dedicated interest in the sport to programs that have no specific method of dealing with medical problems incurred during gymnastics.

The marked variability in age, program design, skill level, training intensity, coaching ability, facilities, medical care, and goals of training undoubtedly accounts in large part for the extreme variability of statistical data on injury reporting within gymnastics.

The basic mechanical activity of gymnastics is common to all programs despite the wide variations noted. Gymnastics require extensive high stress use of the upper extremity. The combination of strength, flexibility, and speed used in the sport subjects the upper extremity to high tension, impact shock, rotational stress, and compression loads. Weight-bearing compression, with or without associated impact, sets gymnastics apart from all other sports. The unavoidable stresses are accentuated by the effort to maintain graceful poise. Hyperextension of the elbow in various positions is considered an integral part of gymnastics (Fig. 38-2).

Acute injuries to the upper extremity are well documented in many sports but, as noted by Matheson et al,[31] stress fractures and other overuse injuries are rare with the exception of specific entities such as little league elbow and shoulder. Contrary to that general pattern in sporting activities, gymnasts do develop overuse injuries of the upper extremity.*

Although gymnastics does inherently place the upper extremity at risk, it is apparent that training techniques and facilities also play a part in the incidence of injury. Any physician dealing with gymnasts would be wise to review the *Gymnastics Safety Manual*[53] and the articles by Ganim[17] and Aronen.[3] Proper attention to flexibility, strength training, and coaching techniques, as well as selection, placement, and maintenance of equipment, play a role in determining the incidence of problems.

Factors in gymnastics injuries

- Flexibility
- Strength training
- Coaching technique
- Equipment
    Selection
    Placement
    Maintenance

---

*References 2-4, 7, 9, 10, 14, 15, 20-22, 28, 29, 31, 32, 34, 36, 38, 41, 43, 48, 55, and 56.

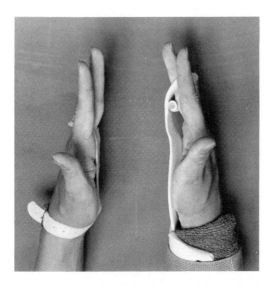

FIG. 38-3. Profile view of traditional grip on left and the doweled grip on the right.

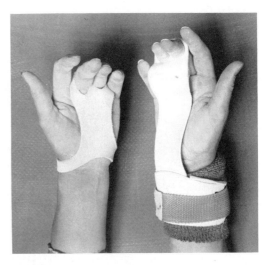

FIG. 38-4. Palmar view of traditional grip on left and the doweled grip on the right.

SHOULDER

Shoulder injuries represent between 0.7% and 16.7% of all gymnastics injuries.[34] They are more frequently related to overuse than to acute injury and are more often encountered in male competitors. This disparity is probably related to the difference in females' flexibility, gymnastics apparatus, and techniques. Women's events are primarily developed to demonstrate grace, rhythm, flexibility, and balance, but the majority of men's events are designed to emphasize power and strength. Maneuvers such as the iron cross, repetitive dislocates on rings, giant swings on the high bar, and programs on the pommel horse, parallel bars, and floor all place high stress on the male gymnast's shoulders. The accentuation of flexibility training in young females who are inherently loose jointed does increase the risk of chronic instability problems in the female gymnast.

As with most overuse syndromes, chronic problems in the gymnast's shoulder may be traced to overtraining, improper technique, inadequate conditioning, inadequate warm-up, inherent anatomic abnormalities, or lack of rehabilitation after acute injury. The most common causes of acute injury are missed moves, falls from the apparatus, and inadvertent contact with apparatus, people, or stationary objects.

Overuse injury etiologies

- Overtraining
- Improper technique
- Inadequate conditioning
- Inadequate warm-up
- Anatomic abnormalities
- Rehabilitation deficiencies following acute injury
- Poor equipment and facilities

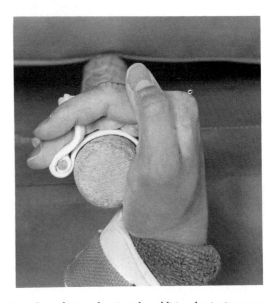

FIG. 38-5. Staged view showing the additional gripping power that the dowel offers.

An aspect of the sport that is in a state of flux at this time is repetitive giant swings, which place stress on the shoulder. Use of this maneuver was relatively limited until the advent of the doweled grip, which allows a much better grip. The increased grip enables the gymnast to perform higher velocity and more frequent giant swings as well as other swinging maneuvers. This problem has primarily been related to male gymnasts because the doweled grip was used only by them until recently. Female gymnasts are now making the transition to the doweled grip on uneven parallel bars, and we can anticipate an increase of shoulder stress phenomena among female gymnasts (Figs. 38-3 to 38-5).

Overuse Problems
Impingement Syndrome

Impingement syndrome is an area fraught with great confusion in the orthopaedic literature today. There are multiple tests that diagnose the syndrome, multiple explanations of its causes and pathophysiology, and therefore, multiple suggestions for treatment. The confusion is caused by attempting to find an acceptable definition and explanation that cross all barriers. The impingement syndrome seen in the 50-year-old nonathletic individual (with a pathologic condition of the rotator cuff and pain on shoulder abduction) is not necessarily the same entity seen in the 14-year-old athlete (with pain on flexion of the internally rotated shoulder). It is possible that a thrower's shoulder (with supraspinatus tendon pain in 30 degrees' flexion and resisted external rotation)[23] is an entirely separate entity.

Despite this controversy, a specific entity is seen in gymnasts that is commonly referred to as impingement syndrome, or rotator cuff inflammatory disease. The general complaint is pain on forward flexion with neutral or internal rotation. The athlete classically has pain when swinging on the bars or rings and in certain positions of handstands. The classic presentation is discomfort initially noted after activities and eventually throughout and after activity. To date I have seen no associated rotator cuff tears or irreversible lesions. It appears that athletes with impingement syndrome are incapacitated early enough with typical Stage I edema, inflammation, and pain that they seek medical help. The use of nonsteroidal antiinflammatory medication in conjunction with activity modification and rehabilitation has uniformly proven to be effective.

Stage I impingement treatment

- Nonsteroidal antiinflammatory medication
- Activity modification
- Rehabilitation

Treatment of impingement syndrome begins with abstinence from all activities that precipitate the primary pain for an initial period of 2 weeks. During that time a trial of nonsteroidal antiinflammatory medication is given, and the patient works on a rehabilitation program that emphasizes symmetric range of motion and selective strengthening. The strengthening component must always include internal and external rotators because of the high probability that impingement syndrome is associated with a subclinical instability component as one of its prime underlying factors. The specific strengthening components are directed to any muscle group that feels detectably weak on manual or Cybex testing. Once the initial symptoms resolve (usually 2 to 4 weeks), the gymnast is allowed to return to the sport with only one modification. I ask them to widen the hand placement on all swinging apparatus, as well as vault. Widening the hand placement by 2 to 3 inches generally makes a significant difference in the impingement symptoms.

Biceps Tendinitis and Subluxation

Although proximal biceps tendinitis may overlap with impingement syndrome, it is occasionally seen as a specific entity in the male gymnast. The athlete complains of pain in the anterior aspect of the shoulder and on examination has tenderness over the biceps groove, a positive Speed test, and equivocal impingement tests. A biceps tendon in subluxation presents as the sensation of something moving within the shoulder during dislocates and power moves on the rings, pommel horse, and parallel bars. The localizing signs are over the biceps tendon, and arthrography occasionally shows a shallow bicipital groove with redundancy of the overlying sheath.

In both biceps tendinitis and subluxation, it appears that faulty technique and inadequate musculature are the primary cause. To date these patients have uniformly responded to conservative rehabilitation efforts; therefore surgical intervention has not been necessary in my practice. A program of rest, ice, nonsteroidal antiinflammatory medication, and range of motion/strengthening exercises has proved effective.[3,23,24]

Chronic Instability

Performing the desired gymnastic maneuvers accentuates hypermobility of the shoulders, allowing the full spectrum of instabilities to be seen. As with other athletes, in gymnasts the most frequent instability is anterior subluxation and the most frustrating is the multidirectional instability seen in loose-jointed females. The natural selection of physiologically hypermobile individuals and the maximum range of motion used in gymnastics increase the risk of developing symptomatic instability. One particular exercise that is routinely performed by gymnasts to increase shoulder mobility causes instability complaints (Fig. 38-6). Those patients with complaints of instability usually have physiologic hypermobility associated with poor technique and/or muscle strength about the shoulder girdle. Rarely is there a history of acute traumatic dislocation or subluxation.

Rehabilitation and minor modification of technique have uniformly proved to successfully alleviate these complaints. The program involves general muscle strengthening of the entire shoulder girdle with accentuation of the internal rotators and modification of warmups to avoid extremes of shoulder motion. The inherent conflict of restricted motion caused by surgical stabilization and the need for extremes of motion in competition mitigate the value of operative intervention. Surgical stabilization of the shoulder is likely to end the athlete's career.

Miscellaneous

There is an entity that treating physicians should be aware of in the male gymnast's shoulder. Fulton, Albright, and El-Khoury[16] originally described **Ringman's shoulder,** which was reported as a radiographic finding on routine shoulder studies. This entity is represented by an area of benign hypertrophy at the humeral insertion of the pectoralis major and latissimus dorsi. It has been described as a corticodesmoid-like lesion on radiographic

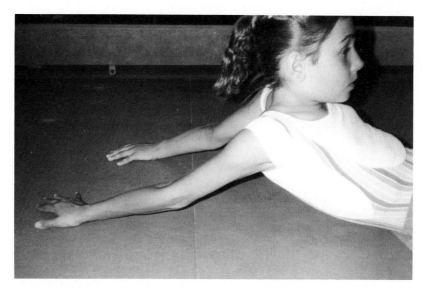

FIG. 38-6. Typical exercise to increase shoulder flexibility. This position may cause symptoms in the gymnast with unstable shoulder.

appearance and is a common finding that has no clinical significance in the male gymnast. One case of a gymnast who had osteochondrosis of the proximal humeral physis or little league shoulder came to my attention.[1] On close questioning the gymnast admitted that he had also been throwing extensively at home with his father in hopes of becoming a pitcher in baseball the next year. I am unaware of any reported cases of gymnastics-related overuse injuries to the proximal humeral physis.

Meeusen and Borms[34] referred to articles by Silvij and Szot that described a high percentage of gymnasts having cystlike shoulder degenerative changes by the end of their careers. My experience and review of the literature have not confirmed this long-term shoulder problem; however, there are no extensive reviews of the adult status of past gymnasts.

Acute Injuries

Contusions and Strains

The most commonly seen acute problems of the shoulder in gymnastics are related to contusion and muscular strain. Contusions are generally the result of a fall from the apparatus or inadvertent contact with an obstacle in the gym. Attention to general safety precautions can prove highly effective in preventing these injuries. Careful arrangement of the apparatus, padding of fixed obstacles, avoidance of horseplay and other distractions in the gym, and generous use of spotting are all beneficial. Strains are, as in most sports, primarily related to inade-

---

Safety precautions to prevent injury

- Careful placement of apparatus
- Padding of fixed obstacles
- Avoidance of horseplay
- Generous spotting

---

quate warm-up, excessive training past the point of fatigue, and inadequate rehabilitation of previous injuries. They are not critical injuries and respond well to the usual conservative measures.

Subluxation or Dislocation

Acute subluxation or dislocation of the shoulder generally is a result of a missed move or a fall from the apparatus. Again, the most effective way to prevent this type of injury is aggressive strength training, avoidance of distractions in the gym, good coaching, and judicious use of spotting during practice.

Treatment

Treatment of the acute problems about the shoulder is relatively standard. Phase I consists of 7 to 14 days of rest, ice massage, and, if necessary for comfort, a sling. Afterward, a formal active and passive range of motion program is started in conjunction with progressive resistance exercises. The gymnast should not be allowed to go back to full-scale activities in the gym until the shoulder has full and equal range of motion as well as normal strength. Before full recovery the gymnast can work out in the gym, go through calisthenics and warm-ups as tolerated, and perform tailored activities that do not put the shoulder into the position of risk. The only exception to this treatment protocol is first time acute dislocation or severe subluxation. Because of the nature of this sport, a minimum of 4 to 6 weeks in a sling and swath should be required before initiating range of motion and strengthening exercises. Conditioning can be maintained during that period either by deep water running with a flotation vest or the use of an exercise bike.

Summary

Although shoulder complaints are not rare in gymnastics, the shoulder joint has not been the site of major

problems. I have not seen the need to operate on the shoulder of any gymnast and have not been aware of any gymnast who has thought it necessary to discontinue the sport because of shoulder problems. Persistent impingement syndrome or recurrent dislocations could necessitate surgical intervention, but the latter would probably be the end of a gymnastics career.

ELBOW

Chronic problems in the gymnast's elbow appear to be related to the use of the extremity for weight-bearing support. Acute elbow injuries are the consequences of falls and high-velocity tumbling. The average female gymnast has extension ranging from 3 to 12 degrees of recurvatum and accentuated valgus inclination of the elbow. It is apparent in motion studies that the female gymnast tends to lock the elbow in a mechanically stable position, taking advantage of that hyperextension to tolerate the load. The male gymnast tends to rely more on the strength of his triceps but still works primarily in full extension. Acute injuries are usually the result of a fall on the outstretched arm and occur more frequently in less experienced gymnasts. Coaches routinely teach gymnasts how to "bail out" when they miss or lose control of a maneuver. The natural reflex is to reach out and break a fall with the outstretched arm. Bailing out replaces that natural reflex with the learned response of tucking the arms in and rolling on impact. Thick pads around the apparatus and generous use of spotting also decrease the frequency of elbow injuries.[40]

Overuse Problems
Benign Problems

Several benign problems occur around the elbow as a result of inadequate conditioning, excessive workouts, or inappropriate training techniques. These include tendinitis at the triceps insertion comparable to a jumper's knee of the elbow, olecranon bursitis caused by repeti-

---

Elbow overuse injuries

- Triceps tendinitis
- Olecranon bursitis
- Chronic synovitis
- Medial epicondylitis
- Lateral epicondylitis

---

tive contact, and chronic synovitis.[19,40] Both medial and lateral epicondylitis is seen, but medial is much more common. This is probably related to the increased valgus causing high-traction forces precipitated by weight-bearing maneuvers. The power moves such as the iron cross and other fixed-support moves used by the male gymnasts also exert high valgus load. All of these overuse problems are treated effectively with ice, strengthening of the elbow and wrist, modification of training techniques, and relative rest during the acute phase.

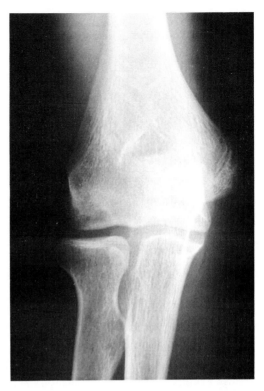

FIG. 38-7. Sixteen-year-old female gymnast with osteochrondritis dissecans lesion visible in the capitellum.

Osteochondritis Dissecans

The most dramatic of the overuse syndromes in the gymnast's elbow is osteochondritis dissecans of the capitellum (Panner's disease). On occasion associated enlargement of the radial head is found, much as is seen in little league elbow. Goldberg,[19] Singer and Roy,[44] and Priest[38,39] have all reported cases of osteochondritis dissecans of the capitellum. Their experience and mine indicate that this entity tends to occur most frequently in successful, aggressive, young gymnasts who are rapidly progressing through the various levels of competitive skills. Although seen in both male and female gymnasts, it is seen predominantly within the female population. (Fig. 38-7).

The presentation of osteochrondritis dissecans is usually pain that is variable in severity and initially noted following activities then gradually progresses to the point that it bothers the gymnast throughout activities. The first complaints are usually related to vault and floor exercise.

Over 50% of the patients I have seen with osteochondritis dissecans of the capitellum have presented at the time of their first visit with mechanical symptoms. They invariably describe several months of aching pain that they ignored before the onset of these symptoms. The presenting complaints are mechanical in the sense of catching, popping, and episodes of locking that require self-manipulation to work the elbow free and regain full motion.

Only 40% of my patients have had the lesion visible

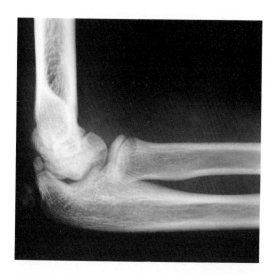

FIG. 38-8. Twelve-year-old female gymnast with osteochrondritis dissecans of the capitellum seen on lateral plain film.

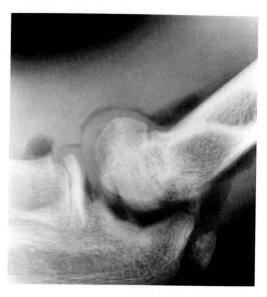

FIG. 38-9. Arthrotomogram of patient in Fig. 38-8 demonstrating a defect in the articular cartilage.

on plain films at the time of the first visit. When it is visible, it is typically centered on the capitellum at the point of radial head contact with the elbow in full extension. The lesion is typically seen as an area of lucency with a sclerotic margin and a sclerotic central fragment in the bed (Fig. 38-8). Occasionally a loose body is actually detected on plain films.

Although magnetic resonance imaging (MRI) is rapidly coming into its own for elbow evaluation, in my practice double contrast arthrotomography or the computed tomography (CT) arthrogram offers the best imaging results. With these techniques the lesion is well defined, loose bodies are highlighted, and the overlying articular surface is reasonably demonstrated (Fig. 38-9). The choice of imaging technique should be made by the treating physician in conjunction with the involved radiologist to select the best method available.

If the study shows no evidence of surface defect, a trial of physical therapy is instituted. Vaulting and tumbling are avoided for 3 to 6 months while the gymnast works on range of motion and strength. Progress is monitored by observation, symptomatology, and radiographs to see if the lesion heals spontaneously.

Arthroscopy is recommended for those patients who are having definite mechanical symptoms or who demonstrate definite loosening of the fragment. The lesion is readily visualized with standard elbow arthroscopic technique. The fragment is excised and the bed curetted down to bleeding bone. Postoperatively the patients are placed in a sling for 7 to 10 days for comfort's sake only, and then started on an active-only range of motion program. As soon as full motion has been obtained, progressive resistance exercises are initiated. Because of the nature of gymnastics, I do not recommend resection of the radial head. In the one case that demonstrated involvement of the radial head, the surface was debrided with a chondral abrader and then the standard postoperative course was followed (Fig. 38-10).

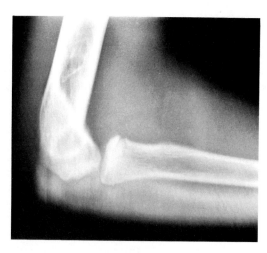

FIG. 38-10. Lateral tomogram of patient who demonstrated a chondral defect on the surface of the radial head.

Singer and Roy[44] reported on seven cases of osteochondritis dissecans of the capitellum in five patients ranging from ages 11 to 13. They noted the change in capitellar vascular supply from poorly collateralized end vessels in ages 5 to 19, to excellent collateral supply in the adult. It was also his belief that cases of this nature are limited to children in that high-risk group of ages 11 to 13. Of the five patients he treated, four returned to full competition and one chose to quit gymnastics rather than undergo treatment.

Chan et al[9] reported on elbow problems in 19 elite gymnasts in 1991. They noted seven cases of osteochondral lesions of the capitellum and seven cases of olecranon fracture or fragmentation. All of the olecranon patients returned to full competition after conservative

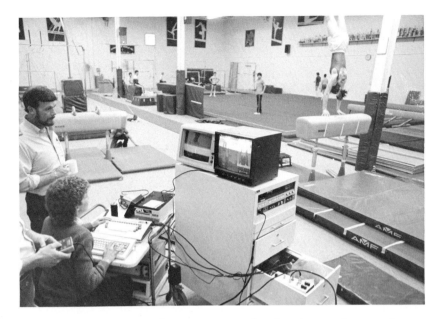

FIG. 38-11. Monitoring system wired to an instrumented vaulting horse to determine forces generated.

treatment. Maffulli, Chan, and Aldridge[29] and Wilkerson and Johns[55] reported olecranon stress fractures that required open reduction and internal fixation. They again had excellent results. None of the capitellum-affected patients reported by Chan et al were able to return to full, preinjury status. Maffulli, Chan, and Aldridge[28] reported essentially the same results in the long-term follow-up of 12 international-level gymnasts with capitellar defects. Neither Chan et al nor Maffulli, Chan, and Aldridge offered their gymnasts aggressive intervention. Their papers represent a study of the natural history of this process and point out that the course is not good.

Jackson, Silvino, and Reiman[22] reported a 2.9-year follow-up of 10 capitellar problems in seven gymnasts. Nine of these had surgical intervention for osteochondritis dissecans of the capitellum after failed conservative treatment. This group also showed poor results and a low rate of successful return to gymnastics.

I have treated 12 female gymnasts with osteochondritis dissecans of the capitellum. One of these had bilateral disease, and five presented with no mechanical symptoms. Evaluation of that five revealed that they had apparently intact articular surfaces. They were treated conservatively with the program previously noted. Three of the five patients healed satisfactorily and returned to full competition without difficulty. Two of the five patients developed mechanical symptoms and underwent surgical intervention with the other seven who presented initially with mechanical symptoms. Of the 10 elbows (in nine females), the first three were treated with diagnostic arthroscopy, arthrotomy, debridement, and curettement. All three of these patients subsequently returned to full competitive symptom-free activity within 6 months. The slowest recovery (6 months) was a patient whose elbow had a large lesion of approximately 1 cm in diameter. After debridement the radial head could be

seen to dip into the defect on extension and then go through a major shift as it rode up and out of the defect. This shift gradually cleared over 6 months, and at the 2-year follow-up, there was normal motion of the elbow and no functional difference between the operated elbow and the nonoperated elbow. The remaining seven procedures were performed arthroscopically and gained full range of motion, full function, and full return to activity within 4 months.

These 12 patients have not been called back for formal reevaluation. The results reported here are based on chart review and anecdotal reports from their various coaches.

CASE STUDY

A male patient with osteochrondritis dissecans sought treatment 18 months after the onset of symptoms. At that point he had an extensive lesion involving nearly 50% of the capitellar surface and associated enlargement and deformity of the radial head. He subsequently saw several other orthopaedic surgeons, all of whom recommended intervention and/or cessation of gymnastics. He and his family elected to stay in the sport without treatment, but after another year he quit because of inability to perform and was lost to follow-up.

Vaulting. My associates and I in the Musculoskeletal Research Department of the Cleveland Clinic Foundation have been evaluating pressure across the upper extremity in vaulting for the past 2 years. Early data gained by coordinating high-speed video and upper extremity forces recorded on an instrumented vaulting horse have demonstrated several interesting facts (Fig. 38-11).[52] The gymnasts exert a force through the upper extremities that averages 2½ to 3½ times their body weight with each vault. The actual force transmitted largely depends on technique. A low angle of attack at the time of contact with the horse markedly accentuates the forces, as

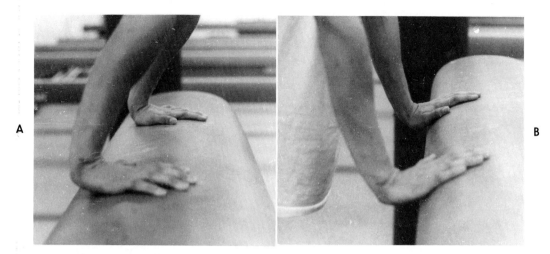

FIG. 38-12. Comparison of contact position on horse. **A,** Correct hand location. **B,** Hands at leading edge.

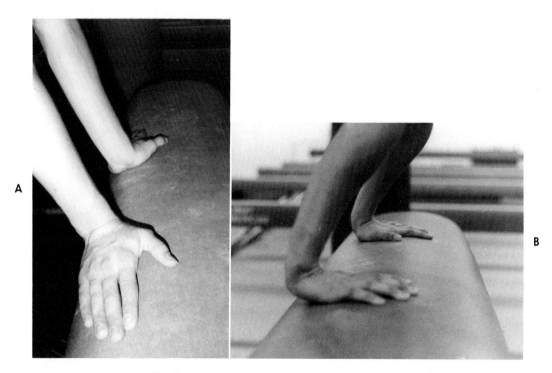

FIG. 38-13. A, Hands in incorrect supinated position. **B,** Hands in correct alignment.

does contact close to the leading edge of the vaulting horse (Fig. 38-12). Vaulting with the elbow fixed in full extension tends to cause higher peak readings than does the technique of slight flexion (5 to 15 degrees) and re-extension on impact. Vaulting with the hands supinated so that the fingers point toward the ends of the horse causes increased load when compared with vaulting with the fingers straight ahead in the line of the body motion (Fig. 38-13). These are all early findings based on a preliminary system of measurement and are not yet in a form satisfactory for formal presentation and publication.

Koh, Grabiner, and Weiker[27] have also looked at the forces of back handspring on floor exercise. That study showed that the average compression load through the elbow was 2.37 times body weight. The valgus moments equaled 0.03 times body weight times body height. Interestingly, the only factor that significantly decreased loads was increased elbow flexion during loading. Regrettably, flexion is considered poor technique and causes a point deduction in the scoring system if the judges can see the elbows bent.

■ ■ ■

All of the anecdotal information relating to osteochondritis dissecans of the elbow is presented to demonstrate several points. First of all, this is a unique entity that is seen almost exclusively in baseball pitchers and gymnasts. Second, body weight and technique are critical in relation to impact loading of the elbow. We anticipate that technique on floor exercise, vault, and beam is equally important in determining the degree of load through the elbow. Third, complaints of chronic elbow pain in the gymnast warrant careful consideration and evaluation. Any gymnast who complains of elbow pain that persists for more than a week should have full and adequate evaluation, including standard radiographs. Fourth, the treatment of this lesion is much easier if the diagnosis is made early. However in those cases in which it is made late, the surgeon should feel comfortable in going ahead with debridement of the lesion and adequate rehabilitation. A high percentage of these athletes should return to full competitive status with appropriate treatment.

Medial Epicondylitis

Use of the upper extremity as a weight-bearing member in athletes with a high degree of valgus elbow alignment causes compression loads across the radiocapitellar joint. It also places chronic traction stress on the medial collateral ligament complex and the medial epicondyle. Chronic medial epicondylitis and medial collateral ligament sprains are a common problem in young gymnasts and are frequently ignored unless a knowledgeable person works closely with the gymnastics program.

Icing, strengthening, stretching, and technique adjustments on floor exercises and vaulting generally allow rapid recovery. It is usually unnecessary to take time out from gymnastics. Treatment should be initiated only after adequate evaluation to rule out osteochondritis dissecans. Goldberg[19] also notes a problem with synovitis in the elbow of these athletes. This again should respond to ice, nonsteroidal antiinflammatory medication, a mild modification of activities to decrease the maximum stresses across the elbow, and a strengthening program.

Acute Injuries
Medial Epicondyle Fracture

Fracture of the medial epicondyle is not a surprising injury in this group of aggressive young athletes with open physeal plates and valgus inclination of the elbow. The best approach to prevention includes proper falling technique to avoid landing on the outstretched arm, thick mats, and liberal use of spotters. Regrettably, when this injury does occur in the gymnast, the medial epicondyle is frequently displaced and trapped. Surgical reduction and fixation are often required.[40] In patients who do not have significant displacement, conservative treatment is appropriate with a brief period of immobilization (10 to 20 days) followed by early range of motion exercises. The rehabilitation program should initially be limited to active range of motion only and progress should be followed closely. Strengthening can begin when the patient has regained motion of no less than 5 degrees to 130 degrees. Resumption of gymnastics is allowed when the patient has achieved full range of motion and full strength comparable to the contralateral side. In Priest's series,[38] over 80% of gymnasts were able to return to competitive activity after major injuries to the elbow.

Two of the gymnasts I have treated in recent years developed ulnar nerve entrapment symptoms. One of these developed 6 months after what appeared to be successful conservative management of a minimally displaced medial epicondylar fracture. The other developed 4 months after conservative treatment for severe second-degree sprain of the medial collateral ligaments. Both of these young women had failed trials of further conservative treatment and subsequently required open neurolysis and transposition of the ulnar nerve. If a gymnast has clinically evident residual laxity after treatment of a third-degree medial collateral ligament sprain, it generally causes symptoms. Operative reconstruction has been necessary in my experience.

CASE STUDY

A gymnast of national caliber was treated conservatively for medial epicondylar fracture and subsequently was unable to regain adequate motion despite intensive physical therapy. At 6 months the radiographs showed a nonunion of part of the medial epicondyle but did not show major displacement or any evidence of entrapment (Figs. 38-14 and 38-15). The elbow was stable on examination but lacked 30 degrees of extension and 20 degrees of flexion. Surgical exploration of the elbow revealed a heavy fibrous band tethering from the nonunion site to the olecranon. When the nonunion was taken down and the band transsected, the patient immediately had full range of motion without restriction. Internal fixation of this fracture and subse-

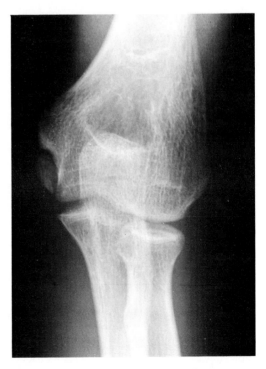

FIG. 38-14. Anteroposterior view of elbow showing nonunion of medial epicondylar fracture after approximately 6 months of conservative care.

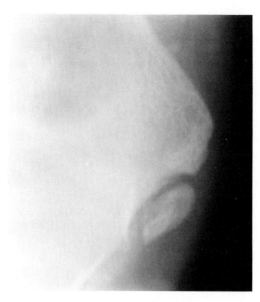

FIG. 38-15. Magnification view of same lesion in Fig. 38-14.

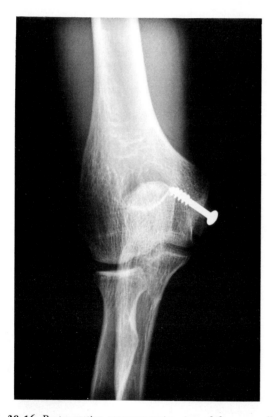

FIG. 38-16. Postoperative anteroposterior view of the same elbow seen in Figs. 38-14 and 38-15.

quent standard postoperative rehabilitation have resulted in essentially full range of motion and return to full competitive level (Fig. 38-16). The standard methods of treatment for the medial epicondylar fracture may be followed in gymnasts, but residual loss of motion warrants surgical exploration.

Supracondylar Fracture

The mechanism of injury, resultant deformity, and associated problems are no different in the gymnast than in any other child sustaining a supracondylar fracture of the humerus. The treating physician should use whatever method of closed reduction and immobilization, closed reduction and internal fixation, or open reduction internal fixation that he or she feels most comfortable with. The only modification from the standard treatment is emphasis on more aggressive early active range of motion. Passive range of motion machines and continuous range of motion machines for the elbow have not proved satisfactory in my experience.

Radial Head Fracture

Fractures of the radial head are rare in gymnasts, but when they do occur they should be treated conservatively but aggressively. The elbow should be rested during the period of initial discomfort and then aggressive active range of motion initiated as soon as it can be tolerated. Operative intervention should be restricted to open reduction and internal fixation with the miniature fragment set if necessary to regain satisfactory anatomic configuration. At all costs, resection of the radial head *should be avoided* in the gymnast. In no case in my personal experience, in my conversations with other orthopaedists who treat gymnasts, or in any literature concerning radial head fracture[38] did a gymnast return to acceptable competitive level after resection of the radial head. This operation should be resorted to only as a salvage procedure if the decision has already been made to withdraw the athlete from gymnastics.

Dislocation

Dislocation of the elbow is usually caused by a fall on the extended arm and is generally lateral or posterolateral. Rarely a straight posterior dislocation is encountered. Patients should be splinted as they lie and transported to an emergency room. Radiographs should be taken and the neurovascular status carefully documented. The elbow can then be carefully reduced by closed technique. Repeat radiographs should be taken to confirm both the reduction and to rule out possible associated fractures. The limb is immobilized in a posterior plaster slab or sling and swath for 7 to 21 days. Josefsson et al[25] reviewed 30 simple dislocations and confirmed the general clinical impression that surgical repair of the ligaments offered no additional stability over the nonoperative treatment. Range of motion was definitely superior in the nonsurgical treatment group. Grossly unstable elbows should be placed in a cast for 2 to 3 weeks and minimally unstable elbows for 1 week. When immobilization is discontinued the patient should be placed on an active-only range of motion program along with ice treatment three to five times a day for 20 to 30 minutes. Frequent monitoring of progress and constant reinforcement are needed to encourage the athlete not to attempt various means of passive motion. Despite the most careful and aggressive treatment, some athletes with this injury fail to regain full extension. Mehloff[35] noted 28% of elbow injuries were dislocations and that the average

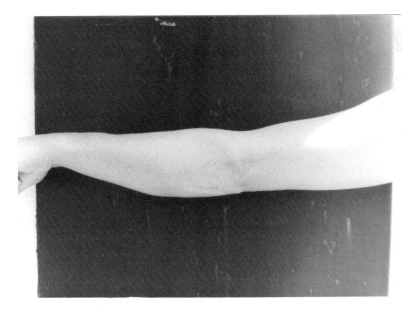

FIG. 38-17. Postoperative extension of elbow in 30-year-old female coach who lacked 30 degrees of extension after conservative treatment of posterolateral elbow dislocation.

adult lost 12.3 degrees of extension after dislocation. Aronen,[3] Josefsson et al,[25] Mehloff,[35] Taylor and Shively and Weise,[46] and Priest[40] all confirmed the need for a shortened period of immobilization and aggressive active range of motion work following the immobilization.

Gymnasts who fail to regain full extension are forced to either drop out of the sport or accept a decreased level of performance. Despite the general teaching to the contrary, it has been my experience that it is possible to regain full extension with surgical intervention (Fig. 38-17). In four elbows explored 9 months or more after dislocation, contracture of the anterior capsule proved to be the limiting factor in all cases. Transverse capsulotomy performed through a lateral incision allows full extension on the operating table. Postoperatively, the elbows are casted in full extension. After 3 weeks in full extension the cast is bivalved and the patient allowed to remove it 3 times a day for active flexion exercises. After 6 weeks the cast is removed and the patient is placed on an active flexion/extension range of motion program. Six months after surgery all four of these patients returned successfully to competitive gymnastics or gymnastics coaching. Two of them have recurvatum of 5 degrees and 3 degrees, which is within 1 degree of the contralateral elbow. One of the patients has full extension of 0 degrees compared with a contralateral elbow that has 5 degrees of hyperextension. The fourth patient lacks 2 degrees of extension compared with a contralateral elbow that has 2 degrees of hyperextension.

Elbow dislocation in the gymnast should be treated as follows: (1) fully evaluate and perform closed reduction, (2) immobilize for 1 to 3 weeks, (3) initiate aggressive active-only range of motion exercises, and (4) perform an anterior capsulotomy if adequate extension has not been obtained by 6 months. In no case has residual instability been a problem.

Treatment of elbow dislocation

- Evaluate carefully and perform closed reduction
- Immobilize 1 to 3 weeks
- Aggressive active-only range of motion program
- Anterior capsulotomy if adequate extension has not been obtained at 6 months

---

Contusions

As with other joints, contusions about the elbow are a frequent occurrence and may involve any aspect of the joint, including the ulnar nerve in its groove. These injuries generally occur secondary to contact with apparatus, floor, stationary obstructions, or other people. They are best avoided by proper layout of the gym, proper attention to technique, avoidance of distractions, and the use of spotters. Treatment is initiated with 1 to 3 days of rest, ice, and use of nonsteroidal antiinflammatory medication. Then active range of motion exercises are instituted until full range of motion is obtained. Progressive resistance exercises are begun once full extension has been achieved and are continued until the athlete has full range of motion and full strength as compared with the contralateral elbow. Only then is the athlete allowed to return to gymnastics.

WRIST

Problems of the wrist are so endemic in gymnastics that dorsal wrist pain has been described as a normal and direct result of the sport.[3] The complexity of the wrist with its multiple bones, joints, bursae, and tendons has resulted in confusion in the literature (see Chapter 21). Injuries are commonly discussed according to subjective

criteria with little objective proof of the underlying pathologic condition. Terms such as *dorsal wrist pain, dorsiflexion wrist jam syndrome, wrist splints, adventitial bursitis, dorsal wrist capsulitis,* and *multiple tendinitis* have appeared in the literature.* The exact pathologic conditions underlying many of the wrist problems have not been well defined.

Although complaints of wrist pain are common in gymnasts, they should not be ignored. A thorough history focusing on the types of maneuvers and the wrist positions that cause the greatest pain should be followed by a thorough physical examination to localize tenderness, identify pain parameters, and demonstrate any of the multiple provocative tests for tendinitis. Routine radiographs and diagnostic local anesthetic injections occasionally offer the answer, but refractory cases require fluoroscopy, arthrography, bone scanning, MRI, CT, cineradiography and/or arthroscopy. The choice of specific techniques for evaluation needs to be individualized according to clinical suspicion.

Overuse Problems
Dorsal Wrist Pain

An entity frequently seen in gymnasts is pain in the dorsum of the wrist with maximum dorsiflexion. The patient usually complains of pain on vaulting, floor exercises, or the pommel horse. He or she had no history of specific acute trauma and frequently no history of a recent technique change. This entity is often described as dorsiflexion jam syndrome, dorsal impaction syndrome, or dorsal capsulitis. The particular problem appears to be primarily endemic in gymnasts; however, it has recently been reported in divers who enter the water with the wrists in dorsiflexion and the hands cupped to decrease their entry splash. It has also been reported in several instances in skaters who have had repetitive falls onto the dorsiflexed hand while practicing skills.

Physical examination reveals diffuse pain over the dorsum of the wrist that is accentuated by active or passive dorsiflexion. Examination, including neurovascular evaluation, yields findings within normal limits. Routine radiographs have consistently proved to be normal, and there have been no reviews in the literature that use MRI

Dorsal wrist pain

- Diffuse dorsal pain
- Pain increased with active or passive dorsiflexion
- Normal results on routine physical examination
- Normal results on routine radiographs

---

or bone scanning in this group of patients. Teitz[47] has noted the presence of dorsal spurs on the lunate and the distal end of the radius that appear to oppose on wrist dorsiflexion. This has not been confirmed in other articles nor in my experience. There is some speculation[42]

*References 3, 7, 8, 11, 13, 20, 21, 26, 30, 31, 33, 35, 39, 41, 48, 51, and 56.

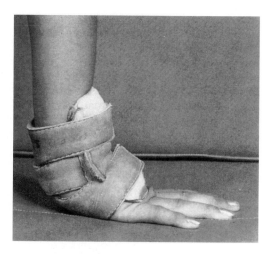

FIG. 38-18. Commercially available dorsiflexion block. (Courtesy R.B.J. Athletic Specialties, Spanish Fork, Utah.)

that this problem is accentuated by the use of overly soft mats, twisting maneuvers such as the Sukahara vault, twisting maneuvers on the beam, and the high repetitions of today's training.

The paucity of experience with more advanced diagnostic imaging and evaluation is related to the frequent occurrence of the problem and relative ease with which it is treated. It is difficult to validate the expense incurred by state of the art testing for a problem that can be adequately managed despite the lack of scientific understanding. Treatment involves a combination of the standard modalities used for overuse syndromes and avoidance of the maximum dorsiflexed position. This is accomplished by decreasing the intensity of training, icing before and after activities, use of nonsteroidal antiinflammatory medication, physical therapy, and use of dorsiflexion blocks. Increased range of motion and strength for wrist extensors and flexors are the primary goals of physical therapy. Limitation of dorsiflexion may be accomplished simply by taping a rectangular piece of ethafoam to the dorsum of the wrist or by a commercial device that straps into place and limits dorsiflexion (Fig. 38-18). In addition, coaches are encouraged to review the gymnast's technique and modify floor, vault, pommel horse, and beam techniques to decrease maximal dorsiflexion loading.

Distal Radius Stress Fracture

Stress fracture of the distal radius, including epiphysis, physis, and metaphysis, have been reported and are receiving increasing attention in the literature.[2,7,13,41-43] This entity is much like dorsiflexion jam syndrome with the gymnast reporting an insidious onset of wrist pain related to weight-bearing and impact-loading activities. Examination reveals volar or dorsal tenderness over the distal radius either at the physis or at the epiphysis. Radiographs in 50% of the cases reported by Roy, Caine, and Singer[42] demonstrated widening of the physeal plate, an epiphyseal fracture line, or sclerosis about the

physeal plate. The other 50% of their cases were diagnosed on the similarity of symptoms without radiographic change. Read[41] noted one difference in clinical presentation when he reported tenderness over the distal radius on the volar aspect. In neither of these studies was the use of bone scans described, so the actual diagnosis of those cases with no specific radiographic changes is open to speculation.

I have found that it is extremely difficult to separate the dorsiflexion jam syndrome from distal radial stress fracture or a continuum phase possibly occurring between the two entities.

Dobyns and Gabel[13] have attempted to define, categorize, and clarify gymnastics wrist injuries. Their article lists 13 osseous and nine soft-tissue diagnoses. The difficulty separating and diagnosing these entities is still intimidating, but the pattern is gradually emerging. Distal radial physis injury is proving to be the most important of all these diagnoses. Multiple authors* have noted premature closure of the physis with resultant ulnar positive variance, volar radial tilt, and tears of the TFCC. Long-term disability from these problems in exgymnasts is yet to be defined, but my experience has shown that these deformities are associated with significant problems in the general population.

The standard treatment is ice, range of motion and strengthening exercises, and partial rest with avoidance of high-impact and twisting loads. All of the reported cases have healed spontaneously without surgical intervention or aggressive treatment. In chronic cases the long-term result and the rate of healing seem to be the same whether or not the wrist is placed at rest.

Injuries that persist over 6 to 8 weeks should be monitored radiographically for evidence of physeal narrowing, asymmetric physeal closure, or the development of the ulnar positive variance. If any of these entities develop, the gymnast should be required to rest the wrist from all compression loading for 8 to 10 weeks and then have it reevaluated.

Chronic Wrist Sprain

Bartolozzi et al[4] recently reported a review of chronic wrist problems in intercollegiate gymnasts. The initial symptoms were similar to those discussed under dorsiflexion jam syndrome and distal radial stress fractures. Radiographic evaluation revealed a tendency toward ulnar drift of the wrist with some degree of aberrant wrist development. The authors speculated that these changes were related to high-impact and weight-bearing loads over a long course of gymnastics during childhood. Arthrography and arthroscopy demonstrated disruption of the radioulnar triangular fibrocartilage. Arthroscopic debridement of the triangular fibrocartilage should alleviate the symptoms. Chronic sprain of the ulnar collateral ligaments presents with localized tenderness over the ulnar styloid and the ulnar side of the wrist. The treatment is the same as that suggested for dorsiflexion jam syndrome.

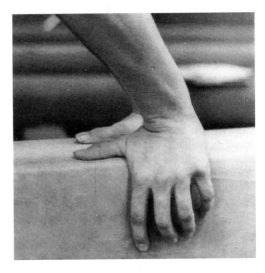

FIG. 38-19. Position of hand on beam that causes symptoms of both ulnar sprains and radial tendinitis.

Tendinitis

Tendinitis about the gymnast's wrist has been found in the abductor pollicis longus, extensor pollicis longus, extensor carpi ulnaris, and the more proximal portion of the abductor pollicis longus. Dorsal radial tendonitis is initially seen as classic de Quervin's tenosynovitis with pain on ulnar deviation and rotational activities of the wrist. On examination there is generally a sense of fullness overlying the tendons and a positive result to Finkelstein's test. The tendinitis variant of the more proximal abductor pollicis longus tendon and associated adventitial bursa[56] has been initially described as localized crepitation proximal to the wrist in addition to the classic findings of de Quervain's tenosynovitis (Fig. 38-19).

All of these entities have been effectively treated with an initial period of complete rest, ice, and nonsteroidal antiinflammatory medication. The gymnast gradually returns to activity while he or she goes through intensive physical therapy to increase the range of motion and strength of the wrist. In the rare refractory case it has been necessary to perform a surgical release of the tendon sheath. In all cases operated on at this institution, recovery has been complete and the gymnasts have resumed full competition.

Carpal Stress Fractures

Tenderness and pain localized over the carpals that are not responsive to the usual conservative measures should be fully evaluated with routine radiographs as well as either bone scan, CT scan, or MRI. Stress fracture and aseptic necrosis of the capitate, carpal scaphoid, and lunate have been described.[32,36,47] A bone scan that shows positive findings for carpal stress fracture should be followed by a period of rest with splinting or casting. After 4 to 6 weeks of protected rest the gymnast is placed on a strengthening, stretching, and graduated return to activity program. Follow-up radiographs should always be obtained to evaluate the healing progress, particularly if avascular necrosis is present.

---

*References 2, 7, 13, 21, 41-43, and 48.

Ganglia

Gymnasts appear to be neither more prone nor more resistant than the general population to the development of ganglia about the wrist. The treatment of a symptomatic ganglion in a gymnast is also the same as generally accepted with the exception that the associated disability may require earlier aggressive intervention. Volar wrist ganglia are initially seen with the classic symptoms of localized pain and tenderness but seldom causes a major problem for the gymnast. Dorsal wrist ganglia are frequently associated with other wrist complaints and present a major problem. The dorsiflexion block braces used for the jam syndrome and distal radial stress fracture put pressure directly on the ganglia, which limits the use of the block braces.

Forearm Splints

Gymnasts occasionally complain of aching pain in the forearm that is exacerbated by activities (particularly weight bearing) in the gym. Deep palpation reveals tenderness between the radius and ulna, and the patient experiences discomfort with maximal dorsiflexion of the fingers and wrist. The pathophysiology of this entity has not been well defined, but it appears to be similar to the shin splint syndrome of the lower extremities. Whether this is traction-related irritation of the radioulnar syndesmosis, periostitis, or myositis is still unknown, but the treatment is definitely conservative. Activity modification to decrease impact loading and weightbearing, ice, and nonsteroidal antiinflammatory medication will initially clear the symptoms. After resolution of the symptoms, strengthening, stretching, short-term circumferential taping, and graduated return to activities are initiated. Forearm splints usually present early in the season and resolve as conditioning is completed. Gymnasts who have experienced this problem in previous years are strongly encouraged to avoid loss of forearm conditioning. They can either work the weight program during the off season or, as is typical in club gymnastics, continue in the sport year-round.

Forearm splints

- Aching forearm pain
- Pain exacerbated by activity
- Seen early in season
- Tenderness found on deep palpation between radius and ulna
- Pain with active wrist and finger dorsiflexion

Acute Injuries

Acute trauma to the gymnast's wrist is not uncommon but is generally not significantly different from that seen in other sports and activities.

Fracture of the Scaphoid

As with other activities, carpal scaphoid fractures generally result from a fall on the dorsiflexed hand with the arm extended and supinated behind the back. Gymnasts should not sustain this injury if they have learned to tuck and roll rather than put their arm back to protect themselves. They present with the classic pain on ulnar and radial deviation as well as pinpoint tenderness over the anatomic snuff-box. Radiographs usually reveal normal findings in the early stages and show delayed visualization of the fracture line in 2 to 3 weeks. Suspicion of carpal scaphoid fracture warrants bone scan or tomography. Treatment, as in other sports, is initiated with a long arm thumb spica cast. This is reduced to a short arm thumb spica cast after 3 weeks and subsequently to a short arm splint or cast at approximately 6 to 8 weeks. Adjustments in timing of cast transitions depend on the radiographic appearance. Return to gymnastics is anticipated at 10 to 12 weeks after the injury, but may well be slower.

Distal Radius Fracture

Colles fractures, reverse Colles fractures, and Salter fractures I through IV have been seen in gymnasts. The treatment is identical to that used for those injuries in any other group of young patients.

Fracture Related to the Doweled Grip

One injury that is unique to gymnastics is the high-speed flexion/rotation fracture-dislocation of the wrist or distal forearm. This particular entity was unheard of until recent years when the doweled grip became popular. This style of grip has a dowel built into it at approximately the level of the middle phalanx (see Figs. 38-3 to 38-5). The dowel allows excellent purchase on the bar and giant swings of greater intensity and frequency than had previously been done. I am aware of several cases reported anecdotally and one in the literature[3] in which the dowel apparently caught on the bar while the gymnast's momentum continued in a giant swing fashion. This resulted in the hand's being trapped to the bar as the body continued to revolve around it, causing a dorsal fracture dislocation of the wrist.

This entity has previously been a unique problem of male gymnasts because only they were using the dowel. It is now becoming common for gyms to convert the uneven parallel bars to the smallest diameter bar allowed by competition rules and to have their female gymnasts use dowel grips also. In one recent case an accomplished 16-year-old female gymnast sustained a comminuted both-bone forearm fracture while performing giant swings on a high bar (Fig. 38-20). Her description of the injury was very clear because she was aware that the grip caught, but was unable to stop her momentum. Treatment of these injuries is beyond the scope of this chapter in that it needs to be individualized to the specific trauma encountered and is best managed by the hand specialist. Precautions against fractures involve being certain that the grips fit the gymnasts correctly, are well cared for, in good repair, and are adequately chalked. The grips need to be carefully fitted according to the manufacturer's directions and frequently checked for any stretching. If they fit too loosely the leather can fold over and lock to the bar (Fig. 38-21). Female gymnasts should *not* be allowed to work out on the men's high bar because of the smaller diameter. Regular cleaning of the

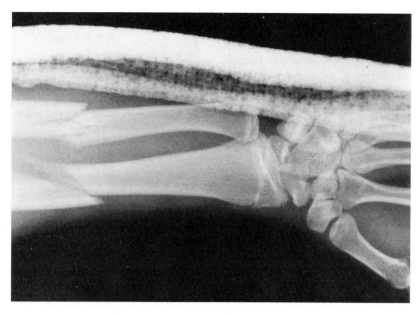

FIG. 38-20. Anteroposterior radiograph of a 16-year-old female gymnast who sustained a comminuted radial and ulnar fracture when her doweled grip caught on the high bar.

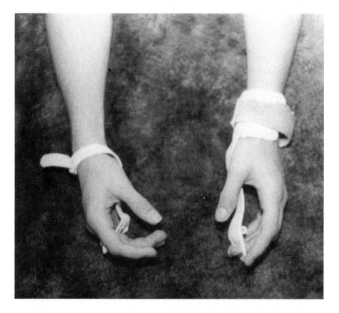

FIG. 38-21. Fit of doweled grip should be tight enough that the fingers cannot reach full extension. There should be no laxity of the grip.

Proper use of chalk

- Chalk hands and grip before each swinging-activity session
- Clean bars of caked chalk to avoid buildup

---

bars to avoid chalk buildup will decrease the likelihood of grip stick.

HAND

With the exception of skin problems, injuries to the hands of gymnasts are neither unique nor particularly frequent.[33] I have seen Bennett fractures, proximal interphalangeal joint fractures and dislocations, mallet finger deformities, metacarpal fractures, gamekeeper's thumb, and jammed fingers in gymnasts. All of these have occurred as unique specific trauma normally related to contact with apparati or the floor. No specific treatment recommendations are required beyond those used for other athletes with comparable injury.

Skin Problems

Skin problems on the hand that are unique to gymnasts warrant consideration. Calluses on the palm and the palmar aspect of the fingers are the natural consequence of the work on bars, rings, and the pommel horse (Fig. 38-22). When the calluses become tender they should be pared with an emory board or sandpaper and massaged with a moisturizing cream after workouts. Grips that are properly fitted, well maintained, and well chalked decrease the friction and therefore the severity of callus formation. Return to the gymnasium after any prolonged period of inactivity predisposes the gymnast to blisters. They are best prevented by gradual return to apparatus and wise use of grips and chalk. When blisters do occur the normal physiologic skin cover should be left in place as long as possible. Once the skin does break, the gymnast should be instructed to keep the hands clean and dry.

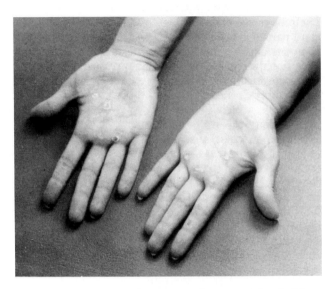

FIG. 38-22. Calluses on palmar aspect of a gymnast's hands. These are typical.

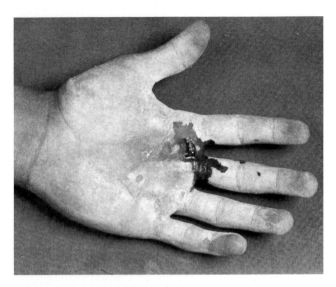

FIG. 38-23. Acute tear on a male gymnast's hands. This occurred while working the pommel horse with no grips and inadequate chalk.

Skin Tears

The primary skin problem of the gymnast's hand is referred to as *tears*. This problem occurs when friction overload causes callused skin to shear loose from its underlying attachments (Fig. 38-23). Prevention of tears is based on a combination of experience and folklore handed down within the gymnastic community. Routine care of the palms includes keeping the calluses trimmed, limiting workouts when so-called hot spots develop, wearing properly fitted and well-maintained grips, and using moisturizing cream after workouts. The proper use of chalk has long been a standard part of gymnastics and has two primary components. First, the hands and grip should be freshly chalked before each use of swinging-type apparatus. Second, the bars should be routinely cleaned to avoid a buildup of caked chalk, which becomes sticky and increases friction.

When a gymnast sustains a tear it is usually a result of continuing to participate despite warning signs. Visible fissuring of the skin or the presence of hot spots, which indicate blistering beneath the callus, require rest. Tears should be kept clean, aggressively moisturized, and monitored for the possibility of infection. Once the tear has sealed and is no longer painful the gymnast then returns to the apparatus with gradual progression to retoughen the hands.

UPPER EXTREMITY PROBLEMS IN THE GYMNASTICS COACH

In most sports the coach is involved primarily on a mental level with instruction and strategy. The gymnastics coach is extensively involved in practice verbally, mentally, and physically. The physical act of spotting to aid maneuver development and protect from injury is a large part of the job. In addition to the well-recognized

low back pain, nasal fractures, and multiple contusions incurred by spotters, we see multiple problems in the upper extremities. It is important to remember that, not only does the coach sustain injuries similar to those of the gymnasts, but also the treatment must be equally aggressive. The coach's ability to perform his or her job requires athletic ability and a sound body.

Shoulder

The coach's shoulder takes a great deal of stress while spotting, especially when working with young, inexperienced gymnasts. Coaches have been treated for biceps tendinitis, supraspinatus tendinitis, chronic acromioclavicular joint arthritis, rotator cuff tears, and acute rupture of the pectoralis major.

Elbow

The crossed-arm position used to spot tumbling tricks puts high stress on the medial side of the elbow.[5] Those stresses are often superimposed on long-standing elbow problems from the coach's days of competition. The coach initially complains of medial epicondylitis types of symptoms or intraarticular symptoms related to long-standing osteochondritis dissecans lesions. Inflammation of the ulnar collateral ligament, de Quervain's tendinitis, and finger injuries are also all common problems among coaches.

The important thing to remember in dealing with this group of individuals is that, although the coaches are not performing the tricks, they are sustaining much the same stresses and loads as the participating gymnasts. Problems need to be taken seriously and treated as aggressively as in the competitive athlete.

CASE STUDY

A 29-year-old college gymnastics coach was spotting a collegiate gymnast who lost control on the vault. He reached in,

broke her fall, and felt something pop in his right elbow. The school trainers treated him for an elbow sprain without success. When the elbow continued to feel weak and painful after 4 months, he came to see me. At that point he was found to have a rupture of the distal biceps tendon insertion with the typical moderate weakness of elbow flexion and extreme weakness of supination. Reconstruction with allograft has allowed him to return to full function and coaching.

SUMMARY

In this chapter we have reviewed multiple problems that occur in the upper extremities of gymnasts. If nothing else is clear, you should be aware that these problems do exist, and many of them have a career-ending potential. The physician involved in sports medicine needs to be aware of the problems and unique characteristics of this group and be readily accessible to the gymnast. The participants are generally young, very enthusiastic, extremely dedicated, subjected to significant peer pressure, and conditioned to accept pain as a normal part of the sport.

Equipment is critical to the prevention of these injuries, and the involved physician should be aware of the following general principles:

1. The gym must be laid out with adequate space between apparatus and adequate padding on all fixed obstacles.
2. Every inch of the floor should be padded with adequate matting and the bases of all apparatus protected with pads.
3. The floor exercise area should have adequate spring to decrease impact loading, but not so soft that it allows abnormal dorsiflexion of the wrists or catching of the hands in rotational maneuvers.
4. The beams must be adequately spaced and their surfaces in excellent repair.
5. Bars and vault must be cleaned frequently to avoid the accumulation of chalk or any other substance that would cause stickiness.
6. Chalk boxes must be readily available and placed throughout the gym.
7. Gymnasts on the swinging apparatus should be wearing well-fitted grips in good repair.
8. Ice should be readily accessible to the gymnasts.

The physician who treats gymnasts should also be aware of the **general principles of training** and monitor the patients under their treatment. The physician should take the following steps to avoid injuries:

1. Encourage logical, graduated progression of training regimens.
2. Encourage strength training throughout the year.
3. Encourage meticulous attention to technique.
4. Encourage the avoidance of distractions within the gym.
5. Recommend modification of intensity in programs as needed for specific problems.
6. Modify individual gymnasts' programs for specific problems.

In the injury incidence studies done thus far the most important factor in prevention of injuries has been the use of spotters.[37,38,40,49] Coaches adequately trained in spotting techniques should be encouraged to routinely spot their athletes during all stages of trick development and the majority of time for established tricks.

REFERENCES

1. Adams JE: Little league shoulder: osteochondrosis of the proximal humeral epiphysis in boy baseball pitchers, *Cal Med* 105:22, 1986.
2. Albanese SA et al: Wrist pain and distal growth plate closure of the radius in gymnasts, *J Pediatr Orthop* 9:23, 1989.
3. Aronen JG: Problems of the upper extremity in gymnasts: symposium on gymnastics, *Clin Sports Med* 4(1):61, 1985.
4. Bartolozzi AR et al: *Wrist pain syndrome in the gymnast: pathogenic, diagnostic, and therapeutic considerations*, Paper presented at American Orthopaedics Society for Sports Medicine, Orlando, June 29 to July 2, 1987.
5. Boone T: Helping hand can equal sore elbow, *Phys Sportsmed* p 41, 1976.
6. Caine D et al: An epidemiologic investigation of injuries affecting young competitive female gymnasts, *Am J Sports Med* 17(6):811, 1989.
7. Caine D et al: Stress changes of the distal radial growth plate, *Am J Sports Med* 20(3):290, 1992.
8. Chambers RB: Orthopaedic injuries in athletes (ages 6 to 17): comparison to injuries occurring in 6 sports, *Am J Sports Med* 7(3):195, 1979.
9. Chan BD et al: Chronic stress injuries of the elbow in young gymnasts, *Br J Radiol* 64:1113, 1991.
10. Cooney WP: Bursitis and tendonitis in the hand, wrist, and elbow: an approach to treatment, *Minn Med* 66(8):491, 1993.
11. Cooney WP III: Sports injuries to the upper extremity: how to recognize and deal with some common problems, *Sports Injuries* 76(4):45, 1984.
12. Dixon M, Fricker P: Injuries to elite gymnasts over 10 years, *Med Sci Sports Exerc* 25(12):1322, 1993.
13. Dobyns JH, Gabel G: Gymnast's wrist, *Hand Clin* 6(3):493, 1990.
14. Dobyns JH, Sim FH, Linscheid RL: Sports stress syndromes of the hand and wrist, *Am J Sports Med* 6(5):236, 1978.
15. Engle A, Busztin-Feldner H: Bilateral stress fracture of the scaphoid, *Arch Orthop Trauma Surg* 110:314, 1991.
16. Fulton MN, Albright JP, El-Khoury GY: Cortical desmoid-like lesion of the proximal humerus and its occurrence in gymnasts (Ringman's shoulder lesion), *Am J Sports Med* 7(1):57, 1979.
17. Ganim RJ: Gymnastics safety for the physician: symposium on gymnastics, *Clin Sports Med* 4(1):123, 1985.
18. Garrick JG: Epidemiology of women's gymnastics injuries, *Am J Sports Med* 8(4):261, 1980.
19. Goldberg MJ: Gymnastics injuries: symposium on sports injuries, *Orthop Clin North Am* 11(4):717, 1980.
20. Hanks GA et al: Stress fractures of the carpal scaphoid, *J Bone Joint Surg* 71A(6):938, 1989.
21. Hermansdorfer JD, Kleinman WB: Management of chronic peripheral tears of the triangular fibrocartilage complex, *J Hand Surg* 16A(2):340, 1991.
22. Jackson DW, Silvino N, Reiman P: Osteochondritis in the female gymnast's elbow, *J Arthroscopic Rel Surg* 5(2):129, 1989.
23. Jobe FW: *Differential diagnosis of the shoulder: the shoulder in the athlete*, Paper presented at American Academy of Orthopaedic Surgeons forty-ninth annual meeting, Los Angeles, August 28, 1983.
24. Jobe FW, Moynes DR: Delineation of diagnostic criteria and rehabilitation program for rotator cuff injuries, *Am J Sports Med* 10(6):336, 1982.
25. Josefsson PO et al: Surgical versus non-surgical treatment of ligamentous injuries following dislocation of elbow joint, *J Bone Joint Surg* 69(4):605, 1987.
26. Kirby RL: Flexibility and musculoskeletal symptomatology in female gymnasts and age-matched controls, *Am J Sports Med* 9(3):160, 1981.

27. Koh TJ, Grabiner M, Weiker G: Technique and ground reaction forces in the back handspring, *Am J Sports Med* 20(1):61, 1992.
28. Maffulli N, Chan D, Aldridge MJ: Derangement of the articular surfaces of the elbow in young gymnasts, *J Pediatr Orthop* 12:344, 1992.
29. Maffulli N, Chan D, Aldridge MJ: Overuse injuries of the olecranon in young gymnasts, *J Bone Joint Surg* 74(2):305, 1992.
30. Markolf KL et al: Wrist loading patterns during pommel horse exercises, *J Biomechanics* 23(10):1001, 1990.
31. Matheson GO et al: Stress fractures in athletes: a study of 320 cases, *Am J Sports Med* 15(1):46, 1987.
32. Mazione M, Pizzutillo PD: Stress fracture of the scaphoid wrist: a case report, *Am J Sports Med* 9(4):268, 1981.
33. McCue FC III et al: Hand and wrist injuries in the athlete, *Am J Sports Med* 7(5):275, 1979.
34. Meeusen R, Borms J: Gymnastic injuries, *Sports Med* 13(5):337, 1992.
35. Mehloff TL: Early mobilization recommended for simple elbow dislocation, *Am Acad Orthop Surg* 6(1):22, 1987 (news bulletin).
36. Murakami S, Nakajima H: Aseptic necrosis of the capitate bone in two gymnasts, *Am J Sports Med* 12(2):170, 1984.
37. Pettrone FA, Ricciardelli E: Gymnastic injuries: the Virginia experience 1982-1983, *Am J Sports Med* 15(1):59, 1987.
38. Priest JD: Sports medicine, fitness and nutrition corner: elbow injuries in sports, *Minn Med*, Sept, 543, 1982.
39. Priest JD: Elbow injuries in gymnastics: symposium on gymnastics, *Clin Sports Med* 4(1):73, 1985.
40. Priest JD, Weise DJ: Elbow injury in women's gymnastics, *Am J Sports Med* 9(5):288, 1981.
41. Read MTF: Stress fractures of the distal radius in adolescent gymnasts, *Br J Sports Med* 15(4):272, 1981.
42. Roy S, Caine D, Singer KM: Stress changes of the distal radial epiphysis in young gymnasts, *Am J Sports Med* 13(5):301, 1985.
43. Ruggels D et al: Radial growth plate injury in a female gymnast, *Med Sci Sports Exerc* May, 393, 1990.
44. Singer KM, Roy SP: Osteochondrosis of the humeral capitellum, *Am J Sports Med* 12(5):351, 1984.
45. Snook GA: Injuries in women's gymnastics: a five year study, *Am J Sports Med* 7(4):242, 1979.
46. Tayob AA, Shively RA: Bilateral elbow dislocations with intraarticular displacement of the medial epicondyles, *J Trauma* 20(4):332, 1980.
47. Teitz CC: Sports medicine concerns in dance and gymnastics, *Clin Sports Med* 2(3):571, 1983.
48. Tolat AR et al: The gymnast's wrist: acquired positive ulnar variance following chronic epiphyseal injury, *J Hand Surg* 17B(6):678, 1992.
49. Weiker GG: Club gymnastics: symposium on gymnastics, *Clin Sports Med* 4(1):39, 1985.
50. Weiker GG: Introduction and history of gymnastics, *Clin Sports Med* 4(1):39, 1985.
51. Weiker GG: Hand and wrist problems in the gymnast, *Clin Sports Med* 111(1):189, 1992.
52. Weiker GG et al: *Pressure across the elbow during gymnastic vaulting,* Unpublished manuscript.
53. Wettsone E (ed): *Gymnastics safety manual,* University Park, 1977, Pennsylvania State University Press.
54. Whiteside JA et al: Fractures and refractures in intercollegiate athletes: an eleven-year experience, *Am J Sports Med* 9(6):369, 1981.
55. Wilkerson RD, Johns JC: Nonunion of an olecranon stress fracture in an adolescent gymnast, *Am J Sport Med* 18(4):432, 1990.
56. Wood MB et al: Abductor pollicis longus bursitis, *Clin Orthop* 93:293, 1973.

CHAPTER 39

Evaluation, Treatment, and Prevention of Upper Extremity Injuries in Golfers

John R. McCarroll

The golf swing is physically demanding and has contributed to various injuries. The person who does not play golf may imagine it is less taxing than other sports.* However, it is not. Injuries are frequent and result in sprained wrists, aching shoulders, and sore elbows; most injuries are related to the golf swing.[3-5]

The frequency of golf injuries to the upper extremity has received little attention in the literature. There have been reports of fractures of carpal bones, especially the hook of the hamate secondary to impact with the end of the club.[10] There are many incidences of ulnar and median neuropathies along with tendinitis as a result of various injuries during different parts of the golf swing.[7,9]

One study of professional golfers reported that in the upper extremity, in right-handed golfers, the left wrist was most frequently injured, followed by the left hand, the left shoulder, and the left elbow (Table 39-1).[3-5]

BIOMECHANICS

To evaluate, treat, and prevent golf injuries, the golfer must understand the golf swing. I like to break the golf swing into three parts: take-away, impact, and follow-through.

Take-Away

Take-away (Fig. 39-1) consists of the setup and movement to the top of the back swing. During this time golfers take their grip, stand properly, and align themselves over the ball. They then rotate the shoulders, trunk, hips, and knees while the head remains stationary. This action is accomplished by hyperabduction of the left thumb in the right-handed golfer, radial deviation of the left wrist at the top of the back swing, and dorsiflexion of the right wrist. The marks in Fig. 39-1 represent areas of stress to the wrist, elbow, and shoulder during this phase of the golf swing.

Impact

Impact (Fig. 39-2) consists of preimpact and impact phases (downswing and acceleration). As the player starts to hit the ball, the right wrist is in maximal dorsiflexion; the left thumb is hyperabducted; the left ulnar nerve, right elbow, and forearm flexors are stretched; and the left hip is rotated. At impact, the left wrist and hand are thrust into the ball, compression occurs at the right wrist, and the left elbow extensor mass contracts.

Follow-Through

The follow-through phase (Fig. 39-3) consists of the time after impact and follow-through. After the player hits the ball while pivoting, the left forearm supinates, the right forearm pronates, the lumbar and cervical areas of the spine rotate and hyperextend, hip rotation is completed, and there is a complete weight shift to the

---

*Editors' note: Walking and swinging golf clubs at an 18-hole, 3-hour pace generate a heart rate increase of approximately 20% on a flat course, and a hilly course can effect a 40% rise in pulse rate (unpublished data, Nicholas Institute of Sports Medicine and Athletic Trauma).

TABLE 39-1 Injuries to the upper extremity in professional golfers

	Men (%)	Women (%)	Total (%)
Left wrist	16.1	31.3	23.9
Left hand	6.8	7.5	7.1
Left shoulder	10.9	3.0	6.9
Left elbow	3.1	4.5	3.8
Left thumb	5.2	1.5	3.3
Right wrist	1.5	4.5	3.1
Right elbow	4.2	1.5	2.8
Right shoulder	0.5	4.5	2.5

Data from McCarroll JR, Gioe TJ: *Phys Sportsmed* 10:64, 1982.

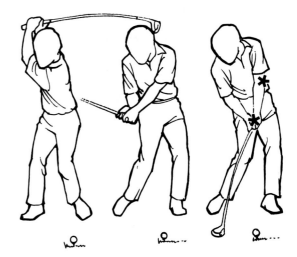

FIG. 39-2. Impact.

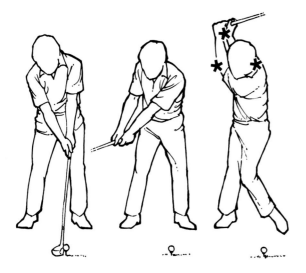

FIG. 39-1. Take-away.

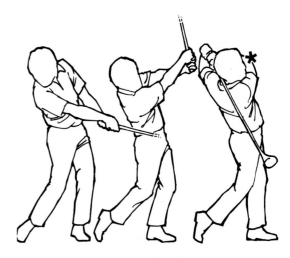

FIG. 39-3. Follow-through.

left side of the body with rotation of the knees to the left and inversion of the left ankle.

EPIDEMIOLOGY

Injuries to the upper extremity may arise in any phase of the golf swing. In a study of professional golfers[5] the wrist and shoulder were the most affected parts of the upper extremity during take-away. The wrist was most affected in the impact phase, followed by the elbow and hand, and the shoulder and elbow were the most affected in the follow-through phase.

The incidence of golf injuries to the upper extremity was reported in two articles. One article[5] on professional right-handed golfers shows that the left wrist was injured in 23.9% of the golfers, followed in incidence by the left hand, left shoulder, left elbow, and left thumb (Table 39-1). In a recently completed but as yet unpublished study I did of recreational golfers, the incidence of injuries to the upper extremity differs, with the elbow being the most commonly injured. This is related to poor swing mechanics (Table 39-2).

The mechanism of injury (Table 39-3) is most commonly related to the golf swing. The most common mechanism of injury is too much play or practice, causing overuse syndrome to the upper extremity. In the professional golfer[5] these injuries are most commonly caused by the repeated stress of practice, but in the recreational golfer these can be the result of poor swing mechanics (Fig. 39-4). Bending of the left elbow on take-away causes the elbow to be extended sharply into the ball at impact, causing increased stress to the forearm and resulting in tennis elbow (Fig. 39-4, *A*). In the middle golfer (Fig. 39-4, *B*) the poor weight shift, or so-called reverse pivot, causes unnecessary stress on the joints, tendons, and muscles of the upper extremity. The golfer on the right in Fig. 39-4, *C*, shows the proper swing that reduces the stress on the upper extremity. Other mech-

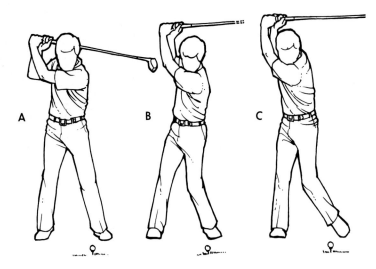

FIG. 39-4. A, Golfer showing bent elbow and poor swinging mechanics. **B,** Golfer showing poor weight shift and poor swinging mechanics. **C,** Golfer showing correct swing position at top of take-away.

TABLE 39-2 Injuries to the upper extremity in recreational golfers

	Men (%)	Women (%)	Total (%)
Left elbow	22.2	28.6	23.2
Left wrist	9.4	5.2	8.7
Left shoulder	7.5	13.0	8.3
Left hand	5.2	6.5	5.4
Right elbow	1.0	3.0	2.2

TABLE 39-3 Mechanisms of injury

Mechanism	Percent
Too much play or practice	21.4
Poor swing mechanics	14.4
Hit ground or large divot	12.8
Pain just starts with no cause	9.2
Hit by ball	8.6
Overswing (swing too hard)	7.9
Poor warm-up	4.9
Hit object other than ball	4.7
Grip or swing change	3.4
Fall	3.1
Twist during swing	2.9
Fell out of golf cart	2.4
Miscellaneous (hit by club, bitten by snake)	4.1

Data from McCarroll JR and Gioe TJ: *Phys Sportsmed* 10:64, 1982.

TABLE 39-4 Treatment of golf injuries

Type	Professional (%)	Recreational (%)	Total (%)
Rest	16.0	30.8	24.7
Physical therapy	16.9	12.0	14.1
Medication	10.7	9.5	9.9
Injection	10.2	9.2	9.6
Ice	6.3	10.8	9.0
Heat	8.5	7.6	8.0
Chiropractor	6.5	0.7	3.1
Braces (tennis elbow)	5.8	8.5	7.4
Surgery	5.8	3.4	4.4
Traction	1.7	0.7	1.2
Acupuncture	1.6	0.4	0.9

Data from McCarroll JR, Gioe TJ: *Phys Sportsmed* 10:64, 1982.

anisms of injury, include hitting trees, roots, or hard ground. These are summarized in Table 39-3.[5]

Just as the incidence, type, and mechanisms of injuries varied, so did the treatment of these injuries. Although specific injuries and their treatment are discussed later, this chapter also summarizes the various types of treatment that these golfers received. In the professional golfer[5] physical therapy was the most commonly prescribed treatment, followed by rest. In the recreational golfer more time was given for rest and physical therapy was second. These findings are summarized in Table 39-4. However, in the professional golfer, 54.3% of the men and 53.7% of the women are still bothered by their injuries.[5] Of the recreational golfers, 44.6% are still bothered by their injury.

SPECIFIC GOLF INJURIES

It would be redundant to repeat the physical findings, treatment, and other tests of such common disorders seen in other parts of this text as carpal tunnel syndrome, rotator cuff impingement, lateral epicondylitis (tennis elbow), and ulnar nerve subluxation or entrapment because these are common injuries in golf and are covered well in other chapters. This discussion emphasizes a few injuries that may be unique to golf.

Fracture of the Hook of the Hamate

The hook of the hamate is a long, thin bone that is subject to injury as it projects toward the palmar surface of the hand. Fractures occur in golf when the grip of the club strikes the hook of the hamate and fractures it. The athlete complains of wrist pain and weak grip. Clinical examination shows tenderness to pressure over the hook of the hamate. Radiographs should include anteroposterior, lateral, and oblique views of the wrist. These routine radiographs often do not show a fracture, and many times a carpal tunnel view of the wrist is needed. If these films do not show a fracture but the injury is still suspected, a bone scan or computed tomography (CT) scan may be helpful. Because the ulnar nerve and flexor digitorum profundus to the small finger are so close to the fracture site, the patient may experience symptoms of ulnar nerve impingement or tendinitis. Fracture of the hook of the hamate may also lead to rupture of the ring finger flexor tendon from chronic inflammatory changes.[10]

In the acute nondisplaced fracture the treatment is a short arm cast and rest for 6 weeks. The incidence of nonunion of this fracture is high, and in a badly displaced fracture or in a nonunion, the excision of the hook itself is indicated.[10]

de Quervain Disease

de Quervain disease is a common condition I have seen in at least five professional golfers as a result of repetitive practice. de Quervain disease is a tenosynovitis of the first dorsal compartment of the wrist. The diagnostic sign of it is the Finkelstein test. This is performed with the thumb and hand forcibly deviated toward the ulnar side of the wrist. There is exquisite pain over the radial styloid process and the common sheath of the abductor pollicis longus and extensor pollicis brevis tendon. This test is also similar to the mechanisms that are involved in hitting the golf ball. Before and upon impact this causes repeated stress and synovitis in golfers. Conservative treatment of de Quervain disease involves splints, ice, and antiinflammatory medication. Only in resistant cases is injection or operative treatment considered.

Traumatic Arthritis

Traumatic arthritis is common in the small joints of the hand, especially in professional and avid golfers because of the constant stress of striking the ball. This can be treated with antiinflammatory drugs and grip changes. However, there are special grips that reduce the torque and stress on the hands and forearms (Fig. 39-5) for those players with these conditions, but these grips are not yet legal under the United States Golf Association's rules.

Miscellaneous Conditions

Other conditions such as tendinitis, ligamentous sprains, and carpal tunnel syndrome may occur in the wrist and hands of golfers. These are discussed in Chapters 26, 27, and 31.

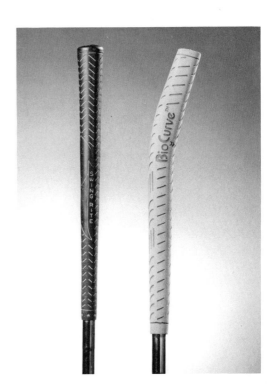

FIG. 39-5. Two golf clubs and their grips. *Left,* The swing right grip is the standard accepted golf grip. *Right,* The Bio-Curve grip is the new curved grip that prevents certain hand, arm, and elbow injuries.

Epicondylitis

The golfer may suffer from two common elbow injuries, medial and lateral epicondylitis. The diagnosis and treatment of these injuries in racquet and throwing sports are well covered (see Chapter 17). Fig. 39-4 shows a golfer with the left elbow bent on the backswing, or take-away. When he tries to hit the ball, he snaps or throws the hand and forearm at the ball, causing excessive and incorrect stress on the extensor muscles of the forearm and their origins at the lateral epicondyle. Also at impact the golfer may roll the wrist or supinate the left forearm, causing increased torque on these muscles and lateral epicondylitis in the left arm of the right-handed golfer. This can be prevented by proper address, take-away, and swing mechanics, as well as the proper medical treatment.

Medial epicondylitis, sometimes referred to as *golfers' elbow,* usually occurs over the medial epicondyle of the right elbow in the right-handed golfer. This is caused by hitting from the top. In this situation, instead of pulling the club through with the left side using the legs, back, shoulder, and other muscles, the golfer throws the club from the top of the backswing, or take-away, down into the ball at impact. This is very similar to hitting a forehand in tennis or a kill shot in racquetball. It causes extreme stress on the flexor muscles, especially at the attachment on the medial epicondyle. Injury to the ulnar nerve must be evaluated during the physical examina-

tion. Treatment is symptomatic, using ice, counterforce bracing, physical therapy, or antiinflammatory medication and injections. Occasionally, surgery is necessary (surgical techniques are discussed in Chapter 17). The need for surgery can often be prevented by correcting the athlete's swing mechanics.

Shoulder Impingement Syndrome

The most common injury to the shoulder in golf is that of rotator cuff impingement syndrome. This problem is discussed in detail in Chapter 8.

PREVENTION OF GOLF INJURIES
Biomechanics

In preventing golf injuries, the instructor should start with the golf swing. As in any sport, proper mechanics are extremely important. The teaching golf professional, using years of experience and such devices as video recording, can correct the mechanisms of the golf swing to prevent injuries and to change abnormal stress applied to various body parts.

Equipment Considerations

The next step in preventing golf injuries is the use of proper equipment. Proper size and shape of the grip are necessary to ensure proper swing mechanics and to relieve torsional stress at impact. The stiffness of the shafts and the length and weight of the club may also play an important role. Many manufacturers are trying to make equipment to relieve specific problems, such as special grips for arthritic or injured golfers. The most recent is the Bio-Curve grip (Fig. 39-5), which decreases torsional stress to the arm and hand. Unfortunately, these clubs have not yet been approved by the United States Golf Association and therefore are not in common use. The club professional is again the expert in these areas and should assist the golfer in these aspects.

Golf equipment considerations

Grip
- Size
- Shape

Club
- Stiffness
- Length
- Weight

Conditioning and Golf

Golf is an activity demanding a high degree of refined motor skills. There are many frustrated golfers trying to play when they are not in shape. The weekend golfer and even the professional golfer must condition the body before going to the course or must assume the risk of injury. Golf is a strenuous game, and weakness in the upper extremity that will not withstand the stress of hitting or swinging at a golf ball will contribute to the oc-

curence of an injury. Too many golfers ruin the entire golf season with injuries to the shoulder, elbow, or wrist, as well as other injuries. Injuries, sore muscles, and frustrating days on the golf course can be eliminated by a preseason, regular season, and off-season conditioning program.

Recent studies add scientific data to the need for a conditioning program. Jobe, Moynes, and Antonelli[1] in a study of bilateral shoulder muscle activity during the golf swing using electromyography and high-speed photography, showed that an understanding of muscle firing patterns might help the golfer prevent injuries and develop appropriate training and conditioning programs. They studied the swings of seven adult male right-handed professional golfers and found that all portions of the deltoid muscles were inactive on the right side during the golf swing. The deltoid was likewise inactive on the left except for a brief spurt from the anterior portion during the milliseconds immediately preceding ball contact.

The rotator cuff muscles on the left, the supraspinatus, fired at a low level throughout the swing as did the infraspinatus. The latter had a slightly larger burst of activity immediately after ball contact. The subscapularis was more active than any other muscle throughout the golf swing. The cuff muscles on the right side showed as much activity overall as those on the left. In addition, the latissimus dorsi and pectoralis major seemed to provide power bilaterally, with marked activity during the preimpact, or acceleration, phase. Jobe, Moynes, and Antonelli[1] also showed that the left shoulder of the right-handed golfer does not provide more drive than the right. To achieve greater distance it seems that a golfer should concentrate on exercising the rotator cuff bilaterally as well as the latissimus dorsi and pectoralis major.

For the golfer to perform at his or her optimal level, to hit the ball farther, to make more consistent contact with the ball, to lessen the chance of injury, and to improve overall endurance, he or she must follow certain types of conditioning programs.

Stretching

Stretching exercises are used to maintain complete range of motion of various body parts, not just the upper extremity. Without maximal attainable range of motion and flexibility, the golfer may be injured when swinging or taking a divot. It is extremely important to have a good warm-up program involving flexibility stretching for the body. These exercises are well illustrated and explained in Jobe and others' works[1,2] and that of Spackman.[8]

Strength

Golf is not only a strength game like many sports; strength in itself will not enable the individual to hit the ball better or longer. However, it allows the skilled player to strike shots with more consistently explosive power over extended periods. Any golfer with a weak area, for example, the shoulder, is at risk for injury. There are various muscles that need to be strengthened to improve basic skills. Driving power involves the buttocks, quadri-

TABLE 39-5 Nautilus workout program for golf

Exercise	Muscles Developed	Skills Involved
Hip and back	Buttocks, lower	Driving power Walking endurance
Leg extension	Quadriceps	Driving power Walking endurance
Leg curl	Hamstrings	Hip turn Driving power
Double shoulder (lateral press)	Deltoids	Club control Impact velocity
Double shoulder (seated press)	Deltoids, triceps	Shoulder turn Club extension
Pullover	Latissimus dorsi	Shoulder turn Club extension
Wrist curl	Forearm flexors	Club head control Impact power Acceleration
Reverse wrist curls	Forearm flexors	Club head control Impact power Acceleration

Data from Peterson J: *Conditioning for a purpose, the West Point way*, West Point, NY, 1977, Leisure Press.

ceps, hamstrings, and lower back muscles. The hip turn involves the lower back muscles and hip flexors. Impact velocity, or swinging the club through the ball, requires well-formed latissimus dorsi and triceps muscles. Control of the club through take-away, impact, and follow-through requires strength in the deltoids, triceps, biceps, forearms, and hand flexors.

A typical Nautilus or Universal gym workout is summarized in Table 39-5.[6] The golfer who does not have specialized exercise equipment can use weighted clubs, chairs, or other household items. These programs are well described by Jobe, Moynes, and Antonelli[1] and Spackman[8] in their monographs.

Cardiovascular Training

Cardiovascular exercise for endurance is another essential part of conditioning. Climbing hills and walking 18 holes are impossible without having the heart and lungs to respond to strenuous exercise, especially in hot, humid weather. Following a preseason conditioning program of jogging and bicycling, walking and staying out of the golf cart will help build endurance and help with overall fitness.

SUMMARY

The golf swing is physically demanding and has contributed to various types of injuries. The wrist, shoulder, and elbow are frequently injured. These injuries may be prevented or reduced by a combination of proper conditioning, treatment, and proper swing mechanics.

REFERENCES

1. Jobe FW, Moynes DR, Antonelli DJ: Rotator cuff function during a golf swing, *Am J Sports Med* 14:388, 1986.
2. Jobe FW, Moynes DR: 30 Exercises to better golf, Inglewood, Calif, 1986, Crampton Press.
3. McCarroll JR: Golf. In Schneider RC, Kennedy JC, Plant ML (eds): *Sports injuries: mechanisms, prevention and treatment*, Baltimore, 1985, Williams & Wilkins.
4. McCarroll JR: Golf: common injuries from a supposedly benign activity, *J Musculoskel Med* 3(5):9, 1986.
5. McCarroll JR, Gioe TJ: Professional golfers and the price they pay, *Phys Sportsmed* 10:64, 1982.
6. Peterson J: *Conditioning for a purpose, the West Point way*, West Point, NY, 1977, Leisure Press.
7. Roberts J: Injuries, handicaps, mashies, and cleeks, *Phys Sportsmed* 6:121, 1978.
8. Spackman RB: *Conditioning for golf*, Murfreesburo, Ill, 1974, Schwebel Printing.
9. Stover CN, Wiren G, Topaz SR: The modern golf swing and stress syndrome, *Phys Sportsmed* 4:42, 1976.
10. Torisu T: Fracture of the hook of the hamate by a golf swing, *Clin Orthop* 83:91, 1972.

CHAPTER 40

Upper Extremity Swimming Injuries

Peter J. Fowler

Injury to the shoulder is the most common problem facing competitive swimmers of all ages. The repeated strong demands made on the upper body stress the shoulder muscles and their tendons far in excess of normal usage and design. Anatomic features and biomechanical forces may combine in the swimmer to produce *swimmer's shoulder*. This term refers to tendinitis of the rotator cuff, usually the supraspinatus or the biceps tendon, and was first used by Kennedy and Hawkins[7] in 1974. However, because inflammation of the rotator cuff

has not been noted, the term *tendinopathy* is a more accurate description.

Earlier papers have indicated that 50% of swimmers have a history of shoulder pain.[7,14] More recent reports cite a 47% to 73% incidence of shoulder pain.[8,10] Intensity of training schedules has increased significantly. This, coupled with biomechanical factors, may be a causal element in the increased incidence of swimmer's shoulder. Awareness of these factors as well as an understanding of the biomechanics of the swimming strokes will assist swimmers and their coaches to plan training programs that reduce the incidence. An informed coach is the best ally a sports physician can have; it is much easier to prevent an injury than to work with an injured athlete.

SWIMMING STROKES

There are four competitive swimming strokes: the front crawl, backstroke, breaststroke, and butterfly. Seventy-five percent of propulsion comes from the arms in the front crawl, backstroke, and butterfly. In the breaststroke the arms and legs contribute equally. The freestyle event in competitive swimming is open to any stroke, usually the front crawl is chosen. In this chapter we use the terms *freestyle* and *front crawl* synonymously.

ANATOMIC FEATURES

The shoulder joint is the most mobile joint in the human body and has little bony support or protection. It relies on its capsule, the surrounding ligaments, and the rotator cuff muscles, as well as larger muscles such as the pectoralis major and the serratus anterior for the stability that allows the arm to function with power and precision throughout its range of motion.

The four rotator cuff muscles work in a force couple combination with the deltoid and long head of the biceps to contain the head of the humerus in the glenoid fossa.

The supraspinatus muscle inserts on the uppermost facet of the greater tuberosity. It acts as a fulcrum for the deltoid during abduction and is active throughout that movement. It also assists the other rotator cuff muscles to resist any upward displacement of the humeral head in other arm actions. The infraspinatus and the teres minor are external rotators. In the horizontal plane

the infraspinatus extends the humerus. The infraspinatus muscle also works in combination with the supraspinatus and the subscapularis to depress the humeral head.

The primary internal rotator of the shoulder is the subscapularis. It stabilizes the head of the humerus by resisting anterior or inferior displacement in the glenoid fossa and, as previously mentioned, exerts a depressive force on the humeral head in combination with the supraspinatus and the infraspinatus.

Active in forward flexion of the shoulder, the long head of the biceps also has an important role in stabilizing the head of the humerus. This function should not be overlooked in shoulder mechanics.

The scapular muscles, the serratus anterior, the rhomboids, and the trapezius work constantly in the swimming arm action. If they fatigue, especially the serratus anterior, the scapula may have relative downward tilt, altering the mechanics of the glenohumeral joint. This in turn can contribute to the onset of impingement tendinitis.

Scapular muscles active in swimming arm action

- Serratus anterior
- Rhomboids
- Trapezius

ROTATOR CUFF TENDINOPATHY
Overwork

The shoulder joint is least stable, and therefore most vulnerable to injury, in the overhead position. Swimming puts continuous repeated demands on the shoulder in this position. The muscles of the rotator cuff may work excessively hard to contain and stabilize the humeral head, and the workload may fatigue them. Superior migration of the humeral head may occur with cuff fatigue, increasing subacromial loading. This, in turn, may be a precipitating factor in the onset of tendinopathy.

Impingement
Soft-Tissue Factors

The supraspinatus and the biceps tendons are particularly susceptible to impingement. Their tendons insert on or cross the humerus directly below the coracoacromial arch, formed by the coracoid process, the rigid coracoacromial ligament, and the anterior acromion. When the arm is in abduction, forward flexion, and internal rotation, the head of the humerus moves under the arch and the tendons may be impinged. This position is assumed in the catch phase of all competitive strokes. Repeatedly the tendons are impinged against the arch, which may result in a mechanical irritation and an inflammatory response or tendinitis.

The inflammation may further compromise the available space under the coracroacromial arch. If untreated, the inflammatory process can go on to include the subacromial bursa and the acromioclavicular ligament.

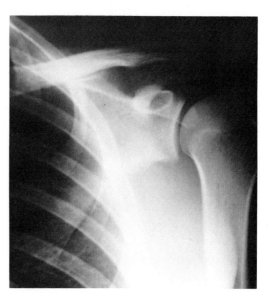

FIG. 40-1. Lateral scapular view taken with the tube directed 10 degrees caudal.

Osseous Contributing Factors

In 1986 Bigliani and his associates[1] reported a study attempting to discover a correlation between acromial shape and full-thickness tears. They examined the acromions of 140 cadavers and classified them according to shape, angle of anterior slope, and the presence of anterior spurs.

Three acromial shapes were identified: Type I, flat; Type II, curved; and Type III, hooked. There were variations in the angle of the slope from 13.1 to 28.7 degrees, and there were rotator cuff tears in 70% of the acromions with bony spurs.

Bigliani and his associates' findings[1] suggested an anatomic factor in refractory tendinitis that does not respond to conservative management. A Type III acromion in a competitive swimmer may precipitate impingement because the dimensions of the coracoacromial arch are already decreased. A tendinopathy would more easily develop and would be more resistant to treatment. The Type III slope described by Bigliani, Morrison, and April[1] can be seen radiographically using a lateral scapular view taken 10 degrees caudally (Fig. 40-1). However, further studies are required to confirm its association with refractory tendinopathy.

Staging

Neer and Welsh[12] have provided clinicians with a chronologic framework for the progression of what they referred to as tendinitis. Stage I, edema and hemorrhage, is most often seen in athletes under 25 years. Stage II, fibrosis and tendinitis, occurs in athletes between 25 and 40 years, whereas Stage III most often develops in those over 40 years. Osteophytes form under the acromion,[11] and tendon ruptures, either partial or complete, can occur. However, in the competitive athlete these stages can occur at any age.

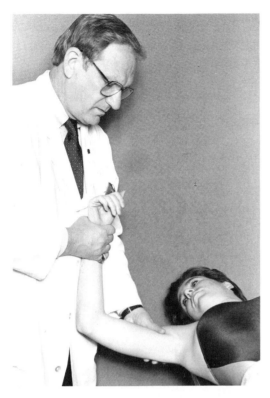

FIG. 40-2. Clinical test for posterior laxity. The abducted position mimics the position of the arm in many sporting activities.

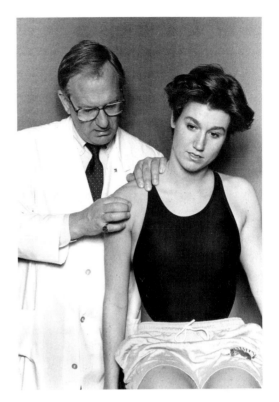

FIG. 40-3. Test for posterior laxity. Ensure that the patient maintains proper posture. Care should be taken when grasping the humeral head; this area may be tender.

Hypovascularity

Rathbun and Macnab's study[13] of the functional relationship between arm position and blood supply to the supraspinatus and the biceps tendon is well known. In adduction and neutral rotation the tendons are stretched tightly over the head of the humerus, and their blood supply is compromised. In abduction the vessels fill, restoring full circulation. This wringing out mechanism, or repeated hypovascularity, may contribute to early degenerative changes in the tendon. It occurs in the area of the tendon most vulnerable to impingement, compounding the potential for damage by repetitive stress.

Increased Shoulder Joint Laxity

Overwork as a factor in rotator cuff tendinopathy in competitive swimmers has already been described. However, if the athlete has loose or lax shoulders, the muscles of the rotator cuff may already be working hard just to contain the humeral head. The added rigor of training makes additional demands on already fatigued or fatiguing muscles. Increased laxity should not be overlooked as a contributing factor in an athlete with resistant tendinopathy.

In 1982 Fowler and Webster[3] evaluated 188 competitive swimmers between 13 and 26 years of age. There was a control group of 50 recreational athletes not bothered by shoulder pain. Each subject had a formal history taken, recording any episodes of shoulder pain. They were assessed for positive signs of tendinopathy and for

posterior, inferior, and anterior instability or increased laxity.

Anterior instability was tested using the apprehension test. A positive response was recorded if the athlete displayed any sign of pain or anxiety. The sulcus sign was used to recognize inferior instability.

Posterior laxity was evaluated using the load and shift test conducted in two positions, sitting and supine. The athlete lies supine on the examining table with the shoulder to be inspected free. The arm is supported in the 90-degree abducted position and force is then applied to the humerus posteriorly (Fig. 40-2). In the second test, with the athlete sitting, the shoulder girdle is stabilized with one hand and forearm while the other hand translates the humerus posteriorly (Fig. 40-3).

The index for posterior laxity was based on the excursion of the humeral head with respect to the posterior glenoid fossa. In many normal asymptomatic individuals the proximal humerus can be translated posteriorly 50% of the glenoid width. Any movement greater than that, in this study, was classified as excessive posterior laxity.

Of the 188 swimmers 50% had a history of shoulder pain. Almost 55% of the swimmers and 52% of the control participants had some degree of posterior laxity in one or both shoulders. These results suggest that *swimming does not predispose an athlete to increased posterior laxity*. Of the swimmers 25% had a history of tendinopathy and increased posterior laxity; the tendinopathy was always in the lax shoulder. There does seem to

TABLE 40-1 Internal-external rotation ratio

Position	Swimmers	Control
90 degrees abduction	62.1	78.2
Neutral	53.7	65.8

TABLE 40-2 Pain during front crawl arm cycle

Position	Percentage
Entry/first half pull phase	44.7
End of pull	14.3
Recovery	23.2
Throughout cycle	17.8

be a relationship between tendinopathy and posterior laxity.

Shoulder Strength Imbalance

Many of these same swimmers demonstrated weakness of the external rotators when gross manual testing was performed. Forty athletes had weakness on one or both shoulders. Thirty-three had weakness and a history of tendinopathy in that shoulder.

This prompted a second study[4] to determine rotation strength about the shoulder. One hundred and nineteen swimmers and 51 controls all between 13 and 26 years of age were tested on the Cybex II dynamometer. The controls were competitive athletes participating in sports that did not primarily require arm rotation strength.

Internal and external rotation strength was measured in neutral, 90 degrees abduction, and 90 degrees flexion. There was a significant difference in the torque ratio between the two groups in abduction and neutral (Table 40-1). The difference in the ratio was attributable to the swimmers' greater strength in internal rotation. There was no significant difference in external rotation strength between the two groups.

Shoulder strength imbalances noted in swimmers

- Very strong internal rotators
- Normal strength external rotators
- Abnormal ratio of internal to external rotators

This study indicated that swimmers have an imbalance in rotation strength ratios when compared with other athletes. This is probably because of the emphasis in their training programs, both swimming and on land, in strengthening the internal rotators and extensors to improve swimming speed and endurance.

Modifying training programs to include external rotation strengthening to restore the normal strength ratio should be a preventive measure against tendinopathy. Evaluation of external rotation strength in swimmers with a resistant tendinopathy can give the clinician added information of value concerning the effectiveness of conservative management.

Impingement Positions in Swimming Strokes

In 1981 Webster, Bishop, and Fowler[14] circulated a questionnaire to age-group swimmers in the province of Ontario. Its aim was to formulate a profile of the athlete with tendinopathy.

Of the 155 responses, 48.4% reported present or past episodes of shoulder pain. Ninety-nine percent used the front crawl as their main practice stroke. Analysis of the

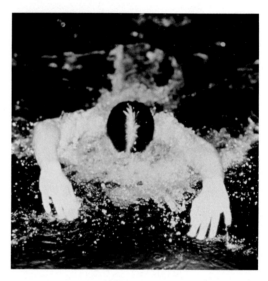

FIG. 40-4. Reach or arm entry position for the butterfly stroke. This arm position is similar for all four competitive strokes.

front crawl arm position at the time they experienced pain seemed to correlate with the biomechanical factors in tendinopathy (Table 40-2).

At entry and the first half of the pull phase, the shoulder is in forward flexion, abduction, and internal rotation. This forces the head of the humerus toward the anterior acromion and coracoacromial ligament and may impinge the supraspinatus and the biceps tendons (Fig. 40-4).

Lateral impingement may be associated with the recovery phase. The shoulder is in abduction and internal rotation, and the head of the humerus comes up against the lateral border of the acromion. This is particularly true when the shoulder leads the rest of the arm. When the head leads the arm through recovery, there is less potential for lateral impingement.

During the end of the pull phase, the shoulder is in adduction and internal rotation, corresponding to the wringing out mechanism (Fig. 40-5).

Summary

Overwork, impingement, and hypovascularity are three main factors that contribute to impingement tendinopathy in the competitive swimmer. Although the anatomic factors predispose some swimmers to tendinopathy, changing training programs and modifying stroke technique can be used effectively both as preventive measures to reduce its incidence and as part of treatment to control its progress.

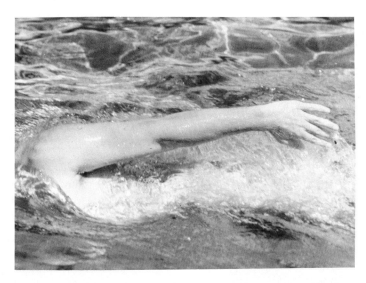

FIG. 40-5. End of the pull phase is similar for all strokes with the exception of the breaststroke. The area of wringing out of the supraspinatus tendon is the same vulnerable area.

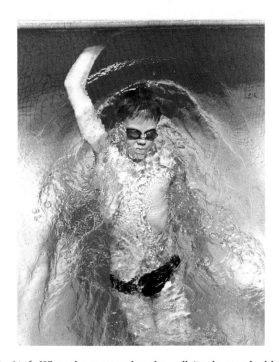

FIG. 40-6. When the arm touches the wall (in the standard backstroke turn, before 1990), the humerus is abducted and externally rotated. The hand remains on the wall around which the body pivots. The head of the humerus may be pried anteriorly if there is anterior laxity.

SHOULDER INSTABILITY
Anterior Instability

Pain from shoulder instability alone is seen in competitive swimmers but not as often. *Anterior instability* is usually secondary to a traumatic incident in another sport. The arm is seldom in the provocative position in any swimming stroke as compared with the throwing

mechanism. Until recently an exception was the usual backstroke turn where the arm could be levered anteriorly (Fig. 40-6). With current rules the backstroker is permitted to roll into a freestyle turn. Because most swimmers take advantage of this option, this problem has been all but eliminated. Anterior instability and its evaluation and treatment are discussed in Chapter 7.

Multidirectional Instability

In contrast to anterior instability, swimmers with frank posterior instability may have pain from dislocating their shoulders in the swimming stroke cycle. The at-risk position of forward flexion and internal rotation occurs in all strokes. Those with multidirectional instability, congenital or acquired, are susceptible to this. This pain must be differentiated from those suffering from painful tendinitis who have concomitant increased laxity.

EVALUATION OF SWIMMERS WITH TENDINOPATHY

Palpation of the supraspinatus tendon medial to its insertion on the greater tuberosity elicits tenderness if the tendon is inflamed. If the long head of the biceps is involved, there will be tenderness over the bicipital groove.

Those with supraspinatus tendinopathy often demonstrate the classic painful arc syndrome. There is pain with active abduction between 60 and 100 degrees. Symptoms of a biceps tendinopathy can be reproduced by resisting forward flexion of the straight arm while the forearm is supinated. The presence of a biceps tendinopathy can be indicative of a refractory supraspinatus tendinopathy.

Clinical pain is often reproduced by placing the shoulder in the impingement aggravated position. In the test described by Neer[11] the examiner further stresses the already forward flexed arm. This test drives the head of the humerus against the anteroinferior border of the acromion.

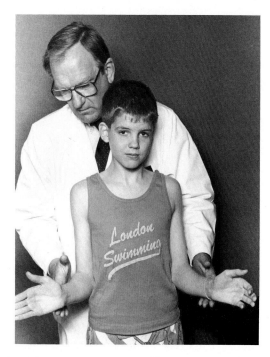

FIG. 40-7. This manual test is appropriate for a gross determination of external rotation muscle strength. A similar resistance test may be performed with the arm abducted to 90 degrees.

A second test, often more appropriate in swimmers, has the examiner internally rotate the arm that is already 90 degrees forward flexed. This pushes the head of the humerus against the coracoacromial ligament, aggravating an inflamed tendon and reproducing pain.

Clinicians should look for muscle weakness about the shoulder, particularly in the external rotators. With the patient's arm in external rotation and adduction and the elbow flexed 90 degrees, the examiner applies an internal rotation force, which the patient resists (Fig. 40-7). Gross weakness is readily apparent. This test is often accompanied by pain.

The generalized laxity of the swimmer is assessed particularly as it relates to the shoulder. Increased laxity or frank instability needs to be documented because it contributes to a tendinopathy progression or may in fact be the total cause of the pain. In anterior instability, the apprehension test is helpful. The patient lies supine on the examining table. The examiner abducts the arm 90 degrees then externally rotates the humerus. A positive sign is when the patient exhibits a feeling of anxiety, often with pain, or will not allow further external rotation. This feeling may be alleviated by applying posterior pressure on the upper arm, keeping the humeral head contained (Fig. 40-8).

Posterior translation can be assessed with the patient supine, while the examiner holds the arm 90 degrees ab-

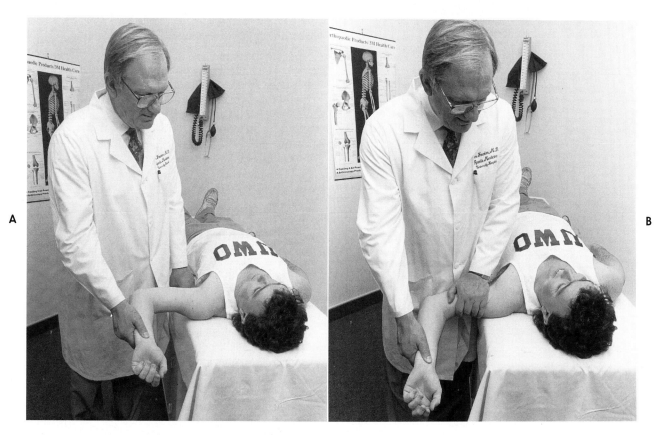

A   B

FIG. 40-8. A, With the arm abducted and externally rotated the humeral head is levered anteriorly. With glenohumeral instability the athlete experiences apprehension or discomfort. B, Reduction of the humeral head in the glenoid fossa relieves the symptoms.

ducted and applies posterior pressure to the upper humerus (Fig. 40-2). Movement of the humeral head 50% of the glenoid width is considered normal, and motion greater than that, while not necessarily abnormal, would influence the mechanics of the shoulder by creating an increased work load to the rotator cuff. If the shoulder is unstable, applying an axial load may reproduce the symptoms the patient is having while swimming. This would be pain from the instability itself.

A second test has the patient sitting while the examiner stabilizes the shoulder girdle with one hand and applies posterior pressure to the humeral head with the other hand. The amount of movement is assessed (Fig. 40-3).

The presence of a sulcus with inferior traction indicates instability in this direction.

The progression of tendinopathy is insidious. Pain becomes generalized about the shoulder and is often present at night or at rest. The athlete tends to avoid painful positions, and subtle changes in stroke mechanics develop to minimize pain. In other activities as well, athletes modify all positions that aggravate the symptoms.

Over time there may be a gradual loss of range of motion at the shoulder followed by muscle weakness. Wasting of the supraspinatus and the infraspinatus may become evident. In a mature athlete this may signal either degeneration of the rotator cuff tendon or a partial cuff tear. Cuff tears are seldom seen in age-group swimmers and are rare in all athletes under 25 years of age.

Clinical classification of tendinitis (tendinopathy) is based on Blazina's[2] categories for jumper's knee. In Grade I tendinitis the athlete has pain after the activity; in Grade II, pain occurs during and after the sport but is not disabling. A Grade III tendinitis describes disabling pain during and after activity, while in a fourth and most serious category the condition is so severe that the athlete has pain with daily activities.

PREVENTION

Stress syndromes about the shoulder are easier to prevent than treat, and the principles for prevention should be incorporated into the athlete's training program early.

The role of the coach in injury prevention cannot be overemphasized. An informed coach plans a training program keeping in mind the dangers of overwork and rotator cuff fatigue. Stroke analysis, performance monitoring, and guidance from stroke errors should all be carried out by coaching staff on an ongoing basis.

Work Load

Overwork is one of the primary causes of tendinopathy and is often the result of increased intensity of the training sets. Putting athletes through rigorous training sessions before they are ready or through an extra hard practice at the beginning of training may do more than show swimmers how much work they need to do. Either of these can trigger the onset of a tendinopathy.

Training should gradually increase the demand on the swimmers as the schedule progresses. Each training ses-

sion can be designed so the difficult portion of the practice is earlier in the workout, before the swimmer begins to overtire. Practice can continue with emphasis on stroke drills, alternating strokes with leg work, and start-and-turn technique to provide the swimmers with relative rest to the structures at risk. With proper instruction, swimmers can learn to guard against the damaging effects of fatigue using increased awareness and good stroke mechanics to minimize the potential for injury.

Strengthening

Imbalance in muscle strength about the shoulder results from emphasis on specific muscle groups during pool and dry-land training, and it contributes to overwork for the cuff muscles. A balanced exercise program that includes external rotation strengthening may reduce the incidence of tendinopathy, particularly that associated with increased posterior laxity (Fig. 40-9). The training program should not overlook exercises for the triceps and the scapular muscle (Fig. 40-10). As in the swimming stroke, the swimmer should avoid painful subacromial loading positions when doing weight training. Using paddles while swimming is a method of increasing re-

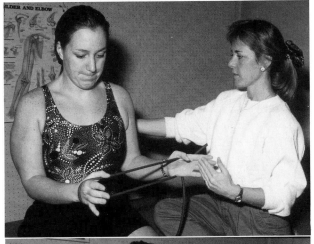

A

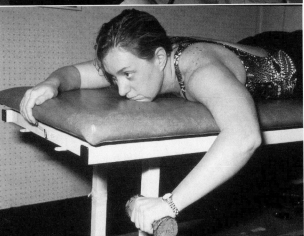

B

FIG. 40-9. Strengthening the external rotators in neutral, **(A),** and 90 degrees of abduction, **(B).**

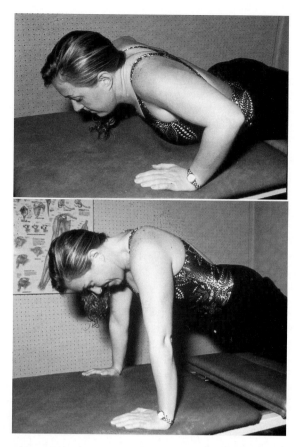

FIG. 40-10. Muscle strengthening for the triceps and scapular muscles is performed.

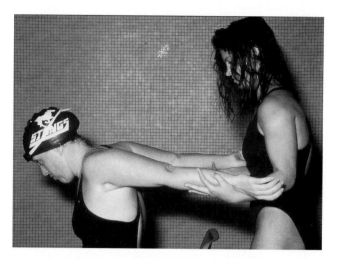

FIG. 40-11. Neuromuscular facilitated stretching with a partner requires a knowledge of proper technique.

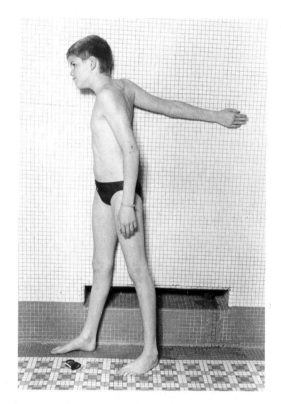

FIG. 40-12. An athlete can accommodate all of the same muscle groups when stretching alone as when stretching with a partner.

sistance. Paddles must be used with caution because the increased leverage can overload the rotator cuff muscles.

Stretching

Stretching should be done regularly as part of the daily training warm-up. Three times weekly is insufficient. In 1981 Griep[5] studied the relationship between shoulder flexibility and the incidence of tendinitis in swimmers. He measured shoulder flexibility in a group of 168 swimmers and recorded the information by gender and by stroke most frequently used. At the end of 6 months Griep was able to predict with 93% accuracy which swimmers would develop tendinitis. Regardless of category, the swimmers with restricted flexibility were more likely to develop a tendinitis than those who maintained flexibility with a stretching program.

Swimmers over age 15 should be sufficiently mature to stretch in pairs (Fig. 40-11). The stretching techniques can be either passive or proprioceptive neuromuscular facilitated (PNF).[6] In the passive type of stretch the partner stretches very slowly to the limit of the pain-free range and then holds the position. In PNF stretching the swimmer to be stretched moves to the limits of range. The partner then maintains that position while the swimmer contracts against the partner's resistance. This is then repeated a variable number of times. Partner stretching has to be done carefully because overstretch-

ing of the soft tissues can increase the irritation to the tendons of the rotator cuff.

Swimmers under the age of 15 are less likely to understand the pitfalls of pairs stretching. For safety reasons they should be taught to stretch on an individual basis (Fig. 40-12).

Stroke Mechanics

Poor stroke mechanics can be a major factor in the onset of shoulder pain. It is important that coaches analyze

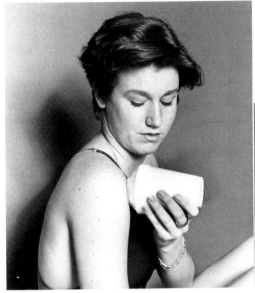
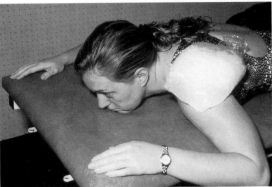

FIG. 40-13. Cold applied to the shoulder is a most effective therapy. Ice cups, crushed ice in plastic bags, or cold packs may be used.

strokes that cause pain and instruct the swimmer on how these should be modified. Swimmers must be made aware of the fact that poor technique not only hinders speed, but also can increase the risk of injury. Any changes in stroke technique during fatigue should be identified as well. Insufficient body roll in freestyle or backstroke can contribute to lateral shoulder impingement. In the freestyle the swimmer may be told to attain a high elbow position during the recovery. The high elbow position must be achieved with body roll rather than muscle activity. Forcing the elbow into a higher position without body roll may induce subacromial humeral head impingement.

In the catch phase of all strokes the swimmer is preparing for maximal propulsion. Overreach with excessive internal rotation may cause undue subacromial loading and excessive activity for the cuff muscles to contain the humeral head. Also, excessive internal rotation at the end of the stroke may intensify the wringing out phenomenon. Effective coaching helps the swimmer alter body roll, reach, and degree of shoulder internal rotation to reduce the frequency and length of time the shoulder is in the provocative position.

There is contradictory evidence that breathing patterns affect the incidence of tendinopathy.[14] Breathing to alternate sides keeps the swimmer from leaning constantly on to the same shoulder.

TREATMENT
Tendinopathy
Grade I

A Grade I tendinopathy responds well to management.[2]

Swimmers are told to increase the time spent in both the prepractice stretch and in the pool warm-up.

Stretches should pay attention to all structures, including the anterior ones. Appropriate stretching can restore lost range of motion, increase the blood flow, and reduce the potential for further impingement injury. In the pool, warm-up should be prolonged, at a very slow pace and in pain-free strokes. Additional arm warm-ups should be done after kicking sets. A swimming warm-down is recommended after the training session.

Treatment of Grade I tendinopathy

- Increase prepractice strength and warm-up times
- Emphasize pain-free strokes
- Encourage swimming warm-down period after training session
- Use cryotherapy to reduce pain and inflammation
- Correct external rotation weakness

After the practice the athlete should ice the sore shoulder for no more than 15 minutes to reduce pain and inflammation. Ice cups or bags are the simplest and most effective way to do this (Fig. 40-13). If the swimmer has weakness of the external rotators this should be corrected. The exercises should work the external rotators beginning in adduction and progressing to varying degrees of abduction (Fig. 40-9). This improves the control of the glenohumeral joint, which in turn results in more efficient muscle work and a better performance potential. The swim practice should be as pain free as possible. If the swimmer has pain only when the work load is too heavy, the load must be reduced for a time and then gradually increased. If only one stroke causes symptoms, the athlete should discontinue it temporarily. Once the symptoms have subsided, the stroke, with any faults

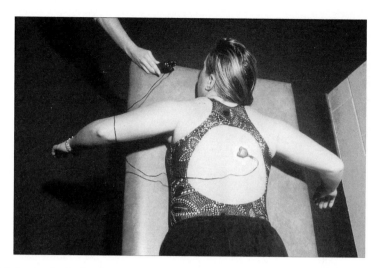

FIG. 40-14. During biofeedback a light signals that a specific muscle is contracting. With repetition as rehabilitation progresses, the athlete learns to use this muscle during swimming.

corrected, can be gradually introduced back into the training program.

Grade II

A Grade II tendinopathy requires rest, physiotherapy, and perhaps medication, in addition to the previous management. Rest does not mean total absence from the sport. The athlete can work on strokes that do not elicit pain or concentrate on leg work. In the latter case, kick boards should not be used because they place the shoulder in the pain-provoking position. For aerobic training, running and cycling can supplement the shorter swim workout.

Treatment of Grade II tendinopathy

- Relative rest (emphasize leg work and pain-free stroke)
- Antiinflammatory medicine
- Physiotherapy modalities (ultrasound, transcutaneous electric nerve stimulation)
- Strengthening program
- Mobilization techniques

A short course of antiinflammatory medication in conjunction with these measures helps improve symptomatic relief.

At this stage or in Grade III tendinopathy the athlete may be referred for physiotherapy. The therapist assesses the athlete's shoulder to determine intensity and duration of pain, range limitations, and any loss of strength in the muscles of the arm and the shoulder girdle.

Treatment is determined by the assessment findings and may include the use of modalities such as ultrasound, interferential therapy, or transcutaneous electric nerve stimulation (TENS). Loss of range is treated with passive mobilization techniques and range of motion exercises. If there is an imbalance in muscle strength or significant weakness in any muscle group, the therapist plans an appropriate strengthening program.

Biofeedback that allows the swimmer to recognize that a certain muscle is working may also be used (Fig. 40-14). Depending on the nature and presentation of the pain, joint range, and weakness, the exercises are isometric, isotonic, or, where possible, isokinetic. However, an effective treatment program can be developed using only free weights or rubber surgical tubing (Fig. 40-10).

The exercises should not reproduce pain. Often the pain is felt only in certain positions and the exercises can be done around such positions. If, however, the exercise is painful throughout range, it should be discontinued or decreased in repetition or resistance to the level at which it is pain free.

If the treatment program is successful, the athlete gradually returns to the full program but is advised to continue with therapy until the preinjury level of activity is attained.

If the tendinopathy is not responding to treatment and there is still painful response to the impingement aggravating test, a steroid injection into the subacromial space may be considered. Such injections should never be used routinely. If the situation merits its use, the athlete's swimming load should be decreased following the injection and gradually return to former levels over 4 to 6 weeks.

Grade III

In some cases none of these measures is successful and the athlete progresses to a Grade III stage or beyond, with the tendinopathy becoming refractory. At this time options available to the athlete include a change of sports or surgery. Unless a high-caliber career is possible at the national or international level, most young swimmers correctly select the former option and in most instances should be encouraged to. Surgical options include resection of the diseased segment of tendon with adjacent subacromial bursal tissue if involved or decompression of the same area.

Before selecting surgery as an option, the clinician should make clear to the athlete that the postoperative

recovery period involves a serious personal commitment. During that time, rehabilitation includes a progressive exercise program to restore range of motion and balance muscle strength. The athlete's cooperation and compliance to the program directly affect its outcome. The return to the pool should begin with slow swimming progressing to interval training and guided stroke modification, as well as an overlap period from formal rehabilitation. The importance of the coach to the athlete's successful return to sport cannot be overemphasized.

Grade IV

A Grade IV clinical presentation, pain with all activity, is most often seen in the mature athlete. It may indicate a tear of the rotator cuff. Conservative treatment may not satisfactorily relieve these symptoms. Although the diagnosis may be made clinically, imaging techniques such as arthrography, ultrasonography, and magnetic resonance imaging (MRI) may give confirmation. Arthroscopy of the shoulder joint and the subacromial space can help identify such lesions as partial thickness tears and thickened subacromial bursae. Although not a frequent cause of pain, particularly in younger swimmers, superior quadrant labral tears, anterior or posterior (SLAP), can cause pain in the swimmer and be successfully treated with arthroscopic excision.[9]

In younger athletes bursectomy alone can provide relief, followed by appropriate rehabilitation. A more radical decompression to include resection of the anteroinferior acromion and a portion of the coracoacromial ligament is usually recommended. Repair of a torn rotator cuff is done to provide symptomatic relief and prevent progressive tearing. This may be noted in the older swimmer competing at the master level. It is unlikely that the athlete will return to the preinjury level of participation, and this should be made clear preoperatively.

Formal physiotherapy plays a significant role postoperatively because range of motion is often lost and muscle strength, endurance, and power deteriorate. Classically the abductors and the external rotators are the weakest groups, but all muscle groups about the shoulder girdle must be included in the program.

Anterior Instability

Although the provocative position is not common in the competitive swimming strokes, factors such as faulty stroke mechanics and fatigue have resulted in clinical anterior dislocation or subluxation. Stroke modification and balance-strengthening exercises are the primary conservative treatments available to the swimmer with anterior instability.

If symptoms do not subside, examination under anesthesia or arthroscopy can assist in diagnosing intraarticular lesions such as the Bankhart or Hill-Sachs lesion. An anterior stabilization procedure can provide relief and return athletes to preinjury levels if they regain their motion and strength.

Multidirectional Instability

Persistence with a nonoperative program is suggested for prolonged periods of multidirectional instability. Stroke modification, correction of strengthening deficits, and alteration of training programs, all designed to minimize the magnitude and incidence of abnormal motion, can be used successfully in most cases. Surgical treatment possibilities include an inferior capsular shift, a reefing procedure to the posterior cuff and capsule, and a glenoid osteotomy. Such procedures should be considered only when nonoperative treatment has been completely exhausted. Restriction of motion by these procedures will undoubtedly terminate a competitive swimming career at a high competitive level. Such treatment can realistically be undertaken to provide symptomatic relief for daily activities and to allow the athlete to participate in recreational swimming and other sports.

SUMMARY

Swimmer's shoulder is most commonly pain experienced from tendinopathy. The etiology of this in a competitive swimmer may be complex. Successful prevention and management require the combined effort and cooperation of the athlete, coach, therapist, and physician.

REFERENCES

1. Bigliani NU, Morrison DS, April EW: The morphology of the acromion and its relationship to rotator cuff tears, *Orthop Trans* 10(2):216, 1986.
2. Blazina ME: Jumper's knee, *Orthop Clinic North Am* 4(3):65, 1980.
3. Fowler PJ, Webster MS: Shoulder pain in highly competitive swimmers, *Orthop Trans* 7(1):170, 1983.
4. Fowler PJ, Webster MS: *Rotation strength about the shoulder: establishment of internal to external strength ratios*, Paper presented at the American Orthopaedic Society for Sports Medicine annual meeting, Nashville, July 1985.
5. Griep JF: Swimmer's shoulder: the influence of flexibility and weight training, *Phys Sport Med* 13(8):92, 1985.
6. Reference deleted in proofs.
7. Kennedy JC, Hawkins RJ: Swimmer's shoulder, *Phys Sports Med* 2(4):35, 1974.
8. Lo YPC, Hsu YCS, Chan KM: Epidemiology of shoulder impingement in upper arm sports events, *Br J Sports Med* 24(3):173, 1990.
9. McMaster WC: Anterior glenoid labrum damage: a painful lesion in swimmers, *Am J Sports Med* 14(5):383, 1986.
10. McMaster WC, Troup J: A survey of interfering shoulder pain in United States competitive swimmers, *Am J Sports Med* 21(1):67, 1993.
11. Neer CS: Anterior acromioplasty for the chronic impingement syndrome in the shoulder, *J Bone Joint Surg* 54A:41, 1972.
12. Neer CS, Welsh RP: The shoulder in sports, *Orthop Clin North Am* 8:585, 1977.
13. Rathbun JB, Macnab I: The microvascular pattern of the rotator cuff, *J Bone Joint Surg* 52B(3):544, 1970.
14. Webster MS, Bishop P, Fowler PJ: *Swimmer's shoulder*, Undergraduate thesis, Waterloo, Ont; 1981, University of Waterloo.

CHAPTER 41

Upper Extremity Injuries in American Football

Michael G. Browne
Stephen J. Nicholas

Approximately 1.5 million young men participate in football in the United States each year, sustaining an estimated 1.2 million injuries annually.[62] The risk of injury is thought by some to be higher in older athletes,[62] whereas others have found a higher injury rate among adolescents.[25] Injuries occur less frequently on teams with more experienced coaches and a greater number of assistant coaches.[62] De Lee and Farney[18] found an incidence of 0.506 injury per athlete per year in 4399 athletes participating in Texas high school varsity football. About 30% of the injuries were to the upper extremity. In general, sprains and strains account for 40%, contusions 25%, dislocations 15%, fractures 10%, and head concussions 5% of all injuries.[62] In 1988 Goldberg et al[25] evaluated the injury frequency in 5128 boys participating in youth football. They found the overall rate of significant injury to be 5%, with 39% of these considered to be major. The upper extremity was more likely to be injured, with fractures the most common injury. Their conclusions pointed out the different pattern between the adolescent and the physically mature football player regarding the rate, site, and type of injury. Luckily, no catastrophic injuries occurred, and permanent disability resulting from injury was rare. Blyth[7] found the following distribution of injuries to the upper body in a large study of high school football injuries: 13% trunk, 13% head and neck, 8% shoulder, and 8% hand. Fewer than 1% were blunt abdominal injuries. Skill level does not correlate with the incidence of injuries.[36]

Injury is the result of forces applied to the body in excess of the body part's ability to tolerate the stress. These forces may be applied instantaneously or repetitively over time. Most sports injuries are essentially the same as those sustained in other activities, but because of the heightened metabolic state of exercising tissue, second-

ary damage (e.g., hematoma formation) may be greater. The severity of injury is affected by the patient's physical and psychologic fitness, his or her morphologic aptitude for the sport, age, sex, and environmental conditions at the time of the injury. Another factor to consider is the higher expectations of the athlete with regard to an accelerated rehabilitation program and the demand of the sport to which he hopes to return. Continued sports activity while injured may produce a second injury via abnormal variations in technique.

Extrinsic injuries are caused by forces generated outside the patient, whereas **intrinsic injuries** are those caused by forces generated within the patient's own body. An example of an intrinsic injury is rupture of the long head of the biceps; an example of an extrinsic cause of injury is a direct blow resulting in a fracture. Generally, extrinsic injuries produce more severe tissue damage than do intrinsic because the forces involved can be substantially greater. The stress may be direct, at the point of application of the force, or indirect when the damage to tissue occurs at a distance.

Injury mechanisms

- Extrinsic—caused by forces generated outside the patient
- Intrinsic—caused by forces generated within the patient

SKIN

Lacerations, abrasions, puncture wounds, and burns are among the possible types of skin injury in football. These all disrupt the skin's integrity and act as a potential portal of entry for environmental contaminants. Prompt and thoughtful treatment prevents these common injuries from becoming serious.

Abrasions/Burns

An abrasion is a partial-thickness injury to the skin involving friction against a surface that is not sharp enough to produce a laceration. A good example is the friction burn **(turf burn)** incurred after a sliding fall on artificial surfaces. Another burn that is unique to sports played on natural grass is a **chemical burn** from the soda lime used to line the field.[5] The powder can collect on areas of the body moistened by perspiration (groin, belt line, collar, or axilla) and cause local irritation if it remains in contact with the skin for a prolonged period. Extensive irrigation of the affected areas with cool water, best performed in a shower, removes the irritant and relieves symptoms.

Unfortunately, the use of ice in the training room is not always judiciously practiced by the unsupervised player, and prolonged therapy frequently results in partial-thickness thermal necrosis of the skin **(ice burn)**. Once the lower temperature induces anesthesia in the injured area, the patient is unaware that prolonged exposure to the ice pack is causing secondary damage to the skin. Using a 20-minute maximum time limit is a good general rule to prevent this injury.

Puncture Wounds, Contusions, and Blisters

Puncture wounds are defined as any laceration in which the depth of tissue penetration is greater than the length. Contusions and superficial hematomas with resultant bruising are routine for every football player. A shoulder pointer is a contusion to the skin and soft tissue overlying the acromion caused by a direct blow. Blisters, when they occur, are the products of new or poorly padded equipment. All attempts should be made to preserve the integrity of the overlying skin as a biologic dressing.

Treatment

Treatment of any injury to the skin first requires careful cleansing and irrigation of the wound. For a turf burn ensure all turf powder has been adequately debrided. Grass burns commonly become secondarily infected, and the pathogens isolated are similar to those seen in olecranon bursitis (see further). If a turf burn shows early signs of infection, antibiotic therapy must include coverage for *Pseudomonas* organisms. Severe breaches of the skin may require closure, in the form of either butterfly bandages or surgical suture to speed the healing process. Treatment of puncture wounds in the athlete is the same as for the general population, with irrigation and exploration if indicated for a foreign body, prophylactic antibiotic coverage, and healing by secondary intention. Close observation on the part of the medical staff is required. All wounds should be securely dressed and protected before return to play.

BURSAE
Olecranon Bursitis

Olecranon bursitis refers to inflammation of either the bursa that lies subcutaneously over the olecranon or the bursa deep to the distal triceps near its insertion. Involvement of the superficial bursa is much more common. The bursitis can be either infectious (septic) or inflammatory (nonseptic).

Olecranon bursitis

- Septic (infections)
- Inflammatory (nonseptic)

Septic bursitis occurs predominantly in males, and approximately 50% of cases are associated with recreational or occupational trauma.[56] Penetrating trauma is by no means a prerequisite.[31] It occurs much less frequently in the young, possibly because cadaveric studies have failed to demonstrate the presence of an olecranon bursa before the age of 7.[13] The bursa increases in size with age, to a length of about 6 cm.[58] The causative pathogen is most commonly *Staphylococcus aureus*, although gram-negative bacteria have been described.[20,41,56] The majority do not require hospitalization and can be effectively treated with oral antibiotics.[56]

Nonseptic olecranon bursitis occurs as an inflammatory process of unknown cause, but is believed to be

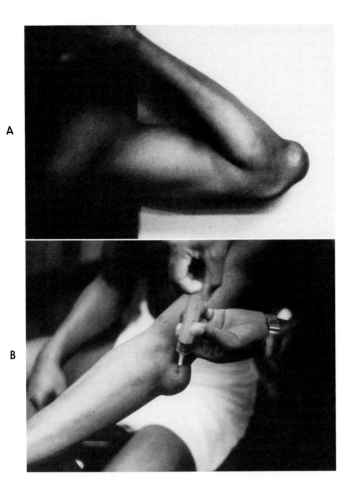

FIG. 41-1. A, Prominent swollen olecranon bursa with aseptic bursitis. It is minimally painful despite its size. **B,** Aspiration technique. Gloves should be worn for all procedures involving potential exposure to bodily fluids.

associated with repetitive microtrauma.[17] From the mechanics of blocking an opponent, or from contact with the ground, every position in football is subject to injury to the elbow area. Linemen are particularly susceptible. Unlike in septic bursitis, the patient develops a painless, slowly expanding fluctuant mass overlying the olecranon, usually on the dominant extremity (Fig. 41-1).[35] Normally the patient cannot recall a specific traumatic event. If a septic process is suspected, diagnostic and therapeutic aspiration can be performed. However, if the inflammation is nonseptic, many authors favor observation, thereby avoiding the potential iatrogenic infection of a sterile bursa. Others promote a diagnostic puncture in all cases: the chance of infection is then definitively ruled out, and methylprednisolone injection can be performed if there is no evidence of infection on Gram stain. According to Smith,[65] local steroids are best used in conjunction with an oral antiinflammatory and are much more effective in reducing both the acute swelling and the recurrence of bursitis than oral antiinflammatory agents alone. Earlier studies, however, contend that there is little advantage to the use of local steroids.[20]

Radiographs of the elbow should be obtained to eval-

uate the olecranon for the presence of a spur and to determine if calcifications are present in the bursa. Bursectomy can be readily performed and is indicated for recalcitrant cases, especially if bony abnormalities are present. Recently endoscopic resection of the offending bursa has been described in the literature. The main advantages to this approach are avoidance of the wound problems associated with open resection and faster return to competition. Limited studies suggest a good outcome with this treatment technique for cases of traumatic etiology.[37,38] We have used this technique for both inflammatory and septic bursitis in 12 patients with good results. Our protocol includes immobilization in a compressive dressing for 5 to 7 days, then return to activities with a protective dressing at 2 weeks. At an average 1-year follow-up there have been no infections, no recurrences of bursitis, and no complaints of scar pain. Football players may return to noncontact activity at 5 days and full contact in 10 days to 2 weeks with appropriate local protection.

With the advent of artificial turf, Larson and Osternig[44] reviewed the experience of the PAC 8 conference and discovered that both olecranon and prepatellar bursitides were much more common on artificial turf. Prophylactic protective padding of the joints at risk greatly reduced the occurrence and the severity of symptoms. Powell,[57] in a study of the National Football League, showed that the injury rate for the upper extremity does not differ from artificial turf to natural grass.

Subdeltoid Bursitis

The shoulder is probably the most common point of high-energy contact between players on the football field, whether directly or indirectly. As a result the shoulder is subject to bursal inflammation from both overuse and trauma. Treatment initially involves cryotherapy and protection from inciting activities in combination with an oral antiinflammatory agent. Passive motion exercises below the horizontal plane are performed to maintain range of motion. Active motion and strengthening are permitted once the acute pain subsides. Modalities of heat and ultrasound are helpful in decreasing symptoms and enhancing the healing process. Local steroid injection may be necessary in the unresponsive case.

Acute traumatic hemorrhagic bursitis of the subacromial bursa may mimic acute rotator cuff tear, prompting further evaluation. This diagnosis should always be considered when symptoms of impingement syndrome or rotator cuff tendinitis are present after acute trauma to the shoulder. Magnetic resonance imaging (MRI) or computed tomographic (CT) arthrography will delineate the injury. Although hemorrhagic bursitis is the less severe injury, it is not unusual for symptoms and disability to last up to 8 weeks, limiting the player's activity.

MUSCLE

Injury to a muscle can be from an extrinsic force such as a blow from another player, or intrinsic force, which occurs when the contractile muscle elements overpower

the supporting soft tissues or bone in response to stress.

A blow to an extremity of any force can cause direct capillary rupture and bleeding. The increase in muscle vascularization that an athlete develops in response to training may at first accentuate the hemorrhage. Capillary permeability is increased in the injured muscle via the usual vasoactive intermediaries of inflammation, causing additional bleeding. Hematoma, muscle spasm, and pain are the early results of injury. The acute effects are best treated with prompt cryotherapy to the injured extremity, inducing local hypothermia and vasospasm, as well as immobilization. The adjacent joints are immobilized so that the injured muscle maintains a lengthened position. In this manner bleeding and the associated swelling and inflammation are kept to a minimum. Injured muscle repairs itself primarily through generation of fibrous scar tissue. Once the scar begins to contract, the involved muscle can shorten considerably, especially if the extent of injury is widespread. In the case of extensive muscle damage, in particular if the muscle has been immobilized in a shortened position, contracture of the adjacent joints may result. Physical therapy to maintain range of motion is imperative during the healing process, within the parameters described in the next section.

Contusions

Myositis Ossificans Traumatica

Myositis ossificans traumatica is a condition in which calcium, and eventually bone, is deposited in muscle in response to trauma, usually as a result of a direct blow. As a rule it does not occur with intrinsic injury. Carlson and Klassen[11] retrospectively reviewed 83 cases of myositis ossificans treated nonoperatively at the Mayo Clinic from 1950 to 1979 in patients younger than 21 years. Thirty-one patients (37%) had upper extremity involvement, 20 of whom were injured playing football. Football was by far the most commonly involved sport in upper extremity myositis (20 of the 31 patients). Although the paper does not specify, the treatments described and the two illustrative case reports given suggest that no elbow dislocations were included. Twenty-three patients were evaluated at an average 13 years after injury (range 2 to 29 years). The brachialis was the muscle most commonly implicated, followed by the biceps brachii. At follow-up two thirds had no symptoms whatsoever. The remaining third had mild complaints, including a lack of elbow extension or tenderness when pressure was placed on the arm in the involved area. Only one patient had late symptoms severe enough to warrant evaluation by a physician, and that patient underwent surgical excision of the ossified tissue.

Blocker's Node

Contusions to the soft tissue of the extremities occur commonly in all contact sports. However, an entity unique to football is the development of a painful nodule on the anterolateral arm called a blocker's node (also blocker's exostosis and tackler's exostosis). The injury occurs primarily in linemen or defensive backs when the player is struck just below the distal extent of the shoul-

der pads, on the anterior or anterolateral aspect of an unprotected arm. The trauma may be a single event, as in an aggressive tackle, or repeated blows to the arm, as occur in day-to-day blocking activities. Poorly fitting shoulder pads have also been incriminated as a causative factor in some cases. The player develops a painful swelling on the anterolateral midportion of the arm, just distal to the deltoid tubercle. Elbow stiffness, pain with range of motion, and weakness are found on examination. As with any extremity injury accompanied by weakness, a careful neurologic evaluation of the affected limb must be performed. After a few weeks a firm, painful mass is palpable in the same area. The pathologic process is calcification of a subperiosteal hematoma of the central third of the humerus, thought by some to be secondary to tearing of the periosteum at the site of the brachialis origin.[42] Radiographically, calcification can be seen as early as 2 weeks after injury[11] or even earlier by ultrasonography.[40] The calcification is in continuity with the thickened cortical bone of the humerus in the affected area (Fig. 41-2). Myositis ossificans of the brachialis or biceps brachii muscles can be an associated injury. It can occur by the same mechanism and even have a similar radiographic appearance. In fact, the term blocker's node is often used interchangeably to describe subperiosteal hematoma and myositis. Differentiating

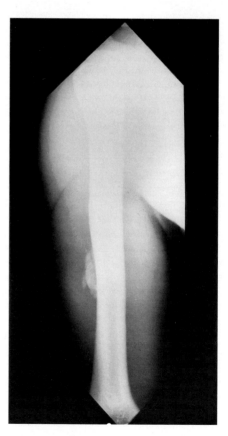

FIG. 41-2. Frontal view of humerus with "blocker's node" anterolaterally. Lucency between the mass and cortex suggests that this lesion represents myositis ossificans of the brachialis. Sequential radiographs have demonstrated complete resorption of the ectopic calcification in some cases.

factors are that myositis ossificans tends to present in the younger athlete, and the calcification is not in direct continuity with the humeral cortex on radiographs.

Treatment

Early treatment of either disorder entails the standard application of ice and possibly a compressive dressing to reduce swelling and inflammation during the first 48 hours. Immobilization in a sling or splint for pain relief is also suggested in the early period after injury. Once swelling and the initial inflammatory period are controlled, the patient can begin gentle active range of motion as pain allows. The greatest concern in this injury is the development of intractable myositis ossificans. Its formation may be induced and potentiated by overly aggressive early treatment, especially with passive stretching, of a muscle with an intramuscular hematoma. Hence passive range of motion and massage are to be avoided. Light active strengthening exercises may be performed only through the pain-free arc of motion. If calcification has been documented, therapy must not progress until complete maturation of the ossification. Although clinical symptoms are helpful measures, the best indicator that the ossification is complete is that the serum alkaline phosphatase level returns to normal. Until full painless range of motion of the shoulder and elbow have been attained, aggressive strengthening should not be undertaken. Return to competition is allowed when the player achieves full range of motion and symmetric upper extremity strength. The affected area should be padded to minimize the risk of further injury.

Strains

When intrinsic injury takes place, a muscle is usually undergoing an eccentric contracture. Muscle strain, or tear, can be classified into two types: complete and partial. Partial tears can then be further divided by the pattern of bleeding. **Interstitial tears** are those in which the bleeding is not contained by the perimysium, allowing subcutaneous or intermuscular tracking of the blood. **Intramuscular tears,** on the other hand, are those in which the hematoma is contained within the structure of the muscle itself. Tears occur when the forceful contraction of a muscle is suddenly blocked or overcome. The severity is often related to the athlete's level of training. As mentioned, bleeding is initially more marked in the conditioned athlete because of the increased capillarization of muscle that occurs in response to training. In the upper extremity complete tears generally occur in the tendinous portion or at the musculotendinous junction. Tears in the substance of a muscle occur much more commonly in the lower extremity and usually in muscles that cross two joints (e.g., hamstring, gastrocnemius). However, the literature contains reports of four cases in which a tear took place in the substance of the triceps muscle.[3,50,55]

TENDONS

Damage to tendons by direct violence in sports is uncommon. Usually the mechanism of injury is intrinsic and most are secondary to overuse. Tendon injuries are readily classified by their local pathology, which is associated with well-defined clinical features.

Anabolic Steroids

In a sport where size and strength are cherished, an additional concern for any physician involved in the care of players is the use and abuse of anabolic steroids. Adverse effects of these short-term performance and size enhancers have been well documented for the hepatic, cardiovascular, hematopoietic, and musculoskeletal systems. Hunter et al [33] have demonstrated statistically significant lower tendon strength-to-failure in mechanical testing of rabbits treated with anabolic steroids relative to an untreated group. These results confirm a detrimental effect of anabolic steroids on connective tissue mechanical properties that previously had only been clinically suspected.

Rotator Cuff and Acute Impingement

The rotator cuff generally becomes a problem only in the throwing athlete or swimmer, who repetitively traumatizes the cuff as it passes under the acromion during overhead motion of the arm. However, it can, like any other tendinous insertion, become traumatically avulsed from its insertion if the force generated overcomes the failure strength of the tissues involved. Traumatic tears of the rotator cuff tendon are rare, but do occur in football. The mechanism is either a fall onto the shoulder with the arm in an adducted position or an indirect force on an abducted arm. This can readily happen in football and has occurred due to acute trauma at the professional level. In general, the player gives a history of having heard a tearing sound or pop. He complains of acute pain and weakness in abduction to a varying degree. In a very strong athlete weakness may not be discernible on physical examination despite considerable loss of strength, so a high index of suspicion must be maintained when given the above history. MRI, ultrasonography, or arthrogram may be used diagnostically. Although arthrogram is the accepted gold standard, a technically good MRI read by an experienced radiologist can be the most sensitive tool available today.[9,52,54] Unfortunately, many professional level football players exceed the size limitations of the standard MRI machine. Ultrasonography is diagnostic in fewer than 40% of patients with a degenerative rotator cuff tear.[49]

Poor vascular supply and retraction of the torn tissue make operative repair of a full-thickness rotator cuff tear the optimal treatment[23] in an attempt to maximize effective healing and recovery. Surgical reconstruction yields excellent pain relief but does not guarantee return to preinjury performance levels, especially in the throwing athlete.[71] Extensive physical therapy is for strengthening, and range of motion is necessary in the postoperative period. It may take 6 months to regain adequate strength before return to competition.

More frequently seen is a syndrome in which the athlete experiences trauma to the shoulder and develops an acute hemorrhagic subacromial bursitis. The symptoms mimic those of a severe impingement syndrome, and the

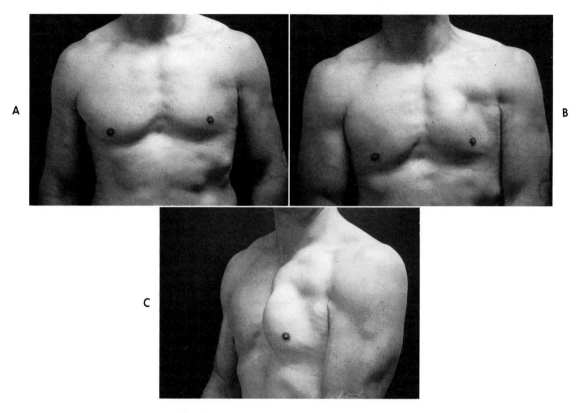

FIG. 41-3. Left pectoralis major avulsion in a lineman. Frontal view with the muscle relaxed, (**A**), and contracted, (**B**). **C,** Oblique view of the contracted muscle, accentuating cosmetic deformity. Player had minimal functional loss.

accompanying weakness makes a rotator cuff tear the primary differential diagnosis. An MRI allays concerns about the integrity of the rotator cuff tendons and demonstrates hemorrhage in the subacromial bursa. Once a tear has been ruled out, therapy can begin (as delineated in the section on bursitis). Despite continuity of the cuff, the injury can be debilitating for 6 to 8 weeks.

Pectoralis Major

Pectoralis major rupture can occur in the weight room or on the playing field. As with the other tendon ruptures, it happens secondary to an intrinsic mechanism. The diagnosis is usually obvious based on history and the palpable (often visible) defect present on physical examination (Fig. 41-3). Most cases constitute a partial rupture and, despite their cosmetic deformity, are rarely of major functional significance. In cases where there is a question of strain versus tear, MRI is a useful diagnostic modality. If functional deficit is a problem, the tendon can be repaired primarily or reattached to its origin lateral to the bicipital groove of the humerus. A recent study has suggested suture anchors as an alternative to the traditional drill hole fixation technique.[48] The decision to operatively reconstruct the pectoralis must not be undertaken lightly in a high level athlete. Prolonged immobilization to protect the repair, muscle atrophy, joint stiffness, and potential failure to regain strength may make the treatment more debilitating than the injury.

Triceps Brachii

The triceps muscle can also suffer a complete or partial tear in the substance of the tendon near its distal insertion into the olecranon. More often the extensor mechanism fails through the bone, and an avulsion fracture is seen. The literature contains an interesting case report of a weight lifter who suffered triceps tendon rupture after multiple local steroid injections for olecranon bursitis.[67] However, history revealed that the patient had also been abusing anabolic steroids so the true detriment to the tendon by the injections is undetermined. Primary repair is required for complete injuries to restore extensor function. The tendon is reapproximated to the olecranon using nonabsorbable braided suture in a modified Kesseler stitch after debriding and abrading the original attachment site. Depending on tissue quality and the adequacy of repair, active flexion and passive extension motion of the elbow can begin at 2 to 3 weeks. A hinged brace with flexion block is used to limit flexion to approximately 90 degrees for another 3 weeks. At 6 weeks after repair light active concentric strengthening is begun, and full range of motion should be obtained. Eccentric strengthening should be avoided for 3 to 4 months after the repair.

Biceps Brachii

An overload of the short head of the biceps brachii usually results in an avulsion fracture at its origin from the coracoid, whereas the long head tears in its tendinous

portion in the bicipital groove of the humerus. Proximal tears occur more commonly (96%) than distal (less than 3%),[24] but the proximal tears are more commonly attritional. Distal ruptures are secondary to a single acute overload with the elbow in 90 degrees of flexion at the moment of rupture. About 80% occur in the dominant arm, and the average age is 50 years (range 20 to 70 years). Distal biceps tendinitis is frequently seen in the weight lifter, and chronic inflammation in this area has been suggested as a cause of tendon attrition associated with later rupture. There is only one documented case of distal biceps rupture in a female described in the literature.[47]

The defect is usually obvious but may be subtle in a very large individual. On clinical examination unequal side-to-side supination strength may be the only finding and warrants further investigation if the patient's history correlates. It is important to check for asymmetric muscular development, although this is infrequently seen in football players, with the possible exception of the quarterback. Other diagnoses to consider are biceps paralysis from musculocutaneous nerve injury, lipoma of the distal biceps, partial rupture of the muscle (Fig. 41-4), and fibrosis of the distal tendon. Treatment can be either open or closed. Studies have shown return to normal strength at 1 year with nonoperative treatment,[12] but others have shown up to a 55% loss of supination strength and an average loss of about 30% of flexion power.[4,51] In a young laborer loss of supination strength (required to drive a screw, for example) may be disabling. Patients who are treated nonoperatively also sometimes complain of chronic antecubital pain.[51]

The currently preferred open technique is the Mayo Clinic modification[19] of the two-incision technique originally described by Boyd and Anderson.[8] The authors favor surgical repair with this technique because of the lower rate of neurologic complications and superior functional results relative to a single anterior incision procedure. There are 98% good to excellent results obtained with surgical repair.[4] If there is significant motor weakness, operative repair has been undertaken with some improvement of strength even long after the initial injury.[51] Our postoperative rehabilitation protocol entails splint immobilization for 4 weeks. Active elbow extension exercises in conjunction with passive flexion are performed for the following 4 weeks. At 2 months after repair the patient may perform active flexion and supination against gravity, with resistance strengthening delayed until 3 months after surgery. Return to sports activity is achieved at 4 to 6 months.

Biceps Tendon Dislocation

Tear of the transverse humeral ligament from its medial attachment on the lesser tuberosity can occur when a quarterback is hit while in the middle of his throwing motion. While the arm is externally rotated, the tension of the proximal biceps tendon peels off the ligament as it dislocates medially over the lesser tuberosity. Players in whom the inclination of the medial wall of the bicipital groove is less than 30 degrees are more susceptible to dislocation of the biceps tendon.[53]

The player complains of anterior shoulder pain and a click or snapping sensation during the throwing motion. When the arm is externally rotated, especially with the biceps actively contracted, the tendon dislocates medially. With internal rotation the tendon returns to the bicipital groove. The bicipital groove is tender to palpation, and the motion of the tendon can often be palpated by internally and externally rotating the humerus while the arm is abducted to 90 degrees. In the past a tunnel view of the groove has been helpful diagnostically if osteophytes are present at the margins. Unfortunately, radiographs are of little value in the acute injury. Although CT arthrogram is also effective, a noninvasive axial T2-weighted MRI is the diagnostic procedure of choice today. In either the acute or chronic injury the position of the low signal tendon is readily apparent in contrast to the bright signal of the joint fluid surrounding the proximal long head of biceps tendon at the proximal humerus.

Initial treatment consists of the standard protocol to combat acute inflammation. The arm is immobilized in adduction and internal rotation to keep the tendon in the groove and allow soft tissue healing to occur. If symptoms persist, operative intervention may be necessary. Options are reconstruction of the transverse ligament and tenodesis of the proximal tendon. Repair of the transverse ligament is most effective in the acute injury and may be combined with deepening the bicipital groove. Tenodesis is the more dependable and more frequently performed procedure. Methods vary from direct suturing to surrounding soft tissues to detaching the proximal tendon origin and forming a sling around the deltoid insertion. With tenodesis of any type, the dynamic function of the biceps as a humeral head depressor is lost.

Flexor Digitorum Profundus

The well-known rugby finger is a traumatic avulsion of the flexor digitorum profundus from its insertion on the volar base of the distal phalanx. This intrinsic injury occurs when a player grabs the opponent's jersey in an attempt to make a tackle. Although any finger may be involved, the ring finger is most susceptible for two rea-

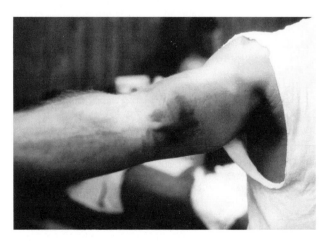

FIG. 41-4. Ecchymosis of the medial arm just above the elbow in association with partial distal biceps rupture.

sons: grip strength is primarily provided by the ulnar side of the hand, and the tip of the ring finger is the most prominent when the fingers are flexed into a grasping fist. As is well described in the hand literature, the tendon, with or without a bony fragment, can retract to various points within its sheath. Early operative repair is the treatment of choice.

NERVE INJURY

Neurapraxia secondary to a direct blow is the most common type of nerve injury in football. A nerve can be compressed between a bony structure and a hard object by a fall on the playing surface or a blow from a helmet. For the ulnar nerve, which is most superficial at the elbow, examples include trauma during the acceleration or follow-through phase of the quarterback's throwing motion and when a defensive lineman performs a swim maneuver to get past a blocker. Athletes with subluxation of the ulnar nerve, rather than frank dislocation, are more vulnerable to this type of injury because the nerve sits directly over the bony humeral epicondyle.[14,15] The radial nerve is well protected as it courses around the posterior aspect of the humerus, but it also becomes fairly superficial at the elbow. Here it is vulnerable to contusion and injury.

A crush injury to a nerve causes numbness and weakness distal to the point of injury in the normal anatomic distribution of the affected nerve. Severe radial nerve injury above the elbow may produce a wrist drop. Treatment involves immobilization with a splint in a position that relieves the injured nerve from stretch, keeps the flaccid or weak joint in a neutral position, and does not put pressure on the nerve in either its injured or subcutaneous segments. A cock-up wrist splint in conjunction with a padded sling is ideal for treating wrist drop. Most of these lesions resolve spontaneously with time, but those with severe hemorrhage within the nerve sheath may develop irreparable nerve damage or possibly fibrosis that causes an intraneural entrapment syndrome. Both of these problems may result in the unwelcome sequela of permanent nerve damage.

Obviously, more severe damage may complicate lacerations, puncture wounds, dislocations, and severe fractures, but discussion of the management of these problems exceeds the scope of this chapter.

Burners

The most usual site for a traction injury is proximal in the brachial plexus itself. The plexus is vulnerable to a traction injury when the shoulder is depressed relative to the thorax, especially when the neck is tilted away from the side receiving the blow. The high-impact positions of offensive and defensive back are susceptible during a shoulder tackle or block. Hyperabduction over an athlete's head can also impart a stretch injury to the nerve plexus.

When shoulder stress by either of these mechanisms results in the sudden onset of ipsilateral neck pain and dysesthesia or paresthesia in the upper extremity, the syndrome is referred to colloquially as a burner or stinger. The pain component of the injury is ephemeral,

lasting no more than a few minutes. Paresthesia or paralysis of the upper extremity can be much longer lasting. The superior roots, C5 and C6, are most likely to be affected, causing predominantly deltoid and biceps weakness. A more extensive injury may compromise lower nerve roots as well.

Initial evaluation includes obtaining an accurate history of the mechanism of injury. If recall is poor, consider head concussion as the primary or associated cause of symptoms. Physical examination should always include accurate evaluation of the neck and shoulder for possible fracture. Careful neurologic examination of the affected extremity defines the level and severity of the lesion.

The injury is generally self-limiting and responds to observation. Severity of symptoms at the time of injury is of little prognostic value.[66] If an athlete recovers sensation and full motor strength, he may return to competition immediately. If weakness persists, the shoulder is immobilized and further work-up is undertaken for occult spinal injury or complete nerve root avulsion. Radiographs, possibly in conjunction with CT, provide accurate evaluation of the bony anatomy. MRI is extremely helpful in evaluating soft-tissue lesions such as a herniated cervical disk. Ice may be applied to the affected side of the neck to decrease inflammation around the nerves. Repeat examination is necessary even if the player returns to the game, since late neurologic changes may occur from hematoma and inflammation.

Electrodiagnostic studies in persistent motor deficits show denervation or reinnervation changes.[28,75,76] Testing is of little value until 3 weeks, and often up to 5 weeks, after injury. Gentle limited passive range of motion is allowed after 48 hours. Once muscle strength has begun to improve, strengthening exercises are begun. Return to competition is allowed once full strength has returned. The concern is not only that the patient may reinjure the nerve before complete healing, but also that he will not be able to protect himself from other potential injuries due to weakness in the upper extremity and neck.

Regular neck and shoulder strengthening may help reduce the likelihood of recurrent injury. A variety of pads and rolls have been used over the years both to protect the plexus from direct trauma and to reduce the range of motion allowed in the player's neck. The reader is referred to Chapter 31 for a more extensive discussion of this topic.

Other specific commonly injured nerves are the supraclavicular (often in association with clavicle fractures), the axillary or musculocutaneous nerves (with shoulder dislocation), the posterior interosseous nerve (entrapment or direct contusion), the median nerve (carpal tunnel syndrome), suprascapular nerve (overuse in overhead activity), transverse scapular nerve (to rhomboids), and radial nerve (with humerus fracture).

VASCULATURE

Isolated vascular injury in football is uncommon. When it does occur, it usually complicates some other injury. Most often vascular lesions occur as the result of

an extrinsic mechanism—a direct blow or penetrating wound. Spontaneous arterial thrombosis has been described but is most likely due to unsuspected intimal damage in association with a minor injury. Aneurysm or arteriovenous fistula may present as late complications of vascular trauma to an extremity. Other than the acute capillary rupture caused by a contusion, thrombosis is the most commonly described venous abnormality. In the study of thrombus formation no specific sites are implicated more frequently than others, but the lower limb is more usually involved. Thrombotic episodes in the athlete are often associated with an episode of overuse, in contrast to those seen in the sedentary population. Some congenital anomalies (e.g., compression of the subclavian vessels by a cervical rib) may predispose to circulatory symptoms in the upper extremity, symptoms which may be subclinical until the patient participates in sports activities. **Paget-Schroetter syndrome,** or effort thrombosis of the subclavian vein, is an exceedingly rare cause of venous thrombosis, especially in an athletic population, but has been described.[64] A simple diagnostic test is to passively raise the athlete's upper extremity overhead; if the superficial veins remain distended, suspect a subclavian vein thrombosis.

JOINTS

In the high-stress environment of contact sports such as football, joint injuries are common. The spectrum of injury varies from a minor strain or sprain to a complete dislocation or fracture. Most joints depend primarily on their bony architecture for stability, with reinforcement in appropriate locations by discrete ligamentous and capsular thickenings. As a general rule, the joints of the upper extremity are more dependent on the support of ligaments than those of the lower extremity (e.g., the glenohumeral joint, which is a ball and socket joint with a very shallow socket). All the joints are synovial, and some contain fibrocartilaginous menisci (each end of the clavicle and the triangular fibrocartilage of the wrist). Traumatic synovitis can occur as the result of a single injury or from repetitive microtrauma to the synovial membrane lining a joint. Severe damage causes an acute hemorrhagic response within the joint, a hemarthrosis, whereas less severe or chronic damage results in a serous effusion.

Sternoclavicular Joint: Subluxation/Dislocation

The incidence of anterior dislocation of the clavicle far exceeds posterior dislocation. Patients experience considerable pain at the time of injury, but the natural course is rapid return to an essentially fully functional upper extremity. Sprains of the capsular ligaments also occur and are treated symptomatically. When an athlete suffers an **anterior dislocation,** the pathology is usually easily recognized by the prominence anteriorly at the base of the neck on the injured side. In the skeletally mature athlete this injury is rarely accompanied by a fracture of the clavicle, but in patients younger than 25 years it may represent a fracture through the proximal ossification center. A Rockwood radiographic view (patient supine with beam angled 50 degrees cephalad to

plane of body) confirms the diagnosis. A variety of treatments have been advocated for this problem. A sling worn as merited by the symptoms is the most conservative modality. Closed reduction is often possible in the acute setting, although it is difficult to maintain. Surgery in this area is fraught with complications, and there is a paucity of evidence in the literature that it improves the functional result. Young patients with a probable fracture through the ossification center (radiographs are of little help because there is no calcification medial to the epiphysis) should be treated closed. Extensive remodeling occurs with no growth abnormality; however, a slowly enlarging, nontender, firm mass at the medial end of the clavicle can develop. Attempted reductions of this "dislocation" are doomed to failure.

Posterior dislocation of the sternoclavicular joint occurs much less commonly. The patient complains of pain or, if the anatomic structures of the anterior neck are impinged upon, dysphagia, hoarseness, and even respiratory distress. The potential injury to the trachea and esophagus is responsible for the greater morbidity associated with this injury. Subcutaneous emphysema of the neck and anterior chest wall has been reported in association with posterior dislocation. Treatment involves closed reduction, which is usually successful and stable if performed soon after the injury. The reduction maneuver requires maximal retraction of the scapula on the affected side so that the proximal end of the clavicle can be levered anteriorly and laterally. A bolster is placed between the shoulder blades with the patient in the supine position, and lateral traction is placed on the arm with the shoulder abducted to 90 degrees. If this is unsuccessful, manipulation with the patient under anesthesia, percutaneous reduction using a towel clip, or open surgical reduction may be necessary.

Acromioclavicular Joint Separation

The scapula is tethered to the clavicle by the joint capsule of the acromioclavicular articulation, as well as the thick coracoclavicular ligaments—the conoid and trapezoid. An injury to this area happens when the arm or the point of the shoulder is struck in such a way as to drive it distally relative to the clavicle. Since the shoulder is one of the primary contact areas in football, acromioclavicular joint separation is very common. Cox[17a] evaluated 164 acromioclavicular joint separations and found that 41% were damaged playing football. The injury is classified in severity by the degree of separation that occurs between the end of the clavicle and the tip of the acromion. A **first-degree injury** occurs when a light blow to the shoulder causes only a strain or partial tear of the acromioclavicular ligaments. In more severe injury **(second degree),** the capsular reinforcements of the acromioclavicular joint are completely ruptured but the clavicular attachments to the coracoid process are preserved. Some inferior displacement of the acromion is usually seen on radiographs, and motion at the joint is clinically palpable. **Third-degree injury** involves complete tear of both the acromioclavicular ligaments and the coracoclavicular ligaments, and the displacement is readily evident on both clinical examination and radiograph. If there is a question of the degree of displace-

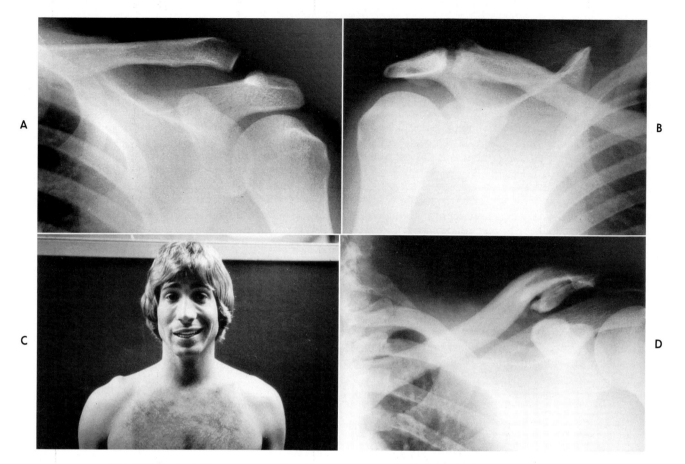

FIG. 41-5. A, Grade II acromioclavicular separation is demonstrated in this anteroposterior (AP) view of left shoulder. Although Grades I and II injuries have less severe ligament damage, they are associated with higher incidence of **chondrolysis, (B),** as seen in this AP view of the right shoulder (in a different player) after a Grade I injury. Note loss of bone density and subchondral erosion at the superior margin of the clavicle. **C,** Prominence over the acromioclavicular joint is caused by residual displacement or osteophyte formation after a Grade II or Grade III injury. **D,** Calcification of the coracoacromial ligaments can be seen as a late sequela of Grade III acromioclavicular separation as observed in this radiograph.

ment, weighted radiographs can be taken in which 10-lb weights are attached to each wrist and AP views of both shoulders are taken for comparison. If the patient holds the weights in his hands, muscular contraction about the shoulder may diminish the degree of separation seen (Fig. 41-5).

Grade I and II injuries are treated with a sling to support the humerus and acromion until symptoms subside, usually in 2 to 4 weeks, depending on the severity of the injury. These injuries are quite painful, and the patient should be instructed to expect occasional exacerbations of pain once regular use of the upper extremity is allowed, especially with activities that involve axial traction and deltoid muscle contraction (e.g., opening a heavy door). Some physicians advocate the use of a sling that not only supports the arm but also applies a downward force to the end of the clavicle to better reduce the joint. The most well-known version commercially available is the Kenny Howard splint. It is most useful in the nonoperative treatment of Grade III acromioclavicular separations but has a high incidence of associated skin

complications. Careful patient selection and instruction, in conjunction with close supervision, are requisite for its safe use.

When the injury is Grade III or higher, some authors advocate the surgical reconstruction of the coracoclavicular ligaments with either local ligament (transfer of the coracoacromial ligament), graft from other areas (semitendinosis, palmaris longus), augmentation with synthetic suture materials, or reduction of the acromioclavicular joint and temporary fixation with either a screw or threaded K-wires across the joint. Surgical treatment of Grade III injuries is controversial but is thought by some to allow quicker return to activity with a better long-term result. However, many athletes function perfectly well with complete dislocation of the acromioclavicular joint. We advocate surgical repair of Grade III separations in the throwing athlete and those unwilling to tolerate the cosmetic deformity.

Ectopic calcification can occur in and around the joint after acromioclavicular subluxation, making a prominent joint even more prominent. It is undetermined whether

the bony hypertrophy is secondary to recurrent capsular damage causing a traction osteophyte or whether it represents early posttraumatic arthritis.

Glenohumeral Dislocation

About 98% of shoulder dislocations are anterior or anteroinferior. In contrast to the direct forces that are responsible for either acromioclavicular joint separation, indirect forces are the standard mechanism for anterior and posterior shoulder dislocations. Anterior dislocations are the result of a fall on an abducted arm with an external rotation stress that can easily occur during a pileup or an arm tackle. The diagnosis is readily apparent on the field, since the arm is held in abduction and external rotation. The humeral head may be readily palpable.

After the diagnosis has been made, we favor immediate reduction of the dislocation before the onset of muscle spasm increases the difficulty of relocation. In cases where reduction is difficult, radiographs should be obtained. If these are normal, reduction should proceed with the assistance of analgesia and muscle relaxants.

The player with a glenohumeral dislocation is placed in a sling for 4 weeks before beginning range of motion and strengthening exercises. MRI may be performed to identify the presence of a soft-tissue Bankart lesion. If a Bankart lesion is present, consideration should be given to operative stabilization of the acute first-time dislocation. Arthroscopic stabilization in this situation requires 4 weeks of immobilization, which is the protocol the patient would be following even without surgery. The advantage of surgery is that the potential for healing without recurrent instability is greatly improved by restoring the ligamentous anatomy of the shoulder. There have been numerous reports in the literature supporting arthroscopic stabilization of acute first-time dislocations, with redislocation rates of between 4% and 20%.[46,74]

The reader is referred to Chapter 7 for a more comprehensive discussion of this subject.

Medial Collateral Ligament of Elbow

The stabilizing structures of the medial aspect of the elbow have been extensively described both anatomically and biomechanically. In brief, the medial collateral ligament is composed of anterior, posterior, and oblique fiber bundles. Functionally the anterior is the most important portion of the ligament. It extends from the medial humeral epicondyle to a small osseous ridge on the medial coronoid process (the sublime tubercle). Like many of the ligaments in the body that stabilize hinge joints with a large range of motion, it has different fascicles that tighten depending on joint position. The most anterior fibers of the anterior portion of the ligament are tight in complete elbow extension, and the more posterior fibers tighten in flexion. The posterior ligament is a thinner fan-shaped structure that takes up tension only in flexion greater than 90 degrees. The oblique portion of the medial collateral ligament attaches at the medial olecranon and medial coronoid process and is of minimal clinical significance.

There are many ways to suffer a valgus stress to the elbow, and a subsequent medial collateral ligament

sprain, on the football field. Any time the hand is fixed against an object, the elbow is vulnerable. A common mechanism is when the outstretched hand is placed on the ground to break a fall or to maintain balance by a running back struggling for a few extra yards. The injury can also be seen in offensive linemen who, while locked up with a defender, are struck on the outside of the elbow by the helmet of a running back who is trying to make a hole where one does not exist.

The injury mechanism can usually be very accurately described by the athlete. Symptoms of severe pain with attempted motion of the elbow are described. The local tenderness over the medial epicondyle is accompanied by obvious swelling. Ligamentous laxity can be best assessed by imparting a gentle valgus stress while flexing the elbow to about 20 degrees. Bony stability while the elbow is fully extended precludes accurate evaluation of the ligament in this position. Radiographs are imperative due to the high incidence of medial humeral epicondyle avulsion with this injury, although one must be aware of normal anatomic variants in this area that can mimic fracture (Fig. 41-6). Associated injuries common to severe medial collateral ligament sprain are radial neck and head fractures, traction injury to the ulnar nerve, and avulsion of the flexor-pronator origin from the humerus.

Treatment acutely requires immobilization and judicious use of ice. Avoid the ulnar nerve when applying ice packs to prevent adding an iatrogenic nerve injury to an isolated ligament injury. Grade I or II sprains are treated with early range of motion. Continuous passive motion machines are helpful in this regard. Grade III sprains are best treated with surgical reconstruction of the ligament. Whether treated operatively or nonoperatively, a lateral brace to prevent valgus stress across the elbow can be worn (if rules permit) to allow earlier return to play (Fig. 41-7).

Ulnar Collateral Ligament of Thumb

Linemen are constantly subjecting their thumbs to an abduction stress, resulting in ulnar collateral ligament insufficiency of the metacarpophalangeal joint. This injury is the same as the original **gamekeeper's thumb** in which repetitive daily microtrauma induces laxity within the ligament. Rarely does this attritional injury warrant reconstruction in the active athlete, since the thumb is quite functional and usually minimally symptomatic. However, acute ruptures do occur. Immobilization and bracing are the initial treatment, with return to play in a brace or thumb spica cast. Reconstruction of the extremely unstable or symptomatic thumb can be undertaken early in the off-season, but many players at the professional level opt for delay until after their active playing days are over because of the prolonged rehabilitation required.

Phalanx Dislocations

Dislocations of the proximal interphalangeal joint are the most common ligament injury to the hand and are thus frequently encountered on the football field. Many times the injury to the proximal joint is simply a mild to moderate sprain or a jammed finger. The joint is painful

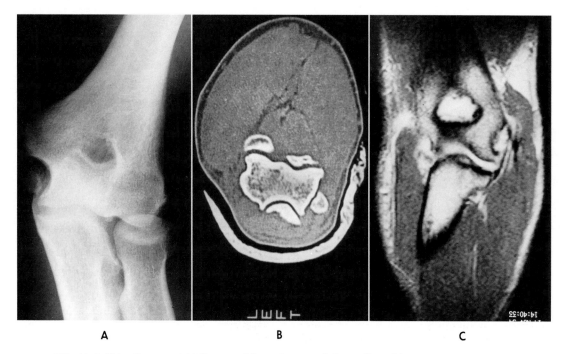

A   B   C

FIG. 41-6. This elbow was initially x-rayed for evaluation of ulnar collateral ligament strain. Because of technically inadequate views, possibility of avulsion fracture was entertained. **A,** True anteroposterior radiograph demonstrates developmental lack of fusion of medial humeral condyle's ossification center, as seen by rounded and dense bony margins. **B,** Axial computed tomography scan confirms diagnosis. Note thick cortical bone of medial humerus and of separate ossification center. **C,** Sagittal magnetic resonance image shows continuity of collateral ligament.

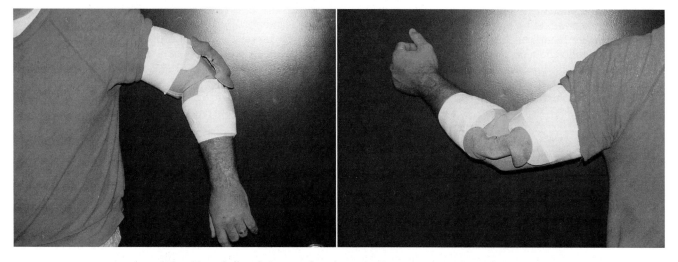

FIG. 41-7. Hinged lateral elbow brace, taped in place over sleeve to protect ulnar collateral ligament against a valgus stress. Blocks on hinge limit motion to prevent full extension and maximal flexion.

and swollen, with decreased range of motion, but does not demonstrate any instability.

Dislocations are described according to the position of the distal component. For the proximal interphalangeal joint they can be dorsal, lateral, or volar, depending on where the middle phalanx lies relative to the proximal phalanx. For a dorsal dislocation usually the mechanism of injury is hyperextension of the joint with some degree of axial load. A complete dorsal dislocation requires in-

jury to the volar plate, and an associated injury to the collateral ligaments to a varying degree depending on the severity of injury. Lateral dislocations occur less frequently and involve direct injury to one of the collateral ligaments and partial volar plate injury. The volar dislocation of the proximal interphalangeal occurs rarely but can be the most problematic if it goes unrecognized or is associated with a central slip injury (Fig. 41-8).

Important factors, other than position, in determining

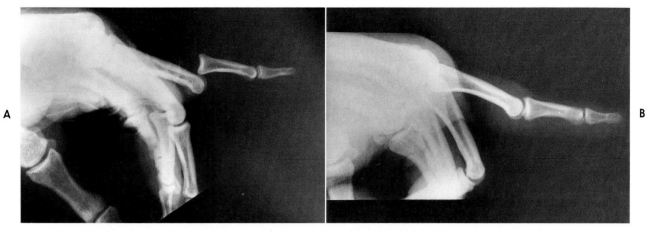

FIG. 41-8. A, Lateral x ray of dorsal dislocation of proximal interphalangeal joint. Bayoneting of distal fragment over proximal fragment necessitates longitudinal traction as first step in any reduction maneuver. **B,** Postreduction lateral confirms congruity of joint surfaces and no evidence of fracture.

the severity of injury and subsequent treatment are whether the dislocation is (1) open or closed, (2) reducible, (3) associated with a fracture, and (4) stable or unstable after reduction. Physical examination at the time of injury includes evaluation of skin integrity and the neurovascular status of the digit. Any glove or tape should be removed before attempting reduction even if the deformity is obvious. Open dislocations, as with any open joint or fracture, are an orthopedic emergency and require immediate irrigation, debridement, stabilization, and the appropriate intravenous antibiotic regimen.

Once the diagnosis is confirmed, closed reduction is immediately attempted. If the dislocation is dorsal, distal traction with an extension moment is applied to the joint. The proximal interphalangeal is then flexed to maintain reduction and keep the injured portions of the volar plate in apposition. Occasionally the condyles of the proximal phalanx buttonhole directly through the volar plate causing a dislocation that cannot be reduced by closed manipulation. Open incision of the volar plate is required to attain reduction of the joint in these rare cases. Lateral dislocations are reduced by gentle traction and realignment of the obvious deformity. Volar dislocations can be difficult to reduce unless the anatomy of the dislocation is appreciated. In this rare dislocation the condyles of the proximal phalanx pass dorsally through the extensor mechanism between the central slip and the ipsilateral lateral band (Fig. 41-9). The lateral bands become volarly displaced. If the digit is extended, the lateral bands tighten around the narrow diaphysis of the proximal phalanx and prevent reduction. Ideally, traction is imparted to the digit with both the proximal and distal phalanges in a flexed position.[70] The wrist may be dorsiflexed to further relax the extensor mechanism and allow reduction.

Dislocations of the phalanges can be associated with fractures in the form of avulsions at the tendinous insertion sites or impaction fractures of the articular surface. Initial treatment of a fracture-dislocation is the same as for a dislocation: immediate attempted closed reduction. Once reduced, whether a fracture is present or not, the joint must be assessed for stability. Evaluation includes

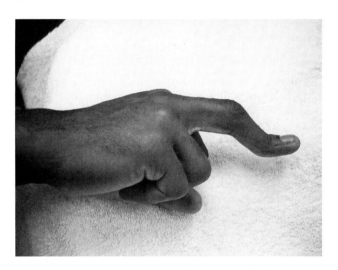

FIG. 41-9. Boutonnière deformity of long finger in defensive lineman. Loss of integrity of central slip extensor tendon with subsequent volar displacement of lateral bands causes flexion at proximal interphalangeal joint and extension of distal interphalangeal joint. This deformity may occur after volar dislocation at proximal interphalangeal joint.

full active range of motion performed by the patient, using local anesthesia if necessary to facilitate pain-free motion. The examiner then performs passive motion throughout the full joint range, including hyperextension and flexion stresses. Varus and valgus stress in extension and flexion is used to evaluate the collateral ligaments. If more than 20 degrees of opening is present on lateral stress, a complete collateral ligament rupture has occurred.[39]

Immobilization for 2 to 3 weeks followed by active range of motion is adequate treatment for either dislocations or fracture-dislocations that are stable after reduction. If irreducible, an open procedure is obviously mandated. Unstable dislocations require a more prolonged course of immobilization with careful supervision to confirm maintenance of the reduction. An unstable fracture-dislocation should undergo open reduction and an appro-

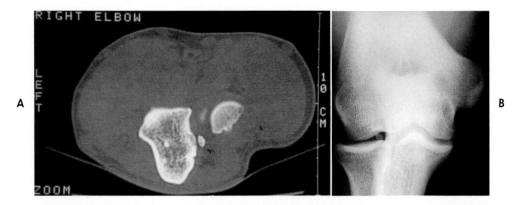

FIG. 41-10. Axial section computed tomography scan, **(A)**, and anteroposterior radiograph, **(B)**, of right elbow demonstrating intraarticular loose body. This lineman was able to play through the season with occasional pain and loss of supination, and he underwent arthroscopic removal immediately after the playing season was over.

priate stabilizing procedure depending on the size of the articular fragment.

Loose Bodies

Fragments of bone or articular cartilage in a joint can result from an acute articular injury or from the fracture of an osteophyte that has occurred in response to instability or a previous injury. As they move about the joint, they may interfere with its mechanical function and cause pain. The classic description of the symptoms is that the joint is fully functional until the sudden onset of a definitive block to range of motion. Often the patient can perform maneuvers such as shaking the affected limb or hyperflexing the joint to relieve the problem. Once suspected, the diagnosis can be confirmed with either radiographs, arthrography, or CT (Fig. 41-10). Treatment of choice is surgical excision, which can be performed arthroscopically in the major joints of the upper extremity. By removing the obstructing loose body, further joint damage by third body wear is prevented.

FRACTURES
Clavicle

The clavicle represents the only bony articulation of the upper extremity with the thorax. As such, the large muscles of the thorax must impart force through it to the upper extremity. The resultant stresses are considerable in all sports, but especially in football, whether the player is a lineman punching out with both hands in an attempt to stand up and control his opponent, or a ball carrier using a straight arm to fend off an impending tackle. Clavicle fractures are the result of either direct or indirect trauma (e.g., a fall on an outstretched hand); they occur most commonly in the midportion of the clavicle (80%), followed by the distal end (15%), and less frequently in the medial portion (5%).[61] When the functional integrity of the clavicle is compromised through a fracture, the strut of the upper extremity is lost and the scapula is allowed to protract and to sag inferiorly. The muscle vector of the sternocleidomastoid pulls the medial segment superiorly. These fractures are particularly

difficult in the mature population because (1) the distal type of fracture occurs more frequently, (2) the coracoclavicular ligaments are more likely to be involved, further destabilizing the fracture site and accentuating the superior displacement of the clavicle, and (3) muscle mass may interfere with anatomic reduction. Treatment involves preventing scapular sag with either a sling or a figure-eight brace while attempting to regain clavicular length. If managed ineffectively, malunion or nonunion can occur. Shortening of the clavicular strut secondary to overlap at the fracture site can result in malfunction of the shoulder. The resulting deformity is both disabling and cosmetically displeasing. Neurovascular injuries are rare, despite the close proximity of the subclavian vessels and the brachial plexus, but must always be considered in the routine examination of clavicle fractures.

Refracture can occur if the patient is allowed to resume activities too early in the healing process. This is especially true if the fracture has poor end-to-end apposition once reduced.

Scapula

Fractures of the scapula are high-energy injuries, usually associated with vehicular trauma, that occur uncommonly in sports. The easiest way to classify them, in ascending order of frequency, is by anatomic location: body of the scapula, spine or acromion process, and the glenohumeral articulation.

Body

Fractures of the body are rare but can be extremely painful. They are associated with a high-energy injury, so damage to other soft tissues such as the large vessels of the thorax must be carefully assessed.[69] Because of the overlying density of the ribs and associated injuries, they are often missed in the emergency department.[26] Body fractures are usually treated nonoperatively, focusing initially on minimizing bleeding and inflammation through the use of cryotherapy and immobilization for the first 48 hours, followed by symptomatic treatment and early motion. Even large displacements are well tolerated once bony healing has been completed.[2,34] **Cora-**

coid process fractures** can occur and are most often due to an avulsion of the short head of biceps with a portion of its bony origin.[6,29] A **fracture of the acromion** usually presents in conjunction with an acromioclavicular joint separation and is minimally displaced. It can be treated in a similar manner. The treating physician must not be fooled by persistent lucent lines that represent unfused centers of ossification and can be easily misleading.

Glenoid

Glenoid fractures most frequently involve the glenoid rim and are associated with an episode of subluxation or frank dislocation. Fracture of the inferior rim of the glenoid can occur after falling on the outside of the shoulder with the arm abducted (e.g., while clutching a football). Treatment is dictated by the resultant stability of the shoulder after a short period of immobilization in a sling for comfort. Large displaced fragments of intraarticular surface may require open reduction and internal fixation, but the results are unpredictable. Cain and Hamilton[10] reported five cases of scapular fractures in four professional football players. All were the result of a direct blow to either the anterior or posterior shoulder, and all involved the glenoid neck. Four of the five had extension into the glenohumeral joint. With nonoperative treatment and early motion only one fracture required electrical stimulation to attain healing at 6 months after injury. Nonoperative treatment with early active motion is the protocol of choice for the minimally displaced glenoid fracture, with or without intraarticular extension.

Humerus
Shaft

Indirect forces, such as rotatory torque, are involved in humerus fractures. They also take place by a direct force when a player falls on a flexed elbow. In the child and adolescent the bone may contain weak areas in the growth plates or in a lesion such as a unicameral bone cyst. Often these lesions are unnoticed until the stress of contact sports creates a pathologic fracture. Diaphyseal humerus fractures in the athlete are treated the same as in the general population, with sling and swathe followed by fracture bracing to allow elbow and shoulder range of motion. Open reduction and internal fixation are generally reserved for a delayed union or a change in neurovascular status with reduction. Early fixation may be considered in the professional athlete seeking rapid return to competition.

Distal Condyles

Osteochondritis dissecans of the capitellum and of the trochlea are possible due to an acute traumatic event or from recurrent injury to the elbow both on the field and in the weight room. If a chondral injury is diagnosed acutely, treatment entails maintaining range of motion of the elbow and avoidance of stress activities for a minimum of 3 weeks. Short-term problems include the development of loose bodies if the cartilage fragment becomes displaced. Long-term, posttraumatic arthritis with pain and stiffness is the predominant sequela.

Olecranon

An olecranon tip fracture is unusual, but when it occurs it is commonly caused by an avulsion of the triceps brachii insertion with a small fleck of bone. Treatment requires surgical repair of the ruptured portion, usually through drill holes in the remaining olecranon. The bone fleck is preserved, if large enough, to allow bone-to-bone healing. The joint should be carefully evaluated for the presence of debris during the case. Early motion in a hinged brace is allowed after 2 weeks. Active motion against gavity may be performed at 4 to 5 weeks, with resisted strengthening beginning after 6 weeks. Strengthening routines that involve eccentric muscle contraction should be avoided for at least 3 months.

Midportion olecranon fractures are the result of a direct blow or fall on the flexed elbow. They are treated as described in the trauma literature, with open reduction and internal fixation as determined by the displacement of the fracture.

The skeletally immature athlete may suffer from osteochondritis of the olecranon epiphysis. Controversy pervades the issue of whether this is a true traction epiphysitis caused by the pull of the triceps tendon or whether a component of the problem is impingement of the posterior cortex of the humerus on the olecranon from repeated forced extension of the elbow joint. The diagnosis is essentially clinical. On plain radiographs the appearance may be misleading; however, a bone scan may help elucidate the diagnosis.

Radial Head and Neck

Radial head and neck fractures occur secondary to axial load with a fall on an outstretched hand. Once again, the treatment is according to an accepted standard espoused in the trauma literature. Most can be treated symptomatically and with early range of motion. If displaced or comminuted, open reduction and internal fixation, or even radial head excision, may be necessary. Initial evaluation must include the distal radioulnar joint for the presence of an Essex-Lopresti lesion. Closed or open treatment may result in some functional loss, and cubitus valgus or varus may be late sequelae.

Forearm

With the possible exception of a nightstick fracture of the ulna, most forearm fractures in the skeletally mature athlete undergo open reduction and internal fixation to decrease the chance of a nonunion, optimize bony alignment, enhance healing, and speed return to athletic activity while allowing early motion of the elbow and wrist (Figs. 41-11 to 41-13).

Much controversy surrounds the question of whether internal fixation devices need to be removed electively from a patient participating in contact sports. An even more important question may be the timing of hardware removal. Most of the studies on forearm plate removal have been performed in the general population and are published in the trauma literature.

The treating physician's primary concern is the potential for complications from removal of internal fixation. Complications can be acute (such as nerve injury or

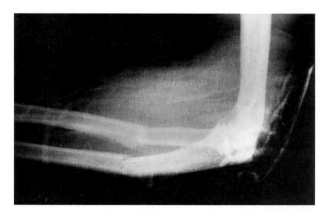

FIG. 41-11. Lateral radiograph of proximal forearm (in a splint) demonstrating transverse fractures of radius and ulna with angulation. Open reduction and internal fixation was performed, with good result. Hardware remained in place until end of player's active career.

A   B

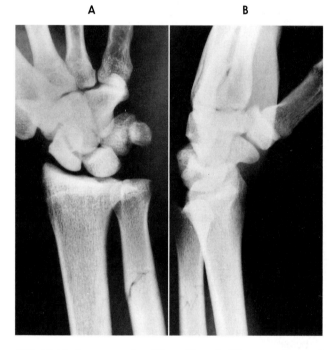

FIG. 41-12. Anteroposterior, **(A),** and lateral, **(B),** views of wrist of running back showing nondisplaced fracture of ulna. Athlete is allowed to perform noncontact workouts in cast until bony healing is seen radiographically and there is no tenderness at fracture site. Return to play is allowed initially with padded splint or cast, as rules allow.

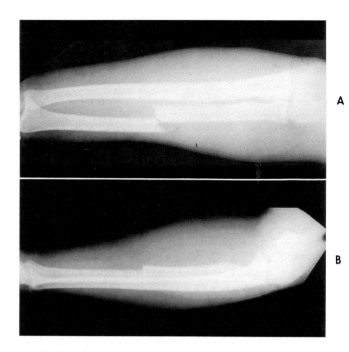

A

B

FIG. 41-13. Displaced midshaft fracture of radius in running back. **A,** Anteroposterior and **B,** lateral views. Open reduction with compression plate fixation is necessary to prevent nonunion. Complete bony healing must be attained before returning to full-contact football.

wound infection) or delayed (such as refracture of the bones under treatment).

First consider the arguments for removal. For the pediatric population various authors have proposed the removal of even asymptomatic internal fixation devices to avoid (1) stress shielding (with resultant osteopenia and incomplete remodeling),[68,72,73] (2) the risk of late infection at a retained implant site,[30] (3) iron toxicity,[77] (4) allergic reaction,[21,45] and (5) possible malignant transformation of the contiguous soft tissues.[22,27,32]

Schmalzried[63] evaluated 152 pediatric cases treated with a variety of internal fixation techniques for multiple disease entities, not only trauma. Of these, 7% were removed for infection at the implant site at a mean interval of 13 months from implantation. Most of the infected cases involved pins (6 of 10) and were located about the knee. The overall operative complication rate for the removal surgery was 11%, with failure of complete removal the most common unfavorable result.

The incidence of symptoms related to implanted hardware varies from 10% to 50%.[1,16,21,43,60] Richards[60] found no correlation between time of implant of forearm plates and the development of symptoms in 88 adults with an average implant period of 28 months (range 3 to 148 months). Of the 31% who were symptomatic, 91% obtained relief after removal of the hardware. Complications occurred in 3% and included one transient superficial radial nerve palsy. There was one refracture that took place 3 weeks after removal of a plate that had been in place for only 15 months.

We advocate removal of forearm plates only if symptomatic, and if so only once they have been in place for an absolute minimum of 18 months. Most professional football players retain the plates through their active career.

Hand

The hand, by both its prominent position and the high functional demands required of it, is particularly susceptible to injury. In addition to the torsional strains to the thumb and digits described in the section on dislocation,

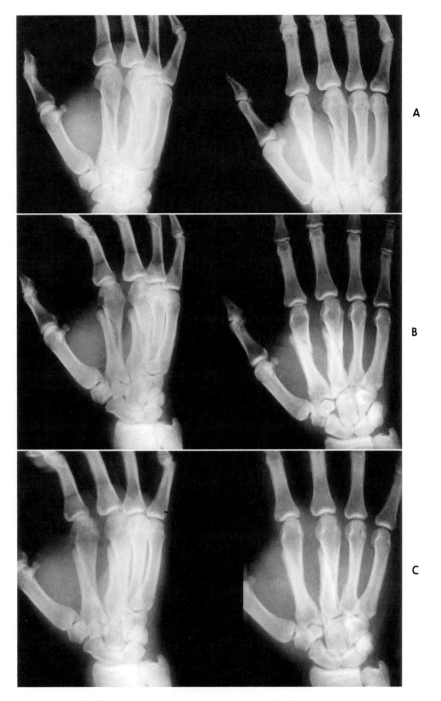

FIG. 41-14. Sequential oblique and anteroposterior views of right hand demonstrating spiral fractures of second and third metacarpal at **A,** injury, **B,** 3 weeks, and **C,** 6 weeks postinjury. Patient was treated nonoperatively with minimal shortening and no rotational deformity.

direct blows and crush injuries are common. Linemen endanger their hands every time they slap an opposing player's helmet or grab at a running back. Hands can be stepped on at any time. Prophylactic taping is used universally to augment the supporting structures of the thumb and fingers and to protect it from injury. A variety of pads can be used to protect the hand.

Once a fracture of the digits occurs, treatment hinges upon the configuration and stability of the fracture pattern (Fig. 41-14 and 41-15). Either surgical or nonoper-

ative treatment entails a period of protection from direct trauma to the hand. During this time the player may participate in noncontact drills. If smooth pins were used to attain fracture fixation, they should be removed before return to full activity. Miniplates may be left in place, but fracture healing should be solid before contact is resumed. The exception to this rule is the lineman, especially offensive linemen who are not supposed to grip the opponent. They can often function with the hand protected in a very well padded mitt that precludes finger

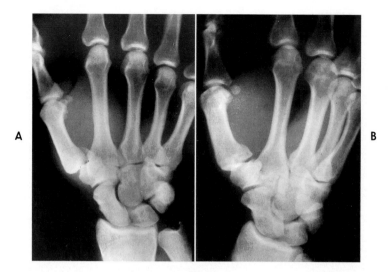

FIG. 41-15. Anteroposterior, **A,** and lateral **B,** radiographs of intraarticular fracture of base of first metacarpal.

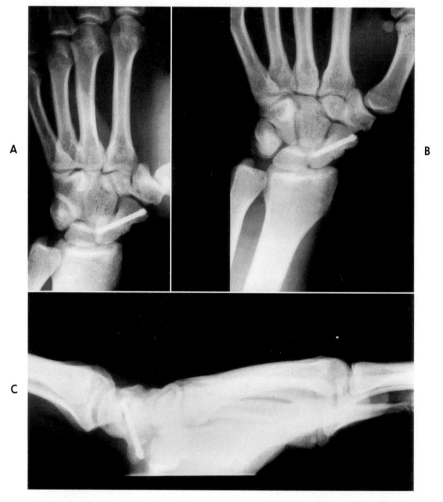

FIG. 41-16. Nondisplaced fracture of body of scaphoid carpal in nondominant hand of professional wide receiver. Player underwent fixation with a **Herbert screw** 4 days after injury and electric stimulation, postoperatively. He returned to full competition 3 weeks after injury in soft thumb spica cast and dorsal splint to prevent hyperextension of wrist. Oblique, **(A),** anteroposterior, **(B),** and lateral, **(C),** views are shown. No fracture line was visible radiographically at 7 weeks, and player had full range of motion with minimal pain after activity at 2 months postoperatively.

motion or grip but allows earlier participation after an injury.

Scaphoid

One of the most common fractures of the hand, as well as one of the most commonly missed fractures, is that of the scaphoid carpal. The mechanism is hyperdorsiflexion of the wrist, and the patient may report having heard a cracking sound. Examination demonstrates tenderness in the anatomic snuff-box and pain with attempted range of motion. A high index of suspicion must be maintained and specific scaphoid views obtained if routine wrist radiographs are indeterminate. Tomograms or CT scan can augment the diagnostic work-up.

Controversy surrounds the treatment of the acute nondisplaced scaphoid fracture in a contact sport athlete. Traditional treatment includes either long or short arm thumb spica casting for a prolonged period, usually not less than 8 weeks. Some sports physicians allow return to play in a modified thumb spica splint after 4 weeks of immobilization. For a professional athlete treatment must consider the athlete's ability to perform at an adequate level while encumbered by a brace, splint, or cast. He must be made aware of the potential complications of nonoperative treatment, including delayed union and possible nonunion as well as avascular necrosis. Extensive discussion is also required of the advantages and disadvantages of surgical intervention. Many players are willing to trade the risks of acute surgical complications for both the financial and potentially career-saving rewards of almost immediate return to a functional level (Fig. 41-16). After consultation with other professional sports physicians, we favor internal fixation of the scaphoid with a Herbert screw in the acute setting even for nondisplaced fractures.[59] This is, of course, only for the athlete at the college or professional level who has been extensively educated as to the pros and cons of the various modes of treatment.

SUMMARY

The upper extremity is subject to a broad variety of injuries in American football. Treatment of these injuries requires an understanding of the mechanical demands and pathophysiology unique to the sport. Through careful diagnosis and educated care, an athlete can be returned to his optimal functional level with minimal time lost from activity.

REFERENCES

1. Anderson L et al: Compression plate fixation in acute diaphyseal fractures of the radius and ulna, *J Bone Joint Surg* 57A:287, 1975.
2. Armstrong C, Van der Spuy J: The fractured scapula: importance and management based on a series of sixty-two patients, *Injury* 15:324, 1984.
3. Aso K, Takehiko T: Muscle belly tear of the triceps, *Am J Sports Med* 12:485, 1984.
4. Baker B, Bierwagen D: Rupture of the distal tendon of the biceps brachii: operative versus non-operative treatment, *J Bone Joint Surg* 67A:414, 1986.
5. Benmeir P et al: Chemical burn due to contact with soda lime on the playground: a potential hazard for football players, *Burns* 19:358, 1993.
6. Benton J, Nelson C: Avulsion of the coracoid process in an athlete, *J Bone Joint Surg* 53A:356, 1971.
7. Blyth C, Mueller F: When and where players get hurt: football injury survey. Part I, *Phys Sportsmed* 2:45, 1974.
8. Boyd H, Anderson L: A method for the reinsertion of the distal biceps brachii tendon, *J Bone Joint Surg* 43A:1041, 1961.
9. Burk DJ et al: Rotator cuff tears: prospective comparison of MR imaging with arthrography, sonography, and surgery, *Am J Roentgenol* 153:87, 1989.
10. Cain TE, Hamilton WP: Scapular fractures in professional football players, *Am J Sports Med* 20:363, 1992.
11. Carlson WO, Klassen RA: Myositis ossificans of the upper extremity: a long-term follow-up, *J Pediatr Orthop* 4:693, 1984.
12. Carroll R, Hamilton L: Rupture of biceps brachii—a conservative method of treatment, *J Bone Joint Surg* 49A:1016, 1967.
13. Chen J et al: Development of the olecranon bursa: an anatomic cadaver study, *Acta Orthop Scand* 58:408, 1987.
14. Childress H: Recurrent ulnar nerve dislocation at the elbow, *J Bone Joint Surg* 38A:978, 1956.
15. Childress H: Recurrent ulnar nerve dislocation at the elbow, *Clin Orthop* 108:168, 1975.
16. Cook S et al: Clinical and metallurgical analysis of retrieved internal fixation devices, *Clin Orthop* 194:236, 1985.
17. Coroso J: Idiopathic or traumatic olecranon bursitis, *Arthritis Rheum* 20:1213, 1977.
17a. Cox JS: The fate of the acromioclavicular joint in athletic injuries, *Am J Sports Med* 9:50, 1981.
18. De Lee J, Farney W: Incidence of injury in Texas high school football, *Am J Sports Med* 20:575, 1992.
19. Failla J et al: Proximal radioulnar synostosis after repair of distal biceps brachii rupture by the two-incision technique: report of four cases, *Clin Orthop* 253:133, 1990.
20. Forovzesh S et al: Septic bursitis, a neglected diagnosis, *Orthop Rev* 10:111, 1981.
21. French H et al: Correlation of tissue reaction to corrosion in osteosynthetic devices, *J Biomed Mater Res* 18:817, 1984.
22. Gaechter A et al: Metal carcinogenesis: a study of the carcinogenic activity of solid metal alloys in rats, *J Bone Joint Surg* 59A:622, 1977.
23. Gartsman GM: Arthroscopic acromioplasty for lesions of the rotator cuff, *J Bone Joint Surg* 72A:169, 1990.
24. Gilcreest EL: The common syndrome of rupture, dislocation, and elongation of the long head of the biceps brachii, *Surg Gynecol Obstet* 58:322, 1934.
25. Goldberg B et al: Injuries in youth football, *Pediatrics* 81:255, 1988.
26. Harris R, Harris J Jr: The prevalence and significance of missed scapular fractures in blunt chest trauma, *Am J Radiol* 151:747, 1988.
27. Heath J, Daniel M: The production of malignant tumors by nickel in the rat, *Br J Cancer* 18:261, 1964.
28. Hershman E et al: Acute brachial neuropathy in athletes, *Am J Sports Med* 17:655, 1989.
29. Heyse-Moore G, Stoker D: Avulsion fractures of the scapula, *Skeletal Radiol* 9:27, 1982.
30. Highland T, LaMont R: Deep late infections associated with internal fixation in children, *J Pediatr Orthop* 5:59, 1985.
31. Ho G et al: Septic bursitis in the prepatellar and olecranon bursae, *Ann Intern Med* 89:21, 1978.
32. Hughes A et al: Sarcoma at the site of a single hip screw, *J Bone Joint Surg* 69B:470, 1987.
33. Hunter M et al: The effect of anabolic steroid hormones on the mechanical properties of tendon and ligaments, *Trans Orthop Res Soc* 11:240, 1986.
34. Imitani R: Fractures of the scapula: a review of fifty-three fractures, *J Trauma* 15:473, 1975.
35. Jaffe L, Fetto J: Olecranon bursitis, *Contemp Orthop* 8:51, 1984.
36. Karpakka J: American football injuries in Finland, *Br J Sports Med* 27:135, 1993.
37. Kerr DR: Prepatellar and olecranon arthroscopic bursectomy, *Clin Sports Med* 12:137, 1993.
38. Kerr DR, Carpenter CW: Arthroscopic resection of olecranon and prepatellar bursae, *Arthroscopy* 6:86, 1990.

39. Kiefhaber T et al: Lateral stability of the proximal interphalangeal joint, *J Hand Surg* 11A:661, 1986.
40. Kirkpatrick J et al: The role of ultrasound in the early diagnosis of myositis ossificans, *Am J Sports Med* 15:179, 1987.
41. Knight JM et al: Treatment of septic olecranon and prepatellar bursitis with percutaneous placement of a suction-irrigation system: a report of 12 cases, *Clin Orthop* 206:90, 1986.
42. Kulund D: *The shoulder: the injured athlete,* Philadelphia, 1988, JB Lippincott.
43. Langkamer B, Ackroyd C: Removal of forearm plates: a review of the complications, *J Bone Joint Surg* 72B:601, 1990.
44. Larson R, Osternig L: Traumatic bursitis and artificial turf, *Am J Sports Med* 2:183, 1974.
45. Mayor M et al: Metal allergy and the surgical patient, *Am J Surg* 139:477, 1980.
46. McIntyre L, Caspari R: The rationale and technique for arthroscopic reconstruction of anterior shoulder instability using multiple sutures, *Orthop Clin North Am* 24:55, 1993.
47. McReynolds IS: Avulsion of the biceps brachii tendon and its surgical treatment, *J Bone Joint Surg* 45A:1780, 1963.
48. Miller MD et al: Rupture of the pectoralis major muscle in a collegiate football player: use of magnetic resonance imaging in early diagnosis, *Am J Sports Med* 21:475, 1993.
49. Misamore GW, Woodward C: Evaluation of degenerative lesions of the rotator cuff: a comparison of arthrography and ultrasonography, *J Bone Joint Surg* 73A:704, 1991.
50. Montgomery A: Two cases of muscle injury, *Surg Clin* 4:871, 1920.
51. Morrey B et al: Rupture of the distal tendon of the biceps brachii: a biomechanical study, *J Bone Joint Surg* 67A:418, 1985.
52. Morrison DS, Ofstein R: The use of magnetic resonance imaging in the diagnosis of rotator cuff tears, *Orthopedics* 13:633, 1990.
53. O'Donoghue D: Subluxing biceps tendon in the athlete, *Am J Sports Med* 6:103, 1973.
54. Palmer WE et al: Rotator cuff: evaluation with fat-suppressed MR arthrography, *Radiology* 188:683, 1993.
55. Penhallow D: Report of a case of ruptured triceps due to direct violence, *NY Med J* 91:76, 1910.
56. Pien FD et al: Septic bursitis: experience in a community practice, *Orthopedics* 14:981, 1991.
57. Powell J: Incidence of injury associated with playing surfaces in the National Football League 1980-1985, *Athl Training* 22:202, 1987.
58. Quayle J, Robinson M: A useful procedure in the treatment of chronic olecranon bursitis, *Injury* 9:299, 1979.
59. Rettig A: Personal communication, Sept, 1994.
60. Richards RH et al: Observations on removal of metal implants, *Injury* 23:25, 1992.
61. Rowe C: Shoulder girdle injuries. In Cave E (eds): *Fractures and other injuries,* Chicago, 1958, Yearbook.
62. Saal JA: Common American football injuries, *Sports Med* 12:132, 1991.
63. Schmalzried TP et al: Metal removal in a pediatric population: benign procedure or necessary evil? *J Pediatr Orthop* 11:72, 1991.
64. Skerker RS, Flandry FC: Case presentation: painless arm swelling in a high school football player, *Med Sci Sports Exerc* 24:1185, 1992.
65. Smith DL et al: Treatment of nonseptic olecranon bursitis: a controlled, blinded prospective trial, *Arch Intern Med* 149:2527, 1989.
66. Speer KP, Bassett FH, III: The prolonged burner syndrome, *Am J Sports Med* 18:591, 1990.
67. Stannard JP, Bucknell AL: Rupture of the triceps tendon associated with steroid injections, *Am J Sports Med* 21:482, 1993.
68. Terjesen T et al: Bone atrophy after plate fixation, *Acta Orthop Scand* 56:416, 1985.
69. Thompson D et al: The significance of scapular fractures, *J Trauma* 25:974, 1985.
70. Thompson J, Eaton R: Volar dislocations of the proximal interphalangeal joint, *J Hand Surg* 2:232, 1977.
71. Tibone JE et al: Surgical treatment of tears of the rotator cuff in athletes, *J Bone Joint Surg* 68A:887, 1986.
72. Uhthoff H, Finnegan M: The effects of plates on post-traumatic remodelling and bone mass, *J Bone Joint Surg* 65B:66, 1983.
73. Walker R: Biomechanics of fractures and of fracture fixation, *Orthop Rev* 12:65, 1983.
74. Wheeler J et al: Arthroscopic versus nonoperative treatment of acute shoulder dislocations in young athletes, *Arthroscopy* 5:213, 1989.
75. Wilbourn A et al: Brachial plexopathies in athletes: the EMG findings, *Muscle Nerve* 9(suppl):254, 1986.
76. Wilbourn AJ: Electrodiagnostic testing of neurologic injuries in athletes, *Clin Sports Med* 9:229, 1990.
77. Winter G: Tissue reactions to metallic wear and corrosion products in human patients, *J Biomed Mater Res* 8:1, 1974.

PART VIII   The Disabled Athlete

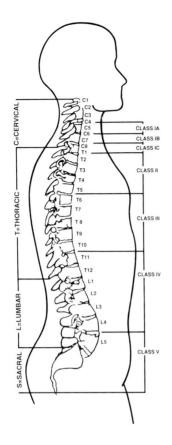

CLASS IA

All cervical lesions with complete or incomplete quadripelgia who have involvement of both hands, weakness of triceps (up to and including grade 3 on testing scale) and with severe weakness of the trunk and lower extremities interfering significantly with trunk balance and the ability to walk.

CLASS IB

All cervical lesions with complete or incomplete quadriplegia who have involvement of upper extremities but less than IA with preservation of normal or good triceps (4 or 5 on testing scale) and with a generalized weakness of the trunk and lower extremities interfering significantly with trunk balance and the ability to walk.

CLASS IC

All cervical lesions with complete or incomplete quadriplegia who have involvment of upper extremities but less than IB with preservation of normal or good triceps (4 or 5 on testing scale) and normal or good finger flexion and extension (grasp and release) but without intrinsic hand function and with a generalized weakness of the trunk and lower extremities interfering significantly with trunk balance and the ability to walk.

CLASS II

Complete or incomplete paraplegia below T1 down to and including T5 or comparable disability with total abdominal paralysis or poor abdominal muscle strength (0-2 on testing scale) and no useful trunk sitting balance.

CLASS III

Complete or incomplete paraplegia or comparable disability below T5 down to and including T10 with upper abdominal and spinal extensor musculature sufficient to provide some element of trunk sitting balance but not normal.

CLASS IV

Complete or incomplete paraplegia or comparable disability below T10 down to and including L5 without quadriceps or very weak quadriceps with a value up to and including 2 on the testing scale and gluteal paralysis.

CLASS V

Complete or incomplete paraplegia or comparable disability below L2 with quadriceps in grades 3-5.

FIG. 42-1. National Wheelchair Athletic Association classification system.

national, and international competitions. The Cerebral Palsy Association for Sport also became active and organized internationally.[17] Thus the 1976 Toronto Games were expanded even more to include blind, amputee, and paralyzed athletes. The International Coordinating Council was formed in 1980 as the governing body for sport for athletes who were disabled for any reason. That same year the Olympic Games for the Physically Disabled were held in Arnaheim, Holland. It was the second largest athletic event that year, with 2500 competitors and the first to include cerebral palsy athletes.[20] Demonstration events by disabled athletes were included in both the Winter Olympic Games in Sarejevo and the Summer Olympic Games in Los Angeles.[18] The first international competition for disabled youth took place at the Pan American Victory Games in 1989 in Tampa, Florida.[41] Today a wide variety of recreational and competitive sports are enjoyed by disabled athletes and are listed in the box on p. 885.*

CLASSIFICATION

To prevent any individual or team from gaining unfair advantage, an equitable medical classification was devel-

oped for the physically disabled. All competitors in the same class should have an equal degree of disability.[18] Classification is done by an international team of doctors who are certified by the sport's governing body. Protests for reclassification occur frequently. The physicians must also be alert for participants who may not cooperate in an attempt to obtain a more severe disability rating, thereby giving them an unfair advantage over their competition.[16]

Physically disabled athletes include those with amputations, blindness, cerebral palsy, dwarfism, spinal cord injuries, and *les autres* (locomotor conditions not encompassed in the other categories).[40] For wheelchair athletics some international controversy exists over the two methods of classifying athletes. The first approach is an anatomic and medical classification based on the site of the spinal cord lesion, the continuing function of diagnostic muscle groups, and the completeness of the spinal cord transsection. The International Stoke-Mandeville Games Federation and The National Wheelchair Athletic Association support this type of system (Fig. 42-1). Other agencies, such as the U.S. National Wheelchair Basketball Association, prefer a functional classification scheme based on the quality and quantity of active muscle and the ability to perform specific tasks (Fig. 42-2). Such a functional approach is thought to

---

*References 2, 11-15, 24, 25, 29, 32, 33, 36, 37, 43, and 44.

CHAPTER 42

Sports Medicine and the Physically Disabled

John G. Yost, Jr.
Daniel W. Schmoll

History

Classification

Technical advances

Benefits of exercise

Injury prevention

Injuries to disabled athletes

Summary

As we enter the twenty-first century, the physically disabled are making an increasingly larger impact on society as a viable and productive force. Before World War II 80% of paraplegics died within 3 years from complications of their disability.[15,17] Today 80% of paraplegics have a normal life expectancy. This remarkable turnaround may largely be credited to Sir Ludwig Guttman, who showed that if the paraplegic is well nursed in the earlier states of the condition, the individual can eventually learn to take care of himself or herself and avoid further sequelae.[15] It is estimated that 0.1% of the entire population of an industrialized nation is wheelchair confined, and preliminary 1990 census results showed 8% of Americans age 16 to 64, approximately 12.6 million people, have a mobility limitation. An additional 6000 spinal cord injuries occur each year.[10,13,38] With this growing number of disabled citizens and the passage of legislation to protect their civil rights, disabled athletes have been able to organize themselves and participate in many recreational and competitive sports. Through their accomplishments and special events like Rich Hansen's Wheel Around the World, the public has become increasingly aware of the disabled athletes and the challenge they offer to the sports medicine community.[19]

HISTORY

Sir Ludwig Guttman used sport as a therapeutic measure in his treatment of paraplegics. Guttman, who was knighted in 1966 for his work with paraplegia, introduced archery in 1948 as a therapeutic measure for the paraplegic war veterans that he treated at the Spinal In-

jury Center at Stoke-Mandeville Hospital in England.[17] In 1950 the first international competition among disabled sportsmen was held when Dutch paraplegic archers competed against the English team. The competition was such a success that it was repeated the next year with more countries invited and more activities added. The International Stoke-Mandeville Game Federation was established in 1952 as the governing body of wheelchair sports.[38]

By 1960 the Stoke-Mandeville Games had reached such popularity that the site was moved to Rome, where the first Wheelchair Olympics followed the regular Olympic Games. The games then moved to Tokyo as the site of the 1964 Olympics but were held in Tel Aviv, Israel, in 1968 when the Mexican government would not support Wheelchair Games. In 1972 1000 competitors met from 38 countries at Heidelberg, West Germany. Meanwhile, a surge of interest from other groups of disabled persons paralleled the development of sports for individuals with spinal paralysis. Amputee athletes were soon included in the Wheelchair Games and developed their own rules and regulations. Blind athletes also became organized on a worldwide basis with local, regional,

---

Sports for disabled athletes

- Fencing
- Equitation
- Basketball
- Swimming
- Archery
- Javelin
- Rugby
- Volleyball
- Tennis
- Water skiing
- Sailing
- Canoeing
- Rowing
- Hockey
- Downhill skiing
- Judo
- Ice picking
- Sledge hockey
- Goalball

- Boccie
- Snooker
- Pistol shooting
- Table tennis
- Bowling
- Fishing
- Triathlon
- Hiking
- Rafting
- Nordic skiing
- Golf
- Weight lifting
- Pentathlon
- Track
- Field
- Rifle shooting
- Slalom
- Wrestling
- Football kicking

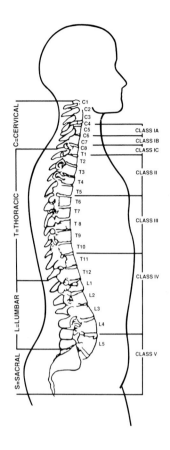

CLASS IA

All cervical lesions with complete or incomplete quadriplegia who have involvement of both hands, weakness of triceps (up to and including grade 3 on testing scale) and with severe weakness of the trunk and lower extremities interfering significantly with trunk balance and the ability to walk.

CLASS IB

All cervical lesions with complete or incomplete quadriplegia who have involvement of upper extremities but less than IA with preservation of normal or good triceps (4 or 5 on testing scale) and with a generalized weakness of the trunk and lower extremities interfering significantly with trunk balance and the ability to walk.

CLASS IC

All cervical lesions with complete or incomplete quadriplegia who have involvment of upper extremities but less than IB with preservation of normal or good triceps (4 or 5 on testing scale) and normal or good finger flexion and extension (grasp and release) but without intrinsic hand function and with a generalized weakness of the trunk and lower extremities interfering significantly with trunk balance and the ability to walk.

CLASS II

Complete or incomplete paraplegia below T1 down to and including T5 or comparable disability with total abdominal paralysis or poor abdominal muscle strength (0-2 on testing scale) and no useful trunk sitting balance.

CLASS III

Complete or incomplete paraplegia or comparable disability below T5 down to and including T10 with upper abdominal and spinal extensor musculature sufficient to provide some element of trunk sitting balance but not normal.

CLASS IV

Complete or incomplete paraplegia or comparable disability below T10 down to and including L5 without quadriceps or very weak quadriceps with a value up to and including 2 on the testing scale and gluteal paralysis.

CLASS V

Complete or incomplete paraplegia or comparable disability below L2 with quadriceps in grades 3-5.

FIG. 42-1. National Wheelchair Athletic Association classification system.

national, and international competitions. The Cerebral Palsy Association for Sport also became active and organized internationally.[17] Thus the 1976 Toronto Games were expanded even more to include blind, amputee, and paralyzed athletes. The International Coordinating Council was formed in 1980 as the governing body for sport for athletes who were disabled for any reason. That same year the Olympic Games for the Physically Disabled were held in Arnaheim, Holland. It was the second largest athletic event that year, with 2500 competitors and the first to include cerebral palsy athletes.[20] Demonstration events by disabled athletes were included in both the Winter Olympic Games in Sarejevo and the Summer Olympic Games in Los Angeles.[18] The first international competition for disabled youth took place at the Pan American Victory Games in 1989 in Tampa, Florida.[41] Today a wide variety of recreational and competitive sports are enjoyed by disabled athletes and are listed in the box on p. 885.*

CLASSIFICATION

To prevent any individual or team from gaining unfair advantage, an equitable medical classification was devel-

*References 2, 11-15, 24, 25, 29, 32, 33, 36, 37, 43, and 44.

oped for the physically disabled. All competitors in the same class should have an equal degree of disability.[18] Classification is done by an international team of doctors who are certified by the sport's governing body. Protests for reclassification occur frequently. The physicians must also be alert for participants who may not cooperate in an attempt to obtain a more severe disability rating, thereby giving them an unfair advantage over their competition.[16]

Physically disabled athletes include those with amputations, blindness, cerebral palsy, dwarfism, spinal cord injuries, and *les autres* (locomotor conditions not encompassed in the other categories).[40] For wheelchair athletics some international controversy exists over the two methods of classifying athletes. The first approach is an anatomic and medical classification based on the site of the spinal cord lesion, the continuing function of diagnostic muscle groups, and the completeness of the spinal cord transection. The International Stoke-Mandeville Games Federation and The National Wheelchair Athletic Association support this type of system (Fig. 42-1). Other agencies, such as the U.S. National Wheelchair Basketball Association, prefer a functional classification scheme based on the quality and quantity of active muscle and the ability to perform specific tasks (Fig. 42-2). Such a functional approach is thought to

PART VIII The Disabled Athlete

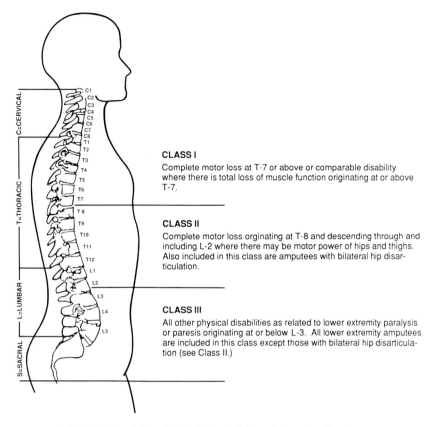

CLASS I

Complete motor loss at T-7 or above or comparable disability where there is total loss of muscle function originating at or above T-7.

CLASS II

Complete motor loss orginating at T-8 and descending through and including L-2 where there may be motor power of hips and thighs. Also included in this class are amputees with bilateral hip disarticulation.

CLASS III

All other physical disabilities as related to lower extremity paralysis or paresis originating at or below L-3. All lower extremity amputees are included in this class except those with bilateral hip disarticulation (see Class II.)

FIG. 42-2. National Wheelchair Basketball Association classification system.

have two main disadvantages. First, it may be abused by participants seeking an unfair advantage by falsifying their actual abilities. Second, it may penalize athletes who have improved their performance through training, developing coordination, and using trick movements to maintain balance. The development of split classifications may be employed in the future based on the advances in knowledge about wheelchair sports and the electromyography of the disabled. For team competition, each member of the team is assessed points based on his or her disability classification. A team classification is then assigned based on the summation of these points.[38] Amputee athletes are subdivided into 12 categories of limb disablement to take into account various combinations of upper and lower extremity losses.[16]

The United States Association for Blind Athletics adopted a three-tiered system for classifying athletes with visual impairments. This classification scheme incorporates both visual acuity and visual field. Studies by Makris et al[27] comparing blind athletes' performance within the current system support it as being valid.

TECHNICAL ADVANCES

Many of the sports in which disabled athletes participate have advanced dramatically with the support of sports medicine pioneers and the technology and development of adaptive equipment. This is best illustrated by the development of skiing for the disabled. The origins of the disabled skiing movement are found in Europe as

---

Classification of blind athletes

B1
- No light perception
  or
- Light perception but no hand motion recognition at any distance

B2
- Hand motion recognition
  or
- Visual acuity of 20/600 and below
  or
- Tubular visual fields of less than 5 degrees

B3
- Visual acuity better than 20/600 up to 20/200
  or
- Tubular visual fields limited from 5 to 20 degrees

---

early as 1935, when the Swiss attempted using underarm crutches for skiing. Siegfried Dreschler, the first "handicapped" skier, skied on one ski following an injury sustained in a downhill race in 1940. Franz Wendel of Germany was the first to compete as a handicapped skier with a leg amputation. He modified crutches by attaching short ski tips, which developed into the outrigger used by disabled skiers today. The Austrian Sepp "Peppi" Zwicknagel further advanced amputee skiing after losing both of his legs in World War II. After becoming a certified instructor, he helped organize demonstrations

of the amputee skiing technique that grew with popularity and culminated in the annual race at Badgastein, Austria.[22] Skiing as a form of rehabilitation for American amputees returning home from World War II was pioneered in 1944 by Gretchen Fraser, the first American skier to win a gold medal.[21] The "granddaddy of handicapped skiing in the U.S." is Paul Leimkuehler, a prosthetist and amputee from World War II.[22] As a pioneer of three-track skiing, using one ski with two outriggers, Leimkuehler was the first handicapped skier inducted into the Skiing Hall of Fame.[22] In 1968 doctors Paul Brown and William Stonek began a rehabilitation ski school that now exists as the Winter Park Handicapped Ski Program in Colorado. Many individuals with various disabilities have been taught skiing and have benefited in rehabilitation of their spinal cord injuries, cerebral palsy, multiple sclerosis, muscular dystrophies, deafness, blindness, and mental retardation.[21]

With the foundation of the disabled ski movement well established, advances in special adaptive skiing equipment continued. As mentioned, three-track skiing uses one full-length ski and two short outrigger skis for balance. It is the most widely known method of skiing for disabled persons and is used by those who have one strong lower extremity and two functional arms. Four-track skiing employs two normal skis and two outriggers. The ski bra, invented in 1974, is often used by four-track skiers, such as patients with cerebral palsy, multiple sclerosis, muscular dystrophy, or myelodysplasia who may have difficulty controlling their skis because of muscle imbalance from the hips or knees. The ski bra consists of a hook attached to one ski tip and an eyelet attached to the other. It allows the skis to move freely but prevents the tips from crossing, making both parallel and snowplow techniques easier. More advanced participants may use a flexible cord arrangement rather than the rigid

ski bra. The toe spreader was developed in 1975 for those who still had problems despite the ski bra. Canting wedges or slant boards inserted under the bindings were developed in 1976 to give a forward, backward, or lateral slant to the stance of those skiers who lacked flexion in their lower extremities.[22] Ski sledding is popular with paraplegics and bilateral short above-knee amputees.

The Arroya Ski Sled was conceived in the handicapped ski program at Winter Park. Careful attention to the seat, backrest, cushioning, and a roll bar resulted in a safe, efficient ski sled. While learning, sit skiers are attached by tether to an able-bodied instructor. Replacing the sit ski as the skiing technique of choice for most patients with paraplegia is the mono ski. This most recent development, consisting of a platform mounted above a single standard downhill ski, was developed in West Germany in 1982 and introduced in the United States in 1985. With the use of short adjustable outriggers for maneuverability, patients with spinal cord injuries as high as T2 have been able to experience the same contact with the snow as able-bodied skiers.[13,22] Blind skiers are able to learn and enjoy skiing working one-on-one with an instructor and may participate safely wearing a specially marked ski vest indicating their disability.[22]

With an efficiency value of less than 10%, the wheelchair is not an efficient mode of transportation.[38] Advances in wheelchair design and technology, however, have benefited those who are confined to the wheelchair. Today's racing wheelchair is built like a racing bicycle with lightweight aluminum frames, pneumatic tubular tires, and large rear wheels with a maximum diameter of 70 cm. Small hand rims, 25 cm in diameter, are used to attain a high gear ratio. The chair thus becomes hard to push but the potential for speed is maximized (Fig. 42-3).[26] No chains, levers, gears, or other mechanical devices are permitted for propulsion in competition. The

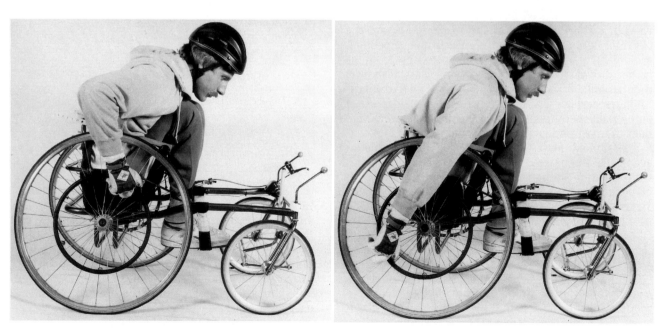

FIG. 42-3. Racing wheelchair with athlete strapped in. Proper propulsion technique for a paraplegic with wrist extension power is demonstrated.

maximum length for racing wheelchairs is 120 cm; no part of the wheelchair can protrude beyond the width of the distance between the outer edges of the hand rims or tires, whichever is widest. No part of the wheelchair can serve the sole purpose of reducing wind resistance.[30] The overall energy cost of movement, however, is less than for walking or running because the body mass is supported throughout. This accounts for the fast times of certain wheelchair marathon competitions, including speeds as high as 35 miles per hour.[38] Changing the position of the rear axle in relation to the athlete's center of gravity affects wheelchair maneuverability, stability, and pushing difficulty. Rear wheel camber, angling the top portion of the wheels inward, adds side stability. Most sport wheelchairs are equipped with antitip devices on the back of the chair, which help prevent the athlete from falling backward should body weight shift during use (Fig. 42-4).

Other advances in disabled sport include the use of energy storing, lighter prosthetic limbs for lower extremity amputees, and shock-absorbing cupped hand prostheses for upper extremity amputees.[13] Another specially developed prosthetic device is the flipper, which allows easier swimming for below-knee amputees.[37]

BENEFITS OF EXERCISE

Of course, the greatest benefit for any athlete is the fun experience of participating in sports and the thrill of competition. Many studies have also focused on the psychologic, physiologic, and social benefits disabled athletes receive from exercising.

Many authors have suggested a relationship between sports participation and improved mental health for the disabled. Research by Super and Block[41] has suggested that athletic participation for the physically disabled is associated with an improved self-esteem and a greater desire to function at the athlete's highest potential. When the profile of mood states was applied to college wheelchair basketball athletes, they reported feeling more vigor and less tension, depression, anger, fatigue, and confusion as compared with similar groups of nonwheelchair college basketball players and nondisabled collegiates.[35] A similar study showed that wheelchair athletes

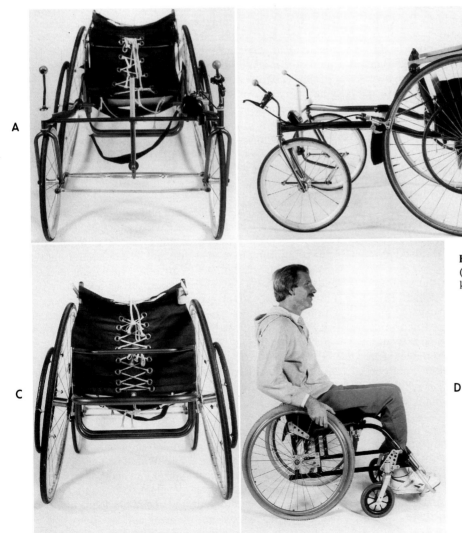

FIG. 42-4. Front, **(A)**, side, **(B)**, and back, **(C)** views of a racing wheelchair. **(D)**, Basketball wheelchair (side view).

had a lower score on the depression scale as compared with wheelchair nonathletes, again implying some value in sports participation in relation to mental health for disabled patients.[34] Other studies have also shown self-concept scores of disabled athletes are similar to those of able-bodied youths.[40] Shephard[39] described wheelchair disabled athletes as more venturesome and tough minded than their inactive peers. They also had a smaller gap between their actual and ideal body image.[39]

The physical benefits of exercise are currently a major interest of researchers. Sports have been employed for the rehabilitation of the disabled since 1948. It may initially be offered to improve stamina, strength, and skill in the use of a wheelchair or as an outlet of competitive desire.[18] Muscular strength and endurance may be improved by exercises, including arm crank training.[7] With habitual physical activity, forearm physical work was increased by 50% in one study. Dynamic strength and endurance of lifting weights increased by 19% and 80%, respectively.[17] Such conditioning helps the disabled patient overcome the difficulties of activities of daily living confined to a wheelchair.[20,28] Trained subjects have been shown to use fewer arm strikes to attain faster speeds against greater resistance, thus demonstrating greater efficiency with reduced metabolic demand.[29]

Interestingly, wheelchair athletes have been shown to possess muscle fibers with larger fiber areas than non-disabled olympic athletes.[42] Relative populations of different fiber types are genetically determined. Wheelchair athletes who have muscles with a high percentage of Type I fibers perform better in marathon racing, whereas those with a higher percentage of Type II fibers, especially Type IIb, are more likely to succeed in wheelchair sprinting.[4,42]

With the increased life expectancy of those with spinal cord injuries, there has grown a concern about their increased risk for cardiovascular disease. Although the upper body musculature of a paraplegic can be trained to increase strength and endurance, this does not necessarily correlate to overall benefits in cardiovascular fitness. It has, in fact, been difficult to accurately assess the cardiovascular fitness of many types of disabled athletes.

Two major physiologic problems hamper the exercise capacity of individuals with a spinal cord lesion and thus their cardiovascular fitness and exercise capacity. The first is that skeletal muscle paralysis reduces the overall muscle mass that is available to perform aerobic exercise. Their exercise capacity is often limited to the smaller arm musculature. This, in turn, is a leading factor for their sedentary life-style resulting in osteoporosis, skeletal and myocardial muscle atrophy, increased total body fat, and decreased lean body mass. The paralysis also promotes blood pooling in the lower extremities from absence of the venous muscle pump with a subsequent decrease in the circulating blood volume. The other major problem encountered by these athletes is a sympathetic nervous decentralization in which they do not have the ability to activate the sympathetic nervous system during exercise. This is seen as a diminished ability of the body to redistribute blood to the active exercising muscles again compounding venous pooling in the upright patient. The pos-

itive cardiac chronotropic and inotropic effects of exercise are also impaired. This inability of the body to mount a hemodynamic response capable of maintaining the increased metabolic demands is defined as circulatory hypokinesis. Thermal regulation is also disrupted. As a result of these two factors it is difficult for the participant to stress his or her cardiovascular system, and the V_{O_2} max may be limited by peripheral factors.[10] Thus the higher the level of the spinal cord lesion, the greater the likelihood for significantly reduced cardiovascular fitness.[8]

Furthermore, it is difficult to accurately assess the cardiorespiratory fitness of an athlete with spinal cord injury. The most frequently used device to estimate V_{O_2} max is the arm crank ergometer. It is economical, portable, easy to use, and is a nonspecific stressor that requires no skill. However, results do not necessarily correlate with useful information about the subject's wheelchair mobility capacity. This testing has also been subjected to criticism by many authors because of the poor reproducibility of predicting the athlete's V_{O_2} max. By contrast, wheelchair ergometry testing is a mobility-specific test of cardiovascular fitness. It may also be used with certain modifications to assess strength and has been shown to be more reliable than arm crank ergometry. Major disadvantages of wheelchair testing include concerns about validity from one device to another, lower mechanical efficiency, lack of commercial availability, and comparative difficulty to use.[8]

Some controversy continues in the literature over whether cardiovascular fitness in paraplegics depends on the sight and severity of the spinal cord injury or the activity level of the individual. In one group of spinal cord injured patients who participated in 4 to 20 weeks of aerobic training, the V_{O_2} max improved 20%.[3] In another study elite wheelchair athletes rated only 9% below able-bodied athletes, again expressed as V_{O_2} max per unit body mass, and 50% above sedentary wheelchair users.[17] There have even been reports of elite wheelchair athletes whose cardiovascular fitness exceeds that of sedentary able-bodied individuals.[28] Some evidence supports the value of training in road racing and basketball in improving cardiovascular fitness.[38] In one wheelchair basketball game, players may wheel as much as 5 km in a 40-minute period with an average speed of 7.2 km per hour.[5] Other investigators have shown a positive correlation of a higher V_{O_2} max with increased frequency and higher quality of exercise.[8]

Currently researchers are working to develop exercise programs that improve the cardiorespiratory status of the spinal cord injured athlete in light of his or her physiologic differences. Attempts are being made to reduce the peripheral limitations in aerobic training through horizontal posturing, lower body compression, sympathomimetic drugs, and electric stimulation of paralyzed lower extremity muscle groups.[10,38] Swimming has been implicated as one of the most appropriate sports for persons with disability because it develops coordination, promotes cardiorespiratory fitness, combats kyphosis, and decreases the risk for contractures and spasticity.[1,20]

The social implications for athletic participation include breaking the barrier of isolation by gaining new ex-

periences and friendships while countering the stigmatization that still may persist about disabled competitors. The community as a whole benefits by getting these disabled individuals back into the work force and allowing them to become more productive members of society.[20]

INJURY PREVENTION

Certain precautions and equipment are necessary for safe, effective training and competition among disabled athletes. Guidelines for equipment, racing protocol, and

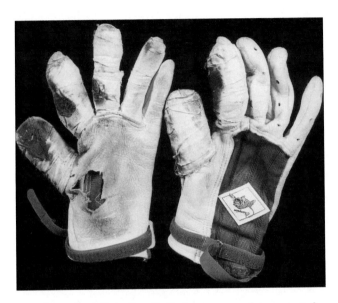

FIG. 42-5. Snug-fitting handball gloves are used to protect the hand. Areas of increased pressure are reinforced with tape, Elastoplast, or cloth friction tape.

safety are set by the National Wheelchair Athletic Association.[30,31] International agreement now exists regarding the specifications of competition wheelchairs. They have a standard foot rest height of 10 cm above the ground and a seat height no greater than 51 cm.[38] The forces applied to the hands during racing are great. Heavily taped gloves are necessary to allow sustained pushing with a minimum of soft-tissue injury. Generally racers wear snug handball gloves heavily wrapped with athletic tape, Elastoplast, or cloth friction tape for padding and adhesion at those points on the hand where the greatest forces are applied (Fig. 42-5).

Contact of the inner aspect of the arm with the top of the tire causes friction burns. This is especially common in the novice competitor. As an athlete becomes more experienced, the best configuration of body position, hand rim diameter, and a camber are found so that friction burns become less of a threat. Athletes wear tube socks or wrist bands to protect the inner aspect of the arm. Strapping is used to add sitting stability for the individual with a relatively high level of paralysis. This consists of a binder or belt around the athlete and the back of the wheelchair. Strapping is also used to control the unwanted motion of spastic lower extremities. Straps can also be used to secure the lower extremities to the wheelchair so that they cannot fall to the ground during road racing. If strapping is not done properly, the feet and legs can be injured and the athlete can be thrown from the chair (Fig. 42-6). A race official is responsible to rule on the safety of the wheelchair and the athlete before any competition. The use of padding on the seats is also helpful in minimizing blisters in long-distance road work. Proper clothing to absorb sweat and protect from adverse environmental temperatures should be worn. Athletes with impaired sensation should inspect their bodies af-

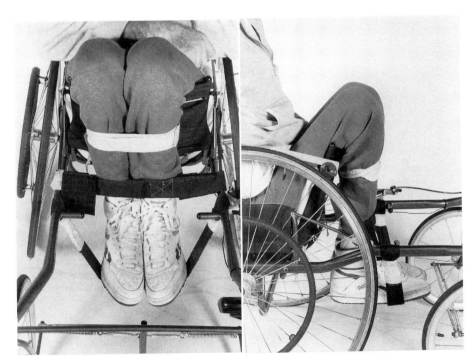

FIG. 42-6. Correct strapping for racing wheelchair. Note position of sacrum and buttocks.

ter each workout for pressure spots, cuts, and abrasions. Care and treatment should be initiated immediately upon recognition of the injury and the causal agent identified so that preventive measures can be taken. In long-distance road racing, with speeds up to 35 miles per hour, helmets should be mandated. Competitors who experience a mishap may be assisted in remounting, provided it is done in such a manner so as not to impede other racers or impart forward assistance to the participant. The rules of long-distance road racing do not allow simultaneous starts with foot runners. Commonly the wheelchair division starts 5 to 15 minutes before the runners. In races with foot runners the ultimate right of way belongs to the runner.

INJURIES TO DISABLED ATHLETES

There have been relatively few series on athletic injuries in this now very active population documented in the literature. However, the number of injuries may be high.[6,9,14-16,23] In one study 72% of all athletes responding to a questionnaire had at least one injury since they started participating. Some athletes reported as many as 14.[15] Yet in another investigation, which had a larger sample size with injury defined as time loss from participation, only 25.8% of the wheelchair athletes reported that they incurred at least one injury. This same study by Ferrara et al[9] also showed that 87% of the total number of injuries occurred to the extremities, with the

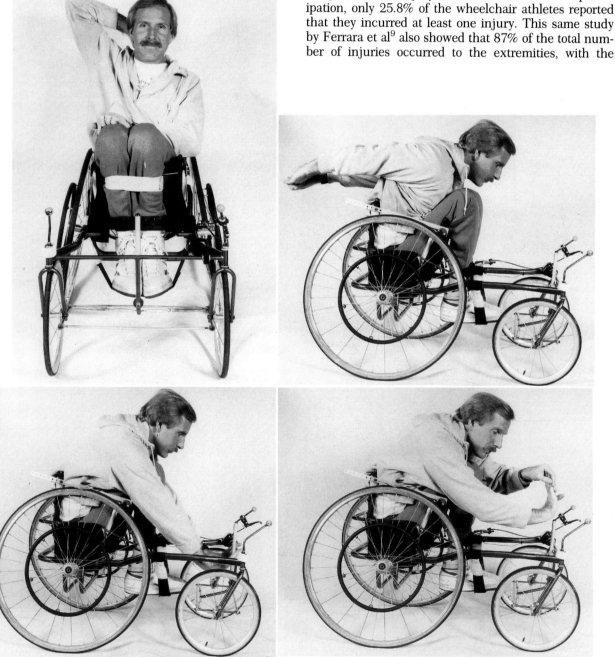

FIG. 42-7. Stretching exercises for the upper extremity with emphasis on shoulders and wrists.

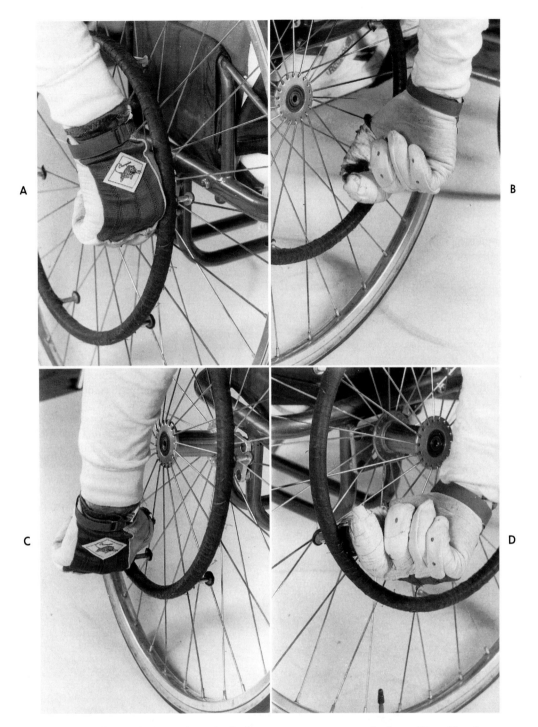

FIG. 42-8. Technique of propelling wheel when wrist extension power is absent. The athlete keeps gloved hand in contact with the rim using biceps power. Propulsion is provided with pistoning motion of shoulders using trapezius muscle. Front (**A** and **C**) and side (**B** and **D**) views.

shoulder, leg, ankle, and knee being the most affected. Many athletes do not seek aid from a physician because of an unsatisfactory experience associated with their original condition.[6] At the 1976 Olympiad more than 1500 athletes participated and 184 were treated for injury or illness. Common problems included muscle strain, headache, abrasions, burns, upper respiratory

tract infections, as well as catheter and colostomy changes.[15,16] This is generally supported by the experience at the 1986 International Flower Marathon for disabled wheelers where strains and sprains, urinary tract infections, and pressure sores were common injuries.[14] Interestingly, studies of snow skiing injuries show no significant differences in the overall injury rate between

disabled and able-bodied skiers; however, the types of injuries sustained do tend to differ between the two groups. Disabled skiers have fewer fractures and lacerations but more abrasions and bruises. One rather large study indicated that the disabled skier was at no greater risk of injury in terms of actual incidence rate or severity when compared with the able-bodied skier.[23] When comparing injuries in the 1989 National Competition of the National Wheelchair Athletic Association, the United States Association for Blind Athletes, and the United States Cerebral Palsy Athletic Association, Ferrara et al[9] did find a greater risk of injury in the blind athletes. In one large series, common sports associated with injuries were track 26%, basketball 24%, road racing 22%, tennis 6%, field events 4%, and swimming 4% of all injuries; 33% of all injuries were soft-tissue injuries, sprains, strains, tendinitis, or bursitis.[6] The shoulder, elbow, or wrist can be involved. Routine stretching with proper warm-up and cool-down for each workout helps prevent chronic overuse injuries (Fig. 42-7).

Improper push techniques with hyperflexion at the wrist cause *tendinitis* and *sprains* of the wrists. The pushing technique for a paraplegic differs from that of a quadriplegic with loss of wrist extension and triceps power (Figs. 42-3 and 42-8). Rest with a wrist splint followed by a rehabilitation program and instruction on proper technique are necessary to treat this injury and prevent recurrence. *Blisters* accounted for 18% of the injuries in one series. The hand and fingers were most commonly involved. The arm is also at risk from tire friction and irritation of the skin at the top of the seat post on the back of the wheelchair. To prevent these blisters, common callus formation is encouraged as initial protection. Taping fingers, wearing gloves, padding over the seat post area, and wrist bands or sleeves on the upper arms should also be used as needed. In this series 17%

of the injuries were *lacerations,* abrasions, or cuts including skin infections.[6] The fingers and thumbs in contact with brakes, metal edges on empty arm rest sockets, spokes, or push rims are at risk for injury (Fig. 42-9). To rule out bone, tendon, or ligament damage, immediate treatment and protection are initiated. Removal of hand brakes eliminates the primary hazard. Filing off the sockets of the arm rests, camber wheels, protective clothing, and gloves also prevents lacerations. *Decubitus sores* are caused by sheer forces in pressure, mainly in those athletes without sensation over the sacrum and buttocks. Friction from the chair, sweat, and newer racing wheelchair design with the knees higher than the buttocks are contributing factors. Decubitus sores require prompt treatment by keeping the area clean and dry and avoiding pressure on that area. Ulcers may require reconstructive surgery with removal of bony prominences and skin flap rotation. To prevent decubitus ulcers, adequate cushioning and padding are needed for the buttocks (Fig. 42-10). Frequent skin checks, shifting weight intermittently, good nutrition and hygiene, and clothing that absorbs moisture help prevent difficult problems.

Carpal tunnel syndrome is caused by median nerve compression at the wrist from constant trauma and compression of the heel of the hand with each arm stroke on the push rim. Carpal tunnel syndrome has also been reported in tennis. Night pain, paresthesia, decreased grip strength, and lack of digit dexterity are the most common symptoms despite a normal physical examination. Acute cases should be splinted, nonsteroidal antiinflammatory medications prescribed, and a carpal tunnel steroid injection considered. If symptoms have not abated after 6 to 10 weeks or if thenar atrophy is present and electromyography and nerve conduction studies confirm the diagnosis, operative decompression should be per-

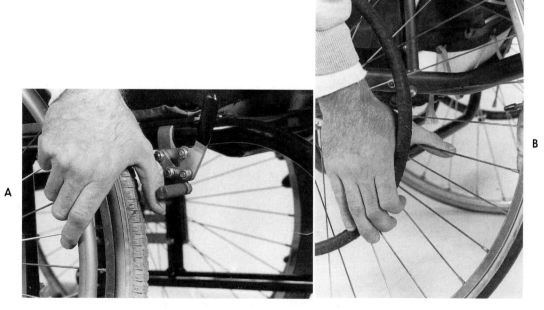

FIG. 42-9. A, Exposed brake handles need to be removed to prevent hand injuries. **B,** Injuries can occur if thumb is caught between spokes and frame.

formed. Decubital tunnel problems have not been reported.

Temperature regulation disorders—hyperthermia or hypothermia—have occurred in road racing and track and field events.[6,14] Athletes with spinal cord injury may have altered sweating responses with an unpredictable result. In the able-bodied runner, evaporative heat loss is enhanced in the legs as they move back and forth, whereas the wheelchair marathoner must rely on evaporative heat loss from the arms. Sweating below the level of the spinal cord injury may also be deficient.[4] A special problem for paraplegic and quadriplegic marathoners is vasomotor paralysis in the absence of active muscles to help pump blood past the valves in the veins to the heart. These problems, when associated with dehydration, can lead to hyperthermia. This can lead to heat exhaustion and sometimes heat stroke. The athlete needs to be rehydrated, moved to shade, and observed. If the skin under the arms of the athlete feels cool, the individual is sweating and probably losing heat adequately. If this skin is hot, the individual is not getting rid of enough heat and requires more fluid, fewer clothes, and cooling of the trunk and extremities. To prevent hyperthermia, the athlete must be well hydrated, wear clothing that allows ventilation, and minimize exposure to high temperatures, humidity, and sunshine. Unlike hyperthermia, which usually occurs during a race, hypothermia may become a problem at the end of the race.[4] When the wheelchair marathoner stops, heat production stops and shivering, which is the natural way to control heat loss, may not occur because of the spinal cord injury. The skin remains vasodilated, hyperemic, and saturated with sweat, allowing heat loss to continue at a high rate, resulting in hypothermia. In cold, rainy, windy conditions, slower competitors can spend more than 5 hours completing a race. To prevent hypothermia, all wet clothing should be removed and dry warm clothing and blankets applied. Adequate hydration is equally important in treating hypothermia and hyperthermia. The disabled sit skier is at increased risk for hypothermia. Because of lack of sensation in the lower extremities, it is important to periodically check the athlete's legs and feet to ensure they are not in danger of frostbite. A double wool sock has proved to be effective for providing warmth and guarding against injury to the stump for those three-track skiers who wear their prosthesis on the slopes.[22]

Racing wheelchair design

- Lightweight aluminum frame
- Pneumatic tubular tires
- Large rear wheels (maximum diameter 70 cm)
- Small hand rim
- Rear wheel camber
- Antitip devices

SUMMARY

Over the last several decades wheelchair athletes have expanded on the international level to take their place next to nondisabled athletes. The benefits for the athletes are physical and psychologic. Disabled athletes are exercising their right to accept the challenges and risks of able-bodied athletes. They are also experiencing many overuse injuries, similar to those of the able-bodied athlete and are at risk for certain injuries unique to their sport or disability. Physicians who treat these athletes

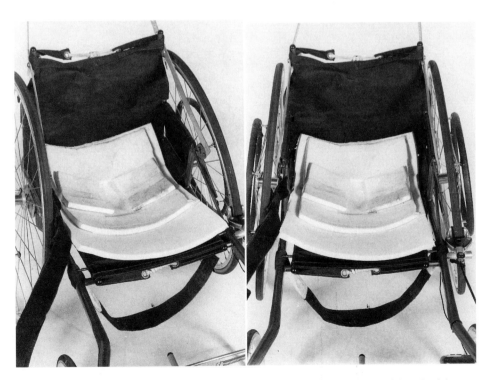

FIG. 42-10. To prevent decubitus sores, special padding is added to the seat of the wheelchair.

Resources

American Blind Bowling Association
c/o Alice Hoover
411 Sheriff Street
Mercer, PA 16137
(412) 662-5748

Aspen Handicapped Skier Services
formerly Blind Outdoor Leisure Development, Inc.
Attn: Edwin H. Lucks
0174 Meadows Road
P.O. Box 5429
Snowmass Village, CO 81615
(303) 923-3294

Handicapped Scuba Association
7172 W. Stanford Avenue
Littleton, CO 80123
(303) 933-4864

Horizons for the Handicapped
P.O. Box 2143
Steamboat Springs, CO 80477
(303) 879-4466

International Committee for Sports for the Deaf (CISSO)
Secretariat CMHSH82
CH-1861
Les Moses, Switzerland

International Stoke-Mandeville Games Federation (ISMGF)
Stoke-Mandeville Sports Stadium
Harvey Road
Aylesbury, Buckinghamshire
England
(296) 436-179

International Wheelchair Road Racers Club
c/o Joseph M. Dowling
30 Myano Lane
Stamford, CT 06902
(203) 325-1429

National Amputee Golf Association
Box 1228
Amherst, NH 03031
(800) 633-6242

National Foundation of Wheelchair Tennis
940 Calle Amanecer, Suite B
San Clemente, CA 92672
(714) 361-6811

National Handicapped Sports
451 Hungerford Drive, Suite 100
Rockville, MD 20850
(301) 217-0960

National Wheelchair Softball Association
1616 Todd Court
Hastings, MN 55033
(612) 437-1792

North American Riding for the Handicapped
Box 33150
Denver, CO 80233
(800) 369-7433

Special Olympics International
1325 G Street NW, Suite 500
Washington, DC 20005
(202) 628-3630

U.S. Association for Blind Athletes
33 N. Institute
Colorado Springs, CO 80903
(719) 630-0422

U.S. Cerebral Palsy Athletic Association
Jerry McCole, Director
3810 West Northwest Highway, Suite 205
Dallas, TX 75220
(214) 351-1510

U.S. Quad Rugby Association
c/o Brad Mikkelsen
1605 Matthews Street
Fort Collins, CO 80521
(303) 484-7395

U.S. Wheelchair Racquet-Sports Association
c/o Chip Parmelly
1941 Viento Verano Drive
Diamond Bar, CA 91765
(909) 861-7312

Wheelchair Sports USA
formerly National Wheelchair Athletic Association
3595 E. Fountain Boulevard, Suite L-1
Colorado Springs, CO 80910
(719) 574-1150

Wilderness Inquiry (offers canoeing, kayaking, and
    dogsledding trips for people of all abilities)
1313 Fifth Street, S.E.
Box 84
Minneapolis, MN 55414
(800) 728-0719

Winter Park Handicapped Ski Program
Hal O'Leary, Director
P.O. Box 36
Winter Park, CO 80482
(303) 726-5514, extension 179 or 286

---

should be aware of potential problems. Disabled athletes are independent, make few complaints, and impress observers with their ability, not disability. A keen awareness of these overuse syndromes and the unique qualities of these athletes with their poor physical image is mandatory for physicians dealing in these areas.

REFERENCES

1. Chatard J-C et al: Physiological aspects of swimming performance for persons with disabilities, *Med Sci Sports Exerc* 24(11):1276, 1992.
2. Compton D et al: Project PAIRS: a peer assisted swimming program for the severely handicapped, *Children Today* 17(1):28, 1988.
3. Compton DM et al: Exercise and fitness for persons with disabilities, *Sports Med* 7:150, 1989.
4. Concoran PJ et al: Sports medicine and the physiology of wheelchair marathon racing, *Orthop Clin North Am* 11(4):697, 1980.
5. Coutts KD: Dynamics of wheelchair basketball, *Med Sci Sports Exerc* 24:231, 1992.
6. Curtis KA: Wheelchair sportsmedicine. Part 4. Athletic injuries, *Sports n Spokes* 8(1):20, 1982.

7. Davis G et al: Gains of cardiorespiratory fitness with arm-crank training in spinally disabled men, *Can J Sport Sci* 16(1):64, 1991.

8. Davis GM: Exercise capacity of individuals with paraplegia, *Med Sci Sports Exer* 25(4):423, 1993.

9. Ferrara MS et al: The injury experience of the competitive athlete with a disability: prevention implications, *Med Sci Sports Exerc* 24(2):184, 1992.

10. Figoni SF: Exercise responses and quadriplegia, *Med Sci Sports Exerc* 25(4):433, 1993.

11. Furst DM et al: Motivation of disabled athletes to participate in triathlons, *Psychol Rep* 72:403, 1993.

12. Glesser JM et al: Physical and psychosocial benefits of modified judo practice for blind, mentally retarded children: a pilot study, *Percep Motor Skills* 74:915, 1992.

13. Hamel R: Getting into the game, *Phys Sportsmed* 20(11):121, 1992.

14. Hoeberigs JH et al: Sports medical experiences from the international flower marathon for disabled wheelers, *Am J Sports Med* 18(4):418, 1990.

15. Jackson RW: What did we learn from the Torontolympiad? *Can Fam Phys* 23:586, 1977.

16. Jackson RW: Sports for the physically disabled, *Am J Sports Med* 7(5):293, 1979.

17. Jackson RW: The value of sports and recreation for the physically disabled, *Orthop Clin North Am* 14(2):301, 1983.

18. Jackson RW: Sport for the spinal paralyzed person, *Paraplegia* 25:301, 1987.

19. Jordon T: Just 7000 miles to go, *Sports n Spokes* 12(3):12, 1986.

20. Klapwijk A: The multiple benefits of sports for the disabled, *Int Disabil Studies* 9(2):87, 1987.

21. Krag MH, Messmer DG: Skiing by the physically handicapped, *Clin Sports Med* 1(2):319, 1982.

22. Laskowski ER: Snow skiing for the physically disabled, *Mayo Clin Proc* 66:160, 1991.

23. Laskowski ER, Murtaugh PA: Snow skiing injuries in physically disabled skiers, *Am J Sports Med* 20(5):553, 1992.

24. Levy AM: The disabled athlete: an approach, *N J Med* 88(9):647, 1991.

25. Madorsky JGB, Curtis KA: Wheelchair sports medicine, *Am J Sports Med* 12(2):128, 1984.

26. Madorsky JGB, Madorsky A: Wheelchair racing: an important modality in acute rehabilitation after paraplegia, *Arch Phys Med Rehabil* 64:186, 1983.

27. Makris VI et al: Visual loss and performance in blind athletes, *Med Sci Sports Exerc* 25(2):265, 1993.

28. Micheo WF, Frontera W: Fitness and the disabled, *Bol Asoc Med P R* 81(11):447, 1989.

29. Molner G: Rehabilitative benefits of sports for the handicapped, *Conn Med* 45(9):574, 1981.

30. National Wheelchair Athletic Association: *A guide for wheelchair sports training,* Colorado Springs, 1986, National Wheelchair Athletic Association.

31. National Wheelchair Athletic Association: *Rules of long distance road racing,* Colorado Springs, 1987, National Wheelchair Athletic Association.

32. Norton B: The best little bass tourney in Texas, *Sports n Spokes* 13(2):8, 1987.

33. Page CJ, Pearson J: Creating therapeutic camp and recreation programs for children with chronic illness and disabilities, *Pediatrician* 17:297, 1990.

34. Paulsen P et al: Comparison of athletes and nonathletes on selected mood states, *Percept Mot Skills* 71:1160, 1990.

35. Paulsen P et al: Comparison of mood states of college able-bodied and wheelchair basketball players, *Percept Mot Skills* 73:396, 1991.

36. Prietz J: Second annual blade run, *Sports n Spokes* 13(1):51, 1987.

37. Saadah ESM: Swimming devices for below-knee amputees, *Prosthet Orthot Int* 16(2):140, 1992.

38. Shephard RJ: Sports medicine and the wheelchair athlete, *Sports Med* 4:226, 1988.

39. Shephard RJ: Benefits of sport and physical activity for the disabled: implications for the individual and for society, *Scand J Rehabil Med* 23:51, 1991.

40. Sherrill C et al: Self-concepts of disabled youth athletes, *Percept Mot Skills* 70:1093, 1990.

41. Super JT, Block JR: Self-concept and need for achievement of men with physical disabilities, *J Gen Psychol* 119(1):73, 1992.

42. Taylor AW et al: Skeletal muscle analysis of wheelchair athletes, *Paraplegia* 17:456, 1979.

43. White E: Leisure and recreation, *Br Med J* 302:461, 1991.

44. Windour R: Canadian ice sports, *Sports n Spokes* 13(2):45, 1987.

Index

Hill-Sachs lesion—cont'd
  recurrent
    anterior dislocations and, 184
    rates of, 184
  reverse, 44
  in shoulder injury, 42, 47
    in throwing, 723
Hinged elbow orthosis, 353
Hip
  flexion of, 821
  Legg-Perthes disease of, 656
History
  in impingement syndrome, 210
  of prior racquet sports injuries, 806
  of sports medicine, 885-886
Home rehabilitation
  in elbow injuries, 344-345
  in hand and wrist injuries, 618
Horizontal abduction
  exercise for, 742
  with outward rotation, 820
  prone, 818, 819
Horizontal adduction, exercise for, 739-742
Horizontal flexion/extension of arm, 700
  muscles in, 703-704
Horizontal flexion/internal rotation of arm, muscles in, 704
Hot packs in hand and wrist therapy, 618
H-plasty, anterior, in multidirectional shoulder instability, 201-204
Humeral head; *see also* Humerus
  abduction of, 217
  elevation of, with large tears of rotator cuff, 216
  excessive translation of, on glenoid fossa, 173
  excursion of, 699
  hypertrophy of, 185, 760
  in impingement, 54, 55
  in injury, 44
  in instability, 46, 47
    physical examination for, 74
  loss of control of, in tennis injuries, 791
  McLaughlin fracture of, 98
  posteriorly forced, 194
  radiographic views of, 76
  retroversion of, 698
  shoulder motion and, 697, 699, 723
  sulcus between acromion and, 49, 50
Humeral osteotomy, 240-241
Humeral vessels, 34, 35
Humeroulnar articulation, 753-754
Humerus; *see also* Humeral head
  aseptic necrosis of, 79
  development of, 23-24
  distal
    anatomy and physiology of, 265-266, 267
    fracture of, in football injuries, 877
  exercise for motion of, 739, 740
  fracture of
    in football injuries, 877
    spontaneous, 222
    supracondylar, in gymnast, 836
  hypertrophy of, 185, 280, 760
  muscles of, 33, 701
  ossification center of, 23-24
  physical examination of, 65-66
  proximal
    anatomy of, 27-28
    tuberosities of, 27
  shoulder motion and, 697, 699
Humpback deformity, 407
HVES; *see* High-voltage electric stimulation
HVPS; *see* High-voltage pulsed stimulation
Hydraulic dynamometer, Jamar, 595, 596
Hydrocollator, 618

Hyperextension
  in cervical spinal injury, 11
  in elbow injury, taping for, 347-350, 351
  in mallet finger injury, 582-583, 600-601
  in wrist injury
    with fracture, 402
    taping in, 849-851
Hyperflexion
  in cervical spinal injury, 11
  in overuse syndromes, 222
Hyperhidrosis, 605
Hyperlaxity, recurrent anterior subluxation and, 185
Hypersupination injuries of wrist, arthroscopy in, 384, 385
Hyperthermia or hypothermia in disabled athlete, 895
Hypertrophy
  bony, of coronoid process of elbow, 780
  of extensor mechanism at metacarpophalangeal joint, 589
  of fibrous band in middle phalanx, 364
  of humerus, 185, 280, 760
Hypothenar hammer syndrome, 604, 690
Hypovascularity in rotator cuff tendinopathy, 853

I

Ibuprofen, 232
Ice burn, 864
Ice therapy
  in cool-down period after shoulder throwing injuries, 727
  in elbow soft-tissue injuries, 773
  in impingement syndrome of shoulder, 221
  in racquet sports injuries, 810
Imaging; *see* Radiography
Immature skeleton; *see* Skeletally immature athlete
Immobilization
  in anterior instability of glenohumeral joint, 184
    rehabilitation and, 251-252
  in blocker's node, 867
  fracture
    in distal radius, 437
    in hamate hook, 425
    in middle phalanx, 540
    in pisiform, 434
    in triquetrum, 427-428
    in wrist, 410-412
  in hand and wrist edema, 608, 610
  for mallet finger, 579
  in olecranon bursitis, 865
  in restoring wrist mobility, 597
  in ulnar collateral ligament injuries, 559
Impact injury of shoulder, 43, 44-45
Impact loading of wrist, 384-386
Impact phase in golf swing, 845, 846
Impingement injection test, 73, 212
  in degenerative disease, 230-231
  in injury, 164
Impingement sign, 72, 211-212, 218, 725
  in tennis injuries, 791
Impingement syndrome, 209-214, 216-222
  with acromioclavicular complex injury, 163-164
  ancillary tests in, 212
  arc of motion evaluation in, 211
  classification of, 727
  clinical evaluation of, 210-212
  diagnosis of, 212
    imaging in, 219-220
  factors contributing to, 210
  in football injuries, 867-868
  golf and, 849
  in gymnasts, 829
  history of, 53-56, 210, 727
  imaging in, 219-220
  impingement sign in, 211-212
  injection test in, 212
  inspection of, 210
  versus instability in throwing injuries, 723-724